Pharmacology
DRUG THERAPY AND NURSING CONSIDERATIONS

Pharmacology
DRUG THERAPY AND NURSING CONSIDERATIONS

THIRD EDITION

Roger T. Malseed, PhD

Adjunct Associate Professor of Pharmacology
University of Pennsylvania School of Nursing
Philadelphia College of Pharmacy and Science
Philadelphia, Pennsylvania

with Nursing Considerations by

Sandra E. Girton, RN, MN
Assistant Professor
Bloomsburg University
Bloomsburg, Pennsylvania

J.B. Lippincott Company   Philadelphia
Grand Rapids   London
New York   Sydney
St. Louis   Tokyo
San Francisco

Acquisitions Editor: Ellen M. Campbell
Coordinating Editorial Assistant: Patricia L. Shear
Project Editor: Grace R. Caputo
Indexer: Alexandra Weir Nickerson
Design Coordinator: Ellen C. Dawson
Interior Designer: Steve Iwanczuk
Cover Designer: Paul Autodore
Production Manager: Carol A. Florence
Production Coordinators: Barney Fernandes and Sharon McCarthy
Compositor: Circle Graphics
Printer/Binder: The Murray Printing Company

Library of Congress Cataloging-in-Publication Data

Malseed, Roger T. (Roger Thomas)
 Pharmacology, drug therapy, and nursing considerations/Roger T.
Malseed; with nursing considerations by Sandra E. Girton.—3rd
ed.
  p. cm.
 Includes bibliographical references.
 ISBN 0-397-54677-7
 1. Pharmacology. 2. Chemotherapy. 3. Nursing. I. Girton,
Sandra Erdene. II. Title.
 [DNLM: 1. Drug Therapy—nurses' instruction. 2. Pharmacology—
nurses' instruction. QV 4 M259p]
RM300.M183 1990
615.5'8'024613—dc20
DNLM/DLC
for Library of Congress   89-13394
                                                                        CIP

3rd Edition

Copyright © 1990, by J. B. Lippincott Company.

Copyright © 1985, 1982, by J. B. Lippincott Company. All rights reserved. No part of this book may be used or reproduced in any manner whatsoever without written permission except for brief quotations embodied in critical articles and reviews. Printed in the United States of America. For information write J. B. Lippincott Company, East Washington Square, Philadelphia, Pennsylvania 19105.

6 5 4 3 2

Any procedure or practice described in this book should be applied by the health-care practitioner under appropriate supervision in accordance with professional standards of care used with regard to the unique circumstances that apply in each practice situation. Care has been taken to confirm the accuracy of information presented and to describe generally accepted practices. However, the authors, editors, and publisher cannot accept any responsibility for errors or omissions or for any consequences from application of the information in this book and make no warranty, express or implied, with respect to the contents of the book.

Every effort has been made to ensure drug selections and dosages are in accordance with current recommendations and practice. Because of ongoing research, changes in government regulations and the constant flow of information on drug therapy, reactions and interactions, the reader is cautioned to check the package insert for each drug for indications, dosages, warnings and precautions, particularly if the drug is new or infrequently used.

*To my students
past and present,
in whose hearts and minds the future of nursing lies*

Contributors

Zoriana Kawka Malseed, PhD
Associate Professor of Anatomy and Physiology
University of Pennsylvania School of Nursing
Philadelphia, Pennsylvania

Freddy Grimm, MS, PharmD
Director of Outpatient Services
Hospital of the University of Pennsylvania
Clinical Associate Professor
Philadelphia College of Pharmacy and Science
Philadelphia, Pennsylvania

Preface

As nurses assume an ever-increasing role in the prescribing and monitoring of drugs, it becomes imperative that their knowledge base regarding the multiplicity of therapeutic agents available be current and broad. The third edition of *Pharmacology: Drug Therapy and Nursing Considerations* is a source from which nurses may readily obtain the necessary information to provide safe and effective drug therapy.

While retaining the overall format and scope of the first two editions of this work, the third edition incorporates many changes that strengthen the nursing content and provide a more patient-oriented approach to pharmacology. As in the previous editions, the content is structured in an outline format, with many comparative tables and charts to aid readers in locating and correlating information easily. The basic design of the book has been retained, enabling the book to serve as both a text and a comprehensive reference. The initial section remains devoted to general principles of pharmacology and has been augmented by the addition of a chapter detailing the legal aspects of drug therapy as they relate to nursing practice. The next nine sections consider the various classes of drugs that affect the different body systems. Most sections begin with a chapter reviewing the physiology of a particular system, a feature that has been well received. Many new drugs have been added, including new classes of antiinfectives, agents for solubilizing gallstones, clot-dissolving drugs, antiulcer agents, and a variety of new antiinflammatory drugs, antihistamines, antidepressants, antihypertensives, and antineoplastic agents. Discussions of diagnostic agents, serums, vaccines and nutrients have been updated. Recent developments in the area of drug abuse, particularly regarding cocaine, have been incorporated into the chapter on drugs of abuse.

The nursing content has been refined and reorganized under the direction of Sandra Girton. Nursing Alerts still are emphasized separately, reflecting their greater importance in properly administering and monitoring drug therapy. A new feature heading is Patient Education, under which information that nurses should provide to patients is clearly delineated. A major addition to the third edition is the inclusion of 12 nursing care plans throughout the text, which relate to the major classes of drugs as well as to topics such as drug compliance and knowledge deficit. These care plans provide comprehensive information on nursing diagnoses, interventions, and expected outcomes to assist the reader in planning and delivering total patient care. They are designed to complement and reinforce the nursing considerations presented for each drug or drug class. The entire nursing content has been thoroughly reviewed and broadened.

Other new inclusions in the third edition of *Pharmacology* are the listing of Canadian as well as American trade names for those drugs that have different trade names when marketed in Canada, and a listing of selected references after each drug chapter for those readers wishing to consult other sources regarding a particular topic or drug discussed in the chapter. As in earlier editions, a general bibliography is presented in the appendix.

Among the unique features of previous editions that have been retained and updated are the extensive tables on antimicrobial drugs of choice for common infections and on combination chemotherapeutic regimens, as well as tables on diagnostic agents, oral contraceptives, and topical corticosteroids. The list of abbreviations in the appendix has been greatly expanded, and a list of FDA pregnancy categories has been added.

In writing *Pharmacology: Drug Therapy and Nursing Considerations*, I have attempted to fashion a comprehensive work that contains relevant, practical information in an easily retrievable format. Extensive use is made of tables comparing similar drugs. Summary tables after most chapters list dosage forms and recommended doses for drugs listed therein. The outline format facilitates quick access to and easy extraction of pertinent information on a particular drug or class of drugs. Whether used as a textbook, a reference book, or both, nurses and other health care professionals should find the book to be a complete source for the information needed to ensure that they are providing the safest, most efficacious drug therapy to their patients.

ROGER T. MALSEED, PHD

Acknowledgments

Many people have been instrumental in bringing this third edition to fruition. In particular, Nancy Mullins and Ellen Campbell, editors in the nursing division of J.B. Lippincott have overseen the bulk of the day-to-day work, and I am greatly indebted to them for their assistance

Grace Caputo, as manuscript editor for production, coordinated the transition from manuscript page to book page with careful attention to detail. I am appreciative of her efforts.

I wish to acknowledge the contributions of Zoriana Malseed and Freddy Grimm, who revised the physiology chapters and the chapter on antineoplastic drugs, respectively. Their work, as always, was complete and current.

Frederick J. Goldstein, Professor of Pharmacology at the Philadelphia College of Pharmacy and Science, shared his expertise in the field of drug abuse and provided much topical information for the chapter on drugs of abuse.

I wish to thank the many users of the first two editions who have provided helpful suggestions and criticisms. The third edition is, I hope, a much better book because of their input.

Finally, to my family, Zoriana, Mark, and Natalie, I convey my love and gratitude for their encouragement and support, and I thank them for the joy that they bring to my every day.

Contents

I
General Principles of Pharmacology 1

1. METHODS OF DRUG ADMINISTRATION 3
2. INTERACTION OF DRUGS WITH BODY TISSUES: PHARMACOKINETICS 11
3. BASIC SITES AND MECHANISMS OF DRUG ACTION: PHARMACODYNAMICS 16
4. PHARMACOLOGIC BASIS OF ADVERSE DRUG EFFECTS 19
5. DRUG INTERACTIONS 26
6. PEDIATRIC PHARMACOLOGY 31
7. GERIATRIC PHARMACOLOGY 37
8. LEGAL ASPECTS OF DRUG THERAPY 41

II
Drugs Acting on the Nervous System 47

9. THE NERVOUS SYSTEM: A REVIEW 49
10. CHOLINERGIC DRUGS 56
11. ANTICHOLINERGIC DRUGS 67
12. ADRENERGIC DRUGS 79
13. ADRENERGIC BLOCKING DRUGS 102
14. ANTIHISTAMINE–ANTISEROTONIN AGENTS 113
15. SKELETAL MUSCLE RELAXANTS 128
16. LOCAL ANESTHETICS 139
17. GENERAL ANESTHETICS 144

18. NARCOTIC ANALGESICS AND ANTAGONISTS 155
19. NONNARCOTIC ANALGESIC AND ANTIINFLAMMATORY DRUGS 170
20. BARBITURATE SEDATIVE–HYPNOTICS 193
21. NONBARBITURATE SEDATIVE–HYPNOTICS 198
22. ANTIPSYCHOTIC DRUGS 205
23. ANTIANXIETY DRUGS 217
24. ANTIDEPRESSANTS 227
25. ANTICONVULSANTS/ ANTIEPILEPTICS 238
26. ANTIPARKINSONIAN DRUGS 253
27. CENTRAL NERVOUS SYSTEM STIMULANTS 262

III
Drugs Acting on the Cardiovascular System 273

28. CARDIOVASCULAR PHYSIOLOGY: A REVIEW 275
29. CARDIOTONIC DRUGS 281
30. ANTIARRHYTHMIC DRUGS 287
31. ANTIHYPERTENSIVE DRUGS 302
32. ANTIANGINAL AGENTS/ VASODILATORS 325
33. PROPHYLAXIS OF ATHEROSCLEROSIS: HYPOLIPEMIC DRUGS 337
34. ANTIANEMIC DRUGS 345
35. ANTICOAGULANT, THROMBOLYTIC, AND HEMOSTATIC DRUGS 351

IV
Drugs Acting on the Renal System ..369

    36   RENAL PHYSIOLOGY: A REVIEW 371

    37   DIURETICS 376

V
Drugs Acting on the Endocrine Glands 393

    38   THE ENDOCRINE GLANDS: A REVIEW 395

    39   HYPOPHYSIAL HORMONES 407

    40   THYROID HORMONES AND ANTITHYROID DRUGS 416

    41   PARATHYROID DRUGS, CALCITONIN, AND CALCIUM 424

    42   ANTIDIABETIC AND HYPERGLYCEMIC AGENTS.........429

    43   ADRENAL CORTICAL STEROIDS.....442

    44   ESTROGENS AND PROGESTINS 454

    45   DRUGS USED IN FERTILITY CONTROL 463

    46   ANDROGENS AND ANABOLIC STEROIDS 474

VI
Drugs Acting on Gastrointestinal Function 481

    47   GASTROINTESTINAL PHYSIOLOGY: A REVIEW 483

    48   ANTACIDS, ANTIULCER DRUGS 490

    49   DIGESTANTS, GALLSTONE SOLUBILIZING AGENTS 500

    50   LAXATIVES 506

    51   ANTIDIARRHEAL DRUGS...........514

    52   EMETICS AND ANTIEMETICS.......520

VII
Drugs Acting on Respiratory Function...............529

    53   RESPIRATORY PHYSIOLOGY: A REVIEW 531

    54   ANTITUSSIVES, EXPECTORANTS, AND MUCOLYTICS 537

    55   BRONCHODILATORS, ANTIASTHMATICS................545

VIII
Antiinfective and Chemotherapeutic Agents 557

    56   ANTIINFECTIVE THERAPY: GENERAL CONSIDERATIONS 559

    57   SULFONAMIDES 573

    58   PENICILLINS, CARBAPENEMS, MONOBACTAMS 582

    59   CEPHALOSPORINS 598

    60   TETRACYCLINES, QUINOLONES......609

    61   ERYTHROMYCINS 619

    62   AMINOGLYCOSIDES...............624

    63   POLYPEPTIDES 632

    64   URINARY ANTIINFECTIVES 637

    65   MISCELLANEOUS ANTIBIOTICS 643

    66   ANTITUBERCULAR AGENTS........655

    67   ANTIMALARIAL AGENTS...........664

    68   ANTHELMINTICS 672

    69   AMEBICIDES 681

    70   ANTIFUNGAL AGENTS 687

    71   ANTIVIRAL AGENTS 699

    72   ANTINEOPLASTIC AGENTS.........708

IX
Nutrients, Fluids, and Electrolytes ...755

- 73 WATER-SOLUBLE VITAMINS: VITAMINS B AND C 757
- 74 FAT-SOLUBLE VITAMINS: VITAMINS A, D, E, AND K 764
- 75 NUTRIENTS, MINERALS, FLUIDS, AND ELECTROLYTES 774

X
Miscellaneous Agents 789

- 76 DIAGNOSTIC AGENTS..............791
- 77 SERUMS AND VACCINES...........803
- 78 MISCELLANEOUS DRUG PRODUCTS......................813

XI
Drug Dependence and Addiction ..833

- 79 DRUGS OF ABUSE: A REVIEW........835

XII
Appendices 843

- 1 COMMON ABBREVIATIONS 845
- 2 FDA PREGNANCY CATEGORIES......846
- 3 DRUG COMPATIBILITY GUIDE.......847

  GENERAL BIBLIOGRAPHY 849

Index

Nursing Care Plans

1	Patients Whose Knowledge of Drug Regimen is Deficient	23
2	Patient Compliance with a Prescribed Drug Regimen	38
3	Patients Treated with Beta-Adrenergic Blockers	109
4	Patients Treated with Antihistamine Drugs	120
5	Patients Treated with H_2-Receptor Antagonists	123
6	Patients Treated with Nonsteroidal Antiinflammatory Drugs (NSAIDs)	179
7	Patients Treated with Benzodiazepine Antianxiety Drugs	219
8	Patients Treated with Nondiuretic Antihypertensive Drugs	306
9	Patients Treated with Diuretic Drugs	379
10	Patients Treated with Antidiabetic Agents	433
11	Patients Treated with Methylxanthine (Xanthine) Bronchodilators	550
12	Patients Treated with Antibacterial Drugs	564

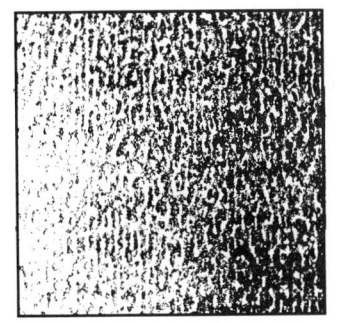

I General Principles of Pharmacology

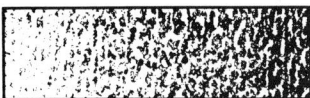

METHODS OF DRUG ADMINISTRATION

Drugs may be administered by several different routes, largely determined by the intended site of action, the rapidity and duration of effect desired, and the chemical and physical properties of the drug itself. *Route of administration* is one of the most important factors influencing the effects of a drug. Some drugs may exert differing actions depending on their routes of administration. For example, diazoxide is a potent, rapidly acting hypotensive agent when given intravenously (IV), but following its oral ingestion, it inhibits the release of insulin from the pancreas and has minimal effects on blood pressure. Magnesium sulfate is a laxative when taken orally, reduces swelling of joints when used as a concentrated soak, and exerts powerful anticonvulsant effects when injected intravenously or intramuscularly (IM).

Although some drugs can be used both locally and systemically, many agents are given by a single mode of administration (i.e., topically, orally, or parenterally). We shall examine the different methods of drug administration and discuss the dosage forms most commonly employed with each route of administration.

TOPICAL APPLICATION

Most topically applied drugs are intended for their local effects and are applied to the surface of the skin or mucous membranes (oral, nasal, vaginal, urethral, anal).

Dermatologic Application

Medications are applied to the skin in several forms: lotions, creams, ointments, sprays, and liquids (wet dressings, baths, soaks). Systemic absorption is limited by the keratinized structure of the skin, which prevents passage of significant amounts of most drugs. Absorption may be enhanced when drugs are applied to damaged skin (wounds, burns). Incorporation of the drug in a fatty vehicle such as waxes or wool fat or the use of a keratolytic agent such as salicylic acid to break down the keratin layer may also increase absorption.

Major uses for dermatologically applied drugs are the following:
1. Antiseptic/antiinfective (antibiotics, antifungal agents, alcohol, hexachlorophene)
2. Antiinflammatory (corticosteroids)
3. Astringent (aluminum acetate, zinc oxide)
4. Antipruritic (local anesthetics, antihistamines)
5. Emollient (vitamins A, D, and E, glycerin, lanolin, mineral oil)
6. Keratolytic (salicylic acid, resorcinol)
7. Vasodilator (nitroglycerin)
8. Antinauseant (scopolamine)

Dermatologically applied drugs may also be used as protectives, absorbents, or counterirritants, and as corrosives to aid in sloughing off or removing damaged tissue. Diseases commonly treated by local application of drugs to the skin surface include acne, psoriasis, allergic dermatoses, skin cancers, infestations of lice, and topical infections. In addition, certain systemic conditions such as angina, or hypertension are amenable to treatment by locally applied drugs that are sufficiently absorbed through the intact skin from specialized dosage forms (e.g., transdermal patches).

Mucous Membrane Application

Absorption of drugs from mucous membranes is generally good, owing primarily to the thinness and vascularity of the membrane. Drugs may be applied to mucous membranes in all the forms used for dermatologic application, as well as in the form of suppositories (rectal, vaginal), powders (nasal), lozenges (oral), and tablets (buccal, sublingual). Because absorption is good, especially from aqueous solution, many drugs exert significant systemic actions following application to mucous membranes. Thus the toxic effects of drugs may be enhanced by systemic absorption, and mucous membrane application must be undertaken more cautiously than dermatologic administration.

Major uses of drugs applied to various mucous membranes are the following:

LOCAL EFFECTS
1. Antiseptic (oral lozenges, sprays, mouthwashes)
2. Antibacterial and antifungal (vaginal creams, suppositories)
3. Decongestant (nasal sprays, drops)
4. Antihemorrhoidal (rectal astringents, local anesthetics, emollients)
5. Contraceptive (vaginal foams, tablets, lotions)

SYSTEMIC EFFECTS
1. Antianginal (sublingual vasodilators)
2. Laxative (rectal suppositories, retention enemas)
3. Migraine relief (sublingual ergotamine)

The rectal route (suppository, retention enema) may also be employed with antiemetics (prochlorperazine), bronchodilators (aminophylline), analgesics (aspirin), sedatives (phenobarbital), and many other drugs that cannot be administered orally because the patient is unconscious or uncooperative, or is vomiting. Rectal absorption is unpredictable, and a small, cleansing enema prior to drug administration may improve absorption.

NURSING CONSIDERATIONS
Dermatologic
1. Remove ointments, creams, or jellies from jar with a sterile tongue depressor or applicator stick—not fingers—to avoid contaminating remainder of jar contents.
2. If the skin is broken or abraded, use aseptic techniques whenever possible and cleanse skin with an antiseptic such as hexachlorophene before application.
3. Apply most ointments and creams (except topical burn preparations) in small amounts; that is, cover area thoroughly with a thin layer of medication, and use firm but gentle pressure.
4. If application stains clothing, instruct patient to take adequate precautions, such as use of a protective covering. Use caution if applying adhesive tape near a wound or an abraded skin area.
5. When using topically applied preparations, monitor for allergic hypersensitivity reactions such as rash, local

edema, or hives (urticaria), and withhold medication and advise drug prescriber if any of these are observed.
6. Seek clarification if local corticosteroids are prescribed for an existing topical infection without concurrent antibiotic therapy, as this may cause the infection to spread.
7. When moist compresses are applied to denuded or oozing skin areas, ensure that aseptic technique is used. Sterile compresses should be wrung out before being applied. If *warm* compresses are needed, do not warm solution to more than body temperature.
8. Provide emotional support to patient and encourage him or her to talk about feelings regarding the skin condition—a sense of rejection, lowered self-image, and a tendency toward isolation are often present. Avoid showing signs of aversion or rejection toward the person because of this condition.

Mucous Membrane

Oral Mucosa

1. Instruct patient taking sublingual or buccal medication or a troche *not* to swallow tablets or take water or food with them.
2. Inform patient that effects of sublingually administered drugs should occur within 5 minutes. If no relief is obtained, advise physician, because dosage adjustment may be necessary.
3. Instruct patient to apply buccal tablets to gums above the upper incisors and to use caution when eating or drinking so that the tablet is not dislodged.

Rectal Mucosa

1. Refrigerate suppositories as indicated, especially in warmer weather, because they tend to soften and become difficult to handle.
2. Assess patient's attitude toward rectal administration. Maintain a professional, straightforward approach to rectal drug administration, explain the procedure completely, and allow the patient privacy to whatever extent possible.
3. If suppository is to be self-administered, be certain patient knows proper technique and depth and can reach anus easily (e.g., arthritic conditions can restrict movement).
4. Urge bowel evacuation, if possible, just before insertion of suppository to aid absorption of systemically acting drug.
5. Inform patient that laxative suppositories generally have a rapid onset of action (10–20 min). Toilet facilities should be nearby.
6. Insert suppository beyond the internal anal sphincter (or assist patient, if necessary). Use gentle, firm pressure with the forefinger. Instruct patient to lie on one side with knees drawn up. Patient should remain on side for 15 minutes to prevent leakage.
7. When possible, give retention enema before a meal and following a bowel movement to enhance drug absorption.
8. Warm the retention enema solution to body temperature, and give small volume (less than 150 mL) slowly with a small-diameter rectal tube to prevent stimulation of peristalsis and subsequent expulsion of rectal contents. Stay with patient and assist to deep breathe if abdominal cramping occurs.

Nasal Mucosa

1. Administer oil-based preparations for nasal application very cautiously. They should usually be avoided because aspiration of oil droplets into lungs may cause severe irritation and lipid pneumonia.
2. Demonstrate head-back position to patient when instilling nasal drops, and instruct patient to hold head in a backward position for several minutes to allow time for drug absorption.
3. Avoid contacting nasal mucosa with tip of dropper because contamination can result or patient may be stimulated to sneeze.
4. Discard any solution remaining in dropper following each administration.

PATIENT EDUCATION

Nasal Mucosa

1. Stress the importance of limiting use of drops containing nasal decongestants (vasoconstrictors) to a period of 3 to 5 days to avoid the development of tolerance, which lessens the effect of the drug and leads to *rebound congestion* (hyperemia, inflammation, and edema of nasal membranes).
2. Warn patient with hypertension or other cardiovascular disorders that systemic absorption of nasal sprays containing vasoconstrictors may elevate blood pressure.
3. Advise patient that excessive use of any nasal preparation may, over a period of time, result in significant systemic absorption, especially if substantial amounts of the drug are swallowed rather than inhaled.
4. Instruct patient to clean nozzle of spray applicator after each use to prevent contamination and possible bacterial growth. Discourage use of same nasal spray bottle by more than one person.

Vaginal Mucosa

1. Explain the technique for insertion of vaginal tablets and suppositories, and assist patient with first insertion as appropriate. Tell patient to remain in bed at least 15 minutes after insertion to allow medication sufficient contact time with target area.
2. Emphasize the importance of taking the medication for the prescribed length of time. Many vaginal infections are difficult to treat and can be very resistant to drugs.
3. If preparation causes stains, suggest wearing a sanitary napkin to prevent staining of clothing or bed linen.
4. Discuss potential harm of excessive douching. If patient douches, provide instructions for mixing, and demonstrate placement of container and tubing to prevent excessive force of flow.
5. If contraceptive foams and jellies are used, ensure that patient understands package instructions regarding timing and method of application. Be prepared to discuss the limitations of their effectiveness, and advise those considering their use to seek expert advice on alternative methods of contraception.

OPHTHALMIC APPLICATION

Drugs intended for use in the eye may be administered as drops, ointments, or washes. In addition, a special type of preparation intended for use in glaucoma is available in the form of sterile insertion units termed Ocuserts. All ophthalmic medications are packaged sterile; thus, aseptic technique is essential when handling these drugs.

Major indications for local administration of drugs in the eye are the following:
1. Glaucoma (miotics, decongestants)
2. Inflammation (corticosteroids)
3. Infection (antibiotics)

Ophthalmic drugs may also be employed to facilitate eye examinations. Mydriatics produce pupillary dilatation, cycloplegics paralyze accommodation, and local anesthetics permit manipulative procedures such as tonometry. Artificial "tears" can be used to provide lubrication.

NURSING CONSIDERATIONS
1. Use aseptic technique in handling ophthalmic drugs. Wash hands before administering; do not allow tip of dropper or ointment tube to come into contact with eyelid; discard any unused portion of each dose.
2. Check solution, suspension, or ointment for expiration date, and make sure solution is clear and free from discoloration.
3. Hold bottle or applicator parallel to the eye, rather than perpendicular, to prevent injury should the patient move or jerk.
4. Have patient look up during administration; place medication in the conjunctival sac, not directly on the cornea; wipe area near the eyes gently with a cotton ball; and instruct patient to lie or sit with head tilted backward.
5. When using ophthalmic ointment, place *small* ribbon of medication into everted lower eyelid and tell patient to close eye. Body heat will cause dispersion of drug over eye surface.

PATIENT EDUCATION
1. Ensure that the patient with glaucoma understands that the drug regimen must be maintained regularly to prevent deterioration of eyesight.

OTIC APPLICATION

Drugs intended for use in the ear are usually administered as drops, although irrigation of the external auditory canal can be performed as well. When the tympanic membrane is intact, sterile technique is not essential.

Principal conditions for which drugs are instilled into the ear are the following:
1. Infections (antibiotics)
2. Inflammation (corticosteroids)
3. Pain (local anesthetics)
4. Obstruction with wax (hydrogen peroxide)

Self-medication should be reserved for those minor conditions (e.g., impacted wax) that can be treated safely. Most patients with ear disorders require professional diagnosis and treatment.

NURSING CONSIDERATIONS
1. Warm ear drops to body temperature before instilling in ear canal.
2. Place patient on his or her side with affected ear uppermost; instruct patient to remain in that position for several minutes after drugs have been administered to allow sufficient time for medication to reach affected area.
3. Use the proper method for instilling drops. *Adults:* Pull external part of lower ear backward and upward and instill drops in the direction of the opening of the ear canal. *Children:* Pull lower part of external ear downward before instilling drops.
4. If cotton is to be inserted into ear after drug administration, insert *loosely.* Cotton should never be packed tightly into ear canal.
5. For irrigation, place tip of special irrigating syringe inside auditory meatus, pull auricle upward and backward, and direct a slow, gentle stream of warmed solution toward the roof of the auditory canal. The patient may sit or lie with head tilted toward the side of the affected ear. Allow fluid to escape freely, and collect it in a basin placed below the ear and against the face. Stop irrigation if pain or dizziness occurs.
6. Following irrigation, place patient with affected ear downward and allow ear to drain. Dry ear when process is completed.

INHALATION APPLICATION

Inhaled drugs are generally intended for their local effects on the respiratory system. In addition, certain drugs, such as general anesthetics exert profound systemic effects when inhaled into the lungs. Many drugs are rapidly absorbed in the alveoli of the lungs because of the large surface area, extensive vascularity, and high permeability of the alveolar epithelium. Thus, although a drug may be given for its local effects in the lungs, systemic absorption can result in undesirable side effects such as cardiac stimulation, and this possibility must be kept in mind. *Particle size* of the delivered drug is the most important factor determining depth of penetration into the bronchial tree, and hence the extent of systemic absorption.

Major indications for inhaled drugs are the following:
1. Anesthesia (general anesthetics)
2. Obstructive pulmonary diseases, such as asthma and emphysema (corticosteroids, bronchodilators, mucolytics, antibiotics)
3. Respiratory aid (oxygen)

Inhalation of drugs is most easily accomplished by use of a metered-dose nebulizer or atomizer, available in prepackaged form, although patients require careful instruction for effective use of this product. Alternatively, an intermittent positive pressure breathing (IPPB) apparatus may be used, most often in a hospital setting. The method provides greater depth and more extensive distribution of the drug in the bronchial tree. Certain powdered drugs (e.g., cromolyn) may be delivered by insufflation, a method in which the powder is blown into the respiratory passages by a pressurized container.

NURSING CONSIDERATIONS
1. Check directions for administering inhaled medications because many must be diluted before use.
2. Carefully observe patient using IPPB machine for signs of dizziness, nausea, or anxiety. Reassure patient who has difficulty mastering the technique.
3. Clean nebulizer or atomizer carefully after each use to prevent obstruction and contamination. Discard unused medication left in nebulizer.

PATIENT EDUCATION
1. Teach patient correct procedure for using metered-dose atomizer or nebulizer (e.g., when to inhale and exhale and how long breath should be held). Directions usually come with containers.
2. Teach patient how to use IPPB machine before drug administration. With patient in an upright position, tell him or her to close lips tightly around mouthpiece and breathe *only* through mouth at normal resting rate.

3. Advise patient using inhalation equipment such as a nebulizer at home to soak it for 30 minutes once every 2 weeks in a solution of equal parts water and white vinegar to prevent pseudomonal contamination.

ORAL ADMINISTRATION

The oral route of drug administration is the simplest, most convenient, and generally the safest and most economical means of administering medications. Commonly employed oral dosage forms are tablets, capsules, and liquids. Most drugs are well absorbed from the gastrointestinal (GI) tract, and absorption is usually enhanced if the drug is in liquid form or is administered with water. Some drugs, such as antiinflammatory drugs, may irritate the GI mucosa and are best given with food, whereas other agents (e.g., penicillins), may be inactivated by the presence of food-induced digestive enzymes and are best given between meals.

It should be recognized that following oral administration of a drug, onset of action is slower and the duration of effect is more prolonged than after sublingual and most forms of parenteral administration. This is of little consequence in most cases, but it becomes significant in emergencies (e.g., acute pain, cardiac arrest, acute asthmatic attacks).

Other important disadvantages of the oral route of administration are the following:

1. Some drugs are rapidly inactivated in the GI tract (e.g., insulin) or are not absorbed (e.g., tubocurarine).
2. Some drugs undergo extensive first-pass hepatic metabolism (i.e., they are largely inactivated in the liver soon after absorption into the portal circulation). Thus, a large fraction of the dose never reaches the systemic circulation. Differences in the rate and extent of hepatic metabolism among patients can lead to significant variations in steady state plasma levels, and hence to widely differing dosage requirements. Sublingual drug administration avoids first-pass hepatic metabolism and generally results in higher plasma levels for those drugs extensively metabolized in the liver.
3. Some drugs have an objectionable odor or taste (e.g., liquid potassium).
4. Some drugs (such as large doses of aspirin) may produce local stomach irritation and cause nausea and vomiting. Drugs that may irritate the stomach can be given in the form of enteric-coated tablets, which dissolve only in the intestine where the environment is more alkaline.
5. Some drugs (such as liquid iron or gastric acids) may stain or destroy the tooth enamel.

In addition, unconscious, uncooperative, or vomiting patients or those without a gag reflex should not be given drugs by the oral route.

NURSING CONSIDERATIONS

1. Know the properties of the drug being administered so that it may be given at the proper time (e.g., at meals or bedtime).
2. Be aware of the intended purpose of the drugs as well as the expected side effects, and observe the response of the patient carefully.
3. Determine the patient's ability to swallow a solid dosage form. If swallowing problems exist, consider use of a liquid preparation or parenteral administration.
4. Instruct patient to take oral medications with a full glass of water to facilitate absorption and to ensure sufficient fluid intake. Carbonated drinks and fruit juices should be avoided, unless necessary to mask a disagreeable flavor of a liquid preparation, because they may alter the absorption rate.
5. Do not attempt to break unscored tablets or divide capsules, because dosage inaccuracies can result.
6. Instruct patient to swallow coated tablets whole and not to chew them, because breaks in the coating will alter dissolution characteristics.
7. Note expiration date on liquid preparations (e.g., antibiotics), and do not use if too old. Potency may be affected.
8. Keep preparations requiring refrigeration cold, and discard unused content at end of period stated on the label.
9. Do not mix liquids together unless so instructed. Incompatibilities may result, affecting the action of the drugs.
10. Do not use liquids that are discolored, exhibit precipitation, or have an unusual odor without consulting the physician or pharmacist.

PATIENT EDUCATION

1. Advise patient to avoid indiscriminate use of over-the-counter (OTC) drugs when taking prescribed oral medications, because many OTC products (such as antacids, laxatives, and cough syrups) can interfere with the other drugs' actions.

ADMINISTRATION OF PARENTERAL MEDICATIONS

Although the term *parenteral* literally means any route other than enteral (by way of the GI tract), it is usually used to refer to the different methods of *injection* of drugs. Parenteral administration requires aseptically prepared drugs and sterile techniques, critical regulation of dosage, careful selection of site and rate of injection, and a certain degree of technical skill not necessary with most other forms of drug usage.

There are often significant differences in onset of drug action, extent of drug effects (local vs. systemic), dosage of drug required, skill in administration, and potential hazards depending on the route of administration selected. We shall examine in more detail several of the more important routes of parenteral administration.

Intravenous

Intravenous administration is accomplished by either direct injection (*bolus*) or slow *infusion*. Direct IV injection is employed primarily in emergency situations because it provides an extremely rapid onset of action. Also, some drugs (e.g., diazoxide) require bolus injection to achieve their desired effect. Because the drug is injected directly into the bloodstream, however, bolus IV injection is also a very hazardous method, and great care must be taken to ensure that the proper preparation and accurate dose have been selected, and to provide prompt antidotal therapy should an overdose occur. Bolus IV injection is most commonly done into the median cubital (antecubital) or basilic vein near the bend of the elbow (Fig. 1-1), although any accessible vein may be used in an emergency.

Irritating substances that cannot be given by other parenteral routes of injection because they produce tissue damage can sometimes be administered by slow IV injection diluted in 100 mL to 200 mL of suitable liquid (e.g., sterile water for injection).

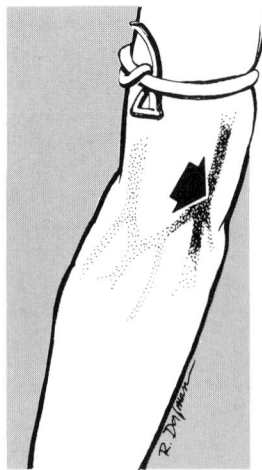

Figure 1–1 The most common bolus IV injection site is into the median cubital (antecubital) or basilic vein near the bend of the elbow (arrow).

The lining of the blood vessels is quite resistant to the irritative effects of many drugs, and the buffering capacity of the blood may reduce local necrosis. This procedure requires selection of a large vein and assurance that the injection is properly placed into the flowing bloodstream.

Slow IV infusions are most commonly employed to replace depleted blood volume, to supply nutrients and electrolytes, to prevent or relieve tissue dehydration, and to administer drugs. The veins of the dorsal venous plexus or the cephalic vein (Fig. 1-2) are commonly used for these purposes. Very large volumes of fluids can be given by IV infusion, although care must be taken to avoid overloading the patient's circulatory capacity. A controlled rate of flow is maintained and may vary depending upon the nature of the drug and the patient's age, weight, and condition. Drugs are either contained in the infusion system itself or added to the flowing infusion.

ADVANTAGES

Major advantages of the IV route of administration are the following:

1. Immediate effect—dosage can be quickly adjusted to response.
2. Fairly constant blood levels can be maintained by a proper rate of infusion.
3. Irritating drugs (such as antineoplastic agents) can often be given with minimal trauma because of the buffering capacity of the blood.
4. Administration can be performed easily in the patient who is unconscious or unable to swallow.

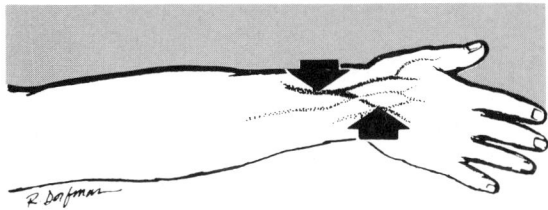

Figure 1–2 The veins of the dorsal venous plexus or the cephalic vein can be used for IV infusions.

DISADVANTAGES

Several disadvantages to IV administration also exist:

1. Rapid action prevents easy antagonism of undesirable drug effects—especially critical in cases of overdosage. Drug is essentially irretrievable once it has been injected.
2. Toxic effects may develop quickly and may be exacerbated by too-rapid injection.
3. Many incompatibilities exist among drugs and IV solutions, because of such variables as pH, temperature of solution, and salt content.
4. IV administration is technically more difficult than most other methods, often causes pain, and may result in infection.

NURSING CONSIDERATIONS

1. Cleanse skin over injection site with alcohol swab; following needle insertion, withdraw plunger slightly. Backflow of blood indicates proper needle placement. Inject solution slowly (e.g., 0.5 mg/min) and steadily, carefully observing patient at the same time.
2. Before beginning IV infusion, check that tubing is unoccluded, all connections are tight, proper drug is being given, and area of needle insertion has been disinfected.
3. Check drug and dosage *carefully* before administering any agent IV.
4. Perform IV injection slowly (1–5 min for most drugs) unless otherwise indicated (some drugs, such as diazoxide, must be given very rapidly). If problems arise during injection (such as with blood pressure, respiratory, or cardiac irregularities), stop injection at once.
5. Observe area immediately around injection or infusion site for any swelling or coldness, which are indications that fluid is leaking from injected vein. If these signs are present, stop injection immediately.
6. Do not inject insoluble materials IV (e.g., suspensions of drugs), because this may cause embolisms.
7. When infusing a drug IV, check flow rate continually (e.g., every 10 minutes initially, then at least every hour or whenever the room is entered for any reason). Be alert for disruption in flow if patient is restless.
8. Remain with patient for 5 to 15 minutes after starting IV infusion to observe for early changes in vital signs or adverse drug effects; recheck patient frequently during the first few hours, especially if the drug is being given for the first time.
9. To check needle placement on IV infusion, lower bottle below level of vein. If blood flows back into needle, vein has been correctly punctured.
10. Assess for indications of extravasation (leakage). These include reduction in flow rate, edema, pain, and coldness at area of infusion. Stop infusion at once if these signs are evident.
11. Monitor for evidence of developing venous phlebitis (pain, tenderness, erythema). Discontinue infusion if present.
12. Discontinue clogged IV system. Flushing should not be attempted because it could dislodge an embolus into circulation.
13. Be alert for symptoms of embolism (cyanosis, tachycardia, hypotension, loss of consciousness), and be prepared to administer oxygen and other necessary drugs; physician should be alerted.
14. Stop infusion or change IV container before container and tubing are completely empty to prevent air from entering system. Prevent development of negative pressure in the

tubing by keeping part of tubing below level of extremity being infused and by placing extremity below level of heart.
15. When terminating IV infusion, clamp tubing, remove dressing around needle or catheter, withdraw needle, and apply firm pressure over site until bleeding ceases. Apply an adhesive bandage tightly to provide continued pressure at needle site.

Intraarterial

Injection of a drug directly into an artery is an infrequently used method of administration, the purpose of which is to perfuse a specific area or organ of the body to achieve a high local concentration of the drug.

Types of drugs most frequently given by the intraarterial (IA) route are the following:
1. Diagnostic agents (x-ray contrast media)
2. Antineoplastic drugs
3. Vasodilators

NURSING CONSIDERATIONS
1. Administer IA drug only if specially trained to do so.
2. Be especially careful to note recommended dilution and rate of administration.
3. Explain diagnostic procedures in detail to patient before beginning injection, and carefully outline any instructions patient must follow.
4. Be alert for development of signs of systemic toxicity. Even though initial drug distribution is local, systemic spread eventually occurs.

Subcutaneous

Subcutaneous (SC) injections are given beneath the skin into the fat and connective tissue underlying the dermis. The most common sites of SC injections are the upper lateral aspect of the arm, the anterior portion of the thigh, and the abdomen (Fig. 1-3). Absorption from these sites through the capillary network is generally rapid (although slower than with IM injection) but can be reduced by local cooling of the area or by the addition of vasoconstrictors to the injection solution. The maximum volume that can comfortably be given by this route is about 2 mL, and the drugs used must be highly soluble and nonirritating to tissues.

In a special form of SC injection termed *hypodermoclysis*, large volumes of fluid are given *very slowly* into the loose connective tissue on the upper surface of the thigh or the outer side of the upper body surface. This procedure can be employed to administer an isotonic sodium chloride solution, glucose, or other parenteral fluids that cannot be given IV for some reason. Hyaluronidase, an enzyme that breaks down the connective tissue matrix, is sometimes added to the mixture to facilitate the spread and absorption of the large volume of injection. It may also reduce the discomfort associated with the injection of such a large volume (500 mL–1000 mL) of fluid.

Compressed pellets can be implanted subcutaneously to provide a "depot" form of a drug, which is continuously and evenly absorbed over a long time. This procedure requires a small incision, and sterility is essential. Absorption from SC sites can also be prolonged by suspending the drug in a protein colloid or gelatin solution.

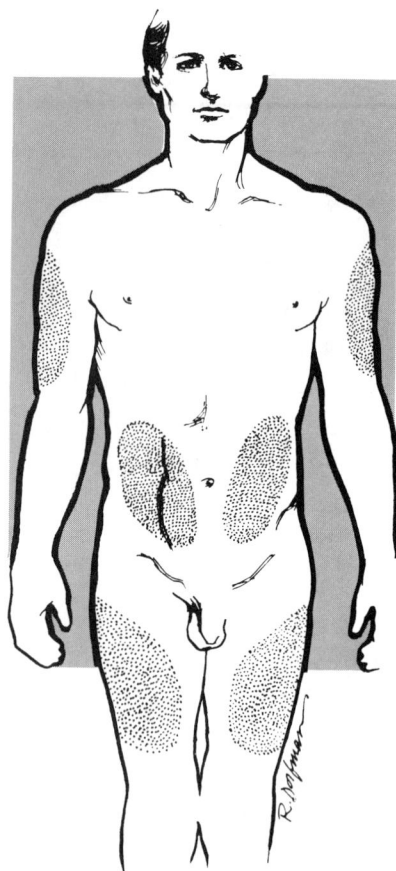

Figure 1–3 The shaded areas show the most common sites for SC injections.

NURSING CONSIDERATIONS
1. Use a fine (25–27 gauge), short ($1/2$–$5/8$ in) needle and a small barrel syringe (1 mL–2 mL). Sterile technique is required.
2. If repeated injections are necessary, vary site of administration to minimize irritation and possible tissue necrosis. Record location of each injection.
3. Grasp and lift skin over injection site, cleanse, and insert needle at a 45° angle with a quick thrust. A 90° angle can be used if the injection site is fatty or when giving insulin or heparin.
4. Before injecting drug, slightly withdraw plunger to aspirate fluid, making sure needle is not in a blood vessel.
5. Inject drug slowly and continuously. When finished, withdraw needle quickly and apply pressure to injection site to retard bleeding.
6. Monitor patient for later development of pain at injection site, which may indicate formation of a sterile abscess. Should this pain occur, report to physician.
7. Assess for appearance of a blister or wheal at injection site, which indicates some drug was given intradermally. Injection may need to be repeated.

Intramuscular

Drug injections can be made into several of the larger muscle masses. Sites most commonly employed are the deltoid muscle (Fig. 1-4A), the gluteal muscles (dorsogluteal and ventrogluteal sites; Fig. 1-4B), and the vastus lateralis (espe-

Methods of Drug Administration

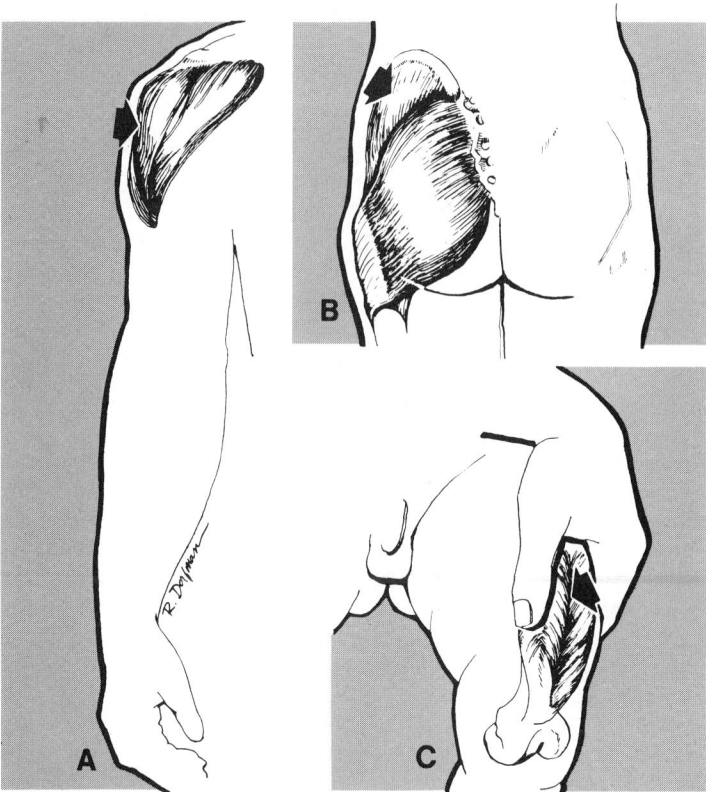

Figure 1-4 Sites most commonly used for drug injections into the larger muscle masses. **A:** The deltoid muscle. **B:** The gluteal muscles. **C:** The vastus lateralis, especially in infants. With gluteal injections, *always* use bony prominences to identify correct injection site (see **Nursing Considerations—IM Administration**).

cially in infants; Fig. 1-4C). Injections are usually made with a longer, heavier needle than that used in SC injections, and larger volumes can be given IM (up to 5 mL at one site) than SC. Absorption is usually rapid because of the vascularity of muscle and the large absorbing surface. The deltoid has perhaps the greatest blood flow of any muscle routinely used for IM injection.

The danger of inadvertent IV administration is increased with an IM injection because of the large number of blood vessels in muscle. Therefore, aspiration of the syringe for blood prior to injecting is essential to ensure proper needle placement. There is also an increased likelihood of nerve damage if the injection is performed incorrectly.

Drugs may be given IM as solutions or suspensions in either water or oil. Aqueous solutions are rapidly absorbed, whereas suspensions or solutions of different drugs (e.g., hormones) in oil provide a depot form from which drug is slowly absorbed for a long-lasting effect. Caution must be exercised when injecting oil-based preparations; some patients may develop allergic reactions to the oil, and in some cases the oil may not be absorbed, requiring excision and drainage.

Depth of needle insertion is very important. It depends mainly on the site and volume of injection and on the condition of the patient (age, weight, extent of body fat).

In small children IM injections are associated with special difficulties, primarily because of the limited muscle mass. Generally, the vastus lateralis (see Fig. 1-4C) on the anterolateral aspect of the thigh is used. Needle lengths should be shorter than with adults, and the child should be restrained to minimize the risk of sudden movement during needle insertion and injection.

Three basic techniques are employed when giving an IM injection: stretching, pinching, and the "Z" method. In *stretch-*

ing, the skin is pressed down and stretched between the thumb and fingers. This method is often used for obese patients to reduce the thickness of subcutaneous fat that must be pierced to reach the muscle. *Pinching* is accomplished by gathering the tissue between the thumb and fingers. This tends to raise the underlying muscle tissue and is helpful with emaciated adults and infants. Finally, the *"Z" method* (sometimes called the Z-track method) is used with medications that might discolor the skin (e.g., iron preparations) or cause subcutaneous irritation should they leak from the underlying muscle. It involves pulling the overlying skin to one side of the injection site, inserting the needle at a right angle to the skin, injecting, and withdrawing the needle quickly while releasing the pulled-back skin at the same time. This maneuver "seals off" the puncture tract.

NURSING CONSIDERATIONS

1. Select appropriate needle size and length depending on site of injection, dosage form of medication, and condition of the patient (age, weight, body fat, scar tissue from repeated injections).
2. Decide on method of injection to be used (stretch, pinch, "Z") and palpate intended site.
3. Place patient in proper position and explain procedure to be followed. For gluteal injections, use location of bony prominences (e.g., greater trochanter, anterior and posterior superior iliac spine) to identify proper site. Keep patient prone and instruct patient to turn toes inward to relax gluteal muscle.
4. After cleansing area, insert needle by means of selected technique usually at a 75° to 90° angle. Aspirate small amount of fluid into syringe to ensure needle is not in a blood vessel. If blood returns in the syringe, withdraw

needle, discard medication, draw up a new dose in a fresh syringe, and inject at a different site.
5. Inject slowly and continuously. Withdraw needle at same angle as insertion and apply pressure. Massage injected site to promote distribution and absorption of drug unless a depot form of drug is used.
6. Do not administer drugs IM when blood supply to the area may be inadequate (as in shock or a paralyzed extremity), because absorption will be impaired and drug effects will be reduced and unpredictable in onset and duration.

Other Parenteral Routes

INTRADERMAL
Drugs may be injected superficially into the outer layers of the skin in very small amounts. Local anesthetics can be given intradermally to facilitate deeper injections, but this method is employed primarily for diagnostic purposes, as in skin testing for allergies or in tuberculin testing. The injection sites commonly employed are the medial forearm area and the surface of the back. Injections are best performed with a small needle (26 gauge) and syringe, and the injection volume is usually 0.5 mL or less. Systemic absorption of intradermally injected agents is very limited, so the method is applicable only to those drugs used locally.

INTRAARTICULAR
This method of injection, directly into a joint, is used primarily for administration of corticosteroids in the treatment of acute local inflammatory conditions. The major advantage is attainment of high local concentrations of steroid in the affected area with minimal systemic absorption, thus reducing toxicity. The procedure requires skill and is painful to the patient.

INTRATHECAL
Intrathecal injections (into the spinal subarachnoid space) are most often employed with local anesthetics, antibiotics, and x-ray contrast media. This technically difficult procedure is usually performed by a physician. It is frequently used to induce localized anesthesia during labor and delivery, although epidural administration of local anesthetics (*outside* the subarachnoid space) is often preferred because of a lower frequency of toxic reactions and less danger of postanesthetic complications.

Several other methods of parenteral administration of drugs are available but are used only infrequently. These are briefly summarized below.

Intraperitoneal. Injection of drugs directly into the peritoneal cavity of the abdomen; widely used in animal experimentation (rapid absorption), but direct injection is not employed in humans because of danger of infection and adhesions. Peritoneal dialysis is performed in cases of renal failure, intractable edema, hepatic coma, azotemia, and uremia and in therapy for peritonitis.

Intracardiac. Direct injection into the heart; occasionally used with epinephrine and isoproterenol for emergency treatment of cardiac arrest.

Intrapleural. Administration of drugs between the lungs and chest wall (pleural cavity). Antibiotics are occasionally given this way.

Intraamniotic. Instillation of drugs into the amniotic sac surrounding the fetus; previously employed with prostaglandin E_2 for second trimester abortion.

NURSING CONSIDERATION
1. After intradermal administration, observe patient for signs of local reaction (swelling, erythema, pain).

PATIENT EDUCATION
1. Following an intraarticular injection, instruct patient not to overuse the affected joint when pain is relieved, because further deterioration of the joint may occur.
2. Caution patient that pain may intensify for several hours after an intraarticular injection before relief is obtained.
3. Warn patient that severe headache may follow intrathecal injection but that it will disappear shortly.

Selected Bibliography
Cockshott W et al: Intramuscular or intralipomatous injections? N Engl J Med 307:356, 1982
DeMoss CJ: Giving intravenous chemotherapy at home. Am J Nurs 80:2188, 1980
Greenblatt D, Koch-Weser J: Intramuscular injection of drugs. N Engl J Med 295:542, 1976
Hanson D: Intramuscular injection injuries and complications. Am J Nurs 73:99, 1973
Hobbs B, Ness S: Rationale for and longterm care of indwelling arterial infusion systems. Oncol Nurs Forum 4:6, 1977
Johnston S, Patt YZ: Caring for the patient on intraarterial chemotherapy. Nursing '81 11(11):108, 1981
Johnston-Early A, Cohen MH, White KS: Venipuncture and problem veins. Am J Nurs 81:1636, 1981
Lenz CL: Make your needle selection right to the point. Nursing '83 13(2):50, 1983
Leutzinger R, Judson A: Drawing blood from a Hickman catheter. Nursing '81 11(12):65, 1981
Nawrocki HR: The ins and outs of administering I.V. bolus injections. Nursing '81 11(11):124, 1981
Newton DW, Newton M: Route, site and technique—Three key decisions in giving parenteral medication. Nursing '79 9(7):18, 1979
Norheim C: Spinal anesthesia. Nursing '86 16(4):42, 1986
Ostrow LS: Air embolism and central venous lines. Am J Nurs 81(11):2036, 1981
Richard C: Nursing implications in the prevention of complications in peritoneal dialysis. Heart Lung 4:890, 1975
Trissel LA: Handbook on Injectable Drugs. Washington, DC, American Society of Hospital Pharmacists, 1980
Vogel TC, McSkimming SA: Teaching parents to give indwelling C.V. catheter care. Nursing '83 13(1):55, 1983
Wong DL: Significance of dead space in syringes. Am J Nurs 82:1237, 1982
Wordell DC: Should you crush that tablet? Nursing '82, 12(9):76, 1982
Wordell DC: Report on intravenous therapy national survey. Nursing '81 11(1):80, 1981

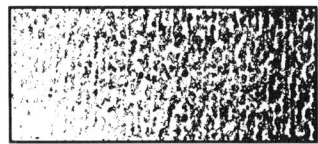

2 INTERACTION OF DRUGS WITH BODY TISSUES: PHARMACOKINETICS

To exert its desired effects, a systemically administered drug must reach its intended site of action. Many factors control the rate and extent to which a drug attains sufficient levels at its site of action. The most important of these factors are the following:

Absorption. The processes involved in transference of drug from its site of administration to the bloodstream, across one or more membranes.

Distribution. The means by which drugs are transported by body fluids to their intended sites of action or to the sites of storage or elimination (liver, kidney).

Biotransformation. The metabolic processes by which a drug molecule is *usually* converted to a less active and more readily excreted form.

Excretion. The mechanisms whereby a drug or its metabolites are removed from the body.

Each of these processes is dependent on many variables and can be modified in several ways. We shall discuss the important aspects of each of these processes and examine how each can be influenced. An outline of the major factors that influence the concentration of a drug at its site of action is shown in Figure 2-1.

To travel from its site of administration to its intended site of action, a drug usually must pass across several body membranes. A typical membrane is composed of phospholipid and protein molecules. The phospholipid molecules are arranged in two parallel rows, termed a *lipid bilayer.* The protein molecules appear to occur randomly, some near the inner or outer surfaces of the membrane and others penetrating the membrane to varying degrees. This arrangement is dynamic; that is, the phospholipid and protein molecules possess the ability to move in conjunction with each other. This concept, which is termed the *fluid mosaic hypothesis,* may help explain the process whereby certain drugs and neurohormones attach to specific receptor areas on the cellular membrane. At different intervals along the membrane, there appear to be breaks in the surface, which may represent the so-called pores in the membrane.

Because cell membranes are largely composed of lipids (fats), the lipid-soluble form of a drug most readily crosses these membranes by means of passive diffusion. Thus, it is essential to understand the lipid membrane concept and how it relates to the different processes involved in the handling of a drug by the body. Many drugs are either weak acids or weak bases, depending on their chemical structure. In solution, they may exist in both the ionized forms and the un-ionized forms. Ionization causes the "splitting apart" of a drug molecule into positively and negatively charged components, and in the *ionized* state, the charged particles are less likely to diffuse across lipid membranes. On the other hand, the *un-ionized* (intact) form of a drug is more lipid-soluble and diffuses most easily across cell membranes. Thus processes such as absorption, distribution, and excretion, which depend upon a drug's ability to diffuse easily through body membranes, are greatly impaired by ionization of the drug molecules.

The ratio of un-ionized:ionized fraction of a drug at any one time is dependent on its ionization (or dissociation) constant (known as the pK_a) and the pH of the aqueous medium in which the drug is present. The pK_a may be defined as the pH at which a drug or other chemical substance exists one half in the un-ionized state and one half in the ionized state. At a pH below the pK_a, acidic drugs will be predominantly un-ionized whereas basic drugs will be largely ionized. Conversely, if the pH of the environment is greater than the pK_a of the drug, acidic drugs will exist predominantly in the ionized state, while basic drugs will be largely un-ionized.

For example, an acidic drug such as aspirin (pK_a 3.5) exists largely in an un-ionized state in the stomach (pH 1.0–3.0) and is well absorbed here. Basic drugs, such as morphine (pK_a 7.9), however, exist predominantly in the ionized state at this site and are not well absorbed. As the drugs travel through the intestinal tract, the pH increases and acidic drugs become more ionized while basic drugs are converted more to the un-ionized state. Therefore, absorption of basic drugs is more extensive in the upper intestinal tract.

The most important factors, then, that control the onset and duration of a drug's effects, are the chemical characteristics of the compound, such as the degree of ionization and the lipid solubility of the un-ionized form. These properties determine the drug's ability to readily traverse body membranes and therefore play a significant role in the movement of drug molecules throughout the body. In general, *un-ionized* drugs are better absorbed, more widely distributed, and less readily excreted than *ionized* drugs.

ABSORPTION

The site and mechanisms involved in the absorption of a drug depend to a large extent on the means of administration.

Absorption From the GI Tract

Drugs may be absorbed from several regions of the gastrointestinal (GI) tract, although most absorption occurs throughout the upper region of the small intestine. The main reasons for this are the presence of many small folds, or *villi,* which greatly increase the absorbing surface area, and the highly permeable nature of the intestinal epithelium. Other factors that make the small intestine the major site for most drug absorption are the presence of special transport systems for absorption of sugars, amino acids, nutrients, and other substances; the fairly rapid gastric emptying of many drugs, which delivers a greater fraction of unabsorbed drug to the upper intestine; and the extensive capillary network of the intestinal villi.

In general, absorption of most drugs from the GI tract is best explained by simple diffusion of the lipid-soluble form of the drug across the mucosal barrier. Some absorption, especially of low molecular weight drugs, also occurs by way of diffusion through aqueous pores in the membrane. With some substances, absorption involves active (energy-requiring) transport mechanisms in which a carrier moves a drug molecule *against* a concentration gradient. For example iodide is absorbed by the thyroid and glucose is reabsorbed by the renal tubules in this manner. Facilitated diffusion is also a carrier-mediated process, but unlike active transport, it does not re-

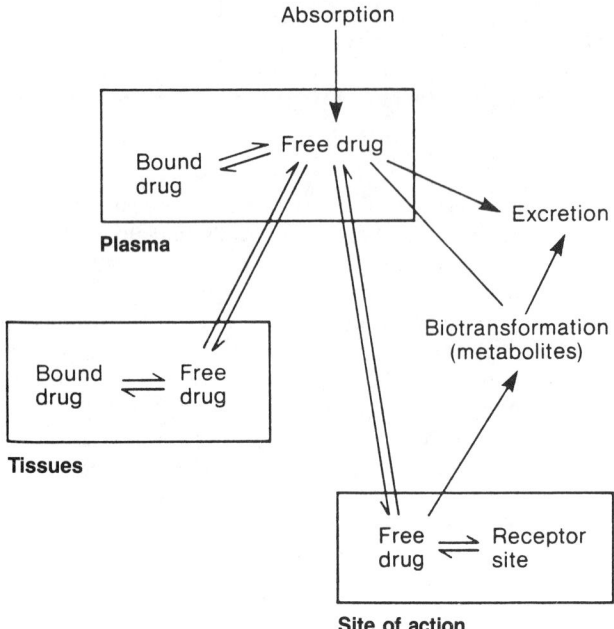

Figure 2–1 Factors influencing concentration of a drug at its site of action.

quire energy and moves *down* the concentration gradient. It is utilized to move less lipid-soluble drugs across the membrane.

Absorption of drugs from the GI tract is influenced by several factors:

NATURE OF THE DRUG

1. Lipid solubility of the un-ionized form, because it is this form that more readily crosses GI membranes
2. Stability of the drug in GI fluid
3. Molecular weight and configuration of the drug, which may influence its passage through the membrane pores. Smaller molecules have a better chance of "squeezing" through the pores

NATURE OF THE DOSAGE FORM

1. Concentration of the drug if administered in solution
2. Dissolution rate of a solid dosage form of the drug
3. Presence of special (enteric) coatings on the drug molecules that resist breakdown and hence prevent absorption in the stomach

NATURE OF THE ABSORBING BARRIER (MEMBRANE)

1. Permeability of the mucosal epithelium
2. Blood flow in the absorbing area
3. pH of the region, which determines the ratio of the un-ionized to ionized form of the drug present
4. Amount of absorbing surface exposed, which is a function of the total surface area present (the length of the absorbing segment, and the presence of surface modifications such as villi)

OTHER FACTORS

1. Length of time the drug is in contact with the absorbing surface. This may depend on peristaltic activity, gastric emptying time, or the presence of inactivating enzymes in the GI tract.
2. Presence of food, which reduces the rate of absorption of many drugs but can increase bioavailability of other drugs, presumably by slowing first-pass hepatic metabolism (see below).
3. Presence of other drugs or substances that can retard absorption by binding free drug molecules or altering GI function (e.g., laxatives, anticholinergics). "Bound" drugs usually cannot be absorbed efficiently.

Absorption From Parenteral Sites

In general, most parenteral sites provide for a more rapid and predictable rate of absorption than the intestinal tract, all other factors being equal. Absorption following subcutaneous or intramuscular injection depends primarily on two factors:
1. Solubility of the drug in the interstitial fluid
2. Area of the absorbing capillary membrane

Drugs in aqueous solution are absorbed more rapidly than drugs in suspension. Often, however, drugs are suspended in certain vehicles to retard their rate of absorption and to provide a prolonged action. Examples of this are some penicillins (benzathine and procaine penicillin G) and long-acting hormones and steroidal agents. Certain types of insulin are combined with proteins or zinc to delay their rate of absorption.

Absorption of drugs from IM sites is usually more rapid than from SC areas because of the more extensive vascular supply per unit area of muscle compared with fatty subcutaneous tissue. The decreased peripheral blood flow present during circulatory failure (as in cases of shock) may significantly reduce the rate of absorption of injected drugs and greatly alter their efficacy. Blood flow to a superficial area can be increased and absorption enhanced by application of heat, local vasodilators, or massage; conversely, decreased blood flow and delayed absorption can result from use of cold packs, a tourniquet, or vasoconstrictors. All these factors can exert a profound influence on the onset, as well as the extent, of a drug's action.

IV administration, of course, provides the most rapid drug action because the drug enters the bloodstream directly without crossing any membranes. The advantages as well as the hazards of this method have been discussed previously.

Absorption From Skin and Mucous Membranes

Absorption of most drugs through the intact skin is very poor, primarily because of the keratinized structure of the epidermis. The underlying dermis, however, is quite permeable, and significant drug absorption can occur if the overlying skin is abraded or denuded. In general, drug absorption occurs to a greater extent through mucous membranes, which present a much thinner and more permeable absorbing surface than the skin. Enhanced absorption of topically applied drugs can be obtained by dissolving the drug in an oily base, by vigorously massaging it into the area of application, or by simultaneously applying a keratin-softening agent such as salicylic acid.

Increasingly, drugs intended for systemic action are being formulated in specialized topical dosage forms, such as transdermal patches, to take advantage of their ability to be consistently absorbed through the skin. Examples of such drugs are nitroglycerin, scopolamine, and clonidine.

Sublingually administered drugs are very rapidly absorbed, owing to the extremely thin epithelial membrane and extensive capillary network in the area of administration.

Absorption of inhaled medication depends to a large extent on the particle size of the drug, which determines the extent of penetration into the alveoli of the lungs. This is the primary site of systemic absorption of inhaled medications, because of the close proximity of capillaries to the alveolar membrane. Although most inhaled drugs are intended for their local effects, systemic absorption may be appreciable, leading to unwanted adverse effects.

DISTRIBUTION

After a drug is absorbed, it is distributed throughout the body by the circulatory system. To produce a significant pharmacologic effect, a drug must reach adequate levels in tissues on which it exerts its principal actions. Because the distribution pattern of a drug is ultimately dependent on its ability to cross body membranes, the principles governing membrane transport of a drug, discussed earlier in the chapter, apply here as well. In general, the initial distribution of a drug is dependent on cardiac output and blood flow to local tissue. In addition, several other factors addressed below can determine the amount of active drug that ultimately reaches the intended site of action.

Binding of the Drug

Drugs may bind either to constituents of plasma (e.g., albumin) or to cells (e.g., nucleoproteins). Binding to plasma proteins slows the disappearance of the drug from the plasma, limits the rate of accumulation in tissues, and prolongs the time that the drug remains in the body. A protein-bound drug is usually inactive, because it is only the free drug that is capable of diffusing across membranes to reach its site of action in the tissues. However, a dynamic equilibrium usually exists between the bound and free forms of a drug (see Fig. 2-1), and some drug will be present in either state. Plasma protein binding may provide a reservoir of drug that gradually dissociates from the binding sites to replace the free drug that has been inactivated.

It is important to keep in mind that the binding capacity of plasma proteins is limited, and saturation may occur, although the amount of drug capable of being bound by plasma proteins is variable and difficult to determine. However, once protein-binding sites are completely occupied, further administration of the drug may increase its effects or produce toxic reactions because of the presence of large amounts of non–protein-bound drug. Similarly, many different kinds of drugs are protein-bound, and *simultaneous* administration of two or more of these drugs can lead to competition for the binding proteins with displacement of active drug and subsequent enhanced drug effects. This type of drug interaction is discussed more fully in Chapter 5.

Lipid Solubility of the Drug

Because most membranes are lipid in nature, drug distribution across these membranes, and ultimately to the site of action, depends to an extent on the lipid solubility of the drug. Moreover, highly lipid soluble drugs tend to localize in adipose (fat) tissue where they may be stored for extended periods because blood flow in these regions is usually sparse. In the case of some drugs, slow release of active drug from these storage sites can result in prolonged subtherapeutic effects (e.g., continued drowsiness following use of a central nervous system depressant that is highly lipid-soluble).

Blood–Brain Barrier

It is well established that some drugs enter the central nervous system (CNS) with relative ease, whereas others do not enter this area at all. These observations have led to the concept of the existence of a blood–brain barrier. The capillaries in the CNS exhibit very tightly joined endothelial cells that lack pores and are enveloped by poorly permeable cells, termed *glial* cells, which impede the access of many water-soluble drugs to the CNS while permitting some highly lipid-soluble drugs to pass. It must be remembered that this is not an absolute barrier but describes a *measurable* difference in the permeability of CNS capillaries to various drugs. For a drug to more easily pass the blood\/brain barrier, it should possess the following properties:
1. Low ionization at plasma pH
2. High lipid solubility of the un-ionized form of the drug
3. Minimal plasma protein binding

Placental Barrier

Although some form of a barrier probably exists between the bloodstream and the placenta, it is very nonselective. Most drugs (except for strongly charged and high molecular weight molecules) are capable of readily entering the placental circulation. During the first trimester of pregnancy, many drugs have a potentially damaging effect on the developing fetus, even though they may not be harmful to the mother. Other drugs, such as alcohol, barbiturates, nicotine, and narcotics, may have untoward effects on both the mother and the fetus. No drug should be taken during pregnancy without consulting the physician, and drugs should be used during pregnancy only when the advantages greatly outweigh the potential risks.

BIOTRANSFORMATION

Although some drugs, such as certain antibiotics, are excreted from the body largely unchanged, most compounds undergo one or more metabolic transformations. These metabolic changes usually occur in the liver by way of hepatic microsomal enzyme systems. These consist of a group of enzymes located on the smooth endoplasmic reticulum of liver cells. The endoplasmic reticulum resembles a series of canals that are continuous with the cell membrane and the membrane of the nucleus. Microsomal enzymes catalyze most oxidative drug metabolism. Metabolites as well as unchanged drugs are then conjugated, for example, with glucuronic acid, which results in the formation of less active, more water-soluble, and hence more easily excreted compounds. Other enzyme systems capable of biotransforming drugs are found in the lungs, plasma, intestine, kidneys, and nerve endings.

Biotransformation does not always lead to formation of *less active* compounds. The metabolic changes occurring with some drugs result in formation of equally active (e.g., imipramine, ephedrine) or more active (e.g., chloral hydrate) products. Similarly, metabolism may bring about formation of a product *more* toxic than the administered agent; an example is ethanol metabolized to acetaldehyde.

Some drugs are administered in the form of an inactive *pro-*

drug, which is then converted to an active metabolite. An example of such a drug is dipivefrin, an eye drop that is converted to epinephrine, the active component, in the eye. Dipivefrin is better absorbed than epinephrine, hence less drug is required.

Biotransformation of drugs usually occurs in two phases. The initial phase involves reactions that produce a chemical change in the drug molecule, such as *oxidation, reduction,* and *hydrolysis*. The second phase involves the coupling of the drug or its metabolic product formed in phase one to another chemical group (e.g., sulfate, acetate) or substrate (e.g., carbohydrate, amino acid). This coupling, or *conjugation,* results in the formation of a more water-soluble and hence more readily excretable product.

There is often considerable variation in the rate at which different individuals metabolize drugs. Several factors are important in determining the capacity of an individual to inactivate a drug:

1. Diseases that alter liver function
2. Age (immature liver functioning in the infant and impaired liver functioning in the geriatric patient)
3. Presence of other drugs, such as barbiturates or pesticides, which may increase liver enzyme function and enhance metabolism or of drugs such as allopurinol, cimetidine, and quinacrine, which inhibit drug-metabolizing enzymes. See Chapter 5 for further discussion of drug interactions based on alterations in liver enzyme function.
4. Genetically determined differences in metabolic activity (which may explain hypersensitivity, resistance, or tolerance to drugs).

A significant factor in determining the efficacy of many orally administered drugs is *hepatic first-pass metabolism*. After absorption from the stomach or intestines, drugs enter the portal circulation and are immediately transported to the liver, where they may be taken up by hepatic cells and metabolized. In some cases, the metabolism of the drug is extensive on first pass, and drugs such as morphine and nitroglycerin, which undergo extensive first-pass metabolism, must be given in higher doses when used orally than when given by other routes of administration that avoid first-pass metabolism, such as subcutaneously or sublingually. Some drugs, such as propranolol, also undergo extensive first-pass metabolism but are converted in part to an active intermediate. Other drugs cleared to a considerable extent by first-pass inactivation include desipramine, reserpine, and verapamil.

EXCRETION

Elimination of a drug or its metabolites from the body is accomplished by several routes including the kidney, lungs, intestine, and, to a lesser extent, the sweat, salivary, and mammary glands. Of these, the most important for the majority of drugs is the kidney.

Kidney

Renal excretion of drugs involves the interaction of three processes: glomerular filtration, active tubular secretion, and tubular reabsorption. The first two of these processes remove drugs from the plasma, whereas tubular reabsorption promotes retention of the drug in the body by returning it to the plasma. The net *excretion* of a drug substance, therefore, depends on the sum total of these three processes.

GLOMERULAR FILTRATION

Glomerular filtration is the process whereby drug molecules diffuse out of the blood perfusing the glomeruli of the nephron and pass into the tubules of the kidney. The drug may then either be reabsorbed into the bloodstream at different segments of the tubule or excreted in the urine. Several factors can influence renal excretion by glomerular filtration.

Molecular size. The amount of drug filtered by the glomerulus depends on its molecular size; smaller molecules are more easily filtered.

Plasma protein binding. Because only free drug can be filtered by the kidney, binding to plasma proteins reduces renal excretion.

Blood level of the drug. The greater the drug concentration in the plasma, the more readily the drug can be filtered and ultimately excreted.

TUBULAR SECRETION

The proximal renal tubule can actively secrete certain drugs, transporting them from the bloodstream directly into the tubular fluid. This process is not significantly affected by protein binding so long as the binding is reversible. Many drugs that are secreted are also filtered by the glomeruli and thus have a very short period of action. An example is penicillin. The tubular secretion process for one drug can be inhibited by another drug. For example, probenecid is often given with penicillin to inhibit its active tubular secretion by competing for a saturable transport system. The duration of action of penicillin in the body is therefore prolonged.

TUBULAR REABSORPTION

Throughout much of the length of the renal tubules, reabsorption of drugs back into the surrounding capillary network occurs, so that a portion of the filtered fraction of drug is retained. Renal tubular reabsorption is in many respects similar to absorption from the gastrointestinal tract; that is, drug molecules are *passively* transported through the tubular epithelial cells. Thus a drug existing in the non-ionized, lipid-soluble state in tubular fluid tends to be more rapidly and more completely reabsorbed than a drug that is highly ionized in tubular fluid. Altering the pH of the urine can markedly affect excretion of a drug. Weak acids such as salicylates, barbiturates, and sulfonamides are excreted more readily as the pH of tubular fluid increases, because weak acids ionize more as the urine is made more basic. Conversely, weak bases like amphetamines, ephedrine, and meperidine are best excreted in an acidic urine because they are largely ionized at a low pH. The techniques of acidification or alkalinization of the urine with drugs such as ascorbic acid and sodium bicarbonate, respectively, can be employed to hasten excretion of certain drugs taken in overdosage. For example, barbiturate intoxication may be managed in part by administration of sodium bicarbonate to raise the urinary pH, thus promoting ionization of the drug molecules in the tubular fluid.

Intestine

Drugs that are not absorbed from the GI tract or drugs or metabolites that are secreted into the GI tract by the bile, salivary glands, and digestive glands can be excreted in the feces. Because many drugs are metabolized in the liver, their metabolites are often secreted into the bile, which passes to the intestine. The metabolite may then be excreted in the feces, but most often it is *reabsorbed* from the intestine into the bloodstream and ultimately excreted in the urine. Thus, biliary and fecal excretion is important mainly for those drugs (such as penicillin or colchicine) that cannot be reabsorbed from the intestine because ionization occurs at the intestinal pH.

Lungs

The lungs are a relatively minor route of excretion. This route is important primarily in the case of the gaseous and volatile-liquid general anesthetics, which can be excreted from the bloodstream across the alveolar membrane into the expired air. Many other volatile substances (including alcohols, paraldehyde, and oils) can appear in the expired air in limited amounts, but they are mainly broken down in the liver and excreted by the kidneys. Enough alcohol can be eliminated unchanged by the lungs to be detected and measured, and this procedure (breathometer) is often used to determine the degree of intoxication.

Mammary Glands

Many drugs can be secreted by the mammary glands, although the amounts present are generally minimal. However, some drugs, such as anticoagulants, barbiturates, corticosteroids, penicillins, and sulfonamides, may be transferred to the infant in breast milk in significant amounts; thus use of such drugs during lactation should be restricted as much as possible. Specific mention of drugs that are likely to appear in milk is made throughout this text.

Selected Bibliography

Atkinson AJ, Kushner W: Clinical pharmacokinetics. Annu Rev Pharmacol 19:105, 1979

Benet LZ: Effect of route of administration and distribution on drug action. J Pharmacokinet Biopharm 6:559, 1978

Benet LZ, Massoud N, Gambertoglio JG (eds.): Pharmacokinetic Basis for Drug Treatment. New York, Raven Press, 1984

Evans WE, Schentag JJ, Jusko WJ (eds): Applied Pharmacokinetics: Principles of Therapeutic Drug Monitoring. San Francisco, Applied Therapeutics, 1980

Garrett ER: Biological responses and pharmacokinetics. Pharm Int 1:121, 1980

Gibaldi M, Levy G: Pharmacokinetics in clinical practice. JAMA 235:1864; 1987, 1976

Gibaldi M, Perrier D: Pharmacokinetics, 2nd ed. New York, Marcel Dekker, 1982

Gibaldi M, Prescott LF (eds). Handbook of Clinical Pharmacokinetics. Sydney, ADIS, 1983

Greenblatt DJ, Koch-Weser J: Clinical pharmacokinetics, Parts I and II. N Engl J Med 293:702; 964, 1975

Gringauz A: Drugs: How They Act and Why. St Louis, CV Mosby, 1978

Mayerson M: Clinical pharmacokinetics: Applying basic principles to therapy. Drug Ther 10:79, 1980

Ritschel WA, Handbook of Basic Pharmacokinetics, 2nd ed. Hamilton, IL, Drug Intelligence Pub., 1982

Shamoo AE (ed): Second International Conference on Carriers and Channels in Biological Systems: Transport proteins. Ann NY Acad Sci 358, 1980

Welling PG: Influence of food and diet on gastrointestinal absorption. A Review. J Pharmacokinet Biopharm 5:291, 1977

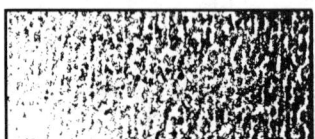

3

BASIC SITES AND MECHANISMS OF DRUG ACTION: PHARMACODYNAMICS

To exert its desired pharmacologic effect, a drug must either act on abnormal parasites or growths (e.g., microorganisms, neoplasms) or modify existing physiologic processes. The actions of a drug in the body must be viewed as the consequence of a complex series of physical and chemical interactions with certain cellular constituents of the living organism. Although much remains to be learned about the molecular basis of a drug's effects, sufficient information exists to establish a fairly detailed picture of the sites at which drugs act and the biochemical mechanisms involved in their actions.

The net result of a drug's action on a biochemical level is an alteration in the normal physiologic functioning of the organism. If this alteration occurs in an abnormal parasite or growth on the body such as bacteria, viruses, or neoplastic tissue, the drug is termed a *chemotherapeutic agent* (e.g., antibiotics, antineoplastics). If the response to a drug consists of a change in the normal physiologic function of the body (e.g., reduction in blood pressure, slowing of the heart rate, or increased urine output), the drug is termed a *pharmacodynamic* agent. Most drugs, of course, fall into the latter category. The effect of a pharmacodynamic agent is strictly quantitative; that is, these drugs are capable of modifying *existing* physiologic functions but are unable to induce a system to perform an action other than a preexisting physiologic one.

Virtually all body tissues are exposed to systemically administered drugs, but certain tissues appear to be affected much more than others. Most drugs exert their *primary* actions at specific sites in the body, although they may affect several tissues or organs depending upon their distribution.

Drugs are believed to produce their effects by combining with cell constituents, thus altering the functioning of the target cell and ultimately the target tissue. This drug–cell constituent combination is believed to be in the form of a chemical bond with reactive sites on the cell constituent. The reactive sites that have an affinity for the drug are termed *receptors*. Although the precise structure of most receptors is still uncertain, several concepts relating to drug-receptor interactions can be stated:

- Drugs exert a quantitative, not a qualitative, effect at receptor sites; that is, drugs alter the *rate* of ongoing physiologic processes but cannot create new functions.
- Receptors have specific molecular conformations, corresponding to certain kinds of drugs (lock and key theory).
- Forces must be present to attract and hold a drug in contact with a receptor so that the drug may exert its effect.
- Drugs "fitting" the receptor may either activate it (*agonists*) or inhibit it (*antagonists*). (See subsequent discussions.)
- Not all receptors on a particular cell need to be occupied for a drug effect to occur; potent drugs may be effective at very low concentrations, occupying only a fraction of the receptors.

In considering drug-receptor interactions, it is important to understand several basic concepts:

1. *Affinity:* the tendency for a drug to bind or attach to its receptor site
2. *Intrinsic activity:* the ability of a drug to produce an effect when bound to the receptor
   A drug that combines with receptors and initiates an effect possesses both affinity and intrinsic activity; it is termed an *agonist.* A drug that combines with a receptor, fails to produce an effect itself, but prevents an agonist from eliciting a response at the same receptor site is termed an *antagonist.* For example, acetylcholine functions as a cholinergic agonist, but its effects are inhibited by atropine, a cholinergic antagonist capable of occupying the same receptor sites but possessing no intrinsic cholinergic activity of its own.
3. *Intensity of effect:* the magnitude of the response to a drug–receptor interaction. The intensity of a drug effect may be explained by two theories:
   a. *Receptor occupation theory:* the intensity is proportional to the fraction of receptors occupied; this probably holds true only to a certain extent and does not account for differences in absolute milligram potency among drugs.
   b. *Rate theory:* the intensity is proportional to the rate at which the drug–receptor combinations occur.

POTENCY VERSUS EFFICACY

Two terms relating to drug action that are often confused are *potency* and *efficacy*. A drug is said to be *potent* when it possesses high intrinsic activity at low unit weight doses. Potencies are compared based on doses that elicit the same intensity of effect, rather than based on magnitudes of effects elicited by the same dose. Knowledge of a drug's potency is important for approximating the appropriate dosage level to be administered but is relatively unimportant in deciding which of two drugs exhibiting the same maximal effect should be used. It makes little difference if the dose of a drug is 5 mg or 500 mg so long as the dosage is convenient to administer. There is no rationale for believing the more potent drug is the clinically preferred drug, as is sometimes implied in drug advertising.

Efficacy, on the other hand, refers to the maximal effect produced by a drug, and it is an important determinant in the drug selection process. For example, oral administration of 4 mg of hydromorphone (Dilaudid) results in much greater pain relief than 65 mg of propoxyphene (Darvon). Therefore, hydromorphone is more effective as well as more potent than propoxyphene.

THERAPEUTIC INDEX

The therapeutic index (TI) for a given drug is a measure of its safety margin and is defined as the TD_{50}/ED_{50}, where the TD_{50} is the dose producing a certain toxic reaction in 50% of an experimental population and the ED_{50} is the dose eliciting the *desired* effect in 50% of an experimental population. The greater the TI, the wider is the safe dosage range for the drug. It is important to recognize, however, that the TI is simply one measure of a drug's safety and has no bearing on the efficacy. Further, the TI must be viewed in general terms, because certain patients display extreme sensitivity to certain drugs and thus have a very low TI for that particular drug. As an example, aspirin is a very safe drug in normal doses in the majority of individuals; however, severe hypersensitivity reactions to small doses of aspirin have occurred in some patients. Therefore, while the TI for aspirin is quite high in the general population, some patients are extremely sensitive to very low doses of aspirin.

NON–RECEPTOR-MEDIATED DRUG EFFECTS

Unlike most drugs, certain agents do not act by combining with receptor sites. For example, *gastric antacids* neutralize the hydrochloric acid secreted by gastric parietal cells, *osmotic diuretics,* (e.g., mannitol) reduce body fluid by increasing the osmolarity of plasma, and *metal chelating agents* such as EDTA can form a chemical complex with heavy metals to prevent poisoning by these substances. The number of drugs acting by non–receptor-mediated mechanisms is small, however, when compared to the number of drugs that owe their action to a drug–receptor complexation.

FACTORS MODIFYING DRUG EFFECTS

In determining the proper drug and dosage to employ, it is important to recognize that many factors can alter an individual's response to a drug. Several important factors follow.

Body Size and Weight

Drug dosages should be adjusted in proportion to the body weight, because the greater the body weight, the more the drug can become diluted in the body. This factor becomes especially critical in infants and small children and will be explored in more detail in Chapter 6. Similarly, the reduced body weight frequently noted in elderly or debilitated persons can increase the effects of drugs (as discussed in Chap. 7).

Age

In general, the pediatric and geriatric patients are very sensitive to the effects of many drugs, principally because of altered metabolic activity, reduced body mass, and decreased excretory capacity.

Sex

Females are thought to be more susceptible to the actions of some drugs, exhibiting either a more intense or a more prolonged effect. This may be due to their smaller body weight and greater proportion of body fat, wherein many drugs are metabolized much more slowly, and possibly also to the influence of hormonal factors.

Route and Time of Administration

Absorption is greatly affected by the route of administration (as discussed in Chap. 2) as well as the time of administration; for instance, greater absorption of most orally administered drugs occurs when the stomach is empty.

Pathologic Conditions

Rates of absorption, metabolism, and excretion can be markedly altered by changes in the normal physiologic state of the individual. Examples include nutritional disorders, thyroid dysfunction (increased sensitivity toward epinephrine), hepatic or renal disease (delayed metabolism and clearance of drugs), cardiovascular impairment and presence of pain (paradoxical excitatory effect with barbiturates), fever, anxiety (decreased analgesic efficacy), or infection.

Drug Idiosyncrasies

Drug idiosyncrasies may take the form of an abnormal drug response or an allergic drug reaction. Many appear to be related to genetically determined enzyme deficiencies that may interfere with the normal metabolism of drugs or increase the vulnerability of certain cells to the adverse effects of drugs. The study of the genetic factors that can influence drug responsiveness is known as *pharmacogenetics,* and the importance of genetic alterations as determinants of drug responsiveness is receiving increasing and well-deserved attention.

Psychological Factors

The attitude and expectations of the person taking the drug can greatly influence its effectiveness. A perfect example of this kind of response is the placebo effect, in which a clinical effect is seen after a dose of a pharmacologically inactive substance is given to a patient who believes he or she is receiving an active drug. The importance of patient reassurance and encouragement in enhancing clinical effectiveness of drugs cannot be overemphasized in this respect.

Repeated Dosage

Variations in the response to an individual drug over time may take several forms:

1. *Cumulative effect:* a progressively increasing response to repeated doses that occurs if the rate of dosing exceeds the rate of excretion; the plasma levels rise until the rate of elimination equals the rate of administration. At that point, a *steady state plasma level* is attained and, all other factors being equal, can be maintained so long as strict adherence to dosing schedules is maintained.
2. *Tolerance:* decreased response to a drug resulting from its repeated administration. Although the mechanism is not entirely understood, it may be related to elevated rates of drug metabolism or cellular adaptation to a drug's local action. It is frequently observed with prolonged use of hypnotics and sedatives. *Rapid* development of tolerance, such that the response becomes progressively less with subsequent doses of drug, is known as *tachyphylaxis.*
3. *Resistance:* impaired response to a dose that normally is effective. It is a type of tolerance usually seen in connection with anti-infective drugs: The microorganism becomes resistant to the bactericidal effects of the antibiotic. The phenomenon of resistance is considered in greater detail in Chapter 56.

Combined Effects of Drugs

Effects of one drug may be modified in several ways by the presence of a second drug.

1. *Synergism:* an enhanced pharmacologic response resulting from the simultaneous use of two drugs
   a. *Additive effect:* the net response is equal to the algebraic sum of the individual drug responses; that is, if the dose of

each were reduced by half, the resultant effect would *equal* that observed with full dosage of either drug alone.
   b. *Potentiation:* the net response is greater than the algebraic sum of the individual drug responses. It is usually seen when two drugs exert the same clinical effect by different mechanisms. For example, the combined antihypertensive effect of hydrochlorothiazide, a diuretic, and propranolol, a beta blocker, is significantly greater than the sum of their individual antihypertensive actions.
2. *Antagonism:* a reduced or abolished drug effect due to the presence of a second drug
   a. *Competitive:* competition for the same receptor sites (e.g., acetylcholine, an agonist, and atropine, an antagonist.)
   b. *Chemical:* inactivation of a drug by formation of a chemical complex (e.g., chelating agents in metal poisoning)
   c. *Physiologic:* use of two drugs having opposing biologic effects (e.g., amphetamine and barbiturates)

MECHANISMS OF DRUG ACTION

Although the *clinical* effects of a drug can be described in terms of alterations in physiologic function, the underlying biochemical and biophysical mechanisms of drug action are less well understood. As discussed earlier in the chapter, the interaction of a drug molecule with a receptor site is the initial event by which the majority of drugs evoke a biological response. This drug–receptor interaction subsequently initiates a chain of biochemical or physiologic events that determine the ultimate therapeutic response to the drug. Several theories have been advanced to help explain how the chemical complexation between a drug molecule and a reactive site in the body can lead to the enormous range of clinical manifestations that constitute the response to drug therapy.

Enzyme Inhibition

Many drugs have been shown to interfere with enzymes necessary for the normal functioning of the organism by combining with the enzyme molecules in much the same way as the normal enzyme substrates. Because practically all biologic reactions are catalyzed by cellular enzyme systems, alteration of normal enzymatic function can significantly accelerate or retard biological functions.

Inhibition of tyrosine hydroxylase or aromatic L-amino acid decarboxylase can decrease catecholamine synthesis, and drugs having these actions have been used as antihypertensives and antiparkinsonian agents. Cholinesterase inhibitors increase functional levels of acetylcholine by slowing its enzymatic inactivation and are effective in treating glaucoma and myasthenia gravis. Inhibitors of hepatic microsomal enzymes can increase the effects of those drugs that depend on microsomal enzymatic function for their metabolic inactivation.

Enzyme Stimulation

Drugs that stimulate the action of adenyl cyclase, the enzyme responsible for the formation of cyclic AMP, have a variety of actions in the body, including bronchodilation, lipolysis, and glycogenolysis. Many drugs can accelerate the activity of the hepatic microsomal enzymes, thus reducing the effectiveness of other drugs, which are then metabolized at a much faster rate by these catabolic enzymes (see Chap. 5).

Alterations in Membrane Permeability

Drugs such as local anesthetics, insulin, or antibiotics may increase *or* decrease permeability of cellular membranes, alter active transport processes, or redistribute the concentration of ions on either side of the cellular membrane, thereby changing its resting potential. As discussed previously, passage of drugs across body membranes is essential for most of the interactions between a drug and body tissues.

Interaction With Neurohormones

Most physiological processes are regulated by neurohormonal activity (e.g., catecholamines, acetylcholine). Drugs may modify the actions of these neurohormones in several ways:

- Altering their rate of synthesis (e.g., carbidopa)
- Interfering with their binding and storage (e.g., reserpine, imipramine, cocaine)
- Varying their rates of release (e.g., guanethidine, amphetamine)
- Interfering with their receptor interaction (e.g., propranolol, atropine)
- Modifying their rate of inactivation (e.g., imipramine, physostigmine)

In addition to the general types of drug mechanisms discussed above, a variety of other mechanisms are responsible for the clinical effects of many drugs. Chemical neutralization of gastric acid, a detergent action on bronchiolar mucus, physical debridement of dead tissue, adsorption of toxins onto the surface of drug particles, and osmotic swelling of muciloids to provide a laxative action are just a few examples of mechanisms of action for other drugs.

Selected Bibliography

Baxter JD, Fonder JW: Hormone receptors. N Engl J Med 301:1149, 1979
Creese I, Sibley DR: Receptor adaptations to centrally acting drugs. Annu Rev Pharmacol Toxicol 21:357, 1981
Fuller RW: Pharmacology of brain epinephrine neurons. Annu Rev Pharmacol Toxicol 22:31, 1982
Kenakin TP: The classification of drugs and drug receptors in isolated tissues. Pharmacol Rev 36:165, 1984
Smythies JR, Bradley RJ (eds): Receptors in Pharmacology. New York, Marcel Dekker, 1978
Snyder SH: Receptors, neurotransmitters and drug responses. N Engl J Med 300:465, 1979
Starke K: Presynaptic receptors. Annu Rev Pharmacol Toxicol 21:7, 1981
Vessell ES: Why individuals vary in their response to drugs. Trends Pharmacol Sci August:349, 1980

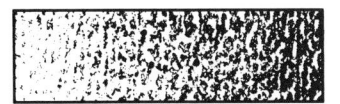

4 PHARMACOLOGIC BASIS OF ADVERSE DRUG EFFECTS

Adverse reactions to drug therapy include any unwanted, undesirable, or potentially injurious consequence of drug administration. Not all adverse reactions, however, are unexpected or unpredictable; some represent a logical extension of a drug's normal pharmacologic spectrum of action. Others can often be predicted on the basis of the patient's condition, the route of drug administration, and the presence of other drugs. Although the distinction is arbitrary and quite flexible, those expected and usually unavoidable untoward drug reactions are termed *side effects,* and while frequently troublesome and annoying, they are rarely serious. Examples are drowsiness, dry mouth, and nausea. In contrast, unpredictable, unusual, unexpected, or potentially serious reactions are generally referred to as *adverse reactions* (e.g., gastric ulceration, ocular damage, respiratory depression, blood dyscrasias). Changing the dose, dosage form, route of administration, or diet can often reduce or abolish minor side effects. Major adverse reactions, however, are frequently dose- and dosage-form independent, and their occurrence frequently is more difficult to control. The propensity for a particular drug to cause reactions, the kind of reactions produced, and the frequency of occurrence will determine the utility of the drug for treating a particular disease state. That is, the possibility of serious toxicity resulting from drug usage is usually acceptable if the condition being treated is serious enough to warrant the risk. Conversely, drugs causing a high degree of adverse effects should not be used to treat trivial or psychosomatic illnesses. For example, chloramphenicol, a highly toxic antibacterial agent, is acceptable in the treatment of certain salmonella or meningeal infections in which other agents have failed or are inappropriate, but the drug should not be used to treat uncomplicated respiratory tract infections. Potent corticosteroids are invaluable in many types of inflammatory conditions but should not be routinely prescribed for such relatively minor ailments as poison ivy or urticaria.

CLASSIFICATION OF ADVERSE DRUG EFFECTS

Classification of adverse drug effects is difficult because a wide range of diverse manifestations can occur. No single classification is adequate to categorize the multiplicity of adverse effects that can follow drug treatment. To discuss adverse effects in a logical format, however, we will classify them in the following manner:

I. Pharmacologic
  A. Extension of therapeutic effect
  B. Nontherapeutic effects
II. Nonpharmacologic
  A. Hypersensitivity
  B. Idiosyncrasy
  C. Photosensitivity
III. Disease-related
IV. Multiple-drug reactions
V. Miscellaneous
  A. Carcinogenicity
  B. Teratogenicity
  C. Drug dependence

A brief review of these different types of adverse drug reactions will aid in their proper identification.

PHARMACOLOGIC ADVERSE EFFECTS

Many adverse drug effects result from a greater than desired intensity of action or elicitation of one or more *secondary* drug effects in addition to the *primary* or intended drug effect.

Primary Actions (Extension of Therapeutic Effect)

Overdosage with a therapeutic agent will usually elicit, among other effects, an excessive reaction to the *primary* effect of the drug. For example, tranquilizers used as daytime sedatives in excessive amounts will generally produce drowsiness and possibly hypnosis. In this case, the adverse reaction usually can be overcome by either reducing the dosage or decreasing the frequency of administration. Other common examples of untoward reactions induced by drug overdosage are superficial hemorrhaging with anticoagulants and excessive electrolyte and water depletion secondary to diuretic therapy.

Secondary Actions (Nontherapeutic—Side Effects)

In many instances, the adverse effects caused by drug administration related to a manifestation of one or more *secondary* actions produced by a drug molecule. In some cases, these secondary drug effects can be largely eliminated by adjusting the dosage carefully in each individual. Many times, however, these adverse reactions are an inescapable consequence of normal therapeutic dosages. For example, normal doses of many antihistamines are associated with a certain degree of drowsiness, a potentially dangerous occurrence. Even in small, therapeutic doses, anticholinergics used for relief of GI spasm and hypermotility usually produce xerostomia (dry mouth), blurring of vision, and some degree of urinary retention and constipation. Other examples of drug-induced secondary reactions include constipation with narcotic analgesics, potassium loss (hypokalemia) with diuretics, and orthostatic (positional) hypotension with antipsychotics.

These secondary effects of a drug usually cannot be controlled by dosage adjustment because minimal therapeutic doses are already being used, but the effects often can be reduced by substituting or adding other drugs to the regimen. For example, the drowsiness seen with many antihistamines can be minimized by using a mild central stimulant such as caffeine, or by switching to an antihistamine possessing minimal CNS depressant actions, such as terfenadine.

Secondary adverse reactions may be quite serious, requiring careful patient monitoring and perhaps changes in the drug regimen. Potentially dangerous secondary effects of drugs include the possibility of thrombotic complications with oral contraceptives, arrhythmias with improper digitalis usage, and GI bleeding and ulceration with aspirin and related drugs.

Most pharmacologic adverse reactions have been extensively documented. Thus, in assessing the suitability of a particular therapeutic regimen, the disadvantages of a drug's known predictable toxicity should be weighed against its potential beneficial effects.

NONPHARMACOLOGIC ADVERSE EFFECTS

Another group of adverse drug effects have little relationship to the pharmacologic effects of a drug. Rather, they are related to an abnormal sensitivity or reactivity to a chemical substance on the part of the drug recipient. This aberrant reaction may be termed a *hypersensitivity* (or allergic) *reaction* or an *idiosyncratic reaction*. A principal hazard of this type of nonpharmacologic adverse reaction is that it cannot be predicted from the profile of drug action, and its onset is often abrupt and unexpected. Fortunately, these types of reactions occur only in a fraction of patients receiving the drug.

Hypersensitivity

Hypersensitivity or allergic reactions are perhaps the largest single group of untoward drug effects. Allergic reactions are usually not dose related and are largely independent of the pharmacologic properties of the drug molecule. These hypersensitivity reactions are associated with an altered reactivity or sensitization of the patient resulting from prior exposure to a drug or chemical that behaves like an allergen. The drug (or metabolite) interacts with a tissue or plasma protein, activating the reticuloendothelial system, resulting in production of antibodies to the drug molecule. A subsequent exposure to the same drug (or in some cases a similar one) elicits an antigen–antibody reaction that produces the symptoms of the allergic response (e.g., itching, edema, congestion, wheezing).

Allergic drug reactions may be classified as either immediate (e.g., anaphylaxis, urticaria) or delayed (e.g., serum sickness).

IMMEDIATE

An immediate allergic drug reaction develops within minutes of drug exposure. The drug–antibody reaction probably releases several vasoactive substances, such as histamine and bradykinin, from their tissue stores. These substances can react with the smooth muscle of many body tissues (blood vessels, bronchioles, GI tract) to produce characteristic signs of the allergic reaction such as bronchoconstriction or vasodilation. The symptoms may be very mild (rash, itching, urticaria) or serious enough (respiratory distress, circulatory collapse) to require immediate attention and swift medical treatment to prevent death. In general, the severity of the reaction is independent of the drug itself but probably depends to a large extent on a patient's sensitivity. It has been documented that even very small doses of common drugs such as aspirin and penicillin can produce violent hypersensitivity reactions in susceptible patients. The grave concern about these kinds of reactions is that often they are totally unpredictable, and quick recognition and proper treatment are essential to minimize serious consequences such as respiratory distress, hypotension, and cardiovascular collapse.

DELAYED

A delayed allergic drug reaction develops slowly following drug challenge. The clinical picture of delayed hypersensitivity often includes a diffuse rash, fever, and swelling and stiffness of the joints. This syndrome is frequently referred to as *serum sickness*. This name derives from the fact that the allergic response results from damage produced by *circulating* immune complexes that may lodge in small vessels and cause the characteristic symptoms. Sometimes the liver, kidney, and bone marrow may become damaged, although the factors that determine specific organ involvement are largely unknown.

Idiosyncrasy

Idiosyncrasy refers to a peculiarity in bodily function that causes an individual to react to a drug in an abnormal manner. Idiosyncratic reactions may manifest themselves as either a quantitative (i.e., over- or under-responsiveness) or a qualitative (e.g., paradoxical excitation) change from the norm.

These reactions are probably not caused by formation of an antigen–antibody complex but are related to a genetically determined defect in the ability of the patient's body to handle a particular drug. The manifestations of idiosyncratic reactions can assume a great number of forms; they may range from the rather mild (erythema, rash, photosensitivity) to the very serious (blood dyscrasias, exfoliative dermatitis, systemic lupus-like reaction, hemolytic anemia, malignant hyperpyrexia). A general description of some of the more important idiosyncratic drug reactions appears at the end of this chapter. A specialized field of study termed *pharmacogenetics* deals with altered drug responses that are under hereditary control; great strides have been made in determining some of the genetic flaws that predispose certain individuals to toxic drug effects. For example, development of hemolytic anemia upon exposure to certain drugs has been linked to a genetic deficiency of the enzyme glucose-6-phosphate dehydrogenase in red blood cells.

Photosensitivity

A unique type of dermatological hypersensitivity reaction following use of many drugs is observed upon exposure to sunlight and is termed *photosensitization*. Two principal types of reactions can occur in people whose skin has been sensitized by either topical or internal use of photosensitizing drugs. A *photoallergic* reaction presents itself as a papular eruption on sun-exposed areas similar to that resulting from contact dermatitis. It is probably due to the photosensitizing drug forming an antigen by absorption of sunlight and subsequent combination with a skin protein. The resultant antibody formation sensitizes the patient to further synthesis of antigen by continued sun exposure.

A *phototoxic* reaction, on the other hand, is characterized by a severe sunburn; as such it is not always viewed as a hypersensitivity reaction. Nevertheless, it is probably caused by a photosensitizing chemical that absorbs ultraviolet radiation energy to such an extent that it becomes toxic to epidermal cells.

A wide variety of clinically useful drugs can produce photosensitization. This fact is noted under the **Significant Adverse Reactions** heading for each of the offending drugs.

DISEASE-RELATED ADVERSE EFFECTS

The pathophysiological state of a patient is a major determinant of the potential for a drug to cause adverse effects. Underlying disease states, often unrecognized, can greatly increase the possibility of drug toxicity. The more common abnormalities are discussed briefly below.

Hepatic Disease

Because the liver plays a major role in the metabolism and inactivation of many drug molecules, impaired liver function may lead to plasma levels of a drug being abnormally high for extended periods. If normal dosing schedules are followed, accumulation of drug in the body can occur, resulting in symptoms of drug overdosage. Because of the tremendous reserve capacity of the liver, however, near-normal metabolic function usually is present except in the most severe forms of hepatic disease.

Renal Disease

The presence of kidney disease can lead to many adverse reactions with those drugs that are eliminated largely through renal excretory processes. In the presence of renal disease, doses of drugs excreted by the kidney, such as the potentially toxic aminoglycoside antibiotics, need to be reduced in order to avoid accumulation and subsequent toxicity. In progressive renal failure, plasma albumin stores may also be diminished, which can reduce the serum protein binding of many drugs, resulting in potentiation of their effects.

Emotional Disorders

Mentally unstable individuals should be monitored carefully during their drug therapy. Too often, emotionally disturbed patients do not comply with proper dosing instructions, and this may lead to overdosage with many prescribed drugs (e.g., hypnotics, antipsychotics) or use of improper drugs. A major problem exists with misuse of, or overmedication with, the antipsychotic group of drugs. Because many individuals taking these drugs are emotionally unstable to some extent, these drug users represent an extremely high-risk group for potential adverse reactions.

Other Disease States

Many other types of existing disease can increase the likelihood for a particular drug to elicit an adverse drug reaction. Use of nonselective beta-adrenergic blockers (e.g., nadolol, propranolol) in patients with asthma may worsen the already impaired ventilatory flow. Beta-adrenergic blockers, as well as the calcium channel blocker verapamil, also should not be given to patients with advanced heart block, because these drugs can reduce myocardial contractility and further slow atrioventricular (AV) conduction. Aspirin and other antiinflammatory drugs are more likely to cause GI bleeding in a person with an active or recent gastric ulcer. Careful assessment of a patient's overall health status is important in ensuring the safest and most effective use of a drug.

MULTIPLE-DRUG REACTIONS

The presence of a second drug may greatly modify the actions of a concurrently administered drug. In many instances, drugs are used together to achieve a better clinical response than either drug could achieve alone. This is an example of a positive clinical interaction. On the other hand, indiscriminate multiple-drug therapy can be quite hazardous; the chance of untoward reactions increases dramatically as additional drugs are added to a therapeutic regimen. This problem becomes especially acute in the elderly or the seriously ill patient, for whom several different drugs may be administered concurrently. Adverse effects due to multiple-drug therapy can be manifested in several ways; this aspect of pharmacotherapy is examined in Chapter 5.

MISCELLANEOUS ADVERSE REACTIONS

A number of other adverse drug effects that do not fall within one of the above groups have been reported with certain drugs, and some of the more important of these are the following:

Carcinogenicity: the ability of a drug or chemical to elicit malignant changes in cells

Teratogenicity: the ability of a drug or chemical to produce structural defects in the developing fetus. The U.S. Food and Drug Administration (FDA) has established five categories indicating the potential of a drug for causing fetal damage (Table 4-1)

Drug Dependence: the ability of a drug or chemical to induce a state of psychological or physical need for itself (see Chap. 79)

NURSING CONSIDERATIONS

1. Recognize that any drug can be potentially toxic, and administer all drugs with respect for their adverse effects as well as their beneficial effects.
2. Carefully assess the seriousness of the condition being treated before using any medications. The potential benefit should outweigh the apparent risk, and less toxic agents should be tried first if at all possible.
3. Always monitor the dose being given to ensure that it is within acceptable limits for the condition and patient being treated.
4. Obtain a careful drug history, including any previous drug allergies, from each patient before administering any pre-

---

Table 4-1
FDA Pregnancy Categories

Category	Description
A	No demonstrated fetal risk in humans during any stage of pregnancy
B	No demonstrated fetal risk in animal studies but no adequate studies in pregnant women *or* Animal studies have shown an adverse effect but studies in pregnant women have not demonstrated a risk during any stage of pregnancy
C	Animal studies have shown an adverse effect on the fetus but there are no adequate studies in humans *or* No animal or human studies are available (use of the drug *may be acceptable* despite the risks)
D	Evidence of human fetal risk but the benefits from use of the drug *may be acceptable* despite the risks
X	Animal or human studies have demonstrated fetal abnormalities or adverse reaction reports give evidence of fetal risk (risk to a pregnant woman clearly outweighs the possible benefit)

scribed medication. This measure reduces the possibility of hypersensitivity reactions.
5. Plan to administer drugs to maximize their intended effects and to minimize their untoward reactions. For example, give diuretics in the morning to reduce need to void at night, and give antihistamines at night to avoid daytime drowsiness.

PATIENT EDUCATION

See **Plan of Nursing Care 1 (Knowledge Deficit Related to Drug Therapy)** in this chapter.

ADVERSE DRUG REACTIONS—A GLOSSARY

Alopecia: loss of hair, sometimes accompanied by extreme drying of the scalp. Alopecia is a side effect of many antineoplastic agents as well as anticoagulants, mephenytoin, methimazole, and others.

Anaphylactic reaction: a severe systemic allergic reaction that develops suddenly, progresses rapidly, and is frequently fatal if not treated. Symptoms range from itching, hives, nasal congestion, abdominal cramping, and diarrhea to dyspnea, hypotension, fainting, choking sensation, cardiovascular collapse, and possibly death. An anaphylactic reaction can theoretically occur with any drug, but it is most commonly observed with drugs that are frequently associated with drug allergies, such as penicillins, sulfonamides, and salicylates.

Blood dyscrasias: abnormal conditions of the formed elements or other clotting constituents of the blood. Several types are commonly observed:

Agranulocytosis: an acute febrile disease characterized by an absence of granulocytes and often a corresponding reduction in monocytes and lymphocytes. Clinical symptoms include chills, fever, and extreme weakness. Because of the lack of white blood cells, the body's defense mechanism is impaired, and severe infection can result. Early warning signs are mucous membrane ulceration, sore throat, skin rash, and fever. Recovery normally occurs within 1 to 2 weeks after drug is withdrawn. Any existing infection should be vigorously treated. Agranulocytosis is the most common drug-induced blood dyscrasia.

Anemia: a reduction in the number of red blood cells, hemoglobin concentration, and volume of packed red cells. The result is a sharp curtailment in the oxygen-carrying capacity of the blood.

Aplastic: results from drug-induced damage to the bone marrow and is marked by a deficiency of red cells, hemoglobin, and granular cells, and a predominance of lymphocytes. Clinical signs include fatigue, tachycardia, bleeding, fever, and increased susceptibility to infection. Aplastic anemia is often fatal owing to hemorrhage and overwhelming infection.

Hemolytic: characterized by a short life span of the red cell. Circulating erythrocytes are destroyed owing to increased hemolytic activity induced by certain drugs or poisons. Especially common in individuals with a glucose-6-phosphate dehydrogenase deficiency. Withdrawal of offending agent usually corrects the condition.

Thrombocytopenia: a lowered blood platelet count, resulting from either platelet destruction or depression of the platelet-forming mechanism in the bone marrow. Onset may be sudden, and symptoms include purpura (petechiae; epistaxis; oral, vaginal, or GI bleeding) and easy bruising. The platelet count returns to normal within a few weeks after cessation of drug therapy, but the count may again rise briefly immediately following withdrawal of the drug. Most severe complications can result from excessive cerebral hemorrhage.

Erythema multiforme: an acute inflammatory skin disease characterized by lesions consisting of concentric circles of erythema, usually appearing on the neck, face, and legs. Occasionally blisters are observed. Often accompanied by fever, malaise, arthralgia, and gastric distress. The most severe variant, *Stevens–Johnson syndrome*, is characterized by high fever, headache, and inflammatory lesions of the mouth, eyes, and genitalia. Often the bronchial and visceral mucosa are involved. Death can occur because of renal impairment.

Exfoliative dermatitis: erythema and scaling of the skin over large parts of the body. Symptoms include itching, weakness, malaise, fever, and weight loss. Exfoliation may include loss of hair and nails as well as skin, and mucosal sloughing can occur. The reaction is generally unpredictable in its duration and recurrence. Relapses are frequent, and secondary infections can be serious. Exfoliative dermatitis may occur secondary to preexisting dermatoses or to contact dermatitis resulting from an underlying carcinoma, or can be caused by drug usage.

Hepatotoxicity: liver damage resulting from either infections or drug hypersensitivity. The most frequently observed drug-induced manifestation is *jaundice,* characterized by hyperbilirubinemia and deposition of bile pigments in the mucous membranes and skin; these pigments impart the typical yellow appearance. At least three main types of jaundice are recognized:

Cholestatic: due to interference with the normal secretion of bile by an obstruction of the biliary passages. It may result from gallstones, tumors, or drug-induced inflammation of the bile channels.

Hepatocellular: due to impairment of the function of liver cells. It is also termed *necrotic jaundice* and closely resembles severe viral hepatitis.

Hemolytic: due to a drug hypersensitivity or a direct toxic effect of the drug on erythrocytes, possibly interference with normal glucose metabolism in the red cells. In addition, a hepatitis-like reaction may be elicited by several kinds of drugs, resulting from either a hypersensitivity to the drug or a direct toxic effect of the drug on liver cells.

Lupus erythematosus (LE): an autoimmune inflammatory disorder that can occur in two forms, one affecting only the skin (discoid LE) and the other, more serious, affecting multiple body organs (systemic LE). The etiology of the naturally occurring disease is unknown, but both forms occur predominantly in young women. Several drugs, for example hydralazine and procainamide, can also cause a lupus-like reaction. Among the many symptoms are diffuse rash; fever; malaise; alopecia; joint symptoms including stiffness, swelling, and synovitis; conjunctivitis; photophobia; pneumonitis; pleurisy; myocarditis; arrhythmias; lymphadenopathy; splenomegaly; and hemolytic anemia. Renal and neurologic features are absent in drug-induced lupus but are seen in the spontaneously occurring form of the disease. Clinical features generally revert slowly toward normal when the offending drug is withdrawn, but altered laboratory values (e.g., ele-

PLAN OF NURSING CARE 1
PATIENTS WHOSE KNOWLEDGE OF DRUG REGIMEN IS DEFICIENT
Nursing Diagnosis: Knowledge Deficit Related to Drug Therapy
Goal: Patient will possess knowledge and skills needed to implement drug regimen and related actions.

Intervention	Rationale	Expected Outcome
Assess patient's readiness to learn, current level of understanding, and factors likely to influence learning.	Learning can be impeded by physical, emotional, or social factors such as pain, extreme anxiety, and cultural background. To help ensure success, teaching should begin at current level of understanding.	
Initiate planning when patient is ready to learn.	Motivation significantly affects learning. Learning is enhanced when information is presented in response to expressed need.	Patient will verbalize awareness of the need to learn and a desire to do so.
Explain the need for and the benefits of learning.		
Determine whether patient is likely to benefit more from individual or group sessions, formal or incidental teaching.	Drug instruction may be provided to individuals or groups. In formal teaching, instruction is the primary activity. Incidental teaching occurs in conjunction with other activities.	
Establish goals and teaching plan with patient.	Identification of objectives, responsibilities, approaches, tools, and sequence of instruction improves teaching/learning efficiency. Patient involvement promotes cooperation and success.	Patient will express satisfaction with the goals and teaching plan.
Involve different senses and include active learning experiences.	Involvement of multiple senses and active learning experiences enhances learning and improves retention.	
Sequence learning from simple to complex.	Learning is easier if content progresses from simple to complex.	
Arrange for significant others to attend teaching sessions.	Significant others can support and reinforce desired behavior and can administer drug if patient is unable to do so.	
Select quiet, private times and environments for teaching.	Distraction and other environmental obstacles impede learning.	
Use terminology patient understands and relate content to patient's own experiences.	The patient may be too embarrassed to acknowledge lack of familiarity with complex terminology. Content that relates to the patient's own experiences is more meaningful and easier to grasp.	
Pace sessions to correspond to patient's attention span and ability to retain information.	Frequent, short teaching sessions may be more effective than a few lengthy ones.	
Teach the following information related to the prescribed drug:		Patient will accurately answer questions regarding the content of the teaching plan.
1. Name of drug and availability of generic preparations	Where generic prescribing exists, the patient needs to know that generic substitutes are available in order to take advantage of them.	
2. Drug action, purpose, response expected, length of time it takes to become effective	Compliance improves when the patient's expectations of results are realistic and the patient accepts susceptibility to or diagnosis of the condition being prevented or treated.	
3. Dosage, route, and schedule of administration (including whether an oral drug is to be taken before or during meals, how much water or other fluid to take with it, and at what intervals it is to be taken)	Prescription labels may not clearly specify all requirements. Absorption of some drugs, for example, is greatly affected by food.	Patient will describe his/her role in drug therapy.

Continued

PLAN OF NURSING CARE 1 (continued)
PATIENTS WHOSE KNOWLEDGE OF DRUG REGIMEN IS DEFICIENT
Nursing Diagnosis: Knowledge Deficit Related to Drug Therapy
Goal: Patient will possess knowledge and skills needed to implement drug regimen and related actions.

Intervention	Rationale	Expected Outcome
4. Importance of adhering to prescribed regimen and impact of deviation on drug effects and the condition being prevented or treated	Rigid adherence to the prescribed dosage schedule is often necessary to maintain stable, effective blood levels and minimize adverse reactions. The patient may believe, for example, that if one dose helps, two may be twice as good, possibly paving the way for adverse reactions.	
5. Technique for administration (see Nursing Considerations sections in Chap. 1 for specific information regarding techniques for particular routes of administration)	Unfamiliar routes of administration may require special explanations (e.g., sublingual tablets and troches). Injections usually require multiple demonstration and practice sessions.	Patient will correctly demonstrate skills required for the drug regimen.
6. Length of time drug is to be taken, risks entailed in premature discontinuation	For some drugs, such as antibiotics, effective use may depend on administration over a period of time even though the patient may feel better before the entire course has been taken. Serious reactions may ensue from sudden cessation of certain drugs, such as some antihypertensives.	
7. Usual side effects and how to manage them	Some side effects may be quite alarming if the patient is unaware of their cause, such as black stools from iron tablets or urine discoloration from other drugs. Also, the patient is less likely to discontinue medication when side effects appear if he/she expects them and knows what to do about them.	
8. Signs of adverse reactions that should be immediately reported and person to whom they should be reported	The patient needs to be evaluated quickly if signs of serious adverse reactions appear. Symptoms of adverse reactions to some drugs may seem relatively innocuous to the uninformed patient (e.g., sore throat, mild fever, itching).	
9. Potential interactions with other prescription drugs, OTC drugs, food, and laboratory tests	Serious interactions and toxic effects can occur when medications are combined, even OTC preparations. This can happen if the patient visits more than one healthcare provider, each of whom may be unaware of drugs prescribed by others. Furthermore, the patient may not consider OTC preparations to be drugs, may take drugs prescribed for someone else, and may be unaware of interactions with food and laboratory tests.	
10. Techniques for monitoring drugs effects and the importance of these	To ensure safe and effective use, some drugs require periodic laboratory tests, such as blood counts or prothrombin times. With certain drugs, such as cardiac glycosides and beta blockers, the patient may need to monitor his/her pulse. The patient receiving hypoglycemics may need to test his/her urine or blood for glucose.	
11. Storage requirements	Some drugs need special handling such as refrigeration or storage in light-resistant containers.	
12. When and where to get prescription filled and obtain other supplies or services		

Continued

PLAN OF NURSING CARE 1 (continued)
PATIENTS WHOSE KNOWLEDGE OF DRUG REGIMEN IS DEFICIENT
Nursing Diagnosis: Knowledge Deficit Related to Drug Therapy
Goal: Patient will possess knowledge and skills needed to implement drug regimen and related actions.

Intervention	Rationale	Expected Outcome
13. Safety measures to prevent injury or poisoning		
Encourage patient to ask questions and verbalize understanding of what is taught.	An atmosphere of trust and rapport facilitates the learning process.	
Provide positive feedback regarding learning progress.	Learning is enhanced when the patient is aware of progress. Rewarded behaviors tend to be repeated.	
Repeat information in various ways.	Repetition improves retention.	
Provide written material to supplement content taught in other ways.	Written material serves as memory aid and reference source.	Patient will possess written information regarding the drug regimen.
Refer patient to appropriate community healthcare agencies for follow-up or further instruction as needed.	The elderly or chronically ill patient or one with few support systems may need additional evaluation or instruction in the home setting.	Patient will be evaluated and receive additional instruction/support in the home setting.

vated antinuclear antibody titer, leukopenia, thrombocytopenia) indicative of the disease may persist for many months.

Nephrotoxicity: damage to the functional units of the kidney, such as the glomerular filtration apparatus, blood vessels, or renal tubular cells, or a dysfunction of the components (e.g., enzymes, transport carriers) involved in the tubular secretory and reabsorptive processes.

Neurotoxicity: damage to different nervous system structures, manifested as a wide range of central and peripheral disturbances. Some of the more important neurotoxic effects of drugs are the following:

Myasthenia-like reaction: extreme muscle weakness due to an impairment in the transmission of impulses at the neuromuscular junction.

Extrapyramidal reactions: disturbances of the extrapyramidal motor-regulating system in the CNS, resulting in abnormal motor function. Common manifestations include immobility (akinesia); fixed positioning of the limbs (rigidity); sudden violent movements of the arms and head (dystonias); restlessness (akathisia); and rhythmic, clonic muscular activity (tremor). Extrapyramidal reactions are frequently associated with use of antipsychotic drugs.

Ototoxicity: progressive hearing loss and tinnitus caused by damage to the eighth cranial nerve. Often accompanied by vertigo and nystagmus if the vestibular branch of the nerve is affected. It is common with the aminoglycoside antibiotics and certain diuretics.

Ocular toxicity: disturbances in the functioning of the eye. The most common manifestation is *blurred vision,* which can occur following use of many drugs, especially those with an anticholinergic action. Other drug-induced ocular disorders include myopia, scotomata, amblyopia, optic neuritis, corneal deposits, pigmentary retinopathy, and cataracts.

Photosensitivity: an altered responsiveness to light, usually eczematous in nature. Common manifestations are itching, scaling, urticaria, and in severe cases multiform lesions.

Purpura: localized hemorrhaging, occurring in the skin, mucous membranes, or serous membranes. The lesions may be petechiae (small blood spots) or ecchymoses (larger areas of bleeding). Purpura is commonly seen in patients with thrombocytopenia caused by increased platelet destruction.

Selected Bibliography

Curtis JR: Drug-induced renal disease. Drugs 18:377, 1979

Jick H, Walker AM, Porter J: Drug-induced liver disease. J Clin Pharmacol 21:359, 1981

Karch FE, Lasagna L: Adverse drug reactions: A critical review. JAMA 234:1236, 1975

Poirier TI: Factors involved in adverse drug reactions. US Pharmacist April:33, 1983

Schiff G: Adverse drug reactions: Recognition of the problem. Facts Compar Drug Newslett 3:49, 1984

Sherlock S: Hepatotoxicity caused by drugs. Ration Drug Ther 22(7):1, 1988

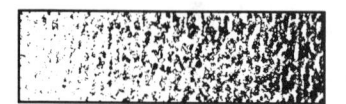

5 DRUG INTERACTIONS

The term *drug interaction* refers to the process whereby the expected therapeutic effect of a drug is modified by the presence of another factor, usually a drug or other chemical agent that may be dietary, environmental, or endogenous. When two drugs are administered in close sequence to each other, they may interact either to enhance or to diminish the intended effect of one or both drugs, or they may produce an unintended and potentially harmful reaction.

Thus, drug interactions may also be viewed as either *beneficial* or *adverse*. The means by which the presence of a second drug can augment or reduce the effects of the initial drug were briefly reviewed in Chapter 3 under **Combined Effects of Drugs.** This chapter offers a more detailed look at why drug interactions occur and the mechanisms that may be involved.

The clinical significance of adverse drug interactions is often greatly understated. When a patient on multiple drug therapy develops an unusual or disturbing symptom, it is often very difficult to determine whether the reaction is caused by an alteration in the disease state being treated, by the presence of a certain drug, by the interaction of two concurrently used drugs, or by some other change in the individual's physiology. What may be a significant drug interaction might simply be viewed as a deterioration in the patient's status or the appearance of a new disease entity. It is apparent, then, that many drug reactions can go completely unheeded or fail to be recognized immediately, especially if the reaction is mild. The clinician must therefore make a careful assessment of *any* change in a patient's condition and possess sufficient knowledge of potential drug interactions to be able to recognize the possibility of a developing drug-interaction problem.

The practice of multiple drug therapy is becoming increasingly prevalent as the median age of the population rises, with an attendant increase in the presence of chronic disease conditions requiring drug treatment. It stands to reason that as the number of drugs used concurrently increases, the *potential* for drug interactions increases to an even greater degree. Thus the benefit-to-risk ratio assumes critical importance in decisions about the number and kinds of drugs to be employed in the management of chronic diseases. Occasional episodes of dizziness or tachycardia may be acceptable consequences of drug combinations used to control severe hypertension. On the other hand, use of aspirin in users of coumarin anticoagulants is totally unwarranted, since other equally effective analgesics that do not interfere with the action of the anticoagulants are readily available. Knowledge of the etiology of drug interactions and the ability to predict possible problems related to drug mechanisms can greatly minimize the toxicity resulting from concurrent drug usage. Of themselves, most drug interactions are usually not serious or life-threatening, but ignorance of them, either through lack of knowledge or because of inadequate observation, can be annoying to the patient and frequently dangerous.

There are numerous reasons why drug interactions occur, yet many interactions can be eliminated or at least minimized by recognizing the probable causative factors and by undertaking appropriate preventive action. Some of the more common reasons are the following:

1. *Insufficient knowledge:* Safe and effective combination drug therapy requires adequate understanding of the mechanisms of action and potential complications of each type of drug employed.
2. *Dietary factors:* Many constituents of an individual's diet can interact with certain drugs. In cases in which such interactions are documented, it is important that the patient be advised to avoid the offending dietary agents. Caffeine increases central nervous system (CNS) excitatory effects of many drugs; licorice produces hypokalemia; calcium retards tetracycline absorption; and tyramine increases the blood pressure response to monoamine oxidase (MAO) inhibitors. These substances, which commonly occur in a variety of different foods, are some common examples of dietary influences in drug interactions.
3. *Physiological state of the individual:* The effect of factors such as age, sex, weight, and genetic abnormalities can greatly influence the occurrence of drug interactions.
4. *Presence of disease states:* The likelihood of a drug interaction is higher in those persons whose pathologic condition (such as liver disease, kidney damage, or altered enzyme systems) may affect the handling of one or more drugs used as part of a therapeutic regimen.
5. *Patient behavioral patterns:* The fairly common practice of seeing more than one physician concurrently can increase the risk of a drug interaction if each prescriber is not fully aware of all the drugs being taken by the patient. Self-medication is likewise responsible for a large number of drug interactions that could easily be avoided with proper counseling.
6. *Environmental factors:* Often overlooked as a contributory factor in drug interactions is the possibility of exposure to pollutants—industrial, agricultural, and other types of chemical agents that are pharmacologically active. Although little direct reliable information exists concerning interactions with these substances, even small amounts of insecticides, fungicides, or industrial wastes can markedly alter the effects of certain therapeutic agents. For example, chlorinated insecticides may stimulate drug metabolism by liver enzymes, whereas pesticides containing cholinesterase inhibitors can cause respiratory distress, muscle weakness, and convulsions.
7. *Dosage form factors:* Incompatibility of different dosage forms or improper preparation of a drug may cause drug interactions on either a physical or a chemical level. Generally, the major concern in this regard is one of bioavailability—that is, what fraction of the dose is available through absorption to the fluids of distribution. In vitro chemical interactions, or in vivo alterations in rate or extent of absorption resulting from the presence of a second drug can significantly influence the response to the initially administered agent. Opponents of generic equivalency (i.e., similar efficacy and safety for the same drug manufactured by different companies) often cite the demonstrated differences in absorption rates, dissolution characteristics, and peak blood levels as evidence that not all forms of the same drug are therapeutically or toxicologically equal. Further, the maintenance of constant plasma levels of a drug for extended periods through use of a sustained-release dosage form can be upset by the presence of another drug that alters GI motility and intestinal transit time; thus, the sustained-release dosage form is eliminated too quickly.

DRUG INTERACTIONS—CLASSIFICATION AND MECHANISMS

Interactions between drugs may occur in vitro or in vivo. An understanding of the basic mechanisms by which drug reactions develop can enable the practitioner to prevent many interactions from occurring or at least to recognize potential interaction problems before they develop into serious complications. Although any classification of drug interactions represents an oversimplification, the following outline will serve as an aid to categorizing many of the important types of drug interactions according to their mechanisms of action.

In Vitro

The term *incompatibility* is often used to designate in vitro drug reactions and may refer to either a physical or a chemical interaction.

1. *Physical:* occurs if the physical state of either drug is altered when the chemicals are mixed. For example, amphotericin will precipitate if mixed with normal saline instead of 5% dextrose. Likewise, the anticoagulant effect of heparin, a negatively charged acid, is antagonized by protamine, a positively charged base.
2. *Chemical:* occurs when the components of a drug mixture interact to form chemically altered products. For example, chemical incompatibilities in solution exist between methicillin and kanamycin, aminophylline and chlorpromazine, and dopamine and sodium bicarbonate.

In most cases, physical and chemical incompatibilities are manifested by a visible change such as precipitate formation or color change. Occasionally, however, in vitro interactions may occur without any observable signs, possibly resulting in undetected loss of potency. Thus, the compatibility of two drugs should always be ascertained by reference to an appropriate source prior to mixing to ensure that the clinical efficacy of each is not impaired by parenteral admixture.

In Vivo

Most drug interactions occurring in the body can be categorized into one of several classes, depending on the mechanisms responsible for the interaction. It should be repeated that drug interactions can be desirable and expected and often purposely caused, or they may be unwanted and unexpected. The interaction may enhance, retard, or abolish the actions of one or both drugs. Several important mechanisms of in vivo drug interactions are discussed, and pertinent examples are given. An understanding of the mechanisms of drug interactions can help the practitioner to recognize many potential problems when two or more drugs are combined, but it is important that the sections of the book pertaining to each individual drug be consulted to obtain a listing of the most likely drug interactions for each agent used. The following classification is intended to serve only as an overview of this tremendously complex field.

ALTERATIONS IN DRUG EFFECTS

Several types of interactions result from alterations in the normal pharmacologic effects of one drug due to the presence of a second drug with similar or different pharmacologic effects.

Similar Pharmacologic Effects

Each of two drugs possessing similar pharmacologic actions will generally enhance the pharmacologic and toxicologic effects of the other. This synergistic interaction can result in either an additive effect or potentiation (see Chap. 3). For example, alcohol and barbiturates are CNS depressants having an additive effect when used in combinations. Anticholinergics and tricyclic antidepressants, which also have significant anticholinergic action, can result in increased side effects such as dry mouth, blurred vision, and urinary retention if used concurrently.

Different Pharmacologic Effects

Administration of two drugs with opposing actions usually significantly reduces or totally abolishes the pharmacologic effects of each. This type of interaction is generally easy to predict if the mechanisms of action of both drugs are known. Examples might be the simultaneous use of a locally acting cholinergic (miotic) in the eye together with an adrenergic (mydriatic) or the administration of epinephrine (a vasoconstrictor) and histamine (a vasodilator).

Competitive Receptor Antagonism

This form of drug interaction is similar to that of administering drugs with opposing actions. The effects of one drug can be cancelled by the concomitant use of a second drug that blocks the access of the first drug to its receptor site of action. Again, this kind of interaction can usually be avoided by an awareness of the mechanisms of action of the two agents. For example, anticholinergic drugs should not be used in patients with glaucoma because they would block the receptor actions of the cholinergic drugs (such as pilocarpine) used to treat this eye disorder. Propranolol, a beta-adrenergic blocking drug, would interfere with the bronchodilatory action of isoproterenol in the treatment of chronic obstructive pulmonary disease.

Blockade of Neuronal Uptake or Release

Drugs interfering with the uptake or release of other agents by the nerve endings can cause significant interactions that usually decrease the effects of one or both drugs. Phenothiazines and tricyclic antidepressants exert an inhibitory effect on uptake of drugs by the nerve endings. These agents nullify the antihypertensive effect of guanethidine, which must be taken up by the nerve endings to produce its intended effect. Because many important endogenous pressor amines, such as tyramine and norepinephrine, are partially inactivated by neuronal uptake, these endogenous substances will be potentiated in the presence of neuronal uptake blockers such as the phenothiazines and the tricyclics. This potentiation can lead to serious consequences such as severe hypertension or cardiac arrhythmias.

Altered Receptor Sensitivity

The sensitivity of a receptor for a particular drug action can be modified by the presence of a second drug. For example, thyroxine may increase the sensitivity of receptors to the anticoagulant effect of the coumarins, so that a dosage adjustment is needed. Long-term use of antipsychotic drugs can lead to a hypersensitivity of central dopamine receptors. This dopamine supersensitivity is thought to be responsible for the appearance of a series of chronic orofacial involuntary movements, known as tardive dyskinesias, that occur with prolonged antipsychotic drug use because the endogenous dopamine is interacting with hypersensitive receptor sites. As a general rule, receptor sensitivity decreases with prolonged stimulation and increases with chronic blockade or disuse. This phenomenon helps explain the action of many drugs that alter receptor sensitivity, and the terms *down-regulation* and *up-regulation* can be applied to drug-induced decreases or increases in receptor sensitivity, respectively. This concept is explained more fully in relation to those drugs acting in this manner under the heading Mechanism of Action throughout the book.

ALTERATIONS IN DRUG HANDLING

Many drug interactions are related to alterations in the handling of one drug that are caused by the presence of other drugs. These interactions may reflect changes in the absorption, distribution, biotransformation, or excretion of one drug that are caused by the actions of a second pharmacologic agent.

Absorption

Any substance capable of altering the normal physiologic processes of the GI tract can markedly impair drug absorption. Alterations in gastric absorption may be caused by the following:

CHANGES IN GASTRIC pH
Drugs (e.g., sodium bicarbonate or antacids) that can raise the pH of the gastric fluid may decrease the absorption of weakly acidic drugs and may increase the absorption of weakly basic drugs. This is based on the concept that un-ionized drug molecules are lipid-soluble and thus cross absorptive membranes more readily. Acidic drugs, such as the salicylates, barbiturates, and oral anticoagulants, are largely ionized at high pH and therefore are less efficiently absorbed. Conversely, basic drugs, such as amphetamines and ephedrine, exist more in the un-ionized state at a high pH and thus are better absorbed than at lower pH.

CHANGES IN INTESTINAL MOTILITY AND FUNCTION
The faster a drug passes through the stomach and intestines, the less it is absorbed. Therefore drugs that slow GI motility (e.g., anticholinergics, opiates, antidiarrheals) may allow for more complete absorption of some drugs, all other factors being constant. If a drug is absorbed more readily from the intestines than from the stomach, however, slowing GI motility can actually decrease the rate of absorption of that drug, as it will remain in the stomach longer before reaching its site of absorption in the intestines.

In contrast, drugs that speed movement of substances through the GI tract, such as laxatives, cholinergic stimulants, or metoclopramide, can reduce absorption of orally administered drugs, since the drugs are in contact with the absorbing membrane for a shorter time. Again, however, if a drug accelerates the emptying of the stomach, it may *enhance* the absorption of those drugs that are largely absorbed from the upper intestines.

CHEMICAL BINDING OF DRUGS
Several classes of agents are capable of forming complexes with many orally administered drugs, thereby impairing their GI absorption. The absorption of tetracyclines is inhibited by the presence of drugs (e.g., antacids) or foods (e.g., milk, cheese) containing calcium, magnesium, or aluminum, substances capable of chemically chelating the tetracycline molecule. Many antacids, as well as cholestyramine (an ionic-exchange resin), may interfere with the absorption of drugs such as warfarin, digitoxin, and phenylbutazone by forming a chemical complex.

SEQUESTRATION
Fat-soluble drugs, including vitamins A, D, and K, will be sequestered in the presence of a fatty vehicle like mineral oil, and absorption may be retarded.

ALTERATION OF INTESTINAL FLORA
Alterations in the microbial population of the GI tract can occur with many antibiotics, causing destruction of vitamin K synthesizing organisms in the intestines, possibly leading to increased activity of oral anticoagulants and increased bleeding episodes. Drug-induced diarrhea can occur in response to changes in intestinal flora, affecting drug absorption as well.

COMPETITION FOR ABSORPTION MECHANISMS
Active transport mechanisms function in the absorption of many drugs and can be inhibited by pharmacologic agents that compete for these active absorptive mechanisms. Phenytoin, for example, impedes absorption of folic acid, leading to megaloblastic anemia in many instances. Certain amino acids compete for the same transport mechanisms involved in methyldopa and levodopa absorption.

MISCELLANEOUS FACTORS
Other factors associated with altered absorption of one drug due to the presence of a second drug include decreased mucosal blood flow, altered volume and content of GI secretions, direct damage to the mucosal surface, and osmotic pressure changes within the intestinal lumen.

Distribution

The distribution of drugs within the body can be significantly altered by the presence of other drugs. Among the more important mechanisms of drug interactions related to drug distribution are the following:

COMPETITION FOR PLASMA PROTEIN BINDING
Drugs bound to plasma proteins are inactive, even though present in the body. When released from the protein-bound stores, the free drug becomes active and is capable of exerting a pharmacologic effect. Many classes of drugs display significant protein-binding capacity, and when two highly protein-bound drugs are employed concurrently, a drug interaction is likely to occur. This interaction results from the fact that one protein-bound drug generally displays a higher affinity for the binding sites than does the second drug. Thus, one drug is capable of displacing the other from its binding sites, thereby increasing the effects of the displaced drug and possibly also accelerating its elimination, since the displaced drug is now subject to metabolism and excretion. This type of drug interaction be-

comes especially significant with very highly protein-bound drugs, since a minimal decrease in the fraction of bound drug may be associated with a substantial increase in the plasma level of free drug. Examples of highly protein-bound drugs that are likely to interact if present at the same time in the plasma are salicylates, barbiturates, oral anticoagulants, oral hypoglycemics, sulfonamides, hydantoins, nonsteroidal antiinflammatory drugs, calcium channel blockers, cyclophosphamide, clofibrate, diazoxide, chloral hydrate, and methotrexate.

DISPLACEMENT FROM STORAGE DEPOTS

Many endogenous substances, including neurotransmitters and hormones, are stored by different means in the body. Many drugs exert their effects either by liberating these substances from their storage sites or by preventing their release. A drug interaction can occur when two drugs affecting storage mechanisms are given concurrently. For example, because of its releasing action on stored catecholamines, amphetamine may interfere with the antihypertensive action of guanethidine but can enhance the stimulatory action of ephedrine.

BLOOD FLOW ALTERATIONS

Pharmacologic agents capable of modifying blood flow to different body organs can greatly influence the distribution and handling of other drugs. For example, epinephrine is often combined with local anesthetics to restrict the spread of the anesthetic by reducing local blood flow. Some cardiovascular drugs can alter blood volume and blood pressure by producing vasoconstriction, thereby restricting the access of other drugs to certain body organs. Reduction in hepatic blood flow by vasoconstrictors likewise can significantly reduce the rate and extent of drug metabolism.

Biotransformation

The process of converting drugs to their respective metabolites is termed biotransformation, and it usually occurs in the liver. These reactions are generally mediated by enzymes; consequently any drug capable of altering the enzymatic processes involved in the metabolism of other drugs can produce a drug interaction.

ENZYME INHIBITION

There are many examples of compounds that interfere with the activity of inactivating enzymes, thereby potentiating other drugs. MAO inhibitors, compounds that inhibit the normal functioning of the endogenous enzyme monoamine oxidase, elevate levels of biogenic amines and may produce severe hypertensive reactions in the presence of pressor amines. Xanthine oxidase inhibitors such as allopurinol raise plasma levels of mercaptopurine by blocking its breakdown. Cholinesterase inhibitors such as physostigmine and neostigmine block degradation of choline esters and can enhance the effects of acetylcholine, succinylcholine, and other cholinergic drugs. Carbidopa competitively inhibits the enzyme dopa decarboxylase in the plasma. This enzyme normally inactivates L-dopa before it reaches its site of action in the CNS. Thus, dopa decarboxylase inhibition elevates the brain level of L-dopa and increases the synthesis of dopamine in the motor-regulating centers of the CNS.

ENZYME ACCELERATION

Certain pharmacologic agents, including barbiturates, hydantoins, meprobamate, griseofulvin, and chlorinated hydrocarbon insecticides, can stimulate hepatic microsomal enzymes involved in the metabolic breakdown of many classes of drugs. This process, known as *enzyme induction,* decreases the therapeutic response to drugs that are metabolized by the microsomal enzymes, because the drugs are being metabolized more rapidly. Literally hundreds of drugs and chemicals can stimulate hepatic enzymes, and the range of potential drug interactions along these lines is enormous. For example, coumarin anticoagulants are metabolized at a much faster rate in the presence of a barbiturate, and an appropriate dosage adjustment must be made. Phenytoin reduces the effects of dexamethasone by inducing the microsomal enzymes responsible for its metabolism. Enzyme induction may be responsible for development of tolerance to certain drugs because some drugs may stimulate their own liver metabolism. Examples of such drugs are barbiturates, meprobamate, and glutethimide.

Excretion

Drug interactions occurring with the excretion of drugs may involve any of the renal excretory processes (glomerular filtration, tubular reabsorption, active tubular secretion). Most clinically important drug interactions are either caused by changes in urinary pH, alterations in the fraction of reabsorbed drug, or competition for active tubular secretory mechanisms.

CHANGES IN URINARY pH

Acidification of the urine by means of agents such as ammonium chloride can potentially reduce the effects of basic drugs (e.g., amphetamine, quinidine) because they will be largely ionized at the acidic pH and readily excreted. Conversely, renal excretion of acidic drugs, such as salicylates, barbiturates, and anticoagulants, will be accelerated by alkalinization of urine with sodium bicarbonate, acetazolamide, or potassium citrate. Alteration of urinary pH is often an effective technique in treating drug overdosage.

COMPETITION FOR TUBULAR MECHANISMS

Many drugs and metabolites are actively secreted from the renal capillary network into the tubules of the kidney and are subsequently eliminated. When any two actively secreted drugs are used together, drug interactions may occur because of competition for the active secretory mechanisms. Drugs that may interact by this means, leading to prolonged therapeutic effects, are salicylates, sulfonamides, penicillins, thiazide diuretics, pyrazolones, dicumarol, indomethacin, probenecid, oral hypoglycemics, acetazolamide, diazoxide, and methotrexate. Small doses of aspirin may impair the uricosuric (uric acid–excreting) action of probenecid by interfering with the active secretion of uric acid into the renal tubules. Aspirin may also inhibit the excretion of methotrexate. Competition for active tubular secretion can be used to therapeutic advantage as well. For example, probenecid may be used with penicillin to delay the normally rapid excretion of the penicillin molecule thereby significantly prolonging the effective duration of penicillin in the body.

ALTERATIONS IN FLUID AND ELECTROLYTE BALANCE

Changes in fluid and electrolyte levels induced by certain drugs can markedly affect the therapeutic effectiveness and toxicity of other drugs, particularly those acting on the heart, kidney, and skeletal muscles. Hypokalemia (low serum potassium levels) produced by many diuretic agents and corticosteroids increases the likelihood of digitalis toxicity and can antagonize the antiarrhythmic effects of quinidine, lidocaine, procainamide, and phenytoin. Potassium loss may also cause prolonged paralysis following use of antidepolarizing skeletal muscle relaxants.

Another interaction of potential clinical significance is the use of drugs that induce sodium and water retention (e.g., pyrazolones or corticosteroids) in combination with antihypertensive or diuretic drugs. These fluid-retaining drugs can negate the action of antihypertensive agents in lowering blood pressure.

MISCELLANEOUS DRUG INTERACTIONS

Alterations in the Immune Response

Certain drugs may alter antibody production. Vaccines and toxoids stimulate antibody production, whereas glucocorticoids such as hydrocortisone can markedly inhibit the immune response and should not be used with vaccines.

Although antibiotics are frequently given in combination, drug interactions can occur if bacteriostatic and bactericidal drugs are given together. For example, penicillins are bactericidal because they interfere with cell wall synthesis in dividing bacteria. They are less effective, however, when used with tetracyclines—drugs that prevent cell division and bacterial growth. This mutual antagonism can cause serious complications when combination therapy is used to treat severe infections.

Residual Drug Effects

A potential source of drug interactions is the prolonged period of therapeutic effectiveness that is often observed even after a drug is discontinued. Drugs with prolonged actions have the potential to interact with newly introduced drugs even though the first drugs are no longer being administered. For example, when MAO inhibitors are given within 2 weeks of tricyclic antidepressants, severe hypertension can occur owing to the residual effects of the MAO inhibitors combined with the effects of the tricyclic antidepressants.

It is difficult to make a simple statement summarizing the overall clinical importance of drug interactions. Some are beneficial. Others represent mild and essentially benign reactions, requiring merely an adjustment in the dosage of one or more drugs, while others are potentially life-threatening interactions requiring immediate action. Recognition of potential drug interactions becomes of critical interest when patients are receiving one or more drugs having a narrow safety margin (e.g., digitalis, lithium, oral anticoagulants) or drugs that are being used to treat serious diseases, such as cancer, diabetes mellitus or cardiac arrhythmias. Clinically significant adverse drug interactions can be minimized by an understanding of the different mechanisms involved in their production, awareness of the presence of predisposing factors, and avoidance, where possible, of multiple-drug usage.

Selected Bibliography

Adverse interactions of drugs. Med Lett 23(5):17, 1981

Albanese JA, Bond T: Drug Interactions: Basic Principles and Clinical Problems. New York, McGraw-Hill, 1978

Caranasos GJ, Stewart RB, Cluff LE: Clinically desirable drug interactions. Annu Rev Pharmacol Toxicol 25:67, 1985

Carr CJ: Food and drug interactions. Annu Rev Pharmacol Toxicol 22:19, 1982

Cohen SN, Armstrong MF: Drug Interactions: A Handbook for Clinical Use. Baltimore, Williams & Wilkins, 1974

Hansten PD: Drug Interactions, 4th ed. Philadelphia, Lea & Febiger, 1979

Holtzman JL: The role of protein binding in drug therapy. Ration Drug Ther 18(9):1, 1984

Shinn AF, Shrewsbury RP: Evaluations of Drug Interactions. 3rd ed. St. Louis, CV Mosby, 1985

Sriwatanakul K, Mehta G: Clinically significant drug interactions. Ration Drug Ther 17(4):1, 1983

Toothaker RD, Welling PG: The effect of food on drug bioavailability. Annu Rev Pharmacol Toxicol 20:173, 1980

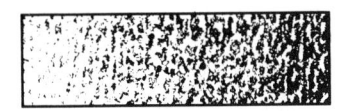

6 PEDIATRIC PHARMACOLOGY

An infant or small child should not be considered a little adult for the purpose of administering drugs. Unique and potentially serious problems exist in the use of pharmacologic agents in the pediatric population, and perhaps nowhere is the choice of the proper dose and route of administration so important as with the small child. Yet critically defined guidelines for safe and efficient use of pediatric drugs do not always exist. Thus, drug therapy in small children is often undertaken simply by scaling down the recommended adult dose, largely on the basis of differences in body weight. However, a small child has many immature physiologic processes that can greatly alter the handling of drugs by the body. Especially important are the lesser metabolic and excretory capacities of the small infant compared to the adult, which may markedly impair the infant's ability to detoxify and eliminate many drugs safely.

Although it is difficult to divide the pediatric population arbitrarily according to age and developmental characteristics, certain stages in a child's growth are important in relation to drug handling. These may be described as follows:

1. *Neonatal period* (0–1 mo): period of marked physiological immaturity and rapid change; a dangerous time for drug administration.
2. *Infancy* (1–12 mo): period of gradually improving capacity of the body to handle drugs efficiently.
3. *Toddler period* (1–3 yr): fairly well-developed metabolic excretory processes; child resists many medications when they are presented; use of rituals and routines (e.g., taking a pill before a favorite TV show) are important at this age.
4. *Preschool age and adolescence* (3 yr and older): few anatomical problems but occasional behavioral problems associated with drug administration; probably the most important consideration for safe drug therapy is body weight.

FACTORS THAT AFFECT THERAPEUTIC RESPONSE

Many factors determine the drug dosage and therapeutic response in infants and children. In one respect, children and adults are similar because each individual has a peculiar biochemical system that handles a drug in its own way. Thus individual differences in drug responses are as apparent in children as adults. However, the pediatric population must contend with more variables in drug handling than the adult population. Such variables may include immaturity of enzymatic processes, incomplete development of metabolic and excretory functions, increased tissue responsiveness to many drugs, and acceptance and ease of drug administration.

The neonatal period, is characterized by rapid physical growth and continual changes in organ functioning that persist through the early years of life, although at a somewhat reduced rate. This period of rapid growth and development represents the most critical time with regard to potential hazards of drug usage. Persons administering drugs to infants and children should recognize the complex nature of the many variables affecting drug activity and attempt to understand as clearly as possible the major determinants of drug responsiveness in the pediatric population.

Absorption

In general, absorption of *orally* administered drugs in infants less than 6 to 9 months old is somewhat slower than that in adults. Young children exhibit slowed GI motility, prolonged gastric emptying time, more acidic gastric pH, decreased absorptive capacity of the various segments, and differences in the composition of intestinal flora. Also, transport mechanisms that carry drug molecules across the intestinal membranes into the bloodstream may be underdeveloped in small infants, resulting in slowed absorption of certain vitamins and nutrients. Of course, the presence of nausea or vomiting can significantly influence the amount of drug absorbed from the intestinal tract.

Conversely, absorption of *topically* applied drugs is often greatly enhanced in small children compared to adults, largely because of a child's reduced keratin layer and thinner epithelium. This can be particularly significant with the prolonged use of topically applied corticosteroids for conditions such as diaper rash and eczema. Significant absorption through the skin can lead to many untoward systemic reactions.

Absorption of drugs from IM injection sites (e.g., vastus lateralis muscles) may be more erratic in small infants than in older children, partly because of the small muscle mass and also because of reduced intramuscular circulation. Drugs used to treat serious illnesses in hospitalized infants are often most effectively given by the IV route, frequently by way of the frontal or superficial scalp veins in very young infants.

Distribution

Differences in drug distribution among different pediatric age groups may depend on circulatory dynamics, extent of body water, binding of the drug in the plasma, membrane permeability, and the specificity of the drug for tissue receptor sites.

CIRCULATORY DYNAMICS
Therapeutic agents generally penetrate highly perfused organs (e.g., liver, kidney, brain) to a greater extent than organs receiving less blood flow (bone and muscle). The growth of these organs progresses at different rates, so the amount of drug distributed to each will change with development of the child. Young infants may have poor peripheral circulation, resulting in slowed absorption of intramuscularly or subcutaneously administered drugs.

BODY WATER
The newborn has a much higher percentage of total body water and extracellular fluid volume (80%–85%) than the older child or adult (60%–65%). Fat content, on the other hand, is markedly reduced in the neonate compared with the older child. Thus, water-soluble drugs diffuse to a greater extent in the very young, often resulting in reduced plasma concentrations compared with older children. An important consideration in this regard is that in states of dehydration, "normal" doses of a drug in the infant can result in very high plasma levels, because the overall extracellular fluid volume may be considerably reduced. Further, because of the reduced fat content of the neonate, lipid-soluble drugs will not exhibit the same distribution pattern as in

the older child, and they may not be stored to the same extent because there is less total adipose tissue.

BINDING

Binding of most drugs to plasma proteins such as albumin and globulins is significantly less in the newborn compared with adults. This may be due to the following causes:

- Lower levels of plasma proteins in the neonate secondary to reduced hepatic synthesis of these proteins
- Altered binding characteristics of neonatal proteins
- Presence of endogenous substances (e.g., bilirubin, steroids, hormones, fatty acids) that compete for plasma protein binding sites during the early days of life

Because reduced protein binding increases the amount of pharmacologically active drug in the plasma, this effect may predispose the child to a greater likelihood of toxic reactions, especially when multiple-drug therapy is undertaken. Among the more important drugs that may exhibit reduced binding in the newborn are salicylates, barbiturates, penicillins, sulfonamides, and phenytoin.

MEMBRANE PERMEABILITY

Delayed maturation of the infant's body membranes, especially the blood–brain barrier, leads to increased distribution of drugs to certain areas of the body, notably the brain. Lipid-soluble drugs (e.g., anesthetics, sedatives, analgesics, antibiotics) readily enter the brain of the neonate and may cause serious harm (respiratory depression or brain damage). However, factors other than lipid solubility are involved in the penetration of many drugs into the brain. Blood chemistry changes (acidosis, hypoxia, hyperglycemia), body temperature fluctuations, and structural alterations in the blood–brain barrier itself (e.g., incomplete myelination) can all affect drug passage into the neonatal brain.

DRUG RECEPTOR SPECIFICITY

Differences in the responsiveness of infants and adults to certain drugs suggest that the sensitivity of some receptor sites is not equal. For example, therapeutic doses of atropine and epinephrine are proportionately greater on a mg/kg basis in the infant than in the adult, presumably because receptor responsiveness is lower in the infant.

Metabolism

Hepatic drug-metabolizing activity is substantially reduced in early neonatal life, and drug-metabolizing enzymes in the liver mature at different rates. Liver function therefore changes very rapidly after birth, and major problems relating to reduced hepatic catabolism of drugs occur primarily in the first few weeks following delivery. The major consequence of the low hepatic drug-metabolizing capacity in the infant is that many drugs have a more prolonged duration of action, and this may predispose the child toward a cumulative toxic reaction.

In contrast, drug metabolism in the neonate may be enhanced by administration of certain drugs—the barbiturates, for example—that function as hepatic-enzyme inducers. That is, certain pharmacologic agents are capable of enhancing the action of liver microsomal enzymes involved in the metabolism of other drugs (see Chap. 5). This effect becomes important when multiple drug therapy is undertaken in the infant, because addition of a second drug can markedly shorten the duration of action of the first drug, greatly reducing its efficacy. In this regard, repeated administration of certain drugs (e.g., barbiturates) to the mother throughout pregnancy may lead to enzyme induction in the neonate. Infants born to such mothers often are capable of metabolizing many drugs at an accelerated rate from the time of birth. Thus, the efficacy and duration of action of drugs that the newborn may require can be dangerously reduced.

Reduced neonatal hepatic functioning also decreases synthesis of plasma proteins, allowing larger amounts of a drug to circulate unbound in the body, possibly leading to more side effects, as discussed under **Binding,** above.

Excretion

Like liver metabolic function, the renal excretory capacity is immature at birth and shows gradual maturation with advancing age. For example, shortly after birth the neonate's renal function is approximately 30% to 40% of that of an adult; however, a substantial increase in renal function occurs in the first week of life, and renal blood flow attains 60% to 70% of adult capacity within that time. Glomerular filtration rates of newborns are approximately one half that of adults but attain comparable levels by 6 months of age. Tubular secretion in infants likewise is about one third less than in adults. By nine months of age, however, renal function of the child is approximately equivalent to that of the young adult.

The significance of reduced renal elimination in the infant with respect to a particular drug depends on whether that drug is excreted largely by the kidney. Many important drugs used in pediatric pharmacology are eliminated predominantly by renal excretory processes (e.g., many antibiotics, salicylates, acetaminophen, aminophylline, digoxin, thiazide diuretics) and thus may exhibit prolonged durations of action in the very young. This is an important factor to consider, especially when determining the frequency of dosage.

DRUG DOSAGE AND ADMINISTRATION

The pediatric population presents unique problems with regard to drug dosage and administration. As we have seen, a number of factors other than age and size can affect drug response. Thus no single rule can be applied to the entire pediatric group with regard to dosage and route. Nevertheless, most therapy is undertaken on the basis of milligrams of drug per kilogram of body weight (mg/kg). This method, of course, considers only one factor (weight) in determining a pediatric dosage, but it is probably the most appropriate method for the majority of drugs prescribed for children.

Dosage

Many rules for pediatric dosing have been described, most of them based on a fraction of the adult dose as determined by some factor (e.g., age, weight, or surface area). The four pediatric dosage rules are given below, with the first three being largely of theoretical interest.

1. *Young's rule* (2 yr and older)

$$\frac{\text{Age (yr)}}{\text{Age (yr)} + 12} \times \text{adult dose}$$

2. *Clark's rule* (infants and young children)

$$\frac{\text{Weight (lb)}}{150 \text{ lb}} \times \text{adult dose}$$

(150 lb = weight of average adult)

3. *Fried's rule* (infant under 1 yr)

$$\frac{\text{Age (mo)}}{150} \times \text{adult dose}$$

4. *Surface area method* (all children except newborns)

$$\frac{\text{Surface area child (m}^2)}{1.7} \times \text{adult dose}$$

(1.7 = average surface area of an adult, in square meters)

The surface area of the child is determined from its height and weight using standard nomograms found in many pharmacology and pediatric texts. Although somewhat unwieldy, it is the most accurate method of pediatric dosage calculation, since surface area reflects the growth of body systems that influence metabolism and excretion.

Dosage must be individualized for the patient, the drug, and the disease, whether the patient is an adult or a child. For example, doses calculated on age alone cannot compensate for the variations in body weight observed among children, especially in the proportion of body fat. Body surface area probably provides a more consistent dose schedule for older children but is not suitable for neonates, because a high percentage of their weight is water. Moreover, this method requires computation and the use of nomograms. On the other hand, rules based on weight *assume* an average adult weight of 150 lb and with many drugs, infants would receive an *underdosage* if given mg/kg doses calculated by this method. Because adult doses should be individually calculated, it is erroneous to base a child's dose on an "average" adult weight.

Although pediatric dosage rules can provide guidelines for the use of drugs in children, they cannot guarantee safety or adequacy of dosage, especially in the newborn. Further, no rule can anticipate all the variables associated with pediatric therapy, especially those caused by individual differences in drug response. Thus drug dosage in children must be critically adjusted for each patient, and the child must be carefully observed during therapy to maximize efficacy and to minimize toxicity.

Administration

The preferred method of drug administration in young children is usually the oral route, in the form of a liquid preparation. Of course, other routes (topical, rectal, parenteral) may be used, depending on the situation. A brief consideration of several routes of administration used in children is presented below.

ORAL
- This is *generally* the preferred route.
- Liquid medications, especially if flavored, may facilitate administration but should also be kept out of the child's reach to prevent self-administration and potential overdosage.
- In small infants, medication may be placed along the side of the tongue by dropper or syringe to avoid its being pushed out by tongue movement.
- Tablets or capsules may be crushed and mixed with honey, syrup, jam, or fruit if the child is unable or unwilling to swallow them whole, although the parents should consult a pharmacist for the proper procedure.

RECTAL
- Can be used when oral route is contraindicated or difficult (e.g., cleft palate, nausea or vomiting)
- Many drugs are erratically absorbed rectally.
- Diarrhea often makes rectal administration impractical.

INTRAMUSCULAR
- Often used for single-dose administration (e.g., vaccines, antibiotics).
- Buttocks and the deltoid muscle should *not* be used in infants and small children (under 2 yr) because of danger of sciatic nerve damage and lack of sufficient muscle mass; vastus lateralis is the preferred site.
- With repeated injections, sites should be rotated.
- Absorption is generally good and fairly rapid.
- Always use bony prominences to identify injection site.

INTRAVENOUS
- Should be used in young children only when other routes have failed or are inappropriate.
- Infants and small children should be restrained so needle is not dislodged once inserted.
- Because of reduced peripheral circulation in the very young, veins in the extremities are difficult to locate; the superficial scalp or frontal veins are used.
- Drug must be properly diluted and drug given at a slow rate (e.g., 0.5 mL/min–2 mL/min), because overdosage is most dangerous with IV route, and adverse reactions can develop quickly.
- Circulatory overload can occur more rapidly in children than in adults. As a general rule, never give more than 250 mL fluid to a child under 2 years, or 500 mL to an older child, unless special conditions warrant (e.g., rapid or severe dehydration, renal impairment).

TOPICAL AND LOCAL (EYE, EAR, NOSE)
- Possibility of significant percutaneous absorption of topically applied drugs must be considered in children, especially with repeated application of lipid-soluble drugs.
- Eye and ear drops may be warmed before instillation.
- Oil-based preparations should not be used in the nose, because aspiration may cause lipid pneumonia.
- In infants, if nose drops are indicated, they should be instilled briefly, then aspirated with a bulb syringe.

Whatever method of drug administration is used in children, perhaps the most important single factor in successful pediatric drug usage is the relationship between the child and the practitioner. Successful and simple drug administration depends to a great extent on the cooperation between the child and the person giving the drug. Establishment of a secure, positive relationship between the drug giver and the drug receiver can overcome many obstacles to successful therapy. Each child has an individual personality that must be used to maximum advantage in administering medications. Honest explanations are essential, and medications should never be portrayed as candy, rewards, or anything less serious or important than they really are. If children are old enough, they should be told why medications are being used and the importance of proper dosage schedules in a manner appropriate to the child's age and level of understanding. A child's fears should be understood and allayed if possible. Pediatric drug administration can be exceedingly difficult and trying at times, and requires not only skill but patience, understanding, and recognition of the child's concerns and feelings.

NURSING CONSIDERATIONS

1. Assess the age and the developmental stage of the child, particularly as these relate to the appropriate route of administration, as well as the child's ability to understand the necessity for drug treatment.
2. Be honest with the child and explain as clearly as possible what is happening. Do not lie (e.g., this shot won't hurt); rather, give truthful information and provide comfort and support. Recognize the child's fears and attempt to allay them as much as possible.
3. Plan the most convenient drug regimen, both in terms of route of administration and frequency of dosage, that is appropriate for the particular child and condition being treated. Stress the importance of compliance with the prescribed drug regimen.
4. Do not offer rewards in the form of candy, ice cream, or other sweets for drug taking, because the child will associate taking medication with something bad or unpleasant that should be rewarded if carried out. Try to develop a *positive* outlook on the part of the child that drug therapy is a beneficial and necessary function.
5. Attempt to disguise disagreeable oral medications whenever feasible. Do not force any drug orally, because pulmonary aspiration can result. Try to gain the child's cooperation, but if this fails, inform physician so that an alternative drug or route of administration can be attempted.
6. Be cautious about mixing disagreeable drugs with foods in the child's normal diet (e.g., milk, cereal, juice) because the child may associate the food with the drug and an eating problem may develop.
7. Avoid mixing a dose of medication in *too large* a volume of fluid or food, because the child will often not consume the entire amount and thus will not receive sufficient medication. Follow drug with fluid if possible.
8. Monitor carefully for development of side effects; recognize that children vary in their ability to give verbal feedback concerning untoward drug effects.
9. Realize that, with very small children, dosing may be facilitated by crushing tablets or emptying capsule contents and mixing with appropriate vehicles such as juice, formula, or milk. Obtain proper directions for mixing before attempting to do this, especially because the properties of the vehicle may alter bioavailability of some drugs.
10. When giving liquid medication to an infant, direct flow from dropper toward inside of the cheek to prevent gagging and stimulation of the cough reflex. Raise the infant's head to prevent aspiration.
11. Recognize that older children sometimes respond best to recognition of their maturity. For example, let children drink unassisted, let them choose which medication to take first if more than one must be given, or let them pour from the bottle unassisted. Always monitor that correct dose is being used and all medication is taken.
12. If child is totally uncooperative in taking oral medication, consider rectal or parenteral administration and discuss with physician.
13. When giving parenteral medication to children, say truthfully that injection will hurt briefly and proceed promptly and smoothly with the procedure.
14. Enlist the aid of one or more individuals to restrain the child, if necessary, to prevent tissue trauma and possible needle breakage.
15. In children under 2 years, give IM injections in vastus lateralis or rectus femoris muscle (see Chap. 1). Gluteal injections in the very young risk sciatic nerve injury, while the deltoid provides insufficient muscle mass.
16. If child will not hold eye open for instillation of drug, place proper number of drops on inner corner of eye while child is recumbent, and wait for child to open eye. Drug will then be dispersed over cornea.
17. With child under 3 years, pull pinna of ear down and back for administration of ear drops. With older child, pull pinna up and back. Gently massage outer area of ear to facilitate entry of drug.
18. With small children, instill nose drops 30 minutes before feeding to facilitate suckling.

PATIENT EDUCATION

1. Provide the patient and family with appropriate information on the effects of the medication, storage of the drug, and administration techniques.
2. Carefully evaluate the knowledge of parents with regard to the child's condition and the rationale for drug therapy. Assess the parents' ability to manage a small child's drug treatment and provide the necessary information as required.
3. Assist parents in planning an administration schedule that is optimal for the family as a whole.
4. Instruct parents about any storage requirements for the drugs being used or any special handling techniques (e.g., shaking the medication, wearing gloves during topical administration).
5. Instruct parents in how to measure liquid doses correctly. Make sure they use calibrated measuring devices and not household spoons, which can differ significantly in volume.
6. Work with parents to provide a safe storage environment for the medications to minimize the danger of accidental poisoning

Selected Bibliography

Chudzik G, Yaffee S: Introduction to the special problems of pediatric drug therapy. Drug Ther, July:17, 1973

Dunne R, Perez R: Reye's syndrome: A challenge not limited to critical care nurses. Iss Comprehens Pediatr Nurs 5(4):253, 1981

Foster S: Administering medications to children. Iss Comprehens Pediatr Nurs 3(5):1, 1978

Gellert E: Psychosocial Aspects of Pediatric Care. New York, Grune & Stratton, 1978

Giacoia G, Gorodisher R: Pharmacologic principles in neonatal drug therapy. Clin Perinatol 2(1):125, 1975

Golden N et al: Maternal alcohol use and infant development. Pediatrics 70(6):931, 1982

Hingson R et al: Effects of maternal drinking and marijuana use on fetal growth and development. Pediatrics 70(4):539, 1982

Howry L, Bindler R, Tso Y: Pediatric Medications. Philadelphia, JB Lippincott, 1981

Hurwitz E, Goodman R: A cluster of cases of Reye syndrome associated with chickenpox. Pediatrics 70(6):901, 1982

Jusko W: Pharmacokinetic principles in pediatric pharmacology. Pediatr Clin North Am 19(1):81, 1972

Masaki B: Physiologic basis for pediatric drug therapy. US Pharmacist Nov/Dec:36, 1978

Ormond E, Caulfield C: A practical guide to giving oral medications to young children. MCN 1(5):320, 1976

Pagliaro LA, Pagliaro AM (eds): Problems in pediatric drug therapy. 2nd ed. Hamilton IL, Drug Intelligence Publications, 1987

Rane A, Sjoqvist F: Drug metabolism in the human fetus and newborn infant. Pediatr Clin North Am 19(1):37, 1972

Trauner D: Reye's syndrome. Curr Probl Pediatr 12(7):5, 1982

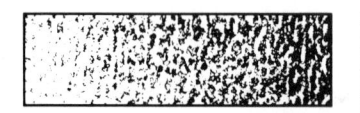

7 GERIATRIC PHARMACOLOGY

With advancing age, the number of cells in most body tissues diminishes, and changes in such cellular activities as metabolism, permeability, and respiration occur. Connective tissue and fat proliferate, and adaptation to stress becomes impaired. Muscle strength, oxygen utilization, and sensory perception decline. These changes in organ and tissue function may alter responsiveness to drugs. Therefore, drug therapy in the aged may have unpredictable effects, and untoward reactions are quite common and often serious. Table 7-1 summarizes the nine important age-associated changes in organ function.

Complicating the picture is the multiplicity of drugs that may comprise an elderly individual's therapeutic regimen. A progressively increasing life span has resulted in a greater proportion of the population reaching advanced age, with a corresponding increase in the use of drugs for treating chronic disease conditions such as congestive heart failure, hypertension, cerebrovascular disease, and carcinomas. It has been estimated that in the United States, the elderly account for almost one third of all drug taking. They often take several drugs concurrently, and close to 90% experience one or more episodes of adverse reactions to these drugs, not to mention the high likelihood of drug interactions with such a multiple-drug regimen. Therefore, constant attention to the drug therapy of the aged individual is essential if maximum benefit is to be derived with minimal adverse effects.

VARIABLES THAT AFFECT RESPONSE TO DRUGS IN THE ELDERLY

The frequent presence of numerous pathologic conditions in the elderly, as well as the wide variability in the development of organ and tissue pathology, can make determination of the proper drug and dosage a difficult matter. The safe and effective use of drugs in the aged depends on individually planned therapy and requires constant reevaluation. A number of variables influence the response to drugs in the geriatric population. In general, drugs tend to be absorbed, distributed, metabolized, and excreted much less efficiently in elderly patients compared with younger adults. Thus the danger of untoward reactions as well as drug interactions is magnified. A brief examination of the changes that can occur in the handling of a drug in the elderly will highlight some of the problems that can be expected.

Absorption

Many changes can occur in the GI tract to impair absorptive capacity: fewer absorbing cells, decreased GI motility, impaired gastric secretory cell function, reduced intestinal mucosal blood flow, and an elevated gastric pH. Such alterations can retard both active and passive absorption. In general, drugs are absorbed at a slower rate and less consistently in the aged; however, the *extent* to which drugs are absorbed is probably not significantly different from that in younger patients.

Distribution

Drug distribution in the elderly may be severely curtailed, in part because of reduced cardiac output and decreased perfusion of body organs. Compromised peripheral blood flow (due to atherosclerosis) can also affect the final distribution of drugs. Other factors that may alter distribution in the geriatric population are smaller body size and lowered proportion of body water, decreased plasma protein binding resulting from lower plasma albumin levels, and increased stores of body fat, leading to the possibility of accumulation of highly lipid-soluble agents (e.g., barbiturates).

Metabolism

Significant changes in liver function generally do not occur until rather late in life (after age 70), partly because of the organ has tremendous reserve capacity. However, reductions in hepatic function may develop at an earlier age secondary to the presence of chronic disease states, and these reductions are frequently implicated in the toxic effects of drugs used to treat these states. Reduced metabolism of drugs in the elderly is often a consequence of progressive loss of liver cells as well as impaired enzyme function but is more commonly related to decreased perfusion of the liver secondary to diminished cardiac output. Hepatic blood flow may be reduced by as much as 50% in the elderly compared to young adults. The important implication here is that doses of many drugs need to be reduced in the elderly, because the retarded rate of metabolism can prolong the duration of action and increase the danger of accumulation. Of course, patients with liver disease (cirrhosis, hepatitis, fatty infiltration) or diminished hepatic blood flow (congestive heart failure, pulmonary hypertension, arteriosclerosis) are extremely sensitive to those drugs that are detoxified primarily by the hepatic enzyme systems.

Excretion

Glomerular filtration diminishes by approximately one third by age 65, largely owing to reduced renal blood flow and loss of functioning nephrons. Tubular reabsorption and active tubular secretion are also somewhat compromised in the elderly. The maximum amount of a drug that can be removed from the blood by the kidney depends largely on the volume of blood presented to the glomeruli—a function of renal blood flow. It is estimated that the blood flow to the kidney is reduced about one half by age 70. This impaired renal perfusion greatly limits the amount of drug that is filtered and excreted at any one time. Because the majority of drugs are eliminated primarily by the kidney through glomerular filtration, dosage of these drugs should be reduced to avoid cumulation and subsequent toxicity. Tests of creatinine clearance using 24-hour urinary excretion as well as serum creatinine levels may be used as a reliable indicator of glomerular filtration in the geriatric patient.

Other Factors

Many other factors contribute to altered drug responsiveness in the geriatric population. Some of the more important of these are:

1. *Altered tissue sensitivity:* Certain drugs (e.g., barbiturates) can produce greatly enhanced effects in a percentage of the elderly population. Although diminished metabolism may account for part of this effect, it appears that altered receptor sensitivity to certain pharmacologic agents occurs as the patient ages. Conversely, some older patients display in-

Table 7-1
Potential Changes in Organ Function with Age

Heart	Lungs
Size ↑	Loss of elasticity
Heart rate ↓	
Cardiac output ↓	**Kidneys**
Impaired adaptation to stress	Renal blood flow ↓
	Glomerular filtration rate ↓
Cardiovascular System	Loss of functioning nephrons
Peripheral blood flow ↓	
Systemic resistance ↑	**Liver**
Loss of vessel elasticity	Enzymatic activity ↓
	Impaired hepatic perfusion
Nervous System	
Loss of neuronal function	**Hormonal**
Brain weight ↓	Loss of gonadal steroidal function
Impaired neuronal conduction	Anabolic activity ↓
Sensory perception (vision, hearing) ↓	
	Gastrointestinal
Musculoskeletal System	Digestive secretions ↓
Osteoporosis	Motility and peristalsis ↓
Loss of muscle mass	Gastric acidity ↓

↓, decreased; ↑, increased

---

creased resistance to the actions of certain drugs, which may be reflective of a reduction in the number or sensitivity of receptor sites.

2. *Presence of chronic disease states:* As mentioned earlier, many elderly patients exhibit one or more chronic pathologic conditions, such as hypertension, diabetes, angina, congestive heart failure, or peripheral vascular disease. These can often markedly affect responsiveness to a particular drug. Altered drug responses may result from interference with one or more of the basic functions discussed above (e.g., absorption) or may be due to reduced compensatory reactions caused by impaired homeostatic mechanisms. For example, orthostatic hypotension is common in the elderly patient. It results from blunted cardiovascular reflex responses normally operative in maintaining blood pressure. This condition may be exacerbated by a number of drugs, including some antihypertensives, vasodilators, and antipsychotics. Obviously, chronic liver or kidney disease can significantly prolong the effects of drugs by reducing their rate of metabolism or excretion.

3. *Hormonal changes:* Many drugs act through hormonal mechanisms and thus may elicit altered responses because of reduced endocrine secretion as the aging process continues. In elderly people, decreases are often observed in thyroid function, glucose tolerance, adrenal cortical activity, and gonadal hormone release. Replacement drug therapy is frequently indicated in these instances, but drug effects may be greatly enhanced early in therapy owing to hypersensitivity of the receptor sites. Atrophic changes in certain structures (bones and genital organs) due to lack of hormonal action may likewise greatly modify a drug's effect or increase its toxicity. For example, use of steroids in the aged can result in marked glucose intolerance, osteoporosis, and susceptibility to infection.

4. *Behavioral changes:* Often overlooked, but critically important as a major determinant of drug responses in the aged, is the mental condition of the patient. Cerebral arteriosclerosis can cause confusion, loss of memory, and even dementia. These behavioral abnormalities may adversely affect physiological functioning. Also, impaired memory and disorientation frequently are responsible for poor dosage compliance, accidental overdosage, and ingestion of the wrong drug.

DRUG THERAPY IN THE ELDERLY

Drug therapy in the geriatric population is at best difficult and in many instances quite hazardous. A thorough understanding of the altered physiology of this age group is essential for proper drug prescribing. In addition, an awareness not only of the expected beneficial effects but also of the potential adverse reactions that are likely to occur in this population is very important. Several other considerations also should be borne in mind when using drugs in the aged.

Necessity of Therapy

Not all health problems of the elderly require drug treatment, and others should be treated only on a short-term basis. Frequent review of patient's drug regimen is essential. Generally, drugs having a profile of potential adverse reactions that are worse than the symptoms described by the patient should be avoided. The benefit:risk ratio assumes critical importance in the geriatric population because of the greater likelihood that these patients will experience untoward reactions.

Duration of Therapy

Equally important as deciding which drug or drugs to prescribe is determining how long therapy with a particular drug should be continued. Many diseases in the elderly (e.g., angina, congestive heart failure, osteoporosis) require prolonged drug treatment. Even so, a critical assessment of an elderly patient's drug regimen can often eliminate one or more drugs that could have potentially deleterious effects, not to mention adverse drug interactions.

Adequacy of Therapy

Overprescribing of medications can be as harmful as inadequate therapy. Because many geriatric patients have numerous diseases, a "shotgun" approach to prescribing is sometimes employed. This greatly increases the danger of drug toxicity and especially drug interactions. In addition, neurosensory loss sometimes associated with aging may make it difficult for the patient to manage multiple-drug therapy. Thus, the fewest number of drugs that are adequate to serve the patient's needs should be prescribed. Complex dosage schedules should be avoided if at all possible, and a thorough assessment of the drug regimen should be undertaken whenever new drugs are added.

Level of Competence

Lastly, the patient's capacity for managing any drug regimen must be assessed before teaching begins and prior to the decision to allow self-medication. The patient's level of alertness, independence in care, memory for recent events, and retention of information are critical factors in planning medication administration and home care. Sometimes, an elderly person's memory deficit will cause problems in compliance. If potential problems are identified early, many methods can be employed to help the person continue the regimen.

NURSING CONSIDERATIONS

1. Anticipate the need for detailed assessment. The elderly often have multisystem problems that may require thorough evaluation prior to initiation of drug therapy.
2. Carefully evaluate drug effects. They are often magnified in the elderly, and serious adverse effects (hypotension, extreme drowsiness, confusion) may occur at normal dosage ranges. Close monitoring of the patient is essential to minimize untoward effects.
3. Carefully evaluate side effects associated with drugs used in the elderly that mimic behavior often present in older people (e.g., weakness, forgetfulness, confusion, anxiety).
4. When an opiate is used to treat pain, monitor respiratory rate. Use the smallest effective dose prescribed, and withhold drug if respiratory rate falls below 10/min. Opiates may induce severe respiratory depression in the elderly.
5. Expect digitalis therapy to begin at very low doses because the elderly patient is extremely sensitive to cardiotonic drugs. Careful monitoring of symptoms and critical dosage adjustment are necessary for maximum therapeutic benefit. Blood levels should be tested regularly (every 6–12 mo) to prevent excessive dosing.
6. Monitor diuretic usage, dietary and fluid intake, and use of laxatives, as severe dehydration and electrolyte imbalances may occur; evaluate hemodynamic status and be prepared to provide potassium supplementation and volume replacement if needed.
7. Evaluate the elderly patient carefully when administering CNS stimulants. These drugs may exaggerate confusion and lead to disordered behavior in some individuals.
8. Monitor anticholinergic drug therapy closely; give liberal fluids to overcome dryness of mucous membranes. Treatment may lead to confusion, delirium, and extreme dryness of the mouth.
9. Monitor clotting time at frequent intervals in patients taking oral anticoagulants, as their effects are often enhanced because of decreased metabolism and excretion and reduced plasma protein binding.

See also **Plan of Nursing Care 2 (Compliance)** in this chapter.

PLAN OF NURSING CARE 2
PATIENT COMPLIANCE WITH A PRESCRIBED DRUG REGIMEN

Nursing Diagnosis: Potential Noncompliance with drug therapy related to patient's emotional, physical, or social status or nature of drug regimen

Goal: Patient will follow prescribed drug regimen.

Intervention	Rationale	Expected Outcome
Assess patient's attitude towards drug therapy; if problematic, attempt to resolve (e.g., values clarification, contracting).	Numerous complex factors affect compliance with drug therapy, including attitudes about drug therapy and the nature of the condition being prevented or treated. Compliance tends to be better when evidence that drugs control symptoms or disease is apparent to the patient, which is more often the case in short-term, acute conditions.	
Assess patient's level of knowledge and skills related to drug therapy: if inadequate, see **Plan of Nursing Care 1 (Knowledge Deficit).**	The patient cannot comply without the knowledge or skills needed to implement the drug regimen.	Patient will verbalize possession of or awareness of the availability of resources needed to comply with the drug regimen.
Ascertain ability to pay for drugs; if problematic, refer patient to appropriate resources.	The elderly and the poor are most likely to need prescription drugs and least able to pay for them.	
Assess ability to remember to take drugs at prescribed times; if problematic, suggest memory aids such as setting an alarm, keeping a daily log, posting reminder notes in places where they will be seen when it is time for drugs to be taken, keeping medications near something that is used when drugs are to be taken (e.g., near toothbrush for bedtime doses), or using color-coded containers that correspond with times drugs are to be taken, containers that hold an entire day's or week's medications, containers with an alarm that can be set to go off each time a dose is to be taken, or calendars on which doses can be written and crossed off each day.	The elderly, in whom memory may be failing, are most likely to require pharmacologic therapy.	

continued

PLAN OF NURSING CARE 2 (continued)
PATIENT COMPLIANCE WITH A PRESCRIBED DRUG REGIMEN
Nursing Diagnosis: Potential Noncompliance with drug therapy related to patient's emotional, physical, or social status or nature of drug regimen
Goal: Patient will follow prescribed drug regimen.

Intervention	Rationale	Expected Outcome
Assess ability to prepare drugs for administration: if childproof caps are too difficult to manage, inform patient that a regular cap may be requested when a prescription is filled. If vision is defective, teach a significant other to prepare the drug or refer patient to a home health care agency, which may be able to prepare multiple doses during a home visit (e.g., a week's supply of daily insulin injections drawn up in syringes).	The patient may have handicaps, such as arthritis or visual impairments, that interfere with appropriate drug usage.	
Determine ability to obtain medications; if problematic, explore options for transporting patient to health care provider who prescribed the drugs and to drugstore (or drug delivery to patient's home). Refer patient to appropriate resources as necessary.	Difficulty going up and down steps to get outdoors; weather that is too hot or too cold; lack of safe, affordable, convenient public transportation; inability to drive a car; and other factors may impede patient visits to either the drug prescriber or the drugstore.	
Assess support systems; if inadequate, suggest to healthcare provider that patient be followed more closely or refer patient for home help.	Support systems affect motivation and ability to use drugs (obtain, remember to take, administer). If inadequate, closer follow-up is indicated (e.g., frequent, short telephone calls from care providers improve compliance, as do short waiting periods for visits to care providers).	
Collaborate with patient, significant others, and persons who prescribed drugs to ensure that the following are as few, as simple, and as convenient as possible:	The simpler the drug regimen and the more conveniently it fits into daily living patterns, the more likely the patient is to comply with it.	Patient will agree that the drug regimen is as simple and as convenient as possible.
1. Numbers of dosage forms (e.g., one-half, one, two)	Most drugs are available in several dosages. Sometimes one preparation can be substituted for two that contain half the dose. Many oral preparations combine two or more drugs in one product (e.g., many antihypertensive drug combinations), reducing the number of different formulations that need to be taken.	
2. Types of dosage forms (e.g., tablet, capsule, solution)	Many patients find it easier to swallow capsules than tablets, easier to swallow liquids than capsules. The dosage form should suit individual needs and preferences to the extent possible.	
3. Numbers of times a day drugs are taken	For a drug with a long half-life, it may be possible to increase the dosage and reduce the number of times a day it is taken; or, a timed-release (sustained-action) preparation, if available, might be used.	
4. Routes of admninistration	Certain routes of administration tend to be more objectionable than others (e.g., rectal, parenteral) and more difficult to fit into certain lifestyles.	
Assist patient to plan a daily dosing schedule for all medications being used.	Many patients take numerous drugs and have difficulty figuring out an appropriate daily dosing schedule.	
Promote patient's faith and trust in the drug presciber.	Faith and trust in the person prescribing the drug tends to improve compliance.	Patient will express confidence in the person prescribing the drug regimen.

PATIENT EDUCATION

1. Give patient taking several drugs concurrently a list of drugs taken to carry at all times. This information may be important in an emergency to determine proper treatment and avoid drug interaction problems.
2. Teach elderly patient taking drugs that may produce hypotension (antipsychotics, antidepressants, antihypertensives, sedatives) measures that help control orthostatic hypotension. See **Plan of Nursing Care 9 (Antihypertensive Drugs)** in Chapter 31 for specific information.
3. Warn patient taking oral anticoagulants that excessive use of aspirin can increase the likelihood of bleeding.
4. Instruct patient to avoid self-medication with proprietary products containing anticholinergics.
5. Advise patient to label all medications clearly, and if two or more drugs have a similar appearance (two green liquids, for example) to place them in different types of containers to avoid confusion.

See also **Plan of Nursing Care 1 (Knowledge Deficit)** in Chapter 4.

Selected Bibliography

Abrams WB: Drugs and the elderly. Ration Drug Ther 19(6):1, 1985

Alford DM, Moll JA: Helping elderly patients in ambulatory settings cope with drug therapy. Nurs Clin North Am 17:275, 1982

Cohen JL: Pharmacokinetic changes in aging. Am J Med 80(Suppl 5A):31, 1986

Coodley EL: Drug metabolism in the aged. Ration Drug Ther 17(12):1, 1983

Dall CE, Gresham L: Promoting effective drug-taking behavior in the elderly. Nurs Clin North Am 17:283, 1982

Greenblatt DJ, Sellers EM, Shader RI: Drug disposition in old age. N Engl J Med 306:1081, 1982

Hayter J: Why response to medication changes with age. Geriatr Nurs 2:411, 1981

Hudson MF: Drugs and the older adult: Take special care. Nursing '84 14(8):47, 1984

Jarvik L (ed): Clinical Pharmacology and the Aged Patient. New York, Raven Press, 1981

Lamy PP: Special features of geriatric prescribing. Geriatrics 36:42, 1981

Mullen EM, Granholm, M: Drugs and the elderly patient. J Gerontol Nurs 7:108, 1981

Pagliaro LA, Pagliaro AM (eds): Pharmacologic Aspects of Aging. St Louis, CV Mosby, 1983

Poe WD, Holloway DA: Drugs and the Aged. New York, McGraw-Hill, 1980

Richey DP, Bender DA: Pharmacokinetic consequences of aging. Annu Rev Pharmacol Toxicol 17:49, 1977

Rowe JW: Health care of the elderly. N Engl J Med 312:827, 1985

Salzman C: Geriatric psychopharmacology. Annu Rev Med 36:217, 1981

Severson JA: Neurotransmitter receptors and aging. J Am Geriatr Soc 32:24, 1984

Sivertson L, Fletcher J: Assisting the elderly with drug therapy in the home. Nurs Clin North Am 17:293, 1982

Vestal RE (ed): Drug Treatment in the Elderly. ADIS Health Science Press, 1984

Ward M, Baltman M: Drug therapy in the elderly. Am Fam Physician 19:143, 1979

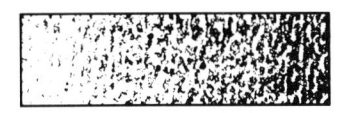

8 LEGAL ASPECTS OF DRUG THERAPY

A number of federal laws have been enacted during the 20th century whose purpose has been to protect the public from fraudulent claims and misbranded medications and to ensure safety as well as efficacy in drug products brought to market. The first part of this chapter examines the most important federal drug laws, including the narcotic drug regulations, and examines the nurse's role in the handling and administration of controlled substances.

The remainder of the chapter is devoted to a discussion of medication orders, including the proper format for prescribing drugs and the responsibilities of the nurse in carrying out medication orders.

DRUG LEGISLATION

The Pure Food and Drug Act

The first important federal law concerning drugs was the Wiley-Heyburn Act, more commonly known as the Pure Food and Drug Act, which took effect in 1907. This act was an attempt to prohibit adulteration and misbranding of food or drugs in interstate commerce. Sale of preparations containing any of the listed narcotic or habit-forming drugs without a proper label that indicated the name of the drug and the quantity contained in the preparation was prohibited. Under this law, however, accurate labeling was all that the federal government could require. Further provisions were the designation of the *United States Pharmacopeia* (USP) and the *National Formulary* (NF) as the *official* standards for establishing the strength, quality, and purity of medications recognized therein when sold in interstate commerce and the establishment of the U.S. Food and Drug Administration (FDA) as the regulatory agency to enforce the law.

Drugs listed in the USP or NF are designated as *official drugs* and conform to the standards of strength, purity, packaging safety, labeling, and so on, that are set by these compendia. Drugs meeting these standards can be identified by the letters USP or NF following their name. In the past, the USP and NF were separated entities, but because of their close similarity in style and content, they were combined into a single publication (USP-NF) in 1980. Because this publication is revised only every 5 years, many new drugs do not appear in the USP-NF until several years after they have become available. Thus, it is important to recognize that even though a new drug may not be classified as *official,* having not yet appeared in the official compendium, this should not be viewed as intimating lack of efficacy, safety, or purity; the term *official* merely connotes inclusion in the USP-NF.

The Sherley Amendment to the Pure Food and Drug Act was passed in 1912, prohibiting use of fraudulent advertising claims. These two pieces of legislation stood for over 30 years as the principal governmental attempt to regulate the sale of drugs.

The Federal Food, Drug and Cosmetic Act

Concern over the safety of drug products eventually led to the passage of the Federal Food, Drug and Cosmetic Act of 1938. This act was quite comprehensive in nature and contained a number of provisions intended to ensure both the safety and the efficacy of drug products. Among the important requirements of this act were that new drugs be demonstrated to be safe before being marketed, that all drugs (prescription and nonprescription) be properly labeled, that certain drugs be designated as "habit-forming" and so labeled, and that "good manufacturing procedures" be followed in the processing of drugs, according to standards set by the FDA

The Durham-Humphrey Amendment

Despite its comprehensive nature, the 1938 act had several deficiencies, and a number of amendments were added in later years. The first amendment, enacted in 1952, was the Durham-Humphrey Amendment. It designated certain drugs as being available by prescription only. These drugs, termed *legend* drugs, must bear the words "Caution: Federal law prohibits dispensing without prescription" on their containers. This amendment also prohibited refilling of such drugs without authorization and presented guidelines about oral and telephone orders for prescription drugs and refills. In addition, the Durham-Humphrey Amendment recognized another class of drugs, namely those that were safe for use without medical prescription, the so-called over-the-counter (OTC) drugs. Proper labeling procedures for OTC drugs were also provided in this amendment.

The Kefauver-Harris Amendment

Despite the existing drug laws, federal control over drug advertising and marketing practices was still inadequate, according to many observers. In 1958 U.S. Senator Estes Kefauver launched a controversial Senate investigation of the drug industry which ultimately culminated in the passage of the Kefauver-Harris Amendment to the Federal Food, Drug and Cosmetic Act in 1962. Among the important provisions of this amendment was the requirement that drugs be proved effective as well as safe before being marketed. The FDA was given authority to oversee and regulate the procedures by which new drugs were tested for safety and efficacy. Prescription drug advertising guidelines were tightened considerably, as were guidelines for investigational use of drugs on humans. Quality control laws for drug manufacturing were upgraded, and the role of the FDA in registering, monitoring, and inspecting drug manufacturers was greatly increased.

Another provision of the 1962 amendment granted the FDA the authority to regulate the efficacy, as well as the safety, of all drugs marketed since 1938, not just the drugs introduced beginning in 1962. Thus drug products marketed between 1938 and 1962 had to be reevaluated to determine their efficacy.

The Drug Efficacy Study Implementation

To facilitate this task, the FDA contracted with the National Academy of Sciences (NAS) and its research division, the National Research Council (NRC), to evaluate the efficacy data and therapeutic claims of the drug products. This study was called the Drug Efficacy Study Implementation (DESI). Based on the results of the evaluation, every drug was classified into one of six categories as follows:

1. *Effective:* Considerable evidence of effectiveness for the designated indications
2. *Probably effective:* More evidence is necessary to conclusively demonstrate effectiveness
3. *Possibly effective:* Little evidence to suggest effectiveness for the recommended indications
4. *Ineffective:* No significant evidence of effectiveness
5. *Ineffective as a fixed combination:* No evidence to suggest all components of the combination are necessary for the claimed effect, although one or more components may be effective if given alone
6. *Effective but:* A restriction or qualification must be added to the labeling

Drugs rated as ineffective were withdrawn from the market. Those rated either probably effective or possibly effective must carry their rating on the label, and their manufacturers are given additional time by the FDA either to substantiate their claims or to withdraw the drugs from the market.

NARCOTIC DRUG LAWS

It was not until 1914 that the first federal law aimed at controlling traffic in so-called illicit drugs was enacted.

The Harrison Narcotic Act

The Harrison Narcotic Act of 1914 established and legally defined the word *narcotic* and established regulations governing the importation, manufacture, sale, or use of opium, cocaine, and their derivatives. Subsequent revisions of the Harrison Narcotic Act provided similar guidelines relative to marijuana and many newer synthetic opiate drugs. This law, with minor periodic revisions, stood for over 50 years, but, unfortunately, gradually became obsolete and was ineffective in rectifying the burgeoning drug-abuse problem.

The Controlled Substances Act

In an attempt to put more teeth into federal control of habituating drugs, Congress, on May 1, 1971, passed the Comprehensive Drug Abuse Prevention and Control Act of 1970, which superseded all previous federal drug laws regulating narcotics and other dangerous drugs. This piece of legislation, commonly referred to as the Controlled Substances Act, was designed to control the manufacturing, distribution, administration, and disposition of narcotics, depressants, stimulants, and other drugs having abuse potential as designated by the Drug Enforcement Administration (DEA), a government agency responsible for enforcing the provisions of the Controlled Substances Act.

Among its many provisions, the Controlled Substances Act classified the various drugs subject to abuse into one of five *schedules* according to their medical usefulness and potential for abuse. The drugs comprising the various schedules are given in Table 8-1. Regulations governing each group of drugs are as follows:

SCHEDULE I
Drugs in Schedule I have a *high* abuse potential and no *accepted* medical use in the United States. They are not available for routine prescription use but may be obtained for investigational studies by proper application to the Drug Enforcement Administration.

SCHEDULE II
Drugs in Schedule II have valid medical indications but exhibit a *high* abuse potential. Misuse of these substances can lead to profound psychologic and physical dependence.

SCHEDULE III
Drugs in Schedule III have a potential for abuse less than those in Schedule I or II; however, misuse can still lead to moderate to low physical dependence and rather high psychologic dependence.

SCHEDULE IV
Drugs in Schedule IV have a lower abuse potential than Schedule III drugs. Misuse most often results in varying degrees of psychologic dependence, with occasional reports of limited physical dependence.

SCHEDULE V
Schedule V drugs consist mainly of preparations containing moderate amounts of opioid drugs, generally for antitussive or antidiarrheal use. Their abuse potential is less than Schedule IV drugs.

Each commercial container of a controlled substance bears on its label a symbol designating the schedule to which it belongs. Symbols are a large red C, either enclosing or followed by one of the Roman numerals I through V referring to the schedule to which the drug belongs.

The following discussion pertains to the requirements for ordering and dispensing controlled substances. The pharmacology of these substances, together with a review of procedures for recognizing and treating drug abuse will be found in Chapter 79.

PRESCRIBING AND DISPENSING CONTROLLED DRUGS

The requirements for dispensing a controlled drug outlined below are the currently mandated federal regulations. However, it should be stressed that in many instances, individual *state* laws are more stringent than the *federal* law and must be observed by all practitioners within a particular state. Persons handling controlled substances must therefore acquaint themselves with those specific state regulations, if any, that supersede the federal law.

All prescription orders for Schedule II drugs must be either typewritten or written in ink or indelible pencil and signed by the physician. No prescriptions for Schedule II drugs may be refilled, and all records and inventory information must be maintained separately from the other pharmacy records. A triplicate order form is necessary for ordering Schedule II drugs. Under certain emergency situations outlined below, a Schedule II drug may be dispensed on oral authorization.

Table 8-1
Schedules of Controlled Drugs

Schedule I	Schedule II	Schedule III	Schedule IV
benzylmorphine	*DEPRESSANTS*	*DEPRESSANTS*	*DEPRESSANTS*
cannabinols (e.g., hashish, marijuana, tetrahydrocannabinol)	amobarbital	aprobarbital	barbital
dihydromorphine	methaqualone	butabarbital	benzodiazepines (alprazolam, chlordiazepoxide, clonazepam, clorazepate, diazepam, flurazepam, halazepam, lorazepam, midazolam, oxazepam, prazepam, temazepam, triazolam)
hallucinogens (e.g., bufotenin, DET, DMT, DOB, DOM, ibogaine, LSD, MDA, mescaline, peyote, PMA, psilocybin, psilocyn)	pentobarbital	glutethimide	
	phencyclidine	hexobarbital	
	secobarbital	metharbital	
	NARCOTICS	methyprylon	
	alfentanil	talbutal	
ketobemidone	codeine	thiamylal	chloral hydrate
levomoramide	etorphine	thiopental	ethchlorvynol
nicocodine	fentanyl	*NARCOTICS*	ethinamate
nicomorphine	hydromorphone	opiates in combination with other nonnarcotic drugs (e.g., Empirin with codeine, Tylenol with codeine, Hycodan)	mephobarbital
racemoramide	levorphanol		meprobamate
	meperidine		methohexital
	methadone		paraldehyde
	opium and opium alkaloids (e.g., morphine, codeine)	paregoric	phenobarbital
		STIMULANTS	*NARCOTICS*
	oxycodone	benzphetamine	pentazocine
	oxymorphone	chlorphentermine	propoxyphene
	phenazocine	phendimetrazine	*STIMULANTS*
	sufentanil		diethylpropion
	STIMULANTS		fenfluramine
	amphetamine		mazindol
	coca leaves		pemoline
	cocaine		phentermine
	dextroamphetamine		
	methamphetamine		### Schedule V
	methylphenidate		buprenorphine
	phenmetrazine		diphenoxylate and atropine (e.g., Lomotil)
	CANNABINOIDS		loperamide
	dronabinol		narcotic drugs in combination with other nonnarcotic agents, generally used as antitussives, where the amount of narcotic (e.g., codeine, dihydrocodeine) is limited
	nabilone		

Orders for Schedule III and IV drugs and those Schedule V drugs requiring a prescription (see below) may be issued either orally or in writing and may be refilled up to five times within 6 months of the original prescription date if so authorized by the physician. Oral prescription orders must be immediately committed to writing. Prescriptions for drugs in Schedule III, IV, or V must be readily retrievable from the files, and if these controlled substances prescriptions are filed with the remainder of the prescription orders (except Schedule II drugs), each prescription for a Schedule III, IV, or V drug must be marked with the letter "C" in red ink to facilitate retrieval. Records must be maintained for at least 2 years.

Each time a prescription for a Schedule III, IV, or V drug is refilled, the date and amount of drug dispensed must be noted on the back of the order blank and initialed by the dispenser. The label of any controlled drug in Schedule II, III, or IV must contain the following statement "Caution: Federal law prohibits the transfer of this drug to any person other than the patient for whom it was prescribed."

Partial Distribution of Controlled Substances

If the full quantity of a Schedule II drug cannot be supplied with the original prescription order, the remaining portion may be dispensed within 72 hours provided the quantity dispensed with the initial order is noted on the face of the written prescription. Additional partial quantities may not be supplied beyond the 72-hour time limit except on a new prescription order.

Partial dispensing of Schedule III and IV drugs is allowed provided the quantity dispensed is noted on the back of the prescription order. The balance of the partial quantities dispensed may not exceed the total amount authorized (that is, original quantity plus allowable refills), nor extend past the 6-month time limit.

Emergency Dispensing of Schedule II Drugs

In the event of an emergency situation, a Schedule II controlled substance can be dispensed on oral authorization provided certain conditions are satisfied. An emergency situation is defined as one in which

- *Immediate* administration of the drug is necessary for proper treatment.
- No appropriate alternative treatment is available.
- A written prescription cannot reasonably be provided by the prescribing physician before the drug is required.

The provisions for dispensing a Schedule II drug under an emergency situation are as follows:

- Quantity dispensed must be limited to the amount necessary to treat the patient during the emergency period.
- Prescription order must be reduced to writing immediately.
- All efforts to verify the identity of the prescriber should be made, in the event that he or she is not known to the dispenser.
- A written prescription with the notation "Authorization for Emergency Dispensing" must be delivered to the dispenser within 72 hours of the oral authorization, or if mailed, postmarked within 72 hours.

Nonprescription Dispensing of Schedule V Drugs

Certain Schedule V preparations may be dispensed without a prescription providing the following conditions are met:

- The dispensing is done only by a pharmacist or pharmacist-intern.
- The purchaser is at least 18 years of age (proof of age is necessary if the purchaser is unknown to the dispenser).
- Not more than 240 mL or not more than 48 solid dosage units of any substance containing opium, nor more than 120 mL or not more than 24 solid dosage units of any other controlled substance may be distributed to the same purchaser within 48 hours.
- The name and address of the purchaser, kind and quantity of substance purchased, date of sale, and pharmacist's initials must be recorded for each sale in a Schedule V record book and records maintained for 2 years.

State and local laws, which often are more stringent with respect to retail distribution of Schedule V substances, must be observed in lieu of the federal law.

A practitioner (physician, dentist, veterinarian) must apply for permission to dispense controlled drugs by registering with the Drug Enforcement Administration and, on approval, receives a seven-digit registration number (DEA number) that must appear on every order for controlled substances. This registration must be renewed annually. Likewise, every pharmacy that dispenses controlled drugs must register annually with the Drug Enforcement Administration, and its DEA number must be available for inspection at the location of business.

THE NURSE'S ROLE IN ADMINISTRATION OF CONTROLLED DRUGS

The nurse is guided in the administration of controlled substances by agency policies, which reflect state and federal regulations.

Administration Within Healthcare Institutions

In any institution, whether acute or extended care, controlled drugs must be kept in a locked cabinet with access to these medications limited to certain personnel. Agency policy states the frequency with which the stock must be counted (usually every shift), who may give the drugs, how the drugs are to be obtained from the central pharmacy, and who bears ultimate responsibility for loss of any of these drugs. State regulatory agencies generally investigate all losses of controlled substances, so such incidents must be accurately reported.

Institutional policies also reflect the frequency with which controlled drugs are to be reordered. The nurse must comply with these policies and ensure that such drugs are reordered promptly. In acute care settings, it may be necessary to reorder some Schedule II drugs every 24 hours to 48 hours, whereas orders for drugs in other categories may be valid for 7 days. In extended care facilities, orders may be written and renewed once every 30 days. Whatever the time limitation, the nurse is responsible for monitoring the response to the drugs administered and for reporting to the physician evidence of change in pain control, development of tolerance, addiction behaviors, or toxic reactions related to the medication. Changes may occur without warning, so the nurse should document the patient's response to the drug each time it is administered.

Administration in Home-Care Settings

In the home-care setting, patients and their families are responsible for obtaining the controlled medication through a local pharmacy. Therefore, the nurse must monitor the patient's response to the drug and report any changes to the physician. If suspicions arise that the patient or another family member has abused the drug, such information should be shared with the physician and the dispensing pharmacist. The frequency of refill requests can then be monitored. Hospice nurses report that this problem occurs occasionally and is best dealt with by professionals—the physician, pharmacist, nurse, and regulatory agencies—rather than by a single person making an accusation.

MEDICATION ORDERS

Proper ordering of medications is essential for safe and effective drug therapy. Transmission of the physician's wishes regarding drug treatment of the patient is usually accomplished by a written order, in either a drug file or a patient chart in the case of hospitalized persons, or in the form of a prescription in the case of an outpatient. Medication orders may be given orally, by telephone, and it is important that such orders be reduced to writing as soon as possible to minimize chance of error.

Generally, persons empowered by state law to write prescriptions include physicians, dentists, and veterinarians. In some states, however, the law has been modified to permit nurse practitioners and physicians' assistants to write prescription orders for certain types of drugs. Since these laws vary from state to state, persons in these situations should acquaint themselves with the regulations in their particular area.

THE NURSE'S ROLE IN CARRYING OUT MEDICATION ORDERS

The nurse has several legal responsibilities in carrying out medication orders written in the hospital. Nurses must accurately transcribe orders to the medication record sheet, which provides a quick reference for all the medications a patient is receiving. This transcription should be clearly written so that all staff personnel will be able to read the order.

Clarifying and Evaluating Written Orders

If the order has not been clearly written, the nurse should question the physician to seek clarification. Legally the standard against which nurses are judged is that they will give the *right* medication in the *right* dose, by the *right* route, at the *right* time, to the *right* patient. That standard makes the nurse liable for giving a wrong medication to a patient even if the physician who ordered it committed the error. Therefore, *when in doubt, question the order.*

There are two steps in the process of assessing the physician's order for a medication: first, an initial reading for clarity, and second, a reading for the appropriateness of the order. What has been written must be understandable and free of ambiguities. Any abbreviations, if used, must be correctly interpreted, and the order must contain all parts and information described above. Secondly, before dispensing the medication, the nurse must evaluate the order for appropriateness, ascertaining for example, whether the dosage form can be conveniently taken by the patient, whether the patient has any underlying condition (e.g., liver or kidney disease) that may alter the effect of the drug, whether the patient is taking other drugs that may interact with the newly prescribed drug, or whether the patient has demonstrated previous allergies to medication.

Telephone Orders

Occasionally, the nurse will be asked to take a telephone order. Institutional policies will identify the context in which this act is permitted. Many institutions require that two nurses listen to telephone orders as they are given to ensure accuracy and appropriateness and to protect the nurse. Telephone orders are most appropriate in emergency situations when the physician cannot be present. The accuracy of a telephone order depends on communication between sender and receiver. To ensure that the order is clear, it is always a good idea to write it down and repeat it to the physician before hanging up the telephone. The physician must cosign the order within 24 hours of giving it. Telephone orders can involve risk if the physician later denies having given the order, or if the nurse misinterprets the order. Most institutions discourage the use of telephone orders for these reasons, and nurses should be cautious about accepting them.

Responsibility for Errors in Administration

Lastly, nurses are responsible for administering most of the medications ordered. In order to meet the legal standard, they must be knowledgeable about the medications given, careful in administration, and alert to potential problems that may result in errors.

Most medication errors made by nurses involve failure to adhere to institutional policies. Policies are designed to protect both the nurse and the patient, so familiarity with them is important. Safe medication administration depends on responsible action by a team of colleagues, all of whom are legally accountable. The interaction of all of these people will determine whether or not the patient receives safe care. Nurses should take an active role in ensuring patient safety by using caution in medication administration and by participating in discussions of committees that formulate guidelines for patient care.

Selected Bibliography

Bell NK: Whose autonomy is at stake? Am J Nurs June:1170, 1981

Bowers JZ, Velo GP (eds): Drug Assessment: Criteria and Methods. New York, Elsevier North Holland, 1979

Cushing M: Drug errors can be bitter pills. Am J Nurs 86:895, 1986

Davis N, Cohen M: Learning from mistakes: 20 tips for avoiding medication errors. Nursing '82 12:65, 1982

Department of Justice: Regulations implementing the Comprehensive Drug Abuse Prevention and Control Act of 1970. Fed Register 36(80):1, 1971

Long G: The effect of medication distribution systems on medication errors. Nurs Res 31(3):182, 1982

A Primer on New Drug Development. Rockville, MD, HEW publication No. (FDA) 74-3021, Department of Health, Education and Welfare, 1974

Slone D, Shapiro S, Miettinen OS, Finkle WD, Stolley PD: Drug evaluation after marketing. Ann Intern Med 90:257, 1979

Wertheimer AI: The placebo effect. Pharm Int 1:12, 1980

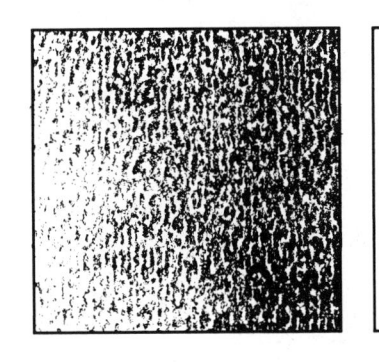

II Drugs Acting on the Nervous System

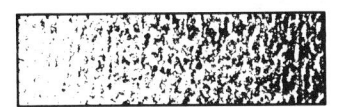

9 THE NERVOUS SYSTEM: A REVIEW

The human nervous system is an immensely complex structure, encompassing more than 12 billion nerve cells or neurons. Along with the endocrine system, it regulates and coordinates the functioning of the organs of the body. The endocrine system provides a slowly developing but long-lasting control, whereas the nervous system evokes rapid changes in body function and therefore provides moment-to-moment control.

The nervous system can be categorized in the following manner:

I. Peripheral nervous system
   A. Somatic system
   B. Autonomic system
      1. Sympathetic division
      2. Parasympathetic division
II. Central nervous system
   A. Brain
   B. Spinal cord

The following brief review of important concepts related to the functioning of the nervous system is presented to provide background sufficient to promote understanding of the subsequent chapters dealing with those classes of drugs affecting neuronal functioning.

PERIPHERAL NERVOUS SYSTEM

The peripheral nervous system consists of the somatic and autonomic branches, and several important differences exist between these two systems as outlined in Table 9-1.

Somatic Branch

The somatic system conveys sensory information about the external environment, such as light, heat, and pressure to the central nervous system (CNS) and mediates the response of skeletal muscles to external environmental stimuli. Thus, the somatic system is viewed as a *voluntary* system—one over which a person exerts conscious control.

Autonomic Branch

In contrast, the autonomic system includes those sensory and motor nerves that primarily innervate organs (smooth muscle, heart, glands) that usually function independently of the individual's will. This system is classified as an *involuntary* system. Although responses of the somatic system, such as contraction of skeletal muscle, are almost always excitatory, those of the autonomic system may be either excitatory (e.g., vasoconstriction) or inhibitory (e.g., bradycardia, bronchodilation), depending on the organ and neurohormone involved.

The autonomic system is further subclassified into *sympathetic* and *parasympathetic* divisions. The characteristics of each division are listed in Table 9-2.

The parasympathetic division is often referred to as a *cholinergic* system because the neurotransmitter at its postganglionic nerve endings is acetylcholine (Ach), whereas the sympathetic system may be termed an *adrenergic* system because its postganglionic neurotransmitter *in most cases* is norepinephrine. Many effector structures are innervated by *both* divisions of the autonomic system, and in dually innervated structures the pharmacologic effects of the two divisions are opposite. That is, if sympathetic activation causes excitation, parasympathetic activation causes inhibition. However, it is important to recognize that the two divisions do not exert equal control over all dually innervated structures. For example, the sympathetic division influences blood vessel tone, and hence blood pressure, to a much greater degree than the parasympathetic system, whereas the reverse is true in the functioning of the GI tract.

A few structures, however, are singly innervated, including the adrenal medulla, sweat glands, certain blood vessels, intrinsic eye muscles, and pilomotor muscles of the skin. The response of these structures is always *excitatory*, irrespective of their innervation. The effects of sympathetic versus parasympathetic stimulation on different structures of the body are outlined in Table 9-3, in which the opposing nature of most responses and the excitatory nature of singly innervated structures is clearly indicated. Note that although the sweat glands and some skeletal-muscle blood vessels are innervated by sympathetic fibers, the neurotransmitter released at the nerve ending is acetylcholine, not norepinephrine.

Moreover, the adrenal medulla receives parasympathetic innervation mediated by ACh, but the postganglionic response is release of epinephrine and norepinephrine from the adrenal chromaffin cells. Thus, peripheral nerves are probably best classified chemically—that is, on the basis of the principal neurohormone released from their nerve endings. Nerves releasing acetylcholine are thus termed *cholinergic,* and those releasing norepinephrine are called *adrenergic.* The mechanisms by which these neurohormones function at nerve endings are reviewed below.

NEUROHORMONAL FUNCTION

The functional unit of the nervous system is the *neuron,* a specialized cell capable of generating and transmitting electrical impulses. The passage of an impulse *along* a neuron, termed *conduction,* is an electrical process involving changes in the potential difference across the neuronal membrane caused by alterations in the flow of ions through the membrane. Drugs such as local anesthetics are capable of interrupting conduction of nerve impulses along a neuron by interfering with ionic flow across the membrane.

In contrast, the transmission of an impulse *between* adjacent neurons is a chemical process mediated by substances termed *neurotransmitters* or *neurohormones* (e.g., acetylcholine, norepinephrine) that are stored within the nerve ending and diffuse from one neuron to another across the interneuronal space, or *synaptic junction.* Remember that the *post*synaptic structure can be either a second neuron or some other type of organ or tissue such as a muscle fiber or gland. The transmission of nerve impulses is an essential step in the functioning of the nervous system, and because it is a chemically (neurohormonally) mediated process, it is readily affected by many different classes of drugs, resulting in a wide range of pharmacologic effects.

To understand how drugs can affect nerve impulse transmission, it is necessary first to review the sequence of events that occur during the transmission of impulses between neurons.

Sequence of Neurotransmission

BIOSYNTHESIS OF NEUROTRANSMITTER

Chemical substances that mediate transmission are formed from precursor substances within the nerve ending. Acetylcholine is synthesized from choline and acetyl coenzyme A by the action of the enzyme choline acetyltransferase. Norepinephrine is formed from the amino acid tyrosine through a series of enzymatic conversions. In the adrenal medulla, as well as in certain brain areas, norepinephrine is further converted to epinephrine.

STORAGE OF NEUROTRANSMITTER

Upon formation, the neurotransmitter is taken up into specialized sites (such as vesicles) within the nerve ending and stored. This allows the neuron to build up a surplus of the transmitter in anticipation of need. Thousands of molecules of acetylcholine are stored in membranous sacs called *vesicles*. Some norepinephrine, the so-called reserve pool, is stored in granules bound to adenosine triphosphate (ATP), whereas other norepinephrine exists in the cytoplasm and is not contained within vesicles. This latter fraction is known as the mobile pool and is not released by a nerve action potential (see below). However, it can be expelled by a number of drugs.

RELEASE OF NEUROTRANSMITTER

With the arrival of a nerve action potential at the nerve ending, depolarization of the *presynaptic* membrane occurs, resulting in release of the neurotransmitter from its storage site into the synaptic junction. Release of the neurohormones is thought to occur in response to influx of calcium ions into the nerve ending, resulting in destabilization of the storage vesicles, subsequent fusion with the terminal plasma membrane, and extrusion of the neurotransmitter into the synaptic cleft.

Table 9-1.
Comparison of the Somatic and Autonomic Nervous Systems

	Somatic	Autonomic
Nature of the response	Voluntary	Involuntary
Centers of neuronal origin in the CNS	Cerebrum, cerebellum, midbrain, basal ganglia, spinal cord	Midbrain, hypothalamus, pons, medulla, spinal cord
Structures innervated by efferent nerve fibers	Skeletal muscles, sensory organs	Smooth muscle, cardiac muscle, exocrine and endocrine glands
Efferent nerve pathways	Single neuron with cell body in CNS and axon terminal at effector structure (e.g., skeletal muscle fiber)	Two-neuron chain, with cell body of *pre*ganglionic neuron in CNS and axon terminal in a peripheral ganglia. *Post*ganglionic neuron has cell body in ganglia (synapses with *pre*ganglionic nerve ending) and axon terminal at effector structure (e.g., heart, GI tract, bronchioles, glands)
Effect of nerve impulse on innervated structures	Excitation (e.g., skeletal muscle contraction)	Excitation (e.g., vasoconstriction, salivation) or inhibition (e.g., bradycardia, bronchodilation)

Table 9-2.
Comparison of the Parasympathetic and Sympathetic Divisions of the Autonomic Nervous System

	Parasympathetic Division	Sympathetic Division
Outflow from CNS	Craniosacral	Thoracolumbar
	Cranial nerves (3, 7, 9, 10; i.e., oculomotor, facial, glossopharyngeal, and vagus) and sacral (S2 to S4) segments of the spinal cord	Thoracic (T1 to T12) and lumbar (L1 to L3) segments of the spinal cord
Ganglia	Near or within structure innervated	Close to spinal cord
Preganglionic fiber	Long and myelinated	Short and myelinated
Postganglionic fiber	Short and nonmyelinated	Long and nonmyelinated
Response to stimulation	Localized to a restricted area	Generalized and widespread
Neurotransmitter at all ganglia	Acetylcholine	Acetylcholine
Neurotransmitter at postganglionic nerve ending	Acetylcholine	Norepinephrine

Table 9-3.
Responses of Effector Structures to Autonomic Nervous System Activation

Effector	Parasympathetic Activation Action	Receptor	Sympathetic Activation Action	Receptor
Heart				
Rate	↓	M	↑	beta$_1$
Contractility			↑	beta$_1$
Blood Vessels				
Coronary			Dilated	
Skeletal muscle			Dilated	M, beta$_2$
Skin and mucosa			Constricted	alpha
Cerebral, pulmonary, abdominal viscera	Dilated		Constricted	alpha
Stomach and Intestine				
Motility and tone	↑	M	↓	beta$_2$
Sphincters	Relaxed	M	Contracted	alpha
Glandular secretion	↑	M	↓	
Urinary Bladder				
Detrusor muscle	Contracted	M	Relaxed	beta$_2$
Trigone and sphincter	Relaxed	M	Contracted	alpha
Other Smooth Muscle				
Bronchial muscle, ureters, gallbladder, and ducts	Contracted	M	Relaxed	beta$_2$
Salivary Glands	Stimulated (profuse, watery secretion)	M	Stimulated (sparse, thick, mucinous secretion)	alpha
Eye				
Radial muscle of iris			Contracted (mydriasis)	alpha
Sphincter muscle of iris	Contracted (miosis)	M		
Ciliary muscle	Contracted (accommodated for near vision)	M	Relaxed (for far vision)	beta
Spleen Capsule			Contracted	alpha
Liver			Glycogenolysis; gluconeogenesis	alpha$_1$, beta$_2$
Uterus (Pregnant)			Relaxed	beta$_2$
Kidney			Renin secretion	beta$_1$
Skin				
Sweat glands			Stimulated	M, alpha
Pilomotor muscles			Contracted	alpha
Pancreas				
Islet cells			Insulin secretion ↓	alpha$_2$
Acinar cells	Enzyme secretion ↑	M		
Adrenal Medulla	Secretion of epinephrine and norepinephrine	N		
Fat Cells			Lipolysis	alpha$_1$, beta$_1$

M, muscarinic; N, nicotinic; ↓, decreased; ↑, increased.

The release of presynaptic stores of norepinephrine can be regulated by a negative feedback mechanism that is mediated by alpha$_2$ receptor sites (see Table 9-4) on the presynaptic nerve ending (see discussion under **Receptor Concept**). When the level of norepinephrine released from the nerve ending becomes excessive, increased activation of presynaptic alpha$_2$ receptor sites on the terminal nerve ending occurs, attenuating further release of norepinephrine. In this way, the neurotransmitter can regulate its own rate of release through a negative feedback mechanism. A number of other clinically useful drugs also influence the release of norepinephrine by either activating (e.g., clonidine) or blocking (e.g., imipramine) presynaptic alpha$_2$ receptor sites. Conversely, activation of presynaptic beta receptor sites is believed to facilitate neurotransmitter release.

Prejunctional regulation of neurotransmitter release is not limited to norepinephrine. Evidence suggests that most substances that function as neurotransmitters, including serotonin, histamine, and polypeptides, can regulate their own release through a negative feedback mechanism.

INTERACTION WITH POSTSYNAPTIC MEMBRANE

The released neurotransmitter diffuses across the synaptic junction and interacts (complexes) with specific reactive areas (receptor sites) on the postsynaptic membrane. This interaction causes either depolarization (activation) or hyperpolarization (inhibition) of the neuron or effector structure, leading to facilitation or blockade of nerve impulse transmission.

INACTIVATION OF NEUROTRANSMITTER

Neurotransmitter action can be terminated in several ways:
1. *Diffusion of the released neurotransmitter away from the synaptic area* is probably important in removing excess or overflow but is of little consequence for terminating the effects of physiologic quantities.
2. *Enzymatic breakdown of neurotransmitter* plays a greater role for acetylcholine than for norepinephrine. Acetylcholinesterase cleaves the neurotransmitter into choline and acetate, thus terminating its action. Two enzymes, monamine oxidase (MAO), which is found in prejunctional nerve endings, and catechol-o-methyl transferase (COMT), which is located postjunctionally, inactivate norepinephrine, but these are of little significance in *initially* terminating the action of the endogenously released hormone.
3. *Uptake of released neurotransmitter,* either into the presynaptic nerve terminal from which it was released (uptake I) or into surrounding nonneural glial or smooth muscle cells (uptake II). Uptake I represents the principal means by which norepinephrine is inactivated after being extruded from the prejunctional nerve ending.

REPOLARIZATION OF POSTSYNAPTIC MEMBRANE

When neurotransmitter action ceases, the postsynaptic receptor area membrane is repolarized—that is, returned to its original ionic polarity and responsiveness.

MECHANISM OF DRUG ACTION ON THE PERIPHERAL NERVOUS SYSTEM

Drugs acting on the nervous system may affect the transmission of impulses at one or more of the preceding steps.

Types of Drug Action

Types of drug action at each step are listed below, along with examples

Table 9-4.
Characteristics of Autonomic Receptor Sites

Type	Location	Activators	Blockers
Cholinergic			
Muscarinic (M)	Sites innervated by postganglionic parasympathetic fibers (heart, smooth muscle cells, exocrine gland); brain; autonomic ganglia (?)	acetylcholine; pilocarpine	atropine
Nicotinic (N)	Autonomic ganglia; neuromuscular endplate of skeletal muscle	acetylcholine; nicotine	trimethaphan (ganglia); d-tubocurare (neuromuscular junction)
Adrenergic			
Alpha$_1$	Most blood vessels, GI tract, pancreas, eye, skin	norepinephrine; epinephrine; phenylephrine	phentolamine; tolazoline
Alpha$_2$	Presynaptic terminal ending of adrenergic nerve fibers; platelets; fat cells; vascular smooth muscle	norepinephrine; epinephrine; clonidine	imipramine
Beta$_1$	Heart; gastrointestinal tract; urinary bladder; eye; adipose tissue; presynaptic sympathetic nerve endings	epinephrine; isoproterenol	propranolol; metoprolol
Beta$_2$	Bronchioles, uterus, skeletal muscle, blood vessels, liver	epinephrine; isoproterenol; metaproterenol	propranolol
Dopamine	Renal, visceral and coronary blood vessels; brain; presynaptic nerve terminals	dopamine	haloperidol

of drugs described in the text that have the particular type of action specified.

- Inhibition of biosynthesis (e.g., carbidopa, metyrosine)
- Interference with intraneuronal binding or storage (e.g., reserpine)
- Interference with transmitter release (e.g., guanethidine, clonidine)
- Enhancement of transmitter release (e.g., amphetamine, amantadine, guanidine)
- Activation of postsynaptic receptor sites (e.g., pilocarpine, isoproterenol, bromocriptine)
- Blockade of postsynaptic receptor sites (e.g., atropine, propranolol, tubocurarine)
- Interference with neurotransmitter inactivation (e.g., physostigmine, imipramine, tranylcypromine)
- Prevention of postsynaptic membrane repolarization (e.g., succinylcholine)

Receptor Concept

A receptor site may be viewed as a chemically reactive area on the surface of a cell membrane that is capable of complexing with specific neurotransmitters. This interaction initiates a sequence of events that alters the ionic permeability of the membrane, eliciting biochemical changes in the postsynaptic structure that either stimulate or inhibit the functional activity of the effector structure, such as a muscle fiber, gland, or neuron. A more extensive discussion of drug–receptor interactions can be found in Chapter 3.

Receptors may be classified on the basis of their location, their selective responsiveness to different activators or blockers, and their differences in effector structure responses. Table 9-4 lists several criteria for distinguishing the different kinds of cholinergic and adrenergic receptor sites found in the peripheral nervous system.

CHOLINERGIC RECEPTORS: M AND N

Cholinergic receptors are differentiated primarily on the basis of their anatomic location and the relative selectivity of cholinergic antagonists. The cholinergic receptor subtypes are named after the alkaloids that were originally used in their identification, and are referred to as muscarinic (M) sites, which respond to the alkaloid muscarine, and nicotinic (N) sites, which are activated by nicotine. *M sites* are located on effector structures innervated by postganglionic parasympathetic and a few sympathetic fibers. They may be found typically in the heart, smooth muscle cells, some glands, and skeletal muscle blood vessels. In addition, M receptors have also been identified in the brain and in autonomic ganglia (see below). *N sites* are situated on postjunctional membranes of all autonomic ganglia (these receptors were previously termed NI sites) and in the neuromuscular endplate of skeletal muscle (these receptors were previously named NII sites). The nicotinic receptors in autonomic ganglia are not identical to those in skeletal muscle, inasmuch as they respond differently to certain agonists and antagonists. Further complicating the picture is the existence of evidence suggesting that muscarinic receptors may be subdivided further into M_1 and M_2 sites according to the selectivity of different cholinergic agonists and antagonists.

ADRENERGIC RECEPTORS: ALPHA, BETA, AND DOPAMINE

Adrenergic receptors have traditionally been classified as *alpha* and *beta* receptor sites according to their location, their differential activation or blockade by various drugs, and the types of responses they mediate. Each receptor type is then further subdivided to reflect differences in location and function. Alpha$_1$ receptors are found postsynaptically in vascular smooth muscle; GI and urinary sphincter muscles; and in the eye, skin, pancreas, and salivary glands. Alpha$_2$ receptors occur on presynaptic nerve endings (where they control the release of norepinephrine) as well as in platelets, fat cells, and possibly also in vascular smooth muscle. Beta$_1$ receptors occur primarily in the heart and adipose tissue, whereas beta$_2$ sites are present in the bronchioles, skeletal muscle vasculature, liver, kidney, and urinary bladder.

A fifth type of adrenergic receptor responds selectively to the neurotransmitter dopamine (DA) and is located on visceral and splanchnic blood vessels, in a number of brain areas, and probably also on presynaptic sympathetic nerve terminals. Dopamine receptors are further classified as DA$_1$ and DA$_2$ sites.

A review of the responses elicited by activation of the different adrenergic receptors is presented in Table 12-1.

OTHER RECEPTOR SITES

In addition to the receptor sites for the cholinergic and adrenergic neurohormones outlined above, other specialized types of receptors exist in peripheral and central structures. For example, two types of histamine receptors (H$_1$ and H$_2$ sites) are present in some body tissues, and these receptors selectively mediate the diverse actions of endogenous histamine on different body organs. A further discussion of histamine receptor sites is found in Chapter 14, which deals with antihistamine drugs. Serotonin, another endogenous neurohormone, interacts with at least two kinds of specific reactive sites to elicit its pharmacologic effects, which can be abolished by agents that are capable of selectively blocking the different serotonin receptor sites. Antiserotonin drugs are also discussed in Chapter 14. Many other putative neurotransmitters, including glycine, glutamic acid, GABA, and bradykinin, are also believed to exert their effects by chemically combining with a corresponding receptor site.

UP-REGULATION AND DOWN-REGULATION

Receptor sensitivity can be significantly altered depending on the degree of activity at a particular receptor site. Persistent activation of a receptor leads to a gradual loss of sensitivity, and probably also an actual decrease in receptor number. Thus, when the agonist is removed, the remaining receptors are less reactive to additional agonists for some time. The term *down-regulation* has been coined to describe this phenomenon, which helps explain the action of several drugs such as the tricyclic antidepressants (for a further description of the mechanisms involved in down-regulation of receptor sites, see Chap. 24). Similarly, persistent receptor antagonism can cause receptor supersensitivity, leading to exaggerated responses once the antagonist is removed. For example, prolonged dopamine blockade by antipsychotic drugs results in hypersensitivity of central dopamine receptors. This dopamine supersensitivity, or *up-regulation* of dopamine receptor sites is believed to be responsible for the appearance of orofacial involuntary movements with long-term antipsychotic drug usage. Presumably, endogenous dopamine acts on hypersensitive receptor sites to elicit altered muscle activity in the facial region.

CENTRAL NERVOUS SYSTEM

The central nervous system is composed of the brain and the spinal cord;

together they integrate and regulate a tremendous range of sensory, motor, and emotional activities. Consequently, drugs that affect central neuronal function have the potential to significantly alter the behavior of an individual. The mechanisms of action of centrally acting drugs are similar to those of peripherally acting drugs, and in fact many drugs exert simultaneous effects on both the central and peripheral nervous systems (e.g., sedation, hypotension). Moreover, because of the complex neuronal interconnections among CNS areas, drugs acting at a specific central locus may exert widespread pharmacologic effects throughout the body and simultaneously alter the functioning of several physiological systems.

The diversity of functions regulated by the CNS can best be illustrated by outlining the major subdivisions of the brain and the principal physiological functions thought to be controlled by each area. Many of these functions are considered in more detail in chapters of this book that deal with drugs capable of influencing one or more of the CNS areas that control the many bodily functions

I. Forebrain
  A. Telencephalon
    1. *Cerebral cortex*
       a. Analysis of sensory input—reception, integration, organization, facilitation of appropriate action (primary sensory areas)
       b. Memory development (temporal lobe)
       c. Storage of short-term information and elaboration of thought (temporal and frontal lobe)
       d. Analysis and control of muscular coordination (superior temporal gyrus and frontal lobe)
       e. Speech (temporal lobe)
       f. Hearing (superior temporal lobe)
       g. Vision (occipital lobe)
    2. *Corpus striatum* (caudate, putamen, globus pallidus)
       a. Planning, programming, and modulation of motor movement
       b. Control of muscle tone
    3. *Corpus callosum*
       a. Connects two hemispheres of the cerebral cortex, permitting functional integration
  B. Diencephalon
    1. *Thalamus*
       a. Relay center for discrimination of incoming sensory signals (e.g., pain, temperature, touch)
       b. Modulation of motor impulses from cerebral cortex
       c. Integration of emotional behavior
    2. *Hypothalamus*
       a. Regulation of cardiovascular function
       b. Regulation of body water
       c. Regulation of temperature
       d. Regulation of food intake and satiety
       e. Control of endocrine functioning
       f. Control of sleep-wake mechanisms
       g. Modification of behavior
II. Midbrain
  A. Mesencephalon
    1. *Corpora quadrigemina* (superior and inferior colliculus)
       a. Relay centers for visual and hearing reflexes
    2. *Cerebral peduncles*
       a. Control of motor coordination and postural reflexes
    3. *Red nucleus*
       a. Regulation of motor functioning
    4. *Substantia nigra*
       a. Regulation of motor functioning
III. Hindbrain
  A. Metencephalon
    1. *Cerebellum*
       a. Coordination of muscle activity (synergia)
       b. Maintenance of equilibrium and posture
    2. *Pons*
       a. Relay center for impulses from the medulla to higher cortical centers
       b. Regulation of respiration
  B. Myelencephalon
    1. *Medulla oblongata*
       a. Control of respiration and cardiovascular function (heart and blood vessels)
       b. Regulation of certain reflex activity (swallowing, salivation, vomiting)
       c. Modulation of GI function

In addition, several groups of CNS structures function as integrated systems to control certain aspects of behavior.

Reticular Formation

The *reticular formation* is a diffuse network of cells and nuclei scattered throughout the brainstem and extending upward into the midbrain. Impulses from spinal-cord ascending pathways (by way of collateral neurons) and the cerebellum impinge on the reticular formation, which in turn makes diffuse connections with the cerebral cortex by way of relay nuclei in many subcortical areas. The reticular formation functions as part of the so-called extrapyramidal system and is capable of modifying motor activity, but its principal role consists of maintaining a state of alertness or arousal. The function of the reticular formation and in fact of the entire reticular activating system (RAS) can be markedly impaired by many classes of drugs, including barbiturates, anesthetics, and antipsychotics, resulting in varying degrees of CNS depression and eventually leading to unconsciousness.

Limbic System

The principal group of structures controlling emotional behavior is collectively termed the *limbic system*. It is composed of several subcortical areas (thalamus, hypothalamus, hippocampus, amygdala, septum, preoptic area, and portions of the basal ganglia) and a surrounding ring of cortical tissue on the medial and ventral surfaces of each cerebral hemisphere. The limbic system has a role in regulating many aspects of behavior, such as feelings of pleasure, anger, rage, and fear. It also functions in regulating biologic rhythms, sexual activity, feeding, and learning. Many portions of the limbic circuit transmit their impulses through the hypothalamus, so their output is frequently expressed in the form of autonomic manifestations such as changes in blood pressure or respiration, hormonal changes, and expressions of pain, anger, and pleasure. Drugs used in the treatment of emotional disorders, such as antipsychotics, antidepressants, and lithium, exert at least a part of their action on the structures of the limbic system.

Basal Ganglia

The *basal ganglia* are composed of three areas in the forebrain—the caudate nucleus, putamen, and globus pallidus—as well as several areas in the midbrain, such as the substantia nigra, red nucleus, and subthalamic nucleus. These structures are important for the integration and regulation of locomotor activity and postural reflexes. Pathologic changes in these ganglia result in the appearance of many types of movement disorders, the most common of which is parkinsonism.

Selected Bibliography

Appenzeller O: The Autonomic Nervous System. Amsterdam, Elsevier, 1982

Cooper JR, Bloom FE, Roth RH: The Biochemical Basis of Neuropharmacology. 4th ed. New York, Oxford University Press, 1982

Cooper JR, Meyer FM: Possible mechanisms involved in the release and modulation of release of neuroactive agents. Neurochem Int 6:419, 1984

Gootman PM: Development of the autonomic nervous system. Fed Proc 42:1619, 1983

Hakanson R, Sundler F: The design of the neuroendocrine system: A unifying concept and its consequences. Trends Pharmacol Sci 4:41, 1983

Hirschowitz BI, Hammer R, Giachetti A, Keirns JJ, Levine RR (eds): Subtypes of muscarnic receptors. Trends Pharmacol Sci (Suppl 1) 1984

Iversen LL, Iversen SD, Synder SH (eds): Handbook of Psychopharmacology. New York, Plenum Press, 1983

Langer SZ: Presynaptic receptors and modulation of neurotransmission: Pharmacological implications and therapeutic relevance. Trends Neurosci 3:110, 1980

Lefkowitz RJ, Caron MG, Stiles GL: Mechanisms of membrane-receptor regulation. Biochemical, physiological and clinical insights derived from studies of the adrenergic receptors. N Engl J Med 310:1570, 1984

Motulsky HJ, Insel PA: Adrenergic receptors in man: Direct identification, physiologic regulation and clinical alteration. N Engl J Med 307:18, 1982

Starke K: Pre-synaptic receptors. Annu Rev Pharmacol Toxicol 21:7, 1981

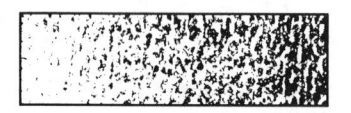

10 CHOLINERGIC DRUGS

Cholinergic drugs are substances capable of evoking biological responses similar to those elicited by the neurotransmitter acetylcholine (ACh). The effects produced by these drugs mimic those evoked by stimulation of cholinergic nerves; thus these drugs are termed *cholinomimetic agents*.

On the basis of their principal mechanisms of action, the cholinergic drugs can be divided into two major groups, the direct acting and the indirect acting.

I. *Direct acting*

These drugs produce their cholinomimetic effects by directly activating cholinergic receptor sites on postjunctional membranes. Drugs in this group can be categorized as one of two types:
   A. Synthetic esters of choline (e.g., bethanechol)
   B. Cholinomimetic alkaloids (e.g., pilocarpine)

II. *Indirect acting*

These compounds exert their effects by elevating the endogenous levels of ACh in the region of the cholinergic receptors. This is accomplished by interfering with the functioning of the cholinesterase enzymes responsible for the inactivation of choline esters such as ACh. These indirect-acting drugs can be categorized further, depending on whether the enzyme inhibition is transient (hours) or prolonged (weeks).

Thus, indirect-acting cholinergic drugs are classified as either:

   A. *Reversible cholinesterase inhibitors* (e.g., physostigmine). Competitive, short-lived receptor blockade; enzymatic function is quickly restored
   B. *Irreversible cholinesterase inhibitors* (e.g., echothiophate). Extremely stable complexation with enzyme; restoration of enzymatic function depends on synthesis of new enzyme, requiring several weeks

Acetylcholine itself is of little clinical usefulness because it is rapidly hydrolyzed by esterase enzymes and therefore has a very short duration of action. Moreover, it is nonspecific, exerting an action at all cholinergic receptor sites in the body and producing a tremendous range of pharmacologic effects (Table 10-1). The therapeutically useful synthetic cholinergic agents are much more resistant to enzymatic hydrolysis and therefore possess a much longer duration of action. In addition, their structural modifications confer a greater degree of selectivity regarding which organ system will be most affected by these synthetic choline esters (Table 10-2).

DIRECT-ACTING CHOLINOMIMETIC DRUGS

Choline Esters

The choline esters are direct-acting cholinergic receptor activators. They are primarily used for their local effects in the eye, although bethanechol can be administered systemically and has selective effects on the GI and urinary tract.

CHOLINE ESTERS FOR TOPICAL ADMINISTRATION

Acetylcholine, intraocular
Miochol

MECHANISM
Contracts smooth muscle of iris sphincter so that pupil constricts and ciliary muscle contracts, accommodating the eye for near vision

USES
During ocular surgery (e.g., cataracts, iridectomy, penetrating keratoplasty) for production of rapid, complete miosis

DOSAGE
0.5 mL to 2 mL of 1% solution administered by instillation into the anterior chamber of the eye, before or after securing one or more sutures

FATE
Rapidly hydrolyzed (duration of action is 10–20 min), so that solution need not be removed from the eye by flushing with saline

COMMON SIDE EFFECTS
Burning, itching, headache

NURSING CONSIDERATIONS
1. Prepare solution immediately before use because aqueous solutions of ACh are extremely unstable. Discard any unused solution.
2. Immerse whole vial (two chambers) in sterilizing solution (e.g., 70% ethanol) 30 minutes prior to use, then mix contents and shake.
3. Instill mixed solution gently, parallel to the face of the iris.
4. In cataract surgery, use only after delivery of the lens.

Carbachol, Intraocular
Miostat
Carbachol, Topical
Isopto Carbachol

MECHANISM
Constricts the pupil and contracts the ciliary muscle of the eye; in glaucoma, facilitates outflow of aqueous humor

USES
Pupillary miosis during surgery (Miostat)
Long-term treatment of open-angle glaucoma especially in cases resistant to pilocarpine (Isopto Carbachol)

DOSAGE
Miostat: 0.5 mL into anterior chamber of the eye before securing sutures
Isopto Carbachol: 2 drops 2 to 4 times/day into lower conjunctival sac

Table 10-1
Pharmacologic Effects of Acetylcholine and Clinical Consequences

Effect	Clinical Consequence
Gastrointestinal Tract	
Peristalsis ↑	Diarrhea
Relaxation of sphincter muscles	
Glandular secretions ↑	
Cardiovascular System	
Heart rate ↓	Hypotension
Vasodilation	
Urinary Tract	
Contraction of detrusor muscle	Urination
Relaxation of trigone and sphincter	
Other Smooth Muscle	
Contraction of bronchiolar smooth muscle	Bronchoconstriction
Contraction of gallbladder and ducts	
Contraction of ureter	
Contraction of sphincter muscle of iris	Miosis
Contraction of ciliary muscle	Accommodation for near vision
Glands	
Stimulation of exocrine gland secretion (lacrimal, sweat, salivary, bronchial)	Sweating Salivation

↓, decreased; ↑, increased.

FATE
Most potent of the direct-acting cholinergic drugs. Onset of miosis is 2 to 5 minutes. Effects persist for up to 8 hours; very slowly hydrolyzed

COMMON SIDE EFFECTS
Headache, hyperemia of conjunctival vessels, ciliary spasm with temporarily decreased vision

SIGNIFICANT ADVERSE REACTIONS
Systemic absorption may cause flushing, sweating, cramping, urinary urgency, and severe headache; usually not present following ophthalmic use in small doses

CONTRAINDICATIONS
Corneal abrasions, acute iritis. *Cautious use* in the presence of asthma, peptic ulcer, GI or urinary distress, hyperthyroidism, cardiac failure, and parkinsonism

INTERACTIONS
Miotic effects may be reversed by atropine or other anticholinergics

NURSING CONSIDERATIONS

Nursing Alert
- Administer carbachol topically *only*, never orally or parenterally.

1. Instill Miostat *gently* into anterior chamber using sterile syringe before or after sutures have been secured.

PATIENT EDUCATION
1. Instruct patient to report any headaches or visual disturbances, as dosage is individually adjusted to minimize them.

CHOLINE ESTERS FOR SYSTEMIC APPLICATION

Bethanechol
Duvoid, Myotonachol, Urabeth, Urecholine

MECHANISM
Activates muscarinic receptors, thereby increasing peristalsis and stimulating micturition and defecation; increases tone of the detrusor muscle; little effect on heart rate, blood pressure, or peripheral circulation

USES
Treatment of acute, nonobstructive urinary retention and neurogenic atony of the urinary bladder
Relief of postoperative abdominal distention and paralytic ileus (essentially obsolete)
Treatment of reflux esophagitis (investigational use only)

DOSAGE
Should be individualized depending on type and severity of condition

Adults: PO—10 mg to 50 mg 2 to 4 times/day; SC—2.5 mg to 5 mg 3 or 4 times/day
Children: 0.6 mg/kg/day in divided doses

Table 10-2
Pharmacologic Properties of Choline Esters

	Muscarinic Receptor Activation			Nicotinic Receptor Activation	Inactivation by Cholinesterase
	GI/Urinary	Cardiovascular	Ocular		
Acetylcholine	Moderate	Moderate	Weak	Moderate	Yes
Bethanechol	Strong	Weak	Moderate	None	No
Carbamylcholine	Strong	Weak	Moderate	Strong	No

FATE
Effects appear within 30 to 90 minutes after oral dose and persist for up to 6 hours; SC administration is effective within 15 minutes

COMMON SIDE EFFECTS
Sweating, flushing, salivation, abdominal discomfort, nausea (usually due to excessive dosage)

SIGNIFICANT ADVERSE REACTIONS
Diarrhea, GI pain and cramping, headache, urinary urgency, hypotension, and asthma-like attacks

CONTRAINDICATIONS
Hyperthyroidism, hypertension, hypotension, peptic ulcer, bronchial asthma, coronary artery disease, AV conduction defects, pronounced bradycardia, urinary obstruction, GI anastomosis, epilepsy, parkinsonism, pregnancy. *Cautious use* following urinary bladder surgery, GI resection, and in the presence of spastic GI disturbances, acute inflammatory lesions of the GI tract, marked vagotonia, and peritonitis

INTERACTIONS
Significant drop in blood pressure can occur if used with ganglionic blocking agents.

Quinidine and procainamide may antagonize the action of bethanechol.

NURSING CONSIDERATIONS

Nursing Alerts
- Administer injectable form SC only, never IM or IV because severe cholinergic overstimulation (hypotension, diarrhea, abdominal cramps, shock, cardiac arrest) can occur.
- Keep a syringe containing 0.6 mg atropine on hand for treatment of symptoms of toxicity. Administer SC as indicated.

1. Administer when stomach is empty. If given after meals, nausea and vomiting can occur.

Cholinomimetic Alkaloids

Cholinomimetic alkaloids produce effects similar to cholinergic nerve stimulation. The only drug of clinical importance in this group is pilocarpine, which is almost exclusively used topically in the eye; significant systemic absorption evokes profuse salivation and sweating.

Pilocarpine

Isopto Carpine, Pilocar, and various other manufacturers
(CAN) Minims, Miocarpine

MECHANISM
Direct cholinergic receptor activation results in contraction of the ciliary muscle and ciliary body; miosis occurs and the outflow of aqueous humor from the anterior chamber is facilitated. Systemic effects include stimulation of sweat, lacrimal and nasopharyngeal secretion, decreased heart rate, vasodilation, bronchoconstriction, and increased GI motility

USES
Open-angle glaucoma

Narrow-angle glaucoma prior to surgery (with other cholinergics or carbonic anhydrase inhibitors)

To reverse effects of cycloplegics and mydriatics following surgery or eye examinations

Treatment of xerostomia in patients with decreased salivary gland function (investigational use: 5 mg orally)

DOSAGE
1 or 2 drops of 1% to 2% solution up to 6 times/day; concentrations greater than 4% are rarely used, although solutions up to 10% are available

Patients with dark pigmented eyes may require higher concentrations because Pilocarpine is absorbed by melanin pigment

To reverse mydriatic/cycloplegic effects of other drugs: 1 drop of a 1% to 2% solution

FATE
Onset of miosis is within 10 to 20 minutes. Duration of miotic effect is 4 to 8 hours, although residual effects can last for 24 hours; excreted in urine as conjugates.

COMMON SIDE EFFECTS
Ciliary spasm, headache, difficulty in focusing, local irritation

SIGNIFICANT ADVERSE REACTIONS
Allergic sensitivity, provocation of acute asthmatic attacks

CONTRAINDICATIONS
Acute iritis and inflammatory conditions of the anterior chamber. *Cautious use* in the presence of asthma

INTERACTIONS
Effects may be reduced by anticholinergics, adrenergics, corticosteroids, and phenothiazines.

NURSING CONSIDERATIONS
1. Avoid touching eyelid with dropper tip because contamination can occur.
2. Protect solutions from light because they are unstable.

PATIENT EDUCATION
1. Instruct patient to report symptoms of sweating, salivation, cramping, and nausea immediately because they may signify onset of systemic toxicity.

Pilocarpine Ocular Therapeutic System
Ocusert Pilo

A continuous release form of pilocarpine (20 µg or 40 µg/h) placed into the lower conjunctival cul-de-sac. Used primarily for continuous therapy of open-angle glaucoma. A system unit is inserted into the conjunctival sac once a week. Release rate of pilocarpine is not affected by presence of other locally acting drugs (e.g., epinephrine, carbonic anhydrase inhibitors). Myopia can occur for several hours following insertion of the system but is usually mild. System can be moved to upper conjunctival sac before sleep to aid in retention during the night.

Use cautiously in presence of infectious conjunctivitis or keratitis. Safety for use in presence of retinal detachments has not been established. Signs of conjunctival irritation, erythema, and increased secretions may occur when first used but tend to lessen after the first week or two. The system is poorly tolerated, however, by many patients, and its usefulness is somewhat limited.

INDIRECT-ACTING CHOLINOMIMETIC DRUGS

Reversible Cholinesterase Inhibitors

Drugs in the group are generally short-acting cholinergic drugs used both topically and systemically. They are capable of increasing the amounts of functional ACh at the postsynaptic receptor site and are primarily indicated for their local effects in the eye and for the diagnosis and treatment of myasthenia gravis. These drugs may be used as antidotes to curariform and atropine-like drugs, to relieve postoperative urinary bladder atony, and to suppress paroxysmal atrial tachycardia.

TOPICAL AND SYSTEMIC USE

Physostigmine, ophthalmic
Eserine, Isopto-Eserine

Physostigmine, systemic
Antilirium

MECHANISM
Competes with ACh for active sites on cholinesterase enzyme, slowing the inactivation of ACh and prolonging its action at cholinergic receptors; highly lipid-soluble and readily penetrates the CNS

USES
Topical (Eye)
  Treatment of open-angle glaucoma (alternative to pilocarpine)
  Reverses cycloplegia and mydriasis caused by anticholinergic drugs
Systemic (Antilirium Only)
  Antidote to toxic neurologic effects caused by drugs (e.g., scopolamine, tricyclic antidepressants) having central anticholinergic activity
  Investigational uses include treatment of respiratory depression due to drug overdosage and treatment of delirium tremens and Alzheimer's disease

DOSAGE
Eserine: 2 drops (0.25%–0.5% solution) 3 or 4 times/day (ophthalmic ointment also available)
Antilirium: Adults—0.5 mg to 2 mg IM or slowly IV; repeat as necessary if life-threatening signs occur. Children—0.5 mg over 1 minute by slow IV injection; repeat in 5 to 10 minutes if needed

FATE
Following topical application, peak miotic effect occurs in 1 to 2 hours, lasting 12 to 24 hours. Systemic doses rapidly metabolized by cholinesterases. IV effects seen in 5 minutes; duration of 1 to 4 hours. Drug readily enters the CNS. Hydrolyzed and inactivated by cholinesterase enzyme

COMMON SIDE EFFECTS
Ophthalmic: decreased visual acuity, eyelid twitching, increased tearing, mild headache
Systemic: sweating, nausea, urinary urgency, cramping, salivation

SIGNIFICANT ADVERSE REACTIONS
Ophthalmic: altered pigmentation of the iris, conjunctival irritation, allergic dermatitis
Systemic: vomiting, diarrhea, muscle weakness, hypotension, bradycardia, bronchospasm, convulsions; respiratory paralysis

CONTRAINDICATIONS
Ophthalmic: inflammation of the iris or ciliary body, narrow-angle glaucoma
Systemic: asthma, gangrene, cardiovascular disease, diabetes, obstruction of intestine or bladder. *Cautious use* in patients with epilepsy, parkinsonism, or bradycardia

INTERACTIONS
Systemic effects may be potentiated by depolarizing neuromuscular blocking agents (e.g., succinylcholine) and choline esters.

NURSING CONSIDERATIONS

Nursing Alerts
- Following systemic administration, observe patient for extreme salivation, vomiting, urination, or defecation, which require discontinuation of the drug. Excessive nausea or sweating requires a dosage reduction.
- Have atropine sulfate injection on hand when giving drug systemically, in case of allergic reaction or accidental overdosage.
- In cases of severe anticholinergic poisoning, be prepared to institute supportive measures (e.g., oxygen or respiratory aids) in addition to use of physostigmine.

1. Apply ointment in a thin ribbon onto lower conjunctival surface. Instruct patient to close eye *gently* and massage area lightly.
2. Administer only clear, colorless ophthalmic solutions of the drug. Avoid exposure to light or excessive heat.

PATIENT EDUCATION
1. Inform patient that vision may be impaired temporarily or localized twitching of the eyelid may occur following instillation of the drops.

TOPICAL USE ONLY

Demecarium Bromide
Humorsol

MECHANISM
Anticholinesterase agent with a duration of action significantly longer than that of other reversible inhibitors; powerful miotic

USES
Treatment of glaucoma
Treatment of convergent strabismus (accommodative esotropia)

DOSAGE

Glaucoma: 1 or 2 drops in conjunctival sac once or twice a day

Strabismus: 1 drop daily; reduce gradually to 1 drop twice a week as condition warrants. Dosage must be titrated and individually adjusted

FATE

Quickly absorbed topically; miosis develops within 30 minutes and is maximal within 2 or 3 hours. Effects are prolonged (up to 1 wk after single administration).

COMMON SIDE EFFECTS

Blurred vision, twitching of eyelid, brow pain, lacrimation

SIGNIFICANT ADVERSE REACTIONS

Photophobia, elevated intraocular pressure, cysts on iris, conjunctival thickening, lens opacities, retinal detachment (rare). Systemic absorption may produce symptoms of cholinergic overdose

CONTRAINDICATIONS

Narrow-angle glaucoma, inflammatory conditions of the eye. *Cautious use* in patients with asthma, ulcers and other GI disorders, bradycardia, hypotension, epilepsy, parkinsonism, and recent coronary occlusion

INTERACTIONS

May potentiate succinylcholine and systemic anticholinesterase drugs used in the treatment of myasthenia gravis.

NURSING CONSIDERATIONS

Nursing Alert
- Observe patient for signs of cholinergic overdosage (e.g., salivation, sweating, diarrhea, or muscle weakness), which require discontinuation of drug.

1. Administer precise dosage and carefully observe patient during initial 24 hours. Frequent tonometer readings are necessary to determine optimal dosage.
2. Compress lacrimal sac immediately after instillation to minimize drainage into nasal chamber and systemic absorption.
3. Question administration prior to ophthalmic surgery, as the drug should be discontinued to reduce danger of bleeding.

PATIENT EDUCATION

1. Advise patient that headache and dimness of vision may persist for up to 1 wk following initiation of therapy.
2. Warn patient of danger of added systemic cholinergic effects if exposed to organophosphorus insecticides or pesticides (e.g., Malathion, Diazinon) when taking this drug.

SYSTEMIC USE ONLY

Ambenonium
Edrophonium
Neostigmine
Pyridostigmine

These four reversible cholinesterase inhibitors are primarily used for the diagnosis and treatment of myasthenia gravis. They all function in a similar manner (i.e., facilitation of cholinergic neurotransmission at the neuromuscular junction), thus alleviating the muscle weakness characteristic of myasthenia. However, significant differences exist among the four drugs with regard to onset and duration of action and incidence and severity of side effects. Table 10-3 lists the onset and duration of each of these drugs when administered by different routes. Since many similarities also exist among these four drugs, they are discussed here as a group. Individual characteristics and dosage ranges are presented in Table 10-4.

MECHANISM

Transiently inhibit cholinesterase enzymes, causing an intensification and prolongation of the actions of ACh at cholinergic receptors throughout the body, including the neuromuscular junction. Neostigmine also exhibits a direct ACh-like stimulating effect at cholinergic receptors on skeletal muscle and may increase the release of presynaptic stores of ACh. These drugs improve muscle strength and delay fatigue; generalized cholinergic responses are frequently noted at the outset of therapy and may require use of a muscarinic antagonist (see Chap. 11) to minimize disturbing side effects; tolerance to the muscarinic effects frequently develops, however

USES

Diagnosis of myasthenia gravis (edrophonium)

Treatment of myasthenia gravis (ambenonium, neostigmine, pyridostigmine)

Symptomatic management of the symptoms of poisoning with

Table 10-3
Comparison of Onset and Duration of Action Among Antimyasthenic Cholinesterase Inhibitors

Drug	Route	Onset	Duration
Ambenonium	PO	30 min	4–8 h
Edrophonium	IM	2–10 min	10–40 min
	IV	<1 min	5–20 min
Neostigmine	PO	30–60 min	2–4 h
	IM	15–30 min	2–4 h
	IV	5–10 min	2–4 h
Pyridostigmine	PO	20–40 min	3–6 h
	IM	10–15 min	2–4 h
	IV	2–5 min	2–4 h

nondepolarizing skeletal muscle relaxants (IV pyridostigmine, neostigmine, or edrophonium)

Relief of postoperative abdominal distention and urinary retention (neostigmine; infrequent use)

DOSAGE
See Table 10-4

FATE
Oral absorption of all drugs is generally poor and erratic. Edrophonium is given by injection only and has a rapid onset and short duration of action. Ambenonium exhibits the longest duration of action with oral administration (see Table 10-3), followed by pyridostigmine and neostigmine; penetration of all drugs into the CNS is minimal; metabolism is by way of hepatic enzymes, and metabolites are eliminated by the kidneys

COMMON SIDE EFFECTS
Nausea, diarrhea, abdominal discomfort, salivation, sweating, urinary urgency, muscle twitching

SIGNIFICANT ADVERSE REACTIONS
CNS: dysphonia, irritability, restlessness, convulsions
Respiratory: increased bronchial secretions, laryngospasm, bronchoconstriction, respiratory paralysis
Ocular: miosis, cycloplegia, diplopia, lacrimation
Cardiovascular: bradycardia, arrhythmias, hypotension
GI: increased salivary, gastric, and intestinal secretions, dysphagia, cramping
Other: muscle weakness, urinary frequency or incontinence, skin rash (neostigmine, pyridostigmine); thrombophlebitis with IV use

Overdosage may lead to a cholinergic crisis characterized by nausea, diarrhea, sweating, increased bronchial and salivary secretions, bradycardia, and increasing muscle weakness. Death can occur due to bronchial airway obstruction and respiratory paralysis.

CONTRAINDICATIONS
Intestinal or urinary obstruction, megacolon, peritonitis. In addition, neostigmine and pyridostigmine are bromide salts and are contraindicated in patients with bromide hypersensitivity. *Cautious use* in patients with bradycardia or bronchial asthma

INTERACTIONS
The actions of the antimyasthenic cholinesterase inhibitors can be antagonized by drugs having a neuromuscular blocking action, such as aminoglycoside antibiotics, general and local anesthetics, and certain antiarrhythmic agents (quinidine, procainamide).

Neostigmine may prolong the action of depolarizing muscle relaxants such as succinylcholine (see Chap. 15).

Neostigmine can antagonize the effects of nondepolarizing neuromuscular blocking agents, such as gallamine, pancuronium, and metocurine.

Magnesium can antagonize the effects of anticholinesterase drugs on skeletal muscle because it exerts a direct muscle-relaxing effect.

NURSING CONSIDERATIONS

Nursing Alerts
- Monitor patient very carefully for signs of cholinergic intoxication (see Significant Adverse Reactions). Warning of overdosage is minimal, and there is a narrow margin between first appearance of side effects and serious toxic manifestations. Report signs of overdosage, as this requires discontinuation of all cholinergic medications and administration of atropine (0.5 mg–1 mg IV).
- Because dosage regulation is difficult, especially with oral administration, observe patient closely for any untoward reaction indicating overdosage. Monitor blood pressure, respiration, and pulse during periods of adjustment.
- Be prepared to assist patient when symptoms prevent self-help (e.g., extreme muscle weakness or difficulty breathing). If extreme muscle weakness develops, an IV test dose of edrophonium may be administered. This helps to determine whether weakness is caused by drug overdosage or patient's condition, as symptoms of excessive cholinergic stimulation (cholinergic crisis) closely resemble those of myasthenic crisis.
- Ensure that emergency measures are readily available (e.g., atropine, oxygen with respirator, suction apparatus) in case a respiratory crisis develops.

1. Monitor patient for signs of CNS toxicity (jitteriness, confusion, dizziness) and inform physician.
2. When drug is used as a curare antidote, be prepared to assist respiration and have atropine available.

PATIENT EDUCATION
1. Instruct patient to take drug before meals if dysphagia occurs when eating.
2. Assist patient to plan a dosing schedule that corresponds with normal periods of stress and fatigue, for example, to take largest portion of total dose before time of expected greatest muscle demands (e.g., eating, shopping).
3. Teach client how to record daily condition carefully, noting changes in muscle strength, respiration, and blood pressure, to assist in developing an optimal therapeutic regimen.

Irreversible Cholinesterase Inhibitors

The irreversible cholinesterase inhibitors are organo-phosphorus compounds that cause phosphorylation of the enzyme cholinesterase, permanently inactivating it. Enzymatic activity remains impaired until new supplies of enzyme can be synthesized, often requiring weeks or even months for full restoration. These compounds were originally developed as chemical warfare agents and are now extensively used as pesticides and insecticides. The major clinical application of the irreversible cholinesterase inhibitors is in the eye, for the production of prolonged miosis and treatment of glaucoma.

Echothiophate
Phospholine Iodide

USES
Treatment of glaucoma (chronic open-angle *and* angle-closure following iridectomy)

Diagnosis and treatment of accommodative convergent strabismus (often with epinephrine or carbonic anhydrase inhibitors)

Table 10-4
Antimyasthenic Cholinesterase Inhibitors

Drug	Preparations	Usual Dosage Range
Ambenonium Chloride Mytelase	Tablets: 10 mg	Adults: 5 mg–25 mg 3 or 4 times/day (up to 75 mg/dose has been used in certain instances but is highly dangerous) Children: 0.5 mg–1.5 mg/kg day in 3 or 4 divided doses
Edrophonium Chloride Tensilon	Injection: 10 mg/mL	*Diagnosis:* Adults: 2 mg IV over 15–30 sec. If no reaction in 45 sec, inject additional 8 mg; alternately, give 10 mg IM if veins are inaccessible. Children: IV—1 mg if weight is less than 75 lb; 2 mg if more than 75 lb; administer within 45 sec, titrate up to 5 mg in small children and up to 10 mg in larger children. IM—2 mg if weight is less than 75 lb; 5 mg if more than 75 lb *Curariform Antagonists* 10 mg IV over 30–45 sec; repeat as necessary to a maximum of 40 mg.
Neostigmine Bromide Prostigmin	Tablets: 15 mg	*Oral:* Adults: 15 mg–30 mg 3 or 4 times/day. Increase gradually until maximum benefit, up to 375 mg/day. Dosage interval must be individualized. Children: 2 mg/kg/day every 3–4 h
Neostigmine Methylsulfate Prostigmin	Injection: 1:1000, 1:2000, 1:4000	*Treatment of Myasthenia SC, IM* Adults: 0.5 mg; repeat as necessary based on response. Children: 10 µg/kg–40 µg/kg every 2–3 h *Diagnosis of Myasthenia:* Adults: 0.022 mg/kg IM Children: 0.04 mg/kg IM *Curariform antidote:* Adults: 0.5 mg–2 mg by slow IV injection. Repeat to a total dose of 5 mg. Children: 0.07 mg–0.08 mg/kg/dose
Pyridostigmine Bromide Mestinon, Regonol	Tablets: 60 mg Sustained-release tablets: 180 mg Syrup: 60 mg/5 mL Injection: 5 mg/mL	*Oral:* Adults: 60 mg–120 mg every 3–4 h initially. Maintenance dose can range from 60 mg–1.5 g/day. Average is 600 mg daily. Children: 7 mg/kg/day in 5 or 6 divided doses *IM, IV:* *Curare antidote:* 10 mg–20 mg *Myasthenia:* 2 mg every 2–3 h

DOSAGE

Glaucoma: 1 drop (0.03%–0.125%) 1 or 2 times/day, individualized to condition

Strabismus: 1 drop 0.06%/day or 0.125% every other day (maximum 0.125%/day)

FATE

Fairly rapid onset of miosis (10 min); effects may persist for several weeks. Intraocular pressure is lowered within 6 hours

COMMON SIDE EFFECTS

Stinging and burning in the eye, temporary blurred vision, lid twitching, hyperemia, browache

SIGNIFICANT ADVERSE REACTIONS

Iris cysts, conjunctival thickening, lens opacities, iritis, retinal detachment (rare); systemic absorption may produce symptoms of cholinergic crisis

Nursing Implications

Longest acting of the orally effective antimyasthenic drugs; lower incidence of GI, respiratory, and CV side effects than neostigmine; cumulative effects have occurred owing to prolonged action; thus, be alert for early signs of overdosage (e.g., salivation, difficulty in chewing or swallowing, muscle weakness); warning of overdosage may be minimal; teach patient and family to contact physician at first sign of side effects; to maximize advantage of drug's prolonged duration of action, instruct patients to take last dose of drug at bedtime so they can sleep through the night without recurrence of symptoms.

Short-acting drug primarily used for differential diagnosis of myasthenia and for reversing neuromuscular block produced by curariform drugs (e.g., tubocurarine, gallamine); not indicated for *chronic* therapy of myasthenia; positive response to diagnostic test is a brief improvement in muscle strength without muscle fasciculations; nonmyasthenic patients evidence transient fasciculations and temporary muscle weakness; patients in cholinergic crisis show further muscle weakness and marked increase in oropharyngeal secretions; atropine sulfate and facilities for respiratory assistance should be immediately available; transient bradycardia can occur, and cardiac arrest has been reported; check pulse frequently during therapy.

Reversible cholinesterase inhibitor that also has a direct agonistic action on cholinergic receptor sites; parenteral form can be used to diagnose myasthenia, but edrophonium is preferred due to more rapid onset and shorter duration; also indicated for symptomatic treatment of curariform drug overdosage; poorly absorbed orally; higher incidence of muscarinic side effects than other orally effective antimyasthenics; monitor changes in muscle strength and side effects in relation to each dose and document accordingly; keep atropine on hand at all times and be prepared to support respiration.

Most commonly used antimyasthenic drug; shorter acting than ambenonium and has slower onset but longer duration of action than neostigmine; lower incidence of GI side effects, salivation, and bradycardia than neostigmine and ambenonium; long-acting tablets are used every 6 h for maintenance therapy but increase the risk of cholinergic crisis; when using sustained-release tablets, instruct patient to take drug at least every 6 h, at same time every day; first signs of overdose may be twitching of muscles around the eyes, mouth, or upper arms; these symptoms should be reported as soon as they occur.

CONTRAINDICATIONS
Narrow-angle glaucoma prior to surgery, inflammatory conditions of the eye. *Cautious use* in patients with asthma, ulcers, hypotension, epilepsy, parkinsonism, cardiovascular disease, and vagotonia

INTERACTIONS
May enhance systemic effects of succinylcholine and other cholinesterase inhibitors.
Effects in eye are readily reversed by atropine.

NURSING CONSIDERATIONS

Nursing Alert
- Evaluate patient for and report early signs of cholinergic overdosage (e.g., salivation, diarrhea, sweating, muscle weakness), as drug should be discontinued if these appear.

1. Facilitate collaboration between patient and drug prescriber to ensure that the lowest concentration that will con-

trol the condition is used and that dosing does not exceed twice a day. Compliance may improve if the total daily dose is instilled at bedtime to minimize the inconvenience of miosis and blurred vision during the day.

PATIENT EDUCATION
1. Inform patient that tolerance may occur with prolonged use. Suggest that patient discuss with drug prescriber the use of drug-free periods or alternate miotics, when possible, to eliminate rapid development of tolerance.
2. Emphasize importance of strict adherence to recommended dosage. The drug's long action increases danger of cumulative systemic toxicity.

Isoflurophate
Floropryl

Isoflurophate is similar to echothiophate in actions, indications, and toxicity. However, because it is insoluble in water, it is available only as an ophthalmic ointment (0.25%), which many patients find inconvenient to use. Following application to the lower conjunctival sac, miosis occurs within 15 to 30 minutes and becomes maximal within 4 hours. Effects may persist for several weeks because of the permanent inactivation of existing cholinesterase. Isoflurophate is unstable in water. Potency is lost if the ointment comes into contact with moisture; thus the tip of the tube should not be allowed to come into contact with any moist surface. The drug is readily absorbed from the skin, and systemic effects have occurred following topical contact. Refer to the foregoing discussion of echothiophate for applicable adverse effects, cautions, and drug interactions.

DOSAGE
Glaucoma: ¼-inch strip of 0.025% ointment every 8 to 12 hours. Frequency of application is then adjusted on the basis of tonometric readings of intraocular pressure. For maintenance therapy, the drug may be applied once every 8 to 72 hours

Accommodative esotropia: not more than a ¼-inch strip of ointment every night for 2 weeks. Dosage is then reduced gradually to once-a-week application as the patient's condition warrants. Therapy may need to be continued indefinitely

Miscellaneous

Guanidine
Guanidine

Guanidine is a unique cholinergic agent that prolongs the action potential in nerve terminals. It alleviates the muscle weakness seen in myasthenia; however, because of its relatively high toxicity its use is generally restricted to the myasthenic syndrome of Eaton–Lambert (carcinomatous myopathy), in which muscle weakness accompanies a malignant disease, particularly bronchogenic carcinoma.

MECHANISM
Enhances the release of acetylcholine following a nerve impulse; may also slow the rates of depolarization and repolarization of muscle cell membranes

USES
Alleviation of the symptoms (muscle weakness, fatigability) of the myasthenic syndrome of Eaton–Lambert

Treatment of severe myasthenia gravis (investigational use only)

DOSAGE
Initially, 10 mg to 15 mg/kg/day in 3 or 4 divided doses. Increase dosage gradually up to a maximum of 35 mg/kg/day

COMMON SIDE EFFECTS
Gastric irritation, nausea, anorexia, flushing, sweating

SIGNIFICANT ADVERSE REACTIONS
GI: diarrhea, abdominal cramping, vomiting
Neurologic: paresthesias, lightheadedness, irritability, nervousness, trembling, ataxia, tremor, confusion, mood changes, hallucinations
Dermatologic: rash, petechiae, purpura, ecchymoses, skin eruptions, scaling of skin
Hematologic: bone marrow depression, anemia, leukopenia, thrombocytopenia
Renal: elevation of creatinine, renal tubular necrosis, interstitial nephritis
Cardiovascular: palpitations, tachycardia, hypotension, atrial fibrillation
Other: sore throat, fever

NURSING CONSIDERATIONS

Nursing Alerts
- Obtain baseline complete blood cell (CBC) and differential counts and perform routine follow-up counts. At first indication of bone marrow suppression, withhold drug and notify prescriber, as drug should be discontinued.
- Monitor renal status, as abnormalities have occurred. Discuss changes with prescriber if indications of malfunction appear.
- Check results of serum creatinine tests, which should be repeated periodically; drug-induced elevations have been noted. Discuss changes with prescriber.
- Ensure that IV atropine (for GI symptoms) and IV calcium gluconate (for neuromuscular and convulsive symptoms) are available to treat cases of overdosage.

1. Be prepared for frequent dosage changes as dose must be carefully titrated in each patient to allow for the possibility of extreme variation in individual tolerance.

PATIENT EDUCATION
1. Instruct patient to notify drug prescriber immediately if sore throat, skin rash, fever, or mucosal ulceration occurs (possible early signs of a developing blood dyscrasia).
2. Instruct patient to report appearance of GI disorders (e.g., anorexia, diarrhea) to drug prescriber, as this often indicates that the dosage is too high and might need to be reduced.
3. Inform patient that the paresthesias that may occur shortly after a dose of guanidine do not indicate that the dosage is excessive.

CHOLINESTERASE INHIBITOR ANTIDOTE

A specific antidote, pralidoxime chloride (PAM), is available primarily for treating overdosage with organophosphorus cholinesterase inhibitors, which usually occurs as a result of insecticide poisoning. It is also capable of antagonizing the effects of the reversible cholinesterase inhibitors (e.g., neostigmine) used in the treatment of myasthenia gravis, although its effectiveness is much less with these compounds. Treatment with PAM should be initiated promptly following poisoning because the enzyme-inhibitor complex that has formed undergoes a fairly rapid process of aging. Thus, within hours, the complex becomes extremely stable and largely resistant to the action of the reactivator PAM.

Pralidoxime Chloride
Protopam, PAM

MECHANISM

Disrupts the bond between the phosphorus group of the enzyme inhibitor and the esteratic site of the cholinesterase enzyme, thus displacing the molecules of the cholinesterase inhibitor from the enzymatic binding sites. Enzyme reactivation diminishes the respiratory paralysis resulting from organophosphate intoxication

USES

Poisoning with pesticides and insecticides of the organophosphate class, e.g., diazinon, malathion.

Antidote to overdosage by anticholinesterase drugs used in treatment of myasthenia gravis

DOSAGE

Insecticide poisoning: Adults—1 g to 2 g as IV infusion in 100 mL saline over 15 to 30 minutes, often with atropine (2 mg–4 mg IV); PO: 1 g to 3 g every 5 hours

Children: 20 mg to 40 mg/kg IV infusion with 0.5 mg to 1 mg atropine. (Most effective if given within a few hours after exposure to poison; usually ineffective if 48 h have elapsed)

Anticholinesterase overdosage: Initially, 1 g to 2 g IV injection; increments of 250 mg every 5 minutes until symptoms subside

FATE

Slowly and erratically absorbed orally; peak plasma levels occur at 5 to 10 minutes IV and 10 to 20 minutes IM; not bound to plasma protein; relatively short-acting (plasma half-life is 2 h) metabolized in the liver and readily excreted in urine, partly as unchanged drug

COMMON SIDE EFFECTS

Dizziness, blurred vision, headache, drowsiness, nausea

SIGNIFICANT ADVERSE REACTIONS

Tachycardia, hyperventilation, laryngospasm, muscle weakness. Excitement and hypomania may occur following recovery of consciousness

CONTRAINDICATIONS

Cautious use in patients with myasthenia gravis

INTERACTIONS

Certain drugs should not be used concurrently with PAM in organophosphate poisoning (morphine, theophylline, succinylcholine, reserpine, and phenothiazines) because enzyme reactivator exerts a depolarizing effect at the neuromuscular junction.

Barbiturates may be potentiated by cholinesterase inhibitors.

NURSING CONSIDERATIONS

Nursing Alerts
- Use infusion control device, if available, to maintain desired flow rate because tachycardia, muscle rigidity, and laryngospasm may occur if infusion is too rapid.
- When drug is used with atropine, monitor patient for indications of atropine toxicity (xerostomia, blurred vision, flushing, excitement) and ensure that atropine administration is terminated at that point.
- Observe patient closely for 72 hours following poisoning. Monitor results of red blood cell and plasma cholinesterase determinations to determine patient's progress.

1. Thoroughly wash skin with alcohol if that is the route of contamination, or prepare patient for gastric lavage following oral ingestion of the poison.
2. Determine what insecticide is involved in the poisoning. Pralidoxime is ineffective in cases of carbamate (Sevin) pesticide poisoning and should not be used for poisoning due to organophosphates lacking anticholinesterase activity.

Selected Bibliography

Blusztajn JK, Wurtman RJ: Choline and cholinergic neurons. Science 221:614, 1983

Drachman DB: Myasthenia gravis. N Engl J Med 298:136; 186, 1978

Drachman DB: The biology of myasthenia gravis. Annu Rev Neurosci 4:227, 1981

Gershon MD: The enteric nervous system. Annu Rev Neurosci 4:227, 1981

Hrovath M: Myasthenia gravis: A nursing approach. J Neurosurg February: 7, 1982

Jeglum E: Ocular therapeutics. Nurs Clin North Am September: 453, 1982

Kaufman PL, Weidman T, Robinson JR: Cholinergics. In Sears ML (ed): Pharmacology of the Eye. Handbook of Experimental Pharmacology, Vol 69, p 149. Berlin, Springer-Verlag, 1984

Lindstrom J, Dau P: The biology of myasthenia gravis. Annu Rev Pharmacol 20:337, 1980

Nilsson E: Physostigmine treatment in various drug-induced intoxications. Ann Clin Res 14:165, 1982

Quail C, Waddleton C: Treating the glaucomas. Nurses' Drug Alert 4:93, 1980

Remis LL, Epstein DL: Treatment of glaucoma. Annu Rev Med 35:195, 1984

Samples JR: Pharmacolgic management of glaucoma. Ration Drug Ther 21(12):1, 1987

Todd B: Using eye drops and ointments safely. Geriatr Nurs Jan/Feb:53, 1983

Watanabe AM: Cholinergic agonists and antagonists. In Rosen MR, Hoffman BF (eds): Cardiac Therapy, p 95. Hingham, MA, Nijhoff, 1983

Webster GD: Advances in treating lower urinary tract dysfunction. Drug Ther 12:113, 1982

SUMMARY. CHOLINERGIC DRUGS

Drug	Preparations	Usual Dosage Range
Direct Acting		
Acetylcholine Miochol	2-mL dual chamber vial containing 20 mg ACh, 60 mg mannitol, and sterile water—yields 1% solution when reconstituted	0.5 mL to 2 mL of 1% solution
Carbachol Carbacel, Isopto Carbachol, Miostat	Miostat: 1.5 mL vials of 0.01% solution Others (Ophthalmic drops): 0.75%, 1.5%, 2.25% and 3.0%	Miostat: 0.5 mL in a single dose Others: 1 or 2 drops 2 to 4 times/day
Bethanechol Duvoid, Myotonachol, Urecholine, Vesicholine	Tablets: 5 mg, 10 mg, 25 mg, 50 mg Injection: 5 mg/mL	PO: 10 mg to 50 mg 2 to 4 times/day SC: 2.5 mg to 5 mg 3 or 4 times/day
Pilocarpine Various manufacturers	Ophthalmic drops: 0.25%, 0.5%, 1%, 2%, 3%, 4%, 5%, 6%, 8%, and 10% Ocular Gel—4%	1 or 2 drops of 1% to 4% solution 3 or 4 times/day
Pilocarpine Ocular Therapeutic System Ocusert	Packets of 8 sterile systems releasing pilocarpine 20 μg or 40 μg/hr	One system placed into conjunctival sac per wk, according to package directions
Indirect Acting		
Physostigmine Antilirium, Eserine, Isopto Eserine	Antilirium: Injection 1.0 mg/mL Others Ophthalmic drops: 0.25%, 0.5% Ophthalmic ointment: 0.25%	*Antilirium:* IM, IV—0.5 mg to 2 mg by slow injection; repeat 1 mg to 4 mg as needed. (Children—0.5 mg by slow IV injection) *Others* Drops: 2 drops 3 times/day Ointment: small ribbon in lower eyelid
Demecarium Humorsol	Ophthalmic drops: 0.125% and 0.25%	1 or 2 drops once or twice a day to twice a wk, depending on condition
Neostigmine Prostigmin and various manufacturers **Ambenonium** Mytelase **Edrophonium** Tensilon **Pyridostigmine** Mestinon, Regonol	*See* Table 10-4	
Echothiophate Iodide Phospholine Iodide	Powder: 1.5 mg, 3 mg, 6.25 mg, and 12.5 mg with 5 mL diluent for ophthalmic use	0.03% to 0.06% (1 or 2 drops) 1 or 2 times/day
Isofluorophate Floropryl	Ophthalmic ointment: 0.025%	*Glaucoma:* 1/4" strip of ointment into eye every 8 to 72 h *Accommodative esotropia:* 1/4" strip of ointment in both eyes every night for 2 wk; gradually reduce frequency of application.
Guanidine Guanidine	Tablets: 125 mg	Initially, 10 mg/kg/day to 15 mg/kg/day in 3 or 4 divided doses; may increase gradually up to 35 mg/kg/day
Antagonist		
Pralidoxime Protopam	Tablets: 500 mg Injection: 1g/20 mL or 1 g powder with one 20-mL vial of diluent	*Insecticide poisoning* Adults: 1 g to 2 g IV in 100 mL saline over 15 to 30 min Children: 20 mg to 40 mg/kg IV *Anticholinesterase overdosage:* 1 g to 2 g IV initially; repeat with 250 mg every 5 min

11 ANTICHOLINERGIC DRUGS

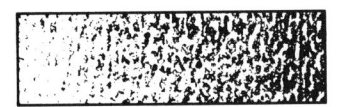

Anticholinergic drugs exert a competitive blocking action at cholinergic receptor sites throughout the body. This diverse group of drugs may be arbitrarily divided into three subgroups based on their *relative* specificity for the different types of cholinergic receptor sites (see Chap. 9) as follows:

I. *Muscarinic blockers* (e.g., atropine, propantheline). These compose the "classic" group of anticholinergic drugs that inhibit cholinergic transmission at postganglionic parasympathetic M (muscarinic) receptor sites, such as those found on smooth muscle, cardiac muscle, and exocrine glands.

II. *Ganglionic blockers* (e.g., mecamylamine, trimethaphan). These drugs inhibit cholinergic transmission at autonomic ganglia N (nicotinic) sites in both parasympathetic and sympathetic nerve fibers.

III. *Neuromuscular blockers* (e.g., tubocurare, pancuronium). These drugs inhibit cholinergic transmission at skeletal neuromuscular junction N (nicotinic) receptor sites.

The term *anticholinergic* has come to be associated primarily with the muscarinic blockers because most of the commonly used anticholinergic drugs exert a relatively selective blocking action at M sites when used at normal dosage levels. Considerable overlap in receptor blocking effects is observed, however, when large doses of any one of the three types of cholinergic blockers are administered. This extension of cholinergic blockade to all cholinergic receptors is frequently responsible for a disturbing range of side effects when any of the cholinergic blocking agents is used in large amounts.

Because the distribution of parasympathetic cholinergic nerves is vast, anticholinergic drugs exert a wide range of pharmacologic effects. Major organs affected by these drugs include the eye, respiratory tract, heart, GI tract, urinary bladder, most nonvascular smooth muscle, exocrine glands, and, to varying degrees, the CNS. The principal pharmacologic actions of the anticholinergic group of drugs are listed in Table 11-1.

Atropine and scopolamine represent the principal naturally occurring anticholinergic drugs; along with hyoscyamine, they are known as the *belladonna alkaloids* (Table 11-2). These compounds are rapidly absorbed orally, exert a relatively selective blocking action at muscarinic receptor sites, and readily enter the CNS, where atropine is primarily a stimulant and scopolamine functions as a depressant. The major disadvantage of the belladonna alkaloids is the wide range of undesirable peripheral and central effects that occur when the drugs are given in dosages sufficient to reduce GI motility and secretions.

For this reason, several tertiary and quaternary ammonium compounds have been synthesized in an attempt to reduce the incidence of side effects while providing a degree of cholinergic receptor site specificity. These goals, however, have only been partially realized.

The synthetic *tertiary amines* may be further subdivided into antispasmodics, mydriatics, and antiparkinsonian drugs (see Table 11-2). The antispasmodics possess little cholinergic blocking action; rather, their effects appear to be related to a direct relaxant effect on GI smooth muscle. Thus, gastric acid secretion is relatively unimpaired, and these drugs are more properly termed *smooth muscle relaxants* rather than anticholinergics. In contrast, the antiparkinsonian tertiary amines exert their anticholinergic action primarily in the CNS.

The *quaternary amine* anticholinergics (see Table 11-2), unlike the belladonna alkaloids and tertiary amines, are poorly and erratically absorbed orally and have a low lipid:water partition coefficient (i.e., are less lipid soluble). Therefore, they do not readily cross lipid membranes, and their distribution to the GI mucosa, eye, and CNS is limited. They are of little value as mydriatics in the eye, and their central effects are minimal. Quaternization of the compounds increases their ganglionic blocking and neuromuscular blocking effects, however, and large doses may affect ganglionic and neuromuscular transmission.

However, in light of the overall similarity of uses, side effects, and clinical implications among the many antimuscarinic drugs, the pharmacology of this group is discussed as a whole. Dosage forms, indications, and specific characteristics for each drug are then listed in Table 11-3. Two anticholinergic agents exhibiting a primary action at autonomic ganglia and therefore more properly termed ganglionic blocking agents are reviewed separately at the end of this chapter. Finally, the several anticholinergic drugs acting at the N receptors on skeletal muscle (i.e., at the neuromuscular junction) are discussed along with other skeletal muscle relaxants in Chapter 15.

ANTIMUSCARINICS

Anisotropine	Isopropamide
Atropine	Mepenzolate
Belladonna	Methantheline
Benztropine	Methscopolamine
Biperiden	Orphenadrine
Clidinium	Oxybutynin
Cyclopentolate	Oxyphencyclimine
Dicyclomine	Oxyphenonium
Ethopropazine	Procyclidine
Glycopyrrolate	Propantheline
Hexocyclium	Scopolamine
Homatropine	Trihexyphenidyl
Hyoscyamine	Tropicamide
Ipratropium	

MECHANISM
Competitive antagonism of acetylcholine (or other direct-acting cholinergic drugs) at postsynaptic muscarinic cholinergic receptor sites. Large doses may block cholinergic transmission at autonomic ganglia and the neuromuscular junction. Certain drugs (e.g., antiparkinsonian agents) may also decrease uptake of dopamine into presynaptic nerve endings (see Chap. 26)

USES
Refer to tabular listing of individual drugs for specific uses of each agent

Table 11-1
Pharmacologic Actions of Anticholinergics

Effects	Clinical Consequences
Cardiovascular	
Heart rate ↓ in small doses (central vagal stimulation)	
Heart rate ↑ in large doses (peripheral vagal blockade)	Prevention of reflex bradycardia
Gastrointestinal Tract	
Motility ↓	Delayed gastric emptying, constipation
Smooth muscle tone ↓	
Secretions ↓	
Urinary Tract	
Relaxation of detrusor muscle	Urinary retention
Contraction of sphincter muscle	
Eye	
Mydriasis (sphincter mucle response ↓)	Blurred vision
Cycloplegia (ciliary muscle response ↓)	
Smooth Muscle	
Slight relaxation of nonvascular smooth muscle (e.g., biliary, bronchiolar, intestinal, uterine)	Relief of biliary or intestinal colic
Exocrine Glands	
Sweat gland secretion ↓	Anhidrosis, xerostomia, hyperthermia
Salivation ↓	
Mucous gland secretion ↓ (nasopharynx and bronchioles)	
Central Nervous System	
Drowsiness, disorientation, hallucinations (large doses)	Treatment of Parkinson's disease
Tremor and rigidity of parkinsonism ↓	Prevention of motion sickness
Vestibular activation ↓	

↓, decreased; ↑, increased.

Production of mydriasis and cycloplegia as an aid to ophthalmic examinations

Preoperative medication to reduce excess salivation and prevent bradycardia (scopolamine additionally produces a tranquilizing effect)

Reduction of GI motility and secretions in cases of peptic ulcer, GI spasms, irritable bowel syndrome, or other GI disorders

Minimization of muscarinic side effects associated with cholinesterase inhibitor treatment of myasthenia

Relief of nasopharyngeal and bronchial secretions accompanying upper respiratory and allergic disorders

Relief of bronchoconstriction due to excessive para-sympathetic nerve activity in bronchial asthma, and other chronic obstructive pulmonary diseases

Prevention and relief of motion sickness

Treatment of enuresis in children and relief of urinary urgency or frequency

Treatment of sinus bradycardia and conduction block due to excessive vagal tone

Production of sedation and amnesia ("twilight sleep") in obstetrics—infrequent use

Antidote to overdosage with cholinergic agents (anticholinesterases, organophosphate insecticides and pesticides)

Relief of symptoms of parkinsonism (especially tremor and rigidity), and control of extrapyramidal disorders resulting from antipsychosis treatment (see Chap. 26)

DOSAGE
See Table 11-3

FATE
Natural alkaloids and most tertiary amines are well absorbed in the GI tract and in the eye. Scopolamine is also absorbed significantly through the postauricular skin when applied in the form of a transdermal patch (see Table 11-3). Quaternary amines are poorly and erratically absorbed orally. The extent of distribution largely depends on lipid solubility; the more lipid-soluble alkaloids and tertiary amines are widely distributed peripherally and centrally, whereas quaternary amines have a more limited peripheral distribution. The duration of action of quaternary amines is somewhat longer than that of tertiary amines

COMMON SIDE EFFECTS
Dry mouth, blurred vision, urinary hesitancy, constipation, palpitations, flushing

Table 11-2
Classification of Antimuscarinic Drugs

Belladona Alkaloids
atropine
hyoscyamine
scopolamine

Tertiary Amine Antispasmodics
dicyclomine
oxybutynin
oxyphencyclimine

Tertiary Amine Mydriatics
cyclopentolate
tropicamide

Tertiary Amine Antiparkinsonian Agents
benztropine
biperiden
ethopropazine
orphenadrine hydrochloride
procyclidine
trihexyphenidyl

Quaternary Amine Anticholinergics
anisotropine
clidinium
glycopyrrolate
hexocyclium
homatropine
ipratropium
isopropamide
mepenzolate
methantheline
methscopolamine
oxyphenonium
propantheline
tridihexethyl

SIGNIFICANT ADVERSE REACTIONS
(Any significant adverse reactions generally result from excessive dosage or individual hypersensitivity.)

GI: vomiting, dysphagia, bloating, paralytic ileus, and possibly gastroesophageal reflux
Cardiovascular: tachycardia, hypertension
CNS: headache, nervousness, drowsiness, confusion, restlessness, insomnia, delirium, hallucinations, elevated body temperature
Ocular: photophobia, cycloplegia, increased intraocular tension
Dermatologic: rash, urticaria, systemic allergic reactions
Other: urinary retention, dysuria, impotence, suppression of lactation, respiratory difficulties, muscular incoordination

CONTRAINDICATIONS
Narrow-angle glaucoma, severe coronary artery disease, urinary or GI obstruction, intestinal atony, paralytic ileus, myasthenia gravis, ulcerative colitis, hiatal hernia, serious hepatic or renal disease. *Cautious use* in patients with glaucoma, asthma, duodenal ulcer, coronary artery disease, arrhythmias, hyperthyroidism, chronic lung disease, and prostatic hypertrophy

INTERACTIONS
The following drugs may increase the side effects of antimuscarinics: antihistamines, tricyclic antidepressants, antipsychotics, antianxiety drugs, meperidine, nitrites and nitrates, methylphenidate, quinidine procainamide, disopyramide, primidone, MAO inhibitors, and amantadine.

Guanethidine, histamine, and reserpine can antagonize the inhibitory effects of antimuscarinics on gastric acid secretion.

Antimuscarinics may enhance the actions of bronchodilators (e.g., adrenergics, theophylline), isoniazid, and methotrimeprazine.

Antacids may impair the GI absorption of antimuscarinics.

Antimuscarinics may decrease the effects of cholinergics (e.g., pilocarpine or physostigmine) used locally in the eye. Concurrent use of antimuscarinics with haloperidol or corticosteroids may elevate intraocular pressure.

The effect of levodopa may be decreased by antimuscarinics owing to accelerated gastric breakdown.

The effect of metoclopramide on GI motility is antagonized by antimuscarinics.

IV administration of antimuscarinics can induce ventricular arrhythmias in patients receiving cyclopropane.

NURSING CONSIDERATIONS

Nursing Alerts
- Observe patient, especially if elderly, for onset of excitement, agitation, and delirium, which are indications for reducing the dosage or considering alternative medication. Notify drug prescriber if they occur.
- Monitor pulse and respiration; report any changes immediately. A dosage adjustment or another drug may be required.
- Ensure that antidotal measures (e.g., cholinesterase inhibitors, barbiturates, levarterenol, respiratory aids, oxygen) are readily available in case of overdosage, especially when drug is used parenterally.

1. Expect to prepare unusual dosages. Many are quite small (e.g., atropine 0.4 mg–0.6 mg), and it is easy to administer an overdose.
2. Use measures to prevent constipation, such as increased intake of fluid and dietary fiber.
3. Monitor urinary output and bowel regularity. Discuss significant changes with drug prescriber.

PATIENT EDUCATION
1. Instruct patient to take oral medication 30 minutes before meals.
2. Explain that certain side effects commonly occur with systemic use of these drugs. These include dry mouth, urinary hesitancy, blurred vision, tachycardia, and possibly constipation. Although they may be minimized by reducing the dosage, they must often be tolerated to obtain the beneficial effects of the drug.
3. Warn patient not to drive or operate machinery if blurred vision, dizziness, or drowsiness occurs.
4. Caution patients, especially the elderly, to take special care during physical activity because the drug may impair coordination.
5. Suggest ways to relieve dry mouth, such as chewing sugarless gum or sucking hard candy.
6. Refer patient to appropriate resources for any dietary instruction needed, especially if medication is used for a GI disorder.

7. Inform patient using drug for symptoms of parkinsonism that optimal effects may take several days to develop. Medication changes or dosage adjustments should be made gradually (see Chap. 26).
8. Inform patient that local irritation, edema, and follicular conjunctivitis may occur if drug is used in the eye for long periods.
9. Instruct patient to stop using drug in the eye and notify physician immediately if a rapid pulse, dizziness, dryness of the mouth, or other signs of systemic toxicity develop.

GANGLIONIC BLOCKING AGENTS

Synaptic transmission at the ganglia of the autonomic nervous system is mediated by acetylcholine (ACh) and thus can be impeded by drugs capable of blocking the actions of ACh at postganglionic cholinergic receptor sites. Specific anticholinergic compounds that act primarily at autonomic ganglia are termed *ganglionic blocking agents*. Although many substances are employed experimentally to alter ganglionic function in the laboratory, only two therapeutically useful agents are currently available: mecamylamine and trimethaphan. Their clinical applicability is restricted to inducing hypotensive states for specialized circumstances. Because the agents are nonselective in their blocking action, they reduce neurotransmission in both sympathetic and parasympathetic ganglia. Thus, in addition to interfering with sympathetic impulses that constrict vascular smooth muscle, the agents likewise block impulses to many other body organs, resulting in a wide range of side effects. Typical effects caused by parasympathetic blockade include decreased GI motility and secretions, dryness of the mouth, urinary retention, constipation, paralysis of ocular accommodation, mydriasis, and impotence. It is evident that the scope of possible untoward reactions greatly limits the clinical utility of these drugs.

Compounds impairing transmission at autonomic ganglia can be categorized by their mechanism of action as either *depolarizing* or *antidepolarizing* blocking agents. Depolarizing blockers, of which the alkaloid nicotine is an example, initially stimulate the postganglionic receptors, then block further receptor activation by persistently occupying the site and preventing repolarization of the postsynaptic membrane. Although of no therapeutic value, nicotine is of considerable toxicologic importance because it is systemically absorbed from tobacco smoke and may be accidentally inhaled from nicotine-containing insecticides. The pharmacologic effects of nicotine are quite variable and depend largely upon the amount absorbed, the extent and level of exposure, and the physiological state of the individual—that is, the presence of underlying pathologic conditions such as peripheral vascular disorders, hypertension, coronary artery disease, or congestive heart failure.

The antidepolarizing group of ganglionic blocking agents, to which the clinically useful drugs belong, function as competitive antagonists of ACh at the postganglionic receptor sites. Their predominant effect is to reduce sympathetic vascular tone, producing marked vasodilation and hypotension (primarily orthostatic) and decreasing venous return to the heart and consequently cardiac output. They are *potent* blood-pressure-lowering agents but are infrequently used today because of their extensive side effects.

Mecamylamine
Inversine

MECHANISM

Competitive antagonism of ACh at cholinergic receptors in autonomic ganglia, producing prolonged (6–12 h) lowering of blood pressure predominantly of the postural type, in both normotensive and hypertensive subjects

USES

Management of moderately severe to severe essential hypertension and uncomplicated malignant hypertension when other antihypertensive drugs have failed

DOSAGE

Initially 2.5 mg twice a day orally, increased by 2.5-mg increments every 2 days until optimal effect is obtained (average dosage 25 mg/day in 2 to 4 divided doses)

FATE

Completely absorbed orally; onset in 30 to 90 minutes; duration 6 to 12 hours; widely distributed; enters CNS; excreted slowly through kidneys, largely in unchanged form; excretion is enhanced in an acidic urine

COMMON SIDE EFFECTS

Dryness of the mouth, constipation, anorexia, weakness, fatigue, mydriasis, and blurred vision

SIGNIFICANT ADVERSE REACTIONS

Abdominal distention, ileus, orthostatic hypotension, dizziness, syncope, urinary retention, and impotence; tremor, confusion, convulsions, and mental aberrations are rare occurrences

CONTRAINDICATIONS

Coronary or renal insufficiency, recent myocardial infarction, uremia, chronic pyelonephritis, pyloric stenosis, and glaucoma. *Cautious use* in patients with cerebral insufficiency; bladder neck or urethral obstruction; prostatic hypertrophy; elevated BUN levels

INTERACTIONS

Hypotensive effect of mecamylamine can be enhanced by alcohol, other antihypertensive agents, diuretics, anesthetics, MAO inhibitors, and bethanechol.

Mecamylamine may potentiate sympathomimetic drugs.

Effects of mecamylamine can be prolonged by urinary alkalinizers (e.g., sodium bicarbonate).

NURSING CONSIDERATIONS

Nursing Alerts
- Monitor patient for manifestations of paralytic ileus (e.g., constipation, abdominal distention, decreased bowel sounds), which is an indication for slowly discontinuing drug.
- Question any sudden discontinuation of drug, as this could lead to hypertensive rebound with the possibility of cerebrovascular accident. The drug should be withdrawn gradually while other antihypertensives are substituted.

1. Administer after meals, if possible, as this permits smoother control. Smaller doses are prescribed for mornings, while larger doses are used later in the day because response is usually greater in early morning.
2. Monitor upright blood pressures and symptoms of postural hypotension at times of maximal drug effect, as effective maintenance dose is determined by titrating to a level just below that which induces orthostatic hypotension, and dosage titration is critical to optimal response.

PATIENT EDUCATION
1. Instruct patient to avoid substances that increase urinary pH (e.g., sodium bicarbonate) and to consult a pharmacist or physician when purchasing OTC medications, particularly antacids. Urinary excretion of mecamylamine is markedly affected by pH: increased pH reduces excretion, thereby possibly intensifying toxicity.
2. Inform patient that bulk laxatives are ineffective if constipation becomes a problem.
3. Advise patient to notify physician if difficulty with urination is experienced. Urinary retention can occur and may necessitate a dosage adjustment.

See also **Plans of Nursing Care 1 (Knowledge Deficit)** in Chapter 4, **2 (Noncompliance)** in Chapter 7, and **8 (Antihypertensive Drugs)** in Chapter 31.

Trimethaphan

Arfonad

MECHANISM
Short-lived, competitive antagonism of ACh at ganglionic receptor sites; may also exert a direct relaxant effect on vascular smooth muscle; causes pooling of blood in peripheral and splanchnic vessels; may also release histamine; blood pressure is markedly reduced and peripheral blood flow is improved

USES
Production of controlled hypotension during surgery
Acute control of blood pressure in hypertensive emergencies
Emergency treatment of pulmonary edema resulting from pulmonary hypertension
Management of dissecting aortic aneurysm or ischemic heart disease in cases in which other agents cannot be used (investigational use only)

DOSAGE
Only by IV infusion—500 mg (10 mL) diluted to 500 mL in 5% dextrose; begin IV drip at 3 mL/min to 4 mL/min and adjust to individual needs; may range from 0.3 mL/min to 6 mL/min

FATE
Onset of action is immediate; duration approximately 10 to 20 minutes; excreted by the kidneys largely as intact drug

SIGNIFICANT ADVERSE REACTIONS
(Primarily due to overdose) Excessive hypotension, rapid pulse, cyanosis, angina-like pain, and vascular collapse

CONTRAINDICATIONS
Conditions in which hypotension may subject the patient to undue risks such as hypovolemia, shock, asphyxia, anemia, respiratory insufficiency, impaired renal function, severe arteriosclerosis, or severe cardiac disease. *Cautious use* in patients with arteriosclerosis; cardiac, hepatic, or renal disease; Addison's disease; degenerative CNS disease; diabetes; allergies; and in the elderly, debilitated, or the very young

INTERACTIONS
Hypotensive effects can be potentiated by antihypertensive agents, anesthetics, vasodilators, and diuretics.

NURSING CONSIDERATIONS

Nursing Alerts
- Monitor blood pressure, pulse, and respiratory rate continuously during infusion and frequently thereafter to ensure that response is stable.
- Have on hand adequate amounts of oxygen, replacement fluids, respiratory aids, and vasopressor agents to treat untoward reactions. Phenylephrine and mephentermine are vasopressor drugs of choice.
- Position patient supine to avoid cerebral anoxia. If pressure fails to drop, raise head of bed carefully to observe response.
- Terminate infusion gradually while closely monitoring blood pressure.

1. Prepare infusion fresh, and discard unused portion. *Do not use trimethaphan infusion as a vehicle for other drugs.*
2. Monitor intake and output, and check for bladder distention because urinary retention can occur.
3. Carefully evaluate patient's response to drug, and report any lessening of effect, as tolerance can develop within 48 hours.
4. In surgical procedures, be prepared to terminate infusion prior to closure of incision to allow pressure to return to normal (usually occurs within 10 minutes).

Selected Bibliography

Greenblatt DJ, Shader RI: Anticholinergics. N Engl J Med 288:1215, 1973

Miletick DJ, Ivankovich AD: Cardiovascular effects of ganglionic blocking drugs. Int Anesthesiol Clin 16:151, 1978

Moree NA: New drugs: Hands on experience. Am J Nurs 85:252, 1985

Price NM, Schmitt LG, McGuire J, Shaw JE, Trobough G: Transdermal scopolamine in the prevention of motion sickness at sea. Clin Pharmacol Ther 29:414, 1981

Salem MR: Therapeutic uses of ganglionic blocking drugs. Int Anesthesiol Clin 16:171, 1978

Shader RI, Greenblatt DJ: Belladonna alkaloids and synthetic anticholinergics: Uses and toxicity. In Shader RI (ed): Psychiatric Complications of Medical Drugs, p. 103. New York, Raven Press, 1972

Table 11-3
Antimuscarinics

Drug	Preparations	Usual Dosage Range
Belladonna Alkaloids		
Atropine several manufacturers	Tablets: 0.4 mg Soluble tablets: 0.3 mg, 0.4 mg, 0.6 mg Ophthalmic drops: 0.5%, 1%, 2%, 3% Ophthalmic ointment: 0.5%, 1% Injection: 0.05 mg/mL, 0.1 mg/mL, 0.3 mg/mL, 0.4 mg/mL, 0.5 mg/mL, 1.0 mg/mL, 1.2 mg/mL Solution for inhalation: 0.2%, 0.5%	*Systemic* Adults: 0.4 mg–0.6 mg every 4–6 h Children: 0.1 mg–0.6 mg depending on weight *Ophthalmic* Adults: 1–2 drops 4 times/day Children: 1 drop 0.5%–1% 1–3 times/day *Refraction* 1–2 drops 1 h before examination *Inhalation (oral)* Adults: 0.025 mg/kg diluted with 3 mL–5 mL saline by nebulizer 3–4 times/day Children: 0.05 mg/mL diluted in saline by nebulizer 3–4 times/day
Belladonna Alkaloids, Levorotatory Bellafoline	Tablets: 0.25 mg Injection: 0.5 mg/mL	*Adults* Tablets: 0.25 mg–0.5 mg 3 times/day Injection: 0.25 mg–0.5 mg SC 1–2 times/day *Children* Tablets: 0.125 mg–0.25 mg 3 times/day
Belladonna Extract	Tablets: 15 mg Liquid: 30 mg belladonna alkaloids/100 mL	Tablets: 15 mg 3–4 times/day Liquid: 0.6 mL–1.0 mL 3–4 times/day
Hyoscyamine Sulfate Anaspaz, Cystospaz, Cystospaz-M, Levsin, Levsinex, Neoquess (CAN) Bellaspaz	Tablets: 0.125 mg, 0.13 mg, 0.15 mg Timed-release capsules: 0.375 mg Elixir: 0.125 mg/5 mL Oral drops: 0.125 mg/mL Injection: 0.5 mg/mL	*Oral/Sublingual* Adults: 0.125 mg–0.25 mg 3–4 times/day Children: 2–10 yr: ½ adult dose *Parenteral* SC, IM, or IV: 0.25 mg–0.5 mg 3–4 times/day
Scopolamine Hydrobromide Isopto Hyoscine, and several manufacturers	Capsules: 0.25 mg Injection: 0.3 mg/mL, 0.4 mg/mL, 0.86 mg/mL, 1.0 mg/mL Ophthalmic drops: 0.25%	*Systemic* Adults: (SC, IM) 0.3 mg–0.6 mg Children: (SC, IM) 0.1 mg–0.3 mg *Ophthalmic* 1–2 drops; adjust dosage to requirements *Motion Sickness* 0.25-mg capsule 1 h before travel; repeat in 4 h if necessary (see transdermal scopolamine below)
Scopolamine Transdermal Therapeutic System Transderm-Scop	Adhesive patch containing 1.5 mg scopolamine and delivering 0.5 mg over 3 days at a constant rate	Apply 1 system to the postauricular skin once every 3 days, several hours before exposure
Tertiary Amine Antispasmodics		
Dicyclomine Hydrochloride Bentyl, and several other manufacturers (CAN) Bentylol, Lomine	Tablets: 20 mg Capsules: 10 mg, 20 mg Liquid: 10 mg/5 mL Injection: 10 mg/mL	*Adults* Oral: 80 mg–160 mg daily in 4 divided doses IM: 20 mg every 4–6 h *Children*: 5 mg–10 mg 3–4 times/day orally
Oxybutynin Chloride Ditropan	Tablets: 5 mg Syrup: 5 mg/5 mL	Adults: 5 mg 2–4 times/day Children: 5 mg 2–3 times/day

Major Uses	Nursing Implications
See general discussion of anticholinergics in text.	Atropine flush due to peripheral vasodilation is a normal effect of the drug; when used in the eye, prevent systemic absorption by compressing lacrimal sac following instillation; do not use in children under 6 yr of age; reduce systemic dose in elderly patients to minimize danger of tachycardia and elevated intraocular pressure; orally inhaled atropine produces a bronchodilatory effect with minimal tachycardia and drying of secretions; ophthalmic drops are available with prednisolone (Mydrapred); IV doses of more than 2 mg may initially cause bradycardia, which will subside within minutes; give oral doses no less than 30 min before mealtimes for best response and give the nighttime dose at least 2 h after the last meal.
Preoperative medication, GI hypermotility, dysmenorrhea, respiratory hypersecretion and bronchial asthma, motion sickness, enuresis, nocturia	Infrequently used preparation; belladonna tincture is also available for GI disturbances (spasms, hypermotility); 0.6 mL–1.0 mL 3–4 times/day.
GI hypermotility, dysmenorrhea, parkinsonism, enuresis, motion sickness	Crude botanical preparation containing hyoscyamine, atropine, and scopolamine; available in combination with phenobarbital (Chardonna-2), or butabarbital (Butibel) and used for GI disorders.
GI spasm and hypersecretion, cholinergic poisoning, dysmenorrhea, urinary spasm, acute rhinitis	Well absorbed orally; may be useful in controlling diarrhea; tablets, elixir, and drops are also available with phenobarbital (Levsin PB).
Preanesthetic medication, motion sickness, spastic states, obstetric analgesia (with narcotics), ophthalmic mydriatic and cycloplegic, hyperhidrosis, excess salivation and secretion	CNS depression can occur with systemic use; overdosage results in excitement, confusion, and delirium; produces amnesia when given with narcotics; may produce delirium if used alone in severe pain; effects generally persist 4–6 h; neostigmine and physostigmine are effective antidotes; initial response to the drug may be a paradoxical excitation that will subside as the patient becomes more sedated; do not be misled by such activity; guard the patient's safety by using side rails and other protective measures as needed.
Prevention of motion sickness	Circular adhesive patch that delivers steady-state blood levels of scopolamine over 3 days; most frequent side effects are dry mouth, blurred vision, and drowsiness; use with caution in the presence of glaucoma, urinary or GI obstruction, impaired liver or kidney function, and in the elderly; safe use in children has not been established; response to this drug will vary from person to person; best results are obtained when the disk is applied the night before motion is experienced; use a new site for a second application.
GI spasm and hyperirritability, ulcerative colitis, infant colic	Usually administered with antacids in GI disorders, since it does not reduce gastric secretions; common side effects are dizziness, abdominal fullness, and slight euphoria; has fewer side effects than atropine but is still contraindicated for any patient with the potential for an adverse response to anticholinergics; it is available with phenobarbital (Bentyl PB).
Urinary incontinence (reflex neurogenic bladder)	Exhibits both a direct smooth muscle relaxing action and a weak antimuscarinic action on smooth muscle; has only one-fifth the anticholinergic activity of atropine but is 5–10 times as potent as an antispasmodic; delays desire to void; do not use in children under 5 yr or in patients with paralytic ileus, colitis, intestinal atony, megacolon, myasthenia, or obstructive uropathy.

Continued

Table 11-3
Antimuscarinics (continued)

Drug	Preparations	Usual Dosage Range
Oxyphencyclimine Hydrochloride Daricon	Tablets: 10 mg	5 mg–10 mg 2–3 times/day
Tertiary Amine Mydriatics		
Cyclopentolate Hydrochloride Cyclogyl, I-Pentolate (CAN) AK-Pentolate,	Ophthalmic drops: 0.5%, 1%, 2%	*Refraction* Adults: 1 drop 1%–2% solution, followed by a second drop in 5 min Children: 1 drop 0.5%–1% solution, followed by a second drop in 5 min
Tropicamide I-Picamide, Mydriacyl, Tropicacyl	Ophthalmic drops: 0.5%, 1%	*Refraction* 1–2 drops of 1%; repeat in 5 min and every 20–30 min as needed to maintain mydriasis *Examination of Fundus* 1–2 drops 0.5% 20–30 min prior to examination
Tertiary Amine Antiparkinson Drugs		
Benztropine Mesylate Cogentin (CAN) Apo Benztropine, Bensylate, PMS Benztropine	Tablets: 0.5 mg, 1 mg, 2 mg Injection: 1 mg/mL	*Parkinsonism* 1 mg–2 mg daily to a maximum of 6 mg *Extrapyramidal Reactions* 1 mg–4 mg 1–2 times/day *Acute Dystonic Reactions* 1 mg–2 mg IM or IV followed by 1 mg–2 mg PO twice/day
Biperiden Akineton	Tablets: 2 mg Injection: 5 mg/mL	*Parkinsonism* 2 mg 3–4 times/day with meals *Extrapyramidal Reactions* 2 mg 1–3 times/day PO or 2 mg IM or IV, repeated every half hour to a maximum of 4 doses
Ethopropazine Hydrochloride Parsidol (CAN) Parsitan	Tablets: 10 mg, 50 mg	Initially 50 mg 1–2 times/day to a maximum of 600 mg/day in severe cases
Orphenadrine Hydrochloride Disipal	Tablets: 50 mg	*Parkinsonism* 50 mg 3 times/day up to 250 mg daily
Orphenadrine Citrate Banflex, Flexoject, Flexon, K-Flex, Marflex, Myolin, Norflex, O'Flex	Tablets: 100 mg Sustained-release tablets: 100 mg Injection: 30 mg/mL	*Muscle Spasms* 100 mg orally twice a day or 60 mg IV or IM every 12 h as necessary
Procyclidine Kemadrin (CAN) PMS Procyclidine, Procyclid	Tablets: 5 mg	*Parkinsonism* 2.5 mg–5 mg 3 times/day *Extrapyramidal Reactions* 2.5 mg–5 mg 3–4 times/day
Trihexyphenidyl Hydrochloride Aphen, Artane, Trihexane, Trihexidyl, Trihexy (CAN) Aparkane, Apo-Trihex, Novohexidyl	Tablets: 2 mg, 5 mg Elixir: 2 mg/5 mL Capsules (sustained release): 5 mg	*Parkinsonism* 1 mg initially, increased by 2-mg increments every 3–5 days to a total dose of 6 mg–10 mg/day; usual maintenance dosage is 6 mg–12 mg daily in divided doses *Extrapyramidal Reactions* 5 mg–15 mg in divided doses
Quaternary Amine Antimuscarinics		
Anisotropine Methyl Bromide	Tablets: 50 mg	Adults: 50 mg 3 times/day

Major Uses	Nursing Implications
Adjunctive treatment of peptic ulcer	May induce CNS stimulation; do not use in children under 12 yr; available with hydroxyzine (Vistrax).
Ophthalmic refraction for diagnostic puposes	Effects can persist for up to 24 h; Pilocarpine (1–2 drops 1% to 2 % solution) reduces recovery time to 3–6 h; can produce behavioral disturbances in children (ataxia, disorientation, restlessness, incoherent speech) if absorbed systemically; ophthalmic drops available with phenylephrine (Cyclomydril) for increased mydriatic effect).
Ophthalmic refraction for diagnostic purposes	Effects occur in 20–30 min; recovery takes 4–6 h; larger doses may be necessary if iris is heavily pigmented.
Parkinsonism, extrapyramidal reactions	If used with L-dopa, adjust dose of each medication accordingly; start with low dose and gradually increase; no significant difference in onset of action IM or IV; sedative effect can occur; withdraw gradually (see Chap. 26).
Parkinsonism, extrapyramidal reactions	Most effective on akinesia and rigidity. May elevate mood. Can produce incoordination following IV or IM use (see Chap. 26).
Parkinsonism, extrapyramidal reactions	Does not potentiate CNS depressants; drug causes high incidence of dose-related side effects, including drowsiness, hypotension, confusion, and GI distress (see Chap. 26).
Parkinsonism, extrapyramidal reactions	Major effect is on rigidity of parkinsonism (see Chap. 26); also available as *citrate* salt for muscle spasms (see below).
Skeletal muscle spasms	Muscle relaxant (probably centrally acting) used to relieve acute musculoskeletal disorders (see Chap. 15); may produce dizziness in addition to normal anticholinergic side effects in large doses.
Parkinsonism, extrapyramidal reactions	Most effective against rigidity; may temporarily worsen tremor. In elderly, may induce confusion and psychotic reactions; note decreased urinary output and reduce dose if necessary (see Chap. 26).
Parkinsonism, extrapyramidal reactions	When used with L-dopa, reduce dose of each drug proportionately; major effect is on rigidity, with minimal effects on tremor; sustained-release capsules are *not* intended for initial therapy but may be used once patient is stabilized; may produce CNS stimulation and excessive drying of the mouth; often given before meals (see Chap. 26).
GI spasms, adjunctive therapy in peptic ulcer	Oral absorption is erratic.

Continued

Table 11-3
Antimuscarinics (continued)

Drug	Preparations	Usual Dosage Range
Clidinium Bromide Quarzan	Capsules: 2.5 mg, 5 mg	2.5 mg–5 mg 3–4 times/day
Glycopyrrolate Robinul	Tablets: 1 mg, 2 mg Injection: 0.2 mg/mL	*Oral* 1 mg–2 mg 2–3 times/day *Parenteral* IM, IV: 0.1 mg–0.2 mg 3–4 times/day *Reversal of Neuromuscular Blockade* 0.2 mg IV for every 1 mg neostigmine or equivalent received *Preanesthetic Medication* 0.004 mg/kg IM 30–60 min prior to anesthesia (children under 12— 0.004–0.008 mg/kg)
Hexocyclium Methylsulfate Tral	Tablets: 25 mg	25 mg 4 times/day
Homatropine Hydrobromide Homatrine, Isopto Homatropine (CAN) Ak-Homatropine	Ophthalmic drops: 2%, 5%	*Refraction* 1–2 drops 2% every 10–15 min if necessary *Iritis* 1–2 drops 2%–5% every 3–4 h
Ipratropium Atrovent	Aerosol: 18 µg per activation	2 inhalations 4 times/day (maximum 12 inhalations/24 h)
Isopropamide Iodide Darbid	Tablets: 5 mg	5 mg–10 mg twice a day (every 12 h)
Mepenzolate Cantil	Tablets: 25 mg	25 mg to 50 mg 4 times/day
Methantheline Bromide Banthine	Tablets: 50 mg	Adults: 50 mg–100 mg 4 times/day Children (less than 1 yr): 12 mg–25 mg 4 times/day over 1 yr: 25 mg–50 mg 4 times/day
Methscopolamine Bromide Pamine	Tablets: 2.5 mg	2.5 mg 3 times/day and 2.5 mg–5 mg at bedtime
Oxyphenonium Bromide Antrenyl	Tablets: 5 mg	10 mg 4 times/day
Propantheline Bromide Norpanth, Pro-Banthine (CAN) Banlin, Novopropanthil, Propanthel	Tablets: 7.5 mg, 15 mg	*Oral* 7.5 mg–15 mg 3 times/day and 30 mg at bedtime Children: 1.5 mg–3 mg/kg/day in 3–4 divided doses
Tridihexethyl Chloride Pathilon	Tablets: 25 mg	Adults: 25 mg–50 mg 3–4 times/day

Major Uses	Nursing Implications
GI hypermotility and hypersecretion	Erratically absorbed orally; reduce dosage in geriatric or debilitated patients; also available in combination with chlordiazepoxide as Librax.
GI disorders, preoperative medication, cholinergic overdosage	Not indicated in children under 12 yr for GI disorders; used preoperatively to reduce salivary, bronchial, pharyngeal, and gastric secretions and to block vagal inhibition of cardiac reflexes during anesthesia; may cause burning at site of injection; do not mix with solutions of sodium chloride or bicarbonate; oral absorption is irregular.
GI hypermotility, hypersecretion	Oral absorption is unpredictable; do not chew tablets; do not use in children.
Refraction, iritis, relief of ciliary spasm, preoperative, cycloplegic, and mydriatic	Cycloplegia may be prolonged and caution in driving is recommended.
Bronchospasm associated with chronic obstructive pulmonary disease	Orally inhaled anticholinergic that relaxes bronchiolar smooth muscle by inhibiting action of parasympathetic nervous system; does not affect volume or viscosity of respiratory secretions; systemic absorption is minimal; *not* indicated for *initial* treatment of *acute* episodes of bronchospasm; most frequent side effects are cough, dryness of oropharynx, and nervousness (see Chap. 55).
GI spasm and hypersecretion, diarrhea	Not for use in children under 12 yr; erratically absorbed orally; iodine skin rash may occur; may alter protein-bound iodine and ^{131}I tests, since drug is an iodide salt.
GI hypermotility, diarrhea, ulcerative colitis	Urinary hesitancy and constipation can occur, especially at larger doses; erratically absorbed orally.
Adjunctive therapy in peptic ulcer	Less effective than many other similar agents; tablets are very bitter; poorly absorbed orally.
GI hypermotility, adjunctive therapy in peptic ulcer	Take drug 30 min before meals; may exert curare-like relaxant effect on smooth muscle.
GI hyperacidity and hypermotility	Erratically absorbed; high incidence of common anticholinergic side effects; not for use in children.
GI spasm and hypersecretion, adjunctive therapy in peptic ulcer	Increased fluid intake may minimize fecal impaction and urinary hesitancy; blurring of vision and dizziness can occur.
Adjunctive therapy of peptic ulcer	Infrequently used.

SUMMARY. ANTICHOLINERGIC AGENTS

Drug	Preparations	Usual Dosage Range
Antimuscarinics	*See* Table 11-3	
Ganglionic Blocking Agents		
Mecamylamine Inversine	Tablets: 2.5 mg	Initially 2.5 mg twice a day; increase by 2.5-mg increments every 2 days to optimal effect (average 25 mg/day)
Trimethaphan Arfonad	Injection: 50 mg/mL	Dilute 500 mg (10 mL) in 500 mL 5% dextrose; begin IV infusion at rate of 3 mL/min to 4 mL/min; adjust to individual (range 0.3 mL/min–6.0 mL/min)

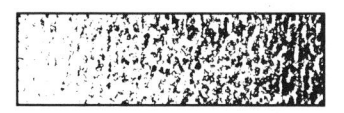

12 ADRENERGIC DRUGS

Adrenergic drugs are compounds, either natural or synthetic, that are capable of eliciting biologic responses similar to those induced by activation of the sympathetic nervous system or by adrenal medullary discharge. For this reason, these agents are also called *sympathomimetic drugs*—that is, drugs that mimic sympathetic neuronal stimulation.

The principal adrenergic compounds naturally occurring in the body are the endogenous catecholamines epinephrine (E), norepinephrine (NE), and dopamine (DA). *Epinephrine* is the major secretory product of the adrenal medulla and is released during periods of physical or emotional stress. It plays an important role in the body's adaptation to the stressful situation. It is also found in other organs of the body where its role is less clear. *Norepinephrine* is found in adrenergic nerve endings and is the principal mediator of transmission at adrenergic neuroeffector junctions. In addition, norepinephrine is found in certain central brain regions and in peripheral sympathetic ganglia, where it probably serves a modulatory function. The principal role of *dopamine* is as a central neurotransmitter involved in regulating motor function and pituitary hormone secretion. It also acts peripherally in certain vascular beds to cause dilation of mesenteric and renal blood vessels.

The adrenergic agents in clinical use comprise a large, heterogenous group of compounds possessing a wide spectrum of pharmacologic actions. Adequate classification of these substances, therefore, is difficult. On the basis of their predominant mechanism of action, adrenergic drugs can be divided into three groups:

I. *Direct acting:* compounds exerting a direct activating effect at the postsynaptic adrenergic receptor site (e.g., norepinephrine, dopamine)
II. *Indirect acting:* compounds acting on the presynaptic adrenergic nerve terminals to promote the release of stored adrenergic neurotransmitters (e.g., tyramine)
III. *Dual acting:* compounds possessing a mixture of direct and indirect actions (e.g., ephedrine, amphetamine)

Qualitative differences in the responses of effector structures to the various groups of adrenergic agents indicate the existence of different kinds of adrenergic receptor sites. A discussion of adrenergic receptors can be found in Chapter 9. It is generally accepted that most adrenergic receptor sites are of two basic types, alpha and beta. Alpha and beta receptors may be further classified, mainly by location. There are two types of alpha receptors, alpha$_1$ and alpha$_2$ and two types of beta receptors, beta$_1$ and beta$_2$. (These names are sometimes written with the Greek letters for which they are named: α_1, β_1, and so on.) In addition, there are receptors specific to the endogenous catecholamine dopamine; these dopamenergic sites are found in the brain and on certain blood vessels. Dopamine can also interact with certain alpha and beta receptor sites and may be further subdivided into DA$_1$ and DA$_2$ sites. Table 12-1 outlines the major adrenergic receptor sites and lists the important pharmacologic effects produced by activation of each type of receptor.

The pharmacologic actions of adrenergic agents depend to a large extent on their affinity and specificity for the different types of adrenergic receptors, as well as their intrinsic activity at each site. An overview of the major pharmacologic effects resulting from activation of the different kinds of peripheral adrenergic receptor sites is presented in Table 12-2.

In addition to their many peripheral actions, many adrenergic compounds exert profound effects on the CNS. Alterations in catecholamine activity in a number of brain structures are believed to be responsible for many affective and motor disorders, and drugs that are useful in treating these conditions function largely by modifying the availability or action of endogenous adrenergic amines. Many noncatecholamine adrenergic drugs (e.g., ephedrine, amphetamine) can easily penetrate the CNS and elicit marked stimulatory effects. These agents are often abused, and they are potentially dangerous drugs. They are considered in Chapter 27 with the other CNS stimulants.

In order to discuss the adrenergic drugs in some reasonable order, the following arbitrary classification is used in this text. Remember that many drugs fall into more than one of the proposed categories:

I. Endogenous catecholamines (e.g., epinephrine, norepinephrine, dopamine)
II. Synthetic catecholamines (e.g., isoproterenol, dobutamine)
III. Vasopressor amines (e.g., metaraminol)
IV. Nasal decongestants (e.g., phenylephrine)
V. Ophthalmic decongestants (e.g., naphazoline)
VI. Bronchodilators (e.g., ephedrine, metaproterenol)
VII. Smooth muscle relaxants (e.g., isoxsuprine, ritodrine)
VIII. CNS stimulants and anorexiants (e.g., amphetamine)

ENDOGENOUS CATECHOLAMINES

The three major endogenous catecholamines, epinephrine, norepinephrine, and dopamine, mediate the functioning of the sympathetic nervous system and are found widely throughout the body. Moreover, many other classes of pharmacologic agents exert their effects by modifying the action of one or more of these endogenous substances, so that the catecholamines participate in the action of a wide range of drugs. Catecholamines can also be prepared synthetically and are widely used in the treatment of many pathologic conditions. The therapeutic indications of the catecholamines are primarily based on their vasoconstrictive, bronchodilatory, and cardiac stimulatory actions.

Epinephrine

Parenteral: Adrenalin, Sus-Phrine
Inhalation: Asthmahaler, Asthmanefrin, Bronitin Mist, Bronkaid Mist, Medihaler-Epi, Micronefrin, Primatene, Vaponefrin
(CAN) Dysne-Inhal
Nasal: Adrenalin
Ophthalmic: Adrenalin, Epifrin, Epinal, Epitrate, Eppy/N, Glaucon

MECHANISM
Direct nonspecific activation of alpha- and beta-adrenergic receptor sites; alpha activation elicits vasoconstriction in many vascular beds; beta$_1$ activation increases the heart rate and the force of myocardial contraction. Beta$_2$ activation evokes bronchodilation and dilation of vessels in skeletal muscles via formation of cyclic AMP; uterine smooth muscle is generally

Table 12-1
Adrenergic Receptor Sites

Alpha₁	Alpha₂	Beta₁	Beta₂	Dopaminergic
Principal Agonists				
Epinephrine Norepinephrine	Epinephrine Norepinephrine	Epinephrine Isoproterenol	Epinephrine Isoproterenol	Dopamine[a]
Major Peripheral Locations				
Vascular smooth muscle GI and urinary sphincters Eye (radial muscles) Pancreas Spleen Salivary glands Skin (sweat glands, pilomotor muscles)	Presynaptic adrenergic and cholinergic nerve terminals Platelets Fat cells Vascular smooth muscle GI tract	Heart Intestinal smooth muscle Adipose tissue	Smooth muscle (bronchiolar, GI, uterine, urinary) Skeletal muscle blood vessels Liver Kidney	Renal, coronary, and visceral blood vessels
Responses				
Excitatory				
Vasoconstriction (rapid onset—short lived) Contraction of GI and urinary sphincters Mydriasis (contraction of radial muscle) Salivary and sweat gland secretion	Platelet aggregation Vasoconstriction (slow onset—long lived)	Cardiac stimulation Lipolysis	Glycogenolysis, gluconeogenesis Increased renin secretion	
Inhibitory				
Pancreatic secretions ↓	Neurotransmitter release ↓ Inhibition of lipolysis GI motility ↓	GI motility ↓	Bronchodilation Uterine relaxation GI motility ↓ Relaxation of urinary bladder Dilation of skeletal muscle vessels	Dilation of renal, coronary, and visceral blood vessels

↓, decreased; ↑, increased.
[a]Dopamine can also activate cardiac beta₁ receptors and vascular alpha₁ receptors in higher doses.

---

contracted, except in the latter stages of pregnancy, when myometrial tone is decreased (beta₂ activation); blood glucose is elevated owing to glycogenolysis and gluconeogenesis. In the eye, epinephrine induces mydriasis and also lowers intraocular pressure by inhibiting formation and stimulating outflow of aqueous humor; effects on the CNS are minimal at normal doses, as the drug does not pass the blood–brain barrier in significant amounts

USES
Symptomatic relief of anaphylactic, allergic, and other hypersensitivity reactions
Pressor agent for acute hypotensive states
Nasal decongestion
Bronchodilation and pulmonary decongestion (relaxes bronchial smooth muscle and constricts mucosal blood vessels)
Restoration of normal cardiac rhythm in cases of cardiac arrest
Management of simple, open-angle glaucoma (decreases production and increases outflow of aqueous humor)
Ocular decongestion (vasoconstriction) and production of mydriasis
Topical hemostasis (controls superficial bleeding)
Potentiation and prolongation of the action of local anesthetics

DOSAGE
I. Parenteral
  A. Cardiac arrest: 5 mL to 10 mL 1:10,000 IV, repeated at 5-minute intervals as required
  B. Intracardiac: 3 mL to 5 mL 1:10,000
  C. Intraspinal: 0.2 mL to 0.4 mL 1:1000 added to anesthetic solution
  D. Bronchospasm: Adults—0.3 mL to 0.5 mL 1:1000 SC or IM; repeat every 20 minutes up to 4 hours *or* 0.1 mL to 0.3 mL of a 1:200 suspension SC. Children—0.01 mg/kg 1:1000 SC; repeat every 20 minutes up to 4 hours.
  E. With local anesthetic: 1:20,000–1:100,000
II. Inhalation
  A. Aerosol: 8 to 15 drops 1%–2% solution from

Table 12-2
Adrenergic Drug Effects

Structure	Response	Receptor Type
Cardiovascular System		
Heart	Rate ↑	Beta$_1$
	Force ↑	Beta$_1$
	AV conduction velocity ↑	
Blood Vessels		
Skeletal	Vasoconstriction	Alpha$_1$, alpha$_2$
	Vasodilation	Beta$_2$
Mucosal	Vasoconstriction	Alpha$_1$
Mesenteric	Vasoconstriction	Alpha$_1$
	Vasodilation	Dopaminergic
Coronary and renal	Vasodilation	Dopaminergic
Bronchioles	Smooth muscle relaxation	Beta$_2$
GI Tract		
Smooth muscle	Relaxation	Beta$_2$
Sphincter	Contraction	Alpha$_1$
Uterus		
Smooth muscle	Relaxation	Beta$_2$
Eye		
Radial muscle	Contraction	Alpha$_1$
Ciliary muscle	Relaxation (weak)	Beta$_1$
Skin		
Pilomotor muscles	Contraction	Alpha$_1$
Sweat glands	Secretion (weak)	Alpha$_1$
Liver	Glycogenolysis	Beta$_2$
	Gluconeogenesis	Beta$_2$
Adipose Tissue	Lipolysis	Beta$_1$
	Inhibition of lipolysis	Alpha$_2$
Pancreas	Insulin secretion ↓	Alpha$_2$
Kidney	Secretion of renin	Beta$_1$
Platelets	Aggregation	Alpha$_2$

↓, decreased; ↑, increased.

---

metered aerosol or nebulizer. Allow 1 to 5 minutes between inhalations, and use least number of inhalations that are effective
III. Topical
  A. Nasal: 1 to 2 drops 0.1% solution every 4 to 6 hours
  B. Hemostatic: 1:1000 to 1:10,000 applied locally
IV. Ophthalmic
  A. Glaucoma: 1 to 2 drops 0.25% to 2% solution (individualized to patient needs)
  B. Ocular mydriasis and hemostasis: 1 to 2 drops 0.1% solution

FATE
Readily absorbed by mucous membranes but rapidly destroyed by digestive enzymes, thus is useless orally. Aqueous solutions are very unstable, oxidize readily (amber or yellow color in solution), and should be used immediately. Effects occur quickly when given SC, IM, intraocularly, or by inhalation. Suspension forms provide more prolonged actions (6–12 h). Drug is usually rapidly inactivated by uptake into adrenergic nerve endings or through enzymatic (MAO, COMT) hydrolysis. Circulating drug is hydrolyzed in the liver, and metabolites, chiefly vanillyl mandelic acid (VMA), are excreted in the urine

COMMON SIDE EFFECTS
Systemic: nervousness, anxiety, nausea, sweating, pallor, palpitations, headache, insomnia
Ophthalmic: headache, stinging, lacrimation, rebound hyperemia
Nasal: burning, mucosal dryness, sneezing, rebound congestion

SIGNIFICANT ADVERSE REACTIONS
Systemic: weakness, dizziness, hypertension, anginal pain, tachycardia and arrhythmias, pulmonary edema, dyspnea, urinary retention, cerebral or subarachnoid hemorrhage, delusions, tremor, psychoses, lactic acidosis
Ophthalmic: conjunctival irritation; pigmentation of eyelids, cornea, or conjunctiva; iritis; shedding of eyelashes; scotomas

CONTRAINDICATIONS
Severe hypertension, arrhythmias, coronary artery disease, shock, porphyria, narrow-angle glaucoma, organic brain damage, during labor (delays second stage), and in combination with general anesthetics, especially halogenated hydrocarbons (increased risk of arrhythmias). *Cautious use* in patients with hypertension, hyperthyroidism, diabetes, parkinsonism, cardiovascular disease, emphysema, psychoneuroses, prostatic hypertrophy, or tuberculosis, and in infants and elderly persons

INTERACTIONS
Epinephrine may be potentiated by other sympathomimetic agents (e.g., phenylephrine, mephentermine), tricyclic antidepressants, MAO inhibitors, antihistamines, thyroxine, guanethidine.

Epinephrine may produce toxic effects when used in combination with digitalis (arrhythmias), general anesthetics (arrhythmias), isoproterenol (arrhythmias), or propranolol (bradycardia).

Epinephrine may induce hyperglycemia, altering the requirements for insulin or oral hypoglycemic agents.

Cardiac and bronchodilatory effects of epinephrine are antagonized by propranolol. Pressor effects are blocked by vasodilators such as nitrites or alpha-adrenergic blockers (e.g., phentolamine) but may be intensified by beta blockers (e.g., propranolol).

Diuretics may increase the vascular pressor response to epinephrine.

NURSING CONSIDERATIONS

Nursing Alerts
- When drug is given IV, take blood pressure and pulse frequently (use cardiac monitor if possible) while a small amount is slowly injected. Injections are repeated only as needed to obtain desired effect. Check blood pressure every 3 to 5 minutes until patient is fully stabilized. Observe for signs of shock (e.g., cyanosis, pallor), and ensure that all emergency equipment and drugs are readily available.
- Carefully check solution *strength* and required dosage before administration. A tuberculin syringe may help ensure dosage accuracy.
- Massage SC or IM injection site to hasten absorption, and rotate injection sites to prevent tissue necrosis related to localized vasoconstriction.
- Avoid simultaneous administration with isoproterenol; serious cardiac arrhythmias can result.

1. Avoid exposing solution to heat, light, or air because deterioration rapidly ensues.
2. Discard solution if it is yellow or amber or contains a precipitate. Drug is readily destroyed by numerous chemical agents.

PATIENT EDUCATION
Systemic
1. Teach patient with a history of acute bronchial asthmatic attacks how to administer epinephrine SC.

Inhalation
1. Instruct patient to use only the fewest number of inhalations needed to relieve symptoms and allow 1 or 2 minutes between them. Excessive use can produce severe adverse systemic effects.
2. Urge patient to consult physician immediately if symptoms are not relieved within 15 to 30 minutes.
3. Instruct patient to reduce dosage if bronchial irritation, nervousness, or insomnia is noted.
4. Instruct patient to rinse mouth with water after inhalation to avoid swallowing residual drug and to prevent excessive mouth-drying effects.

Ophthalmic
1. Suggest taking drug at bedtime, if possible, to minimize photophobia (sensitivity to light) and blurred vision related to mydriasis. Visual perception may be impaired, especially at night.
2. Instruct patient to inform drug prescriber if localized symptoms (stinging, burning, headache, tearing) persist with continued drug use.
3. Instruct patient to stop using drug and consult physician if allergic reaction develops (e.g., itching, edema, watery discharge).
4. Instruct patient to inform the physician in charge of drug use if general surgery is planned. With certain anesthetics (e.g., halothane, other halogenated hydrocarbons), epinephrine should be discontinued prior to surgery to prevent arrhythmias associated with systemic absorption.

Nasal
1. Instruct patient to avoid excessive use because rebound congestion and hyperemia frequently occur.
2. Advise cautious use with elderly person or infant because systemic absorption can produce untoward reactions (e.g., tachycardia, hypertension, anxiety).
3. Inform patient that instillation will sting but discomfort will be temporary.

Dipivefrin
Propine

Dipivefrin is a lipid-soluble *prodrug* of epinephrine; that is, it is converted to epinephrine by enzymatic hydrolysis after it is instilled into the eye. Because of its highly lipophilic nature, its penetration into the cornea is much greater than that of epinephrine itself. Onset of action is within 30 minutes. Dipivefrin is indicated for the control of intraocular pressure in chronic open-angle glaucoma; its use is associated with fewer side effects than conventional epinephrine therapy because it is better absorbed and so less drug is required. Therapeutic response to twice daily administration of dipivefrin is approximately equivalent to that of 2% pilocarpine given 4 times a day; but the miosis and cycloplegia characteristic of cholinergic therapy do not occur. The response is somewhat inferior to that observed with 2% epinephrine however. Because of its mydriatic action, dipivefrin, like epinephrine, is contraindicated in narrow-angle glaucoma.

The side effects associated with dipivefrin therapy are similar to those noted previously for ophthalmic epinephrine administration but occur less often. Burning and stinging following instillation are the most common side effects. In addition, systemic effects (tachycardia, increased blood pressure, arrhythmias) have been reported following ocular administration of epinephrine and can occur with use of dipivefrin as well. Dipivefrin is available as a 0.1% solution, and the usual dosage is 1 drop every 12 hours.

Norepinephrine
Levarterenol, Levophed

MECHANISM
Direct activation of alpha-adrenergic receptor sites on blood vessels, producing powerful vasoconstriction; also possesses slight inotropic action on cardiac beta receptors (increased force of contraction). Increases blood pressure and coronary artery blood flow, but increases workload of the heart as well; in normal doses, little effect on the CNS or on metabolic activity

USES
Restoration of blood pressure in acute hypotensive states
Adjunctive treatment of cardiac arrest and extreme hypotension

DOSAGE
Used by IV infusion—initially, 8 μg/min to 12 μg/min (2 mL/min–3 mL/min) of a 4-μg/mL dilution (4 mg NE/1000 mL 5% dextrose); maintenance dose—2 μg/min to 4 μg/min (0.5 mL/min–1 mL/min)

FATE
Rapid acting; effects disappear within 2 minutes after termination of IV infusion; rapidly inactivated by uptake into sympathetic nerve endings and also by enzymatic hydrolysis; excreted in the urine largely as metabolites

COMMON SIDE EFFECTS
Bradycardia (reflex), headache, palpitation, nervousness

SIGNIFICANT ADVERSE REACTIONS
Hypertension, respiratory distress, tremors, arrhythmias in the presence of certain anesthetics, tissue necrosis following extravasation; large doses may cause chest pain, photophobia, hyperglycemia, vomiting, severe hypertension, cerebral hemorrhage, and convulsions

CONTRAINDICATIONS
Hypovolemic shock, vascular thrombosis; extreme hypoxia or hypercapnia; pregnancy; during general anesthesia when halogenated hydrocarbons (e.g., halothane) are employed. *Cautious use* in persons with hypertension, heart disease, hyperthyroidism, peripheral vascular disorders and in the elderly

INTERACTIONS
The pressor effects of norepinephrine may be potentiated in the presence of tricyclic antidepressants, MAO inhibitors, other sympathomimetic drugs, beta blockers, antihistamines, guanethidine, and methyldopa.
Norepinephrine, together with oxytocic drugs, can cause severe hypertension.
Norepinephrine may precipitate cardiac arrhythmias in the presence of cyclopropane and the halogenated hydrocarbon general anesthetics.
Thiazide and high-ceiling (e.g., bumetanide, furosemide) diuretics may reduce arterial responsiveness to norepinephrine.

NURSING CONSIDERATIONS

Nursing Alerts
- Check blood pressure every 2 to 5 minutes during and following infusion. Attend patient constantly, and carefully monitor skin color and temperature.
- Monitor flow rate continuously. Use microdrip IV administration set and an infusion control device to ensure accuracy.
- Monitor cardiac rate and rhythm. Atropine should be available to treat bradycardia, propranalol to treat other arrhythmias.
- Monitor patient for other early signs of overdosage (headache, vomiting, blurred vision, anginal symptoms) so that dosage can be adjusted appropriately.
- Measure intake and output. Urinary output should be determined frequently to assess renal perfusion.
- Report indications of blood volume depletion. Adequate blood volume must be maintained to prevent tissue ischemia resulting from vasoconstrictive effect of the drug.
- If extravasation occurs (blanching of skin, swelling, hardness), stop infusion. The area should be infiltrated with 10 mL–15 mL saline containing 5 mg–10 mg phentolamine as soon as possible. Once blood pressure and tissue perfusion can be self-maintained, continue monitoring vital signs to ensure circulatory adequacy while therapy is discontinued by *gradual* reduction of infusion rate.

1. Infuse into a large vein if possible, and alternate infusion sites to minimize risk of necrosis. Avoid leg veins, especially in the elderly, because occlusive vascular diseases can result.
2. Avoid use of catheter tie-in arrangement because venous stasis can occur around tubing, increasing local concentration of drug.
3. Administer whole blood or plasma separately. Both are incompatible with norepinephrine.
4. Discard solutions that are colored or contain precipitated matter.
5. Seek clarification before adding to saline *alone* because oxidation and loss of potency can occur rapidly. A 5% dextrose vehicle should be used.

Dopamine
Dopastat, Intropin
(CAN) Revimine

MECHANISM
Direct activation of specific dopaminergic receptors in mesenteric and renal vasculature, resulting in vasodilation and increased renal blood flow; also stimulates myocardial beta receptors, enhancing force of contraction and increasing cardiac output with minimal cardioaccelerator action. In high doses, activates alpha receptors in other vascular beds, causing constriction. Produces less oxygen demand on the myocardium and has a lower incidence of arrhythmias than other catecholamines

USES
Correction of the hemodynamic imbalances associated with different forms of shock (e.g., trauma, heart surgery, myocardial infarction, renal failure, septicemia)

DOSAGE
Initially—2 μg/kg/min to 5 μg/kg/min of diluted solution by IV infusion. May increase by increments of 5 μg/kg/min to 10 μg/

kg/min up to 20 µg/kg/min to 50 µg/kg/min in severely ill patients

FATE

Rapid onset (5 min) and short duration of action (5–10 min); largely inactivated by liver and plasma enzymes and excreted chiefly in the urine as metabolites. A portion is converted to norepinephrine in adrenergic nerve endings; does not cross the blood–brain barrier

COMMON SIDE EFFECTS

Nausea, vomiting, palpitations, tachycardia, slight hypotension, mild respiratory difficulty, and headache

SIGNIFICANT ADVERSE REACTIONS

(Usually occur with high doses) Hypertension, conduction irregularities, azotemia, decreased urinary outflow. Necrosis and tissue sloughing may occur following extravasation

CONTRAINDICATIONS

Ventricular arrhythmias and pheochromocytoma. *Cautious use* in persons with occlusive vascular disease

INTERACTIONS

Pressor effects of dopamine may be potentiated by MAO inhibitors, tricyclic antidepressants, other sympathomimetics, oxytocics, ergot alkaloids, and furazolidone.

Actions of dopamine and diuretics may be mutually additive.

Dopamine may produce arrhythmias in the presence of cyclopropane and halogenated hydrocarbon anesthetics.

Use of phenytoin with dopamine may lead to hypotension, bradycardia, and seizures.

NURSING CONSIDERATIONS

Nursing Alerts

- Carefully monitor blood pressure, heart rate and rhythm, and urine flow during infusion. Rate of flow must be adjusted to maintain desired hemodynamic and renal responses.
- Check infusion flow rate frequently. Use microdrip IV administration set and infusion control device, if available, to help ensure stability and accuracy.
- Monitor for changes in color, temperature, and texture of skin at injection site, indications of possible extravasation. If extravasation occurs, infiltration with 10–15 mL saline containing 5–10 mg phentolamine helps prevent necrosis.
- If high dosages are used, check continually for reduced urine output and monitor for other symptoms of overdosage (hypertension, arrhythmias, change in color of extremities). The dosage must be reduced if such symptoms are noted.

1. Infuse into a large vein (preferably of the antecubital fossa) to minimize danger of extravasation and tissue necrosis.
2. Dilute the solution in the dopamine ampule before using. Add it to a sterile diluent solution (250 mL or 500 mL of sodium chloride, sodium lactate, dextrose 5%, lactated Ringer's), according to package instructions.
3. Protect dopamine solutions from light and discard if discolored.
4. Seek clarification before adding to alkaline IV solutions (e.g., sodium bicarbonate) because dopamine is inactivated by them.

SYNTHETIC CATECHOLAMINES

In addition to the three catecholamines found endogenously, two synthetic derivatives, isoproterenol and dobutamine, are available. They are almost exclusively activators of beta-adrenergic receptor sites. Isoproterenol nonselectively activates all beta receptors, and dobutamine exerts a relatively specific activation of cardiac $beta_1$ receptors.

Isoproterenol

Oral/parenteral: Isuprel
Inhalation: Aerolone, Medihaler-Iso, Norisodrine, Vapo-Iso

MECHANISM

Direct beta-adrenergic receptor activation, resulting in cardiac stimulation, vasodilation, and bronchodilation; also relaxes smooth muscle of the GI tract and uterus, releases free fatty acids, stimulates insulin secretion, and increases glycogenolysis

USES

Relief of bronchospasm associated with respiratory disorders and general anesthesia

Adjunct in management of shock, cardiac arrest, Adams–Stokes syndrome, AV block, and carotid sinus hypersensitivity

DOSAGE

I. Parenteral
  A. Bronchospasm (during anesthesia): 0.01 mg to 0.02 mg IV of a 1:50,000 solution in saline or dextrose 5%
  B. Shock: 0.25 mL/min to 2.5 mL/min of 1:500,000 dilution in Dextrose 5% by IV infusion (0.5 µg/min–5 µg/min)
  C. Cardiac arrest: IV (injection)—1 mL to 3 mL of a 1:50,000 dilution (0.02 mg–0.06 mg); IV (infusion)—1.25 mL of 1:250,000 dilution per minute (5 µg/min); IM, SC—1 mL of 1:5000 solution undiluted (0.2 mg); Intracardiac—0.1 mL of 1:5000 solution (0.02 mg)
II. Sublingual
  A. Bronchospasm: 10 mg to 20 mg 3 or 4 times/day (children—5 mg to 10 mg 3 or 4 times/day)
  B. Heart block: 10 mg initially (range 5 mg–50 mg); maintenance therapy *only*
III. Inhalation
  A. Solution: 3 to 7 inhalations of 1:100 solution or 5 to 15 inhalations of 1:200 solution in a hand-held nebulizer; repeat in 5 to 10 min, if needed; may be given up to 5 times/day.
  B. Aerosol: 1 to 2 inhalations of metered dose aerosol 4 to 6 times/day.

FATE

Readily absorbed when given parenterally or as aerosol; oral and sublingual absorption is unreliable; duration following most forms of administration is 2 to 4 hours (1–2 h with inhalation); metabolites are excreted largely in the urine, within 24 hours following biotransformation in the GI tract, liver, lungs, and other tissues

COMMON SIDE EFFECTS

Nervousness, headache, palpitations, flushing, nausea, dizziness, mild tremors, and dryness of the oropharynx

SIGNIFICANT ADVERSE REACTIONS

Buccal ulcerations (sublingual), bronchial irritation and edema, cardiac distress (tachycardia, dysrhythmias, anginal pain), parotid gland enlargement (rare); overdosage may result in severe bronchoconstriction, cardiac excitability, and possibly cardiac arrest

CONTRAINDICATIONS

Arrhythmias associated with tachycardia, concurrent administration of epinephrine. *Cautious use* in patients with hypertension, cardiac disease, hyperthyroidism, diabetes

INTERACTIONS

Combined use with epinephrine may lead to serious arrhythmias.
Arrhythmias may develop if used with cyclopropane or halogenated hydrocarbon anesthetics.
Effects are specifically antagonized by propranolol and other beta-adrenergic blockers.

NURSING CONSIDERATIONS

Nursing Alerts

- Monitor blood pressure, heart rate and rhythm, and urine flow during infusion and note blood pH and P_{CO_2} results. Rate of flow must be adjusted to maintain stability of these parameters.
- Check infusion flow rate frequently to ensure accuracy. Use microdrip IV administration set and infusion control device if available.
- Closely assess patient in shock during infusion. If heart rate exceeds 110 beats/min, infusion should be reduced or terminated because of the danger of arrhythmias.
- Ensure that oxygen and other respiratory aids are available.

1. Check type of solution carefully while preparing drug. Those intended for oral inhalation cannot be injected.
2. Discard discolored or cloudy solutions.
3. If tablets are to be given rectally, use *sublingual* tablets only.
4. Carefully check dosage and method of inhalation prescribed (e.g., nebulizer, aerosol, powder).

PATIENT EDUCATION

Oral/Sublingual

1. Explain that sustained-release tablets must be swallowed whole.
2. Instruct patient to allow sublingual tablet to dissolve under tongue without sucking tablet or swallowing saliva until drug has been absorbed.
3. Inform patient that mild systemic effects (e.g., flushing, palpitations) may be experienced with sublingual use.
4. Advise patient that prolonged use of sublingual tablets can damage teeth. Suggest rinsing mouth thoroughly after each administration.

Inhalation

1. Teach patient how to use the form of inhalation prescribed.
2. Instruct patient to breathe with normal force and depth, *not* deeply, when using powdered inhalant.
3. Suggest that patient rinse mouth after inhalation to minimize dryness.
4. Inform patient that saliva may appear pink or red following inhalation.
5. Warn patient to avoid excessive use (3–5 treatments within 6–12 h) of inhalation products because tolerance can develop and sudden deaths have been reported.
6. Instruct patient to place no more than a 1-day supply of drug in nebulizer and to rinse mouthpiece thoroughly every day.
7. Instruct patient to notify physician immediately if usual doses do not produce desired relief.

Dobutamine

Dobutrex

MECHANISM

Direct activation of $beta_1$ adrenergic receptors on the myocardium, with minimal action at alpha or $beta_2$ sites; increases contractile force but induces less increase in heart rate and less decrease in peripheral vascular resistance than comparably effective doses of isoproterenol

USES

Short-term treatment of acute heart failure related to depressed contractility

DOSAGE

2.5-μg/kg/min to 10-μg/kg/min IV infusion of a 250-μg/mL, 500-μg/mL, or 1000-μg/mL solution in sterile water or 5% dextrose. Occasionally, infusion rates up to 40 μg/kg/min are required.

FATE

Onset of action within 1 to 2 minutes; short duration of action; plasma half-life of 2 minutes; metabolized in the liver and excreted in urine as conjugates

COMMON SIDE EFFECTS

Tachycardia (5–15 beats/min increase), palpitations, mild hypertension (10–20 mm Hg increase in systolic pressure)

SIGNIFICANT ADVERSE REACTIONS

Premature ventricular beats, anginal pain, headache, dyspnea, nausea, pronounced tachycardia, marked hypertension

CONTRAINDICATIONS

Idiopathic hypertrophic subaortic stenosis. *Cautious use* in persons with arrhythmias, hypertension, or following a recent myocardial infarction

INTERACTIONS

Cyclopropane and halogenated hydrocarbons may increase the incidence of arrhythmias with dobutamine.
Pressor effects of dobutamine can be enhanced by MAO inhibitors, tricyclic antidepressants, other sympathomimetic amines, and oxytocic drugs.

In diabetics, insulin requirements may be increased by dobutamine.

NURSING CONSIDERATIONS

Nursing Alert
- During infusion, continually check blood pressure, heart rate and rhythm, and, where possible, cardiac output and pulmonary capillary wedge pressure. Volume of infusion should be adjusted by coordinating concentration of the solution with patient's fluid requirements.

1. Be prepared to administer volume expanders (e.g., dextran) to the hypovolemic patient before dobutamine is started, as hypovolemia should be corrected before initiating dobutamine therapy.
2. Be prepared to administer digoxin prior to dobutamine in the patient with existing atrial fibrillation and rapid ventricular response.
3. Expect drug effects to terminate shortly after discontinuation of therapy. The drug's duration of action is very brief.
4. Use dilutions for IV use within 24 hours. A color change in the solution during this period indicates slight oxidation, but there is *no* significant loss of potency during the first 24 hours.
5. Seek clarification before diluting in an alkaline solution (e.g., sodium bicarbonate injection) because incompatibility can occur.

VASOPRESSOR AMINES

Sympathomimetic vasopressor agents comprise a group of synthetic substances possessing both direct and indirect adrenergic activity. Their predominant pharmacologic effect is to induce generalized vasoconstriction, and they are primarily indicated for the management of acute hypotensive situations such as those associated with cardiac arrest, circulatory shock, drug reactions, and complications of general anesthesia. They are potent drugs and must be used with extreme care.

The adrenergic amines used for their acute pressor effects include the three endogenous catecholamines discussed previously, in addition to the four vasopressor amines discussed below.

Mephentermine
Wyamine

MECHANISM
Produces both direct adrenergic receptor activation (primarily alpha$_1$) and an indirect action through release of norepinephrine. Pressor effect involves both increased cardiac output (beta activation of the heart) and peripheral vasoconstriction (alpha activation of blood vessels)

USES
Hypotension secondary to ganglionic blockade or spinal anesthesia
Maintenance of blood pressure in shock following hemorrhage while fluid replacement is accomplished

DOSAGE
IM, IV: 30 mg to 45 mg in a single injection (30-mg supplements as needed to maintain blood pressure)

IV infusion: 0.1% (1.0 mg/mL) in 5% dextrose by continuous infusion at a rate of 1.0 mg/min; two 10-mL vials (30 mg/mL) added to 500 mL of 5% dextrose in water

FATE
Rapid onset following IM or IV administration; duration of pressor effect is 2 to 3 hours IM and 30 to 60 minutes IV; readily excreted as metabolites in the urine; minimal effects on the CNS

COMMON SIDE EFFECTS
Occasional anxiety

SIGNIFICANT ADVERSE REACTIONS
(Occasionally with large doses) Tremor, arrhythmias, drowsiness, hypertension, incoherence, and convulsions

CONTRAINDICATIONS
Patients receiving MAO inhibitors, halothane or related anesthetics or chlorpromazine. *Cautious use* in the presence of hypertension, cardiovascular disease, hyperthyroidism, or occlusive vascular disease and in debilitated or severely ill patients

INTERACTIONS
Pressor effects may be potentiated by MAO inhibitors, tricyclic antidepressants, sympathomimetic amines, and oxytocic drugs.
May cause arrhythmias if used in combination with cyclopropane, halothane, or digitalis.
Pressor effects can be antagonized by guanethidine and reserpine
Hypotensive effects of chlorpromazine may be potentiated by mephentermine

NURSING CONSIDERATIONS

Nursing Alerts
- Monitor blood pressure, pulse, and ECG constantly during IV administration (every 2 min until stabilized, then every 5–15 min for duration of drug action). Rate of infusion and duration of therapy are regulated according to patient response. Used to treat hemorrhagic shock only until blood volume is replaced.
- With repeated injections, evaluate patient response to detect development of tolerance. Dosage should *not* be increased to compensate.
- To prevent hypotension, give prescribed IM injection 10 to 20 minutes prior to spinal anesthesia.

Metaraminol
Aramine

MECHANISM
Pressor effect is largely due to peripheral vasoconstriction resulting from a direct alpha-adrenergic receptor agonistic action; cardiac beta stimulation probably plays only minor role in pressor response; reflex bradycardia is common. Drug can also deplete norepinephrine stores in adrenergic nerve endings. Systolic and diastolic blood pressure rises, but perfusion of vital organs may decrease

USES
Acute hypotensive states associated with spinal anesthesia
Adjunctive management of hypotension caused by brain dam-

age, hemorrhage, surgery, drug reactions, septicemia, or cardiogenic shock

DOSAGE

IM, SC: 2 mg to 10 mg (prevention of hypotension)

IV injection: 0.5 mg to 5 mg followed by infusion of 15 mg to 100 mg in 500 mL 5% dextrose

IV infusion (preferred in shock): 15 mg/500 mL to 100 mg/500 mL 5% dextrose; rate adjusted to maintain desired blood pressure (Pediatric: IV—0.01 mg/kg; as a single dose)

FATE

Onset 1 to 2 minutes with IV infusion, 10 minutes with IM and 10 to 20 minutes with SC; effects persist 15 to 60 minutes; partly excreted in the urine and partly taken up by adrenergic nerve endings; weak CNS stimulatory effect

COMMON SIDE EFFECTS

Restlessness, headache, flushing, sweating, palpitations

SIGNIFICANT ADVERSE REACTIONS

(Usually with large doses) Tachycardia, anginal pain, arrhythmias, severe hypertension, convulsions, cardiac arrest, and cerebral hemorrhage. Prolonged use may perpetuate the shock state by preventing volume expansion; hypotension may occur after termination of the drug

CONTRAINDICATIONS

Combined use with halothane or related halogenated hydrocarbon anesthetics or MAO inhibitors, pulmonary edema, metabolic acidosis, use as the sole treatment in cases of hypovolemic shock. *Cautious use* in patients with hypertension, hyperthyroidism, diabetes, cirrhosis, and in patients taking digitalis drugs

INTERACTIONS

Pressor effects may be enhanced by sympathomimetics, MAO inhibitors, tricyclic antidepressants, guanethidine, reserpine, oxytocics, and ergot alkaloids.

Arrhythmias may develop in combination with halogenated hydrocarbon anesthetics or digitalis.

NURSING CONSIDERATIONS

Nursing Alerts

- Monitor blood pressure closely during infusion (every 2–5 min).
- Regulate infusion rate carefully. Use microdrip IV administration set and infusion control device if available. Change flow rate cautiously because drug has a prolonged effect, and accumulation can occur if rate is too rapid.
- Monitor intake and output because renal response may fluctuate. Monitor patient with cirrhosis for excessive water, sodium, and potassium loss because drug may cause diuresis.
- Withdraw drug gradually because severe hypotension often occurs following abrupt termination.

1. Use larger veins whenever possible and avoid extravasation because tissue necrosis and sloughing can occur.
2. Because response may be erratic when shock and acidosis coexist, ascertain whether blood volume is to be corrected before initiating administration.
3. Ensure that atropine is readily available to treat reflex bradycardia.
4. Seek clarification if prescribed for SC administration because necrosis is likely to occur if given SC.

Methoxamine

Vasoxyl

MECHANISM

Direct alpha-adrenergic receptor stimulant, producing extensive vasoconstriction with little or no effects on the heart or the CNS; may induce reflex bradycardia, which is abolished by atropine; reduces renal blood flow

USES

Restoration or maintenance of blood pressure during anesthesia

Termination of paroxysmal supraventricular tachycardia

DOSAGE

I. *Hypotension*
   A. IV: 3 mg to 5 mg by slow injection
   B. IM (usual route): 10 mg to 15 mg just prior to anesthesia; repeat if necessary in 15 minutes
II. *Paroxysmal supraventricular tachycardia*
   A. IV: 10 mg by slow injection

FATE

Onset is 10 to 15 minutes after IM injection; immediately with IV use; duration 1 to 2 hours; not distributed to CNS; excretion is by way of the kidneys

COMMON SIDE EFFECTS

Paresthesias, pilomotor stimulation, bradycardia, coldness in the extremities

SIGNIFICANT ADVERSE REACTIONS

Sustained hypertension, urinary urgency, severe headache, and vomiting

CONTRAINDICATIONS

With local anesthetics to prolong their action; advanced cardiovascular disease. *Cautious use* in patients with hypertension, hyperthyroidism, or myocardial damage, and following parenteral injection of the ergot alkaloids

INTERACTIONS

See metaraminol

NURSING CONSIDERATIONS

Nursing Alert

- Continuously monitor blood pressure and heart rate during and for some time following administration. Be particularly alert for sudden changes when drug therapy is terminated.

1. Measure urinary output and report any significant changes because urinary retention may occur.
2. Ensure that atropine is available to treat severe bradycardia.

Phenylephrine Parenteral
Neo-Synephrine

MECHANISM

Direct, powerful activation of alpha-adrenergic receptors, resulting in marked vasoconstriction and reflex bradycardia; little direct effect on the heart or the CNS; most vascular beds are constricted

USES

Maintenance of blood pressure during spinal and inhalation anesthesia
Treatment of shock or drug-induced hypotension
Treatment of paroxysmal supraventricular tachycardia
Production of vasoconstriction for regional analgesia (added to local anesthetic solution)

DOSAGE
  I. *Hypotension*
     A. SC, IM: 2 mg to 5 mg of a 1% solution
     B. IV: 0.1 mg to 0.5 mg of a 0.1% solution (may repeat in 15 min)
     C. IV infusion: 100 to 200 drops/min of a 1:50,000 solution until pressure is stabilized, then 40 to 60 drops/min for maintenance
     D. Pediatric: 0.1 mg/kg SC or IM
 II. *To prolong spinal anesthesia*
     2 mg to 5 mg added to anesthetic solution
III. *Tachycardia*
     0.5 mg IV injection over 20 to 30 seconds; may increase by 0.1-mg increments as needed

FATE

Rapid acting following injection; duration of effects is 20 to 30 minutes with IV and 45 to 90 minutes with SC and IM

COMMON SIDE EFFECTS

Palpitations, tingling in extremities, reflex bradycardia, and lightheadedness

SIGNIFICANT ADVERSE REACTIONS

Tachycardia, arrhythmias, tremor, dizziness, hypertension, and weakness

CONTRAINDICATIONS

Severe hypertension, cardiac dysrhythmias, and coronary artery disease *Cautious use* in patients with hyperthyroidism, myocardial damage, partial heart block, arteriosclerosis, and severe hypertension, and in elderly patients

INTERACTIONS

See metaraminol

NURSING CONSIDERATIONS

Nursing Alerts
- Check blood pressure and heart rate often during infusion. Maintain desired levels by carefully controlling infusion rate.
- Inform physician if early symptoms of overdosage (fullness in the head, tachycardia, numbness or tingling of extremities) appear.
- Ensure that an alpha-adrenergic blocking agent (e.g., phentolamine) is always on hand to treat a hypertensive emergency.
- Discard cloudy or discolored solutions.

NASAL DECONGESTANTS

Desoxyephedrine	Phenylpropanolamine
Ephedrine	Propylhexedrine
Epinephrine	Pseudoephedrine
Naphazoline	Tetrahydrozoline
Oxymetazoline	Xylometazoline
Phenylephrine	

Adrenergic drugs may be administered either orally or intranasally for the relief of nasal congestion. They provide a prompt decongestant effect, especially when applied topically to the nasal mucosa. They exert a direct vasoconstrictive action on the arterioles in the mucosa, thereby reducing local blood flow, fluid exudation, and mucosal edema. Tolerance to this decongestant effect develops rapidly, however, particularly with use of nasal sprays, and continued use often leads to the appearance of "rebound congestion," characterized by hyperemia and edema of the mucosal membrane. This condition can occur in as short a period as 1 week. Most of the clinically important nasal decongestants have a reasonably long duration of action and are usually used only twice a day. A general discussion of adrenergic nasal decongestants is followed by more specific prescribing information concerning each individual drug in Table 12-3.

MECHANISM

Direct activation of alpha-adrenergic receptor sites on smooth muscle of the nasal mucosal blood vessels; vasoconstriction reduces engorgement of mucosa and fluid exudation, thereby relieving congestion; mucus secretion may also be reduced; orally effective nasal decongestants exert a more generalized vasoconstrictive action and a less intense nasal mucosal decongestant action

USES

Relief of nasal congestion associated with allergic reactions, colds, acute and chronic inflammatory states, and hay fever
Adjunctive therapy in middle ear infections (reduces congestion around eustachian tubes)
Relief of pressure and pain due to ear block during air travel

DOSAGE
See Table 12-3

FATE

Topically applied drugs exert a rapid effect that persists for several hours, up to 12 hours readily absorbed through mucous membranes; large doses may exert systemic effects

COMMON SIDE EFFECTS

Stinging and burning of the nasal mucosa, sneezing, dryness of mucosa, and headache; prolonged use results in rebound congestion

SIGNIFICANT ADVERSE REACTIONS
(Usually observed following systemic absorption of topically applied drugs or with oral use) Palpitations, tachycardia, hypertension, arrhythmias, nervousness, insomnia, dizziness, blurred vision. Severe overdosage and significant absorption may cause marked somnolence, sedation, hypotension, bradycardia, and coma

CONTRAINDICATIONS
Narrow-angle glaucoma, concurrent therapy with MAO inhibitors or tricyclic antidepressants. *Cautious use* in the presence of hypertension, angina, hyperthyroidism, diabetes and arteriosclerosis

INTERACTIONS
Systemic effects may be potentiated by other sympathomimetics, MAO inhibitors, tricyclic antidepressants, antihistamines, and thyroxine.

NURSING CONSIDERATION
1. Instill drops with patient in lateral, head-low position to minimize possibility of swallowing solution and consequent systemic absorption.

PATIENT EDUCATION
1. Explain the importance of adhering to recommended dosage and avoiding prolonged treatment with topical nasal decongestants because rebound congestion is likely to occur. Suggest patient consult health care provider if relief is not obtained within 5 days.
2. Instruct patient to stop using drug and notify health care provider promptly if anxiety, irregular or very fast heartbeat, change in blood pressure, or difficulty in breathing occurs (signs of developing systemic toxicity).
3. Teach patient to keep spray bottle upright to ensure that a fine mist is expelled rather than a liquid stream that can cause overdosage.
4. Instruct patient to blow nose prior to nasal instillation to clear nasal passages.
5. Instruct patient using an inhaler to close one nostril while inhaling through open nostril.
6. Instruct patient to rinse spray or dropper tip in hot water after nasal instillation to prevent contamination from nasal secretions. The same container should never be used for more than one person.

OPHTHALMIC DECONGESTANTS

Epinephrine	Phenylephrine
Hydroxyamphetamine	Tetrahydrozoline
Naphazoline	

Sympathomimetics used in ophthalmology are employed primarily to induce arteriolar vasoconstriction and pupillary dilation by means of their strong alpha-adrenergic effects. Depending on the strength of the different preparations, these drugs have a number of indications. The stronger solutions of phenylephrine (2.5%, 10%) as well as 1% hydroxyamphetamine are used mainly in diagnostic eye examinations, during ocular surgery, and to prevent synechiae formation in uveitis. Medium strength solutions (0.5%, 1%, and 2% epinephrine) are indicated in open-angle glaucoma, whereas the weaker solutions (0.1% epinephrine, 0.012% and 0.02% naphazoline, 0.08%, 0.12%, and 0.15% phenylephrine, and 0.05% tetrahydrozoline) are principally employed for symptomatic relief of minor eye irritations due to allergies, colds, wind, pollens, and so forth. These weaker solutions are available over the counter, whereas the stronger solutions require a prescription.

The principal advantages of these drugs over the anticholinergic preparations that have many of the same actions in the eye are that ophthalmic decongestants do not cause cycloplegia (i.e., paralysis of accommodation) nor do they increase intraocular pressure. Owing to their mydriatic effect, however, they are contraindicated in *narrow-angle* glaucoma because refraction of the iris would further impair the already reduced drainage of aqueous humor resulting from occlusion of the channels by the abnormally positioned iris. A general review of this class of drugs is followed by a listing of individual drugs in Table 12-4.

MECHANISM
Direct activation of alpha-adrenergic receptor sites leading to constriction of small blood vessels and contraction of the radial muscle, producing pupillary dilation (mydriasis); epinephrine also possesses a beta-adrenergic action, which decreases formation of aqueous humor

USES
(Not all drugs used for each indication; see Table 12-4)
Facilitate examination of the fundus of the eye
Reduce the incidence of synechiae formation in uveitis
Treatment of open-angle glaucoma (increases outflow and decreases production of aqueous humor)
Symptomatic relief of minor eye irritations due to colds, hay fever, dust, wind, and so forth
Dilation of the pupil prior to intraocular surgery

DOSAGE
See Table 12-4

FATE
Onset of mydriatic effect is rapid and persists for several hours

COMMON SIDE EFFECTS
Stinging and burning in the eyes, headache, and blurred vision

SIGNIFICANT ADVERSE REACTIONS
Conjunctival irritation; pigmentation of the eyelids, cornea or conjunctiva; maculopathy with a central scotoma; systemic absorption of significant amounts may lead to palpitations, tachycardia, hypertension, anxiety, sweating, insomnia, dizziness, and pallor

CONTRAINDICATIONS
Narrow-angle glaucoma. *Cautious use* in patients with hypertension, heart disease, diabetes, or cerebral arteriosclerosis

INTERACTIONS
Effects may be potentiated by MAO inhibitors, tricyclic antidepressants, or other sympathomimetic drugs.
Mydriatic effects can be reduced by levodopa.

Table 12-3
Nasal Decongestants

Drug	Preparations
Desoxyephedrine Vicks inhaler	Inhaler: 50 mg
Ephedrine Efed II, Efedron, Va-Tro-Nol	Drops: 0.5% Jelly: 0.6% Capsules: 25 mg, 50 mg Syrup: 11 mg/5 mL, 20 mg/5 mL
Epinephrine Adrenalin	Drops: 0.1%
Naphazoline Privine	Drops: 0.05% Spray: 0.05%
Oxymetazoline Afrin, Dristan Long Lasting, Neosynephrine 12 Hour, Sinex Long Lasting, and several other manufacturers (CAN) Nafrine	Drops: 0.025%, 0.05% Spray: 0.05%
Phenylephrine several manufacturers	Drops: 0.125%, 0.16%, 0.2%, 0.25%, 0.5%, and 1% Spray: 0.2%, 0.25%, 0.5% Jelly: 0.5%
Phenylpropanolamine Propagest, Rhindecon, Sucrets Cold Decongestant Lozenge	Tablets: 25 mg, 50 mg Timed-release capsules: 75 mg Syrup: 12.5 mg/5 mL Lozenges: 25 mg
Propylhexedrine Benzedrex	Inhaler: 250 mg
Pseudoephedrine Afrinol, Neosynephrinol, Novafed, Sudafed, and several other manufacturers (CAN) Eltor-120, Pseudofrin, Robidrine	Tablets: 30 mg, 60 mg Repeat-action tablets: 120 mg Capsules: 120 mg (timed release) Liquid: 15 mg/5 mL, 30 mg/5 mL
Tetrahydrozoline Tyzine	Drops: 0.05%, 0.1%
Xylometazoline Chlorohist Long Acting, Neo-Spray Long Acting, NeoSynephrine II, Otrivin	Drops: 0.05%, 0.1% Spray: 0.1%

Usual Dosage Range

1 to 2 inhalations as needed

Topical: 2 to 3 drops or small amount of jelly every 3 to 4 h
Oral: 25 mg to 50 mg every 3 to 4 h

1 to 2 drops every 4 to 6 h

2 drops or sprays each nostril every 3 to 6 h

Adults: 2 to 3 drops or sprays of 0.05% twice a day
Children under 6: 2 to 3 drops of 0.025% twice a day

Adults: 0.25% to 0.5% solution or spray every 3 to 4 h
Children (6–12 yr): 0.25% solution every 3 to 4 h
Infants: 0.125% to 0.2% solution every 2 to 4 h

Adults: 25 mg every 4 h *or* 50 mg every 8 h *or* 75 mg every 12 h
Children: (6–12 yr) 12.5 mg every 8 h
(2–6 yr) 6.25 mg every 8 h

1 to 2 inhalations as needed

Adults: 60 mg every 4 to 6 h *or* 120 mg every 12 h
Children: 15 mg to 30 mg every 4 to 6 h

Adults: 2 to 4 drops 0.1% every 3 to 4 h
Children (2–6 years): 2 to 3 drops 0.5% every 3 to 4 h

Adults: 2 to 3 drops or sprays every 8 to 10 h
Children: 2 to 3 drops 0.05% every 8 to 10 h

Nursing Implications

Avoid excessive use; headache may occur

Avoid swallowing nose drops because systemic effects may occur; do not use drops or jelly longer than 4 days; other uses are discussed under Bronchodilators, Table 12-5

Do not use in children under 6; avoid prolonged or excessive use; *see also* epinephrine under Endogenous Catecholamines and Table 12-4

Insomnia is not a problem, so drug may be given at bedtime; naphazoline is incompatible with aluminum; may produce CNS depression; ophthalmic drops also available; *see* Table 12-4

Long-acting preparation; do not exceed twice-a-day dosage; do not use in children under 2 yr; limit usage to 14 days maximum

Jelly is placed into nasal cavity and gently inhaled; do not use for prolonged periods, especially in children; avoid swallowing solution because systemic effects can occur

Do not exceed recommended dosage, especially in children because side effects are likely to occur; reserpine can antagonize effects of phenylpropanolamine; also available over the counter as an anorexiant of questionable efficacy, either alone or in combination with caffeine; *see* Summary, Section VIII

Do not overuse because CNS stimulation can occur; may induce headache and temporary elevation of blood pressure

Fewer side effects, less pressor action, and longer duration than ephedrine; rebound congestion is minimal; avoid taking drug near bedtime because stimulation can occur; do not use if restlessness, dizziness, tremors, or other signs of CNS excitation are present

Large doses may induce CNS depression; not recommended in children under 2 yr; ophthalmic drops also available; *see* Table 12-4

Effects persist 4 to 8 h; do not use in aluminum containers; do not exceed recommended dosage because systemic effects are likely

Table 12-4
Ophthalmic Decongestants

Drug	Preparations
Epinephrine Several manufacturers	Drops 0.1%, 0.25%, 0.5%, 1.0%, and 2%
Hydroxyamphetamine Paredrine	Drops: 1%
Naphazoline Ak-Con, Albalon, Allerest, Clear-Eyes Comfort, Degest-2, Muro's Opcon, Nafazair, Naphcon, VasoClear, Vasocon	Drops: 0.012%, 0.02%, 0.03%, 0.05%, and 0.1%
Phenylephrine Ak-Dilate, Ak-Nefrin, Isopto Frin, Mydfrin, Neo-Synephrine	Drops: 0.12%, 2.5%, and 10%
Tetrahydrozoline Clear and Bright, Murine 2, Opt-Ease, Soothe Eye, Tetracon, Tetrasine, Visine	Drops: 0.05%

Arrhythmias with digitalis drugs and halogenated hydrocarbon anesthetics (e.g., cyclopropane, halothane) can occur in the presence of sympathomimetics, although the incidence with ophthalmic application is rare.

NURSING CONSIDERATION
1. Check concentration of drops carefully before administration. Stronger concentrations (2.5%–10%) are used for diagnostic eye examinations and during ocular surgery; intermediate strengths (0.5%–2%) are used to treat glaucoma; and weaker concentrations (0.05%–0.1%) are used to treat minor eye irritations.

PATIENT EDUCATION
1. Instruct patient to adhere to recommended dosage because systemic absorption can occur.
2. Inform older patient that blurred vision (i.e., rebound miosis) can occur within 1 day after termination of drug use. If the drug is used again, it may be less effective in eliciting mydriasis.
3. Advise patient that some preparations may stain contact lenses.
4. Instruct patient to discard cloudy or discolored solution.

BRONCHODILATORS

Sympathomimetic bronchodilators are employed in the treatment of bronchial asthma and other chronic obstructive pulmonary diseases (COPDs). Parenteral (i.e., SC, IM) injections of epinephrine are usually effective in relieving respiratory distress (dyspnea, wheezing, chest tightness) during an acute asthmatic attack. However, some patients respond poorly to epinephrine during an acute attack; such patients are often successfully treated by IV infusion of aminophylline, a xanthine bronchodilator discussed in Chapter 55. Continual symptomatic management of chronic asthma may be accomplished with oral or inhaled use of one of the adrenergic bronchodilators, although several other types of drugs (e.g., theophylline, corticosteroids, ipratropium, cromolyn) may be employed as well. These other drugs will also be considered in Chapter 55.

Sympathomimetic agents used as bronchodilators possess prominent *beta*-adrenergic activity that elicits relaxation of the smooth muscle of the bronchioles. This action is primarily due to an elevation in the levels of cyclic AMP resulting from activation of the enzyme adenyl cyclase, which catalyzes formation of cyclic AMP from ATP.

Some drugs in this category (epinephrine, isoproterenol) activate all beta-adrenergic receptor sites, and their use is often associated with a disturbing range of side effects, particularly involving cardiac stimulation. Other adrenergic bronchodilators (e.g., albuterol, metaproterenol) exhibit a greater degree of selectivity with regard to the beta$_2$ receptors located on bronchiolar smooth muscle, and thus elicit a lower incidence of cardiac side effects, although *complete* separation of beta$_1$ and beta$_2$ activity has still not been realized, especially at elevated doses. The relative popularity of the adrenergic bronchodilators is determined by many factors, including the type and severity of the condition being treated, physician preference, patient acceptance, and cost. Epinephrine and isoproterenol are potent bronchodilators whose use is somewhat restricted by their tendency to cause a considerable amount of cardiac excitation in many patients. They have been discussed earlier in

Usual Dosage Range	Nursing Implications
1 to 2 drops 0.1% to 0.25% individualized to condition	*See* general discussion of epinephrine
1 to 2 drops as needed	Pupillary dilation persists for several hours; used for eye exams, ocular surgery, and uveitis
1 to 2 drops every 3 to 4 h	Mainly used as an ocular decongestant; 0.012% to 0.05% solutions available over the counter, 0.1% by prescription only; available in combination with pheniramine (Naphcon-A) and antazoline (Albalon-A, Vasocon-A)
10%: uveitis, open-angle glaucoma, prior to intraocular surgery 2.5%: refraction, ophthalmic exams, prior to surgery 0.02% to 0.15%: ocular decongestion, relief of minor eye irritations	Do not use 10% solution in children; prior instillation of a local anesthetic in the eye may alleviate much of the stinging and burning caused by phenylephrine; the 2.5% solution may be used as a diagnostic test for narrow-angle glaucoma; also available over the counter combined with zinc sulfate (e.g., Zincfrin), or by prescription only combined with pyrilamine (Prefrin-A) or pheniramine (Ak-Vernacon); drug has a narrow safety margin; may cause rebound miosis in the elderly; readministration may be less effective
1 to 2 drops 2 or 3 times/day	Mainly used to relieve minor symptoms of eye irritation; available without perscription

the chapter. Ephedrine is a less potent bronchodilator which exhibits more pronounced central excitatory effects than other adrenergic drugs. It is discussed below, as is ethylnorepinephrine, another nonselective beta agonist. Finally, the selective beta$_2$ agonists are considered as a group and then listed in Table 12-5. Other types of drugs used as bronchodilators (e.g., theophylline) are discussed in Chapter 55.

Ephedrine
(*See also* Table 12-3)

MECHANISM
Direct activation of both alpha- and beta-adrenergic receptor sites, and indirect action through release of norepinephrine from presynaptic nerve terminals; effects include tachycardia, increased blood pressure and cardiac output, mydriasis, and relaxation of bronchiolar and GI smooth muscle; bronchodilation is less intense than that produced by epinephrine but is more prolonged; central stimulatory effects are more pronounced than with epinephrine. Contracts urinary sphincter; may potentiate cholinergic neurotransmission at the neuromuscular junction.

USES
Bronchodilation in milder forms of chronic pulmonary diseases (e.g., bronchial asthma, bronchitis)
Relief of nasal mucosal congestion (see Table 12-3).
Maintenance of blood pressure during spinal anesthesia, and control of postural hypotension (injection only)
Treatment of enuresis (with atropine)
Treatment of narcolepsy
Support of ventricular rate in Adams–Stokes syndrome
Treatment of overdosage with CNS depressants
Adjunctive treatment of myasthenia gravis (with cholinesterase inhibitor)

DOSAGE
Adults: 25 mg to 50 mg PO, SC, IM, or slow IV injection every 3 to 4 hours as necessary (not to exceed 150 mg/24 h)
Children: 2 mg/kg/day to 3 mg/kg/day in 4 to 6 divided doses PO, SC, or IV

FATE
Readily absorbed orally or parenterally; onset of bronchodilation is 30 minutes orally and 10 minutes IM or SC; effects persist 3 to 5 hours orally and 1 to 2 hours IM or SC; crosses blood–brain barrier and exerts a central stimulating effect; excreted largely unchanged in the urine

COMMON SIDE EFFECTS
Similar to epinephrine; in addition, nervousness, anxiety, and insomnia due to central stimulatory properties are common

SIGNIFICANT ADVERSE REACTIONS
Tachycardia, confusion, delirium, tremors (usually observed with large doses); vertigo, sweating, palpitations, urinary retention, arrhythmias; CNS and respiratory depression can occur with overdosage

CONTRAINDICATIONS
Narrow-angle glaucoma, patients receiving MAO inhibitors, severe hypertension, or severe coronary artery disease. *Cautious*

use in persons with chronic heart disease, diabetes, hypertension, and hyperthyroidism

INTERACTIONS

Pressor effects may be increased by ergot alkaloids, MAO inhibitors, furazolidone, and oxytocics.

Ephedrine may reduce the action of guanethidine.

Ephedrine may be less effective in the presence of methyldopa or reserpine.

Arrhythmias can occur if used in combination with halothane and related anesthetics or digitalis drugs.

NURSING CONSIDERATIONS

Nursing Alert
- When drug is given IV, monitor blood pressure frequently until patient is stabilized.

1. Clarify prescription of prolonged-acting forms of high dosages for the elderly because they are more prone to develop hallucinations, convulsions, and CNS depression.

PATIENT EDUCATION

1. Explain the importance of adhering carefully to recommended dosage because central stimulatory effects can lead to abuse.
2. Inform patient that drug effects may diminish with prolonged use. A drug-free interval of several days may be needed to restore effectiveness.
3. Suggest that patient discuss insomnia with drug prescriber if it becomes a problem. Night-time doses and long-acting preparations should be avoided if possible.
4. Urge older patient to notify drug prescriber immediately if difficulty in urinating occurs.

Ethylnorepinephrine

Bronkephrine

Ethylnorepinephrine is an adrenergic bronchodilator similar in most respects to isoproterenol. It primarily activates beta-adrenergic receptor sites; its alpha effect is considerably less than that of epinephrine, hence the effect on blood pressure is less marked.

The principal application of ethylnorepinephrine is relief of bronchospasm; however, it is usually reserved for acute attacks, inasmuch as it must be administered IM or SC. Onset of action is 5 to 10 minutes, and effects last 1 to 2 hours. The adult dose is 1 mg to 2 mg (0.5 mL–1.0 mL), while children receive 0.1 mL to 0.5 mL according to weight. Refer to the discussion of isoproterenol earlier in the chapter for additional information.

SELECTIVE BETA$_2$ AGONISTS

Albuterol	Metaproterenol
Bitolterol	Pirbuterol
Isoetharine	Terbutaline

The selective beta$_2$ bronchodilators preferentially activate beta$_2$ receptor sites on bronchiolar and other smooth muscle at normal dosage levels, leading to relaxation. The absence of significant beta$_1$-receptor activity at recommended dosage reduces the degree of cardiac excitability frequently observed with nonselective beta agonists such as isoproterenol or epinephrine. When beta agonists are administered by inhalation, bronchodilation is comparable to that seen with isoproterenol. Certain beta$_2$ agonists are also available for oral or parenteral use (see Table 12-5) for either long-term (oral) or acute (SC) symptomatic management of bronchial asthma. The beta$_2$ agonists will be reviewed as a group, then detailed individually in Table 12-5.

MECHANISM

In recommended doses, preferentially activate beta$_2$ adrenergic receptors, thereby relaxing bronchiolar, vascular, and uterine smooth muscle to varying degrees; action at cardiac beta$_1$ receptors is generally minimal, thus tachycardia and increased cardiac output are rarely significant

USES

Relief of reversible bronchospasm associated with asthma and other bronchospastic disorders

Delay premature labor (investigational use only)

DOSAGE

See Table 12-5

FATE

Inhaled drugs have a rapid onset of action, generally within 5 minutes; following oral or SC administration, effects are noted within 15 to 30 minutes; duration of action ranges from 2 to 4 hours with inhalation (up to 8 h with bitolterol); effects persist 4 to 8 hours following oral administration; excretion is largely by the kidney, both as unchanged drug and metabolites

COMMON SIDE EFFECTS

(Usually with oral dosage) Nervousness, mild tremor, flushing, sweating, irritability, insomnia, headache, weakness

SIGNIFICANT ADVERSE REACTIONS

Palpitations, tachycardia, arrhythmias, chest discomfort, increased blood pressure, dysuria, nausea, muscle cramping, coughing

CONTRAINDICATIONS

Tachyarrhythmias, severe coronary artery disease; use in combination with halogenated hydrocarbon general anesthetics. *Cautious use* in patients with mild to moderate coronary artery disease, hypertension, hyperthyroidism, diabetes; also in elderly or debilitated persons

INTERACTIONS

Effects of selective beta$_2$ agonists may be potentiated by other sympathomimetics, MAO inhibitors, and tricyclic antidepressants and inhibited by nonselective beta-adrenergic blocking agents (see Chap. 13)

NURSING CONSIDERATIONS

Nursing Alerts
- When drug is used parenterally, assess cardiovascular status periodically because toxicity can occur. Specificity for beta$_2$ sites is observed principally following oral administration.

- If more than one sympathomimetic agent is prescribed, ensure that administration times are alternated. Excessive tachycardia can occur if more than one drug is administered at the same time.

1. Seek clarification before administering more than two SC injections 15 to 30 minutes apart. Other measures should be used if patient does not respond to second injection.

PATIENT EDUCATION
1. Teach patient how to administer an aerosol dose.
2. Stress the importance of adhering to recommended dosage and frequency of use because excess use can result in drug toxicity with serious complications such as acute asthmatic crisis or cardiac arrest.
3. Instruct patient to use only one inhaled medication at a time unless others are specifically prescribed.
4. Instruct patient to notify drug prescriber and stop using drug immediately if breathing difficulty increases with drug use, because severe side effects can develop. Increased airway resistance (paradoxical bronchospasm) sometimes develops after repeated use.
5. Advise patient to notify prescriber if usual dose does not provide relief for a sufficient period. Prolonged use may lead to shorter duration of action (tolerance).
6. Inform patient that a bad taste can occur with oral inhalation, but this will gradually disappear with repeated usage.

SMOOTH MUSCLE RELAXANTS

The ability of several adrenergic drugs to relax smooth muscle has led to their use in the treatment of peripheral vascular insufficiency and premature labor.

Nylidrin and isoxsuprine are two orally effective sympathomimetics that exhibit a beta-adrenergic receptor agonistic action. Activation of beta$_2$ receptor sites in skeletal muscle vasculature can lead to vasodilation of normal vessels. However, the vasodilator effects of nylidrin and isoxsuprine on muscle blood flow are *not* prevented by beta blockers. Thus, these drugs also probably exert a direct relaxant effect on vascular smooth muscle in addition to their beta-agonistic action. Even though blood flow in normal resting skeletal muscle can be increased by these drugs, there is *no* conclusive evidence that they have a beneficial effect in chronic occlusive vascular conditions such as arteriosclerosis or thromboangiitis obliterans. It is probable that skeletal muscle and cerebral vascular beds are dilated by reflexes stimulated by ischemia resulting from a vascular occlusion. This means that peripheral vasodilator drugs primarily increase blood supply to *nondilated, nonischemic* areas that are not in critical need of improved perfusion. Further compromising their efficacy is the fall in blood pressure that frequently accompanies their administration. Thus, their hypotensive effect may actually *reduce* cerebral blood flow and perfusion of vital organs. Therefore, use of nylidrin and isoxsuprine for treating peripheral and cerebral vascular insufficiency should be discouraged.

Isoxsuprine has also been used to delay premature labor, because it also exerts a relaxant effect on uterine smooth muscle. Its effects are nonselective, however, and side effects due to beta-receptor activation elsewhere in the body are frequent. Use of isoxsuprine as a uterine relaxant has been largely supplanted by ritodrine, another beta-agonist that exerts a somewhat more selective effect on beta$_2$ receptors in the uterus. These three sympathomimetic smooth muscle relaxants are discussed below.

Isoxsuprine
Vasodilan

MECHANISM

Activation of beta-adrenergic receptor sites on vascular smooth muscle, diminishing vascular resistance and increasing resting blood flow in skeletal muscles; also exerts a direct relaxant effect on vascular smooth muscle; exhibits some alpha-adrenergic blocking action, and high doses may inhibit platelet aggregation and lower blood viscosity; increases heart rate and contractile force and relaxes uterine smooth muscle

USES

(Clinical effectiveness has not been demonstrated conclusively)

Symptomatic treatment of peripheral vascular insufficiency (e.g., Raynaud's disease, thromboangiitis obliterans) or cerebrovascular insufficiency

Treatment of dysmenorrhea, premature labor, and threatened abortion (experimental uses only)

DOSAGE
Orally: 10 mg to 20 mg 3 or 4 times/day

FATE
Peak effects occur in about 1 hour and persist 2 to 3 hours; largely excreted in the urine

COMMON SIDE EFFECTS
Lightheadedness, lethargy, and flushing

SIGNIFICANT ADVERSE REACTIONS
Hypotension, palpitations, tachycardia, dizziness, nausea, anxiety, abdominal distress, vomiting, and rash

CONTRAINDICATIONS
Arterial bleeding; immediate postpartum use. *Cautious use* in patients with coronary artery insufficiency, thyrotoxicosis, paroxysmal tachycardia, also following a myocardial infarction

INTERACTIONS
Effects may be antagonized by other sympathomimetic drugs (particularly those possessing significant alpha activity).

NURSING CONSIDERATIONS

Nursing Alerts
- Assess peripheral vascular status periodically. Individuals with extensive circulatory impairment may not respond to the drug. Inform physician if condition deteriorates (e.g., numbness, coldness, paresthesias).
- When drug is used for relief of premature labor (experimental use only), carefully monitor pattern of contractions. Dosage and rate of administration are adjusted accordingly.

1. Monitor blood pressure and pulse in standing and lying positions frequently during treatment, especially with IM use.

Table 12-5
Selective Beta₂ Adrenergic Bronchodilators

Drug	Preparations
Albuterol Proventil, Ventolin (CAN) Novosalmol	Inhaler: 90 µg/metered dose Tablets: 2 mg, 4 mg Extended release tablets: 4 mg Syrup: 2 mg/5mL Solution for inhalation: 0.83 mg/mL, 5 mg/mL
Bitolterol Tornalate	Aerosol: 0.8% (delivers 0.37 mg per inhalation)
Isoetharine Arm-a-Med Isoetharine, Beta-2, Bronkometer, Bronkosol, Dey-Dose Isoetharine, Dey-lute, Disorine, Dispos-a Med Isoetharine	Solution for nebulization: 0.062%, 0.08%, 0.1%, 0.125%, 0.14%, 0.167%, 0.17%, 0.2%, 0.25%, 0.5%, 1%
Metaproterenol Alupent, Metaprel	Tablets: 10 mg, 20 mg Syrup: 10 mg/5 ml Aerosol inhaler: 225 mg (0.65 mg/dose) Solution for nebulization: 0.6%, 5%
Pirbuterol Maxair	Aerosol inhaler: 0.2 mg delivered per inhalation
Terbutaline Brethaire, Brethine, Bricanyl	Tablets: 2.5 mg, 5 mg Injection: 1 mg/ml Aerosol: 0.2 mg delivered per dose

PATIENT EDUCATION
1. Teach measures to help control postural hypotension if it occurs. See **Plan of Nursing Care 8 (Antihypertensive Drugs)** in Chapter 31 for specific information.
2. Instruct patient to notify drug prescriber promptly at first sign of a skin rash.
3. Inform patient that beneficial effects may not appear for several weeks. They are usually indicated by cessation of numbness, coldness, or tingling in the extremities.
4. Teach patient how to care for feet and legs (hygiene, measures to minimize trauma).
5. Teach adjunctive measures that may help alleviate condition (e.g., exercise, cessation of smoking, proper footware).

Nylidrin
Arlidin
(CAN) PMS Nylidrin

MECHANISM
Activation of vascular beta receptors, relaxing arteriolar smooth muscle and reducing circulatory resistance; also exerts a direct relaxant effect on vascular smooth muscle; cardiac output is slightly increased and blood pressure is reduced; cerebral blood flow is usually not altered significantly

USES
(Clinical effectiveness has not been demonstrated conclusively)

Usual Dosage Range

Inhalation: 1 to 2 inhalations every 4 to 6 h
Prevention of exercise induced bronchospasm:
  2 inhalations 15 min prior to exercise
Oral: 2 mg to 4 mg 3 to 4 times/day
  (maximum 32 mg/day)
Children (2–6 yr): 0.1 mg/kg 3 times/day
Children (6–14 yr): 2 mg 3 or 4 times/day

2 inhalations at an interval of 1 to 3 min; a third inhalation may be given if necessary
Prevention of bronchospasm: 2 inhalations every 8 h

Solution: 3 to 7 inhalations of undiluted solution by a hand nebulizer *or* 0.25 mL to 0.5 mL of a 0.5% or 1% solution diluted 1:3 with saline or other diluent (lower strength solutions are given undiluted) by oxygen aerosolization or IPPB apparatus
Aerosol nebulizer: 1 to 2 inhalations as needed

Oral:
Adults: 20 mg 3 or 4 times/day
Children (6–9 yr): 10 mg 3 or 4 times/day
Children (under 6 yr): 1.3 to 2.6 mg/kg/day
Inhalation: 10 inhalations of 5% solution by hand nebulizer or 2 or 3 inhalations of metered-dose aerosol inhaler every 3 to 4 h to a maximum of 12 inhalations/day

2 inhalations every 4 to 6 h (maximum 12 inhalations/day)
Oral:
Adults: 2.5 mg to 5 mg 3 times/day (maximum 15 mg/day)
Children over 12 yr: 2.5 mg 3 times/day
SC: 0.25 mg; repeat in 15 to 30 min if needed; if no response after two doses, seek alternate measures
Aerosol: 2 inhalations, 1 min apart, every 4 to 6 h
To delay premature labor: (investigational) 10 µg/min IV infusion titrated upward to a maximum of 80 µg/min

Nursing Implications

Gradually absorbed from the bronchioles; onset occurs within 15 min following inhalation and persists for 3 to 4 h; with oral use, onset is 30 min and effects persist for 4 to 6 h; most common side effects are nervousness and tremor (20%), headache (7%), and tachycardia (5%); may delay preterm labor; drug has displayed a tumorogenic potential in animals at high doses; do not use with other sympathomimetic drugs (danger of increased CV side effects)

Used for prophylaxis or treatment of bronchospasm; effects occur within 5 min and persist up to 8 h; longest acting inhaled beta$_2$ agonist; may be used with theophylline or corticosteroids

Relaxes bronchial smooth muscle by an action on beta$_2$ receptors; may also inhibit histamine release; can be administered by IPPB apparatus—see package instructions; do not use if solution is brown or contains a precipitate; avoid contact with the eyes; oxygen flow rate is adjusted to 4 L/min to 6 L/min over 15 to 20 min for oxygen aerosolization; pediatric dosage has not been established

Effects appear almost immediately with inhalation and within 15 to 30 min orally. Duration is 2 to 4 h with inhaler and 4 to 5 h orally; nervousness, tremor, and weakness are common with oral administration of 20 mg; bad taste can occur with oral inhalation but will gradually disappear with repeated use; overdose can lead to cardiac arrest; encourage adherence to prescribed dose

Rapid-acting bronchodilator; effects occur within 5 min; duration of action is 5 to 6 h

Slowly absorbed orally and parenterally. Effects appear within 15 to 30 min and persist 2 to 4 h with SC injection, up to 6 h with inhalation, and 4 to 8 h with oral administration; muscle tremor common with 5-mg oral dose; used by IV infusion to delay premature labor (investigational use); cardiovascular side effects more common with SC injection

---

Symptomatic relief of peripheral vasospastic disorders (e.g., diabetic vascular disease, acrocyanosis, Raynaud's disease, night leg cramps, ischemic ulcer, frostbite, thrombophlebitis)
Relief of circulatory disturbances of the inner ear (e.g., cochlear cell, macular, or ampullar ischemia; labyrinthine artery spasm)

DOSAGE
Orally: 3 mg to 12 mg 3 or 4 times/day

FATE
Well absorbed orally; maximum effects occur within 30 to 45 minutes and persist for 2 hours; slowly excreted in the urine

COMMON SIDE EFFECTS
Palpitations, nervousness, and weakness

SIGNIFICANT ADVERSE REACTIONS
Dizziness, vomiting, tremors, and hypotension

CONTRAINDICATIONS
Acute myocardial infarction, paroxysmal tachycardia, severe angina, thyrotoxicosis, and uncompensated heart failure. *Cautious use* in the presence of hypertension, cardiac disease, and peptic ulcer

INTERACTIONS
Effects can be antagonized by other sympathomimetic agents having pressor effects.

PATIENT EDUCATION

1. Inform patient that beneficial effects may not appear for several weeks.
2. Instruct patient to report the development of palpitations. If they do not subside during therapy, dosage should be reduced.
3. Teach patient proper care for feet and legs (wound cleansing, hygiene).
4. Teach adjunctive measures that may help alleviate condition (e.g., exercise, cessation of smoking, proper footwear).

Ritodrine

Yutopar

Ritodrine is a fairly selective beta$_2$ adrenergic receptor agonist that can inhibit uterine contractions. It is used in the management of premature labor. It is administered initially by IV infusion to arrest contractions, then orally for as long as necessary to prolong pregnancy to the desired extent. Its overall toxicity is somewhat lower than that of other agents employed in premature labor (alcohol, magnesium sulfate, isoxsuprine).

MECHANISM

Activates beta$_2$ receptor sites on uterine smooth muscle, thus reducing the contractile response; also affects beta$_1$ receptors when given in larger doses. Resulting in tachycardia and blood pressure changes

USES

Management of preterm labor in suitable patients, if the gestation is longer than 20 weeks

DOSAGE

Initially, 0.1 mg/min by IV infusion. May be increased by 50 mg/min every 10 minutes to a maximum of 350 mg/min. Continue infusion for 12 hours after labor has ceased. Administer an oral dose of 10 mg 30 minutes before terminating infusion, then 10 mg every 2 hours for 24 hours, then 10 mg to 20 mg every 4 to 6 hours for as long as necessary. Maximum oral dose is 120 mg/day

FATE

Oral bioavailability is approximately 30% of IV dose. Maximum serum levels following oral ingestion occur in 30 to 60 minutes; effective half-life is 1.5 to 2 hours; metabolized in the liver and excreted primarily in the urine, 90% within 24 hours; crosses placental barrier

COMMON SIDE EFFECTS

(Especially with IV infusion) Alterations in maternal and fetal heart rates and blood pressure, transient elevations in blood glucose and insulin levels, hypokalemia, palpitations, nausea, tremors, headache, and erythema

SIGNIFICANT ADVERSE REACTIONS

(Especially with IV infusion) Vomiting, anxiety, nervousness, chest pain, arrhythmias, dyspnea, sweating, chills, weakness, diarrhea, bloating, rash, anaphylactic shock, lactic acidosis, glycosuria

CONTRAINDICATIONS

Before the 20th week of pregnancy, any condition of mother or fetus in which continuation of pregnancy is dangerous (e.g., antepartum hemorrhage, fetal death, eclampsia, pulmonary hypertension), cardiac arrhythmias, severe bronchial asthma, and pheochromocytoma. *Cautious use* in persons with hypertension, diabetes, or cardiac disease

INTERACTIONS

Combined administration of ritodrine and corticosteroids may lead to pulmonary edema.

Effects of other adrenergic amines may be potentiated by ritodrine.

Nonselective beta blockers reduce the effectiveness of ritodrine.

Ritodrine may increase the hypokalemia observed with a number of diuretics.

NURSING CONSIDERATIONS

Nursing Alerts

- Closely monitor maternal pulse rate and blood pressure as well as fetal heart rate, and observe for indications of maternal pulmonary edema (chest pain, dyspnea, sweating).
- Carefully monitor infusion rate to avoid circulatory overload. Use an infusion control device if available.

1. Be prepared to initiate IV infusion if labor recurs during oral drug therapy.
2. Seek clarification if prescribed earlier than the 20th week of gestation because many fetuses are abnormal when labor begins before this time.
3. Discard solution if it is discolored, cloudy, or contains a precipitate.

CNS STIMULANTS AND ANOREXIANTS

The principal adrenergic drugs used for their central stimulatory effects are the amphetamine derivatives and ephedrine. The major indications for these compounds are control of obesity, relief of depression, and treatment of the attention deficit disorder syndrome in children. Because of their profound central excitatory action, they are an often-abused class of drugs. These compounds are discussed in Chapter 27 (CNS Stimulants), and aspects of their abuse potential are reviewed in Chapter 79 (Drugs of Abuse—A Review).

A number of products containing phenylpropanolamine, a sympathomimetic decongestant, in amounts ranging from 25 mg to 75 mg are promoted as over-the-counter nonprescription diet aids (e.g., Acutrim, Control, Dexatrim, Prolamine). Many of these preparations contain other substances as well, such as vitamins, minerals, and grapefruit extract. Phenylpropanolamine is claimed to exert an anorexiant effect by a central action at the level of the appetite control center in the hypothalamus. However, many health professionals doubt its efficacy as an appetite suppressant, and use of the drug, especially at high dosages, should be strictly controlled. Because of its cardiac-stimulating and blood pressure–elevating effects, phenylpropanolamine should not be used by patients with cardiovascular disease, hypertension, diabetes, hyperthyroidism, glaucoma, or renal impairment. Combined use with other sympathomimetics, MAO inhibitors, and tricyclic antidepressants should also be avoided. Phenylpropanolamine administration must be discontinued at once should palpitations, dizziness, or rapid pulse occur. Recommended doses are 25 mg phenylpropanolamine 3 times a day or 50 mg to 75 mg of the long-acting preparations once daily. Continuous use for longer than 3 months is not recommended. The drug must be used in conjunction with a restricted caloric intake.

Selected Bibliography

Abundis J: Hazards of metered-dose bronchodilator inhalers. J Emerg Nurs 11:252, 1985.

Balkam JA: Allergic rhinitis therapy and the nursing mother. Pediatr Nurs March/April: 47, 1981.

Caritis SN: Treatment of preterm labor: A review of therapeutic options. Drugs 26:243, 1983.

Dixon WR, Mosimann WF, Weiner N: The role of presynaptic feedback mechanisms in regulation of norepinephrine release by nerve stimulation. J Pharmacol Exp Ther 209:196, 1979.

Feely J, DeVane PJ, MacLean D: Beta-blockers and sympathomimetics. Br Med J 286:1043, 1983.

Frederiksen MC: Tocolytic therapy with beta-adrenergic agonists. Ration Drug Ther 17(6):1, 1983.

Goldberg LI: Dopamine—Clinical uses of an endogenous catecholamine. N Engl J Med 291:707, 1974.

Henney HR: Knowledge of nurses and respiratory therapists about using cannister nebulizers. Am J Hosp Pharm 41:2403, 1984.

Hoffman BB, Lefkowitz RJ: Alpha-adrenergic receptor subtypes. N Engl J Med 302:1390, 1980.

Huss P, et al: The new inotropic drug, dobutamine. Heart Lung January/February: 121, 1981.

Kelly RB, Deutsch JW, Carlson SS, Wagner JA: Biochemistry of neurotransmitter release. Annu Rev Neurosci 2:399, 1979.

Langer SZ: Presynaptic receptors and their role in the regulation of transmitter release. Br J Pharmacol 60:481, 1977.

McGrath JC: Evidence for more than one type of post-junctional alpha-adrenoceptor. Biochem Pharmacol 31:467, 1982.

Minneman KP, Pittman RN, Molinoff PB: Beta-adrenergic receptor subtypes: Properties, distribution, and regulations. Annu Rev Neurosci 4:419, 1981.

Motulsky HJ, Insel PA: Adrenergic receptors in man. N Engl J Med 307:18, 1982.

Nelson HS: Betla-adrenergic agonists. Chest 82:335, 1982.

Rogers T: Clinical problems in the adult with asthsma. Nurs Clin North Am June:293, 1981.

Webb-Johnson DC, Andrews JL: Bronchodilator therapy. N Engl J Med 297:476, 1977.

SUMMARY. ADRENERGIC DRUGS

Drug	Preparations	Usual Dosage Range
Catecholamines		
Epinephrine *Several manufacturers*	Solution: 1:1000, 1:10,000 Suspension: 1:200, 1:400 Inhalation: 1%, 1.25%, 2.25% Aerosol: 0.16 mg/dose, 0.2 mg/dose, 0.27 mg/dose Nasal drops: 0.1% Ophthalmic drops: 0.25%, 0.5%, 1%, and 2%	*Parenteral* Cardiac arrest: 5 mL to 10 mL 1:10,000 IV every 5 min as required Intracardiac: 3 mL to 5 mL 1:10,000 Intraspinal: 0.2 mL to 0.4 mL 1:1000 added to anesthetic solution Bronchospasm: 0.3 mL to 0.5 mL 1:1000 SC or IM *or* 0.1 mL to 0.3 mL 1:200 SC (Pediatric—0.01 mg/kg 1:1000 SC) With local anesthetic: 1:20,000 to 1:100,000 *Inhalation* 8–15 drops 1%–2% solution *via* nebulizer or metered aerosol (1–5 min between doses) *Nasal* 1 to 2 drops 0.1% 4 times/day *Ophthalmic* 1 to 2 drops 0.25% to 2%
Dipivefrin Propine (An epinephrine prodrug)	Ophthalmic drops: 0.1%	1 drop every 12 h
Norepinephrine Levophed	Injection: 1.0 mg/mL	8 µg/min to 12 µg/min IV infusion (2 mL/min–3 mL/min) of a 4 µg/mL dilution. Maintenance: 2 to 4 µg/min
Dopamine Dopastat, Intropin (CAN) Revimine	Injection (for dilution): 40 mg/mL, 80 mg/mL, and 160 mg/mL Infusion solution: 80 mg/100 mL, 160 mg/100 mL	Initially: 2 µg/kg/min to 5 µg/kg/min IV infusion of diluted solution; increase by 5 µg/kg/min to 10 µg/kg/min to maximum of 50 µg/kg/min

Continued

SUMMARY. ADRENERGIC DRUGS (continued)

Drug	Preparations	Usual Dosage Range
Synthetic Catecholamines		
Isoproterenol Several manufacturers	Injection: 1:5000 (0.2 mg/mL) Sublingual tablets: 10 mg, 15 mg Inhalation solution: 1:100, 1:200, and 1:400 Aerosol: 0.2%, 0.25% Powder: 10 mg, 25 mg per cartridge	*Parenteral* Bronchospasm: 0.01 mg to 0.02 mg 1:50,000 solution IV injection Shock: 0.25 mL/min to 2.5 mL/min 1:500,000 dilution IV infusion Cardiac arrest: 1 mL to 3 mL 1:50,000 IV injection; 1.25 mL/min 1:250,000 IV infusion; 1 mL 1:5000 IM, SC; 0.1 mL 1:5000 intracardiac injection *Sublingual* 10 mg to 20 mg 3 or 4 times/day (Pediatric—5 mg to 10 mg 3 or 4 times/day) *Inhalation* 1 to 2 inhalations 4 to 6 times/day (dose range 45 µg–250 µg)
Dobutamine Dobutrex	Injection: 250 mg/20 mL	IV infusion: 2.5 µg/kg/min to 10 µg/kg/min of a 250 µg/mL to 1000 µg/mL solution in sterile water or 5% dextrose; maximum 40 µg/kg/min
Vasopressors		
Mephentermine Wyamine	Injection: 15 mg/mL, 30 mg/mL	IM, IV: 30 mg to 45 mg single dose; 30 mg supplements as needed IV infusion: 1 mg/min of a 0.1% solution in 5% dextrose
Metaraminol Aramine	Injection: 10 mg/mL	IM, SC: 2 mg to 10 mg IV injection: 0.5 mg to 5 mg IV infusion: 15–100 mg/500 mL 5% dextrose (Pediatric—IV: 0.01 mg/kg as a single dose
Methoxamine Vasoxyl	Injection: 20 mg/mL	IV injection: 3 mg to 5 mg (hypotension) IV injection: 10 mg (tachycardia) IM: 10 mg to 15 mg prior to anesthesia
Phenylephrine Neo-Synephrine	Injection: 1% (*See also* Tables 12-3 and 12-4)	SC, IM: 2 mg to 5 mg of a 1% solution IV injection: 0.1 mg to 0.5 mg of a 0.1% solution IV infusion: 100 to 200 drops/min of a 1:50,000 solution until stabilized, then 40 to 60 drops/min (Pediatric—SC, IM: 0.1 mg/kg)
Nasal Decongestants *See* Table 12-3		
Ophthalmic Decongestants *See* Table 12-4		
Bronchodilators		
Ephedrine	Capsules: 25 mg, 50 mg Syrup: 11, 20 mg/5 mL Injection: 25, 50 mg/mL (*See also* Table 12-3)	*Oral and Parenteral:* 25 mg to 50 mg every 3 to 4 h as necessary to a maximum 150 mg/24 h (Pediatric: 6–12 yr; 6.25 mg–12.5 mg every 4–6 h; 2–6 yr; 0.3 mg/kg–0.5 mg/kg every 4–6 h)
Ethylnorepinephrine Bronkephrine	Injection 2 mg/mL	SC, IM: 1 mg to 2 mg (0.5 mL–1.0 mL) (Pediatric: 0.1 mL–0.5 ml)
Selective Beta₂ Adrenergic Bronchodilators	*See* Table 12-5	

Continued

SUMMARY. ADRENERGIC DRUGS (continued)

Drug	Preparations	Usual Dosage Range
Smooth Muscle Relaxants		
Isoxsuprine Vasodilan	Tablets: 10 mg, 20 mg	Oral: 10 mg to 20 mg 3 to 4 times/day
Nylidrin Arlidin (CAN) PMS Nylidrin	Tablets: 6 mg, 12 mg	Oral: 3 mg to 12 mg 3 to 4 times/day
Ritodrine Yutopar	Tablets: 10 mg Injection: 10 mg/mL	Initially, 0.1 mg/min IV infusion; increase by 50 µg/min every 10 min to maximum of 350 µg/min; continue for 12 h after labor has ceased; begin oral dosage (10 mg) 30 min before terminating infusion, then 10 mg every 2 h for 24 h, then 10 mg to 20 mg every 4 to 6 h for as long as needed
CNS Stimulants and Anorexiants		
Amphetamines	*See* Chapter 27	
Anorexiants	*See* Chapter 27	
Phenylpropanolamine Acutrim, Dexatrim, and several other manufacturers	Tablets: 25 mg Capsules: 37.5 mg Timed-release capsules: 50 mg, 75 mg Timed-release tablets: 75 mg	25 mg 3 times/day or 50 mg to 75 mg timed-release once daily

13 ADRENERGIC BLOCKING DRUGS

Several types of pharmacologic agents are capable of interfering with the functioning of the sympathetic nervous system as well as the actions of exogenous adrenergic drugs. Certain compounds can either deplete the catecholamine stores in adrenergic nerve endings or retard release of the catecholamine neurotransmitters (e.g., norepinephrine) from the nerve ending. These drugs are often termed *adrenergic neuronal blockers;* they serve primarily as antihypertensive drugs and are considered in Chapter 31. Other antiadrenergic agents antagonize the actions of sympathomimetic amines at adrenergic receptor sites in body tissues. These drugs, termed *adrenergic receptor blockers,* are effective antagonists of either exogenously administered adrenergic compounds or endogenous catecholamines released from sympathetic nerve endings.

Reflecting the accepted classification of adrenergic receptor sites into alpha and beta types, the adrenergic receptor blockers are likewise separated into alpha-adrenergic and beta-adrenergic blocking agents, and the delineation is essentially complete for most of the currently available drugs (i.e., most alpha blockers do not block beta sites and vice versa). However, adrenergic blocking drugs have been developed that display a greater selectivity for alpha and beta receptor subtypes. Thus, while some alpha blockers (e.g., phentolamine, tolazoline) are nonselective and block both alpha$_1$ and alpha$_2$ receptors, others (e.g., phenoxybenzamine, prazosin) are selective for the alpha$_1$ site. Similarly, beta-adrenergic blocking agents can be grouped into selective beta$_1$ blockers (e.g., atenolol and metoprolol) and nonselective (i.e., beta$_1$ and beta$_2$) blockers such as nadolol, propranolol, pindolol, and timolol. With both alpha and beta blockers, the greater specificity of action of the selective blockers reduces many of the undesirable side effects associated with nonselective adrenergic blockade.

ALPHA-ADRENERGIC BLOCKING AGENTS

Compounds capable of blocking the actions of different agonists at the alpha-adrenergic receptor sites are termed *alpha blockers*. Postsynaptic (i.e., alpha$_1$ blocking) agents act primarily on alpha sites located on vascular smooth muscle to antagonize the pressor (vasoconstrictive) effects of epinephrine and norepinephrine. In addition, the shorter-acting drugs (see below) exert a direct relaxant effect on vascular smooth muscle that contributes to the peripheral vasodilation seen with these drugs. They also exert a cardiac stimulant action that may cause tachycardia. Blockade of presynaptic (alpha$_2$) sites on sympathetic nerve endings, like that seen with yohimbine, increases release of norepinephrine from the nerve ending. This action has limited clinical usefulness but is a valuable laboratory tool.

Among the clinically useful drugs with alpha-adrenergic blocking activity are the following:

1. *Prolonged-acting, noncompetitive antagonists* (e.g., phenoxybenzamine): form a stable bond with alpha receptor site; blockade can persist for days or even weeks.
2. *Reversible, competitive antagonists* (e.g., phentolamine, prazosin, terazosin, tolazoline): form a reversible, competitive blockade at alpha site that persists for only a few hours; can be overcome by larger amounts of agonist (e.g., norepinephrine); prazosin and terazosin are selective alpha$_1$ antagonists used as antihypertensive agents and will be reviewed in Chapter 31.
3. *Ergot alkaloids* (e.g., ergotamine): possess some alpha-blocking action but primarily exert a direct *spasmogenic* action on vascular smooth muscle, causing vasoconstriction. Used primarily for relief of vascular headaches; reviewed in Chapter 14.

Phenoxybenzamine
Dibenzyline

MECHANISM

Long-acting, essentially noncompetitive alpha-adrenergic blockade exerted principally at postsynaptic alpha$_1$ sites; forms stable covalent bond with receptor site, possibly inducing structural alterations; increases blood flow to skin, mucosa, and viscera; induces orthostatic hypotension; may exhibit antihistaminic and antiserotonin activity at high dosages

USES

Control hypertension and sweating associated with pheochromocytoma

Improve circulation in vasospastic peripheral vascular diseases (e.g., Raynaud's, acrocyanosis, frostbite; effectiveness not conclusively determined)

DOSAGE

Individually titrated to obtain symptomatic relief with minimal side effects

Initially: 10 mg orally daily. Increase by 10 mg every 4 days. Usual range 20 mg to 60 mg daily (may require several weeks to obtain optimal effect)

FATE

Oral absorption is erratic (20%–30% absorbed in active form); peak effects occur in 4 to 6 hours; may accumulate in adipose tissue at high dosages; excreted largely through the kidney and bile, mostly within 24 hours

COMMON SIDE EFFECTS

Lightheadedness, nasal congestion, dryness of the mouth, flushing, tachycardia, miosis, and GI irritation (if given on empty stomach)

SIGNIFICANT ADVERSE REACTIONS

Dizziness, orthostatic hypotension, weakness, failure of ejaculation; overdosage can cause vomiting, CNS stimulation, and shock

CONTRAINDICATIONS

Congestive heart failure or other conditions when a drop in blood pressure might be dangerous. *Cautious use* in the presence of cerebral, coronary, or renal insufficiency

INTERACTIONS

May increase blood pressure–lowering effects of antihypertensive agents

May enhance the hypotensive and cardiac stimulant effects of epinephrine

NURSING CONSIDERATIONS

Nursing Alerts
- Monitor blood pressure and heart rate and rhythm in both erect and recumbent positions during periods of dosage adjustment and for at least 4 days thereafter. Dosage should not be increased sooner than 4 days following previous increase.
- If severe hypotension occurs and norepinephrine (levarterenol) infusion is used, keep patient flat for 24 hours; apply abdominal binder and support hose or bandages to legs as necessary. Epinephrine should *not* be used because a further drop in blood pressure can occur due to unmasking of the beta effect.
- Use precautions for postural hypotension. See **Plan of Nursing Care 8 (Antihypertensive Drugs)** in Chapter 31 for specific information.

1. Monitor patient for signs of clinical improvement (e.g., increased skin color and temperature, less sensitivity to cold). In patients with pheochromocytoma, reductions in blood pressure and pulse are indications of effectiveness.

PATIENT EDUCATION
1. Teach patient techniques that help control postural hypotension. See **Plan of Nursing Care 8 (Antihypertensive Drugs)** in Chapter 31 for specific information.
2. Inform patient that palpitations, rapid heart rate, and postural hypotension will disappear with continued therapy.
3. Inform patient that beneficial effects may not appear for several weeks.
4. Suggest taking drug with meals to minimize GI irritation.
5. Warn patient that symptoms of respiratory infection may be aggravated by the drug and must be treated with appropriate therapy. The health care provider should be contacted for treatment.

Phentolamine
Regitine

MECHANISM
Reversible, competitive antagonism at presynaptic and postsynaptic alpha receptor sites and direct relaxant action on vascular smooth muscle; decreases peripheral vascular resistance and pulmonary pressure; slightly increases heart rate and cardiac output; GI motility may be stimulated (parasympathomimetic action), and secretion of pepsin and hydrochloric acid (histamine-like action) can be increased

USES
Control of hypertension in patients with pheochromocytoma during stress periods and prior to or during surgical excision of tumor
Prevention of tissue necrosis and sloughing associated with extravasation of norepinephrine or other vasopressors
Diagnosis of pheochromocytoma (measurement of urinary catecholamines is the preferred diagnosis)
Treatment of hypertensive crises or rebound hypertension following withdrawal of antihypertensive drugs (investigational use only)

DOSAGE
Hypertension: IV, IM—5 mg (adults), 1 mg (children)
Prevent necrosis: 10 mg added to each liter IV infusion *or* 5 mg to 10 mg in 10 mL saline infiltrated into area within 12 hours

FATE
Onset is rapid following IV or IM use; effects persist for 15 minutes with IV use and several hours following IM injection; excreted largely as metabolites in the urine

COMMON SIDE EFFECTS
Flushing, nasal congestion, and GI distress

SIGNIFICANT ADVERSE REACTIONS
(Usually following parenteral use) Tachycardia, hypotension, arrhythmias, anginal pain, myocardial infarction, shock, and cerebrovascular occlusion

CONTRAINDICATIONS
Recent myocardial infarction, coronary insufficiency, and angina. *Cautious use* in patients with peptic ulcer, gastritis, coronary artery disease, or congestive heart failure

INTERACTIONS
See **phenoxybenzamine**

NURSING CONSIDERATIONS

Nursing Alerts
- Keep patient supine while drug is given IV. Monitor blood pressure and pulse frequently until stabilized. Overdosage should be treated vigorously and promptly.
- Question the use of epinephrine to treat hypotension resulting from overdosage because unmasking of beta effect may increase drop in blood pressure.
- Use precautions for postural hypotension. See **Plan of Nursing Care 8 (Antihypertensive Drugs)** in Chapter 31.

1. Minimize GI irritation by giving drug with meals or milk.

Tolazoline
Priscoline

MECHANISM
Reversible nonselective blockade of alpha-adrenergic receptor sites and direct relaxant effect on vascular smooth muscle; also exhibits significant beta-adrenergic activity (increased cardiac rate, force, and output), cholinergic activity (increased GI motility), and histaminergic activity (increased gastric secretions)

USES
Adjunctive management of persistent pulmonary hypertension in the newborn when sufficient oxygenation cannot be maintained by usual supportive care
Improved blood flow in spastic peripheral vascular disorders associated with acrocyanosis, arteriosclerosis obliterans, thromboangiitis obliterans, gangrene, and various other conditions. (Efficacy has not been established, and the drug is rated only "possibly effective")

DOSAGE

Pulmonary hypertension: 1 to 2 mg/kg via scalp vein; follow with infusion of 1 to 2 mg/kg/h until arterial oxygen has risen sufficiently

Improve blood flow: 10 mg to 50 mg SC, IM, or IV (infrequently used)

FATE

Maximal effects occur within 30 to 60 minutes IM or SC; duration of action 3 to 4 hours; excreted largely unchanged by the kidney

COMMON SIDE EFFECTS

Flushing, tingling or loss of sensation in extremities, nausea, and reflex tachycardia

SIGNIFICANT ADVERSE REACTIONS

Arrhythmias, anginal pain, orthostatic hypotension, ulcer-like pain, vomiting, epigastric distress, duodenal perforation, apprehension, rash, edema, oliguria, hematuria, pulmonary hemorrhage

CONTRAINDICATIONS

Coronary artery disease, cerebrovascular insufficiency

INTERACTIONS

See **phenoxybenzamine**

NURSING CONSIDERATIONS

Nursing Alerts
- See **phentolamine**. In addition:
- Assess status of patient's skin periodically: Flushing in extremities, increased temperature, and piloerection indicate optimal dosage.
- If hypotension occurs because of overdosage, place patient flat. The best treatment consists of IV fluids and infusion of ephedrine, not epinephrine or norepinephrine.

PATIENT EDUCATION

1. Warn patient that ingestion of alcohol with tolazoline may cause a disulfiram-like reaction (e.g., tachycardia, sweating, dyspnea, vomiting). See Chapter 78.
2. Inform patient that most side effects disappear with continued therapy.
3. Suggest that patient avoid overexposure to cold environments because drug effectiveness is enhanced in warm surroundings.

BETA-ADRENERGIC BLOCKING AGENTS

Acebutolol	Metoprolol
Atenolol	Nadolol
Betaxolol	Penbutolol
Carteolol	Pindolol
Esmolol	Propranolol
Labetalol	Timolol
Levobunolol	

Drugs capable of exerting a reversible, competitive blocking action at beta-adrenergic receptor sites can antagonize the effects of catecholamines released from adrenergic nerve endings as well as from the adrenal medulla. Beta-blocking agents effectively reduce the myocardial stimulant, vasodilator, bronchodilator, and metabolic (glycogenolytic, lipolytic) actions of the catecholamines.

The beta blockers may be classified as nonselective or selective. Nonselective beta antagonists (carteolol, levobunolol, nadolol, penbutolol, pindolol, propranolol, timolol) block both $beta_1$ and $beta_2$ receptor sites, whereas selective beta blockers (acebutolol, atenolol, betaxolol, esmolol, metoprolol) at the dosages usually administered exert their blocking effects *predominantly* at $beta_1$ receptors. The selectivity of certain drugs for cardiac $beta_1$ sites is relative, however, and is dose dependent. That is, in high concentrations, the beta-blocking actions of the "selective" $beta_1$ blockers may also extend to the $beta_2$ receptors, such as those in the bronchioles.

All the available beta-receptor blockers are effective competitive antagonists at the various beta receptors, but a number of differences exist in the properties of the individual drugs. A brief comparison of some of the pharmacologic and pharmacokinetic properties of the beta blockers is presented in Table 13-1. Labetalol, a combined beta and alpha blocker, is included in the table but is considered in greater detail in Chapter 31, as it is used exclusively as an antihypertensive agent. Esmolol, a rapid-acting beta blocker used to control excessive heart rate, is also discussed along with the other beta-blockers.

Although the beta blockers are discussed as a group, characteristics of individual drugs are noted where differences are important. Beta blockers are then individually listed in Table 13-2, along with the dosage ranges and pertinent information regarding each. Additional information relating to the respective uses (e.g., antianginal, antihypertensive, antiarrhythmic) of specific beta blockers can be found in chapters dealing with specific uses. A listing of currently approved as well as investigational uses for beta blockers is presented in Table 13-3.

MECHANISM

Reversible competitive blocking action at beta-adrenergic receptor sites (see Table 13-1 for site specificity), resulting in decreased heart rate and force of contraction, slowed atrioventricular (AV) conduction, decreased plasma renin, and lowered blood pressure; a quinidine-like membrane-stabilizing action is exhibited by propranolol and to a lesser extent by metoprolol and pindolol. Pindolol and carteolol also possess intrinsic sympathomimetic activity (ISA) and consequently reduce the heart rate less than other beta blockers. Central effects of beta blockers are exerted at the level of the vasomotor center in the brainstem to retard the outflow of tonic sympathetic nerve impulses. In the eye, beta blockers reduce formation of aqueous humor without inducing miosis or hyperemia. Platelet aggregation may be impaired, possibly through inhibition of thromboxane A_2 synthesis

USES

See Tables 13-2 and 13-3

DOSAGE

See Table 13-2

FATE

(*See also* Table 13-1) Oral absorption is generally good except for atenolol and nadolol. First-pass hepatic metabolism is signifi-

Table 13-1
Pharmacologic and Pharmacokinetic Properties of Beta Blockers

Drug	Receptor Activity	Oral Absorption	Protein Binding	Elimination Half-Life	Membrane-Stabilizing Activity[a]	Intrinsic Sympatho-mimetic Activity[a]
Acebutolol Sectral	$beta_1$	90%	25%	3 h–4 h	0	+
Atenolol Tenormin	$beta_1$	50%	5%–15%	6 h–9 h	0	0
Betaxolol Betoptic	$beta_1$	(ophthalmic use only)			0	0
Carteolol Cartrol	$beta_1$, $beta_2$	80%	20%–30%	4 h–6 h	0	+ +
Esmolol Brevibloc	$beta_1$		50%–60%	10 min–20 min	0	0
Levobunolol Betagan	$beta_1$, $beta_2$	(ophthalmic use only)			0	0
Metoprolol Lopressor	$beta_1$	95%–100%	10%–15%	3 h–6 h	+	0
Nadolol Corgard	$beta_1$, $beta_2$	30%	30%	18 h–24 h	0	0
Penbutolol Levatol	$beta_1$, $beta_2$	95%–100%	80%–100%	4 h–6 h	0	+
Pindolol Visken	$beta_1$, $beta_2$	95%–100%	40%–50%	3 h–4 h	+	+ + +
Propranolol Inderal	$beta_1$ $beta_2$	90%–100%	90%–95%	3 h–6 h	+ +	0
Timolol Blocadren, Timoptic	$beta_1$, $beta_2$	90%–95%	10%	3 h–4 h	0	0
Labetalol[b] Normodyne, Trandate	$beta_1$ $beta_2$	100%	50%	6 h–8 h	+	0

[a] Refer to the discussion of mechanism of beta blockers in the text for an explanation of these characteristics.
[b] Also possesses $alpha_1$ blocking activity and $beta_2$ agonist activity.

cant for acebutolol, metoprolol, propranolol, and timolol; thus interpatient plasma levels vary widely. Food enhances the bioavailability of propranolol and metoprolol. Protein binding is minimal with the exception of penbutolol and propranolol. Acebutolol, atenolol, carteolol, and nadolol do not readily pass the blood–brain barrier because their lipid solubility is low. Carteolol and nadolol are excreted largely unchanged by the kidney. The remaining beta blockers are metabolized in the liver and are excreted as metabolites and unchanged drug by the kidney. Elimination half-lives are rather short (3–6 h), except for atenolol and carteolol (6–9 h) and nadolol (16–24 h)

COMMON SIDE EFFECTS
(Not all effects seen with all drugs) Drowsiness, lightheadedness, lethargy, nausea, paresthesias, cramping, and bradycardia

SIGNIFICANT ADVERSE REACTIONS
(Not all reactions seen with all drugs)
Cardiovascular: tachyarrhythmias, chest pain, AV block, sinoatrial block, peripheral arterial insufficiency, pulmonary edema, syncope, cerebrovascular accident, cardiac failure
CNS (decreased incidence with acebutolol, atenolol, carteolol, and nadolol): dizziness, vertigo, depression, weakness, behavioral disturbances, agitation, disorientation, memory loss, emotional instability, sleep disturbances, bizarre dreams, hallucinations, catatonia
GI: diarrhea, vomiting, gastric pain, anorexia, bloating, dry mouth, ischemic colitis, hepatomegaly
Respiratory: bronchospasm, dyspnea, cough, rales, nasal congestion
Musculoskeletal: joint pain, muscle cramping
Dermatologic: rash, pruritus, skin irritation, sweating, dry skin, increased pigmentation
Other: hypoglycemia, alopecia, acute pancreatitis, agranulocytosis, thrombocytopenia, eosinophilia, urinary difficulty, fever, sore throat, psoriasis-like rash, blurred vision, elevated BUN, serum transaminase, alkaline phosphatase, lactic dehydrogenase

CONTRAINDICATIONS
Sinus bradycardia, greater than first-degree heart block, right ventricular failure, severe congestive heart failure, cardiogenic shock, in combination with drugs potentiating adrenergic amines (such as MAO inhibitors or tricyclic antidepressants); in addition, nonselective beta blockers are contraindicated in bronchial asthma. *Cautious use* in patients with nonallergic bronchospasm (e.g., chronic bronchitis, emphysema), peripheral vascular insufficiency, history of allergies, allergic rhinitis (especially during the pollen season), impaired renal or hepatic function, diabetes, or myasthenia gravis

INTERACTIONS
Beta blockers can have additive cardiac depressant effects with digitalis, phenytoin, verapamil, and quinidine

(Text continued on page 109)

Table 13-2
Beta-Adrenergic Blocking Agents

Drug	Preparations	Usual Dosage Range	Nursing Implications
Acebutolol *Sectral*	Capsules: 200 mg, 400 mg	*Hypertension:* Initially 400 mg daily in 1 single or 2 divided doses; usual maintenance dose range is 400 mg–800 mg daily *Ventricular Arrhythmias:* 200 mg twice a day initially; increase gradually until optimal response; usual dosage range is 600 mg–1200 mg daily	Selective beta$_1$ blocker used for hypertension and controlling ventricular premature beats; may be taken without regard to meals; reduce dosage in elderly persons because plasma levels are higher; use cautiously in impaired renal or hepatic function; low lipid solubility; does not significantly pass blood–brain barrier
Atenolol *Tenormin*	Tablets: 50 mg, 100 mg	*Hypertension:* Initially, 50 mg once a day; increase to 100 mg once a day if necessary after 1–2 wk *Angina:* 50 mg once a day; may increase to 100 mg once a day if necessary	Long-acting, selective beta$_1$ antagonist; minimal protein binding; dosage may have to be reduced in patients with significant renal failure because drug is excreted unchanged in the urine; does not pass blood–brain barrier; long half-life allows once-daily dosing—drug should be taken same time every day; available with chlorthalidone as Tenoretic
Betaxolol *Betoptic*	Ophthalmic solution: 0.5%	1 drop twice a day	Used for treating ocular hypertension and chronic open-angle glaucoma; may be given alone or in combination with other antiglaucoma drugs; onset of action is 30 min and effects persist up to 12 h; little effect on pupil size or accommodation; discomfort and tearing may occur upon instillation; virtually devoid of systemic side effects
Carteolol *Cartrol*	Tablets: 2.5 mg, 5 mg	*Hypertension:* 2.5 mg–5 mg once daily	Nonselective beta-blocker used for treatment of mild to moderate hypertension; possesses intrinsic sympathomimetic activty, thus heart rate and cardiac output are reduced to a smaller extent than with most other beta-blockers; excreted largely unchanged in the urine—caution in persons with kidney impairment
Esmolol *Brevibloc*	Injection: 10 mg/mL, 250 mg/mL	*Supraventricular tachycardia:* 50–200 µg/kg/min following a loading dose infusion of 500 µg/kg/min for 1 min	Short-acting cardioselective beta blocker indicated for rapid control of ventricular rate in patients with atrial fibrillation or flutter where short-term control of ventricular rate is desirable; usually administered for 24–48 h; venous irritation is associated with infusion concentrations greater than 10 mg/mL; rapidly metabolized by enzymes in red blood cells; plasma half-life is 10–15 min
Labetalol *Normodyne, Trandate*	Tablets: 100 mg, 200 mg, 300 mg Injection: 5 mg/mL	*Hypertension:* *Oral:* Initially, 100 mg twice a day; increase in 100-mg twice-daily increments until desired response; usual maintenance dose is 200 mg–400 mg, twice daily *IV:* 20 mg by slow IV injection initially; repeat at 10-min intervals with 40 mg or 80 mg to a maximum of 300 mg; or 2 mg/min of a 1-mg/mL dilution by IV infusion to a maximum of 300 mg (usual dosage range is 50 mg–200 mg)	Combined nonselective beta blocker and alpha$_1$ blocker; may also exhibit beta$_2$ agonistic activity; used as an antihypertensive in both acute (IV) and chronic situations; does not elicit marked changes in heart rate, renal function, or cardiac output; postural hypotension can occur; complete discussion of the drug is found in Chapter 31
Levobunolol *Betagan*	Ophthalmic solution: 0.5%	1 drop once or twice a day	(*See* betaxolol.) Onset of acton is 30–60 min; effects persist up to 24 h; greater likelihood of systemic side effects than with betaxolol (e.g., bradycardia, hypotension); frequently causes burning or stinging upon instillation in the eyes; headache and dizziness have also been reported

Continued

Table 13-2
Beta-Adrenergic Blocking Agents (continued)

Drug	Preparations	Usual Dosage Range	Nursing Implications
Metoprolol Lopressor	Tablets: 50 mg, 100 mg Injection: 1 mg/mL	*Hypertension:* Initially, 50 mg orally, twice a day; increase at weekly intervals until optimum effect is attained; usual maintenance dose is 100 mg twice a day (range 100 mg–450 mg/day) *Myocardial infarction:* Three IV bolus injections of 5 mg each at 2-min intervals; then 50 mg orally every 6 h thereafter for 48 h, then 100 mg twice a day	Selective beta$_1$ blocker; well absorbed orally but undergoes significant first-pass hepatic metabolism; weakly protein bound; readily enters the CNS; if twice-daily administration does not provide sufficient blood pressure control owing to short half-life of drug, give 3 times/day in divided doses; ingestion of food enhances oral absorption; during early phase of myocardial infarction, treatment should be initiated as soon as possible; if immediate IV administration is not possible or not tolerated, begin oral therapy (100 mg twice/day) as soon as clinical condition allows; treatment may be continued for months if deemed beneficial; prevention of reinfarction is most dramatic in patients suffering first infarction and presenting with left ventricular failure, cardiomegaly, or atrial fibrillation
Nadolol Corgard	Tablets: 20 mg, 40 mg, 80 mg, 120 mg, 160 mg	*Hypertension:* Initially, 40 mg once daily; increase gradually in 40 mg–80 mg increments; usual dosage range 40 mg–80 mg once daily; maximum dose is 320 mg/day *Angina:* Initially, 40 mg once daily; increase at 3–7 day intervals until desired effect; usual dosage range is 40 mg–80 mg once daily; maximum dose is 240 mg/day	Long-acting, nonselective beta blocker; does not enter CNS; excreted essentially unchanged by kidney, therefore dosage may need to be reduced in renal failure; presence of food does not affect rate or extent (approximately 30%) of absorption; if drug is to be discontinued, taper dosage gradually over 1–2 wk; do not administer more often than once a day
Penbutolol Levatol	Tablets: 20 mg	*Hypertension:* 20 mg once daily	Nonselective beta agonist used for treating mild to moderate hypertension; effects occur within 2–4 wk; larger doses do not seem to provide greater antihypertensive effect
Pindolol Visken	Tablets: 5 mg, 10 mg	*Hypertension:* Initially 5 mg 2 or 3 times/day; adjust dosage at 2–3 week intervals in increments of 10 mg to obtain desired reduction in pressure; maximum dose is 60 mg/day	Nonselective beta antagonist with intrinsic sympathomimetic activity, thus exhibits slightly less slowing of heart rate than other beta blockers; rapidly absorbed orally; peak plasma levels in 1 h; short acting; excreted both as unchanged drug and metabolites; no significant first-pass hepatic metabolism; use is frequently associated with slight weight gain
Propranolol Inderal	Tablets: 10 mg, 20 mg, 40 mg, 60 mg, 80 mg, 90 mg Capsules (sustained-release—SR) 60 mg, 80 mg, 120 mg, 160 mg Injection: 1 mg/mL Oral solution: 20 mg/5 mL, 40 mg/s/mL Concentrated solution: 80 mg/mL	*Hypertension:* Initially, 40 mg twice a day *or* 80 mg SR once daily; increase gradually until desired response; usual dosage range is 120 mg–240 mg/day in 2 or 3 divided doses *or* 120 mg–160 mg SR once daily *Angina:* Initially, 10 mg–20 mg 3 or 4 times/day *or* 80 mg SR once daily; increase at 3–7 day intervals; usual dose is 160 mg/day in single or divided doses *Arrhythmias:* 10 mg–30 mg 3 or 4 times/day *Hypertrophic subaortic stenosis:* 20 mg–40 mg 3 or 4 times day *or* 80 mg–160 mg once daily *Migraine:* Initially, 80 mg once daily or in divided doses; usual dosage range is 160–240 mg/day	Widely used, nonselective beta blocker; well absorbed orally (food enhances absorption), but undergoes extensive first-pass hepatic metabolism, and variations in plasma levels among patients are wide; highly protein bound; excreted largely as metabolites in urine; if treatment of angina is to be discontinued, reduce dose gradually as severe angina or myocardial infarction can be precipitated by abrupt termination; if a satisfactory response in treatment of migraine is not achieved within 4–6 wk after reaching the maximum dose (i.e., 240 mg/day), drug should be discontinued; IV injection should be undertaken with extreme caution, and central venous pressure and ECG closely monitored; transfer to oral therapy as soon as possible

Continued

Table 13-2
Beta-Adrenergic Blocking Agents (continued)

Drug	Preparations	Usual Dosage Range	Nursing Implications
Timolol *Oral:* Blocadren *Ophthalmic:* Timoptic	Tablets: 5 mg, 10 mg, 20 mg Ophthalmic drops: 0.25%, 0.5%	*Oral:* *Hypertension:* Initially, 10 mg twice a day; usual maintenance range is 20 mg–40 mg/day in 2 divided doses *Myocardial infarction:* 10 mg twice a day for long-term prophylaxis following acute phase *Ophthalmic:* *Glaucoma:* 1 drop of 0.25%–0.5% solution twice a day	Nonselective beta antagonist used orally for hypertension, as prophylaxis following an acute myocardial infarction, and as eye drops for the management of chronic open-angle glaucoma; oral absorption is good and protein binding is minimal; oral drug is short acting and may have to be given 3 times/day if response is inadequate; effects in eye begin in 30 min, peak in 1–2 h, and persist up to 24 h; do not give more than 1 drop 0.5% twice a day; add other antiglaucoma drugs if necessary (see Chap. 10); when used intraocularly, systemic effects can occur frequently, especially with prolonged use; systemic absorption can be minimized by instructing patients to press gently on the lacrimal duct after drug administraton; ocular use is contraindicated in patients with bradycardia, second or third degree heart block, congestive heart failure, pulmonary edema, or bronchial asthma.

Table 13-3
Approved and Investigational Uses for Beta Blockers

Indication	Drugs
Approved Uses	
Hypertension	acebutolol, atenolol, carteolol, labetalol, metoprolol, nadolol, penbutolol, pindolol, propranolol, timolol (oral)
Angina	atenolol, metoprolol, nadolol, propranolol
Arrhythmias	acebutolol, esmolol, propranolol
Migraine prophylaxis	propranolol
Hypertrophic subaortic stenosis	propranolol
Reduce risk of reinfarction after acute infarct	metoprolol, propranolol, timolol (oral)
Glaucoma	betaxolol, levobunolol, timolol (ophthalmic)
Pheochromocytoma (adjunctive therapy)	propranolol
Hyperthyroidism (to control cardiac stimulation)	propranolol

Investigational Uses

One or more of the beta blockers have been reported to be of benefit in the following conditions:

Acute pain symptoms	Hypothermia	Spastic colon
Alcohol withdrawal	Insulinoma	Tardive dyskinesia
Anxiety	Lithium-induced tremor	Tetanus
Cardiogenic shock	Mitral stenosis	Tetralogy of Fallot
Digitalis intoxication	Narcolepsy	Ureteral colic
Disseminated intravascular coagulation	Narcotic withdrawal Parkinsonism	Urinary incontinence
Dissecting aorta	Phantom limb pain	
Essential tremor	Pulmonary stenosis	
GI bleeding in cirrhosis	Schizophrenia	
Hemorrhagic shock		

The effects of beta blockers can be reversed by norepinephrine, isoproterenol, dopamine, dobutamine, and other sympathomimetic drugs

Plasma levels of propranolol and possibly other beta blockers can be elevated by chlorpromazine, cimetidine, furosemide, and hydralazine

Beta blockers can antagonize the bronchodilating action of theophylline and may reduce its clearance

The hypotensive action of beta blockers can be increased by diuretics and other antihypertensives and reduced by indomethacin or salicylates

Phenobarbital and phenytoin can reduce plasma levels of beta blockers metabolized in the liver by accelerating their hepatic metabolism

Beta blockers may prolong insulin-induced hypoglycemia and mask the symptoms of lowered blood glucose

Beta-adrenergic blockade may increase the incidence of the "first-dose" orthostatic hypotensive response to prazosin (see Chapter 31)

Propranolol or metoprolol may decrease the clearance of lidocaine

Beta blockers may enhance the muscle-relaxing actions of neuromuscular blocking agents

NURSING CONSIDERATIONS

See **Plan of Nursing Care 3** in this chapter. In addition:

Nursing Alerts

- Before initiating administration, determine whether patient has any condition (e.g., asthma, allergies, congestive heart failure) that might be aggravated by beta blockers.
- When drugs are administered IV, use infusion control device and carefully monitor ECG and blood pressure. Have on hand atropine (for bradycardia), vasopressors (for hypotension), and bronchodilators for emergency use. Patient should be transferred to oral therapy as soon as possible.

1. Withhold drug and seek clarification if prescribed for patient who received an MAO inhibitor drug within past 2 weeks.
2. With nadolol and atenolol, seek clarification if prescription exceeds recommended doses because accumulation can occur. These drugs have long half-lives that permit once-daily dosing.

PATIENT EDUCATION

See **Plan of Nursing Care 3** in this chapter. In addition:

1. Advise patient that if drugs are used for prolonged periods, tests may be performed periodically to assess blood, kidney, and liver function.
2. If angina is present, explain that heart rate and rhythm and exercise capacity may be routinely monitored. Beta blockers should not be continued in patients with angina unless they reduce pain and increase work capacity.
3. Instruct patient to take propranolol and metoprolol during meals; other beta blockers should be taken before meals.

Selected Bibliography

Cruickshank JM: The clinical importance of cardioselectivity and lipophilicity in beta blockers. Am Heart J 100:160, 1980

Doxey JC, Smith CFC, Walker JM: Selectivity of blocking agents for pre- and postsynaptic alpha-adrenoceptors. Br J Pharmacol 60:91, 1977

Fischer RG, Byrd HJ: Beta-adrenergic blocking agents. US Pharmacist Aug:46, 1982

Frishman WH: Beta-adrenoceptor antagonists: New drugs and new indications. N Engl J Med 305:500, 1981

Frishman WH, Furberg CD, Friedenwald WT: Beta-adrenergic blockade for survivors of acute myocardial infarction. N Engl J Med 310:830, 1984

Graham RM: The physiology and pharmacology of alpha and beta blockade. J Cardiovasc Med (Suppl) April 1981

Johnson GP, Johanson BC: Beta blockers: An expert's guide to what's on the market. Am J Nurs 83:1034, 1983

McDevitt DG: Beta-adrenergic blocking drugs and partial agonist activity: Is it clinically relevant. Drugs 25:331, 1983

Ople LH: Drugs and the heart. I. Beta blocking agents. Lancet 1:693, 1980

Pritchard BN, Tomlinson B: The additional properties of beta adrenoceptor blocking drugs. J Cardiovasc Pharm 8(Suppl 4):1, 1986

Vedin JA, Wilhelmsson CE: Beta receptor blocking agents in the secondary prevention of coronary heart disease. Annu Rev Pharmacol Toxicol 23:29, 1983

Wood AJJ: How the beta-blockers differ: A pharmacologic comparison. Drug Ther 13:59, 1983

PLAN OF NURSING CARE 3
PATIENTS TREATED WITH BETA-ADRENERGIC BLOCKERS

Nursing Diagnosis: Potential Alteration in Cardiac Output: Decreased secondary to drug therapy with a beta-adrenergic blocking agent

Goal: Patient will receive treatment for early signs of congestive heart failure.

Intervention	Rationale	Expected Outcome
Before administering drug: 1. Take blood pressure. 2. Take apical pulse for a full minute. Withhold dose and notify appropriate person if pulse is below 50–60 beats/min or another established limit. If indicated, teach patient to monitor heart rate:	Among other beta-blocker effects, inhibition of beta$_1$ adrenergic receptors reduces the rate and force of cardiac contractions (negative chronotropic and inotropic effects). Consequently, cardiac output decreases. Decisions about the degree of bradycardia acceptable for continued drug administration should be made individually.	Patient's blood pressure and pulse will remain within acceptable limits.

Continued

PLAN OF NURSING CARE 3 (continued)
PATIENTS TREATED WITH BETA-ADRENERGIC BLOCKERS

Nursing Diagnosis: Potential Alteration in Cardiac Output: Decreased secondary to drug therapy with a beta-adrenergic blocking agent

Goal: Patient will receive treatment for early signs of congestive heart failure.

Intervention	Rationale	Expected Outcome
1. Instruct to count radial pulse before taking drug. 2. Teach how to take radial pulse. 3. Instruct to notify drug prescriber if pulse is slower than usual, below 50 beats/min, or irregular.		
Observe hospitalized patient for signs of fluid retention: 1. Monitor intake and output. 2. Weigh daily. 3. Check for peripheral edema.	Reduced cardiac output lowers blood pressure and reduces glomerular filtration and sodium excretion. Accumulation of excess fluid may signify developing heart failure.	Patient will be treated promptly if congestive heart failure occurs.
Monitor for signs of impending heart failure: 1. Determine whether patient is experiencing dyspnea on exertion, orthopnea, or night cough. 2. Auscultate lungs to detect pulmonary rales. 3. Check for distended neck veins. Monitor vital signs and fluid balance throughout periods of dosage adjustment. Consult prescriber regarding acceptable parameters.	Serious adverse effects can occur from drug-induced reduction in sympathetic tone in patients who need the stimulation of sympathetic impulses to the heart. Congestive heart failure may occur if cardiac function is already compromised or if other cardiac depressant drugs are administered concurrently. Beta blockers with some intrinsic sympathomimetic activity (ISA), such as pindolol, may be used for patients whose cardiac function is already impaired.	
Teach patient early signs of heart failure and instruct to report signs to drug prescriber immediately.	Heart failure requires prompt treatment with appropriate drugs. If no improvement is noted, the beta blocker should be discontinued.	

Nursing Diagnosis: Potential Knowledge Deficit related to beta-blocker drug therapy

Goal: Patient will possess knowledge needed to implement beta blocker drug regimen and related actions.

Intervention	Rationale	Expected Outcome
See also **Plan of Nursing Care 1 (Knowledge Deficit) and 2 (Compliance)** Emphasize factors significant in compliance: 1. The maximal effect of beta blockers may not be seen for several weeks. 2. Dosage must be carefully and individually titrated during follow-up care.	Compliance may improve if patient is aware of course of action.	Patient will explain important factors related to compliance.
3. All doses of the drug should be taken, particularly if drug is to be taken more than once a day.	Some conditions may be aggravated if medication is not taken regularly.	
4. If angina exists or is suspected, the drug prescriber should be notified before the drug is discontinued.	Angina can be markedly aggravated if drug is stopped suddenly, and arrhythmias or myocardial infarction may occur. If usage is to be terminated, the drug should be slowly withdrawn under prescriber supervision by a gradual decrease in dosage.	
5. Enough medication should be on hand at all times to last through weekends, holidays, or vacations. Suggest patient obtain an extra prescription to carry in billfold or purse in case of emergency.	Prescriptions cannot be refilled when drugstores are closed. An extra prescription can be filled if medication runs out or is lost while patient is away from home.	Patient will state precautions that can be taken to avoid unexpectedly running out of medication.

Continued

PLAN OF NURSING CARE 3 (continued)
PATIENTS TREATED WITH BETA-ADRENERGIC BLOCKERS
Nursing Diagnosis: Potential Alteration in Cardiac Output: Decreased secondary to drug therapy with a beta-adrenergic blocking agent
Goal: Patient will receive treatment for early signs of congestive heart failure.

Intervention	Rationale	Expected Outcome
Teach patient precautions appropriate for reduced responsiveness of sympathetic nervous system and rationale for precautions:		Patient will state potential consequences of reduced sympathetic nervous system activity induced by beta blockers.
1. Avoid driving, using machines, or performing other activities that require alertness until reactions to drug are established. Dyspnea, weakness, fatigue, dizziness, drowsiness, lightheadedness, or reduced alertness are potential side effects. If symptoms continue or get worse, discuss them with drug prescriber.	Safety precautions help avoid accidents and injuries.	Patient will explain precautions for diminished sympathetic nervous system responsiveness induced by beta blockers.
2. Dress warmly during cold weather, and avoid prolonged exposure of extremities to cold, such as in winter sports. Hands and feet may feel cool and be more sensitive to cold. Fingers and toes may tingle.	Blockade of beta$_2$ receptors decreases circulation in the skin, fingers, and toes. Existing peripheral vascular insufficiency may be aggravated.	
3. Discuss an appropriate exercise level with drug prescriber. Chest pain from physical exertion is usually reduced or obliterated by beta blockers, and this may lead to overactivity.	Blockade of beta$_2$ receptors impedes adaptive responses to stress (e.g., vigorous exercise, surgery, fever), such as an increase in the heart rate.	
4. Prior to any surgery, inform physician or dentist in charge that beta blockers are in use.		
5. Wear a tag or carry a medical identification card indicating the drug that is being used.	Emergency health care personnel should know if a patient is taking a beta blocker.	
Teach special precautions necessary for diabetic patient:	Ordinarily, hypoglycemia elicits the release of epinephrine to help convert glycogen to glucose by acting on beta-adrenergic receptors in skeletal muscles and the liver. When beta blockers occupy beta adrenergic receptor sites, glucose cannot be mobilized as readily.	
1. Explain that blood sugar levels may fall and signs of hypoglycemia (e.g., increased pulse rate and blood pressure) may be masked.		
2. Teach patient to recognize signs of hypoglycemia not affected by beta blockers: hunger, fatigue, inability to concentrate.		
3. Advise that it may be necessary to adjust dosage of insulin or other hypoglycemic agent.		
Caution nondiabetic patient that prolonged fasting may greatly potentiate hypoglycemic effects of beta blockers.		
Inform patient that smoking may reduce drug effectiveness.	Smoking may reduce the effectiveness of beta blockers, especially propranolol.	Patient will explain how smoking affects drug action.
See also **Plan of Nursing Care 8 (Antihypertensive Drugs).**		

SUMMARY. ADRENERGIC BLOCKING AGENTS

Drug	Preparations	Usual Dosage Range
Alpha-Adrenergic Blocking Agents		
Phenoxybenzamine Dibenzyline	Capsules: 10 mg	Oral: 10 mg initially; increase by 10 mg every 4 days; usual range 20 mg–60 mg daily
Phentolamine Regitine	Injection: 5 mg/mL	IV, IM: Adults: 5 mg–10 mg Child: 1 mg
Tolazoline Priscoline	Injection: 25 mg/mL	1–2 mg/kg via scalp vein; follow with infusion (1–2 mg/kg/h)
Beta-Adrenergic Blocking Agents *See* Table 13-2		

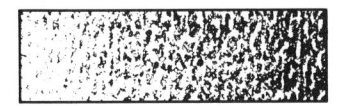

14 ANTIHISTAMINE–ANTISEROTONIN AGENTS

ANTIHISTAMINES

Drugs that competitively block the effects of histamine at various receptor sites in the body are termed antihistamines. Histamine is present in virtually all mammalian tissues, arising from the decarboxylation of the amino acid histidine. Sites of highest histamine concentration in the body include:

- mast cells and basophils, the fixed tissue and circulating histaminocytes, respectively, where histamine is thought to be bound in an inactive complex with heparin and an acidic protein
- gastric mucosal cells, where histamine is not extensively bound
- CNS histamine-containing cells, located primarily in the hypothalamus

Upon release from binding sites or tissue stores, histamine is capable of eliciting a tremendous range of pharmacologic effects, from mild itching to circulatory shock.

The physiologic functions of endogenous histamine (e.g., neurotransmission, gastric acid secretion, tissue growth, repair) remain largely speculative. Its role in several pathologic processes associated with acute and chronic allergic and hypersensitivity reactions is much more clearly established. Histamine can be released from cells by physical and chemical agents, a variety of drugs and toxins, and antigen–antibody reactions; therefore it plays a critical role in the symptomology of many allergic, anaphylactic, and hypersensitivity reactions.

The major pharmacologic actions of histamine are centered on the cardiovascular system, nonvascular smooth muscle, exocrine glands, and the adrenal medulla. The more important pharmacologic effects of histamine are the following:

- arteriolar and venular dilation
- increased capillary permeability
- increased heart rate
- contraction of nonvascular smooth muscle (e.g., bronchoconstriction, GI hypermotility)
- stimulation of gastric hydrochloric acid secretion
- release of catecholamines from the adrenal medulla

These effects of histamine are mediated by an action on two distinct receptors, termed H_1 and H_2 receptor sites. H_1 receptors are those associated with the smooth muscle of the blood vessels, bronchioles, and GI tract, whereas H_2 receptors are found on gastric parietal cells, the myocardium, and certain blood vessels. Thus it appears that the contraction of nonvascular smooth muscle is an H_1 receptor effect, the secretion of gastric acid and acceleration of the heart rate are caused by H_2 receptor activation, and vascular dilation and increased permeability result from a combined action of histamine on both H_1 and H_2 sites.

Clinical uses of histamine are essentially obsolete. Histamine itself and its structural analog betazole (Histalog) were once commonly used in testing for functional achlorhydria (lack of gastric hydrochloric acid), but they have now largely been replaced by a more effective and less toxic diagnostic agent, pentagastrin (Peptavlon), which is discussed in Chapter 76. Histamine phosphate injection (0.275 mg) is occasionally used for presumptive diagnosis of pheochromocytoma (see Chap. 76), but it is a dangerous procedure and should be employed only by persons trained in its administration. The principal importance of histamine lies in its role as mediator of certain pathologic conditions and in the therapeutic value of its antagonism by antihistamine drugs.

Antihistamines are classified as either H_1- or H_2-receptor antagonists, although the H_1 blockers comprise the overwhelming majority of drugs. The term *antihistamine* has come to be associated synonymously with H_1 antagonists. In contrast, the H_2 blockers exert a specific blocking effect on the histamine receptor sites of gastric parietal cells, markedly reducing their output of hydrochloric acid. The clinically available H_2 antagonists are reviewed following the discussion of the H_1 blockers.

H_1 Receptor Antagonists

Astemizole	Diphenhydramine
Azatadine	Diphenylpyraline
Brompheniramine	Doxylamine
Buclizine	Meclizine
Carbinoxamine	Methdilazine
Chlorpheniramine	Promethazine
Clemastine	Pyrilamine
Cyclizine	Terfenadine
Dexchlorpheniramine	Tripelennamine
Dimenhydrinate	Triprolidine

H_1 receptor blockers can be categorized into one of several groups on the basis of their chemical composition (Table 14-1). Certain differences exist among the various groups of H_1 antagonists with regard to the incidence and type of side effects they elicit; these differences are also illustrated in Table 14-1. Clinical efficacy differs significantly from group to group, and certain patients may respond much better to one group of H_1 antagonists than to others.

It is important to recognize that although H_1 antagonists can prevent effector-cell responses to both exogenous and endogenous histamine, they are significantly more effective against the former. Yet *endogenous* histamine is the main cause of most allergic reactions. Moreover, antihistamines are much more useful when given before a histamine challenge rather than after an allergic attack has begun. Finally, antihistamines are effective only to the extent that histamine is the primary causative factor in the allergic response. Therefore, H_1 antagonists are most effective in prevention of seasonal pollinosis and urticaria; somewhat less effective in allergic dermatoses, contact dermatitis, vasomotor rhinitis, serum sickness, and allergic transfusion reactions; and seldom useful alone in bronchial asthma, GI allergies, and systemic anaphylactic reactions.

H_1 receptor antagonists are remarkably similar in most of their actions; therefore, their pharmacology is discussed collectively. A listing of individual drugs is given in Table 14-2.

MECHANISM
Competitive blockade of the actions of histamine at H_1 receptor sites on effector structures (e.g., vascular and nonvascular smooth muscle, salivary and respiratory mucosal glands); also

Table 14-1
Classification of Antihistamines

Chemical Category	Drugs	Characteristics
Alkylamines	brompheniramine chlorpheniramine dexchlorpheniramine triprolidine	Low incidence of drowsiness and moderate GI upset; most widely used antihistamine group
Ethanolamines	carbinoxamine clemastine dimenhydrinate diphenhydramine doxylamine	Moderate to high incidence of drowsiness; minimal GI upset; dimenhydrinate is used for prophylaxis of motion sickness; diphenhydramine and doxylamine used in OTC sleep aids
Ethylenediamines	pyrilamine tripelennamine	Moderately sedating; high incidence of GI upset; pyrilamine used in some OTC sleep aids
Phenothiazines	methdilazine promethazine trimeprazine	High degree of drowsiness; trimeprazine also blocks serotonin; many side effects and contraindications; can be used for motion sickness
Piperazines	cyclizine meclizine	Used principally for prophylaxis of motion sickness
Piperidines	azatadine cyproheptadine diphenylpyraline phenindamine	Sedation is moderate with cyproheptadine and azatadine which also block serotonin
Miscellaneous	terfenadine astemizole	Nonsedating at recommended dosage; long-acting

exert anticholinergic (e.g., drying), antiserotonergic, local anesthetic, and CNS depressent (i.e., sedative) actions

USES

(*Note:* Not all H_1 blockers have *all* of the following indications; refer to Table 14-2 for uses of individual drugs)

Relief of symptoms of certain allergic disorders (e.g., allergic rhinitis, vasomotor rhinitis, uncomplicated urticaria and angioedema, allergic reactions to blood or plasma)

Adjunctive treatment in anaphylactic reactions (with epinephrine and other measures)

Prevention and treatment of motion sickness

Temporary relief of insomnia

Adjunctive therapy for parkinsonism and extrapyramidal reactions due to antipsychotic drug therapy

Relief of coughs caused by colds, allergies, or minor throat irritations

Prevention and control of nausea and vomiting associated with anesthesia or surgery

Adjunct to analgesics for obstetrics and postoperative pain, and for preoperative sedation and relief of apprehension

Local oral anesthesia

DOSAGE

See Table 14-2

FATE

Most drugs are used orally and are well absorbed; onset is normally within 10 to 30 minutes; duration is 3 to 4 hours (sustained-action forms, 8–12 h); metabolized by liver and kidney and excreted largely in the urine, usually as metabolites; readily enter CNS and produce depression; effectiveness not significantly enhanced by parenteral administration; topical forms involve risk of sensitization

COMMON SIDE EFFECTS

Sedation, dizziness, epigastric distress, dryness of mouth, thickened bronchial secretions

SIGNIFICANT ADVERSE REACTIONS

(Frequency and severity vary among different preparations)
Cardiovascular: hypotension, palpitations, tachycardia, arrhythmias
GI: anorexia, nausea, vomiting, diarrhea or constipation
CNS: confusion, restlessness, impaired coordination, blurred vision, vertigo, tinnitus, heaviness and weakness of the hands, nervousness, tremors, paresthesias, irritability, excitation, insomnia, hysteria
Hematologic: hemolytic anemia, thrombocytopenia, leukopenia, pancytopenia, agranulocytosis
Urinary: urinary frequency or retention, dysuria
Respiratory: wheezing, chest tightness, nasal congestion
Hypersensitivity: urticaria, drug rash, photosensitivity, anaphylactic shock
Other: headache, diplopia, sweating, pallor, stinging, or burning at site of injection
With overdosage: fever, ataxia, hallucinations, convulsions, coma, cardiovascular, and respiratory collapse (children are especially susceptible)

CONTRAINDICATIONS

Narrow-angle glaucoma, peptic ulcer, prostatic hypertrophy, GI or bladder obstruction; in premature or nursing infants, elderly or debilitated patients, pregnant or nursing women, patients on

(Text continued on page 119)

Table 14-2
Antihistamines

Drug	Preparations	Usual Dosage Range	Major Uses	Nursing Implications
Astemizole Hismanal	Tablets: 10 mg	Adults and children over 12: 10 mg once a day	Allergic disorders	Long acting largely non-sedating drug; minimal anticholinergic activity; taken on an empty stomach; not recommended in children under 12; can cause headache
Azatadine Optimine	Tablets: 1 mg	1 mg–2 mg twice a day	Allergic disorders	Do not use in children under age 12; has antiserotonin effects as well
Brompheniramine Bromphen, Dimetane, and several other manufacturers	Tablets: 4 mg Tablets: timed-release: 8 mg, 12 mg Elixir: 2 mg/5 mL Injection: 10 mg/mL, 100 mg/mL	*Oral:* Adults: 4 mg–8 mg 3–4 times/day or 8 mg–12 mg timed-release twice a day Children over 6: 2 mg–4 mg 3–4 times/day Children under 6: 0.5 mg/kg daily in divided doses *Parenteral* Adults: 5 mg–20 mg IV, IM, or SC twice a day (maximum 40 mg/day) Children: 0.5 mg/kg/day	Allergic disorders; cough	Keep patient lying down during IV administration; sweating, hypotension, and faintness may occur with IV use; do not use solutions with preservatives IV; may induce agranulocytosis; perform blood counts during prolonged therapy
Buclizine Bucladin-S	Tablets: 50 mg	*Nausea:* 50 mg–150 mg/day *Motion sickness:* 50 mg 30-min before travel, and 50 mg every 4–6 h as needed	Nausea, vomiting, and vertigo; prevention of motion sickness	Tablets may be chewed or swallowed whole—can also be dissolved under tongue; do not use during pregnancy or in small children; may induce headache, nervousness, drowsiness, and dryness of mouth
Carbinoxamine Clistin	Tablets: 4 mg	Adults: 4 mg–8 mg 3 or 4 times/day Children: 2 mg–6 mg 3–4 times/day depending on age	Allergic disorders	Mildly sedating; strong anticholinergic action; good antiemetic
Chlorpheniramine Chlor-Trimeton, Teldrin, and other manufacturers (CAN) Chlorphen, Chlor-Tripolon, Novopheniram	Chewable tablets: 2 mg Tablets: 4 mg Timed-release tablets: 8 mg, 12 mg Timed-release capsules: 8 mg, 12 mg Syrup: 2 mg/5 mL Injection: 10 mg/mL, 100 mg/mL	*Oral:* Adults: 4 mg 3–6 times day or 8 mg–12 mg twice a day (timed-release) Children 6–12: 2 mg 3–6 times/day Children 2–6: 1 mg 3 or 4 times/day *Parenteral* Allergy: 5 mg–20 mg IM, SC (maximum 40 mg/day) Anaphylaxis: 10 mg–20 mg IV	Allergic disorders; transfusion and drug reactions; anaphylactic reactions	May be used prophylactically for blood transfusion; only injection solution used IV is 10 mg/mL; when given IV or added directly to stored blood, do not use solution with preservatives; low incidence of drowsiness and other side effects; has antiemetic, antitussive, and some local anesthetic action; timed-release preparations not recommended in children under age 12; may produce increased sedation in elderly persons

Continued

Table 14-2
Antihistamines (continued)

Drug	Preparations	Usual Dosage Range	Major Uses	Nursing Implications
Clemastine Tavist	Tablets: 1.34 mg, 2.68 mg Syrup: 0.67 mg/5 mL	Adults: 1.34 mg–2.68 mg 2 or 3 times/day (maximum 3 tablets daily)	Allergic disorders	Not recommended in children under age 12; monitor blood levels; can produce hemolytic anemia; use cautiously in the elderly
Cyclizine Marezine (CAN) Marzine	Tablets: 50 mg Injection: 50 mg/mL	*Oral:* 50 mg 30 min before travel; repeat every 4–6 h to a maximum of 300 mg/day (children 6–10 yr—½ adult dose) *IM:* 50 mg every 4–6 h	Prevention and treatment of motion sickness and postoperative nausea and vomiting	Do not use in pregnancy or in children under age 6; produces frequent drowsiness; for postoperative nausea and vomiting give 20–30 min before end of surgery; overdosage may produce hyperexcitability and convulsions; claimed to reduce the sensitivity of the labyrinthine apparatus to motion; store in a cool place; injection may discolor to light yellow—does not affect potency
Dexchlorpheniramine Dexchlor, Poladex, T.D. Polaramine, Polargen	Tablets: 2 mg Repeat-action tablets: 4 mg, 6 mg Syrup: 2 mg/5 mL	Adults: 2 mg 3–4 times a day or 4 mg–6 mg repeat-action tablets twice a day Child: ½ adult dose Infant: ¼ adult dose	Allergic disorders	Low incidence of many common side effects; do not use repeat-action tablets in children; available as an expectorant with pseudoephedrine and guaifenesin
Dimenhydrinate Dramamine, and several other manufacturers (CAN) Gravol, Nauseatol, Travamine	Tablets: 50 mg Liquid: 12.5 mg/mL Injection: 50 mg/mL	*Oral* Adults: 50 mg–100 mg every 4h Children (6–12 yr): 25 mg to 50 mg 3 times/day Children (2–6 yr): up to 25 mg every 6–8 h *IM* Adults: 50 mg as needed Children: 1.25 mg/kg 4 times/day up to 300 mg/day *IV (adults only):* 50 mg in 10 mL sodium chloride given over 2 min	Prevention and treatment of nausea, vomiting and vertigo of motion sickness, radiation sickness, or anesthesia	Drowsiness is common, especially at higher dosages; caution when used in combination with aminoglycoside antibiotics, because it may mask signs of ototoxicity, leading to permanent damage; tolerance develops with continued use; do not mix parenteral solutions with other drugs because many are incompatible; dilute IV solutions with maximum allowable fluid—drug is irritating to veins.
Diphenhydramine Benadryl, and other manufacturers (CAN) Allerdryl, Insomnal	Tablets: 25 mg, 50 mg Capsules: 25 mg, 50 mg Elixir: 12.5 mg/5 mL Syrup: 12.5, 13.3 mg/5 mL Injection: 10 mg/mL, 50 mg/mL Cream: 1% Lotion: 1% Spray: 1%	*Oral* Adults: 25 mg–50 mg 3–4 times/day Children (over 20 lb): 5 mg/kg/day in divided doses *Parenteral—IV or deep IM* Adults: 10 mg–50 mg as needed (maximum 400 mg/day)	Allergic disorders, motion sickness, adjunctive therapy in anaphylactic reactions, prevention of reactions to blood or plasma, sedative in pediatric patients, cough due to colds or allergies, treatment of insomnia, oral anesthesia in	Topical preparations may cause hypersensitivity reactions; high incidence of drowsiness initially, which decreases with use; monitor blood pressure carefully with parenteral use; very low incidence of GI disturbances; found in

Continued

Table 14-2
Antihistamines (continued)

Drug	Preparations	Usual Dosage Range	Major Uses	Nursing Implications
		Children: 5 mg/kg/day in 4 divided doses	dental practice, parkinsonism, acute dystonias	several OTC sleep aids (Sleep-EZE, Sominex 2, Twilite); solution is irritating to tissue—give deep IM and rotate injection sites with every dose.
Diphenylpyraline Hispril	Timed-release capsules: 5 mg	Adults: 5 mg twice a day Children: (over 6): 5 mg daily	Allergic disorders	Do not use in children under age 6
Doxylamine Unisom	Tablets: 25 mg	Adults: 25 mg 20–30 min before bedtime	Insomnia	Drowsiness is common; indicated as a nonprescription sleep aid
Meclizine Antivert, Antrizine, Bonine, Dizmiss, Motion Cure, Ru-Vert M, Wehvert (CAN) Bonamine	Tablets: 12.5 mg, 25 mg, 50 mg Chewable tablets: 25 mg	*Motion sickness:* 25 mg–50 mg 1 h prior to travel; repeat every 24 h *Vertigo:* 25 mg–100 mg daily in divided doses as needed	Motion sickness, vertigo due to disease of the vestibular system	Do not use in pregnancy or young children; commonly causes dry mouth and drowsiness; weak anticholinergic action; tablets are oral or chewable; this drug has a slower onset and longer duration than many others; watch for delayed development of side effects
Methdilazine Tacaryl (CAN) Dilosyn	Chewable tablets: 4 mg Tablets: 8 mg Syrup: 4 mg/5 mL	Adults: 8 mg 2–4 times/day Children: 4 mg 2–4 times/day	Pruritus, urticaria	Tablets may be chewed (4 mg) or swallowed whole (8 mg); structurally a phenothiazine (see Chap. 22 for possible adverse reactions); strong anticholinergic and antiemetic; do not use in children under age 3
Promethazine Phenergan and other manufacturers (CAN) Histantil	Tablets: 12.5 mg, 25 mg, 50 mg Syrup: 6.25 mg/5 mL, 25 mg/5 mL Suppositories: 12.5 mg, 25 mg, 50 mg Injection: 25 mg/mL, 50 mg/mL	*Oral* Adults: 12.5 mg–50 mg every 4–6 h as necessary Children: 6.25 mg–12.5 mg 3 times/day as needed *Rectal* 12.5 mg–25 mg every 4–6 h as necessary *Parenteral (usually IM):* 12.5 mg–25 mg individualized to condition Children: 0.6–1.2 mg/kg When used IV, maximum concentration is 25 mg/mL/min	Allergic disorders and reactions to blood plasma; motion sickness; nausea and vomiting due to anesthesia, drugs, or surgery; preoperative and obstetrical sedation; adjunct to analgesics in postoperative or chronic pain; sedation and light sleep; cough	Phenothiazine derivative (see Chap. 22); potent antihistamine and sedative with prolonged effects; may cause false-positive on urine pregnancy tests (immunologic type); avoid intra-arterial injection because severe arteriospasm can result; irritating to tissue if given SC; give deep IM and rotate sites with every dose; photosensitivity is a problem; caution patient to use dark glasses and avoid bright light; reduce dose of analgesics and other sedative-hypnotics if used in combination with promethazine; injection is incompatible with alkaline drugs; should be diluted with saline

Continued

Table 14-2
Antihistamines (continued)

Drug	Preparations	Usual Dosage Range	Major Uses	Nursing Implications
Promethazine (cont'd)				prior to injection; flush heparin lock with saline prior to and after injecting drug because it is incompatible with heparin; avoid contact with skin or eyes; good antiemetic but may mask vomiting caused by other drugs; protect injectible form from light and do not use if cloudy or darkened; available with expectorant, either plain or with codeine and/or decongestants
Pyrilamine Dormarex	Tablets: 25 mg Capsules: 25 mg	Adults: 25 mg–50 mg 3 times/day *Insomnia:* 50 mg at bedtime	Allergic disorders, insomnia	Not recommended in children under age 6; found in several OTC cough formulations; drug is only mildly sedating and weakly anticholinergic
Terfenadine Seldane	Tablets: 60 mg	Adults and children over 12: 60 mg twice a day	Allergic disorders (especially rhinitis)	Long-acting oral antihistamine used for control of chronic allergic disorders; very minimally sedating
Tripelennamine Pyribenzamine, Pelamine, PBZ	Tablets: 25 mg, 50 mg Long-acting tablets: 100 mg Elixir: 37.5 mg/5 mL	Adults: 25 mg–50 mg every 4–6 h (maximum 600 mg/day or 100 mg 2–3 times/day) Children: 5 mg/kg/day in 4–6 doses (maximum 300 mg/day)	Allergic disorders and reactions to blood or plasma; pruritis and other topical skin disorders; mucous membrane analgesia and anesthesia in the mouth; cough	Do not use 100-mg sustained-acting form in children; used as mouthwash for herpetic gingivostomatitis in children; caution in elderly because dizziness, sedation, and hypotension are more likely to occur; possesses some antitussive and local anesthetic activity
Triprolidine Actidil, Myidil	Tablets: 2.5 mg Syrup: 1.25 mg/5 mL	Adults: 2.5 mg 3–4 times/day Children: (6–12): 1.25 mg 3–4 times/day Children (2–6): 0.6 mg 3–4 times/day Children (under 2): 0.3 mg 3–4 times/day	Allergic disorders	Low degree of drowsiness and most other side effects; rapid onset of action; may cause paradoxical excitation and irritability; combined with pseudoephedrine as Actifed—this combination is also available with codeine and guaifenensin as Actifed-C; children under age 6 should be given syrup only

MAO inhibitor therapy. In addition, phenothiazine antihistamines (methdilazine, promethazine, trimeprazine) are contraindicated in comatose patients; in states of CNS depression due to drug overdosage; in jaundice and bone marrow depression; and in acutely ill or dehydrated children. *Cautious use* in patients with cardiovascular disease, convulsive disorders, renal or hepatic impairment, hypertension, urinary retention, glaucoma, diabetes, asthma, or other chronic lower respiratory disease, and hyperthyroidism, and in young children, elderly, or debilitated patients, and pregnant women

INTERACTIONS
Sedative effects may be enhanced by concurrent use of other CNS depressants (e.g., alcohol, barbiturates, narcotics, antianxiety drugs)

Atropine-like side effects (e.g., dryness of mouth, blurred vision, urinary retention, constipation) are potentiated by other anticholinergics, tricyclic antidepressants, and MAO inhibitors

Effects of epinephrine can be increased by several antihistamines (e.g., diphenhydramine, chlorpheniramine, tripelennamine)

NURSING CONSIDERATIONS
See **Plan of Nursing Care 4** in this chapter. In addition:

Nursing Alerts
- Withhold topical application of antihistamine-containing preparation at earliest sign of dermatologic toxicity. Serious hypersensitivity reactions can occur.
- During parenteral use, observe patient closely. Hypersensitivity reactions are more likely to occur with parenteral rather than with oral administration. Inform patient that brief stinging sensation may occur.

1. Give IM antihistamine deep into large muscle mass to reduce tissue irritation. SC injection should not be used.
2. Apply topical preparation only to intact skin. Avoid broken, exposed, or weeping areas.

PATIENT EDUCATION
See **Plan of Nursing Care 4** in this chapter. In addition:
1. Instruct patient with severe allergy to carry identification stating type of allergy, medication being used, and name of physician.

H₂ Receptor Antagonists

Cimetidine   Ranitidine
Famotidine   Nizatidine

As previously noted, the designation *antihistamine* is generally used synonymously with H₁ receptor antagonists. A second series of compounds act as competitive antagonists of histamine specifically at H₂ receptors. These H₂-reactive sites mediate the gastric acid secretory effects and the cardiac stimulatory action of histamine. Because H₂ antagonists can effectively and almost completely block the secretion of gastric hydrochloric acid in response to most stimuli, it appears that histamine plays a major role in acid secretion from gastric mucosal parietal cells. Clinical studies show substantial reductions in gastric secretory volume, total acidity, and pepsin activity following administration of an H₂ blocker. Therefore, these substances have an important role in the therapeutic management of peptic ulcers and certain other gastric hypersecretory states.

The clinically available H₂ receptor antagonists are similar in many aspects and will be discussed as a group. Certain important differences among the drugs exist, however, particularly with regard to their potential for causing some serious side effects and for interacting with other drugs. These differences are highlighted during the general discussion of the drugs. The individual drugs then are listed in Table 14-3, with specific information regarding their dosage.

MECHANISM
Selective antagonism of the actions of histamine at H₂ receptor sites, especially those in the gastric mucosa; reduce daytime and nocturnal basal gastric acid secretion by 90% to 100%, as well as acid secretion stimulated by food, caffeine, pentagastrin, and insulin; increase gastric pH to 5 or greater for 3 to 4 hours and decrease total pepsin output

USES
Short-term treatment of gastric and duodenal ulcers (up to 8 wk)

Maintenance therapy for duodenal ulcer at reduced dosage following healing of an active ulcer

Treatment of pathologic hypersecretory conditions (e.g., Zollinger–Ellison syndrome, systemic mastocytosis, multiple endocrine adenomas)

Investigational uses include prevention of stress induced ulcers (e.g., in hospitalized patients), prevention of aspiration pneumonitis during general anesthesia, and treatment of gastroesophageal reflux. In addition, cimetidine has been used to treat hirsutism in women because of its antiandrogenic action (see **Significant Adverse Reactions**)

DOSAGE
See Table 14-3

FATE
Oral absorption is generally good, although bioavailability can vary among the different drugs. Peak serum levels usually occur within 1 to 2 hours. Duration of action ranges from 4 to 5 hours with cimetidine and up to 12 hours with nizatidine and ranitidine. Plasma protein binding for all drugs is minimal (15%–35%); elimination half-life is short (2–3 h), and the major route of excretion is in the urine as both unchanged drug and metabolites; the half-life may be significantly prolonged in patients with renal impairment

COMMON SIDE EFFECTS
Headache, transient diarrhea, nausea

SIGNIFICANT ADVERSE REACTIONS
(Not all reactions have been noted with each drug) Dizziness, muscle pain, rash, confusion, constipation, abdominal pain, insomnia, arthralgia, malaise, increased serum transaminases, altered heartbeat, ataxia, delirium, and, rarely, blood dyscrasias. *In addition,* cimetidine has been associated with alopecia, gynecomastia, galactorrhea, impotence, and decreased sperm count because of its antiandrogenic activity

PLAN OF NURSING CARE 4
PATIENTS TREATED WITH ANTIHISTAMINE DRUGS
Nursing Diagnosis: Potential for Trauma related to sedation from antihistamine drug therapy
Goal: Patient will not be injured as a result of sedation.

Intervention	Rationale	Expected Outcome
Protect safety of hospitalized patient: 1. Instruct unsteady patient to seek assistance when getting out of bed. 2. Supervise ambulation. 3. Use side rails for elderly or debilitated patient.	Most antihistamines depress the CNS, causing sedation. A drowsy patient is prone to injury. The elderly or debilitated patient is particularly likely to experience dizziness, sedation, confusion, and hypotension.	Patient will not be injured.
Warn patient of danger associated with activities that require mental alertness and motor coordination (e.g., driving, operating machinery) while taking antihistamines. Children should also avoid activities that could lead to injury (e.g., climbing).		Patient will express awareness of precautions for sedation.
Caution patient about additive sedative effects of antihistamines, alcohol, and other CNS depressant drugs, both OTC and prescription (e.g., sedatives, hypnotics).	Drugs with additive effects magnify the sedation induced by antihistamines.	Patient will state the effect of combined usage of CNS depressants.
Inform patient that drowsiness usually lessens or disappears with continued drug use.	Compliance may improve if patient knows that side effects are temporary.	
Encourage patient to report sedation to appropriate person if it becomes a problem to determine whether: 1. A different antihistamine can be used 2. The dosing schedule can be altered	Subclasses of antihistamines vary in the degree of sedation they induce. Once-daily doses at bedtime minimize sedative effects. Even with divided doses, a bedtime dose may reduce late-day sedation. Dosage schedule may depend, however, on half-life and other drug characteristics.	Patient will verbalize feeling more alert. Patient will appear more alert.

Nursing Diagnosis: Potential Knowledge Deficit related to antihistamine drug therapy
Goal: Patient will possess knowledge needed to implement antihistamine drug regimen and related actions.

Intervention	Rationale	Expected Outcome
See also **Plan of Nursing Care 1** (Knowledge Deficit) Teach patient potential, frequently occurring side effects and appropriate corresponding actions: 1. Nausea may be minimized by taking drug with meals or small snack. 2. Thickened bronchial secretions, which make expectoration more difficult, may be loosened by increasing fluid intake, humidifying room air, deep breathing, and coughing. 3. Constipation may be alleviated by increasing fluid intake, adding roughage and fiber in the diet, and exercising daily. 4. Urinary retention may be averted by voiding immediately after taking the drug. If retention occurs, drug prescriber should be notified. 5. Blurred vision should be reported to the drug prescriber. 6. Paradoxical excitation, which occurs most often in children, should be reported to drug prescriber.	Taking the drug with food decreases gastric irritation. Because of their structural similarity to anticholinergic drugs, many antihistamines induce anticholinergic effects.	Patient will state potential side effects of antihistamines. Patient will discuss appropriate responses to side effects.

Continued

PLAN OF NURSING CARE 4 (continued)
PATIENTS TREATED WITH ANTIHISTAMINE DRUGS

Nursing Diagnosis: Potential for Trauma related to sedation from antihistamine drug therapy
Goal: Patient will not be injured as a result of sedation.

Intervention	Rationale	Expected Outcome
Encourage patient to report continuing side effects to drug prescriber.	Many side effects can be eliminated by reducing the dosage or changing to a different antihistamine.	Patient will express awareness of option of changing drug if side effects continue.
Instruct patient using an antihistamine for motion sickness to take first dose at least 30 minutes prior to travel and several times a day during travel if necessary, preferably before meals.	Usage should correspond with duration of onset to control motion sickness.	Patient will explain timing of drug use for treatment of motion sickness.
Warn patient to keep antihistamines out of the reach of children.	Overdosage in children may result in hallucinations, convulsions, and possibly death.	Patient will indicate awareness of need to keep antihistamines away from children.

Nursing Diagnosis: Potential Alteration in Oral Mucous Membrane related to dry mouth (xerostomia) from antihistamine drug therapy
Goal: Patient will avoid complications and experience minimal discomfort from dry mouth.

Intervention	Rationale	Expected Outcome
Suggest measures to reduce mouth dryness: 1. Suck hard candy or ice chips 2. Chew sugarless gum 3. Frequently rinse the mouth 4. Increase fluid intake 5. Use a commercial saliva substitute 6. Avoid overuse of commercial mouthwashes 7. If dentures are worn, remove several times a day when rinsing mouth to moisten all oral tissues	Mouth dryness can be uncomfortable and can interfere with eating, talking, and other emotionally important physical and social activities. It may also interfere with compliance. Most commercial mouthwashes contain alcohol, which tends to aggravate the dryness.	Patient will discuss measures that alleviate mouth dryness.
Discuss oral hygiene routines (timing) and techniques (flossing, soft toothbrush for brushing, fluoride toothpaste) and their importance.	A bad taste in the mouth often accompanies mouth dryness. In addition, dental disorders (e.g., caries) are more likely to occur with xerostomia.	Patient will explain oral hygiene routines and techniques and their purpose.

CONTRAINDICATIONS
No absolute contraindications. *Cautious use* in the presence of impaired renal or hepatic function, in very ill or debilitated patients, and in pregnant or nursing women. In addition, cimetidine must be used cautiously in persons with altered endocrine function

INTERACTIONS
Antacids and metoclopramide may impair oral absorption of H_2 blockers if administered simultaneously

Cimetidine may lengthen the half-life of certain benzodiazepine drugs (alprazolam, chlordiazepoxide, diazepam, flurazepam, triazolam), beta blockers, caffeine, theophylline, lidocaine, salicylates, phenytoin, quinidine, and other drugs metabolized in the liver as a consequence of slowed hepatic metabolic functioning

Cimetidine or ranitidine may increase the pharmacologic effects of procainamide by reducing its renal clearance

Concurrent use of cimetidine and morphine may lead to muscle twitching, confusion, and apnea

The effectiveness of sucralfate may be reduced by H_2 blockers because sucralfate requires an acid medium to be most effective

Decreased oral absorption of ketoconazole may occur in the presence of H_2 blockers because of increased pH

Increased effects of carbamazepine have been reported when it was given in conjunction with cimetidine

Concurrent administration of cimetidine and digoxin has reduced serum levels of digoxin

NURSING CONSIDERATIONS
See **Plan of Nursing Care 5** in this chapter. In addition:

Nursing Alerts
- Screen patient's medication record for potential drug interactions before administering cimetidine because it increases the half-life of many drugs.
- Monitor patient receiving cimetidine and interacting drugs for possible overdosage. Dosage of potentiated drugs may need to be reduced.

Table 14-3
H₂-Receptor Antagonists

Drug	Preparations	Usual Dosage Range	Nursing Implications
Famotidine Pepcid	Tablets: 20 mg, 40 mg Powder for oral suspension: 40 mg/5 mL Injection: 10 mg/mL	*Oral* Duodenal ulcer: 40 mg once a day for 6–8 wk; maintenance therapy: 20 mg once a day Hypersecretory conditions: 20 mg every 6 h *IV:* 20 mg every 12 h	Long-acting H₂-receptor antagonist used for short-long-term treatment of duodenal ulcer; antacids may be given concomitantly if needed; does not affect hepatic metabolism of other drugs (as seen with cimetidine); no antiandrogenic activity has been reported; IV solutions stable for 48 h at room temperature
Cimetidine Tagamet (CAN) Apo-Cimetidine, Novocimetine, Peptol	Tablets: 200 mg, 300 mg, 400 mg, 800 mg Liquid: 300 mg/5 mL Injection: 300 mg/2 mL, 300 mg/50 mL	*Oral* Duodenal ulcer: Initially, 300 mg 4 times/day *or* 400 mg twice a day *or* 800 mg at bedtime for 4–6 wk; reduce to 400 mg at bedtime for maintenance therapy as necessary to prevent recurrence Hypersecretory conditions: 300 mg 4–6 times/day to a maximum of 2400 mg/day *Parenteral* IM injection: 300 mg every 6 h IV injection: 300 mg diluted to 20 mL in saline and injected over 1–2 min every 6 h IV infusion: 300 mg in 50 mL 5% dextrose, infused over 15–20 min every 6 h (maximum 2400 mg/day)	Used in treating both acute and chronic gastric and duodenal ulcers; drug has been administered up to 5 yr in some patients; not recommended in children under 16; possesses antiandrogenic action that may cause some side effects over time (e.g., gynecomastia, impotence); reduces hepatic metabolism of many drugs (*see* Interactions) by impairing cytochrome *P*450 pathway in the liver; antacids should *not* be taken concurrently; injectable solutions stable up to 48 h at room temperature; reduce dosage in patients with severely impaired renal function
Nizatidine Axid	Capsules: 150 mg, 300 mg	*Active duodenal ulcer:* 300 mg once daily at bedtime *or* 150 mg twice daily *Maintenance therapy:* 150 mg once daily at bedtime	Long-acting competitive H₂-receptor antagonist; dosage must be reduced in patients with renal insufficiency; does *not* inhibit hepatic enzymes nor possess antiandrogenic activity; most common side effects are drowsiness and sweating
Ranitidine Zantac	Tablets: 150 mg, 300 mg Injection: 25 mg/mL	*Oral* Initially: 150 mg twice a day *or* 300 mg once daily at bedtime Maintenance therapy: 150 mg at bedtime *IM:* 50 mg undiluted every 6 h *IV injection:* 50 mg every 6–8 h diluted to a volume of 20 mL and given over 5 min *IV Infusion:* 50 mg in 100 mL given over 15–20 min every 6–8 h	Used to treat gastric and duodenal ulcers and other hypersecretory conditions; may be given without regard to meals and with antacids; does not generally reduce hepatic metabolism of other drugs; may slow clearance of warfarin or procainamide; no reported antiandrogenic activity; reduce dosage in persons with severely impaired renal function; transient pain can occur at injection sites; solutions stable for 48 h

1. Observe patient with renal impairment for signs of overdosage. Dosage should be reduced for patient with renal failure.
2. Discard injectable form added to commonly used IV solutions after it has been at normal room temperature for 48 hours, the length of time it is stable.

ANTISEROTONIN AGENTS

Many antihistamine drugs exert varying degrees of serotonin-blocking activity, although in most cases this activity is too weak to be clinically significant. A few drugs, however, exert considerable serotonin antagonism, and these drugs are employed in several disease states in which overactivity of serotonin may be the primary etiologic factor. It is important to recognize, however, that drugs classified as antiserotonin agents possess many other pharmacologic actions as well (e.g., antihistaminic, anticholinergic, local anesthetic, oxytocic, vasoconstrictor), and that their clinical effects cannot always be ascribed solely to their serotonin-blocking action. Antiserotonin drugs are mainly used for symptomatic management of allergic conditions, especially to relieve itching, for prophylaxis of migraine and other vascular headaches, and to reduce diarrhea and abdominal cramping in the treatment of the carcinoid syndrome.

PLAN OF NURSING CARE 5
Patients Treated with H_2-Receptor Antagonists
Nursing Diagnosis: Potential Knowledge Deficit related to H_2 blocker drug therapy
Goal: Patient will possess knowledge needed to implement H_2 blocker drug regimen and related actions.

Intervention	Rationale	Expected Outcome
See also **Plan of Nursing Care 1 (Knowledge Deficit) and 2 (Compliance)**		
Teach patient about drug regimen (*cimetidine only*):		Patient will explain how drug should be taken.
1. If several doses are prescribed, it is best to take them with meals and at bedtime.	Food delays absorption and thus prolongs drug effect. Also, if drug is taken with meals, peak blood levels coincide with gastric acid secretion induced by food. Bedtime doses help control nocturnal gastric acid secretion. Thus, appropriate timing of administration may promote faster healing.	
2. A single daily dose is most often taken at bedtime.		
3. If concurrent antacids are prescribed, allow an hour between taking antacid and taking cimetidine.	H_2 blockers may not begin to relieve gastric pain for several days. Concurrent administraton of antacids helps lessen gastric acidity and relieve pain, but simultaneous administration of antacid interferes with oral absorption of cimetidine.	
Teach patient about side effects:		Patient will discuss drug side effects and related actions.
1. Inform patient that side effects are uncommon, but the following occasionally occur: reversible sexual impotence (*cimetidine only*, especially with high dosage over prolonged time), breast swelling or tenderness in females and males (*cimetidine only*), diarrhea, dizziness, headache, muscle cramps or pain, skin rash.	The incidence of adverse effects during short-term treatment is relatively small. Minor reactions occur more frequently with prolonged therapy. Cimetidine is chemically different from other H_2 blockers and causes different side effects. It has antiandrogenic effects that may cause gynecomastia.	
2. Inform patient that any side effects may diminish with continued drug use. Suggest that patient check with drug prescriber if they continue or are bothersome.		
3. Instruct patient to notify drug prescriber as soon as possible if the following rare drug reactions occur: confusion, sore throat and fever, unusual bleeding or bruising, unusual tiredness or weakness.	Granulocytopenia has been reported with cimetidine use.	
4. Advise patient who is elderly, has kidney or liver disease, is very ill, or is using very high doses to be very cautious until effects of drug are known; these patients are particularly susceptible to dizziness and confusion.		
Instruct patient not to combine cimetidine with any other drug, including OTC drugs, without consulting drug prescriber.	Cimetidine reduces the hepatic metabolism and thus potentiates the effects of numerous drugs. If any of these drugs are used, the dosage should be reduced and the patient should be monitored for possible overdosage.	Patient will express awareness of: 1. The need to consult drug prescriber before using any other drugs if cimetidine is taken 2. The effect of smoking on drug control of ulcer disease 3. The need to complete full course of treatment
Advise patient that smoking interferes with drug control of peptic ulcer disease.	Ulcer recurrence is greater in smokers.	
Encourage patient to complete full course of therapy even though symptoms may subside.	The drug regimen must usually be continued for 4 to 8 wk unless ulcer healing is demonstrated earlier. Single bedtime doses are sometimes used prophylactically, as significant recurrences have been noted when drug is stopped.	

Cyproheptadine

Periactin

MECHANISM

Competitive antagonism of serotonin, histamine, and possibly acetylcholine at postsynaptic receptor sites; structural analog of the phenothiazines; exhibits mild CNS depressant activity; may impair platelet aggregation; may stimulate the appetite, possibly by acting on the hypothalamus

USES

Relief of several allergic disorders, especially rhinitis, allergic conjunctivitis, and allergic skin manifestations (e.g., cold urticaria, pruritus, angioedema)
Prevention or reduction of allergic reactions to blood and plasma
Adjunctive therapy for anaphylactic reactions
Relief of pruritus resulting from drug or serum reactions, physical allergies, or insect bites
Treatment of carcinoid syndrome
Investigational uses include appetite stimulation in underweight or anorexic patients, treatment of vascular cluster headaches, and prophylaxis of migraine

DOSAGE

Adults: 4 mg 3 or 4 times/day (usual range is 12 mg–16 mg/day; maximum dose 32 mg/day)
Children: (2–6 yr) 2 mg 2 to 3 times/day (maximum 12 mg/day); (7–14 yr) 4 mg 2 to 3 times/day (maximum 16 mg/day)

FATE

Absorption is adequate; onset of action is within 60 minutes; duration 4 to 6 hours

COMMON SIDE EFFECTS

Sedation; dryness of mouth, nose, and throat; dizziness; gastric distress; and thickening of bronchial secretions

SIGNIFICANT ADVERSE REACTIONS

Urinary difficulty, skin rash, excitation, impaired coordination, tremor, irritability, confusion, ataxia (CNS effects occur especially in children), hypotension, and tachycardia

CONTRAINDICATIONS

Urinary retention, bladder obstruction, lower respiratory disease, narrow-angle glaucoma, peptic ulcer, prostatic hypertrophy, elderly or debilitated patients, newborn or premature infants, nursing mothers, and combination with MAO inhibitors. *Cautious use* in bronchial asthma, glaucoma, hypertension, hyperthyroidism, cardiovascular disease, and in young children, pregnant or nursing women

INTERACTIONS

MAO inhibitors or anticholinergics may intensify many of the side effects of cyproheptadine
Cyproheptadine has additive CNS depressant effects with other depressants (e.g., alcohols, narcotics, barbiturates)

PATIENT EDUCATION

1. Warn patient to avoid activities requiring alertness and coordination in early stages of therapy because drowsiness is common, although it usually disappears in several days.
2. Caution patient to guard against injury resulting from dizziness and hypotension, which may also occur, particularly in the elderly.
3. Warn patient to avoid using other substances that add to CNS depressant effects (e.g., alcohol, narcotics, barbiturates).
4. Advise parents to observe children for early signs of stimulation. They may experience an excitatory state (e.g., agitation, confusion, possibly hallucinations).

Ergotamine

Ergomar, Ergostat, Medihaler-Ergotamine, Wigrettes
(CAN) Gynergen

Ergotamine is an ergot alkaloid used principally for relief of pain associated with vascular headaches. It is reviewed below, together with its structural analog dihydroergotamine and another ergot alkaloid, methysergide. Additional ergot alkaloids discussed elsewhere in this text are ergonovine (Chap. 39), bromocriptine (Chap. 26), and LSD (Chap. 79).

Because prolonged use of ergotamine is not recommended, and migraine is usually a chronically recurring condition, it is important to identify the underlying psychological and physical factors that contribute to the etiology of a migraine attack. Drug therapy, per se, is rarely curative and often dangerous, owing to a wide range of drug-induced adverse reactions. Alternative measures such as relaxation therapies, stress-reduction techniques, and changes in diet should be explored.

MECHANISM

Direct spasmogenic effect on smooth muscle of peripheral and cerebral arteries; constricts the vessels and thereby reduces the pressure exerted on sensory nerve endings by the strong pulsations of the dilated arteries; also exhibits an alpha-adrenergic blocking and a serotonin-blocking action; *not* a true analgesic and specific only for the pain of vascular headaches; large doses have an oxytocic effect on the myometrium

USES

Relief of pain associated with vascular headaches, such as migraine and histamine cephalgia (most effective if given early in an attack)

DOSAGE

Sublingual: 1 tablet (2 mg) at onset of attack; repeat at 30-minute intervals to a maximum of 3 tablets/24 h or 10 tablets/wk
Inhalation: 1 inhalation at onset of attack; repeat at 5-minute intervals to a maximum of 6 inhalations/24 h
Note: Ergotamine is also available with caffeine as oral tablets and suppositories (e.g., Cafergot, Wigraine). These products do *not* provide as rapid relief as sublingual or inhalation modes of administration

FATE

Incompletely and erratically absorbed from GI tract; sublingual absorption is more predictable; prolonged duration of action, up to 24 hours; metabolized in the liver and excreted in the bile

COMMON SIDE EFFECTS

Numbness or tingling in extremities, muscle weakness, cold hands or feet, GI discomfort, diarrhea

SIGNIFICANT ADVERSE REACTIONS

Hypertension, bradycardia, angina-like pain, intermittent claudication, depression. Prolonged use of high doses can lead to ergotism, with vomiting, convulsions, weak pulse, confusion, cold and cyanotic skin, or gangrene due to severe peripheral vasoconstriction. Severe vasoconstriction can be overcome by a vasodilator such as nitroprusside (Nipride—see Chap. 31)

CONTRAINDICATIONS

Occlusive or vasospastic coronary or peripheral vascular disease, hepatic or renal disease, hypertension, severe pruritus, sepsis, infectious states and malnutrition, pregnancy, and young children. *Cautious use* in elderly persons and in nursing mothers

INTERACTIONS

Vasoconstrictor action of ergotamine may be enhanced by beta blockers, vasopressor amines, alpha$_1$-adrenergic agonists, and other peripheral vasoconstrictors

Effects of ergotamine may be potentiated by nitroglycerin (increased bioavailability) and troleandomycin (decreased metabolism)

NURSING CONSIDERATIONS

1. Assist patient to identify, where possible, underlying emotional or physical stressors that may precipitate headaches.

PATIENT EDUCATION

1. Explain that the drug is more effective if taken early in an attack. If visual impairment, paresthesias, nausea, or other early symptoms ("aura") of vascular headache occur, the initial dose should be taken right away.
2. Suggest using sublingual tablets, if possible, early in an attack because onset of action is more rapid than with oral or parenteral forms.
3. Instruct patient to watch for onset of early signs of drug-induced vascular insufficiency, such as numbness, coldness, and weakness in extremities, or a tingling sensation. Stopping the drug for 2 or 3 days usually overcomes circulatory problems.
4. Urge patient to adhere to recommended dosage because adverse reactions are much more common at high dosage levels.
5. Suggest that, when feasible, patient lie down in a dark, quiet room after taking drug to expedite pain relief.
6. Discuss relaxation and coping techniques, avoidance of stress, importance of diet, and adequate rest to deter onset of headaches.

Dihydroergotamine

D.H.E. 45

An ergot alkaloid possessing pharmacologic and toxicologic properties similar to those of ergotamine, with a weaker vasoconstrictive and oxytocic action and a slightly lower incidence of nausea and vomiting; given IM in a dose of 1 mg (1 mL), repeated at 1-hour intervals to a total dose of 3 mg, or IV for a more rapid onset in a dose of 1 mg, to be repeated once. Effects occur within 15 to 30 minutes following IM injection and persist for up to 4 hours.

Methysergide

Sansert

MECHANISM

Primarily acts as a serotonin-receptor antagonist; also possesses moderate agonistic action at serotonin receptors and may exert direct smooth muscle stimulation as well; has little direct vasoconstrictive action itself but appears to interact with serotonin in such a way as to facilitate its vasoconstrictive activity on cranial arteries, thus reducing excessive pulsations; strictly a prophylactic drug; does not abort an acute attack of migraine

USES

Prevention or reduction in frequency of vascular (migraine-type) headaches, especially if frequency exceeds once a week or if severity is intense

DOSAGE

(Not for use in children)

Adults: 4 mg to 8 mg daily in divided doses (if no response in 3 wk, effects are unlikely to develop)

Discontinue drug in 3- to 4-week intervals every 6 months in patients on long-term therapy to minimize danger of fibrotic complications (see **Significant Adverse Reactions**)

FATE

Well absorbed orally; onset of optimal effect is 1 to 2 days; metabolic fate not clearly established

COMMON SIDE EFFECTS

GI distress, abdominal pain, drowsiness, lightheadedness, flushing, muscle and joint pains

SIGNIFICANT ADVERSE REACTIONS

WARNING

Fibrotic complications may occur with prolonged use of methysergide, these include retroperitoneal fibrosis (associated with fatigue, weight loss, fever, backache, urinary obstruction, lower limb vascular insufficiency), pleural fibrosis (dyspnea, chest tightness, pleural effusion), and cardiac fibrosis (thickening of aortic root, aortic and mitral valves). Therapy must be suspended for 3- to 4-week intervals every 6 months to minimize the danger of fibrotic complications

Cardiovascular: chest or abdominal pain, numbness in extremities, paresthesias, peripheral edema, postural hypotension, tachycardia, thrombophlebitis, claudication

GI: nausea, vomiting, constipation, increased gastric acid

CNS: insomnia, euphoria, feelings of dissociation, hallucinations, nightmares (may be related to vascular headache and not the drug)

Dermatologic/hematologic: nonspecific rash, telangiectasia, alopecia, neutropenia, eosinophilia

Other: weight gain, weakness, scotomas

CONTRAINDICATIONS

Peripheral vascular disease, phlebitis, arteriosclerosis, hypertension, coronary artery disease, pulmonary disease, impaired liver or renal function, collagen diseases, valvular heart disorders, pregnancy, debilitated states, and serious infections. *Cautious use* in patients with cardiac or renal disease and in nursing mothers

INTERACTIONS

Antimigraine effects may be antagonized by cerebral vasodilators (e.g., nylidrin, papaverine)

NURSING CONSIDERATION

Nursing Alert
- Carefully evaluate patient's understanding of instructions. This is a very dangerous drug. Fibrotic complications (formation of scar tissue) can occur in any patient on long-term therapy.

PATIENT EDUCATION
1. Suggest taking drug with meals to minimize GI distress.
2. Stress the urgency of reporting any sign of coldness or numbness in extremities; leg cramps; edema; girdle, flank, or chest pain; dysuria; or other early signs of developing toxicity.
3. Teach patient how to check for edema, and instruct to maintain low salt intake and adjust caloric intake if edema or weight gain is noted.
4. Advise patient that cardiac status, kidney function, blood status, and pulmonary function are carefully monitored during therapy since adverse effects are usually reversible if drug is discontinued early enough.
5. Teach measures to control orthostatic hypotension. See **Plan of Nursing Care 8 (Antihypertensive Drugs)** in Chapter 31 for specific information.
6. Inform patient that abrupt discontinuation of drug may cause headache rebound. The drug should be withdrawn *gradually* over a period of 2 to 3 weeks.
7. Discuss the importance of adjunctive measures (e.g., relaxation, proper exercise, avoidance of stressful situations) in dealing with migraine-type headaches.

Trimeprazine
Temaril

MECHANISM

Antagonism of the receptor actions of histamine and serotonin; structurally related to the phenothiazines (see Chap. 22); exerts some anticholinergic activity

USES

Relief of pruritus in urticaria and other dermatologic disorders
Preoperative sedation in children (investigational)

DOSAGE

Adults: 2.5 mg 4 times/day or 5 mg (sustained-release capsules) every 12 hours
Children: (over 3 yr) 2.5 mg 3 times/day as needed (6 to 3 yr) 1.25 mg 3 times/day

FATE

Onset of action in 30 to 60 minutes; duration is 3 to 6 hours; sustained-release forms persist for 8 to 12 hours; excreted in the urine as metabolites and intact drug

COMMON SIDE EFFECTS

Drowsiness, lightheadedness, dryness of the mouth, blurred vision, GI distress, and weakness

SIGNIFICANT ADVERSE REACTIONS

Allergic skin reactions, extrapyramidal reactions, orthostatic hypotension, tachycardia, urinary difficulty, blurred vision, dryness of bronchial and other secretions, respiratory difficulties; see also phenothiazines (see Chap. 22)

CONTRAINDICATIONS

Excess CNS depression, bone marrow depression, newborn or premature infants, pregnancy, acutely ill or dehydrated children (danger of adverse effects [e.g., dystonias] is increased). *Cautious use* in persons with renal or hepatic disease, asthma, CNS disorders, hypertension, prostatic hypertrophy, history of convulsive disorders, narrow-angle glaucoma

INTERACTIONS

Anticholinergic effects are intensified by MAO inhibitors, tricyclic antidepressants, thiazide diuretics
Phenothiazine-related adverse effects may be intensified by reserpine, nylidrin, oral contraceptives, progesterone
Drug may potentiate depressant and analgesic effects of narcotics, barbiturates, alcohol, and similarly acting drugs

NURSING CONSIDERATION
1. Observe patient for possible phenothiazine-related toxic effects (see Chap. 22) because drug is a structural analog of the phenothiazines.

PATIENT EDUCATION
1. Warn patient to avoid hazardous activities because drug induces marked drowsiness, especially during first few days. Advise particular caution for elderly patient because hypertension, syncope, confusion, and excessive sedation may occur.
2. Explain that depressive effects of other drugs can be potentiated by trimeprazine.

Selected Bibliography

Aghajanian GK, Wang RY: Physiology and pharmacology of central serotonergic neurons. In Lipton MA, DiMascio A, Killam KF (eds): Psychopharmacology: A Generation of Progress, p 171. New York, Raven Press, 1978

Ambielli MP: Drug stop. J Neurosurg Nursing 15:370, 1983

Berde B: Ergot compounds: A synopsis. Adv Biochem Psychopharmacol 23:3, 1980

Diamond S, Solomon GD: Pharmacologic treatment of migraine. Ration Drug Ther 22(10):1, 1988

Green JP, Johnson CL, Weinstein H: Histamine as a neurotransmitter. In Lipton MA, Dimascio A, Killam KF (eds): Psychopharmacology: A Generation of Progress, p 319. New York, Raven Press, 1978

Hirschowitz BI: H-2 histamine receptors. Annu Rev Pharmacol Toxicol 19:203, 1979

Kunkel RS: Pharmacologic management of migraine headaches. Ration Drug Ther 21(6):1, 1987

Moree NA, et al.: How do the new drugs measure up? Am J Nurs 84:902, 1984

Raskin NH: Pharmacology of migraine. Annu Rev Pharmacol Toxicol 21:463, 1981

Sanowski RA: Complete management of the patient with peptic ulcer disease. Mod Med 55(8):28, 1987

Todd B: Drugs and the elderly: Antiulcer preparations. Geriatr Nurs (New York) March/April:122, 1983

Zakusov VV (ed): Pharmacology of Central Synapses: 5-hydroxytryptamine Antagonists, p 143. New York, Pergamon Press, 1980

Zimmerman TW, Schenker S: A comparative evaluation of cimetidine and ranitidine. Ration Drug Ther 19(4):1, 1985

SUMMARY. ANTIHISTAMINE–ANTISEROTONIN DRUGS

Drug	Preparations	Usual Dosage Range
H_1-Receptor Antagonists	See Table 14-2	
H_2-Receptor Antagonists	See Table 14-3	
Antiserotonin Agents		
Cyproheptadine Periactin	Tablets: 4 mg Syrup: 2 mg/5mL	*Adults:* 4 mg 3 or 4 times/day (usual range 12–16 mg/day; maximum 32 mg/day) *Children:* (2–6 yr) 2 mg 2 or 3 times/day; maximum 12 mg/day; (7–14 yr) 4 mg 2 or 3 times/day; maximum 16 mg/day
Ergotamine Ergomar, Ergostat, Medihaler-Ergotamine, Wigrettes (CAN) Gynergen	Sublingual tablets: 2 mg Aerosol: 9 mg/mL (0.36 mg/dose)	*Sublingual:* 2 mg–6 mg per attack at 30-min intervals; (maximum 10 mg/week) *Inhalation:* 1 inhalation (0.36 mg) 5 min apart until pain is relieved (maximum 6 inhalations/day)
Dihydroergotamine D.H.E. 45	Injection: 1 mg/mL	*IM:* 1 mg at 1-h intervals to a total of 3 mg *IV:* 1 mg; repeat if needed (maximum 2 mg)
Methysergide Sansert	Tablets: 2 mg	*Adults only:* 4 mg to 8 mg/day (if no effects in 3 wk, discontinue drug); allow 3–4 wk drug-free interval every 6 mon
Trimeprazine Temaril	Tablets: 2.5 mg Sustained-release capsules: 5 mg Syrup: 2.5 mg/5 mL	*Adults:* 2.5 mg 4 times/day or 5 mg every 12 h *Children:* (over 3 yr) 2.5 mg 3 times/day; (6 mo to 3 yr) 1.25 mg 3 times/day

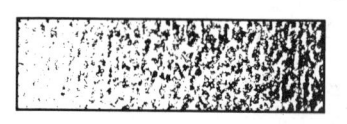

15 SKELETAL MUSCLE RELAXANTS

Skeletal muscle activity can be affected by a diverse group of pharmacologic agents capable of acting either at the neuromuscular junction or at various levels within the spinal cord and brain stem. Those agents that interfere with transmission of cholinergic impulses at the neuromuscular junction generally induce *paralysis* of the skeletal muscles involved. Those drugs that act either directly on the contractile mechanism of the skeletal musculature or on transmission within spinal cord motor reflex pathways elicit varying degrees of skeletal muscle *relaxation*. Agents that induce paralysis are employed mainly as adjuncts to general anesthetics and in minor surgical procedures or shock therapy. Agents that induce relaxation are used to afford a degree of relief from muscle spasms and hyperreflexia associated with such conditions as inflammation, anxiety, stress, and neurologic disorders.

According to their site of action, skeletal muscle relaxants may be classified in the following manner:
I. Peripherally acting muscle relaxants
   A. Neuromuscular blocking agents
      1. Antidepolarizing blockers (e.g., tubocurarine, atracurium, gallamine)
      2. Depolarizing blockers (e.g., succinylcholine)
   B. Direct myotropic acting agents (e.g., dantrolene)
II. Centrally acting muscle relaxants (e.g., carisoprodol, methocarbamol)

PERIPHERALLY ACTING MUSCLE RELAXANTS

Neuromuscular Blocking Agents

Drugs in this category interfere with the transmission of cholinergic impulses between somatic motor neurons and skeletal muscle fibers—that is, at the neuromuscular junction. Two mechanisms may be involved in the inhibition of transmission at this junction, both involving the postsynaptic receptor site. One group of drugs, typified by *d*-tubocurarine, function as *antidepolarizing* agents, competitively antagonizing the action of acetylcholine at the receptor site and preventing depolarization of the postsynaptic membrane. The second group of drugs, exemplified by succinylcholine, act as *depolarizing* agents, producing an initial activation (depolarization) of the receptor followed by a persistent occupation that markedly delays repolarization, thereby blocking further receptor stimulation. These mechanisms are essentially similar to those displayed by the ganglionic blocking agents, in which both antidepolarizing (e.g., trimethaphan) and depolarizing (e.g., nicotine) blocking actions are also evident.

Neuromuscular blocking agents are essentially anticholinergic agents; however, their specificity for the neuromuscular junction is realized only at normal therapeutic dosages. If present in excessive amounts, their cholinergic antagonism may extend to additional sites, namely autonomic ganglia and postganglionic parasympathetic (atropine-sensitive) endings. This overlapping of effects is responsible for certain untoward reactions exhibited by these drugs at high dosage levels (e.g., cardioacceleration, arrhythmias, hypotension). On the other hand, these drugs do *not* effectively penetrate the blood–brain barrier at therapeutic concentrations, so their CNS effects are minimal. Finally, these agents release histamine from intracellular stores, and the increased levels of circulating histamine may cause varying degrees of bronchospasm, salivary and mucosal secretions, hypotension, and other unwanted effects.

The skeletal muscles are not all equally susceptible to the paralytic effects of neuromuscular blocking agents. The smaller muscles of the eye and eyelids, along with the muscles involved in talking and swallowing, are the first to be affected, followed by progressive weakening of the muscles of the neck and extremities. Fortunately, the muscles of respiration (intercostals, diaphragm) are the most resistant. However, differences in sensitivity among many of the muscles are very slight, and the margin between the effective dose and the potentially toxic dose of most neuromuscular blocking drugs is quite small. Therefore, these drugs should only be used by individuals trained and experienced in their use.

Because there is a very small margin between the dose eliciting clinically useful skeletal muscle relaxation and the dose producing muscle paralysis, a slight overdose can cause serious impairment of respiration and severe hypotension. Overdosage with neuromuscular blocking agents is therefore treated by artificial respiration with oxygen and use of vasopressors (e.g., levarterenol). Cholinesterase inhibitors (e.g., edrophonium) may also be employed in cases of poisoning with *anti*depolarizing blockers (tubocurarine, gallamine, metocurine, pancuronium) to overcome the competitive blockade, but the inhibitors are contraindicated in cases of overdosage with depolarizing blockers (e.g., succinylcholine) because they would further stimulate the cholinergic receptors, and thus may intensify the muscle paralysis.

ANTIDEPOLARIZING BLOCKERS

Drugs belonging to the group classified as antidepolarizing blocking agents are also known as nondepolarizing, stabilizing, or curariform drugs. This latter designation derives from the fact that the first antidepolarizing muscle relaxant was the alkaloid *d*-tubocurarine, the active principle of a group of South American arrow poisons collectively called curare. Several synthetic and semisynthetic products have since been developed that all possess, like *d*-tubocurarine, a quaternary nitrogen structure. These quaternary nitrogen compounds function as reversible competitive antagonists of ACh at postsynaptic, neuromuscular cholinergic (nicotinic) receptor sites. Skeletal muscle contraction in response to somatic nerve stimulation is therefore blocked, and a temporary state of muscle paralysis develops.

Because considerable differences exist among the antidepolarizing agents with regard to potency, duration of action, and incidence and type of side effects, the drugs are discussed individually.

Atracurium

Tracrium

MECHANISM
Blocks cholinergic neurotransmission at the neuromuscular junction by competitively binding to cholinergic receptor sites

on the motor end plate; less likely to release histamine than metocurine or *d*-tubocurarine, and hypotensive effect is minimal at recommended doses

USES
Relaxation of skeletal muscles during surgery, as an adjunct to general anesthesia

Facilitation of endotracheal intubation or mechanical ventilation

DOSAGE
Initially, 0.4 mg/kg to 0.5 mg/kg as an IV bolus injection; maintenance doses during prolonged surgical procedures are 0.08 mg/kg to 0.2 mg/kg given every 15 to 45 minutes; alternatively, maintenance during prolonged procedures may be accomplished by IV infusion at a rate of 5 µg to 10 µg/kg/min. If atracurium is administered under isoflurane or enflurane anesthesia, the dosage should be reduced by one third

FATE
Maximum neuromuscular blockade occurs within 2 to 5 minutes of IV injection; recovery begins within 20 to 30 minutes and is nearly complete within 1 hour after injection. Time of onset is shorter and duration of effect is longer as dosage increases; repeated doses have no cumulative effect on the duration of neuromuscular blockade if recommended dosage intervals are followed; rapidly inactivated in the plasma, with an elimination half-life of about 20 minutes; half-life is *not* altered by impaired renal function

COMMON SIDE EFFECTS
(Especially at high doses) Flushing, mild hypotension

SIGNIFICANT ADVERSE REACTIONS
(Mostly due to histamine release at high doses) Erythema, itching, urticaria, wheezing, hypotension, tachycardia. Rarely, apnea and cyanosis

CONTRAINDICATIONS
No absolute contraindications. *Cautious use* in patients with myasthenia gravis, electrolyte disturbances, asthma, cardiovascular disease, or systemic allergies, and in pregnant or nursing women

INTERACTIONS
The muscle relaxing action of atracurium can be enhanced by halothane, enflurane, isoflurane, aminoglycosides, polymyxins, lithium, magnesium salts, quinidine, procainamide

The muscle relaxing effects of atracurium may be antagonized by cholinergic drugs, cholinesterase inhibitors, and potassium

Concurrent administration of succinylcholine with atracurium may accelerate the onset and increase the depth of neuromuscular blockade

NURSING CONSIDERATIONS

Nursing Alerts
- Use atracurium only if skilled in respiratory management. Equipment for endotracheal intubation and respiratory assistance must be readily available.
- Administer IV only and only after unconsciousness has been attained. Severe tissue irritation can result from IM use. Adequate analgesia is required because drug has no effect on consciousness or pain threshold.

1. Avoid mixing injection solution with alkaline solutions (e.g., barbiturates) in the same syringe or administering simultaneously during IV infusion through the same needle because atracurium may be inactivated.

Gallamine
Flaxedil

MECHANISM
Competitive antagonism of ACh at the neuromuscular junction; less potent than *d*-tubocurarine but has no significant effect on the bronchioles, autonomic ganglia, GI tract, or blood pressure, and does not release histamine

USES
Production of skeletal muscle relaxation as an adjunct to general anesthesia

Facilitate management of patients undergoing mechanical ventilation

Reduce intensity of muscle contractions during electroshock or chemoshock therapy

DOSAGE
1 mg/kg by slow IV injection to a maximum of 100 mg; may be reinjected after 30 to 40 minutes at a dose of 0.5 mg/kg to 1 mg/kg depending on patient status

FATE
Onset of action is immediate; maximal effect in 2 to 3 minutes; duration is 20 to 30 minutes; drug may accumulate in the body with repeated injections; excreted largely unchanged in urine

COMMON SIDE EFFECTS
Tachycardia, dizziness

SIGNIFICANT ADVERSE REACTIONS
(Usually an extension of its pharmacologic action) Profound muscle weakness, respiratory depression, apnea, and hypersensitivity reactions

CONTRAINDICATIONS
Myasthenia gravis, shock, impaired renal function, cardiac disease, hypertension, hyperthyroidism, sensitivity to iodides (drug is the triethiodide salt), infants under 11 pounds (5 kg). *Cautious use* in the presence of impaired pulmonary function, collagen diseases, severe coronary artery disease, renal impairment, or history of allergies, and in elderly, debilitated, or dehydrated patients

INTERACTIONS
Muscle relaxant effects may be potentiated by inhalation anesthetics, aminoglycoside antibiotics, amphotericin, clindamycin, lincomycin, lithium, potassium-depleting diuretics, antiarrhythmics (quinidine, procainamide, propranolol), phenothiazines, diazepam, calcium and magnesium salts, trimethaphan

Effects may be antagonized by cholinergic drugs, anticholinesterases, and potassium

Tachycardia may be enhanced by anticholinergic agents (e.g., atropine, phenothiazines, antihistamines, tricyclic antidepressants)

NURSING CONSIDERATIONS

Nursing Alerts
- Administer only if experienced in proper usage. Ensure that facilities are on hand for intubation, artificial respiration, and oxygen administration as well as proper antidotes (cholinesterase inhibitors, antihistamines, atropine).
- Verify results of renal function tests and serum electrolyte studies before administering. Drug effects may be increased in the presence of hypokalemia, hypermagnesemia, or decreased renal clearance capacity.
- Monitor vital signs continuously until recovery from drug effects is complete. Use precautions for possible residual muscle weakness caused by accumulation of drug in some individuals.

1. If succinylcholine has been administered, allow time for effects of succinylcholine to dissipate before giving a curariform drug.

PATIENT EDUCATION
1. Inform the patient that a rapid heartbeat may occur immediately following administration but will decline gradually.

Metocurine
Metubine

MECHANISM
Competitive antagonism of ACh at nicotinic receptor sites on skeletal muscle; approximately 2 to 3 times more potent than *d*-tubocurarine; releases histamine upon IV injection less frequently than *d*-tubocurarine and produces minimal ganglionic blockade

USES
Adjunct to general anesthesia to induce adequate skeletal muscle relaxation
Assist patients undergoing mechanical respiration
Reduce intensity of muscle contractions during chemo- and electroshock

DOSAGE
Anesthesia adjunct: size of initial dose dependent on general anesthetic used; usual range 0.2 to 0.4 mg/kg by IV injection over 30 to 60 seconds; repeat at 0.5 mg to 1 mg every 60 minutes as needed
Electroshock/Chemoshock: 2 mg to 3 mg IV, injected slowly

FATE
Onset within 3 minutes; duration of effect 30 to 90 minutes (average 60 minutes); half-life is 3 to 4 hours; excreted rapidly by the kidney, approximately 50% unchanged

COMMON SIDE EFFECTS
Dizziness

SIGNIFICANT ADVERSE REACTIONS
Bronchospasm, hypotension, profound muscle weakness, respiratory depression, apnea, circulatory depression, hypersensitivity reactions, and increased secretions

CONTRAINDICATIONS
Patients in whom histamine release poses a definite hazard (e.g., asthmatic patients, allergic individuals), myasthenia gravis, and sensitivity to iodides. *Cautious use* in persons with impaired pulmonary, cardiovascular, renal, endocrine, or hepatic function, hypotension, thyroid or collagen disorders, or history of allergies, and in elderly or debilitated patients and pregnant or nursing women

INTERACTIONS
See **gallamine**. In addition: Precipitate may form whenever drug is combined with thiopental or methohexital because drug is unstable in alkaline solutions

NURSING CONSIDERATIONS
See **gallamine**. In addition:

Nursing Alert
- Ensure that vasopressors and fluid replacement are on hand to combat hypotension should it occur.

1. Monitor physical signs of anesthesia cautiously because metocurine can mask some of these signs

Pancuronium
Pavulon

MECHANISM
Competitive antagonism of ACh at the neuromuscular junction; approximately 5 times as potent as *d*-tubocurarine; little ganglionic blockade or histamine release; high doses produce tachycardia and mild hypertension probably through a vagal blocking action

USES
Adjunct to anesthetics during surgery
Assist patients receiving mechanical ventilation

DOSAGE
Initially 0.04 mg/kg to 0.1 mg/kg IV; increments of 0.01 mg/kg given as needed; children's dose same as adults, except for neonates, who should receive a test dose of 0.02 mg/kg to measure sensitivity

FATE
Onset about 1 minute; maximal effects in 5 minutes, persisting approximately 60 minutes; excreted largely unchanged by the kidneys

COMMON SIDE EFFECTS
Tachycardia, muscle weakness, salivation

SIGNIFICANT ADVERSE REACTIONS
Profound muscle weakness, apnea, acne-like skin rash, hypertension

CONTRAINDICATIONS
Myasthenia gravis, bromide hypersensitivity, severe coronary artery disease, and other conditions in which tachycardia is undesirable. *Cautious use* in patients with impaired pulmonary, renal, or cardiovascular function or electrolyte imbalances, in debilitated or dehydrated patients, and in children

INTERACTIONS

See **gallamine**. In addition: Use with cardiac glycosides may result in additive cardiotoxic effects

NURSING CONSIDERATIONS
See **gallamine**. In addition:
1. Although drug may be used in obstetric surgery, be prepared for delayed reversal of effects in patient receiving magnesium sulfate for convulsions because magnesium enhances neuromuscular blockade.

Tubocurarine

Tubocurarine
(CAN) Tubarine

MECHANISM

Antagonism of cholinergic transmission at nicotinic receptor sites on skeletal muscle, blocking nerve impulse activation of muscle fibers; also possesses ganglionic blocking and histamine-releasing effects possibly leading to hypotension and bronchospasm

USES

Adjunct to general anesthetics to provide adequate muscle relaxation

Reduction in intensity of muscle contractions during shock therapy

Facilitation of patients mechanical ventilation

Diagnosis of myasthenia gravis (when results of other tests are inconclusive)

DOSAGE

Anesthesia: 40 to 60 units (6 mg–9 mg) IV at time of incision; supplements of 20 to 30 units (3 mg–4.5 mg) as needed

Shock therapy: 0.5 units/lb (1.1 units/kg) of body weight by slow IV injection prior to induction of shock

Diagnosis of myasthenia: $1/15$ to $1/5$ of average adult electroshock dose IV

FATE

Immediate onset of action; duration of paralysis 30 to 90 minutes; has a cumulative effect in the body; half-life is 1 to 3 hours; moderately (40%) bound to plasma proteins; irregular and unpredictable absorption when given IM; excreted largely through the kidney, approximately half is unchanged form

COMMON SIDE EFFECTS

Dizziness, muscle weakness, sensation of warmth

SIGNIFICANT ADVERSE REACTIONS

Bronchospasm, hypotension, profound muscle weakness, respiratory and circulatory depression, increased bronchial and salivary secretions, hypersensitivity reactions, and malignant hyperthermia

CONTRAINDICATIONS

Myasthenia gravis, persons in whom release of histamine is a hazard, hyperthermia, and electrolyte imbalance or acidosis. *Cautious use* in the presence of reduced pulmonary, renal, cardiovascular, endocrine, or hepatic function; hypotension; thyroid disorders; or history of allergies, and in debilitated or dehydrated patients

INTERACTIONS

See **gallamine**. In addition: Concurrent use of tubocurarine and diazepam may increase the possibility of malignant hyperthermia

NURSING CONSIDERATIONS
See **gallamine**. In addition:

Nursing Alerts
- Monitor fluid intake and output to determine renal status because renal dysfunction may greatly prolong and intensify drug effects.
- Critically observe patient during diagnostic test for myasthenia (positive response is a clinically apparent increase in muscle weakness) because very small doses can elicit an exaggerated response. Have antidotal measures on hand.

1. Administer IV only. Absorption is unpredictable with IM route.
2. Give injection in a syringe separate from that used for thiopental or methohexital because precipitate will form if drugs are mixed.

Vecuronium

Norcuron

MECHANISM

Competitively blocks cholinergic receptors at the motor end plate in skeletal muscle; onset of action is faster and duration of paralysis is longer with increasing doses; hemodynamic function is largely unchanged at recommended dosage

USES

Adjunct to general anesthesia to provide skeletal muscle relaxation during surgery or mechanical intubation

DOSAGE

Initial adult dosage: 0.08 to 0.1 mg/kg given as an IV bolus. During prolonged procedures, additional doses of 0.01 to 0.015 mg/kg may be given at 15- to 25-minute intervals as necessary

Children over 10: same as adult dosage

Children under 10: may require a slightly higher initial dosage and more frequent supplementation

Not recommended for neonates

FATE

Maximal neuromuscular blockade occurs within 3 to 5 minutes; recovery is nearly complete within 45 to 60 minutes; repeated doses have little cumulative effect; drug is approximately 75% protein bound; elimination half-life is 60 to 75 minutes, and vecuronium is eliminated in both urine and bile

SIGNIFICANT ADVERSE REACTIONS

Excessive muscle weakness, respiratory insufficiency, apnea

CONTRAINDICATIONS

No absolute contraindications. *Cautious use* in patients with myasthenia gravis or other neuromuscular disorders, hepatic disease (prolongs recovery time), electrolyte imbalances, obesity (may impair normal ventilation), cardiovascular disease, edema, and in elderly persons and pregnant or nursing women

INTERACTIONS
See **gallamine**

NURSING CONSIDERATIONS
See **gallamine**.

DEPOLARIZING BLOCKERS

The action of the depolarizing neuromuscular blocking agents is biphasic: an initial depolarization of the muscle end plate, inducing an immediate but short-lived activation (depolarization) of the muscle fibers followed by a persistent occupation of the receptor site, which prevents repolarization and essentially desensitizes the receptor site to ACh. This "second phase" block persists for 10 to 30 minutes depending on the drug and dose used. During this time, the muscle remains paralyzed to motor nerve stimulation. The major difference between these drugs and the antidepolarizing blockers discussed previously is that, owing to the initial depolarization phase, transient muscle contractions (fasciculations) occur immediately following administration of the depolarizing drug. Contractions are followed rapidly by a flaccid paralysis similar to that observed with the antidepolarizing agents. There is also some evidence that the neuromuscular blockade following a depolarizing drug may persist beyond the actual presence of the drug at the receptor; this suggests the possibility of desensitization of the receptor caused by conformational changes of the reactive area.

One means of delaying enzymatic hydrolysis of succinylcholine and prolonging its effects is the prior administration of hexafluorenium, a potent, relatively selective inhibitor of plasma cholinesterase. Hexafluorenium is discussed following succinylcholine.

Succinylcholine

Anectine, Quelicin, Sucostrin, Sux-Cert

MECHANISM
Depolarizing neuromuscular blockade leading to initial muscle contraction (fasciculations), followed quickly by flaccid paralysis; rapidly hydrolyzed by plasma cholinesterases; slightly increases intraocular pressure; may produce altered heart rhythm and slightly elevated blood pressure

USES
Skeletal muscle relaxation as an adjunct to general anesthesia
Reduction of the intensity of muscle contractions during shock therapy
Facilitation of intubation procedures
Assisting mechanical respiration

DOSAGE
Adults: 0.3 mg/kg to 1.1 mg/kg IV given over 10 to 30 seconds which produces muscle paralysis lasting approximately 5 to 10 minutes; prolonged muscle relaxation is achieved by subsequent IV injections of 0.04 mg/kg to 0.07 mg/kg at appropriate intervals
Children: 1 to 2 mg/kg by IV injection *or* 2.5 to 4 mg/kg IM; IM injections should be given deep into the deltoid muscle

FATE
Onset following IV use within 1 minute; maximum effects last 2 to 4 minutes and return to normal within 8 to 10 minutes; quickly hydrolyzed by plasma cholinesterases; onset with IM injection 2 to 3 minutes; duration 10 to 20 minutes; excreted through kidneys, both as metabolites and small amounts of unchanged drug

COMMON SIDE EFFECTS
Muscle twitching, bradycardia (especially in children)

SIGNIFICANT ADVERSE REACTIONS
Prolonged muscle weakness, muscle pain, tachycardia, hypertension, arrhythmias, respiratory depression, apnea, excessive salivation, increased intraocular pressure, hyperkalemia, rash, myoglobinemia, decreased GI motility, anaphylactoid reactions, and cardiac arrest; abrupt onset of malignant hyperthermia, a hypermetabolic disease of skeletal muscle, can occur with succinylcholine; early signs include muscle rigidity, tachycardia, rising body temperature, and metabolic acidosis

CONTRAINDICATIONS
History of malignant hyperthermia, severe respiratory depression, acute narrow-angle glaucoma, penetrating eye injury, and genetically determined deficiency of plasma pseudocholinesterase. *Cautious use* in patients with renal, cardiovascular, hepatic, pulmonary, or metabolic disorders; severe burns, electrolyte imbalance, glaucoma, spinal cord injury, degenerative neuromuscular diseases, fractures, respiratory depression, or in patients with low levels of plasma pseudocholinesterase (e.g., dehydrated or anemic patients; patients exposed to neurotoxic insecticides; patients with liver disease, cancer, collagen disorders, or myxedema; and patients receiving certain other drugs (see **Interactions**)

INTERACTIONS
Neuromuscular blocking action of succinylcholine may be enhanced by aminoglycosides, beta blockers, chloroquine, furosemide, lidocaine, lithium, isoflurane, magnesium salts, oxytocin, phenothiazines, polymyxin antibiotics, procainamide, quinidine, and trimethaphan

Effects of succinylcholine may be prolonged and intensified by drugs that interfere with the action of plasma pseudocholinesterase enzyme (e.g., cholinesterase inhibitors, cyclophosphamide, thio-TEPA, MAO inhibitors, procaine, antimalarial drugs, oral contraceptives, pancuronium, and chlorpromazine)

Diazepam may reduce duration of neuromuscular blockade elicited by succinylcholine

Succinylcholine may cause arrhythmias in the patient receiving digitalis or quinidine by causing a sudden release of potassium from muscle cells

Concurrent administration of an antidepolarizing muscle relaxant may reduce the effectiveness of succinylcholine

NURSING CONSIDERATIONS

Nursing Alerts
- Administer only if trained in proper usage.
- Ensure that facilities are available for treating respiratory distress. Overdosage can cause complete respiratory paralysis for which oxygen with artificial ventilation is the only effective countermeasure. Use of cholinesterase inhibitors may worsen muscle paralysis.
- Verify results of laboratory studies before administering. Drug actions are intensified by dehydration, hypothermia, renal disease, carcinomas, and electrolyte imbalances (especially potassium, calcium, and magnesium).

- To avoid patient distress, administer only after unconsciousness has been attained with anesthesia.
- Monitor body temperature during administration because drug may precipitate malignant hyperthermia, especially in presence of general anesthetics.
- Be prepared for the possibility of transient apnea at onset of maximal effect. If spontaneous respiration does not return within a few minutes, initiate controlled ventilation with oxygen.
- Monitor vital signs during and immediately following administration. Keep airway clear of secretions. Be alert for postprocedural muscle weakness and assist patient as necessary.

1. When giving IM, inject deep into muscle, preferably the deltoid.
2. Use only freshly prepared solutions; succinylcholine is rapidly hydrolyzed in solution and quickly loses potency.
3. Be prepared for lengthy paralysis following prolonged use or high dosage. The drug is initially metabolized to succinylmonocholine, a weaker-acting blocker. Because this compound is slowly hydrolyzed, it may accumulate if administration is prolonged or dosage is high.
4. Observe for development of tachyphylaxis (loss of drug response) with repeated use.
5. Question simultaneous administration with an antidepolarizing blocker, which may prolong effects.
6. Seek clarification before mixing succinylcholine with solutions of barbiturates or other alkaline drugs because these agents are incompatible.

PATIENT EDUCATION
1. Inform patient that muscle pain and stiffness may be present for some time following recovery, owing to the initial stimulatory response.

PLASMA CHOLINESTERASE INHIBITOR

Hexafluorenium
Mylaxen

MECHANISM
Reversible inhibition of plasma cholinesterases; does not affect intracellular cholinesterase as do other cholinesterase inhibitors; used exclusively with succinylcholine to delay enzymatic hydrolysis

USES
To prolong succinylcholine-induced muscle relaxation, and to reduce initial muscle fasciculations

DOSAGE
0.4 mg/kg IV 3 minutes before a dose of succinylcholine (0.2 mg/kg)

In long surgical procedures, may repeat at doses of 0.1 mg/kg to 0.2 mg/kg at necessary intervals (e.g., 60–90 minutes)

FATE
Onset of action is rapid (2–3 min); duration is approximately 30 minutes and is unaffected by general anesthetic

COMMON SIDE EFFECTS
None (see below)

SIGNIFICANT ADVERSE REACTIONS
(Primarily due to increased succinylcholine activity) Bronchospasm, hypotension, arrhythmias, hyperthermia, increased intraocular pressure, respiratory depression, apnea, and prolonged and profound muscle paralysis

CONTRAINDICATIONS
Bromide hypersensitivity

INTERACTIONS
Effects of other muscle relaxants can be enhanced if hexafluorenium–succinylcholine combination is used

NURSING CONSIDERATIONS

Nursing Alert
- Administer only if facilities for artificial respiration, intubation, and oxygen are immediately available.

1. Verify plasma cholinesterase levels prior to administration. Drug use should be avoided if cholinesterase titer is low or pattern is atypical.

Direct Myotropic Acting Blocking Agent

A different type of peripherally acting skeletal muscle relaxant is typified by the drug dantrolene; unlike the classic neuromuscular blocking agents, dantrolene does not interfere with transmission of impulses between somatic motor nerves and skeletal muscle. Its action appears to occur through a direct effect on the skeletal muscle fibers that interferes with their contractile mechanisms. Specifically, the drug retards the release of a contraction-activating substance, probably calcium, from its binding sites in the sarcoplasmic reticulum. Dantrolene is available in oral form for treatment of muscle spasticity resulting from chronic neurologic disorders such as cerebral palsy, multiple sclerosis, or stroke, and as an IV injection for the emergency managment of malignant hyperthermia such as that resulting from general anesthesia.

The principal danger with dantrolene therapy is hepatotoxicity, especially with high doses (i.e., above 400 mg/day) or long-term treatment. The risk of hepatic injury appears to be greater in females, in patients over 35 years of age, and in patients taking additional medications.

Dantrolene
Dantrium

MECHANISM
Direct relaxation of skeletal muscle fibers through interference with the release of calcium ions from the sarcoplasmic reticulum; impairs catabolism within muscle cells by blocking increases in myoplasmic calcium and therefore prevents abnormal rise in body temperature; may possess some CNS action as well, resulting in drowsiness, dizziness, and weakness

USES
Relief of muscle spasticity associated with chronic neurologic disorders—cerebral palsy, stroke, spinal cord injury, or multiple sclerosis (most effective where spasticity is painful and limits muscle performance)

Emergency treatment of malignant hyperthermia (IV injection)
Preoperative prophylaxis of malignant hyperthermia in high-risk patients (orally)

DOSAGE
Muscle spasticity
Adults: initially 25 mg orally once daily; increase gradually in 25-mg increments to a maximum of 100 mg 2 to 4 times/day; maintain each dose for 4 to 7 days before increasing
Children: initially 0.5 mg/kg orally twice a day; increase by 0.5 mg/kg increments to a maximum of 3 mg/kg 2 to 4 times/day
Malignant hyperthermia (adults and children)
Treatment: initially 1 mg/kg IV; if abnormalities persist or reappear, repeat up to a cumulative dose of 10 mg/kg; usual required dose is 2 mg/kg to 5 mg/kg
Prophylaxis: 4 mg/kg to 8 mg/kg/day orally in 3 or 4 divided doses for 1 to 2 days prior to surgery (last dose given 3–4 h before start of surgery)

FATE
Oral absorption is slow and incomplete but consistent; significantly bound to plasma proteins; optimal effects with oral use may take several days to become manifest; half-life is 8 to 9 hours with oral administration and 5 hours after IV injection; metabolized primarily in the liver, and both metabolites and unaltered drug are excreted in the urine

COMMON SIDE EFFECTS
(Oral use only)
Drowsiness, dizziness, weakness, malaise, fatigue, diarrhea

SIGNIFICANT ADVERSE REACTIONS
(Oral use only)
GI: constipation, bleeding, cramping, anorexia, difficulty in swallowing, gastric irritation, severe diarrhea
CNS: headache, lightheadedness, insomnia, visual and speech disturbances, taste alterations, seizures, depression, confusion, nervousness
Cardiovascular: tachycardia, phlebitis, erratic blood pressure
Urinary: urinary frequency, crystalluria, incontinence, nocturia, urinary retention, impotence
Dermatologic: abnormal hair growth, rash, pruritus, urticaria, eczema-like reaction, photosensitization
Other: hepatitis, backache, myalgia, lacrimation, chills, fever, respiratory distress

CONTRAINDICATIONS
Hepatic disease, conditions in which spasticity is necessary to sustain upright position or balance. *Cautious use* in presence of impaired pulmonary function, cardiac impairment caused by myocardial disease, a history of hepatic dysfunction, in pregnant or lactating women, children under age 5, and in patients over 35 years of age at high risk for developing hepatotoxicity

INTERACTIONS
Estrogens may increase the danger of hepatotoxicity.
CNS depression may be potentiated by other tranquilizing agents.
Warfarin and clofibrate reduce the protein binding of dantrolene and may potentiate its effects.

NURSING CONSIDERATIONS

Nursing Alerts
- Closely observe patient for signs of developing toxicity. The drug can cause serious hepatotoxicity, especially with long-term therapy (more than 60 days) and should be used only in conjunction with appropriate and frequent monitoring of hepatic function (e.g., SGOT, SGPT, alkaline phosphatase, total bilirubin).
- Carefully evaluate patient's response to drug. Dantrolene should be discontinued if no observable benefit occurs within 45 days because the danger of liver damage increases with prolonged use.

1. If drug is withdrawn for 2 to 4 days to confirm subtle improvement, watch for signs of exacerbation of spasticity, an indication that the drug is providing some clinical benefit.

PATIENT EDUCATION
1. Provide support and encouragement, inform patient that beneficial effects may be delayed 1 to 2 weeks but that, conversely, side effects will lessen with time.
2. Caution patient to avoid hazardous situations (e.g., driving, operating machinery) until response to drug is known because drowsiness is likely to occur in early stages of therapy.
3. Urge patient to be alert for appearance of skin rash, itching, black or bloody stools, and yellowish skin discoloration and to report these developments immediately.
4. Advise patient to avoid prolonged exposure to sunlight because photosensitivity reactions may occur.
5. Assist patient to develop a total therapeutic regimen, including an exercise program and use of proper braces if prescribed.

CENTRALLY ACTING MUSCLE RELAXANTS

Baclofen	Cyclobenzaprine
Carisoprodol	Metaxalone
Chlorphenesin	Methocarbamol
Chlorzoxazone	Orphenadrine

The purpose of the centrally acting muscle relaxants is to decrease skeletal muscle tone and involuntary movement without loss of voluntary motor function or consciousness. Many CNS depressants (e.g., alcohol, barbiturates) elicit varying degrees of muscle relaxation but are of little use clinically because they also produce marked sedation and other undesirable effects. Attempts to dissociate this CNS depressant action from the muscle-relaxing effect by synthesis of centrally acting muscle relaxants has met with very limited success, and most currently useful central muscle relaxants evoke a degree of sedation that makes long-term use of these drugs undesirable.

According to their mechanism of action, these agents have been classified as either *interneuronal* or *polysynaptic* blocking drugs. These compounds act at different levels within the CNS (i.e., brain stem or spinal cord interneurons) to depress synaptic transmission in motor reflex pathways. They appear to exert a weak synaptic blocking action between neurons of these motor circuits, the degree of impairment being proportional to the number of synapses involved in the pathway. In addition to their neuronal blocking action, most of these drugs also directly depress higher centers (e.g., basal ganglia) that function in the regulation of motor activity. This CNS depressant action probably contributes a significant amount to the muscle relaxant effects of most of the centrally acting drugs.

With the exception of baclofen and diazepam (see Chap. 23), the drugs comprising the centrally acting muscle relaxants are remarkably similar in their pharmacology and toxicology. No single agent possesses a significant therapeutic advantage over any other agent, and for the most part choice of a drug is a personal preference.

Because these drugs share many common properties, they will be discussed as a group. Individual drugs are then described in Table 15-1.

MECHANISM

Interfere with transmission of impulses in polysynaptic motor reflex pathways at the level of the spinal cord, brainstem, and probably basal ganglia; prolong synaptic recovery time and decrease repetitive spinal interneuronal discharges; no effect on contractile mechanism of muscle fibers or on the motor endplate of skeletal muscles; CNS depressant action probably contributes to the muscle-relaxant effect; baclofen and diazepam also appear to facilitate the action of GABA, an inhibitory neurotransmitter, in the brainstem and at the level of spinal cord interneurons

USES

Relief of pain and discomfort of muscle spasms associated with acute musculoskeletal disorders (e.g., inflammatory states, peripheral injury [sprains, strains], connective tissue disorders)

Alleviation of spasticity resulting from multiple sclerosis, spinal cord disease, and other neurologic conditions (baclofen and diazepam only)

DOSAGE
See Table 15-1

FATE
Well absorbed orally; maximum effects usually occur in 1 hour to 4 hours and persist for several hours; most of these drugs are metabolized by the liver and are excreted in the urine

COMMON SIDE EFFECTS
Drowsiness, fatigue, dizziness, lightheadedness, dry mouth, and GI upset; in addition, other anticholinergic side effects (e.g., blurred vision, urinary hesitancy) are common with cyclobenzaprine and orphenadrine

SIGNIFICANT ADVERSE REACTIONS
(Not all effects noted with all drugs)

GI: anorexia, nausea, diarrhea, hiccups, bleeding, abdominal pain
CNS: ataxia, headache, blurred vision, insomnia, confusion, irritability, paresthesias
Cardiovascular: tachycardia, hypotension, flushing, thrombophlebitis, chest pain, palpitations, syncope
Urinary: urinary retention, dysuria, enuresis
Hematologic: petechiae, leukopenia, pancytopenia, thrombocytopenia, agranulocytosis, hemolytic anemia
Hypersensitivity: rash, erythema, pruritus, fever, asthma-like reaction, dermatoses, angioedema, anaphylactic reactions
Hepatic: abnormal liver function tests, jaundice
Respiratory: nasal congestion, dyspnea
Other: dysarthria, dyspepsia, tremors, euphoria, metallic taste, pain or sloughing at site of injection, increased intraocular tension, conjunctivitis, tinnitus, slurred speech

CONTRAINDICATIONS
See Table 15-1. *Cautious use* in patients with impaired renal or hepatic function or respiratory depression, in persons who must drive or operate machinery, in patients taking other CNS depressants, in young children, in elderly or debilitated patients, and in pregnant or lactating women; in addition, orphenadrine and cyclobenzaprine should be used cautiously in the presence of glaucoma, urinary retention, arrhythmias, and tachycardia, because they possess significant anticholinergic activity

INTERACTIONS
CNS depressive effects of centrally acting muscle relaxants and other CNS depressants (e.g., alcohol, barbiturates, narcotics, antianxiety agents) are additive

MAO inhibitors may increase the toxicity of cyclobenzaprine

Atropine-like side effects may be intensified by use of anticholinergic drugs with cyclobenzaprine and orphenadrine

Cyclobenzaprine may interfere with the antihypertensive action of guanethidine and similarly acting compounds

NURSING CONSIDERATIONS
(For additional information, see Table 15-1.)

1. If drug is abruptly terminated after prolonged use, observe patient for symptoms of withdrawal (cramping, nausea, chills, weakness). CNS effects of these compounds may lead to dependence.
2. When administering IV or IM, expect the dosage to be reduced. Parenteral use enhances the potency of these drugs.

PATIENT EDUCATION

1. Caution patient to avoid engaging in any hazardous activity while taking one of these drugs because drowsiness is common and often severe.
2. Suggest taking last dose at bedtime because drowsiness may aid sleep.
3. Advise patient to avoid concomitant use of other CNS depressants while taking one of these drugs.
4. Emphasize the importance of immediately reporting signs of developing hepatotoxicity (e.g., abdominal pain, high fever, nausea, diarrhea) or blood dyscrasias (e.g., fever, sore throat, malaise, mucosal ulceration, petechiae).

Selected Bibliography
Bowman WC: Non-relaxant properties of neuromuscular blocking drugs. Br J Anaesth 54:147, 1982
Davidoff RA: Pharmacology of spasticity. Neurology 28:46, 1980

Dennis MJ: Development of the neuromuscular junction: Inductive interactions between cells. Annu Rev Neurosci 4:43, 1981

Feldman S: Neuromuscular blocking drugs. In Churchill-Davidson HC, Wylie WD (eds): A Practice of Anesthesia, 5th ed, p 727. Chicago, Year Book Medical Publishers, 1984

Fraulini KE, Gorski DW: Don't let preoperative medications put you in a spin. Nursing 83 13:26–30, December 1983

Herrold RK: The drug connection. Am J Nurs 84:1389, November 1984

Miller RD, Savarese JJ: Pharmacology of muscle relaxants, their antagonists, and monitoring of neuromuscular function. In Miller RD (ed): Anesthesia, p 487. Churchill Livingstone, 1981

Young RR, Delwaide PJ: Spasticity (2 parts). N Engl J Med 304:28, 96, 1981

Zaimis E (ed): Neuromuscular Junction. Berlin, Springer-Verlag, 1976

Table 15-1
Centrally Acting Skeletal Muscle Relaxants

Drug	Preparations	Usual Dosage Range	Nursing Implications
Baclofen Lioresal	Tablets: 10 mg, 20 mg	5 mg 3 times/day; increase by 5 mg every 3 days to optimal effect (maximum 80 mg/day)	Primarily used for relief of spasticity due to multiple sclerosis or spinal cord diseases; sedation is usually transient; absorption is variable and reduced at higher doses; give with milk to decrease GI distress; may increase urinary frequency; do not use in patients with stroke or rheumatic disorders, in children under 12, pregnant women, nursing mothers; cautious use in epileptics and in presence of renal impairment; reduce dose slowly to avoid possibility of hallucinations on abrupt withdrawal; may alter laboratory tests for SGOT, alkaline phosphatase, and blood glucose
Carisoprodol Rela, Soma, Soprodol	Tablets: 350 mg	350 mg 4 times/day	Also available in combination with aspirin as Soma Compound; contraindicated in acute intermittent porphyria, children under 12, and meprobamate sensitivity; allergic reactions may develop early in regimen (rash, erythema, pruritus, eosinophilia)—stop drug and treat symptomatically; carefully monitor urine output and avoid overhydration; use cautiously in addiction-prone individuals; withdrawal symptoms can occur following prolonged use
Chlorphenesin Maolate (CAN) Mycil	Tablets: 400 mg	Initially 800 mg 3 times/day; may reduce to 400 mg 3 or 4 times/day if effective	Do not use in pregnancy, children, liver disease, or for periods exceeding 8 wk; discontinue at first sign of allergic reaction; paradoxical excitation may occur but is usually controlled by dosage reduction; blood dyscrasias may occur—instruct patient to have routine blood counts
Chlorzoxazone Paraflex, Parafon Forte DSC	Tablets: 250 mg, 500 mg	Adults: 250 mg to 500 mg 3 or 4 times/day; reduce gradually as improvement is noted Children: 125 mg to 500 mg 3 or 4 times/day; may be crushed and mixed with food or other vehicle	Also available with acetaminophen as tablets and capsules. Use cautiously in pregnancy, history of drug allergy, hepatic dysfunction; may discolor urine but is *not* nephrotoxic; give with meals to minimize GI irritation
Cyclobenzaprine Flexeril	Tablets: 10 mg	10 mg 3 times/day to a maximum of 60 mg/day (not in children under 15)	Do not use for longer than 2 to 3 wk; *not* effective in spasticity due to cerebral or spinal cord disease or cerebral palsy; contraindicated in hyperthyroidism, arrhythmias, congestive heart failure, acute recovery phase of myocardial infarction, or with MAO inhibitors; similar to tricyclic antidepressants in action (see Chap. 24), and may have similar central effects; high incidence of drowsiness, dry mouth, and dizziness; possesses anticholinergic activity, responsible for atropine-like side effects and interactions (see Chap. 11); caution in glaucoma and urinary retention; reduce dose slowly—withdrawal symptoms can occur
Metaxalone Skelaxin	Tablets: 400 mg	800 mg 3 or 4 times/day (not in children under 12)	Contraindicated in anemia, renal or hepatic impairment, nursing mothers; liver function studies should be done regularly; cautious use in epilepsy, pregnancy, allergic states; GI upset is common as are headache, nervousness and irritability; may interfere with Benedict's and cephalin flocculation tests

Continued

Table 15-1
Centrally Acting Skeletal Muscle Relaxants (continued)

Drug	Preparations	Usual Dosage Range	Nursing Implications
Methocarbamol Delaxin, Marbaxin-750, Robaxin, Robomol	Tablets: 500 mg, 750 mg Injection: 100 mg/ml	*Oral* Adults: 1.5 g 4 times/day initially; reduce to 750 mg to 1000 mg 4 times/day Children: 60 to 75 mg/kg/day *IM:* 0.5 g to 1 g every 8 h *IV:* 300 mg/min to a total daily dose of 1 g to 3 g for maximum 3 days *IV infusion:* 1 g (10 mL) diluted to 250 mL saline or 5% dextrose given by IV drip *Tetanus:* 1 g–3 g directly into IV tubing every 6 h (children 15 mg/kg every 6 h)	IV use may control neuromuscular manifestations of tetanus; substitute oral administration as soon as possible; avoid extravasation because irritation and thrombophlebitis can result; do *not* give SC; contraindicated in renal dysfunction (vehicle may cause acidosis and urea retention), children under 12, epilepsy (especially IV); keep patient recumbent during and at least 15 min after IV usage to minimize orthostatic hypotension and other side effects; may interfere with laboratory tests for 5-HIAA and VMA; too-rapid IV injection may cause CNS side effects (e.g., dizziness, vertigo, syncope, headache, blurred vision) as well as bradycardia, hypotension, flushing, and anaphylactic reaction; cautious use in myasthenia gravis; check IV infusion for proper flow to minimize danger of thrombophlebitis and sloughing; may darken urine; also available with aspirin as Robaxisal
Orphenadrine citrate Banflex, Flexon, Flexoject, K-Flex, Marflex, Myolin, Neocyten, Norflex, O'Flex, Orphanate	Tablets: 100 mg Sustained-release tablets: 100 mg Injection: 30 mg/mL	*Oral:* 100 mg twice a day *IV, IM:* 60 mg every 12 h (give IV over 5 min with patient supine)	Available with aspirin and caffeine as Norgesic; strong anticholinergic with high incidence of atropine-like side effects (see Chap. 11); contraindicated in glaucoma, myasthenia, duodenal obstruction, ulcers, prostatic hypertrophy, bladder obstruction, pregnancy, children; periodic monitoring of blood, renal, and liver function recommended with prolonged use; caution in urinary retention, tachycardia, coronary insufficiency, arrhythmias; also available as the HCl salt (Disipal) for control of parkinsonism (see Chap. 26); narrow safety margin—monitor for signs of toxicity (e.g., flushing, fever, blurred vision, dry mouth)

SUMMARY. SKELETAL MUSCLE RELAXANTS

Drug	Preparations	Usual Dosage Range
Peripheral Neuromuscular Blockers		
Antidepolarizing Agents		
Atracurium Tracrium	Injection: 10 mg/mL	*Initially:* 0.4 mg/kg to 0.5 mg/kg IV bolus injection; maintenance dose is 0.08 mg/kg to 0.2 mg/kg at 15- to 45-min intervals as needed *or* 5 to 10 µg/kg/min by IV infusion
Gallamine Flaxedil	Injection: 20 mg/mL	1 mg/kg IV (maximum 100 mg); repeat as needed (0.5 mg/kg–1 mg/kg) every 30 to 40 min
Metocurine Metubine	Injection: 2 mg/mL	0.2 to 0.4 mg/kg IV over 30 to 60 sec depending on anesthetic used; repeat as needed (0.5 mg–1 mg) every 60 min
Pancuronium Pavulon	Injection: 1 mg/mL, 2 mg/mL	*Initially:* 0.04 to 0.1 mg/kg IV; may supplement with 0.01 mg/kg as needed (children other than neonates; same as adults)

Continued

SUMMARY. SKELETAL MUSCLE RELAXANTS (continued)

Drug	Preparations	Usual Dosage Range
Peripheral Neuromuscular Blockers		
Antidepolarizing Agents		
Tubocurarine Tubocurarine	Injection: 3 mg/mL	*Anesthesia adjunct:* 40 to 60 units (6 mg–9 mg) IV initially, followed by supplements of 20 to 30 units (3 mg–4.5 mg) as needed *Electroshock:* 0.5 unit/lb (1.1 units/kg) body weight IV over 60 to 90 sec prior to shock. *Diagnosis of myasthenia:* 1/15 to 1/5 of adult electroshock dose, IV
Vecuronium Norcuron	Powder for injection: 10 mg/5 mL vial	*Initially:* 0.08 mg/kg to 0.1 mg/kg as an IV bolus; then 0.01 mg/kg to 0.015 mg/kg at 20- to 40-min intervals
Depolarizing Agents		
Succinylcholine Anectine, Quelicin, Sucostrin, Sux-Cert	Injection: 20 mg/mL, 50 mg/mL, 100 mg/mL Powder: 500 mg/unit, 1000 mg/unit	*Initially:* 0.3 mg/kg to 1.1 mg/kg IV over 10 to 30 sec followed by supplements of 0.04 to 0.07 mg/kg as needed *Children:* 1 mg/kg to 2 mg/kg IV injection *or* 2.5 mg/kg to 4 mg/kg IM
Plasma Cholinesterase Inhibitor		
Hexafluorenium Mylaxen	Injection: 20 mg/mL	*IV:* 0.4 mg/kg 3 min prior to 0.2 mg/kg succinylcholine; repeat at doses of 0.1 mg/kg to 0.2 mg/kg as needed in prolonged surgical procedures, at intervals of 60 to 90 min
Direct Myotropic Acting Blocking Agent		
Dantrolene Dantrium	Capsules: 25 mg, 50 mg, 100 mg Powder for injection: 20 mg/vial	*Muscle spasticity* Adults: Initially 25 mg orally daily; increase to a maximum of 100 mg 2 to 4 times/day in 25-mg increments every 4 to 7 days Children: Initially 0.5 mg/kg daily; increase by 0.5 mg/kg-increments to a maximum of 3 mg/kg 2 to 4 times/day *Hyperthermia (adults and children)* Treatment: Initially, 1 mg/kg IV; may repeat up to a cumulative dose of 10 mg/kg Prophylaxis: 4 mg/kg/day to 8 mg/kg/day orally in 3 or 4 divided doses for 1 or 2 days prior to surgery (last dose 3–4 h before start of surgery)
Centrally Acting Muscle Relaxants	*See* Table 15-1	

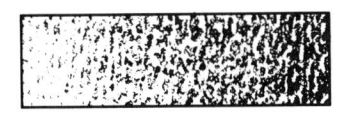

16 LOCAL ANESTHETICS

Local anesthetic agents induce a reversible blockade of impulse conduction along all sensory, motor, and autonomic nerve fibers. Loss of sensation may be accompanied by other physiological changes as well, such as muscle relaxation (motor nerve paralysis) and hypotension (sympathetic nerve blockade). When these agents are administered in the region of mixed nerve fibers, differences in onset and recovery occur, depending on the size and state of myelination of the nerve fibers. In general, small nonmyelinated C fibers (e.g., dorsal root and sympathetic postganglionic) mediating pain and vasoconstrictor impulses are affected first by local anesthetics, followed by the small, myelinated A-delta fibers mediating pain and temperature. Larger fibers carrying sensory impulses (e.g., A-alpha, A-beta) are blocked next, and finally motor nerves (e.g., A-gamma) are anesthetized, resulting in decreased skeletal muscle tone. Recovery proceeds in the opposite direction: Motor function is restored before sensory function.

Although the predominant effects of local anesthetics are confined to the circumscribed area adjacent to the site of injection or application, systemic absorption does occur to varying degrees and may produce undesirable reactions. Large doses or inadvertent intravascular injection of local anesthetics may lead to cardiovascular effects such as hypotension or cardiac depression, or to central nervous system effects such as stimulation and convulsions followed by depression. Systemic absorption of local anesthetics can be minimized by adding a local vasoconstrictor (e.g., 1:200,000 epinephrine) to the injection solution to constrict the vessels in the immediate area and prevent spread of the administered anesthetic. Vasoconstrictors also prolong the duration of local anesthesia and reduce the amount of drug needed. If surgery is performed, they may help slow local hemorrhaging.

A local anesthetic first must be able to *penetrate* the nerve membrane before it can exert its effects. Therefore it must be in the un-ionized state. Most drugs are injected as weak bases in the form of water-soluble cationic salts and must be converted to the free base (nonionic, lipid-soluble form) in order to reach their sites of action. The uncharged, nonionic fraction of drug diffuses across the nerve membrane, then reequilibrates between the nonionic and cationic forms within the nerve fiber. This reequilibration is believed essential to the pharmacologic activity of local anesthetics because it is the cationic form of the drug that *acts* within the nerve fiber. Thus, penetration to the site of action depends on the presence of a sufficient amount of lipid-soluble, nonionic drug; once that drug crosses the nerve membrane, however, activity depends on conversion to the cationic state. (This relationship explains why local anesthetics are frequently much less effective when injected into regions of inflammation. Such sites have a low extracellular pH because of the presence of acidic cellular breakdown products. The low pH favors ionization of the basic drug to the cationic form in the extracellular fluid, thereby interfering with penetration into the nerve fiber.) The cationic form of the local anesthetic drug stabilizes the nerve membrane by decreasing its permeability to sodium, thus increasing the threshold for excitation. It does so by competing with calcium ions bound to phospholipids for a site in the nerve membrane where the passage of sodium across the membrane and into the cell is controlled. The drugs thus block the initial event in the generation of a nerve action potential, namely depolarization.

Classification of local anesthetics can be based either on chemical structure or principal clinical usage. Structurally, most local anesthetic drugs belong to one of three categories:
I. Esters of benzoic or aminobenzoic acid (e.g., procaine)
II. Amides (e.g., lidocaine)
III. Ethers (e.g., pramoxine)

The individual drugs belonging to each of these classes are listed in Table 16-1. The ester-type local anesthetics are usually very short-acting because they are rapidly hydrolyzed by plasma cholinesterases. Amide drugs, however, are primarily inactivated in the liver, although there is considerable variation in the rates of hepatic degradation. Thus, lidocaine and prilocaine exhibit the shortest duration of action, whereas etidocaine and bupivacaine have a significantly longer duration. Impairment of hepatic function can greatly prolong the half-lives of the amide local anesthetics dependent on the liver for metabolism, and can result in a higher incidence of adverse effects.

Local anesthetics have several clinical applications, both topically and parenterally, and thus can also be classified as follows:
I. *Surface anesthetics*: skin and mucous membrane, eye, ear (e.g., benzocaine, cocaine)
II. *Infiltration anesthetics*: local intradermal or subcutaneous injection (e.g., procaine, lidocaine)
III. *Spinal anesthetics*: subarachnoid injection (e.g., procaine, tetracaine)
IV. *Epidural anesthetics*: injection into area surrounding the dura mater of spinal cord (e.g., lidocaine, mepivacaine)

Although some local anesthetics are used only by one route of administration, several of the drugs can be given by more than one route.

The general pharmacology and clinical implications of local anesthetics are discussed as a group. Specific characteristics of individual drugs are then detailed in Table 16-2 along with prescribing information (including the recommended routes of administration) and available preparations.

Local Anesthetics

Benoxinate	Etidocaine
Benzocaine	Lidocaine
Bupivacaine	Mepivacaine
Butamben	Pramoxine
Chloroprocaine	Prilocaine
Cocaine	Procaine
Cyclomethycaine	Proparacaine
Dibucaine	Tetracaine
Dyclonine	

MECHANISM
Stabilize neurons by blocking passage of sodium ions across the membrane; prevent initial depolarization and generation of nerve action potential; compete with calcium for a site on the nerve membrane controlling the passage of sodium, thus blocking propagation of the nerve impulse

Table 16-1
Chemical Classification of Local Anesthetics

Esters of Benzoic or Aminobenzoic Acid	Amides
benoxinate	bupivacaine
benzocaine	dibucaine
butamben	etidocaine
chloroprocaine	lidocaine
cocaine	mepivacaine
cyclomethycaine	prilocaine
dyclonine	
procaine	**Ether**
proparacaine	pramoxine
tetracaine	

USES
(See Table 16-2 for indications for individual drugs)

Relief of pain, soreness, irritation, and itching associated with skin and mucous membrane disorders (e.g., minor burns, rashes, wounds, allergic conditions, fungus infections, skin ulcers, hemorrhoids, fissures)

Production of corneal and conjunctival anesthesia to facilitate ophthalmic procedures such as tonometry, gonioscopy, removal of foreign bodies, and minor ocular surgery

Production of infiltration, nerve block, spinal, epidural, or caudal anesthesia in surgery, obstetrics, or dental work

Management of cardiac arrhythmias (see Chap. 30)

DOSAGE
See Table 16-2

FATE
(See Table 16-2 for specific information)

Absorption depends largely on site of administration, dosage, degree of vasoconstriction, and blood flow to the area. Onset of action is usually rapid (5–10 min with most injections); duration is variable and may range from 1 hour (procaine) to 4 to 6 hours (bupivacaine, dibucaine, etidocaine). Some agents are rapidly hydrolyzed by plasma cholinesterases (e.g., procaine) or liver enzymes (e.g., lidocaine), while others are more resistant to inactivation. Excreted primarily in the urine mainly as metabolites, but some unchanged drug as well.

COMMON SIDE EFFECTS
Topical: sensitization reactions, stinging or burning in the eyes
Injection: (rare at low doses) slight hypotension, anxiety

SIGNIFICANT ADVERSE REACTIONS
(Vary from drug to drug—usually related to excessive dosage or high sensitivity to drug)

Topical: hyperallergenic corneal reaction, keratitis, corneal opacities, allergic contact dermatitis with fissuring of fingertips, urticaria, cutaneous lesions, edema, anaphylactic reactions, urethritis with swelling, irritation, sloughing, and necrosis

Injection: (mainly due to systemic absorption) CNS stimulation (dizziness, blurred vision, confusion, irritability, tinnitus, convulsions, tremors) followed by CNS depression (drowsiness, unconsciousness, respiratory arrest), difficulty in speaking, hearing, swallowing, or breathing, muscle twitching, hypotension, myocardial depression, bradycardia, cardiac arrest

Epidural or caudal injection: may provoke spinal block, urinary retention, incontinence, loss of sexual function, paresthesias, headache, or backache

Spinal anesthesia: may cause hypotension, severe headache or backache, respiratory depression, or nerve root damage

CONTRAINDICATIONS
Spinal: inflammatory conditions of the spine, septicemia, meningitis, lumbar tuberculosis, metastatic lesions of the spine

Epidural: placenta previa, abruptio placentae

In addition, prilocaine is contraindicated in methemoglobinemia and bupivacaine should not be used for obstetrical paracervical block (see also Table 16-2). *Cautious use* in patients with heart block, liver or kidney disease, hyperthyroidism shock, malignant hyperthermia, and inflammation at the intended site of injection; vasoconstrictor-containing preparations should be used cautiously in patients with hypertension or peripheral vascular disease; caution is also warranted when performing spinal anesthesia in patients with chronic backache, frequent headache, or a history of migraine or hypotension

INTERACTIONS
Certain anesthetic drugs (e.g., lidocaine) may enhance muscle-relaxing effects of neuromuscular blocking agents

Additive cardiac depressant effects may occur when some local anesthetics and other cardiac depressant drugs (e.g., quinidine, propranolol, phenytoin) are given together

Solutions of local anesthetics containing a vasoconstrictor such as epinephrine may produce blood pressure alterations in combination with MAO inhibitors, tricyclic antidepressants, phenothiazines, and pressor agents

Vasoconstrictors in local anesthetic solutions may precipitate arrhythmias in combination with halothane and related general anesthetics

Procaine, chloroprocaine, and tetracaine may retard action of sulfonamide antibiotics

Injected local anesthetics may have additive effects with sedatives or other CNS depressants

The metabolism of the ester-type local anesthetics may be slowed by cholinesterase inhibitors

NURSING CONSIDERATIONS

Nursing Alerts

Topical
- If there is a possibility of systemic involvement (e.g., large doses, elderly or debilitated patients, debrided or traumatized areas), ensure that resuscitative equipment and antidotal medications are on hand (e.g., respirators, vasopressors, IV fluids).
- Observe patient for early signs of sensitivity reactions or irritation. Terminate drug administration and initiate appropriate symtomatic measures if reaction occurs.
- Withhold all oral intake for at least 1 hour following application to oral mucosa, as swallowing may be impaired.

Injection
- Ensure that facilities and drugs for respiratory and cardiovascular assistance are on hand at all times.

- Expect the lowest dose capable of inducing effective anesthesia to be administered to minimize the danger of systemic effects. Dosage should be reduced in children and in elderly, debilitated, or acutely ill patients, and the drug should be injected slowly to reduce danger in case an allergic or other systemic reaction develops. The syringe should be aspirated before injecting to prevent intravascular administration.
- Monitor fetal heart rate closely with paracervical block because fetal bradycardia and acidosis can occur. The recommended dosage should not be exceeded.

Topical
1. Avoid contact of topical local anesthetics with the eyes (unless ophthalmic solution is used) and avoid inhalation of mist from aerosol sprays.
2. Administer without touching eyelid, and do not rub eye during period of anesthesia.
3. Withhold drug and notify prescriber if sensitivity reaction or irritation develops.
4. Monitor vision and wound healing if ocular use is prolonged. Visual loss and possible delayed local wound healing could occur.

Injection
1. Assess potential injection site for evidence of infection. Local anesthetic should not be injected into infected areas because effectiveness is greatly diminished, systemic toxicity may be enhanced, and drug (e.g., procaine) may interfere with action of sulfonamide antimicrobials.
2. Place patients receiving spinal anesthesia in proper position to avoid diffusion of drug toward respiratory muscles.
3. Be prepared to provide assistance with movement to patient receiving spinal or epidural anesthesia. Sensation in lower areas of the body may not return for several hours.
4. With repeated injections of certain slowly metabolized drugs, observe patient for evidence of prolonged adverse reactions.
5. Use only solutions that do not contain preservatives for spinal or epidural injection.
6. Discard unused portions of solutions not containing preservatives.

PATIENT EDUCATION
Topical
1. Instruct patient receiving anesthetic eye drops to avoid touching the eye area until effects have dissipated. Alert patient that eye will probably be covered with a patch, since blink reflex is temporarily absent.
2. Warn patient that symptoms of middle ear infection may be masked by anesthetic ear drops.
3. Advise patient to avoid prolonged use of any local anesthetic preparation. Proper treatment should be sought for the *cause* of the condition.

Selected Bibliography
Catteral WA: The molecular basis of neuronal excitability. Science 223:653, 1984

Covino BG: Toxicity of local anesthetics. Adv Anesth 3:37, 1986

Covino BG: Pharmacology of local anesthetic agents. Ration Drug Ther 21(8):1, 1987

Fink BR (ed): Progress in Anesthesiology: Molecular Mechanisms of Anesthesia, Vol 2. New York, Raven Press, 1980

Floyd CC: Drugs for childbirth: Your guide to their benefits and risks. RN 41:May 1977

Grad RK, Woodside J: Obstetrical analgesics and anesthesia: Methods of relief for the patient in labor. Am J Nurs 77:242, February 1977

Nicolls ET, Corke BC, Osthermer GW: Epidural anesthesia for the woman in labor. Am J Nurs 81:1826, October 1981

Strichartz GR (ed): Local Anesthetics. Handbook of Experimental Pharmacology. Berlin, Springer-Verlag, 1985

Tucker GT: Pharmacokinetics of local anesthetics. Br J Anaesth 58:717, 1986

Wildsmith JA: Peripheral nerve and local anesthetic drugs. Br J Anaesth 58:692, 1986

Table 16-2
Local Anesthetics

Drug	Preparations	Usual Dosage Range	Nursing Implications
Benoxinate and Sodium Fluorescein Fluress	Drops: 0.4% benoxinate and 0.25% sodium fluorescein	Tonometry and removal of sutures and foreign bodies: 1–2 drops before operation Ophthalmic anesthesia: 2 drops 90 sec apart for 3 instillations.	Short-acting anesthetic with possible bacteriostatic action; no effect on pupil size or accommodation; minimal stinging or burning; fluorescein sodium stains abraded or ulcerated areas, facilitating visualization of foreign bodies
Benzocaine Several manufacturers	Ointment: 2%, 5%, 20% Cream: 1%, 5%, 6% Lotion: 0.5%, 10% Aerosol solution: 3%, 5%, 9.4%, 20% Oral liquid: 2%, 20% Otic solution: 1.5%, 5%, 20% Gel: 7.5%, 10%, 20% Candy: 6 mg Gum: 6 mg	Apply to area several times a day as required; *rectal ointment* given morning and night, and after each bowel movement *Gel:* used as a lubricant (e.g., catheters, specula) *Liquid, gel, or aerosol* for oral mucous membrane anesthesia in dentistry or topical anesthesia *Candy/gum* as an aid in weight loss: 6 mg–15 mg just prior to food consumption (maximum 45 mg/day);	Slowly absorbed from mucous membranes—exerts a fairly prolonged action; drug is a component of many combination products (e.g., oral, anorectal, otic, topical); produces hypersensitivity reactions in some individuals; stop drug at first sign of allergic response; avoid contact with eyes; may be used for temporary relief of toothache and in dental procedures; not recommended for use teething child; employed to lubricate catheters, endoscopic tubes, sigmoidoscopes, proctoscopes, and vaginal specula; also used as gum or candy (Ayds, Slim-Line) to decrease taste sensation as an adjunct in weight-reduction programs

Continued

Table 16-2
Local Anesthetics (continued)

Drug	Preparations	Usual Dosage Range	Nursing Implications
Bupivacaine Marcaine, Sensorcaine	Injection: 0.25%, 0.5%, 0.75% alone or with 1:200,000 epinephrine	Infiltration: 0.25% Epidural/caudal: 0.25%–0.5% Peripheral nerve block: 0.25%–0.5% Retrobulbar block: 0.75% Sympathetic block: 0.25%; Dental block: 0.5%	Onset slower than lidocaine, but more prolonged duration; widely used for nerve block, epidural or caudal, for long surgical or obstetrical procedures, and relief of pain during labor (*caution:* 0.75% concentration should not be used for obstetrical anesthesia; cardiac arrest and death have occurred); maximum dose 400 mg (with epinephrine) in 24 h; do not use for spinal block; not for use in children under 12
Butamben Butesin	Ointment: 1%	Apply 2 or 3 times/day as needed	Used mainly for minor burns and skin irritations
Chloroprocaine Nesacaine	Injection: 1%, 2%, 3%	Infiltration/nerve block: 1%–2% Caudal/epidural: 2%–3%	Onset within 10 min; effects persist 30–90 min; available without preservatives for caudal or epidural block; more rapid-acting and less toxic than procaine; IV use may cause thrombophlebitis; prior use of chloroprocaine may interfere with subsequent use of bupivacaine
Cocaine Several manufacturers	Soluble tablets: 135 mg Topical solution: 40 mg/mL, 100 mg/mL	Surface anesthesia: 1%–4%	Class II controlled substance (see Chap. 8); central stimulant that can lead to overwhelming psychological dependence when repeatedly inhaled or ingested; causes vasoconstriction when applied to mucous membrane; not used by injection or in the eyes; onset of acton is rapid when applied locally, and duration is about 1–2 h; widely abused drug (see Chap. 79)
Dibucaine Nupercainal	Ointment: 1% Cream: 0.5%	Apply locally 2–3 times/day	Onset about 15 min and duration 3 h–4 h
Dyclonine Dyclone	Solution: 0.5%, 1%	Apply topically to skin or mucous membranes	Used prior to endoscopic procedures to block the gag reflex; also used to relieve pain of oral or anogenital lesions; onset is about 10 min, duration approximately 60 min; may be used in patients hypersensitive to other local anesthetics
Etidocaine Duranest	*Injection:* 1% alone or 1% and 1.5% with 1:200,000 epinephrine	Infiltration: lumbar, central nerve block—1% Caudal: 1% Cesarean, intraabdominal: 1%–1.5% Maxillary: 1.5%	Onset of action within 3–5 min; duration up to 8 h with epinephrine (caution in ambulatory patients); induces profound motor blockade when given peridurally; not for use in children under 14 yr; use caution in elderly persons
Lidocaine Xylocaine, several other manufacturers (CAN) Xylocard	*Ointment:* 2.5%, 5% *Jelly:* 2% *Solution:* 2%, 4%, 10% *Injection:* 0.5%, 1%, 1.5%, 2%, 4%, 10%, 20% alone; 0.5%, 1%, 1.5%, 2% with epinephrine; 1.5% with 7.5% dextrose; 5% with 7.5% glucose	Apply topically as needed; solution for pain and inflammation of mouth, throat, pharynx, and urethra, as needed. Injection: Infiltration—0.5%–1% Nerve block: Dental—2%; intercostal—1%; brachial—1.5% paracervical—1% Epidural: thoracic—1%; lumbar—1%–2% Caudal: obstetric—1%; surgical—1.5%; spinal—5% with glucose; saddle block—1.5% with dextrose	Slightly more potent than procaine; rapid onset of action (1–2 min) lasting up to 2 h; widely used as antiarrhythmic agent (see Chap. 30); do not use solution with epinephrine for arrhythmias or solutions with preservatives for spinal or epidural block; oral solutions can interfere with swallowing reflex; caution in pediatric and geriatric patients; can enhance muscle relaxing action of neuromuscular blocking agents; contraindicated in persons with blood dyscrasias
Mepivacaine Carbocaine, Isocaine, Polocaine	Injection: 1%, 1.5%, 2%, 3% alone; 2% with 1:20,000 levonordefrin	Nerve block: 1%–2% Paracervical block: 1% Caudal/epidural: 1%–2% Infiltration: 1% Analgesia: 1%–2% Dental block—3% alone or 2% with levonordefrin	Twice as potent as procaine with comparable onset but more prolonged duration of action; possesses some vasoconstrictive action, so does not usually require a vasoconstrictor; injection containing levonordefrin used in dental procedures *only;* not used topically; less drowsiness and depression than observed with lidocaine; use with caution in renal dysfunction and with elderly patients

Continued

**Table 16-2
Local Anesthetics (continued)**

Drug	Preparations	Usual Dosage Range	Nursing Implications
Pramoxine Pramegel, Prax, Proctofoam, Tronothane	Cream: 1% Lotion: 1% Suppositories: 1% Aerosol foam (rectal use): 1% Rectal ointment: 1%	Apply topically or rectally 2 or 3 times/day as needed.	Not used by injection, or applied to the eye or nasal mucosa; component of many anorectal preparations (e.g., ointments, foams, suppositories); used mainly to relieve pain and itching, especially of hemorrhoids, and to facilitate endotracheal, intragastric, and rectal intubation procedures
Prilocaine Citanest	Injection: 4%; 4% with 1:200,000 epinephrine	Nerve block infiltration in dental procedures: 4%	Similar to lidocaine in its actions, but has a slower onset; may induce drowsiness and sleepiness; associated with some cases of methemoglobinemia; use is largely restricted to dental procedures
Procaine Novocain	Injection: 1%, 2%, 10%	Infiltration: 0.25%–0.5% Nerve block: 0.5%–2% Spinal block: 10%	Not employed topically; rapidly eliminated, short-acting (30–60 min), little central stimulation; relatively nontoxic but fairly high incidence of allergic reactions; metabolic product may interfere with actions of sulfonamides, and other local anesthetics should be used in presence of sulfonamide antibiotics; amide of procaine is an effective antiarrhythmic agent (see Chap. 30)
Proparacaine Aktaine, Alcaine, I-Paracaine, Kainair, Ophthaine, Ophthetic	Ophthalmic drops: 0.5%	Cataract surgery: 1 drop every 5–10 min Removal of sutures: 1–2 drops 2–3 min prior to surgery Foreign bodies: 1–2 drops prior to extraction Tonometry: 1–2 drops before measurement	Used in the eye exclusively; causes minimal irritation; may produce allergic contact dermatitis with drying and fissuring of fingertips
Tetracaine Pontocaine (CAN) Minims	Cream: 1% Ointment: 0.5% Oral solution: 2% Opthalmic ointment: 0.5% Opthalmic solution: 0.5% Injection: 1% alone; 0.2%, 0.3% with 6% dextrose Powder: 20 mg in Niphanoid (instantly soluble) ampules	Apply locally (0.5%–2%) as needed for pain, burning, itching Cataract surgery: 1 drop (0.5%) every 5–10 min Suture removal: 1 or 2 drops (0.5%) 2–3 min prior to procedure Foreign bodies: 1 to 2 drops prior to operating Tonometry: 1–2 drops before measurement Ophthalmic inflammation: apply ointment 2–3 times/day Spinal anesthesia: 0.2%–1% Caudal anesthesia: 0.2%–0.3% with dextrose Nasal or pharyngeal anesthesia: 2% solution	More potent (8–10 times) and longer-acting than procaine, but more toxic; onset of action relatively slow with duration 2–3 h; employed in rather low concentrations for surface anesthesia of eye, nose, and throat, as well as spinal and caudal anesthesia; induces prolonged spinal anesthesia for operations requiring 2–3 h; doses exceeding 15 mg are rarely required; do not reuse leftover autoclaved ampules because crystals may form

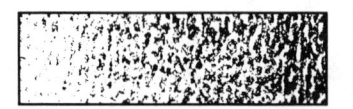

17 GENERAL ANESTHETICS

Drugs classified as general anesthetics are agents that, in sufficient amounts, are capable of inducing analgesia, decreased muscle reflex activity, and ultimately loss of consciousness. General anesthetics have varying degrees of potency, and distinct advantages as well as disadvantages exist among the many drugs used to induce anesthesia. Consequently, no single drug represents an "ideal" general anesthetic in terms of potency, stability, safety, and efficacy. Rather, several drugs are often used in combination to provide smooth induction, sufficient depth and duration of anesthesia, adequate muscle relaxation, and minimal hazards to the vital systems.

Several interesting theories have been proposed to explain the mechanism of action of the general anesthetics, but no single theory appears adequate to describe the effects observed with all of these agents. Parallels have been observed between the action of general anesthetics and their lipid solubility, their ability to inhibit glucose metabolism in the brain by blocking utilization of high-energy compounds such as ATP, and their capacity to combine with intracellular water, thereby interfering with cellular function and nerve transmission. It is likely that general anesthetics in some way alter the structure or function of nerve cell components, thereby reducing neuronal excitability and increasing the firing threshold.

An important site of action of these compounds is the reticular formation in the brainstem, which is the first area of the CNS to be affected by the general anesthetics. By reducing the number of impulses transmitted from this area of the brainstem to the cerebral cortex, these drugs progressively reduce sensory awareness, and when a sufficient concentration of anesthetic is present, consciousness is lost. Cells of the dorsal horn of the spinal cord are also quite sensitive to general anesthetics, resulting in an interruption of incoming sensory (e.g., pain) impulses.

As the degree of general anesthesia deepens, a series of physiological changes ensue. These provide an indication of the depth of depression of the CNS. Traditionally, these changes have been categorized into four stages (I–IV), which were originally described for diethyl ether, a drug having a very slow onset of action, and thus exhibiting a distinct separation between the succeeding stages. In modern anesthesiology, however, the distinctive signs of each stage of anesthesia are frequently obscured because many currently used general anesthetics have a very rapid onset of action and quickly bypass the early stages. In addition, mechanical respiratory assistance eliminates the variability in respiratory rate and depth seen with progressive deepening of anesthesia. Finally, certain characteristic signs of the different stages (e.g., pupillary diameter, tear secretion, and muscle relaxation) can be influenced by the use of preanesthetic medications like anticholinergics and skeletal muscle relaxants. Therefore the delineation of anesthesia into distinct stages is imprecise at best with most modern-day general anesthetics, and the appearance and duration of the effects noted in each stage vary widely, depending on the choice of anesthetic, speed of induction, and technique of the anesthesiologist. Table 17-1 presents a review of the principal physiological changes that occur as the patient passes through the stages of general anesthesia. Most surgery is performed at plane 2 or 3 of stage III, because muscle relaxation is usually optimal at this depth.

Safe, effective general anesthesia depends in part on proper preparation of the patient. In addition to the anesthetic drug itself, several other drugs are used routinely before, during, and after surgical procedures.

PREANESTHETIC MEDICATION

The purposes of preanesthetic medication and examples of drugs used are the following:

I. Relief of anxiety (sedatives such as benzodiazepines, e.g., diazepam, midazolam)
II. Reduction in salivary and mucous secretions (anticholinergics)
III. Inhibition of undesirable side effects (e.g., bradycardia and muscle spasms) occurring reflexly in response to the anesthetic agent (anticholinergics, peripherally acting skeletal muscle relaxants)

The use of narcotics for preoperative sedation and analgesia is subject to some controversy, inasmuch as they may depress respiration and cough, prolong the anesthetic state, and induce postoperative nausea and vomiting. Their use is largely a matter of physician preference.

Antiinfective agents such as cefazolin or metronidazole are often administered prior to and for a brief period following certain types of surgery (e.g., intraabdominal, vaginal hysterectomy, cesarean section) associated with a higher than average likelihood of infection.

ADJUNCTIVE ANESTHETIC MEDICATION

Drugs given during the surgical procedure depend upon the type and length of procedure and the patient's status. Neuromuscular blocking agents (e.g., succinylcholine) are commonly administered during the operation while the patient is still at a relatively light level of anesthesia. These agents provide an additional degree of skeletal muscle relaxation and therefore allow a lower dose of general anesthetic to be used, reducing the incidence of untoward reactions. Since they are all relatively short-acting drugs, good control of skeletal muscle activity can be maintained by an experienced anesthesiologist or anesthetist. For a more complete description of the peripherally acting skeletal muscle relaxants, see Chapter 15.

POSTOPERATIVE MEDICATION

Principal indications for use of drugs postoperatively are:

- Nausea and vomiting (antiemetics such as prochlorperazine)
- Abdominal distention and urinary retention (cholinergics such as bethanechol)
- Pain (analgesics)
- Constipation (laxatives and stool softeners, e.g., docusate, bisacodyl)

Judicious use of pre- and postoperative anesthetic medications can greatly facilitate induction and maintenance of the anesthetic state and recovery from them.

Table 17-1
Stages and Characteristics of Anesthesia

Stage/Plane	Respiration	Cardiovascular	Muscle Tone	Reflexes	Other
Stage I	Regular	Normal	Normal	Normal	Analgesia, euphoria, amnesia
Stage II	Rapid, irregular	Heart rate ↑ Blood pressure ↑	Tense Struggling	Swallowing Retching Gagging Vomiting	Mydriasis, roving eyeballs, loss of consciousness, diminished eyelid reflex
Stage III Plane 1	Regular	Heart rate and blood pressure normal	Smaller muscles relaxed	Lid and pharyngeal (gag) reflexes absent	Increased lacrimation, miosis, some eye movement, increased respiration and blood pressure with incision
Plane 2	Regular but shallow	Normal	Large muscles relaxed	Corneal and laryngeal reflexes absent	Eyes stilled, miosis, decreased lacrimation, no response to incision
Plane 3	Shallow and mainly abdominal	Blood pressure falls slightly; some tachycardia	Complete relaxation	Pupillary (light) and cough reflex disappear	Mydriasis, decreased lacrimation
Plane 4	Abdominal and very shallow	Hypotension and some tachycardia	Complete relaxation	No reflexes	Mydriasis; no lacrimation
Stage IV	Respiratory paralysis	Marked hypotension and failing circulation	Complete relaxation	No reflexes	Extreme mydriasis, medullary paralysis, and eventual death

The clinically useful general anesthetics may be classified in the following manner:

I. Inhalation anesthetics
  A. Gases (e.g., nitrous oxide, cyclopropane)
  B. Volatile liquids (e.g., halothane, methoxyflurane, isoflurane)
II. Intravenous anesthetics
  A. Ultrashort-acting barbiturates (e.g., thiopental, methohexital)
  B. Hypnotics (e.g., etomidate)
  C. Dissociative agents (e.g., ketamine, fentanyl/droperidol— may also be given IM)

Although the clinical pharmacology of each general anesthetic drug is reviewed briefly here, anyone who routinely handles these drugs should become thoroughly familiar with the advantages and disadvantages of each preparation and the procedures for its proper administration (i.e., open-drop, semiclosed, or complete rebreathing methods) by consulting specific literature pertaining to each agent. The following discussions of the more widely used drugs should not be viewed as a complete description of the pharmacologic properties and clinical implications of the compounds.

INHALATION ANESTHETICS

The inhalation anesthetics include gases and volatile liquids. Both types enter the circulation rapidly upon inhalation and are transported through the bloodstream to the CNS. Eventually, most are again returned to the lungs and excreted (exhaled) essentially unchanged. Halothane and methoxyflurane, however, are metabolized to a significant extent in the liver. A potential danger with most of the potent, lipid-soluble inhalational anesthetics is malignant hyperthermia, an acute condition characterized by a sudden, drastic elevation in body temperature that is often fatal unless treated immediately and vigorously. This condition is also associated with the use of many neuromuscular blocking agents, especially when given concurrently with inhalation anesthetics. When these drugs are used together, the patient must be carefully monitored. Treatment consists of injections of dantrolene (see Chap. 15) or possibly one of the calcium channel blockers (see Chap. 32).

Gases

Three gases are currently available for use as general anesthetics, and of these only nitrous oxide is used extensively. In fact, it is one of the most widely used of all general anesthetics, most often as part of a total anesthetic regimen that also includes sedatives, other anesthetics, narcotics, barbiturates, and muscle relaxants; such a regimen is termed *balanced anesthesia*. This type of drug combination usually produces rapid induction with minimal adverse effects, and it allows a significant reduction in the amount of each drug required. The other two gases, cyclopropane and ethylene, are infrequently used today and will be considered only briefly below.

Cyclopropane

Cyclopropane is an anesthetic gas with a rapid onset of action and a good safety margin. It produces satisfactory analgesia and skeletal muscle relaxation in full anesthetic doses. It is explosive, so it must be administered in a closed rebreathing system with oxygen. Respiratory irritation is minimal, although laryngospasm has occasionally occurred. Blood pressure is well maintained during anesthesia. However, the drug sensitizes the myocardium to the arrhythmogenic effects of catecholamines, and this can cause sudden death; maintenance of adequate ventilation minimizes the possibility of arrhythmias. Postoperative nausea, vomiting, and headaches occur frequently following use of cyclopropane. Malignant hyperthermia has been associated with its administration.

For induction, concentrations up to 50% have been employed, whereas maintenance levels are usually 10% to 20%. If emergence excitement occurs, it can be reduced by administering a sedative or narcotic prior to discontinuing the drug. Extreme caution such as use of antistatic equipment must be exercised during administration of cyclopropane to prevent an explosion. The drug is essentially obsolete today.

Ethylene

Ethylene is a highly volatile gas that produces rapid induction and recovery, exhibits low toxicity, and possesses a wide safety margin. It is similar to, but slightly more potent than nitrous oxide; however, unlike nitrous oxide, it is highly explosive and has an unpleasant odor. Muscle relaxation is poor. Ethylene must be given in high concentrations (80%) with oxygen in a closed system, and the major danger is hypoxia. Since more potent and less hazardous general anesthetics are available, the use of ethylene today is almost nonexistent.

Nitrous Oxide (N_2O)

Nitrous oxide, also known as laughing gas, is a nonexplosive gas that displays a rapid onset of action and correspondingly short duration of action. It is a poor skeletal muscle relaxant and, owing to its lack of potency, can induce only a very light plane of anesthesia. It cannot elicit sufficient depth of anesthesia to allow performance of most surgical procedures when used alone. Nitrous oxide is most often employed as a component of balanced anesthesia in conjunction with other, more potent inhalational anesthetics and preanesthetic medication

USES
Induction of anesthesia
Supplemental maintenance of general anesthesia
Production of analgesia for minor surgical or dental procedures: analgesia is approximately equivalent to that induced by morphine

DOSAGE
(Always used in an oxygen mixture)
Induction anesthesia: 70% to 80% N_2O for brief periods
Maintenance anesthesia: 50% to 70% N_2O to prolong anesthetic state
Analgesia: 20% to 30% N_2O
Note: Hypoxia will occur if concentrations of N_2O greater than 80% are used for any length of time—at least 20% oxygen must be provided whenever N_2O is used

FATE
Rapid onset and short duration of action; excreted primarily by exhalation from the lungs

SIGNIFICANT ADVERSE REACTIONS

WARNING
Nitrous oxide is considerably more soluble in blood than is nitrogen; thus it will enter pockets of trapped gas, replacing nitrogen and expanding the volume of gas. This situation can occur in the bowel, lung, or middle ear, leading to possible damage to the organs as a consequence of rapid expansion. Likewise, a significant elevation in cerebrospinal fluid pressure has occurred with nitrous oxide following injection of air into the cerebral ventricles during a pneumoencephalogram.

Dizziness, vivid dreaming, and possibly hallucinations; if a state of hypoxia persists for any length of time, cyanosis, convulsions, leukopenia, and bone marrow depression can occur. Very high concentrations of nitrous oxide may cause vomiting, myocardial and respiratory depression, and ultimately death.

NURSING CONSIDERATIONS

Nursing Alert
- Ensure that oxygen is available for use with N_2O. No more than a few undiluted (without oxygen) breaths should be administered. Hypoxia will occur if concentrations greater than 80% are employed for any length of time.

1. Expect supplemental drugs (muscle relaxants, barbiturates, other general anesthetics) to be administered when N_2O is employed in anesthesia because it is a rather weak anesthetic and muscle relaxant.

PATIENT EDUCATION
1. Warn patient that dizziness, confusion, vivid dreams, and hallucinations may occur with N_2O use but will disappear when the drug is stopped.
2. Caution patient receiving N_2O to use care in driving car or operating other machinery until effects of drug have completely disappeared.

Volatile Liquids

The volatile liquid anesthetics are administered by inhalation of the vapors given off by the liquid along with adequate amounts of oxygen. The depth of anesthesia can be fairly well controlled by varying the concentration, because these agents are generally short-acting. Recovery begins as soon as the drug is removed because most drugs are excreted largely through the lungs. These agents must be used cautiously in patients with pulmonary diseases, because excretion may be impaired and accumulation toxicity can result.

Enflurane
Ethrane

A potent, volatile liquid anesthetic widely used for many surgical procedures; induction and recovery are rapid, skeletal muscle relaxation is good (only minimal amounts of muscle relaxants are needed for more extensive surgery), and the drug is nonflammable; salivary and bronchial secretions are increased; myocardial contractility is somewhat depressed but heart rate is unchanged; blood pressure is usually reduced; high concentrations of enflurane have a CNS stimulant effect and can lead to increased muscle contractions and seizures; frequently given in combination with nitrous oxide, which allows use of a smaller amount of enflurane and hence less danger of CNS excitation;

releases fluoride ion, and thus large amounts may damage kidneys.

USES
Induction and maintenance of general anesthesia, usually in combination with minimal amounts of skeletal muscle relaxants

Provide analgesia for vaginal delivery or supplement other anesthetics for cesarean section (high levels may relax uterus)

DOSAGE
Induction: 2.0% to 4.5% for 7 to 10 minutes
Maintenance: 0.5% to 3.0%

FATE
Rapid onset of action and recovery; excreted largely (85%–90%) through the lungs, the remainder metabolized by the liver and excreted in the kidney

COMMON SIDE EFFECTS
Slight hypotension

SIGNIFICANT ADVERSE REACTIONS
Decreased myocardial contractility, CNS stimulation with prolonged use, renal damage, and malignant hyperthermia

CONTRAINDICATIONS
No absolute contraindications. *Cautious use* in patients with impaired kidney function, history of epilepsy or other convulsive states, cardiac disease or arrhythmias

INTERACTIONS
An increased potential for arrhythmias related to effects of catecholamines on the myocardium may occur in the presence of enflurane

Additive myocardial depression can occur when enflurane is used in combination with beta blockers, quinidine, procainamide, disopyramide, digitalis drugs, and verapamil

Enflurane may potentiate the muscle relaxing effects of antidepolarizing neuromuscular blockers

NURSING CONSIDERATIONS
1. Expect only minimal doses of neuromuscular blocking agents to be used if additional relaxation is desired. Muscle relaxation is generally sufficient for most operations.
2. Question rationale if sympathomimetic agents are prescribed during enflurane administration because arrhythmias can result.

Ether (diethyl ether)
Diethyl ether was the first clinically useful volatile liquid anesthetic. It possesses a good safety margin, excellent skeletal muscle relaxing ability, minimal effects on the cardiovascular system, and substantial analgesic effect. However, the drug's disadvantages include a noxious odor, slow and often unpleasant induction, prolonged emergence, respiratory irritation, increased salivary and bronchial secretions, high incidence of postoperative nausea and vomiting, and extreme flammability; it is therefore rarely used in contemporary practice.

Ether is *occasionally* used where sophisticated patient monitoring equipment is not available, primarily because of its good safety margin. The stages of anesthesia (see Table 17-1) are well delineated with ether owing to its slow induction and recovery, and the level of anesthesia can be fairly well controlled by observation of the patient.

Concentrations of 5% to 10% have been used to induce anesthesia, although the induction process is slow and uncomfortable, and the drug is rarely used for this reason. Good surgical anesthesia can be maintained with concentrations of 3% to 5% in combination with other general anesthetics.

NURSING CONSIDERATIONS

Nursing Alert
- Be prepared for the possibility of prolonged paralysis if additional muscle relaxants are used. They should be used cautiously with ether because the drug has good muscle relaxant actions of its own.

1. Because nausea and vomiting are common during recovery, turn patient's head toward one side to avoid aspiration of vomitus.
2. During recovery, avoid remarks that may upset patient, even if he or she is still unconscious. As with any general anesthetic, *hearing* is one of the earliest senses to return.
3. Use only unopened, sealed containers of ether for anesthesia.

Halothane
Fluothane
(CAN) (Somnothane)

A potent, nonflammable, pleasant-smelling volatile liquid anesthetic, halothane is one of the most widely used anesthetic drugs. It is nonirritating to the respiratory tract and does not increase salivary or bronchial secretions. Muscle relaxation is only fair with halothane, however, and a skeletal muscle relaxant is almost always used. Cardiac output, contractile force, and blood pressure all decrease following administration; in addition, the drug sensitizes the myocardium to the arrhythmogenic effects of catecholamines, and serious arrhythmias can result if a catecholamine is used in the presence of halothane. Respiratory depression is marked, and apnea, hypoxia, and acidosis may develop during deep anesthesia. Postanesthetic nausea and vomiting are rare. Halothane has been associated with liver dysfunction (hepatitis, jaundice), especially in persons with prior hepatic disease or previous exposure to halothane.

USES
Induction and maintenance anesthesia

DOSAGE
(Usually with oxygen or oxygen–nitrous oxide mixture)
Induction: 1% to 4%
Maintenance: 0.5% to 1.5%

FATE
Quickly absorbed; largely excreted through the lungs, but up to 20% may be converted to metabolites and excreted in the urine

COMMON SIDE EFFECTS
Hypotension, rapid and shallow respiration, transient bradycardia

SIGNIFICANT ADVERSE REACTIONS
Arrhythmias (in presence of sympathomimetic agents), vomiting, hypoxia, respiratory difficulty, postoperative shivering,

liver damage, increased intracranial pressure, and malignant hyperthermia (rare)

CONTRAINDICATIONS
Obstetrical anesthesia (drug is a potent uterine relaxant), severe hepatic or biliary disease. *Cautious use* in persons with cardiac disease or preexisting liver damage and during pregnancy

INTERACTIONS
Halothane may potentiate the effects of antidepolarizing muscle relaxants (e.g., curare, gallamine) and ganglionic blocking agents

Arrhythmias may be produced by the combination of halothane and catecholamines

NURSING CONSIDERATIONS

Nursing Alerts
- Notify anesthetist/anesthesiologist if patient's history shows evidence of liver damage (fever, anorexia, nausea, vomiting) following previous halothane administration because it should not be used again. Incidence of serious hepatic damage increases with progressive use. Although not absolutely contraindicated, administration of halothane in patients with preexisting liver disease should be undertaken cautiously.
- Have on hand atropine to treat bradycardia and vasopressors (e.g., ephedrine, phenylephrine) to treat marked hypotension resulting from halothane.

1. Keep patient warm postoperatively to minimize shivering.
2. Be prepared for the possibility that the uterine-relaxant effect of halothane may not respond to ergot drugs or oxytocin.

Isoflurane
Forane

A volatile liquid anesthetic structurally similar to enflurane, isoflurane has a rapid onset and quick recovery. It does not sensitize the heart to catecholamines, and produces good muscle relaxation. CNS excitation is minimal, but respiratory depression may be significant, and blood pressure progressively decreases with depth of anesthesia.

USES
Induction and maintenance of general anesthesia

DOSAGE
Induction: 1.5% to 3% for 5 to 10 minutes
Maintenance: 1.0% to 2.5% with nitrous oxide

FATE
Induction and recovery are rapid; less than 1% of the total dose absorbed systemically is metabolized; primarily excreted through the lungs

COMMON SIDE EFFECTS
Mild hypotension

SIGNIFICANT ADVERSE REACTIONS
Respiratory depression, tachycardia, malignant hyperthermia

CONTRAINDICATIONS
No absolute contraindications. *Cautious use* in patients with respiratory disease or congestive heart failure

INTERACTIONS
The muscle relaxant effect of isoflurane can be increased by concomitant use of other skeletal muscle relaxants

Increased respiratory depression can occur in combination with barbiturates, narcotics, and other respiratory depressants

NURSING CONSIDERATIONS

Nursing Alert
- Monitor respiration closely, because drug is a potent respiratory depressant. Have respiratory assistance immediately available.

1. Have vasopressors available to treat hypotension should it develop.

Methoxyflurane
Penthrane

A very potent inhalation anesthetic, with slow onset and recovery, methoxyflurane produces fair muscle relaxation and significant analgesia at light levels of anesthesia. Incidence of arrhythmias is low, but profound circulatory depression can occur at higher concentrations. The drug is associated with liver and especially kidney damage due to accumulation of free fluoride ion as a metabolic byproduct of methoxyflurane.

USES
Maintenance of surgical anesthesia of less than 4-hour duration (usually with nitrous oxide and oxygen)

Production of analgesia in obstetrics and minor surgical procedures

DOSAGE
I. *Analgesia:* 0.3% to 0.8% (may be used with hand-held inhalers, e.g., Analgizer, Cyprane)
II. *Anesthesia*
   A. Induction: up to 2% for 2 to 5 minutes
   B. Maintenance: 0.1% to 2.0% with at least 50% nitrous oxide

(Use lowest effective concentration at all times)

FATE
Slow onset often associated with excitement; high lipid solubility leads to prolonged emergence if not discontinued 30 to 40 minutes before end of surgery; up to 70% of the drug is metabolized in the liver; remainder is excreted through lungs and kidneys

COMMON SIDE EFFECTS
Mild hypotension, nausea, postanesthetic drowsiness

SIGNIFICANT ADVERSE REACTIONS
Renal dysfunction, hepatic dysfunction (jaundice, necrosis), respiratory depression, prolonged postoperative sedation, delirium, malignant hyperthermia, and cardiac arrest (rare)

CONTRAINDICATIONS

Renal disease, vascular surgery near the renal vessels, patients receiving the drug within the previous month, cirrhosis, viral hepatitis, and patients showing jaundice or unexplained fever with other inhalation anesthetics. *Cautious use* in patients with liver disease, diabetes, for surgical procedure lasting more than 4 hours (increased likelihood of fluoride ion accumulation), and during pregnancy

INTERACTIONS

- Use of methoxyflurane with certain nephrotoxic antibiotics (e.g., vancomycin, aminoglycosides, amphotericin) may cause fatal renal toxicity
- Muscle-relaxing action of antidepolarizing neuromuscular blocking agents may be augmented by methoxyflurane. Reduce dose of each accordingly

NURSING CONSIDERATIONS

Nursing Alert

- **Carefully monitor urinary output and laboratory tests for possible renal dysfunction (e.g., creatinine, electrolytes). Nephrotoxicity is dose related and probably due to liberation of the fluoride ion as a metabolic byproduct. The lowest effective dose should be used to minimize danger of renal damage.**

1. Monitor heart rate and rhythm if catecholamines or related drugs, which should be used carefully, are administered because arrhythmias can develop in the presence of methoxyflurane.
2. Monitor respirations when barbiturates or narcotics are given as adjunctive medication. Conservative dosage should be used to avoid additive respiratory depression.

INTRAVENOUS ANESTHETICS

The general anesthetics administered IV include three ultrashort-acting barbiturates. These are used mainly for induction of anesthesia but may also be employed as the sole anesthetic agent in short surgical procedures associated with minimal pain, and to supplement other anesthetic agents during longer procedures.

They are rapidly taken up by the brain following IV injection and are almost as rapidly redistributed to other parts of the body. Therefore, within 5 minutes after injection, the brain level of the barbiturate has declined to about one half of its peak attained shortly (30–45 sec) after injection. At 30 minutes following injection only about one tenth of the initial concentration remains in the brain because the drug has been redistributed to other fatty stores in the body. Emergence occurs during this period of declining brain levels, even though the rate of metabolism and excretion of the drug from the body is quite constant and rather slow (10%–15%/h).

A rapid-acting nonbarbiturate hypnotic, etomidate, is also available for IV use as an induction anesthetic and for supplementing other anesthetics such as nitrous oxide. It is reviewed below.

Two other drugs that can be administered either IV or IM are categorized as *dissociative anesthetics* because they induce a neuroleptic-like effect that is characterized by analgesia, quietude, and detachment from the environment without loss of consciousness. These two drugs, ketamine and a combination of the narcotic fentanyl and the neuroleptic droperidol differ slightly in some of their pharmacologic properties and are discussed separately.

Ultrashort-Acting Barbiturates

The barbiturates employed in general anesthesia are those having an extremely rapid onset and relatively short duration (15–30 min) of action. The response of the CNS to these drugs is essentially the same as that following an inhalation anesthetic: in succeeding order, loss of consciousness, diminished reflexes, loss of motor tone, and ultimately failure of the vital medullary centers. Recovery proceeds in the reverse direction.

The major advantages of the IV barbiturates as compared with many inhalation anesthetics are rapidity and smoothness of onset, absence of salivation, greater patient acceptance (no occlusive face mask), short duration (allowing better control), speedy recovery, nonflammability, lower degree of irritation, and little danger of arrhythmias.

Disadvantages of the IV anesthetics include higher incidences of respiratory and circulatory depression, laryngospasm, bronchospasm, and if leakage occurs, the danger of tissue necrosis. Prolonged or repeated administration may lead to cumulative toxicity, because the drugs are removed slowly from the body.

As there are many similarities among the three anesthetic barbiturates, they are discussed as a group. Dosages and specific information pertaining to each drug are given in Table 17-2.

Methohexital
Thiamylal
Thiopental

MECHANISM

Intravenous barbiturates exert a CNS-depressant effect to produce hypnosis and anesthesia without analgesia. Muscle relaxation is generally inadequate, even with deep anesthesia. These drugs are potent respiratory depressants, and the degree of respiratory depression is dose-dependent. Large doses can also decrease cardiac output and lower arterial blood pressure by means of a direct myocardial-depressant action. Hepatic blood flow and glomerular filtration rates may be temporarily reduced

USES

Induction of anesthesia

Supplementation of other general anesthetics

Production of anesthesia for short surgical procedures with minimal painful stimuli

Induction of hypnosis

Control of convulsive states during and following general or local anesthesia or other causes (thiopental)

Aid to narcoanalysis and narcosynthesis in psychiatric disorders (thiopental)

DOSAGE

See Table 17-2

FATE

Induction is smooth and rapid; onset of anesthesia occurs within 30 seconds to 60 seconds following IV injection; drugs quickly cross the blood–brain barrier but are then rapidly

Table 17-2
Intravenous Barbiturate Anesthetics

Drug	Preparations	Usual Dosage Range	Nursing Implications
Methohexital Brevital (CAN) Brietal	Powder for injection: 500 mg, 2.5 g, 5 g	*Induction:* 5 mL–12 mL of 1% solution by infusion at 1 mL/5 sec *Maintenance:* 2 mL–4 mL of 1% solution every 4–7 min	Shortest-acting IV barbiturate, poor muscle-relaxing ability; proper preanesthetic medication should be given; sterile water for injection is the preferred diluent; do *not* use dilutions that are not clear and colorless; dilutions in sterile water are stable at room temperature for 6 wk; do *not* mix with acid solutions or allow contact with silicone; incompatible with lactated Ringer's solution
Thiamylal Surital	Powder for injection: 1 g, 5 g, 10 g	*Induction:* 3 mL–6 mL of 2.5% solution at a rate of 1 mL/5 sec *Maintenance:* 2.5% solution by intermittent IV injection as needed *or* 0.3% solution by continuous drip	Similar to methohexital with a longer duration of action (10–30 min); do not mix with atropine, tubocurarine, or succinylcholine; do not reconstitute with Ringer's solution or solutions containing bacteriostatic agents or buffers; sterile water for injection is the preferred diluent for IV injection solutions; continuous-drip solutions are prepared with 5% dextrose or isotonic sodium chloride to avoid hypotonicity; use only clear solutions; stable at room temperature for 24 h and refrigerated for 6 days
Thiopental Pentothal	Injection: 250-mg, 400-mg, 500-mg syringes Powder for injection: 500 mg, 1 g, 2.5 g, 5 g Rectal suspension: 400 mg/g of suspension	Anesthesia: *Induction:* 2 mL–3 mL of 2.5% solution IV at 20–40 sec intervals *Maintenance:* 1 mL–2 mL 2.5% solution as needed (IV drip—0.2%–0.4%) Convulsions: 3 mL–5 mL of 2.5% solution Psychiatry: 4 mL–5mL 2.5% solution (IV drip—0.2% at 50 mL/min) Preanesthetic sedation: 1 g/75 lb (30 mg/kg) rectally to a maximum of 1.5 g for children and 4 g for adults	Most widely used IV barbiturate anesthetic; rectal administration may cause irritation, diarrhea, cramping, and bleeding; do not give rectally in presence of inflammatory, ulcerative, or bleeding lesions of the lower bowel; do not use concentrations less than 2% in sterile water for injection for IV administration, because hemolysis can occur; use freshly prepared solutions; discard unused portions after 24 h; avoid mixing with other solutions having an acid pH (e.g., tubocurarine or succinylcholine solutions)

redistributed to other parts of the body, first to highly vascular organs, subsequently to fatty tissue, where they are stored; duration of anesthesia with methohexital is 5 to 8 minutes compared with 15 to 30 minutes with thiamylal and thiopental; rectal absorption of thiopental is good, and onset occurs within 10 minutes; plasma half-life of the drugs ranges between 4 and 8 hours; repeated dosing or continuous infusion leads to accumulation of the drug in lipid storage sites, causing prolonged drowsiness and respiratory or circulatory depression

COMMON SIDE EFFECTS
Respiratory depression, hypotension, sneezing, coughing, hiccups, yawning

SIGNIFICANT ADVERSE REACTIONS
(Not all reactions occur with all drugs; most are noted with prolonged administration)

CV: myocardial and circulatory depression, arrhythmias, thrombophlebitis, pain on injection, necrosis or sloughing of tissue upon extravasation, arteriospasm upon inadvertent intra-arterial injection

Respiratory: laryngospasm, bronchospasm, apnea, dyspnea
CNS: prolonged somnolence, headache, emergence delirium, anxiety
Other: nausea, vomiting, allergic reactions (pruritus, urticaria, rhinitis), abdominal pain, salivation, shivering, muscle twitching

CONTRAINDICATIONS
Latent or manifest porphyria, absence of suitable veins for IV administration; thiopental contraindicated in status asthmaticus. *Cautious use* in persons with severe cardiovascular disease, bronchial asthma, hypotension, shock, Addison's disease, hepatic or renal dysfunction, myxedema, increased blood urea, severe anemia, increased intracranial pressure, and myasthenia gravis

INTERACTIONS
CNS depressant effects may be additive to those of other depressants, including alcohol, sedatives, and narcotics
Orthostatic hypotension may be elicited by combined use with bumetanide, furosemide, or ethacrynic acid

NURSING CONSIDERATIONS
(For additional information, see Table 17-2.)

Nursing Alerts
- Be prepared for possibility of respiratory depression. Have appropriate resuscitative equipment and respiratory aids on hand.
- Observe vital signs continually during administration. If possible, a small test dose of thiopental should be given initially to determine sensitivity.
- If shivering or facial twitching occurs with thiopental, warm patient with blankets, maintain room temperature near 26°C, and administer appropriate prescribed medications (e.g., chlorpromazine or methylphenidate) if needed.
- Assess injection site frequently for indications of extravasation, which may cause tissue necrosis.
- If extravasation occurs, follow established protocol. To alleviate pain, 1% procaine may be injected locally. Heat may be applied to minimize irritation.
- With methohexital anesthesia, closely monitor patient postoperatively because drug may have extended action owing to slow metabolism.

1. Because thiopental solution contains no bacteriostatic agent, use aseptic technique in preparing and handling solution to prevent contamination. Do *not* sterilize by heating. Use sterile water, saline, or 5% dextrose to prepare solutions.
2. Dilute stock solutions of methohexital before injection. Follow diluting instructions carefully; do not use diluents containing bacteriostatic agents. Discard solutions in saline after 24 hours at room temperature, the length of time they are stable.

Nonbarbiturate Hypnotic

Etomidate
Amidate

Etomidate is a rapid-acting hypnotic but is not an analgesic; it is used principally IV for induction of general anesthesia. The drug has minimal effects on heart rate, cardiac output, or peripheral circulation but produces frequent myoclonic muscle movements and transient venous pain upon injection

USES
Induction of general anesthesia
Supplemental anesthesia during short operative procedures
Prolonged sedation of critically ill patients

DOSAGE
Induction: 0.2 mg/kg to 0.6 mg/kg IV over 30 to 60 seconds
Maintenance: 0.1 mg/kg to 0.3 mg/kg as needed in combination with nitrous oxide and oxygen

FATE
Onset is usually within 1 minute, and effects persist for 3 to 5 minutes; rapidly metabolized in the liver and primarily excreted by the kidney; highly lipid soluble and widely distributed in the body

COMMON SIDE EFFECTS
Transient venous pain, myoclonic skeletal muscle movements, tonic muscle activity, eye movements

SIGNIFICANT ADVERSE REACTIONS
Hypotension, tachycardia, arrhythmias, hyperventilation, transient apnea, laryngospasm, hiccups, postoperative nausea and vomiting

CONTRAINDICATIONS
Children under 10. *Cautious use* in patients with respiratory disease or skeletal muscle hyperactivity states and pregnant or nursing women

INTERACTIONS
An additive CNS depressant effect can occur in combination with narcotics, sedatives, and other depressants

NURSING CONSIDERATIONS

Nursing Alerts
- Be alert for development of myoclonic (and occasionally tonic) skeletal muscle activity following injection.

1. Advise patient that pain at the injection site may occur but is usually transient.
2. Be aware that etomidate is compatible with most commonly used preanesthetic medications.

Dissociative Agents

Two drugs, ketamine and fentanyl/droperidol (Innovar) can be used in certain situations in which an anesthetic-like state is desired but unconsciousness might prove disadvantageous. These agents are employed alone for certain indications or are combined with other anesthetics or analgesics. They differ sufficiently in their actions and pharmacologic properties; thus, they will be discussed separately.

Ketamine
Ketalar

Ketamine is a rapid-acting anesthetic producing a state of dissociation, characterized by profound analgesia, normal skeletal muscle tone and laryngeal reflexes, and variable cardiovascular and respiratory stimulation. The patient is awake but does not respond to pain nor remember the experience. Ketamine possesses a rather wide margin of safety and is compatible with commonly used general and local anesthetics. Emergence from ketamine anesthesia is prolonged (several hours), and in 10% to 15% of patients is marked by psychological manifestations ranging from pleasant (dream-like states, vivid imagery) to quite disagreeable (nightmare-like effects, hallucinations). These may be accompanied by confusion, excitement, and irrational behavior

MECHANISM
Actions are presumed to result from an interruption of association pathways in the brain prior to an effect on specific sensory pathways. Blood pressure is usually elevated within a few minutes after injection but returns to normal within 15 minutes

USES

Diagnostic and short surgical procedures not requiring skeletal muscle relaxation (e.g., treatment of burns)

Induction of anesthesia before administration of other general anesthetics

Supplementation of low-potency agents such as nitrous oxide

DOSAGE

Induction: 1 mg/kg to 4.5 mg/kg IV injection over 60 seconds, or 6.5 mg/kg to 13 mg/kg IM. Alternatively, 1 mg/kg to 2 mg/kg by slow IV injection (0.5 mg/kg/min) in combination with diazepam (2 mg–5 mg IV over 60 sec) in a separate syringe

Maintenance: increments of one half- to full-induction doses repeated as needed, titrated to patient's needs

FATE

Onset of surgical anesthesia is 30 seconds with IV injection and 3 to 4 minutes for IM; duration lasts 5 to 10 minutes IV and 15 to 25 minutes IM. Recovery time is dose-dependent; metabolites are excreted primarily in the urine

COMMON SIDE EFFECTS

Elevated blood pressure, tachycardia, and respiratory stimulation, increased muscle tone

SIGNIFICANT ADVERSE REACTIONS

Pain at injection site, laryngospasm, rash, diplopia, nystagmus, intensified muscle tone (tonic or clonic convulsions); large doses may produce respiratory depression, hypotension, or arrhythmias. Upon recovery, CNS effects such as excitement, delirium, hallucinations, vivid dreams, nightmares, confusion, and irrational behavior may occur. See **Nursing Considerations**

CONTRAINDICATIONS

Individuals for whom an elevation in blood pressure may prove dangerous; drug should not be used without additional muscle relaxants in surgical or diagnostic procedures involving the pharynx, larynx, or bronchial tree. *Cautious use* in patients with hypertension, elevated cerebrospinal fluid pressure, in alcoholics, and in pregnant women

INTERACTIONS

Barbiturates or narcotics may prolong ketamine recovery time

Severe hypertension and tachycardia can occur in the presence of thyroid drugs

Ketamine may increase the neuromuscular blocking effects of nondepolarizing muscle relaxants (e.g., tubocurarine, attracurium, vecuronium)

NURSING CONSIDERATIONS

Nursing Alerts

- Continually monitor blood pressure and respiration during ketamine use. Be prepared to provide assistance with mechanical ventilation if respiratory depression occurs.
- During recovery period, minimize verbal, visual, and tactile stimulation to reduce danger of irrational behavior and other disturbing psychological manifestations. A rapid-acting barbiturate may be given to control severe emergence reactions, which are less likely to occur in the very young (under 15), the elderly (over 65), and when the drug is used IM rather than IV.

1. When drug is given IV, expect it to be administered slowly (over 1 min) to avoid excessive respiratory depression and hypertension. For IV injection, dilute 100 mg/mL concentration in sterile water, saline, or dextrose.
2. Be prepared for the occurrence of tonic–clonic movements during ketamine anesthesia. These do *not* signify a light plane of anesthesia and do *not* indicate a need for additional drug.
3. Use separate syringes to administer ketamine and barbiturates because they are chemically incompatible.
4. Read product literature for specific recommendations for application of ketamine. These recomemndations are quite numerous and encompass many different types of procedures.

Fentanyl/Droperidol

Innovar

This drug is a combination of a narcotic analgesic (fentanyl) and a neuroleptic or major tranquilizer (droperidol), that produces an effect termed *neuroleptanalgesia*, characterized by general quiescence, reduced motor activity, and profound analgesia; complete loss of consciousness usually does not occur with Innovar alone. It can elicit mild to moderate hypotension and bradycardia, respiratory depression, and muscle rigidity. Anesthesia can be induced following Innovar by administration of 65% nitrous oxide in oxygen.

USES

Production of tranquilization and analgesia for diagnostic and minor surgical procedures

Induction of anesthesia or anesthetic premedication

Adjunct for the maintenance of general and regional anesthesia, with nitrous oxide and oxygen

DOSAGE

(1 mL contains 0.05 mg fentanyl and 2.5 mg droperidol)

Premedication: 0.5 mL to 2.0 mL IM 45 to 60 minutes prior to surgery (Children—0.25 mL/20 lb IM)

Induction: 1 mL/20 to 25 lb by slow IV injection (3–5 min), or 10 mL/250 mL 5% Dextrose by IV drip (Children—0.5 mL/20 lb IM; initial dose should be reduced in elderly, debilitated, or other poor risk patients)

Diagnostic: 0.5 mL to 2.0 mL IM 45 to 60 minutes before procedure; increments of 0.5 mL to 1.0 mL IV may be used for prolonged procedures as needed. Dosage must be individually determined and then adjusted according to need. Vital signs must be monitored during administration

FATE

The drug combination exhibits a fairly slow onset and prolonged duration, although each component has different characteristics. Fentanyl possesses an onset of 5 to 10 minutes and a duration of 30 to 60 minutes. Droperidol has a slower onset (30 min) and prolonged action (up to 6 h)

COMMON SIDE EFFECTS

Muscle rigidity, hypotension, postdrug drowsiness

SIGNIFICANT ADVERSE REACTIONS

Extrapyramidal symptoms (see Chap. 22), dizziness, laryngospasm, bronchospasm, respiratory depression, shivering, tachycardia, vomiting, delirium, and hallucinations

CONTRAINDICATIONS

Presence of MAO inhibitors, children under 2, and parkinsonism. *Cautious use* in persons with arrhythmias, chronic obstructive pulmonary disease, liver or kidney dysfunction and in trauma patients (increased likelihood of muscle rigidity)

INTERACTIONS

CNS depressants (e.g., barbiturates, narcotics, alcohol) may have additive CNS effects with Innovar

NURSING CONSIDERATIONS

Nursing Alerts

- Because one component of the drug is a narcotic, have appropriate resuscitative equipment and narcotic antagonists (naloxone) on hand.
- Expect IV injection to be given *slowly* to minimize the occurrence of muscle rigidity. If it should occur, respiratory assistance and a neuromuscular blocking agent are used.
- Ensure that fluids and pressor agents are available in case they are needed to manage hypotension.

1. When Innovar is used for procedures such as bronchoscopy, anticipate administration of an appropriate topical anesthetic, which is still needed.

Selected Bibliography

Andrews DR, Taylor C: Documenting post-anesthesia recovery. Am J Nurs 85:290, 1985

Cohen EN: Toxicity of inhalation anesthetic agents. Br J Anaesth 50:665, 1978

Dripps RD, Eckenhoff JE, Vandam LD: Introduction to Anesthesia: The Principles of Safe Practice. Philadelphia, WB Saunders, 1982

Fink BR (ed): Molecular Mechanisms of Anesthesia. New York, Raven Press, 1980

Ngai SH: Effects of anesthesia on various organs. N Engl J Med 302:564, 1980

Roth SH: Physical mechanisms of anesthesia. Annu Rev Pharmacol Toxicol 19:159, 1979

Smith RM: Anesthesia for Infants and Children. St. Louis, CV Mosby, 1980

White MJ, Wolf-Wilets VC: Memory loss following halothane anesthesia. AORN 26:1053, December 1977

White PF, Way WL, Trevor AJ: Ketamine: Its pharmacology and therapeutic uses. Anesthesiology 56:119, 1982

SUMMARY. GENERAL ANESTHETICS

Drug	Preparations	Usual Dosage Range
Inhalation Gases		
Cyclopropane	Orange cylinders	Induction: up to 50% Maintenance: 10%–20%
Ethylene	Red cylinders	Anesthesia: 80%
Nitrous oxide	Blue cylinders	Induction: 70%–80% Maintenance: 50%–70% Analgesia: 20%–30%
Volatile Liquids		
Enflurane Ethrane	125-mL, 250-mL bottles	Induction: 2.0%–4.5% Maintenance: 0.5%–3.0%
Ether	Containers of several sizes	Induction: 5%–10% Maintenance: 3%–5%
Halothane Fluothane	125-mL, 250-mL containers	Induction: 1%–4% Maintenance: 0.5%–1.5%
Isoflurane Forane	100-mL, 125-mL, 250-mL bottles	Induction: 1.5%–3% Maintenance: 1.0%–2.5% with nitrous oxide
Methoxyflurane Penthrane	15-mL, 125-mL bottles	Induction: 2% Maintenance: 0.1%–2% Analgesia: 0.3%–0.8%

Continued

SUMMARY. GENERAL ANESTHETICS (continued)

Drug	Preparations	Usual Dosage Range
Intravenous		
Ultrashort-Acting Barbiturates	See Table 17-2	
Nonbarbiturate Hypnotic		
Etomidate Amidate	Injection: 2 mg/mL	0.2 mg/kg–0.6 mg/kg IV over 30–60 sec
Dissociative Agents		
Ketamine Ketalar	Injection: 10 mg/mL, 50 mg/mL, 100 mg/mL	*Induction:* 1 mg/kg–4.5 mg/kg IV over 60 sec *or* 6.5 mg/kg–13 mg/kg IM *Maintenance:* half to full induction dose repeated as needed
Fentanyl/droperidol Innovar	Injection: 2-ml, 5-ml ampules (0.05 mg fentanyl and 2.5 mg droperidol per ml)	*Premedication:* 0.5 mL–2.0 mL IM 45–60 min prior to surgery (children: 0.25 mL/20 lb IM) *Induction:* 1 mL/20 lb–25 lb by slow IV injection *IV drip:* 10 mL/250 mL 5% dextrose *Diagnosis:* 0.5 mL–2.0 mL IM 45–60 min before procedure Increments of 0.5 mL–1.0 mL IV as required

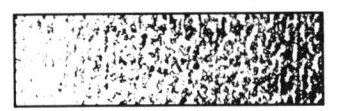

18 NARCOTIC ANALGESICS AND ANTAGONISTS

The narcotic analgesics encompass a group of both naturally occurring and synthetic agents capable of interacting with specific receptor sites in the CNS to relieve pain in conscious persons. Conversely, narcotic antagonists are compounds capable of occupying these same receptor sites but acting to interfere with many of the actions of the narcotic analgesics.

NARCOTIC ANALGESICS

Because the prototype of the narcotic analgesics is morphine, which is obtained from the seeds of the opium poppy, these compounds are probably more properly termed *opiates*. The naturally occurring alkaloids of opium (morphine, codeine) are commonly used, but they may also be modified chemically to form semisynthetic derivatives that are significantly more potent in some cases than the two natural alkaloids. In addition, a group of purely synthetic opiate compounds elicit many pharmacologic effects similar to those of morphine but differ slightly in some of their actions.

Classification of Narcotic Analgesics

Drugs possessing an opiate-like action may be classified as belonging to one of two broad categories, the narcotic agonists and the narcotic agonist–antagonists. The agonists consist of those clinically useful opiates that exert only an agonistic action at narcotic receptor sites (see discussion of opiate receptors, below). The agonist–antagonist compounds exert both an agonistic *and* a partial antagonistic effect at certain receptors. Within each of these broad categories, subclassifications are based on the chemical structure of the individual drugs. Even within each subclass, representative drugs are characterized by different potencies and toxicities. For example, morphine and codeine belong to the same chemical grouping (i.e., phenanthrenes), but morphine is quite potent and highly addicting, whereas codeine is less potent and less habituating.

The narcotic analgesics may be classified in the following manner:
I. Narcotic agonist analgesics
   A. Phenanthrenes
      1. Naturally occurring opium alkloids (morphine, codeine)
      2. Semisynthetic derivatives of morphine (hydromorphone, oxymorphone)
      3. Semisynthetic derivatives of codeine (hydrocodone, oxycodone)
   B. Methadones (methadone, propoxyphene)
   C. Morphinans (levorphanol)
   D. Phenylpiperidines (alfentanil, fentanyl, meperidine, sufentanil)
II. Narcotic agonist–antagonist analgesics
   A. Phenanthrenes (buprenorphine, nalbuphine)
   B. Morphinans (butorphanol)
   C. Benzomorphans (pentazocine)

Pharmacologic Actions of Opiate Drugs

The pharmacologic effects of therapeutic doses of the narcotic analgesics extend to many different systems of the body. The more important actions of the opiates are outlined in Table 18-1. However, not all of these effects are exhibited to the same degree by all of the narcotic agents (see Table 18-3). Moreover, many of the actions are dose dependent and therefore may be more intense at high dosages.

The opiate drugs exert their effects by combining with certain narcotic receptor sites in the CNS, each mediating distinctive actions. Sites of high receptor concentration include the dorsal horn of the spinal cord and several subcortical brain areas, such as the periaqueductal gray matter, hypothalamus, thalamus, locus coeruleus, and raphe nuclei.

Characterization of opiate receptors is based on the type of responses mediated by interaction of a narcotic drug at each receptor site, as outlined in Table 18-2.

The narcotic drugs bind to the different receptors to varying degrees, and the relative preference of an opiate for certain receptor types over others determines the overall pharmacologic profile of the drug. Of great clinical importance is the finding that receptors responsible for many of the opiate side effects *differ* from those that mediate the analgesic actions of these drugs; thus it may be possible to separate undesirable from desired opiate effects. For example, most narcotic agonists have agonistic activity at *mu* (μ), *kappa* (κ), and possibly also *delta* (δ) receptors and therefore elicit the characteristic narcotic actions. The mixed agonist–antagonist drugs, however, appear to bind preferentially to the *kappa* and possibly *sigma* (σ) receptors and may act as partial *antagonists* at the *mu* sites. This differential receptor action of the mixed agonist–antagonist drugs may help explain their lower abuse potential, reduced euphoric effects, and greater sedative action compared to the narcotic agonists. In addition, antagonism of the *mu* receptors can at least partially reverse the effects of other narcotic agonists acting at these sites, leading to the appearance of withdrawal symptoms should a mixed agonist–antagonist be given in the presence of an agonist.

Recent evidence has suggested the presence of subtypes of mu receptors; for example, respiratory depression and constipation are thought to be mediated by the mu_2 receptor, whereas supraspinal analgesia is believed to result from mu_1 receptor interaction. Morphine is capable of activating both mu_1 and mu_2 receptors. Conversely, some endogenous opiates (see below), such as enkephalins, activate only mu_1 sites and may not be associated with the degree of respiratory depression noted with morphine and its analogs.

ENDOGENOUS OPIATES

Electrical stimulation of certain CNS areas evokes potent analgesia that can be attenuated by administration of narcotic antagonist drugs. This phenomenon suggests the presence of endogenous substances that interact with opiate receptors to produce effects similar to those of exogenously administered opiates.

Table 18-1
Pharmacologic Effects of Analgesics

CNS
Analgesia
Sedation
Euphoria
Emesis (*anti*emetic at very high doses)
Depressed cough reflex
Respiratory depression (depression of medullary respiratory center)

Cardiovascular
Orthostatic hypotension (depression of medullary vasomotor center; peripheral vascular dilation)

GI Tract
Peristalsis and stomach motility decreased
Delayed gastric emptying time
Constipation

Smooth Muscle
Increased tone of most nonvascular smooth muscle (e.g., GI, urinary, biliary)

Urinary System
Urinary tract spasm
Contraction of urinary sphincter
Release of antidiuretic hormone
Decreased renal blood flow (?)

Eye
Miosis

Neuroendocrine
Release of prolactin and somatotropin
Decreased release of luteinizing hormone and thyrotropin

Table 18-2
Opiate Receptors

Receptor	Pharmacologic Effects
mu (μ)	Supraspinal analagesia Euphoria Respiratory depression Addiction
kappa (κ)	Spinal analgesia Sedation Miosis
delta (δ)	Spinal analgesia Affective behavior
sigma (σ)	Dysphoria Hallucinations Respiratory/vasomotor stimulation

The three distinct groups of endogenous opioid-like peptides that have been isolated are called *endorphins, enkephalins,* and *dynorphins.* Each group is derived from a distinct precursor polypeptide and exhibits a characteristic distribution pattern in the CNS.

Beta-endorphin is a 31-amino-acid peptide derived from a larger peptide that also produces ACTH and alpha melanocyte-stimulating hormone. It occurs predominantly in the pituitary gland and may influence a variety of behavioral and physiological responses to pain.

Enkephalins are pentapeptides, the two most extensively studied being methionine-enkephalin and leucine-enkephalin. The enkephalins are located in nerve endings throughout the central nervous system and are particularly abundant in the brainstem and the dorsal horn of the spinal cord, as well as the basal ganglia and portions of the limbic system. Enkephalins are believed to act by modifying impulse transmission in pain pathways by combining with opiate receptor sites in a manner similar to that of the narcotic analgesics. Enkephalins may be released by a variety of stimuli and appear to provide the body with a natural mechanism for pain control and other behavioral modifications. Activity of enkephalins may also be enhanced by the presence of narcotic drugs, and these pentapeptides may play a major role in eliciting the analgesia associated with use of exogenous opiate drugs.

Dynorphins are derived from still another precursor and are located in neurons throughout the brain. Their precise role in pain modulation or behavior remains to be established.

The endogenous opioid peptides display differing affinities for the opioid receptor sites. For example, enkephalins appear to bind to both delta and mu_1 sites with approximately equal affinity. Beta-endorphin likewise binds predominantly to mu and delta sites although it can interact with more specialized sites as well. Dynorphins appear to interact primarily at kappa sites, although some may bind to mu and delta receptors as well. The clinical significance of this differential receptor interaction among the endogenous opiates remains to be established.

Although both the endorphins and the enkephalins can mimic the action of opiate drugs in pharmacologic test systems, they are of little clinical value because they are not absorbed orally and are rapidly degraded by metabolizing enzymes in the brain, blood, and other tissues. Their precise function in central adaptation to pain and stress as well as their role in the analgesic and addictive properties of the narcotic drugs has not been conclusively determined. Replacing the second amino acid in the enkephalin molecule appears to confer greater stability to inactivation, and several synthetic enkephalins are being tested for their analgesic activity.

Narcotic analgesics can modify the actual *sensation* of pain through their effect on pain pathways in the spinal cord and brain. They can also modify the *perception* of pain through their effect on higher cortical areas. Thus, the transmission of a painful stimulus from the site of origin to the sensory cortex is reduced, while the painful sensation is perceived as being less intense or bothersome. The resultant tranquility and release from tension often lead to a state of euphoria and an exaggerated sense of well-being, and it is this euphoric state that is frequently responsible for the desire to repeat the drug, ultimately leading to habituation in many chronic users.

The principal *acute* toxic effect of morphine and related narcotic agonists is respiratory depression, characterized by slow, shallow, irregular respiration and cyanosis. Other important adverse effects include hypotension, decreased urinary output, and hypothermia. Treatment includes mechanical ventilation and use of a narcotic antagonist. Conversely, use of narcotic agonists-antagonists may induce sedation at normal doses, and higher doses may elicit sweating, nausea, and dizziness. However, the extent of respiratory depression is less at elevated doses than with comparable doses of pure narcotic agonists.

Long-term use of opiate drugs often leads to the development of tolerance, habituation, and eventually physical dependence. Useful diagnostic signs of dependence are miosis, constipation, superficial infections, itching and, of course, needle marks, scars, and abscesses in the abuser. Abrupt termination of a narcotic drug following prolonged use or administration of a narcotic antagonist to a chronic opiate user leads to a fairly predictable pattern of withdrawal reactions. Lacrimation, rhinorrhea, sweating, yawning, chills, and goose pimples usually occur within 8 hours to 16 hours after the last dose. Peak withdrawal effects are generally observed within 36 hours to 48 hours; they include abdominal cramping, muscle aching, nausea, vomiting, diarrhea, hyperthermia, and hyperventilation. Most symptoms subside within 3 days to 5 days, but some may persist for much longer periods of time. Further attention is directed to the problem of narcotic abuse in Chapter 79.

Most of the narcotic drugs exhibit qualitatively similar actions and adverse effects; they differ primarily in potency, analgesic efficacy, addictive liability, and their likelihood of eliciting different adverse effects. A comparison of the properties of the opiates is presented in Table 18-3. Specific information relating to preparations, dosage, and characteristics of individual drugs is given in Table 18-4.

Narcotic Agonists

Alfentanil	Morphine
Codeine	Opium
Fentanyl	Oxycodone
Hydromorphone	Oxymorphone
Levorphanol	Propoxyphene
Meperidine	Sufentanil
Methadone	

Narcotic Agonist–Antagonists

Buprenorphine	Nalbuphine
Butorphanol	Pentazocine

MECHANISM
Actions of narcotic drugs are complex and involve multiple sites and several mechanisms of action: elevation of the pain threshold, alteration in perception of pain, blunting of the anxiety or apprehension associated with the presence of pain, and induction of somnolence and clouding of mentation. Mechanisms may include (1) direct activation of opiate receptor sites in the spinal cord, brainstem, and subcortical brain nuclei; (2) potentiation of the effects of endogenous opiates; and (3) activation of descending spinal cord pathways, which reduces the level of incoming sensory pain impulses at different segmental levels of the cord. Narcotics can reduce calcium influx into neuronal cells, thereby impairing release of a neurohormone substance P, found in primary sensory afferent nerve endings, especially in the spinal cord. Substance P may function as an excitatory neurotransmitter at nerve endings transmitting painful sensations. Narcotics also decrease sensitivity of the medullary respiratory center to carbon dioxide, resulting in dose-dependent respiratory depression; depress responsiveness of alpha-adrenergic receptors, leading to visceral pooling of blood and orthostatic hypotension; reduce GI peristalsis by direct relaxant effect on intestinal smooth muscle; increase tone of the urinary-bladder sphincter; and stimulate the chemoreceptor trigger zone in the brainstem, causing nausea and vomiting

USES
Relief of moderate to severe pain (e.g., myocardial infarction, carcinomas, burns, fractures, postsurgical trauma)
As preoperative medication to reduce anxiety and to enhance effects of general anesthetics
Relief of persistent cough (especially codeine and hydrocodone)
Relief of severe diarrhea and cramping
Immediate (short-term) relief of dyspnea associated with pulmonary edema or left ventricular failure by reduction of left ventricular workload
Obstetrical analgesia

DOSAGE
See Table 18-4

FATE
Absorption from SC and IM injection sites as well as GI mucosa is generally good. Some drugs undergo significant first-pass hepatic metabolism; their effective oral dose is considerably higher than the parenteral dose (see Table 18-3). Widely distributed in the body and localize in highest amounts in the liver, kidneys, lungs, and spleen. Brain concentrations are usually low as compared with other body organs; highly lipophilic drugs (e.g., fentanyl) cross the blood–brain barrier more readily than weakly lipophilic agents such as morphine. Analgesic effects are noted within 30 minutes after oral administration and 5 to 15 minutes following parenteral injection. Duration of analgesia differs among individuals with narcotic drugs (see Table 18-3). Drugs are mostly converted to polar metabolites, which are readily excreted by the kidneys. Small quantities of unchanged drug may also be eliminated in the urine and feces

COMMON SIDE EFFECTS
Dizziness, lightheadedness, sedation, nausea, sweating, flushing

SIGNIFICANT ADVERSE REACTIONS
CNS: euphoria or dysphoria, headache, agitation, tremor, disorientation, delirium, uncoordinated movements, and transient hallucinations
Cardiovascular: bradycardia, palpitations, hypotension, syncope, and phlebitis (IV injection only)
GI: dry mouth, anorexia, constipation, vomiting, biliary tract spasm
Respiratory: respiratory depression (observed in fetus and newborn as well)
Genitourinary: urinary hesitancy or retention, dysuria, antidiuretic effect, loss of potency or libido
Hypersensitivity: urticaria, pruritus, sneezing, edema, hemorrhagic urticaria, wheal and flare at IV injection site
Other: pain at injection site, local tissue irritation, porphyria
Acute overdose: extreme miosis, hypothermia, oliguria, bradycardia, hypotension, deep sleep, marked respiratory depression, pulmonary edema, coma, cardiac arrest

CONTRAINDICATIONS
Convulsive states, severe respiratory depression, increased intracranial pressure, acute asthma, undiagnosed acute abdomi-

Table 18-3
Comparative Pharmacologic Properties of Opiates

	Equianalgesic Doses (mg)[a] PO	Equianalgesic Doses (mg)[a] SC, IM	Onset of Action (min)[b]	Duration of Action (h)[b]	Analgesic Efficacy	Addictive Liability	Antitussive Activity	Respiratory Depression	Sedation	Emesis
Morphine MS Contin, Roxanol	60	10	10–20	4–6	High	High	Strong	Moderate	Moderate	Moderate
Fentanyl Sublimaze	—	0.1–0.2	5–15	1–2	High	High	—	Weak	—	—
Sufentanil Sufenta	—	—	2–4 (IV)	0.5–1	High	High	—	—	—	—
Hydromorphone Dilaudid	8	1–2	15–30	4–5	High	High	Strong	Moderate	Weak	Weak
Oxymorphone Numorphan	6	1–1.5	5–10	3–5	High	High	Weak	Strong	—	Strong
Levorphanol Levo-Dromoran	4	2–3	15–30	4–6	High	High	Moderate	Moderate	Moderate	Weak
Methadone Dolophine	20	7–10	10–15	4–6	High	High	Moderate	Moderate	Weak	Weak
Oxycodone	30	15	15–30	3–5	Medium	Medium–High	Strong	Moderate	Moderate	Moderate
Alfentanil Alfenta	—	—	2–4 (IV)	0.5–1	High	High	—	—	—	—
Meperidine Demerol, Pethadol	300	75–100	10–20	2–4	Medium	High	Weak	Moderate	Weak	—
Codeine	200	120	15–30	3–5	Low	Medium	Strong	Weak	Weak	Weak
Propoxyphene[c] Darvon	—	—	15–30 (PO)	4–6	Low	Low	—	Weak	Weak	Weak
Agonist–Antagonists										
Buprenorphine Buprenex	0.3		10–15	4–6	High	Low	—	Moderate	Moderate	Weak
Butorphanol Stadol	2–4		5–10	3–4	High	Low	—	Weak	Moderate	Weak
Nalbuphine Nubain	10		10–15	3–6	High	Low	—	Moderate	Moderate	—
Pentazocine Talwin	150	30–60	15–30	3–4	Medium	Medium–Low	—	Moderate	Moderate	Weak

[a] All doses as stated are approximately equivalent to 10 mg morphine IM or SC; note that long-term administration of narcotics alters pharmacokinetics and reduces the parenteral:oral dose ratio, for example, with morphine the ratio is reduced from 6:1 to 2:1.
[b] Onset and duration of action based on IM or SC administration.
[c] Propoxyphene is a very weak analgesic that cannot be compared to other opiates in equianalgesic doses.

nal conditions, severe ulcerative colitis, and hepatic cirrhosis. *Cautious use* in persons with adrenal insufficiency, hypothyroidism, cerebral arteriosclerosis, prostatic hypertrophy, acute alcoholism, impaired renal or hepatic function, supraventricular tachycardia, diabetic acidosis, severe obesity, and in elderly, debilitated, pregnant, or lactating patients

INTERACTIONS

CNS depressant effects of narcotics may be potentiated or prolonged by concurrent use of other CNS depressants (e.g., barbiturates, alcohol, anesthetics, phenothiazines, sedatives, tricyclic antidepressants).

Muscle relaxation and respiratory depression may be intensified by concurrent use of narcotics and neuromuscular blocking agents (e.g., succinylcholine)

Symptoms of acute narcotic overdose, possibly causing death, may occur with use of *meperidine* within 14 days of a MAO inhibitor

Withdrawal symptoms may occur in patients addicted to narcotics if the narcotic agonist–antagonists (see Table 18-3) are added, because they may antagonize the effects of the pure agonists

Meperidine has anticholinergic effects that may be additive with those of other drugs (e.g., atropine-like agents, tricyclic antidepressants, quinidine)

Phenytoin or rifampin may reduce blood concentrations of methadone to such an extent as to precipitate withdrawal symptoms

Orthostatic hypotension may be intensified by concurrent use of narcotic analgesics and high-ceiling diuretics such as furosemide, bumetanide, and ethacrynic acid

The analgesic efficacy of opiates may be enhanced by concurrent use of hydroxyzine, amphetamines, and tricyclic antidepressants; however, chronic (i.e., 2–3 wk) use of tricyclic antidepressants during opiate treatment may obtund the analgesic response

NURSING CONSIDERATIONS

Nursing Alerts

- Assess pain experience (e.g., patient's mood, affect, and functional ability, the process eliciting pain, characteristics of the pain) prior to administration. Appropriate use varies greatly in different circumstances (e.g., acute, chronic, terminal illness).
- Maintain balanced perspective toward drug dependence, which may occur with repeated administration of opiates. Excessive fear of dependence on the part of both patient and clinicians is often manifested by undermedication. Patients *rarely* abuse drugs as a result of hospital experiences, and dependence is irrelevant in terminal illness.
- Collaborate with patient and health care team to plan dosing schedule that will optimally provide desired degree of pain relief. Usage at fixed intervals usually provides better control with smaller total dosage than administration only on request (PRN).
- Maintain appropriate concern about toxicity. Tolerance develops to nearly all drug effects, including side effects (except constipation and miosis), although at different rates.
- To attain maximal analgesic effect, administer *before* pain becomes intense.
- Check rate and depth of respirations, pupil size, and degree of alertness before administration. If early signs of toxicity (respiratory rate below 12/min and shallow; miosis, deep sleep) are observed, withhold drug, advise physician, and be prepared to administer narcotic antagonist.
- When administering IV bolus, give dilute solution by *slow* injection because severe toxic effects (e.g., respiratory depression, hypotension, circulatory collapse, cardiac arrest) can occur quickly with rapid injection. A narcotic antagonist and measures for respiratory assistance should always be at hand.
- With IV infusion, use microdrip administration set and infusion monitoring device to ensure accurate, stable flow rate.
- Continually evaluate adequacy of drug regimen. Dosage and timing should be carefully titrated to correspond with response to drug and need for pain control.
- Advocate dosage increases in appropriate situations. Repeated requests for more medication may signal development of tolerance, increased pain, or different pain, all of which may require additional drug.
- Be prepared to assist with management of severe withdrawal symptoms when an antagonist is administered to a drug-dependent individual. Supportive measures (e.g., oxygen, IV fluids, vasopressors) should be at hand, and the smallest possible dose of antagonist should be used.
- Closely observe patient dependent on opiates if a narcotic agonist–antagonist (e.g., pentazocine) is administered because the drug's antagonist properties may precipitate withdrawal.
- Administer cautiously in obstetrics because drugs easily cross the placental barrier and can induce respiratory depression in the fetus and neonate.

1. Assess need for analgesic in patient unable to speak or nonalert (especially postsurgically). Signs include elevated respiratory rate and pulse, grimacing, restlessness.
2. Administer narcotics frequently during first 24 hours after major surgery to prevent pain from interfering with rest, increasing anxiety, and decreasing ability to engage in important activities (e.g., turning, coughing, ambulating).
3. Assist postoperative patient receiving narcotic to cough, deep breathe, and change positions frequently to prevent atelectasis and other respiratory difficulties. Drugs will depress cough and sigh reflexes.
4. Employ appropriate nursing interventions (e.g., anxiety reduction, touch, positioning) for pain relief as adjuncts to medication.
5. Protect patient from injury. Ambulation may induce dizziness and transient hypotension. Assist with ambulation; keep side rails up while patient is in bed.
6. If nausea and vomiting occur, assist patient to lie flat and still to avoid the exacerbation caused by motion and an upright position.
7. Monitor intake and output, periodically remind or assist patient to void (e.g., help male to stand), and notify physician if patient is unable to void: urinary retention can occur.
8. Use preventive measures for constipation (e.g., ambulation, increased intake of fluid and dietary fiber), and monitor bowel regularity and bowel sounds because constipation and paralytic ileus can occur.

9. If flushing, sweating, itching, feelings of warmth, visual or auditory distortions, or dysphoria occur, reassure patient that they are not uncommon, they will disappear shortly, and they are not a cause for alarm. Keep patient quiet and reduce sensory stimulation as much as possible.
10. Discuss possible fear of dependence if patient is reluctant to take appropriate analgesic. Reassure as needed, explain risks and benefits of opiate use and pain reduction.
11. Learn regulations governing handling and dispensing of all classes of controlled substances (see also Chap. 8). Keep proper records of all narcotic drugs used.

PATIENT EDUCATION

1. Caution patient that mental or physical abilities may be impaired, making tasks involving use of machinery (e.g., driving) hazardous.
2. Explain that other CNS depressants should not be used concurrently without professional consultation because of their additive effects.
3. Warn patient that orthostatic hypotension can occur. Advise gradual rising to a sitting and standing position to minimize dizziness.

(Text continued on page 167)

Table 18-4
Narcotic Analgesics

Drug	Preparations	Usual Dosage Range	Nursing Implications
Narcotic Agonists			
Phenanthrenes			
Morphine Astramorph PF, Duramorph-PF, MS Contin, MSIR, Roxanol, Roxanol SR, RMS (CAN) Epimorph, Morphitec, M.O.S., Statex	*Soluble tablets:* 10 mg, 15 mg, 30 mg *Oral tablets:* 15 mg, 30 mg *Sustained-release tablets:* 30 mg, 60 mg *Oral solution:* 10 mg/15 mL, 20 mg/5 mL, 20 mg/10 mL *Injection:* 0.5 mg/mL, 1 mg/mL, 2 mg/mL, 4 mg/mL, 5 mg/mL, 8 mg/mL, 10 mg/mL, 15 mg/mL *Drops:* 20 mg/mL *Suppositories:* 5 mg, 10 mg, 20 mg, 30 mg	*Oral:* 10 mg–30 mg/4–6 h *or* 30 mg–60 mg sustained release every 8–12 h *SC, IM:* (Adults) 5 mg–20 mg/4 h (usual 10 mg); (Children) 0.1 mg/kg–0.2 mg/kg *IV:* 4 mg–10 mg injected slowly *Rectal:* 10 mg–20 mg/4 h *Epidural:* 5 mg in lumbar region once daily or 2 mg–4 mg by continuous infusion over 24 h *Intrathecal:* 1/10 of epidural dose	Principal opium alkaloid, and standard to which other opiates are compared; most effective parenterally because oral availability may be somewhat limited; commonly produces drowsiness and relief from anxiety—large doses induce deep sleep and profound respiratory depression; oral form (especially sustained-release tablets) is very effective in controlling chronic pain when given on a regular schedule; oral solution may be combined with other medications (sedatives, alcohol, amphetamine, phenothiazines) as a "cocktail" for relief of severe pain—such mixtures have been termed Brompton's mixtures; however, use of a single opiate in sufficient dosage is as effective in controlling pain with fewer side effects (Schedule II)
Codeine (CAN) Paveral	*Soluble tablets:* 15 mg, 30 mg, 60 mg *Tablets:* 15 mg, 30 mg, 60 mg *Injection:* 30 mg/mL, 60 mg/mL	*Analgesia* Adults: 15 mg–60 mg 4 times/day orally; SC, IM, or IV Children: 0.5 mg/kg every 4–6 h orally, SC, or IM *Antitussive* Adults: 10 mg–20 mg/4–6 h to a maximum of 120 mg/24 h Children: (6–12 yr) 5 mg–10 mg/4–6 h (maximum 60 mg/day); (2–6 yr) 2.5 mg–5 mg/4–6 h (maximum 30 mg/day)	Less potent and less abuse potential than morphine; widely used in cough medications; suppresses cough by direct depressant effect on medullary cough center; as an analgesic, most frequently used in combination with aspirin, acetaminophen, or other analgesics; high doses (e.g., 60 mg) may cause restlessness and excitement; rapid onset of action following oral administration (10–15 min) and effects persist for up to 6 h; used in combination with centrally acting muscle relaxants for pain of muscle spasm and rigidity (Schedule II)

Continued

Table 18-4
Narcotic Analgesics (continued)

Drug	Preparations	Usual Dosage Range	Nursing Implications
Narcotic Agonists			
Hydromorphone Dilaudid	*Tablets:* 1 mg, 2 mg, 3 mg, 4 mg *Injection:* 1 mg/mL, 2 mg/mL, 3 mg/mL, 4 mg/mL, 10 mg/mL *Suppositories:* 3 mg	SC, IM: 2 mg–4 mg/4–6 h (may also be given by slow IV injection) Oral: 2 mg–4 mg/4–6 h Rectal: 1 suppository every 6 h–8 h	Very potent (8× to 10× morphine) analgesic, producing less sedation, vomiting, and nausea than morphine; elicits marked respiratory depression; therefore, use smallest dose possible; suppositories may give prolonged effect; high abuse potential and popular "street drug" owing to extreme potency and lack of strong hypnotic effect; oral form useful in treating severe chronic pain but drug is relatively short-acting (Schedule II)
Oxycodone Roxicodone (CAN) Supeudol	*Tablets:* 5 mg *Oral solution:* 5 mg/5 mL	5 mg/6 h	Moderately potent, orally effective narcotic, commonly used in fixed combinations with aspirin (Percodan, Codoxy) or acetaminophen (Percocet, Tylox) (Schedule II)
Oxymorphone Numorphan	*Injection:* 1 mg/mL, 1.5 mg/mL *Suppositories:* 5 mg	SC, IM: 1 mg–1.5 mg/4–6 h IV: 0.5 mg as needed Rectal: 5 mg/4–6 h Analgesic during labor: 0.5 mg–1 mg IM/4–6 h	Rapid-acting potent (5× to 10× morphine) analgesic; used for preoperative sedation, obstetrical analgesia, and relief of anxiety in patients with dyspnea due to pulmonary edema or left ventricular failure; high incidence of nausea, vomiting, and euphoria; little constipation or antitussive action; not recommended in children less than 12 yr (Schedule II)
Opium Paregoric, Pantopon	*Injection (Pantopon):* 20 mg opium alkaloids hydrochlorides/mL (equivalent to 15 mg morphine/mL) *Tincture:* 10% opium in 19% alcohol *Camphorated tincture:* (Paregoric): 2 mg morphine equivalent/5 mL with 45% alcohol	*Injection* IM, SC: 5 mg–20 mg/4–5 h *Tincture* 0.6 mL (6 mg morphine) 4 times/day *Camphorated tincture:* Adults: 5 mL–10 mL (2 mg–4 mg morphine) 1–4 times/day Children: 0.25 to 0.5 mL/kg 1–4 times/day	Activity is primarily due to morphine content; has been largely replaced by morphine or other narcotics, except for paregoric, which is widely used orally for cramps and diarrhea and also topically for teething pain in infants; discontinue drug once diarrhea has been controlled to prevent excessive dosage; do *not* confuse paregoric (camphorated opium tincture containing 2 mg morphine/5 mL) with opium tincture itself (50 mg morphine/5 mL); absorption of drug from GI tract is improved if diluted in a little water (injection and tincture are Schedule II; camphorated tincture is Schedule III)
Methadones			
Methadone Dolophine	*Injection:* 10 mg/mL *Tablets:* 5 mg, 10 mg *Oral solution:* 5 mg/5mL, 10 mg/5 mL	*Analgesia* IM, SC, orally: 2.5 mg–10 mg/3–4 h (Children: 0.7 mg/kg/day)	May be used to relieve severe pain, usually orally or IM; SC administration may be painful; longer acting and less sedating

Continued

Table 18-4
Narcotic Analgesics (continued)

Drug	Preparations	Usual Dosage Range	Nursing Implications
Narcotic Agonists			
Methadone (cont)	*Dispersible tablets:* 40 mg (for detoxification only) *Liquid:* 10 mg/mL	*Chronic pain regimen:* 5 mg every 12 h to 20 mg every 5 h; start with 5 mg every 5–6 h and titrate according to patient's needs *Narcotic detoxification* (highly individualized depending on severity of withdrawal symptoms): 15 mg–20 mg orally (up to 40 mg) to suppress symptoms; treatment not to exceed 21 days, during which time the dosage is gradually reduced *Maintenance therapy:* 20 mg–120 mg daily, individualized to control abstinence symptoms without inducing sedation or respiratory depression	than morphine, especially when given long-term; exerts a similar degree of respiratory depression and addiction liability as morphine; not recommended for obstetrics or as an analgesic in young children except in cancer-related pain, for which it is very effective; also used for detoxification and maintenance in approved programs for narcotic addiction; administered orally on a daily basis—abstinence syndrome is qualitatively similar to morphine, but onset is slower, course is more prolonged, and symptoms are less severe; with prolonged oral use, most side effects disappear, but constipation and sweating often persist; euphoria is much less prominent with methadone, and addict may eventually overcome compulsive need for the narcotic "high"; should be used in combination with psychiatric and social counseling (see Chap. 79) (Schedule II)
Propoxyphene Darvon, Dolene, Doxaphene, Profene 65 (CAN) Novopropoxyn, 642	*Capsules:* 32 mg, 65 mg (HCl salt) *Tablets:* 100 mg (napsylate salt) *Suspension:* 10 mg/mL (napsylate salt)	Adults: 65 mg–100 mg every 4 h *Note:* 65 mg of the HCl salt is equivalent to 100 mg of the napsylate salt	*Very weak* analgesic, structurally related to methadone; little antitussive activity; has many of the side effects of narcotics and is associated with habituation and physical dependence to approximately the same degree as codeine; restlessness, tremor, and mild euphoria commonly occur; usually administered in fixed combination with aspirin and caffeine (e.g., Darvon Compound), acetaminophen (e.g., Darvocet, Dolene AP, Wygesic), or aspirin (e.g., Darvon w/ASA); will potentiate CNS depressant effects of alcohol and tranquilizers—such combinations are a major cause of drug-related fatalities; avoid prolonged or excessive dosage and concurrent use of tranquilizers or alcohol; maximum recommended doses are 390 mg/day of the HCl salt and 600 mg/day of the napsylate salt (Schedule IV)

Continued

Table 18-4
Narcotic Analgesics (continued)

Drug	Preparations	Usual Dosage Range	Nursing Implications
Narcotic Agonists *Morphinans* **Levorphanol** Levo-Dromoran	Injection: 2 mg/mL Tablets: 2 mg	2 mg–3 mg orally or SC/4–6 h	Very potent analgesic (4× to 5× morphine); almost as effective orally as parenterally; used preoperatively to potentiate and prolong general anesthesia and to shorten recovery time; also is a useful supplement to nitrous oxide–oxygen anesthesia; low incidence of nausea, vomiting, and constipation but strong sedative and respiratory depressant; slow onset of peak effect (60–90 min) but prolonged duration (6–8 h); reduce dose in pediatric and geriatric population and in poor-risk patients; has a bitter taste; protect from light (Schedule II)
Phenylpiperidines **Meperidine** Demerol, Pethadol	Injection: 10, 25, 50, 75, or 100 mg/mL Tablets: 50 mg, 100 mg Syrup: 50 mg/5 mL	*Analgesia* IM, SC, orally: 50 mg–150 mg/3–4 h Children: 1–2 mg/kg IM, SC, or orally every 3–4 h *Preoperative medication* Adults: 50 mg–100 mg IM or SC 30–90 min before anesthesia Children: 1–2 mg/kg IM or SC *Obstetrical analgesia* 50 mg–100 mg IM or SC; repeat at 1–3 h intervals	Moderately potent analgesic (1/10 morphine) with weak antitussive activity; less spasmogenic and constipating than most other narcotics; more rapid onset and shorter duration of action (2–4 h) compared to morphine; significantly less effective orally than parenterally; frequent dizziness and occasional tremors, uncoordinated muscle movements, and other signs of CNS excitation can occur; attains high levels in breast milk; used for moderate pain, often associated with diagnostic procedures, minor surgical procedures, or obstetrics; also for preanesthetic medication and by slow IV infusion (1 mg/mL) for support of anesthesia; solutions of meperidine and barbiturates are incompatible; prolonged therapy may cause elevated normeperidine levels (detectable by plasma sample) which can lead to CNS symptoms ranging from shakiness to seizures (Schedule II)
Fentanyl Sublimaze	Injection: 0.05 mg/mL	*Preoperative* 0.05 mg–0.1 mg IM *General anesthesia* Induction: 0.05 mg–0.1 mg IV (repeat at 2–3 min intervals) Maintenance: 0.025 mg–0.1 mg IV or IM as needed	Very potent (100× morphine) analgesic used for short durations (e.g., preoperative, intraoperative, or postoperative to relieve pain and anxiety and as an anesthetic agent with oxygen in selected high-risk

Continued

Table 18-4
Narcotic Analgesics (continued)

Drug	Preparations	Usual Dosage Range	Nursing Implications
Narcotic Agonists **Fentanyl** (cont)		*Adjunct to general anesthesia* 0.002–0.05 mg/kg as needed *Postoperative* 0.05 mg–0.1 mg IM/1–2 h for pain, tachypnea, and delirium Children (2–12 yr): 0.02–0.03 mg/20–25 lb	operations such as open-heart surgery, complicated neurologic procedures); rapid onset (10–15 min IM) and short duration (1–2 h); respiratory depression often outlasts analgesia; have antidotal measures (e.g., oxygen, endotracheal tube, narcotic antagonist, muscle relaxant) on hand; rapid IV administration may cause muscle spasm or rigidity; also available in combination with the neuroleptic droperidol as Innovar, which is used for analgesia and tranquilization (neuroleptanalgesia) for short surgical and diagnostic procedures (see Chap. 17); combination may cause restlessness, hallucinations, extrapyramidal symptoms, and postoperative drowsiness; vital signs should be monitored continually during use (Schedule II)
Alfentanil Alfenta	Injection: 0.5 mg/mL	*Analgesia adjunct* 8–50 µg/kg IV, followed by increments of 3–15 µg/kg as required (maximum 75 µg/kg) *Induction anesthetic* 130–245 µg/kg IV followed by 0.5–1.5 µg/kg/min IV infusion	Rapid-acting narcotic used IV as an analgesic adjunct during N_2O/O_2 barbiturate anesthesia; also used as a primary induction anesthetic in general surgery if intubation and mechanical ventilation are required; base dosage on *lean* body weight in obese individuals; reduce dosage in elderly or debilitated persons; not recommended in children under 12; vital signs must be closely monitored (Schedule II)
Sufentanil Sufenta	Injection: 50 µg/ml	*Adults* For general surgery in which intubation and mechanical ventilation are required: 1–2 µg/kg with N_2O/O_2; maintenance dose of 10 µg–25 µg as analgesia lightens For more complicated surgery: 2–8 µg/kg with N_2O/O_2; maintenance doses of 25 µg–50 µg as needed For complete anesthesia: 8–30 µg/kg with 100% O_2 and a muscle relaxant; maintenance doses of 25 µg–50 µg as anesthesia lightens	Can induce and maintain anesthesia with 100% O_2 in patients undergoing major surgical procedures such as cardiovascular surgery or neurosurgery in the sitting position; also used as an analgesic adjunct at doses less than 8 µg/kg to maintain balanced general anesthesia; dosage should be based on lean body weight and reduced in the elderly or debilitated; doses above 8 µg/kg induce sleep; catecholamine release is suppressed at doses up to 25 µg/kg, and sympathetic

Continued

Table 18-4
Narcotic Analgesics (continued)

Drug	Preparations	Usual Dosage Range	Nursing Implications
Narcotic Agonists			
Sufentanil (cont)		*Children* (under 12) 10–25 μg/kg with 100% O₂ for general anesthesia in children undergoing cardiovascular surgery	responses are attenuated at doses between 25 μg/kg and 35 μg/kg; postoperative mechanical ventilation required because of extended respiratory depression (Schedule II)
Narcotic Agonist–Antagonists			
Phenanthrenes			
Nalbuphine Nubain	Injection: 10 mg/mL, 20 mg/mL	*SC, IM, IV:* 10 mg/70 kg individual; repeat every 3–6 h as necessary; maximum 160 mg/day	Chemically related to oxycodone and naloxone, and possesses both agonistic activity at kappa and delta receptors and weak antagonistic activity at mu receptors; analgesia is approximately equivalent to morphine on a milligram basis, with somewhat lower abuse potential (less than that of codeine or propoxyphene); may precipitate withdrawal symptoms in patients on chronic narcotic therapy; use ¼ normal dose initially in these patients; high incidence of sedation; does not increase systemic vascular resistance or cardiac workload like other narcotic agonist–antagonists; at usual adult dose, respiratory depression is equal to that seen with morphine—larger doses (i.e., above 30 mg), however, do not appreciably increase respiratory depression, unlike morphine; duration of analgesia ranges from 3–6 h; do not use in pregnant women or in children under 18 yr (Not a controlled drug)
Buprenorphine Buprenex	Injection: 0.3 mg/mL	*Adults and children over 12 yr:* 0.3 mg–0.6 mg IM *or* slow IV every 6 h as needed	Semisynthetic derivative of thebaine that has a high affinity for mu receptors and dissociates from them slowly; exhibits a long duration of action (up to 6 h) and low degree of dependence; approximately 20–30 times more potent than morphine; possesses antagonist activity equal to that of naloxone; may reduce blood pressure and heart rate and produces respiratory depression equal to that of morphine at normal dosage ranges; sedation is very common; use cautiously in elderly or debilitated patients, or patients with

Continued

Table 18-4
Narcotic Analgesics (continued)

Drug	Preparations	Usual Dosage Range	Nursing Implications
Narcotic Against–Antagonists			
Buprenorphine (cont)			impaired hepatic, renal, or pulmonary function; may precipitate withdrawal symptoms in narcotic-dependent patients (Schedule V)
Morphinan			
Butorphanol Stadol	Injection: 1 mg/mL, 2 mg/mL	IM: 2 mg/3–4 h (maximum 4 mg/dose) IV: 1 mg/3–4 h	Potent analgesic (4×–7× morphine on a weight basis); respiratory depression with 2-mg dose is equivalent to that achieved with 10 mg morphine, but does not increase appreciably at 4 mg; possesses weak narcotic antagonistic activity (considerably less than that of naloxone); use with caution in patients dependent on narcotics because withdrawal symptoms can occur; most frequent side effect is sedation; peak analgesia occurs in 1 h with IM use and persists for 3–4 h; not recommended in children less than 18 yr or in nursing mothers; use cautiously in the presence of liver or kidney disease, coronary artery insufficiency (increases cardiac workload) and respiratory impairment; not a controlled substance
Benzomorphan			
Pentazocine Talwin	Tablets: 50 mg Injection: 30 mg/mL	Oral: 50 mg/3–4 h (maximum dose—600 mg/day) IM, SC, IV: 30 mg every 3–4 h (maximum dose—360 mg/day) Obstetrics: 30 mg IM *or* 20 mg IV/2–3 h	One-third as potent as morphine parenterally; possesses some narcotic antagonist activity as well, therefore, can antagonize effects of other opiates and may elicit withdrawal symptoms in patients who have been taking other narcotics regularly; onset is 15–30 min after IM, SC, or oral use and 2–3 min IV; duration from 2–3 h parenterally and up to 5 h with oral use; has sedative activity and may be used preoperatively in obstetrics as well as for moderate to severe pain; addiction liability about equal to codeine; tablets are marketed as Talwin-Nx and contain 0.5 mg naloxone, a potent narcotic antagonist; although inactive orally, naloxone has profound antagonistic actions against narcotics when injected, and its inclusion in the tablet is intended to curb a form of

Continued

Table 18-4
Narcotic Analgesics (continued)

Drug	Preparations	Usual Dosage Range	Nursing Implications
Narcotic Against–Antagonists Pentazocine (cont)			pentazocine abuse in which the tablets are dissolved and injected; can induce tachycardia, hypertension, confusion, hallucinations, bizarre thought processes, and other CNS effects in large doses; abrupt discontinuation of drug may lead to muscle cramping, chills, restlessness, anxiety, and other symptoms of narcotic withdrawal; do *not* mix with soluble barbiturates because a precipitate will form; rotate injection sites if used chronically to minimize sclerosis of skin and subcutaneous tissues; severe respiratory depression is treated with naloxone and other supportive measures (Schedule IV)

NARCOTIC ANTAGONISTS

Drugs capable of reversing the effects of the narcotic agonists are termed *narcotic antagonists*. Both of the drugs in this category, naloxone and naltrexone, are viewed as "pure" antagonists because, unlike the mixed agonist–antagonist drugs discussed previously, they possess no intrinsic agonistic activity.

Naloxone is a rapid-acting drug given parenterally to reverse (or prevent, in some cases) the effects of opioid drugs, especially in the event of overdosage. It is capable of reversing the respiratory-depressant, sedative, hypotensive, analgesic, and psychotomimetic effects of opiate drugs. In the absence of narcotics, naloxone exhibits essentially no pharmacologic activity. The drug is specific for poisoning with opiate drugs and will not reverse the respiratory depression induced by other types of CNS depressants (e.g., barbiturates, anesthetics). Naloxone is relatively short-acting (i.e., 15–30 min) and must be administered at frequent intervals if the patient is severely intoxicated.

Naltrexone is an orally administered narcotic antagonist that can attenuate or block the subjective effects of opioid drugs and reduce the physical dependence on these agents. It is used as an adjunct in maintaining an opioid-free state in detoxified former addicts.

Naloxone
Narcan

MECHANISM
Competitive antagonism of narcotic drugs at opiate receptor sites; displaces opiate drugs from receptor sites, thereby reversing respiratory depression, sedation, hypotension, and analgesia seen with opiates; can also reverse the dysphoric effects of agonist–antagonist narcotic drugs such as pentazocine; when administered in the absence of narcotics, produces no analgesia, respiratory depression, miosis, or other effects noted with narcotic drugs; no tolerance or dependence has been reported

USES
Reversal of respiratory depression and other untoward effects induced by narcotic agonists and narcotic agonists–antagonists

Diagnosis of suspected narcotic overdosage

Investigational uses include reversal of alcoholic coma and improvement of circulation in refractory shock

DOSAGE
I. Narcotic overdosage (known or suspected)
   A. *Adults:* 0.4 mg to 2.0 mg IV (preferred), IM, or SC; may be repeated IV at 2- to 3-minute intervals for 2 to 3 doses, then at 1- to 2-hour intervals as needed to a total of 10 mg
   B. *Children and neonates:* 0.01 mg/kg IV, IM, or SC initially; may repeat with 0.1 mg/kg if needed
II. Postoperative narcotic depression—0.1 mg to 0.2 mg IV at 2- to 3-minute intervals until desired degree of reversal is attained

FATE
Onset of action is 2 to 5 minutes; duration of action depends on dosage and route of administration, but effects generally last from 1 to 4 hours; metabolized in the liver and excreted as conjugated products in the urine; virtually inactive when given orally

SIGNIFICANT ADVERSE REACTIONS
(Occur with excessive dose or too rapid reversal of narcotic depression) Nausea, vomiting, hypertension, tachycardia, hyperventilation, and tremors

CONTRAINDICATIONS
Respiratory depression due to nonnarcotic drugs. *Cautious use* in the presence of cardiac instability, during pregnancy, and in known or suspected narcotic addicts

NURSING CONSIDERATIONS

Nursing Alerts
- Ensure that additional supportive measures (e.g., respiratory assistance, vasopressors) are available when drug is used.
- Observe patient for signs of pain (e.g., sweating, tachycardia, grimacing, vomiting). If these are noted, the antagonist should be stopped. Large doses may reverse the analgesic as well as the respiratory-depressant effect of narcotics. Dose should be titrated according to patient response.
- Expect severity of withdrawal symptoms to vary with amount and type of opiate used. They are particularly severe with methadone. In contrast, they will not occur when a narcotic antagonist is administered to a meperidine abuser unless person is habituated to extremely large doses (1.6 g or more/day).
- Monitor patient carefully after positive response. Naloxone has relatively short duration of action, and its effect may wear off before effects of the opiate have been sufficiently reversed.
- Be prepared for administration of up to 3 doses. After 3 doses, lack of significant improvement suggests that depressant effects may be partly or wholly due to drugs other than narcotics (e.g., barbiturates).
- Administer diagnostic test for narcotic dependence only in presence of a physician, and inform patient of risks involved and possible untoward reactions.

Naltrexone
Trexan

MECHANISM
Competitively blocks the effects of opiates at opioid receptor sites; attenuates the euphoria and other subjective effects of opiate drugs and assists in maintaining an opioid-free state; blockade can be surmounted by large doses of opiates, therefore drug is only used in conjunction with proper counseling and other supportive measures.

USES
Adjunctive therapy, as an aid in the maintenance of an opioid-free state in detoxified former addicts

DOSAGE

WARNING
Naltrexone should not be administered until a person has remained opioid free for at least 7 days to prevent precipitation of withdrawal symptoms.

Initially, 25 mg orally; if no withdrawal signs are noted, an additional 25 mg is given; thereafter, 50 mg once daily. Alternatively, 100 mg every 2 days or 150 mg every 3 days if patient is stabilized

FATE
Following oral administration, peak blood levels occur within 1 hour. Naltrexone undergoes extensive first-pass hepatic metabolism, and some of the metabolites are active antagonists as well. Effects persist from 24 hours to 72 hours and are apparently independent of dosage. Naltrexone and its metabolites are excreted principally by the kidneys

SIGNIFICANT ADVERSE REACTIONS
(Result from withdrawal from opiate effects) Anxiety, nervousness, insomnia, abdominal pain and cramping, nausea, vomiting, joint and muscle pain, nasal congestion; also, liver damage, skin rash, anorexia, dizziness, chills, increased thirst

CONTRAINDICATIONS
Persons receiving opioid drugs or in acute opioid withdrawal, acute hepatitis, or liver failure. *Cautious use* in persons with liver dysfunction and in pregnant women or nursing mothers

NURSING CONSIDERATIONS

Nursing Alerts
- Administer only after withdrawal program and 7- to 10-day opioid-free interval have been completed.
- Expect small initial amount to be used. If no withdrawal symptoms occur, remainder of dose is given. Maintenance doses may be administered every 1 to 3 days.

1. Support and encourage patient's attempt to remain opiate-free. Effective therapy requires very high motivation because drug does not suppress urge to experience opiate-induced euphoria ("high").

PATIENT EDUCATION
1. Discuss danger of overdosing with an opiate. A dose large enough to produce a high by overcoming naltrexone action would be dangerous, possibly fatal.
2. Instruct patient to promptly report signs of liver damage (e.g., jaundice, dark urine, itching) because drug is a direct hepatotoxin.
3. Instruct patient to inform physician or dentist of naltrexone use. If administration of an opioid is unavoidable, dosage will need to be high, and respiratory depression will be deeper and more prolonged than usual.
4. Instruct patient to wear identification tag indicating naltrexone use.

Selected Bibliography
Akil H, Watson SJ, Young E et al: Endogenous opioids: Biology and function. Annu Rev Neurosci 7:223, 1984

Bloom FE: The endorphins: A growing family of pharmacologically pertinent peptides. Annu Rev Pharmacol Toxicol 23:151, 1983

Brena SF: Chronic pain: A structured approach to drug therapy. Mod Med 52:124, 1984

Chang KJ, Cuatrecasas P: Heterogenicity and properties of opiate receptors. Fed Proc 40:2729, 1981

Chapman CR, Bonica JJ: Acute Pain, Current Concepts. Upjohn, 1983

Collier HOJ, Hughes J, Rance MJ et al (eds): Opioids: Past, Present and Future. London, Taylor and Frances, 1984

Fraser DG: Intravenous morphine infusion for chronic pain. Ann Intern Med 93:781, 1980

Iwamoto ET, Martin W: Multiple opiate receptors. Med Res Rev 1:411, 1981

Martin WR: Pharmacology of opioids. Pharmacol Rev 35:283, 1983

Martinson IM et al: Nursing care in childhood cancer: Methadone. Am J Nurs 82:432, 1982

McCaffery M: Narcotic analgesia for the elderly. Am J Nurs 85:296, 1985

McCaffery M: Problems with meperidine. PRN Forum 3:1, 1984

McCaffery M: Placebos for Pain? Nursing 12:80, 1982

Muller RA, Pelczynski L: You can control cancer pain with drugs. Nursing 12:50, 1982

Panayotoff K: Managing pain in the elderly patient. Nursing 12:531, 1982

Pasternak GW: Multiple morphine and enkephalin receptors and the relief of pain. JAMA 259(9):1362, 1988

Pert CB, Snyder SH: Opiate receptor: Demonstration in nervous tissue. Science 179:1011, 1973

Portenoy RK: Continuous infusion of opioids. Am J Nurs 86:318, 1986

Rogers A: Analgesic consultation. Am J Nurs 85:296, 1985

Schechter NL: Pain and pain control in children. Curr Probl Pediatr 15:1, 1985

Verebey K (ed): Opioids in mental illness. Ann NY Acad Sci 398:1, 1982

Wall PD, Melzack R (eds): Textbook of Pain. New York, Churchill-Livingstone, 1984

Woolverton WL, Schuster CR: Behavioral and pharmacological aspects of opioid dependence: Mixed agonists-antagonists. Pharmacol Rev 35:33, 1983

Yaksh TL, Noveihed R: The physiology and pharmacology of spinal opiates. Annu Rev Pharmacol Toxicol 25:433, 1985

SUMMARY. NARCOTIC ANALGESICS AND ANTAGONISTS

Drug	Preparations	Usual Dosage Range
Narcotic Analgesics	*See* Table 18-4	
Narcotic Antagonists		
Naloxone (Narcan)	Injection: 0.02 mg/mL, 0.4 mg/mL	*Narcotic overdosage (known or suspected)* Adults: 0.4 mg–2.0 mg IV, IM, or SC; repeat IV at 2–3-min intervals for 2–3 doses Children and neonates: 0.01 mg/kg IV, IM, or SC *Postoperative narcotic depression* 0.1 mg–0.2 mg IV at 2–30-min intervals until desired degree of reversal is attained
Naltrexone (Trexan)	Tablets: 50 mg	50 mg once daily *or* 100 mg every other day *or* 150 mg every third day

19 NONNARCOTIC ANALGESIC AND ANTIINFLAMMATORY DRUGS

Nonnarcotic analgesics are a large group of drugs that possess analgesic or antiinflammatory actions but are devoid of many of the undesirable effects (e.g., respiratory depression, habituation) of the narcotic agents. They have a variety of uses, principally relief of mild to moderate pain, reduction of elevated body temperatures (antipyresis), reduction in the symptoms of inflammation, and prevention or relief of the manifestations of gout. Aspirin has also been found to be useful in preventing recurrent transient ischemic attacks (TIAs) and other thromboembolic conditions. In addition, certain of these agents (e.g., salicyclic acid, methyl salicylate) are employed topically as keratolytics, counterirritants, and astringents.

Aspirin (acetylsalicylic acid) is the most widely used and least expensive of the nonnarcotic analgesics. Because it is so readily available, however, aspirin is often viewed with something less than the respect such an important drug deserves. In fact, aspirin is the leading cause of drug poisoning in young children; only barbiturates, alcohol, and carbon monoxide are responsible for more accidental fatalities among the general population. Other nonnarcotic analgesics (e.g., acetaminophen) may offer some advantages over aspirin (e.g., decreased GI irritation, reduced effect on blood coagulation) and are frequently used in its place, especially in small children and in aspirin-intolerant persons. However, no single agent represents the "ideal" analgesic, and each drug possesses certain distinct disadvantages for different drug-taking populations.

The large number and chemical diversity of agents possessing analgesic and antiinflammatory action makes classification of these drugs quite arbitrary. This chapter considers these compounds in the following order:

I. Salicylates (e.g., aspirin, choline salicylate)
II. Para-aminophenol derivatives (e.g., acetaminophen)
III. Pyrazolones (e.g., phenylbutazone)
IV. Nonsteroidal antiinflammatory agents (e.g., ibuprofen, naproxen, tolmetin)
V. Gold compounds (e.g., aurothioglucose, auranofin)
VI. Miscellaneous antiinflammatory agents (e.g., penicillamine)
VII. Anti-gout drugs (e.g., colchicine, probenecid, allopurinol)

SALICYLATES

Aspirin	Salicylamide
Choline salicylate	Salicylic acid
Diflunisal	Salsalate
Magnesium salicylate	Sodium salicylate
Methyl salicylate	Sodium thiosalicylate

Drugs in this category are derivatives of salicylic acid and possess analgesic, antipyretic, and antiinflammatory actions. In addition, some of these drugs are capable of inhibiting platelet aggregation and, in large doses, can decrease prothrombin production and impair renal tubular reabsorption of uric acid.

Since most differences among the salicylates are largely quantitative, they are considered as a group. Characteristics of individual drugs are given in Table 19-1.

MECHANISM

Analgesia: block prostaglandin synthesis by interfering with the activity of the enzyme cyclooxygenase (Fig. 19-1), thus reducing sensitivity of peripheral pain receptors to mechanical or chemical activation; may enhance reabsorption of fluid from swollen, inflamed tissues and possibly interfere with transmission of pain impulses at subcortical brain centers (e.g., thalamus)

Antipyresis: reduce outflow of vasoconstrictor impulses from hypothalamus, thus promoting vasodilation, sweating, and heat loss; decrease production of prostaglandin E in response to endogenous pyrogens

Antiinflammatory: decrease capillary permeability and leakage of fluid into surrounding tissues; interfere with release of tissue-destructive lysosomal enzymes; inhibit synthesis of prostaglandin E, an endogenous substance thought to mediate the inflammatory reaction by causing swelling and sensitization of peripheral pain receptors

Reduced platelet aggregation: block formation of platelet thromboxane A_2, a prostaglandin derivative that facilitates platelet aggregation and causes vasoconstriction. Platelet aggregation appears to be markedly inhibited by aspirin but not by other salicylates. This difference is due to the acetyl group in the aspirin molecule, which irreversibly inhibits platelet cyclooxygenase and thereby thromboxane synthesis; this effect persists for the life of the platelet. Low doses of aspirin are apparently more effective in reducing platelet aggregation than are higher doses. It is thought that this dosage-related difference in effectiveness is related to the drug's having a greater inhibitory action on the formation of platelet thromboxane A_2 than on the formation of vessel-wall prostacyclin (a prostaglandin vasodilator and inhibitor of platelet aggregation). Further, the *prolonged* effect of aspirin suggests that *daily* dosing may be too frequent. The *precise dose* of aspirin that is most effective in blocking platelet aggregation remains to be definitively established. The effects on platelet aggregation suggest a potential clinical value for these compounds in protecting against certain thrombotic events thought to be associated with cerebrovascular and ischemic heart diseases

Other actions: decrease prothrombin formation (high doses only), decrease excretion of uric acid (small doses), increase excretion of uric acid (high doses), and decrease glucose tolerance

USES

Relief of mild to moderate pain, especially that associated with inflammatory states (e.g., myalgia, neuralgia, cephalgia)

Reduction of elevated body temperature

Symptomatic treatment of certain inflammatory conditions (e.g., rheumatoid and osteoarthritis, bursitis, rheumatic fever)

Prophylaxis of thromboembolic complications (e.g., venous emboli, cerebral ischemia) associated with cardiovascular disorders and reduction in the risk of recurrent transient ischemic attacks (*no* benefit in treating completed strokes)

Prevention of acute myocardial infarction (investigational use for aspirin)

DOSAGE
See Table 19-1

FATE
Absorbed essentially intact from stomach and upper intestine; peak serum levels occur within 1 to 2 hours; rapidly hydrolyzed to salicylic acid (except diflunisal) and excreted either free or as conjugates in the urine; rate of excretion is inversely related to blood level, larger doses being eliminated more slowly than small doses; salicylic acid is highly (70%–90%) protein bound; alkalinization of the urine increases the rate of excretion of salicylates by favoring ionization in the renal tubules, which decreases reabsorption

COMMON SIDE EFFECTS
Gastric distress, heartburn, and occasional nausea

SIGNIFICANT ADVERSE REACTIONS

> **WARNING**
> Use of salicylates, especially aspirin, in children with influenza or chickenpox has been associated with occasional development of Reye's syndrome, an acute, life-threatening condition marked by initial severe vomiting and lethargy and progressing to delirium, coma, and death. Mortality rate is 20% to 30%, and permanent brain damage frequently occurs in survivors. Although a *definite* causal relationship to salicylates has not been confirmed, aspirin and other salicylates should not be given to children with influenza or chickenpox.

(Generally dose related—more common at high doses or with prolonged use). Salicylism (headache, nausea, tinnitus, dizziness, confusion, sweating, palpitations, hyperventilation, diarrhea, impaired hearing or vision); idiosyncratic hypersensitivity reactions (bronchoconstriction, urticaria, edema, asthma-like attacks, shock); renal or hepatic impairment; GI bleeding or ulceration; anemia; anorexia; and elevations in serum amylase, SGOT, and SGPT

Severe intoxication may lead to CNS stimulation (delirium, hallucinations), respiratory alkalosis followed by acidosis, acid–base disturbances, petechial hemorrhaging, hyperthermia, hypokalemia, oliguria, convulsions, respiratory failure, and coma

CONTRAINDICATIONS
History of severe GI disorders (ulcer, hemorrhage, gastritis), severe anemia, deficiency of vitamin K, and hemophilia. *Cautious use* in persons with gastric ulcers, anemia, impaired hepatic function, chronic renal insufficiency, asthma or nasal polyps, in persons taking anticoagulants, and in pregnant or nursing women

INTERACTIONS
Effects of aspirin may be enhanced or prolonged by drugs that acidify the urine (e.g., ammonium chloride, ascorbic acid), and decreased by urinary alkalinizers (e.g., absorbable antacids, sodium bicarbonate)

By competing for protein binding sites, the salicylate metabolite of aspirin may enhance the actions and toxicity of oral anticoagulants, heparin, naproxen, oral hypoglycemic drugs, phenytoin, thiopental, indomethacin, methotrexate, thyroid hormones, sulfonamide antibiotics, valproic acid, and penicillins

Aspirin in small doses can inhibit the uricosuric effects of probenecid and sulfinpyrazone

Aspirin may increase the risk of bleeding in persons taking anticoagulants and drugs that interfere with platelet aggregation

Phenobarbital may decrease aspirin's efficacy by enzyme induction

The antihypertensive action of beta blockers may be blunted by concurrent use of salicylates, possibly because of prostaglandin inhibition

The incidence of GI distress and bleeding may be increased by steroids, alcohol, indomethacin, pyrazolones, and other antiinflammatory drugs

Furosemide may decrease salicylate excretion so that toxicity occurs at lower doses

Salicylates in high doses have a hypoglycemic action and may potentiate the effects of insulin and sulfonylurea hypoglycemics

Antacids and activated charcoal reduce the oral absorption of aspirin

Aspirin may lower the clinical effectiveness of nonsteroidal antiinflammatory agents

NURSING CONSIDERATIONS

Nursing Alerts
- Be prepared for possible development of hypersensitivity reactions, especially in patient with asthma, polyps, or a history of allergic reactions. Have epinephrine, antihistamines, and other supportive measures (e.g., oxygen, respiratory aids) at hand.
- In cases of aspirin intoxication, be prepared to assist with treatment: prompt emesis or gastric lavage, administration of fluids and electrolytes, oxygen with artificial respiration, and dialysis in cases of *severe* intoxication.
- Administer carefully and do not give for prolonged periods to children with fever and dehydration because they may be especially likely to develop toxic effects even with small doses.

1. Inform physician if patient is vomiting or otherwise incapable of taking drug orally. Suppositories may be used, but absorption is more variable than with oral route.

PATIENT EDUCATION
1. When high doses are used, instruct patient to be alert for early signs of overdose (e.g., tinnitus, dizziness, impaired vision or hearing) and to report their occurrence to appropriate health care provider.
2. Instruct patient taking large doses of aspirin for its anti-inflammatory effects to maintain a constant dosage schedule to minimize fluctuations in plasma levels.
3. Caution individual with aspirin hypersensitivity to read labels of OTC medications (e.g., cold preparations) carefully because many contain aspirin or other salicylates.

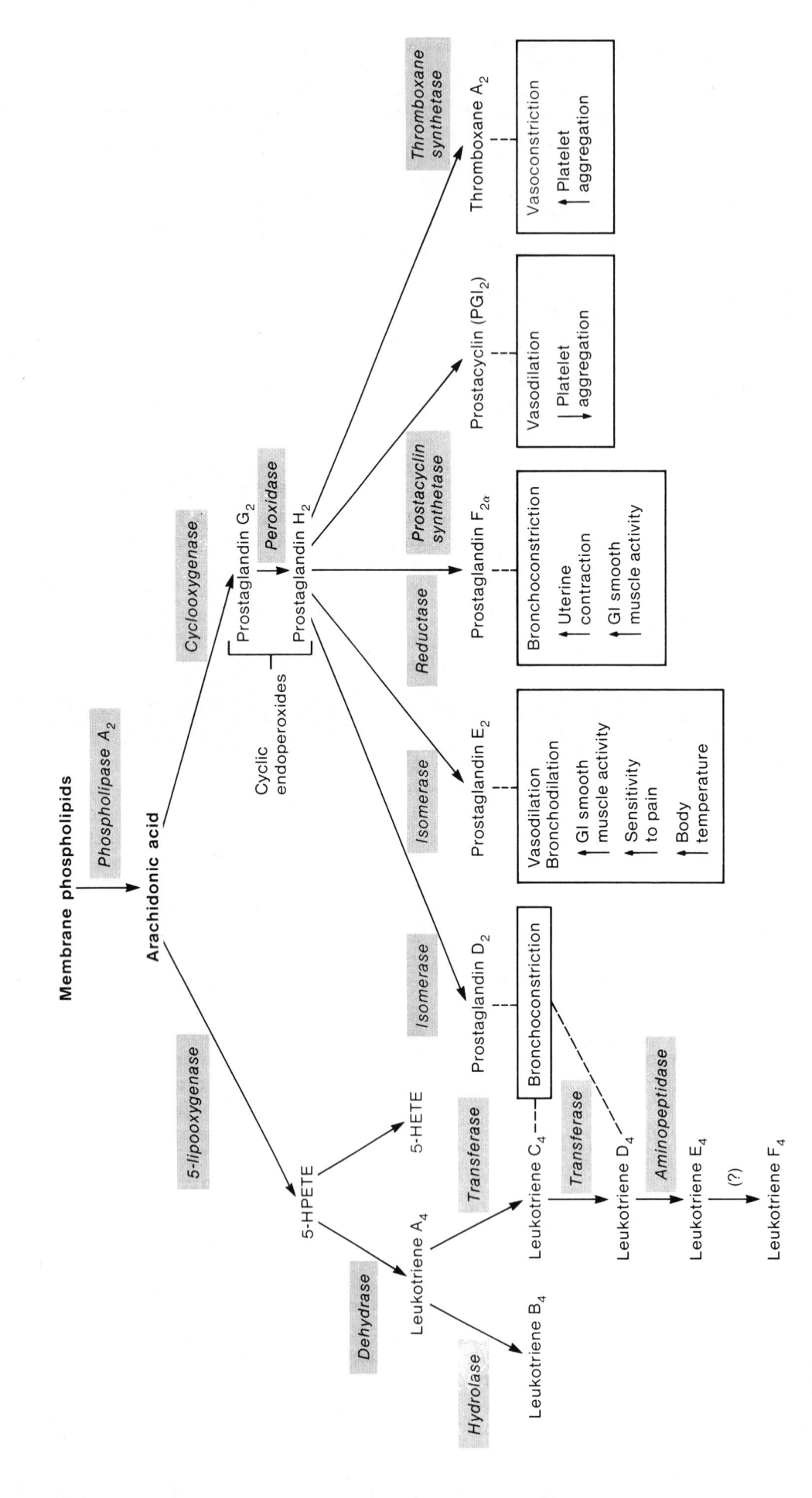

Figure 19–1 Synthesis of eicosanoids and their principal pharmacologic actions.

4. Warn patient on anticoagulant therapy to use aspirin cautiously. Teach patient to observe carefully for appearance of signs of increased anticoagulant effects (e.g., mucous membrane bleeding, bruising, petechiae). If signs appear, physician should be notified because the anticoagulant dosage may need to be reduced.
5. Warn patient that continual self-medication with aspirin for fever or pain may obscure more serious underlying conditions. Advise against prolonged use unless directed by a health care professional.
6. Advise cardiac patient that, although effervescent preparations (e.g., Alka Seltzer) may be more rapidly absorbed and less irritating to the GI tract, repeated use may be hazardous because of their high sodium content. They also may alkalinize the urine.
7. Inform patient who experiences GI upset with aspirin, even when taken with food or milk, that enteric-coated tablets are available (e.g., Easprin, Ecotrin) that resist breakdown in the stomach and therefore may eliminate much gastric distress.
8. Explain that combinations of aspirin and other nonnarcotic analgesics (e.g., acetaminophen, salicylamide) are probably no more effective than aspirin alone and may result in a higher incidence of adverse effects. Such combinations should be avoided.
9. Inform patient that commercially buffered aspirin is probably no less irritating to gastric mucosa than plain aspirin taken with food, milk, or a full glass of water.
10. Instruct patient to keep tablets in a cool, dry place. Exposure to moisture or excessive heat hastens hydrolysis and causes loss of potency. Tablets should not be used if a vinegar-like odor is detectable.
11. Urge patient to keep drug out of reach of all children at all times. See **Warning** under **Significant Adverse Reactions.**

PARA-AMINOPHENOL DERIVATIVES

The only para-aminophenol derivative of interest in clinical medicine is acetaminophen, a widely used analgesic and antipyretic. Acetaminophen is commonly used as an aspirin substitute and has several advantages over aspirin:

- Lower incidence of GI upset and bleeding
- Lower incidence of hypersensitivity reactions
- No significant interaction with oral anticoagulants or uricosuric drugs
- Availability in a palatable liquid form for pediatric use

The principal disadvantage of acetaminophen relative to aspirin is that acetaminophen possesses no significant antiinflammatory action, presumably because it has no inhibitory effect on prostaglandin synthesis in the periphery. In addition, excessive doses of acetaminophen can cause hepatotoxicity, and liver damage may occur with long-term use in alcoholics and patients with impaired hepatic function (see **Significant Adverse Reactions**).

Acetaminophen

Datril, Tempra, Tylenol, and various other manufacturers
(CAN) Atasol, Exdol, Robigesic

MECHANISM
The precise analgesic mechanism of action has not been completely established; elevates the pain threshold, possibly by blocking prostaglandin synthesis in the CNS; reduces elevated body temperature by an action on the hypothalamic heat-regulating center, leading to vasodilation and sweating, and also possibly by inhibiting the action of endogenous pyrogens; possesses no significant antiinflammatory action, presumably because it has no inhibitory effect on *peripheral* prostaglandin synthesis; unlike aspirin, exhibits no uricosuric, platelet antiaggregatory, ulcerative, or prothrombin-inhibitory activity

USES
Relief of mild to moderate pain, such as that of musculoskeletal origin, headache, toothache, teething, dysmenorrhea, "flu," tonsillectomy
Reduction of elevated temperatures associated with colds and other bacterial and viral infections

DOSAGE
Adults: 325 mg to 650 mg 3 to 4 times/day (maximum 4.0 g/day for short-term therapy)
Children:
Under 1 year: 40 to 80 mg 4 to 5 times/day
1 to 3 years: 120 to 160 mg 4 to 5 times/day
4 to 8 years: 240 to 320 mg 4 to 5 times/day
9 to 12 years: 400 to 480 mg 4 to 5 times/day

FATE
Well absorbed from the GI tract; onset 15 to 30 minutes; duration 3 to 5 hours; protein binding is variable but usually not clinically significant; metabolized in the liver, and 80% to 90% is excreted in the urine as conjugated metabolites; a minor intermediate metabolite is converted to a hepatotoxic substance but is normally rapidly detoxified by conjugation with glutathione via sulfhydryl groups and excreted as the conjugated product; large acute doses or chronic dosing with acetaminophen can deplete hepatic stores of glutathione, the substance that quickly detoxifies the potentially hepatotoxic intermediate; in these situations, hepatic necrosis can occur (see below)

COMMON SIDE EFFECTS
None with occasional usage

SIGNIFICANT ADVERSE REACTIONS
(Usually with long-term use of high doses) Urticaria, hypoglycemia, CNS stimulation, cyanosis, methemoglobinemia, hemolytic anemia, leukopenia, kidney damage, and psychological changes; *acute* poisoning characterized by chills, diarrhea, emesis, fever, skin eruptions, palpitations, weakness, sweating, and CNS stimulation (excitement, delirium, toxic psychosis) followed by CNS depression, vascular collapse, convulsions, and coma

Hepatotoxicity can occur with overdosage or long-term high dosage (5 g–8 g/day), especially in adults. Initial signs are nausea, vomiting, malaise, sweating, diarrhea, and abdominal pain. The degree of liver damage following acute overdosage can be estimated by determining the serum half-life or the plasma levels of acetaminophen. Hepatic damage is likely if the half-life is greater than 4 hours *or* if plasma levels exceed 250 to 300 μg/mL 4 hours after ingestion or 50 μg/mL 12 hours after ingestion

(Text continued on page 176)

Table 19-1
Salicylates

Drug	Preparations	Usual Dosage Range	Nursing Implications
Aspirin Several manufacturers	Chewable tablets: 65 mg, 75 mg, 81 mg Tablets: 325 mg, 500 mg Gum tablets: 227.5 mg Enteric-coated tablets: 325 mg, 500 mg, 650 mg, 975 mg Timed-release tablets: 650 mg, 800 mg Suppositories: 60 mg, 120 mg, 125 mg, 130 mg, 195 mg, 200 mg, 300 mg, 325 mg, 600 mg, 650 mg, 1200 mg	*Adults:* Pain, fever: 325 mg–650 mg every 4 h Inflammation: 3.6 to 5.4 g/day Transient ischemic attacks: 40–325 mg/day (highly variable—see text) Prevention of myocardial infarction: 325 mg every other day *Children:* Pain, fever: 65 mg/kg/day in divided doses Inflammation: 90–130 mg/kg/day in divided doses at 4–6 h intervals	*See* general discussion of salicylates. In addition: keep in a cool, dry place; do not use if vinegar-like odor is detectable because potency is likely to be reduced; use of suppositories may be best route if patient is vomiting, but absorption will be more variable; do not use controlled-release preparations for short-term analgesia or antipyresis, because the onset of action is slow.
Choline salicylate Arthropan (CAN) Teejel	Liquid: 870 mg/5 mL (870 mg equivalent to 650 mg aspirin)	890 mg–1740 mg 4 times/day	Liquid preparation provides more rapid absorption and less gastric irritation than aspirin; useful in patients with difficulty in swallowing tablets or capsules, in patients who experience gastric distress with regular aspirin, and in patients who should avoid sodium-containing salicylates; taste may be objectionable—drug can be mixed with fruit juice or other vehicle if desired; do not give with antacids.
Diflunisal Dolobid	Tablets: 250 mg, 500 mg	Pain: 500 mg–1 g initially, followed by 250 mg–500 mg every 8–12 h Rheumatoid arthritis/osteoarthritis: 500 mg to 1 g daily in 2 divided doses (maximum 1500 mg/day)	A salicylic acid derivative *not* metabolized to salicylic acid; used for mild to moderate pain and osteoarthritis; long-acting (used twice a day) analgesic comparable in potency to aspirin or acetaminophen at a dose of 500 mg and equivalent to acetaminophen plus codeine at a dose of 1 g; platelet-inhibitory effect is dose-related and usually transient and reversible; at 1 g/day, bleeding time is only slightly increased; antiinflammatory efficacy is equal to 2–3 g/day of aspirin, with less GI distress in some patients; do *not* use in children under age 12; *use cautiously* in patients with impaired cardiac function or hypertension, because fluid retention can occur; do not administer or take aspirin, acetaminophen or a nonsteroidal antiinflammatory drug with diflunisal
Magnesium salicylate Doan's Pills, Magan, Mobidin	Tablets: 325 mg, 500 mg, 545 mg, 600 mg	650 mg 4 times/day *or* 1090 mg 3 times/day; increase to 3.6 to 4.8 g/day in 3 or 4 divided doses as needed; up to 9.6 g/day has been used in rheumatic fever	*Not* recommended in children under age 12; a sodium-free salicylate having a somewhat lower incidence of GI upset than regular aspirin; use with caution in patients with impaired renal function; contraindicated in advanced renal insufficiency

Continued

Table 19-1
Salicylates (continued)

Drug	Preparations	Usual Dosage Range	Nursing Implications
Methyl salicylate (oil of wintergreen)	10% to 50% in ointment and linaments	Applied topically as a counterirritant to relieve pain associated with muscular and rheumatic conditions	Significant absorption can occur through the skin and may produce untoward effects; toxic if orally ingested, especially by children; liquids containing more than 5% methylsalicylate must be in child-resistant containers; use cautiously on irritated skin
Salicylic Acid Calicylic, Compound W, Derma-Soft, Freezone, Gordofilm, Hydrisalic, Keralyt, Mediplast, Occlusal, Off-Ezy, Oxyclean, Salacid, Salonil, Wart-off (CAN) Saligel, Sebcur, Soluver	Cream: 2.5%, 10% Ointment: 25%, 40%, 60% Gel: 6%, 17% Soap: 3.5% Liquid: 13.6%, 17% Plaster: 40%	Applied to affected area, usually at night, and washed off in the morning; following remission, used occasionally to maintain clearing effect	Primarily used topically as a keratolytic agent for conditions such as psoriasis, keratosis, acne, fungal infections, or any other condition requiring removal of excessive dead skin; skin should be hydrated with wet packs or soaks at least 5 min prior to use; may cause irritation and burning of skin; systemic absorption can occur to a significant extent; also may be applied as an ether-alcohol or a colloidian solution (Freezone, Compound W, Occlusal, Off-Ezy, Wart-off) for removal of corns, warts, and calluses; *use cautiously* in children under 12; avoid contact with eyes or mucous membranes
Salsalate Artha-G, Disalcid, Mono-Gesic, Salsitab, Salflex	Tablets: 500 mg, 750 mg Capsules: 500 mg	3 g/day in divided doses	Primarily used for relief of signs and symptoms of rheumatoid arthritis and other rheumatic conditions; minimal effect on platelet aggregation; following absorption, drug is hydrolyzed to two molecules of salicylic acid; drug is insoluble in gastric juice and not absorbed until it reaches small intestine; low incidence of GI upset; not for use in children under age 12; do *not* combine with other salicylates
Sodium salicylate Uracel (CAN) S-60	Tablets: 325 mg, 650 mg Enteric-coated tablets: 325 mg, 650 mg Injection: 1 g/10 mL	325 mg–650 mg/4h as needed	Less effective than an equal dose of aspirin; irritating to GI mucosa because free salicylic acid is liberated; use cautiously in renal dysfunction or in individuals on a low-sodium diet; sodium bicarbonate given concurrently may reduce gastric irritation but increases rate of excretion as well; when giving injection, avoid extravasation because drug will cause sloughing and necrosis of tissues
Sodium thiosalicylate Asproject, Rexolate, Tusal	Injection: 50 mg/mL	Analgesia: 50 mg–100 mg daily or alternate days Rheumatic fever: 100 mg to 150 mg every 4–6 h for 3 days, then 100 mg twice/day Acute gout: 100 mg every 3–4 h for 2 days, then 100 mg/day	Readily absorbed following IM administration; occasionally used in inflammatory conditions and acute stages of rheumatic fever

Treatment of acute overdosage includes emesis, gastric lavage, and activated charcoal. Hepatic damage can be minimized or prevented by administration of acetylcysteine *within the first 10 to 12 hours* after ingestion of acetaminophen (see Chap. 54). A loading dose of 140 mg/kg is given initially either IV or orally followed by 70 mg/kg every 4 hours for 17 doses

CONTRAINDICATIONS

Glucose-6-phosphate dehydrogenase deficiency. *Cautious use* in patients with impaired liver or kidney function or for periods longer than 10 days

INTERACTIONS

The rate of absorption of acetaminophen may be slowed by anticholinergics, narcotics, activated charcoal, and antacids

Oral contraceptives may increase the hepatic metabolism of acetaminophen

Concurrent use of diflunisal has resulted in increased plasma levels of acetaminophen

Chronic alcohol ingestion increases the likelihood of toxicity with large doses of acetaminophen

Caffeine increases the analgesic effectiveness of acetaminophen

NURSING CONSIDERATIONS

Nursing Alerts

- If ingestion of a toxic dose is suspected, observe patient carefully for signs of hepatic damage (nausea, vomiting, abdominal pain, diarrhea). Hepatic damage may not be evident for several days.
- Observe prolonged users of the drug for possible signs of methemoglobinemia (cyanosis, dyspnea, vertigo, weakness, angina-like pain), hemolytic anemia (pallor, palpitations), and kidney damage (albuminuria, hematuria).

PATIENT EDUCATION

1. Caution against indiscriminate, excessive, or prolonged use. Urge patient to keep drug away from children because many liquid preparations are pleasantly flavored and may be consumed in large amounts.
2. Explain that drug should be used cautiously in arthritis or rheumatic conditions because it lacks antiinflammatory action. If pain persists for more than 10 days or if redness is present, a physician should be consulted because additional medication may be indicated.

PYRAZOLONES

The pyrazolones are currently represented by three drugs (phenylbutazone, oxyphenbutazone, and sulfinpyrazone) that have pharmacologic effects similar to those of the salicylates, but are more potent antiinflammatory agents. Sulfinpyrazone, however, is a much more effective uricosuric drug than it is an antiinflammatory agent and is employed in the maintenance therapy of gout. It is discussed later in the chapter.

Phenylbutazone and oxyphenbutazone are very effective antiinflammatory agents, but they are highly toxic compounds. Therefore their use should be restricted to short-term therapy of severe acute inflammatory conditions not alleviated by other less toxic agents such as the salicylates. Although they possess analgesic and antipyretic actions as well, the pyrazolones should never be used in place of aspirin or acetaminophen as a general-purpose pain reliever or fever reducer.

Phenylbutazone and its metabolite oxyphenbutazone are quite similar in their actions and are reviewed together.

Phenylbutazone

Azolid, Butazolidin

(CAN) Apo-Phenylbutazone, Intrabutazone, Novobutazone, Phenbuff

Oxyphenbutazone

(CAN) Oxybutazone, Tandearil

MECHANISM

Not completely established; interfere with the synthesis of prostaglandins and mucopolysaccharides in cartilage; inhibit leucocyte migration and activity of lysosomal enzymes; exert a weak blocking effect on uric acid reabsorption by renal tubular cells; produce significant retention of sodium and water

USES

Relief of acute symptoms of active rheumatoid arthritis, ankylosing spondylitis, osteoarthritis, psoriatic arthritis, and painful shoulder conditions (e.g., peritendinitis, bursitis, capsulitis)

Symptomatic treatment of acute superficial thrombophlebitis

Short-term treatment of acute attacks of degenerative joint disease of the hips and knees

Treatment of acute gout (short-term use only; not for maintenance therapy)

DOSAGE

(For both drugs)

Arthritis, spondylitis, painful shoulder: Initially—300 mg to 600 mg in divided doses (maximum 600 mg/day); maintenance dose—100 mg to 400 mg/day

FATE

Rapidly and completely absorbed from GI tract; onset of action in 30 minutes; highly bound (90%–98%) to plasma proteins with a half-life of 75 to 85 hours; therefore prolonged duration (3–5 days); slowly metabolized in the liver and excreted in the urine

COMMON SIDE EFFECTS

Nausea, vomiting, gastric discomfort, skin rash, diarrhea, vertigo, insomnia, nervousness, blurred vision, water and electrolyte retention

SIGNIFICANT ADVERSE REACTIONS

WARNING

Aplastic anemia and agranulocytosis can occur with use of these drugs, especially with prolonged administration or in elderly patients; regular hematologic examinations must be performed in all patients receiving the drugs longer than 1 week

GI: ulceration of the esophagus, stomach, small intestine, and bowel; occult GI bleeding, gastritis, abdominal distention; hematemesis

Hematologic: blood dyscrasias, bone marrow depression

Allergic/dermatologic: (requires prompt withdrawal of drug) petechiae, toxic pruritus, erythema nodosum, erythema multiforme, exfoliative dermatitis, Stevens–Johnson syndrome (see Chap. 4), serum sickness, polyarteritis, urticaria, arthralgia, fever, anaphylactic shock

Renal/metabolic: proteinuria, hematuria, oliguria, anuria, glomerulonephritis, renal stones, tubular necrosis, ureteral obstruction, sodium and chloride retention, edema, metabolic acidosis, hyperglycemia, thyroid hyperplasia, toxic goiter

Cardiovascular: hypertension, pericarditis, myocarditis with muscle necrosis, cardiac decompensation

Ocular/otic: diplopia, optic neuritis, retinal hemorrhage, retinal detachment, hearing loss

CNS (seen primarily with overdose): agitation, confusion, lethargy, depression, hallucinations, convulsions, psychosis, hyperventilation

CONTRAINDICATIONS

GI inflammation; ulceration or persistent dyspepsia; blood dycrasias; hypertension; thyroid disease; renal, hepatic, or cardiac dysfunction; temporal arteritis; polymyalgia rheumatica; patients receiving anticoagulants or potent chemotherapeutic agents; children under 14 years; senile patients. *Cautious use* in alcoholics, patients with chronic obstructive respiratory disease, visual disturbances, edema, unexplained bleeding, glaucoma, during pregnancy or nursing, and in older persons

INTERACTIONS

Pyrazolones may potentiate the effects of other protein-bound drugs (oral anticoagulants, sulfonamides, phenytoin, oral hypoglycemics, other antiinflammatory drugs such as salicylates and indomethacin)

Pyrazolones may decrease the effects of digitoxin

Effects of pyrazolones may be decreased by tricyclic antidepressants and by cholestyramine, which inhibits pyrazolone absorption

The effects of insulin and oral hypoglycemics can be enhanced by pyrazolones

Enzyme inducers (e.g., phenobarbital, phenytoin) may shorten the half-life of the pyrazolones

NURSING CONSIDERATIONS

Nursing Alerts

- Before initiating administration, ensure that a detailed history and complete physical and laboratory examinations have been performed. Laboratory examinations should be repeated at regular, frequent intervals during therapy.
- Carefully monitor laboratory studies and patient for indications of adverse reactions. These drugs should not be used as *first choice* in inflammatory states; they are indicated only when other less toxic agents are ineffective or poorly tolerated, and they should be discontinued if any significant change in white cell count occurs. Hematologic status should be monitored for several weeks following termination of therapy because the occurrence of blood dyscrasias remains a possibility for some time after discontinuation.

PATIENT EDUCATION

1. Stress importance of adhering to recommended dosage because incidence of adverse effects increases *sharply* at high dosage levels.
2. Suggest taking with meals or milk to minimize gastric irritation.
3. Because drugs induce sodium retention, instruct patient to restrict salt intake to avoid edema, especially if patient is hypertensive.
4. Urge patient to report appearance of early signs of possible blood dyscrasias (fever, sore throat, mouth ulceration), as well as epigastric pain, unusual bruising or bleeding, black or tarry stools, skin rash, blurred vision, pruritus, or significant edema or weight gain. If any of these appear, the drug should be discontinued immediately.
5. Advise patient that drug will probably be discontinued if no therapeutic effect is observed within 1 week. If improvement is noted, dosage should be reduced promptly to lowest effective level.
6. Explain the need to comply with frequent requests for blood tests. Hematologic status should be monitored frequently during prolonged therapy, especially in patients over 40.

NONSTEROIDAL ANTIINFLAMMATORY AGENTS

Diclofenac	Meclofenamate
Fenoprofen	Mefenamic acid
Flurbiprofen	Naproxen
Ibuprofen	Piroxicam
Indomethacin	Sulindac
Ketoprofen	Tolmetin

Effective antiinflammatory drugs that are less toxic than many of the older, established agents have long been sought. Several organic acids have demonstrated a somewhat lower incidence of side effects (e.g., tinnitus, GI distress) than comparably effective doses of the salicylates or pyrazolones. These compounds have been termed the *nonsteroidal antiinflammatory drugs* (NSAIDs). They are approximately equal to large doses of aspirin in relieving most types of inflammation; however, they have been reported to be *more* effective in certain inflammatory states such as psoriatic arthropathy or ankylosing spondylitis.

Like aspirin, NSAIDs also possess analgesic and antipyretic activity, but they should not be used for the relief of minor headache pain or reduction of elevated body temperature in place of more commonly prescribed drugs (aspirin, acetaminophen). However, with the exception of indomethacin and meclofenamate, they are often quite effective in relieving other types of mild to moderate pain such as dysmenorrhea, postextraction dental pain, postsurgical episiotomy, and soft-tissue athletic injuries.

Their action in inflammatory states is to reduce joint swelling, pain, and stiffness, and to improve the functional capacity of the joint; however, they do *not* alter the progressive course of the underlying pathologic condition. Since these compounds are expensive, there is little justification for their use in treating inflammatory states in persons who can tolerate the large daily doses of salicylates needed to control inflammation and who are capable of complying with such a regimen. Rather, these compounds are logical alternatives to the salicylates in patients unable to take large doses of aspirin-like drugs on a continual basis. They should be used as aspirin substitutes instead of the more toxic pyrazolones and corticosteroids. The long duration of action of several of the NSAIDs permits once- or twice-daily dosing, another advantage over the multiple daily doses of aspirin.

These drugs (other than indomethacin and meclofenamate) exhibit a somewhat lower incidence of the *milder* forms of GI distress than commonly occur with high-dose salicylate use. It must be noted, however, that most of the other untoward reactions and drug interactions associated with large doses of aspirin and related compounds are also evident to a similar degree with the NSAIDs. In addition, aspirin itself should not be given with these nonsteroidal drugs because it can reduce their blood levels and their activity. Likewise, combinations of the nonsteroidal drugs with low doses of corticosteroids are probably not significantly more effective than either drug alone, in most patients.

The NSAIDs are discussed as a group; individual drugs are listed in Table 19-2.

MECHANISM

Not completely established; block synthesis and possibly release of prostaglandins, thereby lowering sensitivity of peripheral pain receptors and reducing capillary leakage; reduce sensitivity of hypothalamic temperature-regulating center; decrease contractions of the myometrium by inhibiting prostaglandin activity in the uterus

USES

Relief of symptoms of rheumatoid arthritis, osteoarthritis, ankylosing spondylitis, and psoriatic arthropathy (not recommended in class IV disease, in which patient is incapacitated, largely bedridden, and capable of little or no self-care)

Relief of mild to moderate pain associated with dysmenorrhea, dental extractions, episiotomy, and athletic injuries such as strains and sprains (*except* meclofenamate)

Treatment of acute gout and gouty arthritis (especially naproxen or indomethacin)

Treatment of juvenile rheumatoid arthritis (tolmetin and naproxen are the *only* agents approved)

DOSAGE

See Table 19-2

FATE

Rapidly and almost completely absorbed; food generally delays absorption but does not affect total amount absorbed. Peak serum levels are usually attained within 2 to 3 hours, except piroxicam (3–5 h) and tolmetin (0.5–1 h). Half-lives differ greatly, with piroxicam having longest duration of action (24 h), followed by naproxen and sulindac (8–12 h). All drugs are highly bound to plasma proteins and are excreted largely as metabolites through the kidney. Some biliary excretion also occurs

COMMON SIDE EFFECTS

GI upset, dizziness, headache, tinnitus, constipation

SIGNIFICANT ADVERSE REACTIONS

(Incidence and severity differ among individual drugs; see Table 19-2)

GI: nausea, vomiting, cramping, diarrhea, bloating, epigastric pain, peptic ulceration, ulcerative stomatitis, bleeding, proctitis

Allergic: pruritus, skin rash, urticaria, erythema multiforme (rare), purpura (rare)

CNS: drowsiness, nervousness, insomnia, confusion, depression, tremor, muscle weakness

Eye/ear: blurred vision, diplopia, diminished hearing

Cardiovascular: palpitation, tachycardia, edema, prolonged bleeding time, arrhythmias, chest pain

Hepatic: cholestatic hepatitis, jaundice

Renal: dysuria, proteinuria, cystitis, oliguria, fluid retention, glomerular and interstitial nephritis, renal papillary necrosis (*Note:* Indomethacin and fenoprofen appear to be the most nephrotoxic)

CONTRAINDICATIONS

Aspirin sensitivity, active peptic ulcer; in addition, mefenamic acid is contraindicated in patients with ulceration or chronic inflammation of the GI tract and in those with significantly impaired renal function. *Cautious use* in the presence of epilepsy, parkinsonism, psychotic disturbances, GI pain or bleeding, coagulation defects, hypertension, infections, and in elderly or debilitated persons

INTERACTIONS

Effects of other protein-bound drugs (e.g., hydantoins, sulfonamides, oral hypoglycemics, oral anticoagulants, pyrazolones) may be increased by NSAIDs

GI adverse reactions may be intensified by concurrent administration of indomethacin, pyrazolones, salicylates, and corticosteroids.

Aspirin and other salicylates may reduce the blood level of nonsteroidal drugs

Barbiturates may lower the effects of fenoprofen by promoting its metabolism by the liver.

Plasma levels of NSAIDs can be raised by probenecid

Diuretics and antihypertensive drugs may be less effective because of the fluid retention associated with some NSAIDs

NURSING CONSIDERATIONS

See **Plan of Nursing Care 6 (Nonsteroidal Antiinflammatory Drugs [NSAIDs])** in this chapter. In addition:
1. If renal function is impaired, monitor results of creatinine clearance tests, which should be performed often. These drugs should be used very cautiously in patients with renal impairment.
2. Note that additional therapeutic benefit can be obtained with these drugs in combination with gold salts, but usually not with salicylates or corticosteroids.

GOLD COMPOUNDS

Injectable preparations containing about 50% elemental gold have been used for many years as part of the regimen for treating severe rheumatoid arthritis. Aurothioglucose and gold sodium thiomalate are two preparations used primarily in active arthritis that progresses despite adequate rest, physical therapy, and other drug treatment. In addition, auranofin is an orally effective compound containing 29% gold used for the management of active severe rheumatoid arthritis. These gold compounds can temporarily arrest the progression of bone destruction in involved joints, but there is no substantial evidence that they can repair damage caused by previously active disease. Gold compounds are potentially highly toxic, so persons receiving them must be carefully and continually observed for adverse reactions.

PLAN OF NURSING CARE 6
Patients Treated With Nonsteroidal Antiinflammatory Drugs (NSAIDs)
Nursing Diagnosis: Potential Impaired Tissue Integrity related to gastrointestinal effects of NSAID therapy.
Goal: Patient will experience minimal impairment of tissue integrity related to GI irritation from NSAID therapy.

Intervention	Rationale	Expected Outcome
Administer drug with food or antacid (*except* for fenoprofen).	GI irritation caused by a NSAID is minimized when drug is taken with meals.	Patient will state that no symptoms of GI irritation have occurred.
Instruct outpatient to take drug with food or antacid (*except* for fenoprofen).		Patient will explain how drug should be taken.
Teach patient symptoms of gastric intolerance such as nausea, vomiting, anorexia, abdominal cramps, epigastric pain.	Prostaglandins protect gastric mucosa and inhibit gastric acid secretion. When present in the stomach, NSAIDs, which interfere with prostaglandin synthesis, may eliminate this effect.	Patient will name symptoms of gastric intolerance to be reported.
Instruct patient to report symptoms of GI distress to drug prescriber, particularly if a history of GI problems exists.	The patient with a history of upper GI disease should be followed very closely, as NSAIDs may induce ulceration.	
If persistent GI distress occurs, consult with drug prescriber about: 1. use of another drug that causes less GI irritation 2. more frequent dosing with smaller quantities of drug (same total daily dosage) 3. reduction of total daily dosage (with same frequency of dosing)	More frequent dosing permits administration of same total daily dosage with smaller amount of drug ingested with each dose, thus reducing concentration delivered to gastric mucosa. Smaller total daily dosage with same frequency of dosing also reduces quantity of drug delivered to stomach with each dose.	Patient will report that GI distress is reduced with altered drug regimen.
Instruct patient to report a change in color or consistency of stools to drug prescriber.	Incidence of diarrhea is quite high with some NSAIDs. Black (tarry) stools indicate presence of GI bleeding.	Patient will express awareness of need to report change in stool color/consistency.
When indicated, test stools periodically for presence of occult blood.	Small amounts of GI bleeding may be present without frank signs of blood loss.	Occult GI bleeding will be detected early.

Nursing Diagnosis: Potential Sensory-Perceptual Alterations: Visual and Auditory related to neurological side effects of NSAID therapy.
Goal: Patient's sight and hearing will remain unimpaired by NSAID therapy.

Intervention	Rationale	Expected Outcome
Assess visual and auditory function prior to initiation of therapy.	Minor neurologic reactions are among the most common side effects of NSAIDs. Baselines should be established before therapy is initiated.	Baseline visual and auditory function will be established.
Instruct patient to report any visual changes to drug prescriber.	Decreased visual acuity, blurred vision, changes in color vision, and corneal deposits may occur.	Patient will express awareness of the need to: 1. Report any visual changes that occur
With patient on long-term therapy discuss the need to obtain periodic ophthalmologic evaluations.	If eye problems manifest during therapy, the drug should be discontinued until their cause has been determined.	2. Obtain periodic ophthalmologic examinations
Instruct patient to report any auditory changes to drug prescriber.	Tinnitus and hearing loss are potential side effects.	3. Patient will report any auditory changes that occur
If hearing loss is suspected, instruct patient to obtain audiometric tests at regular intervals.	Audiometric tests may be indicated to monitor hearing capacity.	4. Patient will obtain recommended audiometric tests

Continued

PLAN OF NURSING CARE 6 (continued)
Patients Treated With Nonsteroidal Antiinflammatory Drugs (NSAIDs)

Nursing Diagnosis: Potential Knowledge Deficit related to NSAID therapy.
Goal: Patient will possess knowledge needed to implement NSAID regimen and related actions.

Intervention	Rationale	Expected Outcome
See also Plan of Nursing Care 1 (Knowledge Deficit) and 2 (Compliance)		
Explain the following aspects of drug regimen:		Patient will verbalize understanding of factors affecting drug regimen.
1. In management of arthritis, better results are obtained if drug is taken routinely, as ordered, rather than intermittently.	Stable blood levels provide more consistent results.	
2. Improvement in condition may not occur for up to 2 wk. At that time, dosage may begin to be decreased gradually to lowest effective level.	The likelihood of compliance increases when patient's expectations are realistic.	
3. Some persons respond to only one of several available NSAIDs. Different derivatives may be tried at 2- to 3-wk intervals before concluding that NSAIDs are ineffective.		
Teach patient potential side effects and related actions:		Patient will name drug side effects and related actions.
1. Sedation and dizziness: Warn patient to perform potentially dangerous mechanical tasks cautiously until effects of drug are known.	NSAIDs often cause CNS side effects. Mechanical tasks should be performed cautiously to avoid injury.	
2. Headache: Advise patient to consult health care provider for appropriate treatment if headache becomes problematic. Discourage self-medication with aspirin or other salicylates.	Headache is a frequent CNS side effect. Salicylates may reduce the NSAID's effectiveness. Acetaminophen may, however, be used without significant problems in this regard.	
3. Fluid retention: Instruct patient with compromised cardiac function, hypertension, or renal impairment to weigh self daily. Instruct patient to report weight gain in excess of 2 to 5 pounds (as determined by health care provider).	Prostaglandin inhibition causes a reduction in renal blood flow, glomerular filtration, and salt and water excretion. Salt and water retention may occur. Rapid weight gain is an early sign of developing edema and fluid retention.	
4. Unusual bleeding, bruising, or petechiae: Instruct patient to report appearance of unusual signs of bleeding to drug prescriber.	NSAIDs have anticoagulant effects related to inhibition of prostaglandin synthesis.	
5. Skin rash: Instruct patient to report appearance of skin rash to drug prescriber.	Skin rash and other side-effects may necessitate adjustment of drug regimen.	
Discuss the importance of informing physician or dentist of NSAID usage prior to elective surgery.	Because NSAIDs can inhibit platelet aggregation, they should be discontinued for 1 wk prior to surgery to minimize risk of postoperative bleeding.	Patient will express awareness of need to notify health care personnel of NSAID usage prior to elective surgery.

Injections are normally given at weekly or longer intervals for prolonged periods, occasionally with rest periods if remission has occurred. Because of the long course of therapy, the need for repeated injections, and the necessity for periodic laboratory tests to detect toxicity, patients often have difficulty complying with this form of therapy. The oral gold preparation appears to be nearly as effective as the injectable drugs, with the advantage of a lower incidence of adverse reactions and better patient compliance.

Auranofin
Ridaura

Aurothioglucose
Solganal

Gold Sodium Thiomalate
Myochrysine

(Text continued on page 184)

Table 19-2
Nonsteroidal Antiinflammatory Agents

Drug	Preparations	Usual Dosage Range	Nursing Implications
Diclofenac Voltaren	Enteric coated tablets: 25 mg, 50 mg, 75 mg	100 mg–200 mg/day in 3 or 4 divided doses	Chemically unique drug used for rheumatoid and osteoarthritis and ankylosing spondylitis; short plasma half-life, but drug persists for extended period of time in synovial fluid; may inhibit synthesis of leukotrienes as well as prostaglandins (see Fig. 19-1); incidence of side effects is similar to most other nonsteroidal drugs; may be useful in mild to moderate pain, acute painful shoulder and juvenile rheumatoid arthritis
Fenoprofen Nalfon	Capsules: 200 mg, 300 mg, 600 mg Tablets: 600 mg	Arthritis: 300 mg–600 mg 4 times/day (maximum 3200 mg/day) Mild to moderate pain: 200 mg/4–6 h	Administer 30 min before or 2 h after meals unless GI distress occurs, then give with milk; perform periodic auditory function tests during chronic therapy; *not* recommended for children under 14; periodic liver function tests are advised, as drug can elevate serum transaminase, LDH, and alkaline phosphatase; drowsiness and headache are common; urinary toxicity is more common than with other similar drugs
Flurbiprofen Ansaid, Ocufen	Tablets: 50 mg, 100 mg Ophthalmic solution: 0.03%	Rheumatoid and osteoarthritis: 200 mg–300 mg/day in 2–4 divided doses Prevention of intraoperative miosis—1 drop every 3 min beginning 2 h before surgery	Used orally for treating arthritis and also as an eye drop for preventing miosis due to contraction of iris sphincter during surgery; may also be useful in mild to moderate pain and primary dysmenorrhea; low doses have been shown to retard bone loss in periodontal disease; side effects are similar to those observed with other nonsteriodal drugs
Ibuprofen Advil, Motrin, Nuprin and several other manufacturers (CAN) Amersol, Novoprofen	Tablets: 200 mg (OTC), 300 mg, 400 mg, 600 mg, 800 mg	Arthritis: 400 mg to 800 mg 3–4 times/day (maximum 3200 mg/day) Mild–moderate pain: 400 mg/4–6 h Dysmenorrhea: 400 mg/4 h OTC for aches, pain, fever: 200 mg every 4–6 h to a maximum of 1200 mg/day	Available OTC (200-mg tablets) and for prescription-only use (all other strengths); not to be used more than 10 days for pain or 3 days for fever; slightly more effective than aspirin as an antiinflammatory drug and for relief of dysmenorrhea; minimal interaction with oral anticoagulants; if blurred or diminished vision occurs, discontinue drug; perform periodic ophthalmologic examination

Continued

Table 19-2
Nonsteroidal Antiinflammatory Agents (continued)

Drug	Preparations	Usual Dosage Range	Nursing Implications
Indomethacin Indameth, Indocin (CAN) Apo-Indomethacin, Indocid, Novomethacin	Capsules: 25 mg, 50 mg, 75 mg Sustained release capsules: 75 mg Oral suspension: 25 mg/5 mL Suppositories: 50 mg Powder for injection: 1 mg per vial	Chronic inflammation: 25 mg 2–3 times/day to a maximum daily dose of 200 mg; 75 mg sustained-release capsules may be used once or twice daily Acute gout: 50 mg 3 times/day for 3–5 days Patent ductus arteriosus: 0.2 mg/kg initially IV, followed by 0.1–0.25 mg/kg for 2 succeeding doses at intervals 12–24 h	Potent antiinflammatory agent used in moderate to severe rheumatoid and osteoarthritis and acute gouty arthritis; also for aiding closure of patent ductus arteriosus in premature infants; most frequent side effects are headache, stomach pain (always given with meals) nausea; discontinue drug if significant improvement has not occurred in 2–3 wk; give largest portion of dose at bedtime if morning stiffness or persistent night pain is encountered; drug is given IV *only* in infants for closure of ductus and only if, after 48 h following birth, usual medical management is ineffective; IV administration may significantly reduce urinary output and can precipitate renal insufficiency
Ketoprofen Orudis	Capsules: 50 mg, 75 mg	Arthritis: 75 mg 3 times/day or 50 mg 4 times/day (maximum 300 mg/day) Mild–moderate pain; dysmenorrhea: 50 mg 3–4 times/day	Principally indicated for rheumatoid arthritis and osteoarthritis; recurrent peptic ulcers have occurred during prolonged use; dyspepsia, GI distress, and headache are quite common; initial dose should be reduced ⅓ to ½ in elderly patients with impaired renal function; drug may be removed by dialysis in cases of poisoning with renal failure
Meclofenamate Meclomen	Capsules: 50 mg, 100 mg Tablets: 50 mg, 100 mg	Arthritis: 200 mg–400 mg/day in 3–4 divided doses Mild–moderate pain: 50 mg–100 mg every 4–6 h	*Not* recommended for children under 14; should *not* be used as initial therapy for rheumatoid arthritis or osteoarthritis because of high incidence of diarrhea (10%–30%), vomiting (10%–12%), and other GI disorders (10%); administer with meals, milk, or antacids; periodic hemoglobin/hematocrit determinations are recommended during extended therapy
Mefenamic acid Ponstel (CAN) Ponstan	Capsules: 250 mg	Acute pain: Initially 500 mg; then 250 mg/6 h Dysmenorrhea: Initially 500 mg, then 250 mg every 6 h for 2–4 days	Short-acting drug used to relieve moderate pain of brief duration and to treat symptoms of primary dismenorrhea; diarrhea occurs frequently and necessitates discontinuation of therapy; administer with food and do not exceed 1 wk of treatment; maximum duration for dysmenorrhea is 3–4 days; *do*

Continued

Table 19-2
Nonsteroidal Antiinflammatory Agents (continued)

Drug	Preparations	Usual Dosage Range	Nursing Implications
			not use in patients with a history of renal impairment or chronic inflammation or ulceration of the GI tract, discontinue drug if skin rash, petechiae, dark stools, or hematemesis is noted; *contraindicated* in children under 14
Naproxen Naprosyn (CAN) Apo-Naproxen, Naxen, Novonaprox **Naproxen sodium** Anaprox	Tablets: 250 mg, 375 mg, 500 mg Oral suspension: 125 mg/5 mL Tablets: 275 mg, 550 mg (equivalent to 250 mg and 500 mg of naproxen base)	Arthritis: 250 mg–500 mg twice a day (maximum 1000 mg/day) Mild–moderate pain: 550 mg (sodium salt) initially, then 275 mg every 6–8 h Acute gout: 750 mg followed by 250 mg every 8 h until attack has subsided Juvenile rheumatoid arthritis: 10 mg/kg/day in 2 divided doses	Prolonged half-life (13 h) in the body allows only twice-a-day administration, which may aid patient compliance; sodium salt is more quickly absorbed, giving a faster onset of action; duration of action is equal to base, however; drug may have to be used for up to 1 month to obtain a significant clinical response; readily crosses placental barrier and is excreted in significant concentrations in breast milk
Piroxicam Feldene (CAN) Apo-Piroxicam, Novapirocam	Capsules: 10 mg, 20 mg	Initially, 20 mg once daily; maintenance dosage is 10 mg–20 mg once daily	Long-acting drug used in rheumatoid and osteoarthritis; steady state plasma levels are generally attained within 1–2 wk; antacids do not affect plasma levels, but aspirin can reduce blood levels of piroxicam to 80% of normal; GI side effects are experienced by 20% of patients; *not* recommended for use in children
Sulindac Clinoril	Tablets: 150 mg, 200 mg	150 mg–200 mg twice a day (maximum 400 mg/day)	Long-acting drug used twice a day; useful in rheumatoid arthritis, osteoarthritis and gouty arthritis, spondylitis, and acute painful shoulder; may allow a gradual reduction in corticosteroid dosage if used concurrently; liver function test abnormalities can occur; *not* indicated for use in children; high incidence (10%) of GI pain and other GI symptoms; administer with food
Tolmetin Tolectin	Tablets: 200 mg Capsules: 400 mg	Adults: Initially, 400 mg 3 times/day (maximum 2000 mg/day); maintenance doses are 600 mg–1800 mg/day in 3–4 divided doses. Children (over 2 yr): 20 mg/kg/day in 3–4 divided doses (maximum 30 mg/kg/day)	May be used in juvenile rheumatoid arthritis in children over 2; minimal interaction with oral anticoagulants; if GI intolerance occurs, give with food, milk, or antacids other than sodium bicarbonate; sodium and water retention can occur; *caution* in cardiac patients; headache is observed in 10% of patients

MECHANISM

Largely speculative; in animals, gold reduces macrophage phagocytosis, increases collagen cross-linkages, inhibits lysosomal enzymes, decreases formation of glucosamine-6-phosphate in connective tissue, inactivates the first component of complement, prevents prostaglandin synthesis, interferes with binding of tryptophan to plasma proteins, and suppresses the anaphylactic release of histamine

USES

Adjunctive treatment of active adult and juvenile rheumatoid arthritis not adequately controlled by other less toxic agents (greatest benefit in the early, active stages)

Investigational uses include treatment of pemphigus (with steroids) or psoriatic arthritis in persons for whom nonsteroidal antiinflammatory agents are ineffective

DOSAGE

Aurothioglucose

Adults: Weekly IM injections; first week, 10 mg; second and third week, 25 mg; thereafter 50 mg. If improvement is noted, continue with 50-mg injections at 2- to 4-week intervals as necessary. Cessation of treatment depends on individual response

Children (6–12 yr): One fourth of adult dose; maximum 25 mg/week to children under 12

Gold Sodium Thiomalate

Adults: weekly injections; first week, 10 mg; second week, 25 mg; third and subsequent weeks, 25 to 50 mg until major clinical improvement or toxicity occurs. Injections of 25 mg to 50 mg may be given every third or fourth week indefinitely if clinical improvement remains stable.

Children: 1 mg/kg, not to exceed 50 mg on a single injection; schedule is same as for adults.

Auranofin

6 mg a day orally, in a single or divided dosage; may increase to 3 mg 3 times/day after 6 months if response is inadequate

FATE

Injectable drugs show slow absorption from injection site; peak effects occur in 4 to 6 hours after IM administration and within 1 or 2 hours of oral ingestion; serum half-lives vary but increase up to several months with repeated injections; gold is well distributed throughout the body; arthritic joints appear to concentrate more gold than nonarthritic joints; injected gold is excreted mainly in the urine (70%), whereas gold administered orally is eliminated predominantly in the feces

COMMON SIDE EFFECTS

(25%–50% incidence) Erythema, dermatitis, pruritus, stomatitis, metallic taste, flushing, dizziness, sweating, and proteinuria; in addition, diarrhea occurs in over half of patients receiving oral gold

SIGNIFICANT ADVERSE REACTIONS

Dermatologic: papular, vesicular, or exfoliative dermatitis; alopecia, chrysiasis

Mucous membrane: gingivitis, pharyngitis, gastritis, colitis, upper respiratory tract inflammation, vaginitis

Hematologic: blood dyscrasias (rare)

Renal: glomerulitis, hematuria, nephritis

Allergic: syncope, bradycardia, angioedema, difficulty in swallowing or breathing, anaphylactic shock

Other: GI distress (nausea, cramping, vomiting, colic), iritis, corneal ulcers (rare), hepatitis, acute yellow atrophy, peripheral neuritis, synovial destruction, EEG abnormalities, pulmonary fibrosis

Laboratory signs of gold toxicity include leukopenia (less than 4000 WBC/mm^3), fall in hemoglobin, proteinuria, platelet count less than 100,000/mm^3, and a granulocyte count less than 1500/mm^3. Close monitoring of laboratory values is essential to ensure safe and effective therapy.

CONTRAINDICATIONS

Uncontrolled diabetes, renal disease, hepatic dysfunction, severe hypertension, cardiac failure, systemic lupus, history of blood dyscrasias, eczema, colitis, severely debilitated states, recent radiation therapy, elderly patients, and pregnancy. *Cautious use* in individuals with a history of allergies, compromised cerebral or coronary circulation, or moderate hypertension

INTERACTIONS

Incidence of blood dyscrasias or hematologic toxicity may be increased by concurrent use of pyrazolones, antimalarial drugs (e.g., hydroxychloroquine), immunosuppressants (e.g., azathioprine), or cytotoxic drugs

Corticosteroids can reduce the effectiveness and increase the toxicity of gold salts

NURSING CONSIDERATIONS

Nursing Alerts

- Monitor results of laboratory studies. Differential, white blood cell, erythrocyte, and platelet counts; hemoglobin determination; and urinalysis should be performed before therapy is initiated and after every second injection. The drug should be discontinued if proteinuria, hematuria, markedly reduced hemoglobin, leukopenia, or platelet count below 100,000/mm^3 occurs.
- Have dimercaprol (BAL) available as a specific antidote to gold overdosage.

1. Shake vial well, and do not use if color is darker than pale yellow. Inject deep into gluteal muscle with patient lying down. Instruct patient to remain lying for 20 minutes after injection to eliminate possibility of dizziness.

PATIENT EDUCATION

1. Carefully explain the need to be aware of early signs of developing toxicity (e.g., mouth sores, pruritus, GI upset, dermatitis, rash, bleeding gums, petechiae, fever, chills, weakness, sore throat, dysphagia) and the need to immediately report any signs to drug prescriber.
2. Inform patient that periodic blood and urine tests will be required.
3. Inform patient that beneficial effects may take several months to become evident but that their duration will be prolonged once they occur.
4. Discuss use of proper oral hygiene to reduce risk of stomatitis and other mouth disorders.
5. Suggest that patient avoid exposure to sunlight as much as possible during therapy because dermatologic toxicity may be increased.
6. Advise patient to continue to observe closely for possible adverse effects after therapy has been completed because toxic effects can occur for months afterwards.

PENICILLAMINE (CUPRIMINE, DEPEN)

Penicillamine is a chelating agent that has been successfully used to remove excess copper in patients with Wilson's disease and to decrease cystine excretion in cystinuria. It is also approved for the treatment of severe forms of rheumatoid arthritis. Because of its potential to elicit *serious* adverse effects, however, its use should be restricted to those patients with progressive rheumatoid disease that is unresponsive to other less toxic antiinflammatory agents.

MECHANISM

Largely unknown; may inhibit lysosomal enzyme release in connective tissue; suppresses T-cell activity in vitro, and lowers IgM rheumatoid factor titer. Other actions ascribed to penicillamine are degradation of collagen, inhibition of lymphocyte transformation, and reduction of circulating immune complexes. Drug is also capable of combining with copper, thus removing excess amounts of the substance from patients with Wilson's disease. It reduces cystine excretion in cystinuria, probably by forming a substance more soluble and hence more readily excretable than cystine

USES

Treatment of severe, active rheumatoid arthritis resistant to other conventional forms of therapy, including rest, exercise, salicylates, nonsteroidal antiinflammatory drugs, and corticosteroids (up to several months may be needed to obtain a suitable clinical response)

Promotion of copper excretion in patients with Wilson's disease (hepatolenticular degeneration)

Promotion of cystine excretion in patients with cystinuria

Investigational uses include treatment of primary biliary cirrhosis and scleroderma

DOSAGE

Rheumatoid arthritis: initially, 125 mg to 250 mg/day for 4 weeks; increase at 4- to 12-week intervals by 125 mg to 250 mg/day depending on response and tolerance; maximum 1000 mg to 1500 mg/day for 3 to 4 months; if no response at this level, discontinue drug; usual maintenance range is 500 mg to 750 mg/day (dosage may be reduced *gradually* if patient has been in remission for at least 6 months)

Wilson's disease: Initially, 250 mg 4 times/day, increased to 500 mg 4 times/day as needed

Cystinuria: Adults—250 mg to 500 mg 4 times/day; Children—30 mg/kg/day

FATE

Well absorbed orally if given on an empty stomach; peak plasma level in 1 to 2 hours; serum half-life is approximately 2 hours; excreted in the urine, almost completely within 24 hours

COMMON SIDE EFFECTS

Loss of sense of taste, indigestion, epigastric pain, nausea, anorexia, rash, pruritus, and proteinuria

SIGNIFICANT ADVERSE REACTIONS

GI: vomiting, diarrhea, oral ulceration, activation of peptic ulcer

Hematologic: leukopenia, thrombocytopenia, bone marrow depression, agranulocytosis, aplastic anemia

Allergic: arthralgia, lymphadenopathy, pemphigoid reaction, urticaria, exfoliative dermatitis, colitis, synovitis, thyroiditis

Renal/hepatic: hematuria, hepatic dysfunction, cholestatic jaundice, pancreatitis, glomerulonephritis (Goodpasture's syndrome)

CNS: tinnitus, optic neuritis

Other: thrombophlebitis, myasthenia-like reaction, hyperpyrexia, polymyositis, systemic lupus–like syndrome, mammary hyperplasia, epidermal necrolysis, alveolitis, obliterative bronchiolitis

CONTRAINDICATIONS

Renal insufficiency; pregnancy; young children; history of penicillin sensitivity or blood dyscrasias; concurrent use with other antiinflammatory drugs (pyrazolones, gold compounds), antimalarials, or cytotoxic agents. *Cautious use* in persons with a history of allergies or respiratory disease

INTERACTIONS

Penicillamine may potentiate the neurotoxicity of isoniazid

Effects of penicillamine can be reduced by the presence of iron, antacids, or food, which can decrease absorption

Risk of blood dyscrasias and renal toxicity may be increased by concomitant use of antimalarial drugs, antineoplastics, gold compounds, or pyrazolones

Penicillamine can lower serum levels of digoxin

NURSING CONSIDERATIONS

Nursing Alerts

- Monitor results of laboratory studies. Urinalyses, differential blood cell counts, hemoglobin determinations, and direct platelet counts should be performed every 2 weeks for the first 6 months of therapy and monthly thereafter. If WBC counts are below 3500 or platelet counts below 100,000, therapy should be discontinued.
- Monitor patient carefully for indications of proteinuria or hematuria, possible early signs of developing glomerulonephritis. Drug should be discontinued if proteinuria exceeds 2 g/24 hours, or if gross or persistent microscopic hematuria develops.

PATIENT EDUCATION

1. Assist patient to plan dosing schedule so that drug is taken on an empty stomach, at least 1 hour apart from any other drug, food, antacid, or milk.
2. Instruct patient to promptly report early signs of possible developing blood dyscrasias (e.g., fever, sore throat, chills, bruising, abnormal bleeding, malaise) to appropriate person. Blood studies should be performed immediately. Drug-induced fever is an indication for discontinuing the drug.
3. Instruct patient to be alert for appearance of allergic manifestations (e.g., fever, arthralgia, lymphadenopathy, rash, intense pruritus) and to advise physician immediately. Reduction in dosage and use of antihistamines can usually eliminate early rash and pruritus.
4. Prepare patient for the possibility of increased skin friability, especially at pressure points (e.g., elbows, knees, buttocks), because the drug increases soluble collagen. External bleeding or vesicles containing blood may appear, and skin wrinkling can occur. These effects are not progressive and do not require discontinuance of drug; they may disappear with dosage reduction.

5. Instruct patient to watch for signs of increasing muscle weakness because drug can cause a myasthenia-like syndrome. Symptoms will usually disappear following drug withdrawal.

ANTIGOUT DRUGS

Gout is a metabolic disorder of purine metabolism characterized by an excess of uric acid in the blood (hyperuricemia) that results from either overproduction or a defect in elimination. When the solubility of uric acid salts is exceeded in body fluids, monosodium urate crystals begin to precipitate out of the blood and are deposited in joints, skin, kidney, and other tissues, resulting in the appearance of symptoms of acute gout—pain, swelling, tenderness, and other signs of inflammation. The pharamcotherapy of gout, therefore, involves controlling the serum levels of uric acid to prevent attacks, and providing relief of the symptoms of an acute attack of gouty arthritis. Drugs used as anti-gout agents may be classified as one of the following:

- *Antiinflammatory agents:* relieve the pain and inflammation associated with an acute attack of gout
- *Hypouricemic (uricosuric) agents:* reduce the blood levels of uric acid with prolonged administration

The drugs that may be used to relieve the symptoms of an acute attack are indomethacin, phenylbutazone, oxyphenbutazone, naproxen, sulindac, and colchicine. The first five were discussed previously in this chapter, because they are also used to control symptoms of rheumatoid arthritis and osteoarthritis. Colchicine is reviewed in detail in this section. Hypouricemic agents either interfere with the synthesis of uric acid (e.g., allopurinol) or promote the urinary excretion of uric acid by blocking its renal tubular reabsorption (e.g., probenecid, sulfinpyrazone). These drugs are also discussed in this section.

Colchicine

An alkaloid capable of dramatically relieving pain and inflammation associated with acute attacks of gouty arthritis within 12 hours to 24 hours, colchicine is also useful but somewhat less effective in the treatment of chondrocalcinosis (pseudogout). It is nonanalgesic and nonuricosuric, and is specific for the symptoms of gout, being effective in up to 90% of patients if given at the first sign of an attack. Although once it was exclusively the drug of choice, colchicine has now been largely replaced by indomethacin, sulindac, or phenylbutazone because of its extremely high incidence of GI side effects.

MECHANISM
Reduces leukocytic production of lactic acid, thereby decreasing acid deposition; impairs phagocytic breakdown of white blood cell membrane and release of tissue-damaging enzymes; also binds to microtubular cellular proteins, thereby arresting mitosis at metaphase and interfering with movement of mobile cells (e.g., leukocytes)

USES
Relief of pain and inflammation of acute gout and pseudogout
Limiting the destruction of joint cartilage and reducing the incidence of acute attacks (not an approved indication)
Other experimental uses include symptomatic treatment of leukemia, adenocarcinoma, sarcoid arthritis, mycosis fungoides, acute calcium-dependent tendinitis, and familial Mediterranean fever

DOSAGE
Oral: 1 mg to 1.2 mg initially, at earliest sign of acute attack, followed by 0.5 mg to 1.2 mg every 1 to 2 hours until pain is relieved or diarrhea occurs (4 mg–8 mg total dose usually required for acute attack; prophylaxis—0.5 mg to 0.6 mg orally 3 or 4 times/week; severe cases—0.5 mg–1.8 mg daily)
IV: 1 mg to 2 mg initially, followed by 0.5 mg every 6 hours (maximum 4 mg/24 h)

FATE
Rapidly absorbed orally; relatively short-acting (half-life 20 min); partially metabolized in the liver; both metabolites and unchanged drug are recycled into the GI tract through the bile and intestinal secretions; mainly eliminated in the feces, with 10% to 20% excreted in the urine; drug may persist for up to 9 days in leukocytes after single IV dose

COMMON SIDE EFFECTS
Nausea, vomiting, abdominal pain, diarrhea

SIGNIFICANT ADVERSE REACTIONS
(Usually observed at high doses or with hepatic dysfunction) Severe diarrhea, muscle weakness, dermatitis, hematuria, oliguria, generalized vascular damage, alopecia; prolonged use may lead to agranulocytosis, aplastic anemia, and peripheral neuritis. Overdose may be characterized by vomiting, diarrhea (profuse and bloody), burning in the throat, stomach or skin, hematuria, shock due to extensive vascular damage, marked muscle weakness, delirium, and convulsions

CONTRAINDICATIONS
Severe renal, GI, cardiac, or hepatic disease; IV use contraindicated with vascular damage. *Cautious use* in elderly or debilitated persons, especially those with renal, hepatic, GI, or heart disease

INTERACTIONS
Effects of colchicine are enhanced by alkalinizing agents (e.g., sodium bicarbonate) and inhibited by acidifying agents (e.g., ascorbic acid)
Colchicine may increase the response to CNS depressants and sympathomimetics
Prolonged use of colchicine may reduce GI absorption of vitamin B_{12}

NURSING CONSIDERATIONS

Nursing Alerts
- Inform physician if oral administration is associated with excessive GI toxicity. The IV route may be used, but overdose occurs more commonly with IV use, and extravasation can cause pain and necrosis of tissues.
- If parenterally administered, use IV route only, not SC or IM. Observe injection site for signs of localized irritation (pain, swelling, erythema) because thrombophlebitis may occur.
- Monitor intake and output, and force fluids to maintain urine output of at least 2000 mL/day to promote urate excretion and reduce danger of uric acid deposition in kidneys and ureters.

1. When colchicine is used with probenecid to treat chronic gouty arthritis complicated by frequent, recurrent attacks,

advocate use of fixed combination (Col-Benemid, Proben-C), if appropriate, to increase likelihood of compliance.

PATIENT EDUCATION

1. Instruct patient to take with meals or milk to reduce GI irritation.
2. Instruct patient to note and report early signs of toxicity (nausea, vomiting, diarrhea, abdominal discomfort, weakness). Drug should be discontinued until symptoms subside, then carefully resumed.
3. Instruct patient to note and report early signs of bone marrow depression. Drug should be discontinued if sore throat, bleeding gums, fever, or weakness occurs.
4. Instruct patient to immobilize affected joints and avoid applying heat or pressure to involved areas during an acute attack.
5. Instruct patient to inform physician or dentist of diagnosis of gout prior to any surgery. Before and after any surgical procedure (including dental), 0.5 mg to 0.6 mg should be administered 3 times a day for 3 days because surgery may precipitate an acute attack of gout.
6. Explain that colchicine may be needed in the *initial stages* of therapy with uricosuric agents because these drugs can mobilize large quantities of uric acid and thus increase the incidence of acute attacks during the early phase of therapy.
7. Discuss adjunctive measures (e.g., diet control, weight reduction, increased fluid intake, avoidance of alcoholic beverages in large amounts) that may help reduce the incidence and severity of attacks.

Probenecid

Benemid, Probalan
(CAN) Benuryl

A uricosuric agent that enhances the excretion of uric acid through the kidneys, probenecid has no analgesic or antiinflammatory action and thus is of no value in treating acute attacks. The drug also inhibits renal tubular *secretion* of penicillins and cephalosporins and is often used to increase the plasma level of penicillins by two to four times, thus enhancing their effects.

MECHANISM
Inhibits the renal tubular reabsorption of urates, increasing excretion of uric acid and reducing plasma uric acid levels; decreased serum urate concentration retards further urate deposition and increases resorption of urate deposits in tissues; competitively inhibits tubular secretion (i.e., plasma to renal tubule) of many weak organic acids, especially penicillins

USES
Treatment of hyperuricemia associated with gout and gouty arthritis
Adjuvant to therapy with penicillins and cephalosporins to elevate and prolong plasma levels of antimicrobial

DOSAGE
Gout: 0.25 g twice a day for 1 week, then 0.5 g twice a day thereafter; may increase if necessary by 0.5 g/day every 4 weeks to a maximum of 2 g/day
Penicillin therapy:
Adult—2 g daily in divided doses
Children—40 mg/kg/day in divided doses; (over 50 kg—adult dosage may be given)

Gonorrhea: 1 g probenecid given together with 4.8 million units of penicillin G or 3.5 g ampicillin

FATE
Completely absorbed orally; peak effects in 2 to 4 hours; half-life is 8 to 10 hours; highly bound to plasma protein (85%–95%), metabolized in the liver; slowly excreted in urine primarily as metabolites and some unchanged drug; excretion increased by alkalinization of the urine

COMMON SIDE EFFECTS
GI irritation, nausea, skin rash, headache, and worsening of symptoms of acute gout for first few days

SIGNIFICANT ADVERSE REACTIONS
Abdominal discomfort, diarrhea, sore gums, urinary frequency, flushing, dizziness, hypersensitivity reactions (dermatitis, fever, pruritus, anaphylaxis), anemia. Hepatic necrosis, nephrotic syndrome, and aplastic anemia are rare

CONTRAINDICATIONS
Age under 2 years, blood dyscrasias, uric acid kidney stones, an acute gouty arthritis attack, severe renal impairment. *Cautious use* in persons with peptic ulcer, acute intermittent porphyria, and glucose-6-phosphatase deficiency

INTERACTIONS
Probenecid prolongs the action of penicillins and cephalosporins and may enhance the action of methotrexate, clofibrate, oral anticoagulants, oral hypoglycemics, naproxen, indomethacin, sulfinpyrazone, sulfonamides, and thiazide diuretics
Salicylates can antagonize the uricosuric effect of probenecid, especially in small analgesic doses
Xanthines (e.g., caffeine, theophylline) and pyrazinamide may antagonize the uricosuric effect of probenecid

PATIENT EDUCATION

1. Instruct patient to take drug with milk or meals to minimize GI upset.
2. Caution patient to follow prescribed dosage regimen carefully. Reduction in dosage level may lead to sharp elevation of serum uric acid levels and precipitation of acute attacks.
3. Inform patient that frequency of acute attacks may increase during first few months of therapy with probenecid. Prophylactic doses of colchicine or indomethacin may be indicated during initial stages of probenecid therapy (colchicine and probenecid are available in combined form as Col-Benemid or Proben-C).
4. Discuss the need to maintain a high fluid intake (2–3 L/day) and to alkalinize the urine to help retard formation of uric acid kidney stones. Sodium bicarbonate, potassium citrate, or other urinary alkalinizers may be prescribed.
5. Warn patient of the danger of taking aspirin or related drugs while on probenecid therapy: clinical effects of the uricosuric drug may be greatly reduced.
6. Instruct patient to notify physician if an acute attack occurs while taking the drug. The drug should not be discontinued, but colchicine or indomethacin may be added to the regimen. Therapy with probenecid should

not, however, be initiated during an acute attack because symptoms may worsen.
7. Although there is no firm evidence that excessive dietary intake of purines is a primary cause of gout, suggest that patient restrict high-purine foods such as liver, meat extracts, peas, meat soups, broth, and alcohol during early stages of therapy, at least until uric acid levels have stabilized.

Sulfinpyrazone

Anturane

(CAN) Antazone, Apo-Sulfinpyrazone, Novopyrazone, Zynol

A pyrazolone derivative with relatively weak antiinflammatory action, indicated primarily for the maintenance therapy of hyperuricemia, this drug also inhibits platelet aggregation, and some studies suggest that it is effective in reducing the incidence of cardiac death in patients with recent myocardial infarction. This effect may be related to an inhibition of platelet synthesis of thromboxane A_2, protection of the vascular endothelium from injury, and diminished release of ADP and possibly serotonin.

MECHANISM

Inhibits the active renal tubular reabsorption of uric acid, thereby increasing its urinary excretion and reducing serum urate levels; decreases platelet aggregation, although the mechanism is not completely established (see above); very small doses may interfere with active tubular *secretion* of uric acid (transport from blood to renal tubule) thereby causing retention of serum urates

USES

Maintenance therapy in hyperuricemia to reduce the incidence and severity of acute attacks of gouty arthritis

Prevention of cerebrovascular and ischemic heart disease and transient ischemic attacks, and reduction in fatalities following myocardial infarction (experimental use only)

DOSAGE

Initially: 200 mg to 400 mg daily in divided doses; increase gradually to an optimal dose (maximum 800 mg/day); continue without interruption, even during an acute attack, which can be treated with colchicine, phenylbutazone, or indomethacin

To decrease platelet aggregation: a dosage of 200 mg 4 times/day is recommended

FATE

Well absorbed orally; onset in 30 to 60 minutes; duration 4 to 6 hours, perhaps up to 10 hours; highly bound to plasma proteins (98%–99%); excreted primarily unchanged (90%) in the urine

COMMON SIDE EFFECTS

Nausea, epigastric pain, burning, dyspepsia

SIGNIFICANT ADVERSE REACTIONS

Activation of peptic ulcer, dizziness, tinnitus, skin rash, fever, blood dyscrasias, jaundice, precipitation of acute gout (early stages of therapy), urolithiasis, and renal colic

CONTRAINDICATIONS

Active peptic ulcer or GI inflammation. *Cautious use* in impaired renal function, unexplained GI pain, pregnancy

INTERACTIONS

Sulfinpyrazone may potentiate the effects of anticoagulants, sulfonylurea hypoglycemic agents, sulfonamides, penicillins, insulin, allopurinol, indomethacin, and nitrofurantoin

The uricosuric effects of sulfinpyrazone may be reduced by salicylates (low doses) and xanthines (e.g., caffeine, theophylline)

Serum urate levels may be elevated by diuretics, alcohol, diazoxide, and mecamylamine, necessitating higher sulfinpyrazone dosage

Incidence of blood dyscrasias may be increased with combined use of sulfinpyrazone and colchicine, other pyrazolones, or indomethacin

NURSING CONSIDERATION

1. Monitor results of prothrombin times carefully in patient taking sulfinpyrazone and an oral anticoagulant. Adjustment in dosage may be needed.

PATIENT EDUCATION

1. Instruct patient to take drug with food or milk to reduce GI irritation.
2. Inform patient that rigid adherence to dosage schedule is important because *minor* fluctuations in serum levels can lead to untoward reactions.
3. Discuss the need to maintain a fluid intake of at least 2000 mL per day to reduce danger of urate deposition and to alkalinize the urine to increase uric acid solubility (sodium bicarbonate, potassium citrate, or other urinary alkalinizers may be prescribed).
4. Instruct patient to be alert for appearance of fever, sore throat, mucosal lesions, malaise, joint pains, sudden bleeding, or skin rash. Often early signs of blood dyscrasias, these are indications for discontinuing the drug.
5. Instruct patient not to alter sulfinpyrazone dosage schedule during an acute attack. Colchicine or other anti-inflammatory drugs should be *added* to the regimen.
6. Caution patient to avoid aspirin-containing medications because effects of sulfinpyrazone may be reduced.
7. Explain to patient on long-term therapy that blood counts and renal function tests should be performed periodically to avert blood dyscrasias and renal colic.

Allopurinol

Lopurin, Zurinol, Zyloprim

(CAN) Apo-Allopurinol, Noropurol, Purinol

The drug of choice for controlling hyperuricemia resulting from *overproduction* of uric acid, allopurinol is especially effective in preventing development of uric acid stones. By reducing the serum urate level, reabsorption of deposits of urate crystals from tissues is enhanced. Use of allopurinol must be undertaken cautiously because the incidence of untoward reactions, some rather severe, is fairly high.

MECHANISM

Competitively inhibits the action of xanthine oxidase, the enzyme responsible for converting the natural purine hypoxanthine to xanthine, and xanthine to uric acid; substantially reduces both serum and urinary levels of uric acid even in the presence of renal damage; has no analgesic, anti-inflammatory, or uricosuric activity

USES

Treatment of gout, either primary or secondary to the hyperuricemia associated with blood dyscrasias and their treatment

Treatment of primary or secondary uric acid nephropathy

Treatment of recurrent uric acid stone formation

Prevention of urate deposition and uric acid nephropathy in patients receiving cancer chemotherapy (see Nursing Alerts) or radiation for leukemia and other malignancies

Note: Usually given with colchicine or a uricosuric drug at the outset of therapy to prevent acute attacks of gouty arthritis (see under **Side Effects** and **Significant Adverse Reactions**)

DOSAGE

Chronic gout/hyperuricemia: 200 mg to 600 mg/day in divided doses depending on severity of condition

Prevention of uric acid nephropathy during antineoplastic therapy: 600 mg to 800 mg/day for 2 to 3 days with high fluid intake; reduce slowly to minimum effective maintenance levels.

Children (hyperuricemia secondary to malignancy only): 6 to 10 years—300 mg/day; under 6 years—150 mg/day

FATE

Fairly rapidly absorbed orally; peak plasma levels in 2 hours to 6 hours; short half-life (2–3 h) of the parent compound in plasma; widely distributed in body, except for the brain; largely converted to oxypurinol (also a xanthine oxidase inhibitor) that is slowly excreted in the urine (half-life of 18–30 h); small amounts excreted unchanged in urine (10%–30%) and feces (10%–20%)

COMMON SIDE EFFECTS

Skin rash, pruritus

SIGNIFICANT ADVERSE REACTIONS

WARNING
Acute attacks of gouty arthritis may occur early in the course of therapy with allopurinol because urate crystals are mobilized from tissues when plasma urate levels are reduced. Mobilization is followed by recrystallization in the plasma and precipitation in joints. Colchicine may be given during the initial period of allopurinol therapy to minimize these acute attacks

Hypersensitivity reactions (fever, chills, malaise, nausea, muscle pain, eosinophilia, leukopenia, reversible acute interstitial nephritis)

Dermatologic: exfoliative, urticarial, or purpuric skin lesions; erythema multiforme; alopecia; dermatitis

Hematologic: blood dyscrasias, bone marrow depression, vasculitis, necrotizing angiitis

GI: vomiting, diarrhea, abdominal pain

Other: peripheral neuritis, cataract formation, acute gouty attacks (early in therapy), hepatotoxicity, drowsiness, vertigo

CONTRAINDICATIONS

Children other than those with hyperuricemia secondary to malignancy, and nursing mothers. *Cautious use* in patients with liver or kidney disease and during pregnancy

INTERACTIONS

Allopurinol may potentiate the action of oral anticoagulants, oral hypoglycemic agents, azathioprine, and 6-mercaptopurine. The drug is a *nonspecific* enzyme inhibitor and therefore can potentially alter the metabolism of a wide range of drugs dependent on hepatic metabolism for clearance

The effects of allopurinol may be reduced by thiazide and loop diuretics, salicylates, sulfinpyrazone, probenecid, and xanthines

Allopurinol may increase iron absorption and hepatic iron stores. Do not administer oral iron to patients taking allopurinol or use the two drugs together

Increased incidence of skin rash may occur with combinations of ampicillin (and possibly other penicillins) and allopurinol

Allopurinol may increase serum levels of theophylline

NURSING CONSIDERATION

1. Although allopurinol is employed during cancer chemotherapy to prevent hyperuricemia and uric acid nephropathy caused by certain antineoplastic agents, expect the dosage of purine analogs (e.g., 6-mercaptopurine) to be reduced when it is used with them. Allopurinol retards inactivation of these particular antineoplastic drugs and thus increases their toxicity.

PATIENT EDUCATION

1. Warn patient to *continually* observe for signs of skin rash, often an early sign of hypersensitivity. Rash may be followed by severe hypertension or more serious dermatologic disorders (e.g., exfoliative dermatitis, Stevens–Johnson syndrome, toxic epidermal necrolysis). Patient should discontinue drug and notify physician if rash develops.
2. Discuss the need to maintain a fluid intake of at least 2000 mL/day to reduce danger of urate deposition and to alkalinize the urine, thereby increasing uric acid solubility (sodium bicarbonate, potassium citrate, or other urinary alkalinizers may be prescribed).
3. Caution user against engaging in activities requiring alertness because drug may cause drowsiness and vertigo during early stages of therapy.
4. Inform patient that effects may take several weeks to develop. Caution against changing dosage levels unless instructed to do so.
5. Explain the need for blood counts and liver and kidney function tests, which should be performed before therapy is initiated and periodically during therapy, particularly if patient has preexisting liver disease.
6. When allopurinol is substituted for a uricosuric agent, inform patient that the transfer will probably be gradual. Dosage of the uricosuric should be reduced slowly while the dose of allopurinol is simultaneously increased over several weeks.
7. Suggest that patient restrict high-purine foods (e.g., kidney, liver, dried beans, meat extracts) and reduce weight as adjunctive measures to control hyperuricemia. Dietary intake of purines has *not,* however, been firmly linked to the etiology of gout.

Selected Bibliography

Beaver WT: Analgesic efficacy of dextropropoxyphene and dextropropoxyphene-containing combinations: A review. Hum Toxicol 3:1915, 1984.

Bloomfield SS: Analgesic management of mild to moderate pain. Ration Drug Ther 19(9):1, 1985.

Bunch TW, O'Duffy JD: Disease-modifying drugs for progressive rheumatoid arthritis. Mayo Clin Proc 55:161, 1980.

Chan WY: Prostaglandins and nonsteroidal anti-inflammatory drugs in dysmenorrhea. Annu Rev Pharmacol Toxicol 23:131, 1983.

Clive DM, Stoff JS: Renal syndromes associated with nonsteroidal anti-inflammatory drugs. N Engl J Med 310:563, 1984.

Cooper SA: New peripherally-acting oral analgesic agents. Annu Rev Pharmacol Toxicol 23:617, 1983.

Hart FD, Huskisson EC: Non-steroidal anti-inflammatory drugs. Current status and rational therapeutic use. Drugs 27:232, 1984.

Huskisson EC (ed): Anti-rheumatic Drugs. New York, Praeger Publishers, 1983.

Koch-Weser J: Drug therapy: Acetaminophen. N Engl J Med 295:1297, 1979.

Larsen GL, Henson PM: Mediators of inflammation. Annu Rev Immunol 1:335, 1983.

Lyle WH: Penicillamine. Clin Rheum Dis 5:569, 1979.

Markenson JA: Antiarthritic drugs. A comparative overview. Drug Ther 2:45, 1981.

Moncada S, Vane JR: Mode of action of aspirin-like drugs. Adv Intern Med 24:1, 1979.

Simon LS, Mills JA: Drug therapy: Nonsteroidal anti-inflammatory drugs (2 parts). N Engl J Med 302:1179, 1237, 1980.

Spruck M: Gold therapy for rheumatoid arthritis. Am J Nurs 79:1246, 1979.

Symposium for Rational Pharmacotherapy: The non-steroidal antiinflammatory drugs (NSAID's). Drug Intell Clin Pharm 18:34, 1984.

Toxicity of nonsteroidal anti-inflammatory drugs. Med Lett Drugs Ther 25:15, 1983.

Vane J, Botting R: Inflammation and the mechanism of action of antiinflammatory drugs. FASEB J 1(2):89, 1987.

SUMMARY. NONNARCOTIC ANALGESICS

Drug	Preparations	Usual Dosage Range
Salicylates	See Table 19-1	
Para-aminophenols		
Acetaminophen Several manufacturers	Tablets: 160 mg, 325 mg, 500 mg, 650 mg Capsules: 325 mg, 500 mg Chewable tablets: 80 mg Wafers: 120 mg Suppositories: 120 mg, 125 mg, 325 mg, 600 mg, 650 mg Elixir: 80 mg/5 mL, 120 mg/5 mL, 160 mg/5 mL, 325 mg/5 mL Liquid: 160 mg/5 mL, 500 mg/15 mL Drops: 100 mg/mL, 120 mg/2.5 mL	Adults: 325 mg–650 mg 3–4 times/day Children under 1 yr: 40 mg–80 mg 4–5 times/day 1–3 yr: 120 mg–160 mg 4–5 times/day 4–8 yr: 240 mg–320 mg 4–5 times/day 9–12 yr: 400 mg–480 mg 4–5 times/day
Pyrazolones		
Oxyphenbutazone Several manufacturers	Tablets: 100 mg	Initially: 300 mg–600 mg daily in divided doses Maintenance: 100 mg–400 mg daily
Phenylbutazone Azolid, Butazolidin	Tablets: 100 mg Capsules: 100 mg	Initially: 300 mg–600 mg daily in divided doses (maximum 600 mg/day) Maintenance: 100 mg–400 mg daily *Acute gout:* 400 mg initially then 100 mg every 4 h for 3–4 days
Nonsteroidal Antiinflammatory Agents	See Table 19-2	
Gold Compounds		
Aurothioglucose Solganal	Injection: 50 mg/mL	IM: 10 mg first week; 25 mg second and third weeks; 50 mg on subsequent weeks until benefit is observed;

Continued

SUMMARY. NONNARCOTIC ANALGESICS (continued)

Drug	Preparations	Usual Dosage Range
		continue with 25 mg–50 mg every 2–4 weeks as patient's condition warrants Children: One fourth of adult dose (maximum 25 mg/wk)
Gold Sodium Thiomalate Myochrysine	Injection: 25 mg/mL, 50 mg/mL	Adults: 10 mg IM first week, 25 mg second week, then 25 mg–50 mg thereafter at weekly intervals until significant clinical improvement or toxicity Children: 1 mg/kg/wk, not to exceed 50 mg on a single injection
Auranofin Ridaura	Capsules: 3 mg	6 mg/day in a single or divided doses
Penicillamine		
Penicillamine Cuprimine, Depen	Capsules: 125 mg, 250 mg Tablets: 250 mg	*Rheumatoid arthritis:* Initially 125 mg–250 mg/day for 4 weeks; increase by 125 mg–250 mg/day at 4- to 12-wk intervals to maximally tolerated dose; do not exceed 1000 mg–1500 mg/day for longer than 4 mo; usual maintenance dose 500 mg–750 mg/day *Wilson's disease* Adults: 250 mg–500 mg 4 times/day *Cystinuria* Adults: 250 mg–500 mg 4 times/day Children: 30 mg/kg/day
Antigout Drugs		
Colchicine	Tablets: 0.5 mg, 0.6 mg Injection: 1 mg/2 mL	*Acute attack* Oral: 1 mg–1.2 mg initially; repeat with 0.5 mg–1.2 mg every 1–2 h until pain is relieved or diarrhea occurs (control usually accomplished with 4 mg–8 mg total dose). IV: 1 mg–2 mg initially, followed by 0.5 mg every 6 h (total dose 4 mg/24 h) *Prophylaxis* Oral: 0.5 mg–0.6 mg 3–4 times/week (severe cases 0.6 mg–1.8 mg daily)
Probenecid Benemid, Probalan	Tablets: 0.5 g	Gout: 0.25 g twice a day for 1 wk, then 0.5 g twice a day; increase to a maximum of 2 g/day Penicillin therapy: 2 g daily in divided doses (children under 50 kg: 40 mg/kg/day in divided doses) *Gonorrhea* 1 g given with 4.8 million units penicillin G or 3.5 g ampicillin
Sulfinpyrazone Anturane	Tablets—100 mg Capsules—200 mg	Initially: 200 mg–400 mg/day in divided doses Maintenance: 200 mg–800 mg/day adjusted to patients needs (do not interrupt during acute attacks)

Continued

SUMMARY. NONNARCOTIC ANALGESICS (continued)

Drug	Preparations	Usual Dosage Range
Allopurinol Lopurin, Zurinol, Zyloprim	Tablets—100 mg, 300 mg	*Control of gout* 200 mg to 600 mg/day in divided doses *Prevention of uric acid nephropathy* Adults: 600 mg–800 mg/day for 2–3 days; reduce to effective maintenance levels based on serum urate levels Children (6–10 yr): 300 mg/day Children (under 6 yr): 150 mg/day

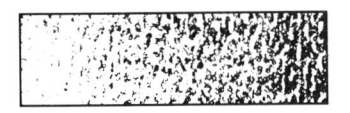

20 BARBITURATE SEDATIVE–HYPNOTICS

Many drugs are capable of eliciting varying degrees of CNS depression, and one such group of agents is commonly referred to as sedative–hypnotics. The central effects associated with these drugs range, with increasing doses, from mild sedation through hypnosis (induction of sleep) to complete loss of consciousness or anesthesia. Drugs possessing these actions are generally classified into two broad categories: *barbiturates*—derivatives of barbituric acid, and *nonbarbiturates*—a group of drugs structurally unrelated to barbituric acid but possessing many of the pharmacologic actions of barbiturates. Chapter 20 addresses the barbiturate sedative–hypnotics and Chapter 21 their nonbarbiturate counterparts.

Barbiturates elicit a general CNS depression, the magnitude of which depends on the dose. Although occasionally employed in small doses for daytime sedation in anxiety states, barbiturates are principally used at full therapeutic dose for the induction of sleep. Certain individual barbiturates are also indicated as antiepileptics (see Chap. 25), general anesthetics (see Chap. 17), and in certain types of psychoanalysis.

The major pharmacologic action of these drugs is a reduction in overall CNS alertness. They appear to act at several levels of the CNS; with increasing dosage they can depress many centrally mediated functions, including motor activity and respiration. All are effective anticonvulsants in large doses, and the longer-acting derivatives are employed as specific antiepileptic drugs as well (see Chap. 25). Barbiturates are not effective analgesics in subanesthetic doses and generally do not produce significant hypnosis in patients with severe pain. Conversely, when combined with a potent analgesic, they are capable of potentiating its ability to relieve pain.

The most important adverse reactions occur with either overdose or prolonged use of the drugs. *Overdose* is characterized by marked respiratory depression, lowered body temperature, circulatory collapse, and eventually coma; it is an acute medical emergency. Conversely the principal danger associated with *prolonged* use of the barbiturates is habituation and addiction. Withdrawal from barbiturates should be accomplished gradually because sudden withdrawal can result in severe anxiety, tremors, marked excitement, convulsions, and delirium. Repeated use of barbiturates also decreases the time spent in the REM (rapid eye movement) phase of sleep, the phase associated with dreaming. Personality changes have been noted in persons deprived of REM sleep for long periods, and signs of irritability, confusion, aggressiveness, and decreased attention may be observed with prolonged use of barbiturates.

Conversely, cessation of barbiturate use after prolonged periods can lead to "rebound REM" manifested by increased dreaming (often of a bizarre nature), nightmares, and hallucinations.

The clinically useful barbiturates have been categorized into one of four groups based upon their duration of action. These groups are

- Long-acting (6–8 h): mephobarbital, metharbital, phenobarbital
- Intermediate-acting: (4–6 h): amobarbital, aprobarbital, butabarbital, talbutal
- Short-acting (2–4 h): pentobarbital, secobarbital
- Ultrashort-acting (10–30 min): methohexital, thiamylal, thiopental

Although this classification is convenient, remember that differences in duration of action among the first three categories depend on several factors other than the drug itself, such as dosage form, route of administration, presence of pathologic conditions (e.g., liver or kidney dysfunction), and length of treatment.

The ultrashort-acting barbiturates are indicated principally as induction anesthetics and are discussed in Chapter 17. The remaining barbiturates are reviewed as a group, and specific information relating to each drug is given in Table 20-1.

Barbiturates

Amobarbital	Pentobarbital
Aprobarbital	Phenobarbital
Butabarbital	Secobarbital
Mephobarbital	Talbutal
Metharbital	

MECHANISM

Act at several sites in the CNS; interfere with the transmission of impulses at synapses in the reticular formation of the brainstem and thalamus, thereby decreasing overall impulse transmission to the cortex; may increase the threshold for electrical excitation of the motor cortex; appear to facilitate GABA-induced inhibition of neuronal function; produce no analgesia alone and may intensify reaction to painful stimuli in small doses; reduce analgesic requirements by approximately 50% when combined with potent analgesics and administered together; have minimal effects on autonomic or cardiovascular system in normal therapeutic doses; depress the respiratory center in a dose-dependent fashion

USES

Short-term treatment of insomnia (tolerance develops within 3 wk)
Control of acute convulsive states (IV, IM)
Treatment of various forms of epilepsy
Pre- and postoperative sedation
Daytime sedation for the relief of anxiety, tension, and nervousness (obsolete use)
Induction anesthesia and brief, minor surgical procedures (ultrashort-acting drugs; see Chap. 17)
As aid in psychoanalysis (narcoanalysis and narcotherapy)
Management of catatonic and manic reactions (IV, IM)

DOSAGE

See Table 20-1

FATE

Variably absorbed from GI tract and IM injection sites; soluble sodium salts are absorbed more rapidly than free bases, especially on an empty stomach; widely distributed in the body and bound to plasma proteins to varying degrees; lipid solubility is a major determinant of distribution; highly lipid-soluble drugs more readily penetrate body tissues; thus, drugs with low lipid solubility (e.g., phenobarbital) have a slow onset and long duration and vice versa. However, lipid-soluble drugs are quickly redistributed from active CNS sites to fatty tissue stores, from which the drug may be slowly released. Because the pharmacologic effects often disappear before the drug is totally eliminated from the body, too-frequent dosing can lead to cumulation toxicity. Most drugs are metabolized in the liver and excreted in the urine, principally as metabolites, except for aprobarbital and phenobarbital, which are excreted in part unchanged

COMMON SIDE EFFECTS
Drowsiness, ataxia, hangover (especially with longer-acting derivatives)

SIGNIFICANT ADVERSE REACTIONS
Oral: skin rash, vertigo, lethargy, nausea, diarrhea, jaundice (rare), hypersensitivity reactions (fever, urticaria, hives, serum sickness), muscle and joint pain; paradoxical excitation occasionally seen, especially in children and older people; prolonged use may lead to tolerance, habituation, and addiction
IV: see *Oral;* in addition, respiratory depression, coughing, hiccuping, laryngospasm, bronchospasm, hypotension, pain at injection site, thrombophlebitis, and blood dyscrasias (rare)
Overdose: respiratory depression, hypothermia, depressed reflexes, anuria, rapid pulse, pulmonary edema, anoxia, cyanotic skin, stupor, and coma

CONTRAINDICATIONS
Latent or manifest porphyria, marked liver impairment, severe respiratory disease or obstruction, uncontrolled pain, impaired renal function, and early pregnancy. *Cautious use* in pediatric, elderly, debilitated, or nursing patients or in the presence of fever; hyperthyroidism; diabetes; hepatic, renal, or cardiac impairment; as well as severe anemia and alcoholism

INTERACTIONS
Barbiturates may potentiate the CNS and respiratory-depressant effects of alcohol, narcotic analgesics, other sedative–hypnotics, phenothiazine and other antipsychotic drugs, antihistamines, anesthetics, antidepressants, antianxiety agents, centrally acting muscle relaxants, and reserpine
Barbiturates, especially phenobarbital, increase the activity of liver metabolic enzymes and therefore may decrease the effects of drugs metabolized by those enzymes, such as oral anticoagulants, corticosteroids, diphenhydramine, digitalis glycosides, methyldopa, lidocaine, griseofulvin, estrogens, progestogens, androgens, pyrazolones, tricyclic antidepressants, and tetracyclines
The effects of barbiturates may be increased by MAO inhibitors, chloramphenicol, valproic acid, sulfonamides, acidifying agents, anticholinesterase drugs, and disulfiram
Barbiturates may inhibit GI absorption of griseofulvin.
Concurrent administration of barbiturates and furosemide can produce or aggravate orthostatic hypotension
Chloramphenicol may impair the metabolism of phenobarbital

NURSING CONSIDERATIONS

Nursing Alerts
- Monitor vital signs continuously when drug is given IV. The drug should be administered *slowly* to prevent respiratory depression, laryngospasm, and hypotension, and resuscitative equipment and other supportive measures (e.g., IV fluids, vasopressors) should be on hand in case respiratory or circulatory depression occurs.
- Observe IV injection site for evidence of extravasation (swelling, pain), which may cause tissue necrosis.
- Maintain appropriate perspective toward administration: Use of barbiturates for prolonged periods, even at therapeutic levels, is associated with a high incidence of dependence and abuse. Barbiturates with the shortest onset of action are most often abused. Discourage long-term use of any barbiturate for daytime sedation.
- Monitor patient for signs of excessive dosage (e.g., mental clouding, impaired coordination). If these occur, dosage should be reduced accordingly.
- Observe patient for signs of developing tolerance (e.g., more frequent usage, requests for larger doses, decreased drug effects). Advise physician if signs appear, as *gradual* drug withdrawal should be considered.
- When drugs are used as hypnotics, carefully evaluate patient response. Barbiturates generally lose effectiveness as hypnotics within 2 weeks of continued usage. Dosage should *not* be increased in an attempt to regain effectiveness.

1. Be prepared to deal with an initial period of excitement or confusion in the patient given barbiturates, especially the very young or elderly. Attempt to calm patient and prevent injury.
2. Assess patient for signs of decreased response to concurrently administered drugs. Because barbiturates enhance the activity of hepatic enzymes, they may diminish effects of drugs metabolized by those enzymes (see **Interactions**). Dosages of such drugs may need to be increased.
3. Always give in combination with an analgesic when pain is present. Given to a patient with severe pain, barbiturates may produce anxiety, restlessness, and an intensified reaction to the pain.
4. Because all barbiturates are controlled substances, follow regulations for handling and dispensing agents in different schedules (see also Chaps. 8 and 79).

PATIENT EDUCATION
1. Warn patient to avoid hazardous activities during therapy because drowsiness and impaired motor coordination are often present.
2. Warn patient that "hangover" effects are common. Suggest rising slowly from bed and walking cautiously until equilibrium is established.
3. Warn patient of dangers of additive CNS depression if combined with alcohol, antihistamines, tranquilizers, and other central depressants.
4. Explain potential consequences of abrupt discontinuation of therapy following prolonged use. Withdrawal symptoms, which can be quite serious (e.g., tremors, convulsions, delirium) may occur.
5. Instruct long-term user to note and report the appearance of sore throat, fever, superficial bleeding, bruising, rash, and jaundice, signs of possible hematologic toxicity.
6. Advise patient *not* to keep more than one night's supply by the bed at night. Drowsiness may cause patient to forget that a dose was taken, and mistaken repeated dosage may result in accidental overdose if large quantities of medication are readily available at the bedside.

Table 20-1
Barbiturates

Drug	Preparations	Usual Dosage Range	Nursing Implications
Short-acting			
Pentobarbital Nembutal (CAN) Nova-Rectal, Novopentobarb, Pentogen	Capsules: 50 mg, 100 mg Elixir: 20 mg/5 mL Suppositories: 30 mg, 60 mg, 120 mg, 200 mg Injection: 50 mg/mL	Oral Sedation: *Adults*—20 mg 3–4 times/day *Children*—2 mg/kg–6 mg/kg/day in divided doses Hypnosis: (*Adults*)—100 mg Rectal: *Adults:*—120 mg–200 mg *Children*—30 mg–120 mg based on age and weight IM *Adults*—150 mg–200 mg *Children*— 25 mg–80 mg IV *Adults*—100 mg initially; repeat at 50–100 mg increments to a maximum of 500 mg	Used for preoperative sedation, for minor diagnostic or surgical procedures, and for emergency control of convulsions; hypnotic effects show rapid tolerance; parenteral solution is highly alkaline; avoid extravasation as necrosis can occur; do *not* give more than 5 mL at one IM site; administer slowly IV, and wait at least 1 min before giving subsequent injections; potent respiratory depressant; can cause bronchospasm, hypotension, and apnea if injection is too rapid; IM injections should be made deep into large muscle mass (e.g., gluteus) (Schedule II)
Secobarbital Seconal	Capsules: 50 mg, 100 mg Tablets: 100 mg Injection: 50 mg/mL	Oral Preoperative: *Adults*—200 mg–300 mg 1 h–2 h before surgery *Children*—50 mg–100 mg Hypnosis: *Adults*—100 mg Rectal *Adults*—120 mg–200 mg *Children*—15 mg–120 mg based on age and weight IM Hypnosis: *Adults*—100 mg–200 mg *Children*—3 mg/kg–5 mg/kg IV Convulsions: 5.5 mg/kg at a rate of 50 mg/15 sec; repeat every 3–4 h as needed Anesthesia: 50 mg/15 sec slow IV injection until effect is attained (maximum 250 mg)	Used for insomnia, to provide basal hypnosis for anesthesia, in the emergency control of convulsions, and for dental and minor surgical procedures; tolerance develops quickly (within 2 wk) to the hypnotic effect; aqueous solutions for injection must be freshly prepared with sterile water for injection; make sure drug dissolves completely, and use solution within 30 minutes because it is very unstable; injectable form is also available in a more stable aqueous-polyethylene glycol vehicle that should be refrigerated; use of this latter vehicle is contraindicated in patients with renal dysfunction or insufficiency because it is irritating to the kidneys; give *slowly* IV and monitor patient continually; also available in fixed combination with amobarbital as Tuinal
Intermediate-acting			
Amobarbital Amytal (CAN) Isobec, Novamobarb	Tablets: 30 mg, 100 mg Capsules: 65 mg, 200 mg (sodium salt) Powder for injection: 250 mg, 500 mg powder with diluent	Oral Sedation: 30 mg–50 mg 2–3 times/day Hypnosis: 100 mg–200 mg Preoperative: 200 mg 1–2 h before surgery Labor: 200 mg–400 mg initially; repeat at 1–3 h intervals to a maximum of 1 g IM and IV Individually titrated according to condition, age, weight; usual adult range is 65 mg to 500 mg by deep IM injection or slow IV injection	Used as sedative, hypnotic, preanesthetic medication, as anticonvulsant, and for the management of catatonic or manic reactions; prepare solutions with sterile water and use within 30 min after opening vial; do not use if solution is not clear; inject deeply IM or by slow IV (1 mL/min maximum IV rate) available in fixed combination with secobarbital as Tuinal (Schedule II)

Continued

Table 20-1
Barbiturates (continued)

Drug	Preparations	Usual Dosage Range	Nursing Implications
Aprobarbital Alurate	Elixir: 40 mg/5 mL	Sedation: 40 mg 3 times/day Hypnosis: 40 mg–160 mg depending on severity	Only used orally for daytime sedation or relief of insomnia (Schedule II)
Butabarbital Butalan, Buticaps, Butisol, Sarisol (CAN) Barbased, Day-Barb	Tablets: 15 mg, 30 mg, 50 mg, 100 mg Capsules: 15 mg, 30 mg Elixir: 30 mg, 33.3 mg/5 mL	Sedation: *Adults:* 15 mg–30 mg 3–4 times/day *Children:* 7.5 mg–30 mg/day Hypnosis: *Adults:* 50 mg–100 mg *Children:* based on age and weight	Used as mild sedative, for insomnia, and preoperatively; similar to phenobarbital in most respects (Schedule III)
Talbutal Lotusate	Tablets: 120 mg	120 mg 15–30 min before bedtime	Infrequently used for relief of insomnia (Schedule III)
Long-acting			
Mephobarbital Mebaral	Tablets: 32 mg, 50 mg, 100 mg	Sedation: *Adults*—32 mg–100 mg 3–4 times/day *Children*—16 mg–32 mg 3–4 times/day Epilepsy: *Adults*—400 mg–600 mg/day *Children*—16 mg–64 mg 3–4 times/day depending on age	Used for daytime sedation in various anxiety states, and primarily as adjunctive treatment of grand mal and petit mal epilepsy (see Chap. 25); similar to phenobarbital in most respects but is very weak hypnotic and produces minimal drowsiness; dosage alterations should be made gradually in epileptic states to avoid precipitation of convulsions (Schedule IV)
Metharbital Gemonil	Tablets: 100 mg	Epilepsy: *Adults*—initially 100 mg 1–3 times/day; increase to optimal level *Children*—5 mg–15 mg/kg/day based on age and weight	Used in several forms of epilepsy (grand and petit mal, myclonic, and mixed seizures), either alone or more frequently combined with other drugs; not as effective as phenobarbital and produces more sedaton (see Chap. 25) (Schedule III)
Phenobarbital Several manufacturers	Tablets: 8 mg, 16 mg, 32 mg, 65 mg, 100 mg Capsules: 16 mg Timed-release capsules: 65 mg Elixir: 15 mg/5 mL, 20 mg/5 mL Injection: 30 mg, 60 mg, 65 mg, 130 mg/mL Powder for injection: 120 mg/vial	Oral Sedation: *Adults*—16 mg–32 mg 2–4 times/day *Children*—1 mg–3 mg/kg/day Hypnosis: *Adults*—100 mg–320 mg Epilepsy: *Adults*—100 mg–300 mg/day *Children*—3 mg–5 mg/kg/day IV Convulsions: *Adults*—300 mg to 800 mg initially, then 120 mg to 240 mg every 20 min, as needed (maximum 2 g/24 h) *Children*—20 mg/kg initially, then 6 mg/kg every 20 min as needed IM Preoperative and postoperative: *Adults*—32 mg–200 mg *Children*—8 mg–100 mg	Widely used for sedation and in grand mal and focal seizures, either alone or combined with other antiepileptic drugs; used IV in acute convulsive states (see Chap. 25); solutions should be freshly prepared with sterile water for injection, and used within 30 min after preparation; do *not* use if solution is not clear after 5 min of mixing; some injectable forms contain alcohol and propylene glycol and are more stable than aqueous solutions; drug has a long half-life (2–5 days), and too-frequent dosing can cause accumulation toxicity (Schedule IV)

7. Inform patient using oral contraceptives that their efficacy may be reduced by prolonged use of barbiturates.
8. Discuss adjunctive interventions (e.g., warm bath, back rub, quiet atmosphere, mild analgesic, avoidance of coffee at night) that aid in sleep induction.

Selected Bibliography

Harris E: Sedative-hypnotic drugs. Am J Nurs 81:1329, 1981.
Hartmann E: Drugs for insomnia. Ration Drug Ther 11:1, 1977.
Ho IK, Harris RA: Mechanism of action of barbiturates. Annu Rev Pharmacol Toxicol 21:83, 1981.
Kales A, Soldatos DR, Bixler EO, Kales JD: Rebound insomnia and rebound anxiety: A review. Pharmacology 26:121, 1983.
Perry SW, Wu A: Rationale for the use of hypnotic agents in a general hospital. Ann Intern Med 100:441, 1984.
Richter JA, Holman JR: Barbiturates: Their in vivo effects and potential biochemical mechanisms. Prog Neurobiol 18:275, 1982.
Rickels K: Clinical trials of hypnotics. J Clin Psychopharmacol 3:133, 1983.
Solomon F, White CC, Parron DL, Mendelson WB: Sleeping pills, insomnia and medical practice. N Engl J Med 300:803, 1979.
Sullivan JT, Sellers EM: Treating alcohol barbiturate and benzodiazepine withdrawal. Ration Drug Ther 20(2):1, 1986
Todd B: Drugs and the elderly: Why are some drugs withdrawn slowly? Geriatr Nurs 4:393, 1983.
Todd B: Drugs and the elderly: Precautions with hypnotics. Geriatr Nurs 3:343, 1982.

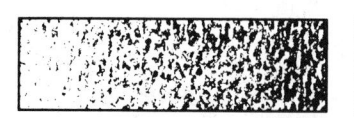

21 NONBARBITURATE SEDATIVE–HYPNOTICS

In addition to the barbiturates, a variety of other drugs are used for many of the same indications, such as daytime sedation and relief of insomnia. Much confusion exists, however, about the terminology used to describe these other sedative–hypnotic drugs. For the purposes of our discussion, drugs reviewed in this chapter will be termed *nonbarbiturate sedative–hypnotics* because, while occasionally employed to provide temporary relief from preoperative anxiety, they are primarily used for short-term treatment of insomnia. A distinction can be made between most of these nonbarbiturate sedative-hypnotics and the minor tranquilizers or antianxiety agents, to be discussed in Chapter 23. Specifically, the benzodiazepine antianxiety agents, of which the prototype is diazepam (Valium), are widely used for relief of simple anxiety states. They are generally not classified with other sedative–hypnotic drugs because of their more favorable pharmacologic profile and their greater safety margin. Table 21-1 compares some important properties of nonbarbiturate sedative–hypnotics and benzodiazepine antianxiety agents. This table is useful as a general guide, but it is important to recognize that the information in it is based on the actions of these agents at recommended doses for short periods (i.e., 1–2 weeks). The differences cited in Table 21-1 become less distinct when the antianxiety drugs are used in large doses or for prolonged periods. Moreover, certain nonbarbiturate sedative–hypnotics, such as chloral hydrate and paraldehyde, are less sedating and less addicting than other agents like glutethimide or methyprylon and thus do not evidence as sharp a contrast with the benzodiazepine antianxiety drugs.

Many of these nonbarbiturate drugs were developed in an attempt to dissociate the undesirable properties of the barbiturates (e.g., respiratory depression, enzyme induction, habituation) from their desirable qualities (e.g., relief of insomnia, anticonvulsive activity). These attempts have been largely unsuccessful, and most clinically available nonbarbiturate sedative–hypnotics share many common properties with barbiturates. However, one group, the benzodiazepine hypnotics, exhibit several advantages over barbiturates, such as absence of enzyme induction, little effect on REM sleep, and lowered abuse potential, and have become the most widely prescribed hypnotics in clinical medicine.

In general, the nonbarbiturate sedative–hypnotics induce sleep in therapeutic doses and produce significant drowsiness and motor retardation in small doses. The difference between the calming or sedative dose and the hypnotic or sleep-inducing dose is often minimal, and likewise the difference between the therapeutic (hypnotic) dose and the toxic dose is quite small. Therefore, most of these drugs, again with the exception of the benzodiazepine hypnotics, offer no advantage over the barbiturates in terms of either efficacy or safety. Habituation and addiction are as much a problem with continued use of these drugs as with the barbiturates, with only occasional exceptions that are noted below.

Classification of nonbarbiturate sedative–hypnotics is difficult, owing to the variety of chemical structures possessed by these agents. However, they all share a common action—that is, the ability to depress the CNS in a dose-related fashion. The mechanism of this action, however, is not completely understood in all cases. Several older drugs, once frequently used, have been rendered essentially obsolete by development of more effective agents, and these older drugs are addressed only briefly in this chapter. A detailed account, however, is given of those drugs currently used on a more frequent basis.

In addition to the nonbarbiturate sedative–hypnotics to be reviewed in this chapter, several antihistamines are found in various over-the-counter sleep aids, in which they provide a small degree of drowsiness to assist the user in falling asleep. The recommended doses are 25 mg to 50 mg diphenhydramine (e.g., Compoz, Nytol, Sleep-Eze, Sominex, Twilite), and 25 mg doxylamine (e.g., Unisom). Maximum recommended dosages are 100 mg/24 hr. Use of antihistamine-containing sleep aids is recommended for short periods only (7–10 days). These preparations should not be given to children, pregnant women, or patients with asthma, prostate enlargement, or glaucoma (see Chap. 14).

The nonbarbiturate sedative–hypnotics are reviewed individually, except for the benzodiazepine hypnotics. Drugs that are essentially obsolete will be considered only briefly.

Acetylcarbromal
Paxarel

A derivative of urea with short-acting sedative–hypnotic properties, acetylcarbromal acts by releasing free bromide ion and therefore can give rise to bromide intoxication (see discussion of bromides later in the chapter). Acetylcarbromal is largely an obsolete drug that provides no advantage over most other sedative–hypnotics. Large doses may cause excessive drowsiness, narcosis, and respiratory depression. Prolonged use may cause decreased reflexes, stupor, skin rash, joint pain, and psychotic behavior. Toxicity is best treated by intake of large amounts of sodium chloride and water to promote bromide excretion. The drug is habit forming and should not be used for long-term administration.

BENZODIAZEPINE HYPNOTICS

Flurazepam   Temazepam
Triazolam

Most benzodiazepine drugs are used for the relief of simple anxiety (see Chap. 23). The above three benzodiazepines, however, are intended primarily for the short-term management of insomnia and should not be given during the day to control anxiety states.

The benzodiazepine hypnotics and the barbiturates are probably equally effective for the short-term treatment of insomnia, but the benzodiazepine hypnotics display a greater safety margin, do not significantly alter REM sleep time, and are free of enzyme-inducing effects. Thus they are the preferred hypnotics for relief of insomnia.

MECHANISM
Primary mechanism of action of benzodiazepines is facilitation of the action of the inhibitory neurotransmitter gamma-

Table 21-1
Comparison Between Nonbarbiturate Sedative–Hypnotics and Antianxiety Drugs

	Nonbarbiturate Sedative–Hypnotics	Benzodiazepine Antianxiety Agents
Major Indications	Insomnia	Stress, tension, and other psychoneuroses
Sedative: hypnotic ratio	Low	High
Drowsiness, psychomotor impairment, and confusion	Moderate to severe	Mild
Dependence liability	High	Moderate to high
Central skeletal muscle–relaxing effect	No	Yes

aminobutyric acid (GABA); also, binding of GABA to its receptors may be enhanced by the ability of benzodiazepines to antagonize a protein that can inhibit GABA–receptor interaction; principal loci of action in the CNS appear to be the limbic system, thalamus, and midbrain reticular formation; unlike the barbiturates, these drugs do not exert a significant effect on higher cortical centers; they possess a hypnotic and anticonvulsant action but exert little suppression of REM sleep and no enzyme induction; hangover effects can occur, especially with flurazepam

USES
Short-term relief of insomnia

DOSAGE
See Table 21-2

FATE
Oral absorption is good; sleep usually occurs within 15 to 45 minutes with all drugs; peak plasma levels are attained at 30 to 60 minutes with flurazepam, 2 to 3 hours with temazepam, and 1 to 1.5 hours with triazolam. Flurazepam is converted to an active metabolite with a half-life of 50 to 100 hours; thus it has the longest duration of action and can elicit a prolonged hangover effect. Temazepam exhibits a plasma half-life of 9 to 12 hours and is metabolized to inactive compounds in the liver. Triazolam is also converted to inactive metabolites and has a plasma half-life of only 1.5 to 3 hours; therefore it is very short acting, and early morning awakening has occurred. All three drugs are excreted largely in the urine

COMMON SIDE EFFECTS
Occasional drowsiness, dizziness, headache (especially triazolam), ataxia, and lightheadedness (more common in older adults)

SIGNIFICANT ADVERSE REACTIONS
(Rare at normal dosage levels) Lethargy, disorientation, slurred speech, faintness, confusion, anorexia, nervousness, apprehension, weakness, irritability, palpitation, joint pain, nausea, vomiting, diarrhea, heartburn, abdominal and urinary discomfort, memory impairment, and depression

CONTRAINDICATIONS
Pregnancy. *Cautious use* in patients with renal or hepatic disease, depression, or a history of drug abuse and in elderly or debilitated persons

INTERACTIONS
An additive CNS-depressive effect can occur when benzodiazepines are used concurrently with other CNS depressants, such as alcohol, barbiturates, and antihistamines
Concurrent use of antacids may delay the oral absorption of the benzodiazepines

NURSING CONSIDERATIONS
1. Monitor results of laboratory studies. Periodic blood counts and liver and kidney function tests should be performed during prolonged therapy.
2. With repeated use, especially of larger doses, observe patient for indications of habituation. Although abuse liability is lower than with most similar drugs, dependence may occur. Drugs are classified in schedule IV.

PATIENT EDUCATION
1. Caution patient to use care in driving or performing hazardous tasks until effects of drug have been determined.
2. Warn patient that sedative effects of long-acting drugs may persist for several days after termination of use, and that daytime carryover effects are enhanced by alcohol, antianxiety drugs, and other CNS depressants.

Chloral Hydrate
Aquachloral Supprettes, Noctec
(CAN) Novochlorhydrate

MECHANISM
Depressant effect on cerebral cortex, with minimal involvement of lower brain centers regulating respiration and blood pressure; metabolized quickly to trichloroethanol, considered to be the active metabolite; little hangover or depressant after effects, and good safety margin; no suppression of REM sleep

USES
Temporary relief of insomnia
Preoperative and postoperative sedation

Table 21-2
Benzodiazepine Hypnotics

Drug	Preparations	Usual Dosage Range	Nursing Implications
Flurazepam Dalmane, Durepam (CAN) Apo-Flurazepam, Novoflupam, PMS-Flurazepam	Capsules: 15 mg, 30 mg	15 mg–30 mg at bedtime (15 mg in elderly or debilitated patients)	Longest acting benzodiazepine hypnotic; major metabolite is *N*-desalkyl-flurazepam, which is an active hypnotic with prolonged half-life (50–100 h); daytime carryover effects may include decreased alertness, impaired coordination, confusion, and subtle personality changes; maximum hypnotic effectiveness may not be achieved for several nights; residual effects can persist for days following discontinuation of therapy; not recommended to children under 15; do not discontinue drug abruptly after prolonged usage.
Temazepam Razepam, Restoril, Temaz	Capsules: 15 mg, 30 mg	15 mg–30 mg at bedtime (15 mg in elderly or debilitated patients)	Intermediate acting benzodiazepine (plasma half-life of 9–12 h); no accumulation of metabolites; hangover effects are minimal and early morning wakening is reduced; use in children under 18 is not recommended; transient sleep disturbances can occur for several nights following discontinuation of therapy.
Triazolam Halcion	Tablets: 0.125 mg, 0.25 mg, 0.5 mg	0.25 mg–0.5 mg at bedtime (0.125 mg–0.25 mg in elderly or debilitated patients)	Short-acting hypnotic; plasma half-life is 2 to 4 h; metabolites are inactive; elicits few daytime hangover effects but may lead to increased wakefulness during the last third of the night; not recommended for children under 18

DOSAGE
Adults:
Hypnosis—500 mg to 1000 mg at bedtime
Sedation—250 mg 3 times/day
Children:
Hypnosis—50 mg/kg (maximum 1000 mg)
Sedation—25 mg/kg/day in divided doses

FATE
Quickly absorbed orally or rectally and converted to trichloroethanol; onset of effect in 30 to 60 minutes; duration is 4 to 8 hours; metabolite is conjugated in the liver and excreted chiefly in the urine, and in lesser amounts in the bile

COMMON SIDE EFFECTS
Unpleasant taste, gastric distress, and lightheadedness

SIGNIFICANT ADVERSE REACTIONS
Drowsiness, vertigo, motor incoordination, allergic reactions (erythema, urticaria, dermatitis), nightmares, paradoxical excitement and delirium, reduction in white cell count; prolonged use—gastritis, skin eruptions, renal damage, habituation, and addiction

CONTRAINDICATIONS
Hepatic or renal impairment, gastritis, severe cardiac disease, history of allergic reactions, and nursing mothers. *Cautious use* in patients with cardiac arrhythmias, asthma, history of drug dependence, and during pregnancy

INTERACTIONS
Effects of other CNS depressants may be potentiated by chloral hydrate

May potentiate the action of acidic, protein-bound drugs (e.g., anticoagulants, salicylates, oral hypoglycemics) by displacing them from protein-binding sites

Effects of chloral hydrate can be potentiated by MAO inhibitors and phenothiazines

Use of IV furosemide with chloral hydrate may cause sweating, tachycardia, and hypertension owing to displacement of thyroid hormone from its bound state

NURSING CONSIDERATIONS

Nursing Alerts
- Observe for signs of chronic intoxication (e.g., gastritis, skin eruptions); if present, supervised *gradual* withdrawal should be started. Supportive treatment should be available (e.g., respiratory aids, pressor agents).
- In patient with severe pain, administer only after pain is controlled with analgesics. Otherwise, delirium and excitement may occur.

1. Administer drug in capsules or well-diluted liquid form with meals, to minimize GI irritation.
2. Follow proper procedures for handling a Schedule IV drug.

PATIENT EDUCATION
1. Caution patient to avoid alcohol while taking drug because combination can induce flushing, tachycardia, hypotension, headache, and loss of consciousness.
2. Warn patient about possible consequences of prolonged use. Chronic users may suddenly exhibit intolerance resulting in hypotension, respiratory depression, and possibly death.
3. Advise patient to avoid hazardous activities because excessive drowsiness may occur.

Ethchlorvynol

Placidyl

MECHANISM

Not established; short-acting hypnotic with anticonvulsant and muscle-relaxing effects; shortens sleep latency and decreases REM sleep time; dependence is common with prolonged therapy; safety margin is comparable to that of the barbiturates

USES

Short-term treatment of insomnia (most effective in patients having difficulty falling asleep rather than having frequent awakenings)

DOSAGE

500 mg to 1000 mg at bedtime; a single 200-mg supplement may be given if awakening occurs (not recommended for children)

FATE

Rapidly absorbed orally; onset in 20 to 30 minutes; duration usually 4 to 5 hours; widely distributed and localized in body lipids; less than 0.1% of the dose excreted in the urine within the first 24 hours; extensively metabolized by the liver and slowly excreted

COMMON SIDE EFFECTS

Dizziness, blurred vision, facial numbness, unpleasant aftertaste, and mild hangover

SIGNIFICANT ADVERSE REACTIONS

Nausea, hypotension, skin rash, urticaria, jaundice (rare), ataxia, and giddiness if absorption is rapid, idiosyncratic reactions (excitement, hysteria, prolonged hypnosis, muscle weakness, syncope); prolonged use—tremors, incoordination, confusion, slurred speech, hyperreflexia, diplopia, and muscle weakness

CONTRAINDICATIONS

Porphyria, early pregnancy (first 6 months), and in children. *Cautious use* in depressed patients and those with a history of or potential for drug abuse

INTERACTIONS

Additive depressant effects may occur if used with other CNS depressants or MAO inhibitors

Drug may reduce the effects of oral anticoagulants by decreasing prothrombin time

Delirium can occur if used in combination with tricyclic antidepressants

NURSING CONSIDERATIONS

Nursing Alerts

- Observe for signs of dependence. Drug should be *slowly* discontinued in patient on prolonged therapy. Abrupt withdrawal may precipitate barbiturate-like withdrawal symptoms.
- In patient with pain, administer only after pain is first controlled with analgesics.

1. Administer with food or milk to slow absorption and to prevent giddiness and ataxia resulting from rapid absorption.
2. Follow proper procedures for handling a Schedule IV drug.

PATIENT EDUCATION

1. Advise patient to avoid activities requiring alertness and to avoid concomitant use of alcohol because excessive drowsiness may occur.

Ethinamate

Valmid

Ethinamate is a urethane derivative possessing a nonspecific CNS depressant action. It may be employed as a short-acting hypnotic, but it has no significant advantage over barbiturates or other nonbarbiturate hypnotics, and there has been some question about its effectiveness. Onset of sleep occurs within 20 to 30 minutes, but effects persist for only about 4 hours, thus nocturnal awakening is common. The hypnotic effect is transient, and the drug rapidly becomes ineffective within 7 to 10 days. However, prolonged use can lead to psychologic and in some cases physical dependence, and the abstinence syndrome is similar to that seen with barbiturates. Ethinamate is infrequently used today and of minimal clinical interest.

Glutethimide

Doriden, Doriglute

MECHANISM

Depressive effects are similar to those of the barbiturates, including decreased REM sleep; has no analgesic or anticonvulsant actions; possesses significant anticholinergic activity, most pronounced in the iris (mydriasis) but also affecting the GI tract (decreased motility) and salivary glands (reduced secretions); little respiratory depression in normal doses; stimulates hepatic microsomal enzymes; high degree of dependence and popular drug of abuse

USES

Short-term relief of insomnia

DOSAGE

Insomnia: 250 mg to 500 mg at bedtime; may repeat once if necessary; maximum dose is 1000 mg/night

FATE

Erratically absorbed orally because of poor water solubility; onset usually within 30 minutes; duration is 4 to 8 hours; about 50% is bound to plasma proteins; quickly distributed to fatty tissues; less than 2% excreted unchanged; most is metabolized by the liver, where it is conjugated and then slowly excreted in the urine; plasma half-life is about 10 hours

COMMON SIDE EFFECTS

Skin rash, hangover, dizziness, ataxia, blurred vision; osteomalacia with long-term use

SIGNIFICANT ADVERSE REACTIONS

Anorexia, nausea, vomiting, urticaria, exfoliative dermatitis, hypotension, hypersensitivity reactions, blood dyscrasias, peripheral neuropathy, and porphyria

Acute overdose: CNS depression (possibly coma), shock, hypothermia (may be followed by fever), depressed reflexes, bladder atony, cyanosis, tachycardia, and sudden apnea; requires immediate treatment. Perform gastric lavage (1:1 mixture of castor oil and water) immediately in cases of overdose. Forced diuresis and urinary alkalinization are *not* recommended. Have adjunctive measures at hand, including vasopressors and mechanical respiratory aids. Do *not* use analeptic drugs to treat overdose.

Chronic intoxication: ataxia, tremors, irritability, slurred speech, hyporeflexia, memory impairment, confusion, delirium; withdraw drug *gradually*

CONTRAINDICATIONS
Intermittent porphyria, pregnancy, and in children under 12. *Cautious use* in patients with glaucoma, prostatic hypertrophy, stenosing peptic ulcer, bladder obstruction, and arrhythmias and in elderly or debilitated persons (danger of paradoxical excitation)

INTERACTIONS
Effects of other CNS depressants (e.g., alcohol, barbiturates) may be enhanced

Drug induces liver microsomal enzyme activity so that effects of anticoagulants, antihistamines, corticosteroids, griseofulvin, meprobamate, phenytoin, and other drugs metabolized by these enzymes may be reduced

May exert an additive anticholinergic effect with tricyclic antidepressants and other anticholinergic drugs

NURSING CONSIDERATIONS
See **ethchlorvynol.** In addition:

Nursing Alert
- After treatment for overdose, monitor patient for prolonged or recurrent signs of overdosage. A lethal dose in some individuals is as low as 5 g. The drug is highly lipid soluble and can persist in the body for long periods. As drug is removed from the bloodstream (e.g., dialysis), more is gradually released from fat storage back into the bloodstream. This phenomenon can prolong symptoms of overdosage or cause them to recur after dialysis is terminated.

1. Observe for appearance of skin rash. If one occurs, the drug should be discontinued.
2. Monitor bowel regularity and urinary output because drug may reduce intestinal motility and cause urinary retention. Provide fluids and roughage as needed.
3. Follow proper procedures for handling a Schedule III drug.

PATIENT EDUCATION
1. Warn patient that the danger of psychological and physical dependence is high with prolonged or excessive usage.
2. Advise patient to take glutethimide no later than 4 hours before expected arising because residual effects may persist during the day.

Methyprylon
Noludar

MECHANISM
Largely speculative; may increase brainstem firing threshold; similar to glutethimide in most aspects; suppresses REM sleep and induces hepatic microsomal enzymes

USES
Short-term treatment of insomnia

DOSAGE
Adults: 200 mg to 400 mg at bedtime
Children (over 12 yr): 50 mg to 200 mg at bedtime

FATE
Onset of action is 30 to 45 minutes, and duration lasts 5 to 8 hours; almost completely metabolized in the liver and 60% excreted in the urine, mostly as conjugated metabolites

COMMON SIDE EFFECTS
Hangover, GI upset, and dizziness

SIGNIFICANT ADVERSE REACTIONS
(Usually rare) Vomiting, diarrhea, skin rash, paradoxical excitation, esophagitis, neutropenia, and thrombocytopenia

Overdose: confusion, somnolence, hypotension, pulmonary edema, respiratory depression, miosis, elevated body temperature, shock, and coma. Treat overdose with gastric lavage, assisted respiration, IV fluids, and pressor agents. If excitement is present, a rapid-acting barbiturate can be given. Closely monitor vital signs and urinary output. Hemodialysis may be performed if necessary

CONTRAINDICATIONS
Porphyria, or in children under 3 months. *Cautious use* in the presence of renal or hepatic dysfunction, severe pain, and in pregnant or nursing women or drug abusers

INTERACTIONS
See **glutethimide**

NURSING CONSIDERATIONS
See **ethchlorvynol.** In addition:
1. Follow proper procedures for handling a Schedule III drug.

PATIENT EDUCATION
1. Instruct patient to notify drug prescriber if fever, rash, sore throat, or petechiae (early indications of possible blood dyscrasias) occur.
2. Prepare patient for the possibility of REM rebound (nightmares, insomnia, hallucinations) if drug is discontinued after prolonged use.
3. Inform patient that periodic blood counts are advisable with prolonged use.

Paraldehyde
Paral

MECHANISM
Nonspecific CNS depression, with minimal effects on respiration and blood pressure; large doses can abolish convulsions and delirium

USES
General sedative and hypnotic
Emergency treatment of tetanus, eclampsia, status epilepticus, and poisoning with convulsive drugs
Basal anesthesia, especially in children (rectally)

DOSAGE
(1 mL liquid or injection equals 1 g paraldehyde)
Oral (adults): 4 mL to 8 mL in milk or fruit juice to mask taste and odor

Rectal (adults): 10 mL to 20 mL with one to two parts of olive oil or isotonic sodium chloride to minimize rectal irritation

IM, IV

Hypnosis (adults): 10 mL IM in 2 divided doses or 10 mL IV, diluted with 200 mL 0.9% sodium chloride injection at a rate not exceeding 1 mL/min; (children): 0.3 mL/kg IM

Sedation (adults): 2 mL to 5 mL IM or 5 mL IV diluted with at least 100 mL of 0.9% sodium chloride injection at a rate not exceeding 1 mL/min; (children): 0.15 mL/kg IM

FATE

Well absorbed by all routes; onset of sleep is within 10 to 15 minutes; duration is 8 to 10 hours; largely metabolized by the liver (70%–80%) or exhaled unchanged through the lungs (11%–28%)

COMMON SIDE EFFECTS

Oral or rectal mucosal irritation, unpleasant taste and odor on breath, and pain at IM injection site

SIGNIFICANT ADVERSE REACTIONS

Metabolic acidosis, GI irritation, skin rash, necrosis or sterile abscess at injection site; IV use may cause severe coughing

Overdose: Respiratory difficulty, pulmonary edema, marked hypotension, gastritis, renal and hepatic damage (albuminuria, oliguria, nephrosis, azotemia, toxic hepatitis, fatty liver), right-side heart dilatation, and cardiovascular collapse

CONTRAINDICATIONS

Bronchopulmonary disease, GI ulceration, and hepatic insufficiency. *Cautious use* in the presence of severe pain or cough, in pregnant or nursing women, and in persons with a history of drug abuse

INTERACTIONS

Effects of other CNS depressants may be potentiated by paraldehyde

Paraldehyde may antagonize the antibacterial activity of sulfonamides by increasing their rate of metabolism, possibly causing crystalluria

Tolbutamide (Orinase) may potentiate the hypnotic action of paraldehyde

Disulfiram (Antabuse) used with paraldehyde may cause a toxic reaction due to excessive blood levels of acetaldehyde

NURSING CONSIDERATIONS

Nursing Alerts
- Expect drug to be discontinued gradually after prolonged use because delirium, hallucinations, and tremors can occur with rapid withdrawal.
- Do not administer paraldehyde if pain is present because it may induce delirium or excitement.
- Discard solution if it has a brownish color or an odor of acetic acid, indications of decomposition. Fatal poisoning or extreme tissue damage can result from administration of decomposed solution. Discard unused contents of container within 24 hours.

1. Give oral drug well chilled in fruit juice or milk to mask objectionable odor and taste and to reduce GI irritation.
2. When injecting drug, use *glass* syringe because paraldehyde is incompatible with most plastics.
3. When giving IM, inject *deeply.* Injections are usually painful.
4. Dilute drug to be administered rectally in 2 volumes of olive or cottonseed oil (retention enema) or in normal saline to reduce mucosal irritation.
5. Keep room well ventilated to minimize odor. Inform patient that breath will have a characteristic odor for several hours after administration.
6. Interpret results of certain laboratory tests cautiously. Paraldehyde may produce false positive plasma and urinary ketone findings and can interfere with urinary steroid measurements.
7. Follow proper procedures for handling a Schedule IV drug.

Propiomazine
Largon

Propiomazine is a phenothiazine derivative–possessing sedative, antihistaminic, and antiemetic effects. It is occasionally used IV or IM in a hospital setting as a sedative for the relief of apprehension either prior to or during surgery, and as an adjunct to analgesics during labor. Peak effects occur within 15 to 30 minutes following IV injection, and within 30 to 60 minutes with IM administration. Effects persist 4 to 6 hours with a single injection. Mild elevations in blood pressure and heart rate have been noted, and dizziness, confusion, and restlessness have occurred.

IV injection can cause thrombophlebitis and therefore drug should be injected only into undamaged vessels, with care being taken to avoid extravasation. Subcutaneous injection is likely to cause tissue irritation, and intraarterial administration may cause vascular spasm. Because propiomazine can markedly enhance the action of other CNS depressants (e.g., barbiturates, narcotics), their dosage should be reduced by one third to one half when used concurrently with propiomazine. Dosage generally ranges from 20 mg to 40 mg and is frequently combined with 50 mg of meperidine (Demerol). For sedation during surgery with local or spinal anesthetics, a dosage of 10 mg to 20 mg is sufficient. Children have been given 0.25 mg to 0.5 mg per pound for presurgical or postsurgical sedation.

NURSING CONSIDERATIONS
1. Discard solution if it is cloudy or contains a precipitate.
2. Observe elderly patient carefully following administration, and assist ambulation as necessary because dizziness and confusion may occur.
3. Expect norepinephrine to be used if a pressor agent is required because of excessive hypotension. Epinephrine should *not* be used because hypotension (epinephrine reversal) can occur.

Selected Bibliography

Bliwise D, Seidel W, Karacan I, Mitler M, Roth T, Zorick F, Dement W: Daytime sleepiness as a criterion in hypnotic medication trials: Comparison of triazolam and flurazepam. Sleep 6:156, 1983

Chartier D: Glutethimide and codeine overdose. J Emerg Nurs 9:307, 1983

Erman MK: Insomnia: Treatment approaches. Drug Ther 14:43, 1984.

Greenblatt DJ, Divoll M, Abernethy DR, Shady RI: Benzodiazepine hypnotics: Kinetic and therapeutic options. Sleep 5:518, 1982.

Harris B: Sedative-hypnotic drugs. Am J Nurs 81(7):1329, 1981

Kales A, Kales J: Sleep laboratory studies of hypnotic drugs: Efficacy and withdrawal effects. J Clin Psychopharmacol 3:140, 1983

Lader M, Petursson H: Long-term effects of benzodiazepines. Neuropharmacology 22:527, 1983

Simon C: Benzodiazepine hypnotics for insomnia. Am J Nurs 83(9):1330, 1983

Wincer MZ: Insomnia and the new benzodiazepines. Clin Pharmacokinet 1:425, 1982

SUMMARY. NONBARBITURATE SEDATIVE–HYPNOTICS

Drug	Preparations	Usual Dosage Range
Acetylcarbromal Paxarel	Tablets: 250 mg	250 mg–500 mg 1–4 times/day
Benzodiazepine hypnotics	See Table 21-2	
Chloral hydrate Aquachloral Supprettes, Noctec	Capsules: 250 mg, 500 mg Syrup: 250, 500 mg/5 mL Suppositories: 325 mg, 500 mg, 650 mg	*Adults* Hypnosis: 500 mg–1000 mg Sedation: 250 mg 3 times/day *Children* Hypnosis: 50 mg/kg Sedation: 25 mg/kg/day
Ethchlorvynol Placidyl	Capsules: 200 mg, 500 mg, 750 mg	Hypnosis: 500 mg–1000 mg as required; supplement of 200 mg may be given once nightly upon awakening
Ethinamate Valmid	Capsules: 500 mg	Hypnosis: 500 mg–1000 mg
Glutethimide Doriden, Doriglute	Tablets: 250 mg, 500 mg Capsules: 500 mg	Hypnosis: 250 mg–500 mg (may repeat if needed)
Methyprylon Noludar	Tablets: 50 mg, 200 mg Capsules: 300 mg	*Hypnosis* Adults: 200 mg–400 mg Children: 50 mg–200 mg
Paraldehyde Paral	Liquid (oral, rectal, injection): 1 g/mL	*Hypnosis* Adults: 4 mL to 8 mL orally *or* 10 mL to 20 mL rectally; 10 mL IM; 10 mL/200 mL sodium chloride IV at a rate of 1 mL/min Children: 0.3 mL/kg IM *Sedation* Adults: 2 mL to 5 mL IM *or* 5 mL IV Children: 0.15 mL/kg IM *Anticonvulsant* 5 mL IM; 3 ml–5 mL/100 mL sodium chloride IV
Propiomazine Largon	Injection: 20 mg/mL	Preoperatively: 20 mg–40 mg IM or IV During regional anesthesia: 10 mg–20 mg IM or IV Obstetrics: 20 mg–40 mg IM or IV with 50 mg meperidine; repeat at 3–4-h intervals

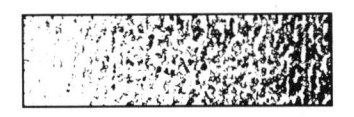

22 ANTIPSYCHOTIC DRUGS

The antipsychotic drugs, represented by several chemically distinct groups of compounds, are capable of improving the mood and calming the disturbed behavior of psychotic patients without causing marked sedation or habituation. Although the term *tranquilizer* is often used to describe these drugs, it is a misnomer because these agents fundamentally are *not* CNS depressants. Rather, they appear to act principally at lower brain centers to improve the disturbed thought processes of the psychotic individual and therefore create a more favorable mental state for other forms of psychotherapy. In fact, the development of effective antipsychotic drugs revolutionized the institutional practice of psychiatry and saved countless thousands of patients from lives of confinement in locked psychiatric wards.

Distinction must be made between antipsychotic drugs, used to treat acute and chronic psychoses, and antianxiety drugs or minor tranquilizers (see Chap. 23) indicated primarily for the relief of anxiety and tension associated with psychoneurotic or psychosomatic disorders. Antipsychotic drugs are significantly more potent than antianxiety agents in their actions on the CNS and are considerably more toxic as well. Yet, despite the greater potency and toxicity of these drugs, prolonged use of antipsychotic drugs is not associated with development of habituation or addiction—a major problem with chronic use of the antianxiety agents.

Chemically, the antipsychotic drugs may be divided into five groups (Table 22-1). In addition, several other drugs that affect central neuronal functioning in different ways are discussed in this chapter. They are *lithium*, used in the control of manic-depressive psychoses; *pimozide*, used to control the erratic behavior of Gilles de la Tourette's syndrome; *droperidol*, a unique tranquilizer; and *methotrimeprazine*, an analgesic.

The *phenothiazines* constitute the largest and most widely used group of antipsychotic drugs. Based on their structural configuration, they are divided into three groups: (1) aliphatics, (2) piperazines, and (3) piperidines. These groups differ in certain respects, outlined in Table 22-1. The piperazines are the most potent derivatives and have the highest incidence of extrapyramidal side effects, whereas the aliphatics and piperidines possess the greatest sedative and hypotensive action. Antiemetic potency generally parallels antipsychotic potency, the only major exception being thioridazine, which is a potent antipsychotic essentially devoid of antiemetic activity. The aliphatics exhibit the greatest anticholinergic activity of the phenothiazines, whereas the piperazines are only weak anticholinergics. Anticholinergic activity leads to a wide range of side effects (xerostomia, blurred vision, urinary hesitancy) but also may reduce the incidence of extrapyramidal reactions.

Thioxanthene derivatives are chemically and pharmacologically similar to the phenothiazines, so the two classes can be used interchangeably. Clinical evidence of an antidepressant action for the thioxanthenes suggests that these agents might be more beneficial than phenothiazines in certain types of withdrawn, retarded, or apathetic psychotic states.

Haloperidol, a butyrophenone derivative, is a potent antipsychotic agent providing an alternative to the phenothiazines in psychotic states characterized by agitation, aggressiveness, or hostility. Its toxicity is quite high, comparable to that of the piperazine group of phenothiazines, but it is only a weak anticholinergic and generally does not cause significant hypotension.

Newer drugs used to control psychotic symptoms are chemically unrelated to other antipsychotic drugs but are pharmacologically and toxicologically similar. *Molindone* and *loxapine* may provide alternatives to the other antipsychotics in unresponsive or intolerant patients but have no distinct advantages over any of the older compounds, except in a somewhat lower incidence of certain side effects.

A comparison of the potencies and incidence of common side effects among the various classes of antipsychotic drugs is presented in Table 22-1. Although distinct *quantitative* differences in milligram potency and toxicologic properties are evident among the different groups, no significant *qualitative* differences exist regarding the effectiveness of each drug; that is, when the drugs are used in therapeutically equivalent doses, their clinical efficacy is essentially equal. Choice of an antipsychotic drug, therefore, is based largely on the desire to minimize particular types of side effects in different psychotic populations (e.g., reduced sedative effects in persons operating machinery, or reduced hypotensive effects in older patients).

The pharmacologic actions of the antipsychotic agents are quite complex. In addition to their behavior-modifying effects, the agents have a range of other central and peripheral effects, the extent of which differs among the various chemical groups. An outline of the principal pharmacologic actions of the antipsychotic drugs is presented in Table 22-2.

Because many similarities are evident among the antipsychotic drugs, they are reviewed as a group. Specific information pertaining to individual drugs is then given in Table 22-3. Several antipsychotic-related drugs (e.g., lithium, pimozide, droperidol, methotrimeprazine) with different indications are considered at the end of the chapter.

ANTIPSYCHOTIC DRUGS

Acetophenazine	Perphenazine
Chlorpromazine	Prochlorperazine
Chlorprothixene	Promazine
Fluphenazine	Thioridazine
Haloperidol	Thiothixene
Loxapine	Trifluoperazine
Mesoridazine	Triflupromazine
Molindone	

MECHANISM
Complex and not completely understood; act primarily at several subcortical brain sites, including the limbic system, hypothalamus, and brain stem; among the known effects of the drugs are reduction of intraneuronal levels of cyclic AMP in brain regions associated with emotion and behavior, and decreased cortical sensory input from ascending spinal tracts by way of collateral nerves to the reticular formation. Biochemical mechanisms of action may include dopamine receptor blockade (primary action), increased dopamine turnover, inhibition of neuronal uptake of norepinephrine and serotonin, and suppression

Table 22-1
Antipsychotic Drugs—Comparison of Effects

	Approximate Potency Relative to Chlorpromazine	Relative Incidence of Side Effects			
		Extrapyramidal Symptoms	Sedation	Hypotension	Anticholinergic
Phenothiazines					
Aliphatics					
Chlorpromazine	1	++	+++	+++	++
Promazine	0.5	++	++	++	+++
Triflupromazine	4	++	+++	++	+++
Piperazines					
Acetophenazine	5	+++	++	+	++
Fluphenazine	50	+++	+	+	+
Perphenazine	12	+++	+	+	++
Prochlorperazine	10	+++	++	+	+
Trifluoperazine	25	+++	+	+	+
Piperidines					
Mesoridazine	2	+	+++	++	++
Thioridazine	1	+	+++	+++	+++
Thioxanthenes					
Chlorprothixene	1	++	+++	+++	++
Thiothixene	25	+++	+	++	+
Butyrophenone					
Haloperidol	50	+++	+	+	+
Indolone					
Molindone	5	+++	++	++	++
Dibenzoxazepine					
Loxapine	5	+++	++	++	+

+++—frequent
++—occasional
+—infrequent

of acetylcholine release. No appreciable direct cortical depression is evident. These drugs elicit varying degrees of sedation, antiemesis, hypothermia, and altered pituitary hormone release in addition to an antipsychotic action. Other peripheral actions that are responsible for many of the observed side effects include antiadrenergic (alpha-blocking effect) and anticholinergic activity, as well as some degree of antiserotonergic, local anesthetic, and a quinidine-like cardiac depressant effect.

USES
(See Table 22-3 for specific indications of each drug)

Management of acute and chronic psychoses, either organic or drug-induced
Control of the manic phase of manic–depressive psychoses (lithium)
Relief of severe nausea and vomiting
Control of intractable hiccups
Relief of anxiety, apprehension, and agitation associated with a variety of somatic disorders, or prior to surgery
Facilitation of alcohol withdrawal
Adjunctive treatment of tetanus and acute intermittent porphyria
Control of aggressiveness in disturbed children
Control of tics and vocal utterances of Gilles de la Tourette's disease (haloperidol, pimozide)

DOSAGE
See Table 22-3

FATE
Adequately absorbed orally and well absorbed parenterally; widely distributed to most body tissues and found in high concentrations in the brain; onset and duration of action largely dependent on dosage form and route of administration; clinical effects may not be attained for several weeks after initiation of therapy; most drugs are significantly protein-bound, and metabolism and excretion are generally slow; metabolized by the liver and excreted in both the urine and feces; many metabolites are biologically active and contribute to the prolonged effects of some drugs. Enzyme inducers (e.g., barbiturates, meprobamate) can accelerate phenothiazine metabolism. Excretion is by way of the kidneys and the enterohepatic circulation

COMMON SIDE EFFECTS
(Most common in early stages of therapy) Drowsiness, orthostatic hypotension (dizziness, weakness), dry mouth, blurred vision, constipation, nasal stuffiness, and palpitations

Table 22-2
Antipsychotic Drugs—Pharmacologic Effects

Central Nervous System

Antipsychotic effect: reduced agitation, emotional quieting, decreased paranoid ideation, and lessening of hallucinations and disturbed thought processes.
Antiemetic effect: decreased sensitivity of chemoreceptor trigger zone (CTZ) in medulla to activation by drugs or toxins and direct depression of brain stem vomiting center in large doses
Impaired temperature regulation: hypothermia caused by increased heat loss and decreased compensatory heat production
Endocrine effects: inhibition of FSH and LH release, and increased release of LTH (prolactin), resulting in abnormal lactation. Hormonal effects are due to the blocking action of antipsychotic drugs on dopamine receptors either in the hypothalamic–pituitary pathway or on anterior pituitary cells themselves.
Motor effects: increased involuntary muscle activity (e.g., tremors, dyskinesias, akathisias) caused by dopamine blockade in motor-integrating areas of the CNS

Peripheral Nervous System

Antiadrenergic effects: blockade of central and peripheral alpha receptors, and possibly inhibition of catecholamine uptake by nerve endings, leading to orthostatic hypotension and reflex tachycardia
Anticholinergic/antihistamine effects: blockade of cholinergic (largely muscarinic) and histaminergic activity

Other

Antiarrhythmic effects: quinidine-like depressant action on the myocardium, and local anesthetic action
Diuretic effect: depression of ADH release and inhibition of water and electrolyte reabsorption (weak effect)

SIGNIFICANT ADVERSE REACTIONS
(Incidence varies among different drugs)

CNS: neuroleptic malignant syndrome (high fever, sweating, muscle rigidity, tachycardia, confusion, delirium), lowering of convulsive threshold, hyperactivity, bizarre dreams, insomnia, depression, cerebral edema
Neuromuscular: extrapyramidal reactions, akathisia (motor restlessness), dystonias (muscle spasms of the face or throat, difficulty in speech or swallowing, extensor rigidity of the back muscles, upward rotation of the eyeballs), pseudoparkinsonism, tardive dyskinesias (involuntary orofacial movements such as chewing, protrusion of the tongue, puffing of the cheeks and puckering of the mouth—developing slowly over 6 to 24 mo), hyperreflexia
Cardiovascular: tachycardia, fainting, ECG changes, cardiac arrest (rare)
Hematologic: blood dyscrasias (agranulocytosis, leukopenia, leukocytosis, anemias, thrombocytopenic purpura, pancytopenia)
Hypersensitivity: urticaria, itching, eczema, photosensitivity, contact dermatitis, angioneurotic edema, anaphylactic reaction, exfoliative dermatitis, cholestatic jaundice
Endocrine: abnormal lactation, breast engorgement, gynecomastia, changes in libido, amenorrhea, glycosuria and hyperglycemia, increased appetite
Autonomic: fecal impaction, adynamic ileus, urinary retention, enuresis, incontinence, impotence
Ocular: ptosis, photophobia, pigmentary retinopathy, lens opacities
Respiratory: laryngospasm, bronchospasm, dyspnea
Other: skin pigmentation, polydipsia, aggravation of peptic ulcers, fever, systemic lupus–like reaction, psychotic flare-up

CONTRAINDICATIONS

Bone marrow depression, blood dyscrasias, parkinsonism, jaundice, liver damage, renal insufficiency, cerebral arteriosclerosis, coronary disease, circulatory collapse, mitral insufficiency, severe hypotension, chronic alcoholism, comatose states, and subcortical brain damage. *Cautious use* in the presence of glaucoma, prostatic hypertrophy, epilepsy, diabetes, severe hypertension, ulcers, cardiovascular disease, chronic respiratory disorders, liver impairment, in pregnant or lactating women, in children under 6 months of age, and in persons exposed to extreme heat, phosphorus insecticides, or pesticides

INTERACTIONS

Antipsychotic drugs may potentiate the effects of other CNS depressants (e.g., alcohol, barbiturates, general anesthetics, antianxiety agents, narcotic analgesics)
Additive anticholinergic effects may be observed with concomitant use of antipsychotic drugs and other agents having anticholinergic activity (e.g., antihistamines, tricyclic antidepressants, antiparkinsonian drugs)
Effects of antipsychotics may be enhanced by estrogens, progestins, anticholinesterases, furazolidone, and MAO inhibitors
Hypotensive action of antipsychotic drugs can be increased by antihypertensives, epinephrine, thiazide diuretics, and tricyclic antidepressants
Antipsychotic drugs may decrease the effectiveness of amphetamines, oral anticoagulants, heparin, anticonvulsants (lowering of seizure threshold), oral hypoglycemics, levodopa, and other antiparkinsonian drugs
The hypoglycemic effect of insulin may be potentiated by antipsychotics
Absorption of antipsychotic agents can be impaired by antacids and antidiarrheal preparations
Lithium and other antipsychotic drugs may exert additive hyperglycemic effects
The combination of antipsychotic drugs and griseofulvin may precipitate acute porphyria
Narcotic analgesics may increase the respiratory-depressant action of the antipsychotics
Antipsychotics can reduce the effectiveness of guanethidine by interfering with its neuronal uptake
Antipsychotic drugs can potentiate muscle relaxants, possibly resulting in prolonged apnea
Additive cardiac depressant effects may occur with quinidine and antipsychotic drugs
Antipsychotic-induced extrapyramidal effects can be intensified by anticholinergic antiparkinsonian drugs and piperazine, and can be reduced by diphenhydramine

NURSING CONSIDERATIONS

Nursing Alerts

- Monitor patient frequently for appearance of fine, worm-like movements of the tongue, an early sign of tardive dyskinesia, which usually develops only during long-term (6–24 mo) treatment. Symptoms (see **Significant Adverse Reactions**) may be irreversible; prompt cessation of therapy at onset of the developing syndrome can minimize severity. Antiparkinsonian drugs do *not* alleviate these symptoms and may, in fact, aggravate them.
- Be alert for onset of acute dystonic reactions (i.e., neck spasms, eye rolling, dysphagia, convulsions), especially in

children with acute illnesses (e.g., mumps, measles, severe infections) or who are dehydrated, as they are more susceptible than adults. These reactions are very frightening to most patients. If one occurs, advise physician, remain with patient to provide reassurance, and be prepared to discontinue drug.
- Assist with periodic evaluation of patient on long-term therapy. Dosage should be kept as low as possible, and drug-free intervals should be employed where possible to minimize incidence of untoward reactions, particularly extrapyramidal syndromes. Antiparkinsonian medication should not be used to *prevent* extrapyramidal reactions. If symptoms appear during therapy, an attempt should be made to eliminate them by reducing the dose of the antipsychotic drug. If symptoms persist, the antiparkinsonian drug should be carefully titrated so that the smallest dose that relieves the symptoms is used (see Chap. 26).
- Monitor blood pressure of hospitalized patient before each dose during initial treatment period. Employ appropriate interventions to protect patient from injury due to orthostatic hypotension. See **Plan of Nursing Care 8 (Antihypertensive Drugs)** in Chapter 31 for specific information.
- Keep patient flat for at least 1 hour after parenteral administration of nondepot form, and monitor blood pressure often. Marked hypotension can be treated by placing patient in head-low position and, if necessary, using volume expanders and pressor agents such as levarterenol or dopamine. Epinephrine is *contraindicated*: It can have a reverse effect and aggravate hypotension.

1. Supervise emotionally disturbed patient to ascertain that medication is swallowed. Syrup, injection, or depot injection forms may help ensure that patient receives prescribed dose.
2. Implement measures to prevent constipation (increased intake of fluid and dietary roughage), and monitor bowel and bladder function during prolonged therapy because constipation and urinary retention can occur. A dosage reduction should be considered if these conditions become problematic.
3. If patient is on long-term therapy, monitor results of renal function tests. If serum creatinine is elevated, drug dosage may need to be reduced.
4. Monitor diabetic patient for signs of altered carbohydrate metabolism such as glycosuria, weight loss, and polyphagia. Dosage alterations or dietary changes may be warranted.
5. Avoid drug contact with skin or mucous membranes because contact dermatitis can occur.
6. Discard discolored injectable solutions. Do not mix other solutions in same syringe. Give deep IM injection.
7. Store oral liquid preparations in dark bottles because they are light sensitive.
8. Cautiously interpret results of laboratory tests for pregnancy, I^{131} uptake, urinary catecholamines, urinary ketones, bilirubin, and steroids because phenothiazines may interfere with these tests.

PATIENT EDUCATION
1. Discuss the importance of maintaining a regular dosing schedule, especially during initial stages, because it sometimes takes several weeks for beneficial effects to become manifest. Stress the need for regular follow-up care.
2. Encourage patient to continue long-term therapy. Another person may need to assume responsibility for ensuring that patient takes medication. *Abrupt* stoppage, particularly if dosage is high, could cause gastritis, vomiting, dizziness, tremors, insomnia, and psychotic behavior. The drug should be withdrawn gradually over several weeks (e.g., 10%–25% reduction in dosage every 2 wk).
3. Reassure patient that many side effects (drowsiness, dry mouth) are common early in therapy but usually disappear. Others, such as orthostatic hypotension, extrapyramidal reactions, and sedation, may be minimized by selection of proper agent.
4. Warn patient that no other drugs, including OTC preparations, should be taken without consulting the health care provider or pharmacist.
5. Teach patient early signs of blood dyscrasia (fever, sore throat, mucosal irritation, fatigue, upper respiratory infection) that need to be reported to physician immediately.
6. Caution patient not to operate dangerous machinery during initial stages of therapy because drowsiness is common.
7. Teach patient measures that help control orthostatic hypotension. See **Plan of Nursing Care 8 (Antihypertensive Drugs)** in Chapter 31 for specific information.
8. Instruct patient to inform physician if fever, abdominal pain, rash, itching, diarrhea, or yellowing of skin (signs of developing jaundice) appear.
9. Suggest interventions to alleviate mouth dryness. See **Plan of Nursing Care 4 (Antihistamines)** in Chapter 14 for specific information. Stress meticulous oral hygiene to prevent development of oral candidiasis, especially if oral concentrate is used.
10. Explain endocrine disturbances that could occur: menstrual irregularities, gynecomastia, breast engorgement, impotence, and altered libido. Reassure patient that it may be possible for physicians to minimize such changes by adjusting the dosage or substituting another drug.
11. Instruct patient to be alert for indications of decreased visual acuity, photophobia, and brownish discoloration of objects in visual field, symptoms which call for immediate ophthalmologic examination.
12. Advise patient to avoid direct sunlight and to use sunscreen lotion because photosensitivity reactions can occur.
13. Inform patient that drug may discolor the urine (pink to red brown). Explain that this is not serious and does not necessitate interruption of therapy.

Lithium

Cibalith-S, Eskalith, Lithane, Lithobid, Lithonate, Lithotabs
(CAN) Lithizine, Carbolith, Duralith

An alkali metal ion effective in the control of the manic phase of manic–depressive psychoses, lithium is capable of calming the agitated patient and smoothing out the wide swings in mood between mania and depression. Its toxicity is very closely related to its serum levels, and the effective therapeutic dose in many instances is near the toxic level. Therefore, repeated and

(Text continued on page 213)

Table 22-3
Antipsychotic Drugs

Drug	Preparations	Usual Dosage Range	Nursing Implications
Phenothiazines			
Aliphatics			
Chlorpromazine Thorazine and several other manufacturers (CAN) Chlorpromanyl, Largactil, Novochlorpromazine	Tablets: 10 mg, 25 mg, 50 mg, 100 mg, 200 mg Sustained-release capsules: 30 mg, 75 mg, 150 mg, 200 mg, 300 mg Syrup: 10 mg/5 mL Concentrate: 30 mg/mL, 100 mg/mL Suppositories: 25 mg, 100 mg Injection: 25 mg/mL	*Adults* *Psychoses* Oral: Initially 50 mg–100 mg/day; increase until desired effect occurs; usual maintenance range is 300 mg–400 mg/day IM: Initially 25 mg; increase gradually up to 400 mg every 4–6 h until patient is quiet and cooperative; substitute oral dosage when possible *Nausea/vomiting* Oral: 10 mg–25 mg every 4–6 h IM: 25 mg–50 mg every 3–4 h Rectal: 50 mg–100 mg every 6–8 h *Preoperative sedation* Oral: 25 mg–50 mg IM: 12.5 mg–25 mg *Porphyria* Oral: 25 mg–50 mg 3–4 times/day IM: 25 mg 3–4 times/day *Tetanus* IM, IV: 25 mg–50 mg 3–4 times/day *Hiccups* Oral: 25 mg–50 mg 3–4 times/day IM: 25 mg–50 mg IV: 25 mg–50 mg diluted in 500–1000 mL saline by infusion *Children* Oral: 0.25 mg/lb 2–4 times/day Rectal: 0.5 mg/lb every 6–8 h IM: 0.125 mg–0.25 mg/lb every 6–8 h IV: 0.25 mg/lb	Used in acute and chronic psychoses, manic phase of manic–depressive psychoses, for pre- and postoperative sedation, intractable hiccups, acute intermittent porphyria, tetanus, and control of severe nausea and vomiting resulting from drugs, surgery, or toxins; plasma levels following IM injection are several times higher than following oral administration; duration of action ranges from 3–6 h; high incidence of drowsiness, dizziness, and hypotension, especially during first few weeks of therapy and in older patients; IV solution should be diluted to 1 mg/mL in saline and administered at a rate of 1 mg/min; doses in excess of 1000 mg/day for prolonged periods are *not* recommended
Promazine Sparine, Prozine	Tablets: 25 mg, 50 mg, 100 mg Syrup: 10 mg/5 mL Injection: 25 mg/mL, 50 mg/mL	*Adults* Initially: 50 mg–150 mg IM Maintenance: 10 mg–200 mg every 4–6 h orally *or* IM as required *Children* (over 12): 10 mg–25 mg every 4–6 h	Used primarily for management of psychotic disorders; the preferred parenteral route is IM; IV administration is recommended only in hospitalized patients; when used IV, injections should be given slowly in diluted solutions (25 mg/mL or less); concentrate for oral use should be diluted in fruit juice or other flavored vehicle (2 tsp of diluent for every 25 mg of drug); less potent and equally toxic compared to chlorpromazine
Triflupromazine Vesprin	Injection: 10 mg/mL, 20 mg/mL	*Adults* *Psychoses* IM: 60 mg–150 mg/day *Nausea/vomiting* IM: 5 mg–15 mg every 4 h IV: 1 mg–3 mg *Children* (over 2 yr) *Psychoses* IM: 0.2 mg–0.25 mg/kg (maximum 10 mg) *Nausea/vomiting* IM: 0.2 mg–0.25 mg/kg (maximum 10 mg)	Effective in psychotic disorders (other than psychotic depression) and for control of nausea and vomiting; sedation and extrapyramidal reactions are common, especially in the elderly and debilitated; has been used as an adjunct for pre- and postoperative management
Piperazines			
Acetophenazine Tindal	Tablets: 20 mg	*Adults:* 20 mg 3 times/day (80 mg to 120 mg/day in hospitalized patients) *Children:* 0.8 mg–1.6 mg/kg/day	Used for management of psychotic disorders. In patients with insomnia, last tablet should be taken 1 h before bedtime; infrequently used

Continued

Table 22-3
Antipsychotic Drugs (continued)

Drug	Preparations	Usual Dosage Range	Nursing Implications
Phenothiazines *Piperazines* **Fluphenazine** Permitil, Prolixin (CAN) Apo-Fluphenazine, Modecate, Moditen	Tablets: 1 mg, 2.5 mg, 5 mg, 10 mg Elixir: 2.5 mg/5 mL Concentrate: 5 mg/ml Injection: HCl—2.5 mg/mL Enanthate—25 mg/mL Decanoate—25 mg/mL	*Oral* Initially: 2.5 mg–10 mg/day; (maximum 20 mg) Maintenance: 1 mg–5 mg/day *IM* HCl: 1.25 mg 2–4 times/day (range 2.5 mg–10 mg/day in divided doses) Enanthate/decanoate (esters in a sesame oil vehicle): 12.5 mg–25 mg every 2–3 wk (may also be given SC); range—12.5 mg–100 mg at 1–3-wk intervals	Used for control of psychotic manifestations; oral dosage forms and HCl injection are rapid acting and can be used initially to stabilize patient; enanthate and decanoate salts are released slowly from tissue sites and thus have a prolonged effect (1–4 wk); indicated for maintenance therapy in patients who cannot be relied upon to follow a regular oral dosage schedule; if given cautiously in *low doses*, may be useful in patients who are hypersensitive to other phenothiazines; very potent drug with high incidence of extrapyramidal reactions and mental depression; decanoate may have a lower incidence of extrapyramidal side effects than other dosage forms; monitor renal function and blood picture periodically in patients on long-term therapy; protect solutions from light and use dry syringe and needle for injection because moisture may cloud the solution; avoid use of antacids with oral dosage forms, because GI absorption is impaired; owing to prolonged effects of enanthate and decanoate salts, advise patients to report appearance of side effects *immediately; not indicated in children*
Perphenazine Trilafon (CAN) Apo-Perphenazine, Phenazine, PMS Levazine	Tablets: 2 mg, 4 mg, 8 mg, 16 mg Repeat-action tablets: 8 mg Concentrate: 16 mg/5 mL Injection: 5 mg/mL	*Oral* Psychoses: 8 mg–16 mg 2–4 times/day (maximum 64 mg/day) initially; reduce to 4 mg–8 mg 3 times/day for maintenance Anxiety and tension states: 2 mg–4 mg 3 times/day Nausea and vomiting: 8 mg–16 mg/day in divided doses IM: Initially 5 mg–10 mg; repeat every 6 h (maximum 30 mg/day); switch to oral therapy as soon as possible IV (severe vomiting only): 1 mg/min infusion of an 0.5 mg/mL dilution (maximum 5 mg)	Effective in psychoses and in the control of severe nausea and vomiting due to surgery or other acute situations; may also be effective in the management of anxiety and tension due to severe neurosis; *do not use* in children under 12; high incidence of extrapyramidal reactions; transient hypotension can occur, especially IV; keep patient recumbent and monitor pulse and pressure; oral concentrate should be diluted (2 oz diluent/5 mL concentrate) with fruit juice, milk, carbonated beverage, or other liquid (tea is *not* recommended)
Prochlorperazine Chlorpazine, Compazine (CAN) Stemetil	Tablets: 5 mg, 10 mg, 25 mg Capsules: (sustained-release) 10 mg, 15 mg, 30 mg Syrup: 5 mg/5 mL Suppositories: 2.5 mg, 5 mg, 25 mg Injection: 5 mg/mL	*Adults* *Psychoses* Oral: 10 mg 3–4 times/day, increased gradually until maximum effect (usually 100 mg–150 mg/day) IM: 10 mg–20 mg initially; repeat in 2–4 h; switch to oral form as soon as possible *Nausea/vomiting* Oral: 5 mg–10 mg 3–4 times/day Rectal: 25 mg 2 times/day IM: 5 mg–10 mg; repeat every 3–4 h to a maximum of 40 mg/day IV (severe vomiting): 5 mg–10 mg IV injection or 20 mg added to 1 L IV infusion 15–30 min before induction of anesthesia *Children (over 2 yr and 20 lb)* *Psychoses* Oral/rectal: 2.5 mg 2–3 times/day IM: 0.06 mg/lb	Used for control of psychotic manifestations in adults and children over 2 years and for relief of nausea and vomiting; widely used pre- and postoperatively; do not use in short-term vomiting in children or for vomiting of unknown cause; discontinue if signs of restlessness or excitement occur; inject deeply IM (avoid SC use) and do not mix solution with other agents in same syringe; do not confuse *2.5-mg* child suppository with *25-mg* adult suppository; use cautiously in the elderly or debilitated patients and in children who are dehydrated or who have an acute illness because extrapyramidal reactions are common; monitor blood pressure during IV use because hypotension is likely to occur; supervise ambulation following parenteral use

Continued

Table 22-3
Antipsychotic Drugs (continued)

Drug	Preparations	Usual Dosage Range	Nursing Implications
Phenothiazines			
Piperazines			
Trifluoperazine Stelazine, Suprazine (CAN) Apo-Trifluoperazine	Tablets: 1 mg, 2 mg, 5 mg, 10 mg Concentrate: 10 mg/mL Injection: 2 mg/mL	*Nausea/vomiting* Oral/rectal: 2.5 mg–5 mg 1–2 times/day based on weight IM: 0.06 mg/lb *Adults* Oral: Initially 2 mg–5 mg twice a day (maximum 40 mg/day); maintenance: 1 mg–2 mg twice a day IM: 1 mg–2 mg every 4–6 h (maximum 10 mg/day) *Children* (over 6 yr) Oral: 1 mg 1–2 times/day (maximum 15 mg/day in older children) IM: 1 mg 1–2 times/day	Indicated for treatment of psychotic disorders and for controlling manifestations of severe psychoneuroses; very potent agent with high incidence of extrapyramidal reactions; maximum response may be delayed 2–3 weeks; increase dosage very slowly in elderly or debilitated patients; prolonged action of the drug allows once-a-day dosing in many less severe cases; dilute concentrate in 60 mL of appropriate vehicle (liquid or semisolid) to aid palatability; do not give IM injections more frequently than every 4 h because of danger of cumulation
Piperidines			
Mesoridazine Serentil	Tablets: 10 mg, 25 mg, 50 mg, 100 mg Concentrate: 25 mg/mL Injection: 25 mg/mL	*Psychoses* Oral: Initially 25 mg–50 mg 3 times/day (range 100 mg–400 mg/day) IM: 25 mg; repeat in 30–60 min if necessary (range 25 mg–200 mg/day) *Neuroses* Oral: 10 mg 3 times/day (range 30 mg–150 mg/day) *Alcoholism* 25 mg twice a day (range 50 mg–200 mg/day)	Used for treatment of schizophrenia, chronic brain syndrome, and psychoneuroses, and as adjunctive therapy in acute and chronic alcoholism; weak antiemetic; low incidence of extrapyramidal reactions but very sedating; may reduce hyperactive behavior associated with mentally deficient states; *not recommended in children under 12*; concentrate should be diluted prior to use
Thioridazine Mellaril (CAN) Apo-Thioridazine, Novoridazine, PMS Thioridazine	Tablets: 10 mg, 15 mg, 25 mg, 50 mg, 100 mg, 150 mg, 200 mg Concentrate: 30 mg/mL, 100 mg/mL Suspension: 25 mg/5 mL, 100 mg/5 mL	*Adults* *Psychoses* Initially: 50 mg–100 mg 3 times/day; maintenance 200 mg–800 mg/day in 2–4 divided doses *Depressive neuroses* Initially: 25 mg 3 times/day Maintenance: 20 mg–200 mg/day in 3–4 divided doses *Children* (over 2 yr): 0.5–3.0 mg/kg/day depending on severity of condition	Indicated for psychotic disorders and short-term treatment of depressive neuroses; possibly useful in hyperactive or aggressive children, alcohol withdrawal, intractable pain, and senility; low incidence of extrapyramidal reactions and no antiemetic action, but strong anticholinergic effect and highly sedating; abnormal ECG readings have occurred, especially at high doses; may be potentially cardiotoxic; frequently produces dryness of the mouth, constipation, urinary retention, and impotence in early stages of therapy; discontinue drug or reduce dosage if visual changes (reduced or brownish vision, impaired night vision) occur; periodic blood and liver function tests should be performed during prolonged therapy; dilute oral concentrate immediately prior to use with fruit juice or water
Thioxanthenes			
Chlorprothixene Taractan (CAN) Tarasan	Tablets: 10 mg, 25 mg, 50 mg, 100 mg Concentrate: 20 mg/mL Injection: 12.5 mg/mL	*Adults* Oral: Initially 25 mg–50 mg 3–4 times/day; increase to optimal level (maximum 600 mg/day) IM: 25 mg–50 mg 3–4 times/day; substitute oral therapy as soon as possible *Children* Oral: 10 mg–25 mg 3–4 times/day IM: over 12 yr, same as adult dose	Effective in acute and chronic schizophrenia; produces significant sedation and orthostatic hypotension; when used IM, keep patient recumbent during administration; do *not* give IM in children under 12, or orally in children under 6; anticholinergic side effects are prominent

Continued

Table 22-3
Antipsychotic Drugs (continued)

Drug	Preparations	Usual Dosage Range	Nursing Implications
Thioxanthenes			
Thiothixene Navane	Capsules: 1 mg, 2 mg, 5 mg, 10 mg, 20 mg Concentrate: 5 mg/mL Injection: 2 mg/mL, 5 mg/mL	Oral: Initially 2 mg–5 mg 2–3 times/day; maintenance 20 mg–60 mg/day in divided doses IM: 4 mg 2–4 times/day (usual range 16 mg–20 mg/day)	Used for management of acute and chronic schizophrenia; *not* for use in children under 12; high incidence of extrapyramidal reactions and drowsiness in early stages of therapy; therapeutic effects may take several weeks to develop with oral administration; do not withdraw drug abruptly because delirium can occur; dosage may need to be adjusted when switching from IM to oral administration
Butyrophenone			
Haloperidol Haldol, Halperon (CAN) Apo-Haloperidol, Novoperidol, Peridol	Tablets: 0.5 mg, 1 mg, 2 mg, 5 mg, 10 mg, 20 mg Concentrate: 2 mg/mL Injection: 5 mg/mL Depot injection: 50 mg/mL	*Adults* Oral: 0.5 mg–5 mg 2–3 times/day depending on symptoms (maximum 100 mg/day) IM: 2 mg–5 mg (up to 30 mg if necessary); repeat at 4–8-h intervals as needed Depot injection: 10×–15× daily oral dose IM every 4 weeks *Children* (3–12 yr) 0.5 mg/day initially in 2–3 divided doses; increase at 0.5-mg increments every 5–7 days until desired effect (range is 0.05 mg/kg/day–0.15 mg/kg/day)	Indicated in psychotic disorders, manic phase of manic–depressive psychoses, and for management of tics and vocal utterances of Gilles de la Tourette's disease; very potent antipsychotic with high incidence of extrapyramidal reactions; strong antiemetic; less sedation and hypotension than many other similar drugs; do *not* use in children under 3 or in parkinsonian patients (drug is a potent dopamine-blocking agent); use cautiously in epileptic individuals because drug may lower convulsive threshold; when used for manic episodes, be alert for reversal to severe depression which may invite suicidal attempts; concomitant use with lithium may elicit dyskinesias, parkinsonian-like symptoms, or dementia; observe patients closely, and provide emotional support as necessary; peform periodic liver function and blood studies; depot injection is for *chronic* psychoses only
Indolone			
Molindone Moban	Tablets: 5 mg, 10 mg, 25 mg, 50 mg, 100 mg Concentrate: 20 mg/mL	Initially: 50 mg–75 mg/day Maintenance: 5 mg–25 mg 3–4 times a day depending on symptoms (maximum 225 mg/day)	Used for control of schizophrenia; not recommended in children under 12; provides an alternative drug to the phenothiazines and thioxanthenes in unresponsive patients, although actions are essentially identical to other classes of antipsychotics; high degree of initial drowsiness; resumption of menses in previously amenorrheal women has been reported; no ophthalmologic complications have occurred; tablet contains calcium, which may interfere with GI absorption of phenytoin and tetracyclines
Dibenzoxazepine			
Loxapine Loxitane (CAN) Loxapac	Capsules: 5 mg, 10 mg, 25 mg, 50 mg Concentrate: 25 mg/mL Injection: 50 mg/mL	Initially 10 mg orally twice a day; increase to optimal levels (usually 60 mg–100 mg/day; maximum 250 mg/day) IM: 12.5 mg–50 mg every 4–6 h to control acutely agitated patients	Indicated for manifestations of schizophrenia; elicits strong sedation in early therapy, lowers convulsive threshold, produces hypotension, and is an anticholinergic of moderate potency; has antiemetic activity and may produce ocular toxicity; not recommended in children under 16; produces frequent extrapyramidal reactions, usually parkinsonian-like in nature; no endocrine abnormalities have been reported; concentrate should be mixed with orange or grapefruit juice before administration

accurate serum lithium levels should be determined in all patients taking the drug (see **Dosage**)

MECHANISM

Specific mechanism for control of mania is unknown. The drug can alter sodium transport at the nerve ending, thereby changing the electrophysiologic characteristics of nerve cells. It promotes neuronal uptake of norepinephrine, thereby causing more rapid inactivation, and may also reduce norepinephrine release and inhibit catecholamine-activated cyclic AMP formation; also appears to increase serotonin-receptor sensitivity

USES

Control of symptoms of acute mania (i.e., motor hyperactivity, talkativeness, restlessness, poor judgment, grandiose ideation, aggressiveness, and possibly hostility)

Prophylaxis of recurrent manic–depressive episodes in patients with classic bipolar affective disorder

Adjunctive therapy of psychoses associated with excitement

Investigational uses include management of violent, aggressive behavior in prisoners; prophylaxis of cluster headache and frequent, cyclic migraine attacks; and improvement of the neutrophil count in patients with chronic neutropenia or cancer chemotherapy–induced neutropenia

DOSAGE

Acute mania: 600 mg 3 times/day (desired serum level is 1 mEq/L–1.5 mEq/L); adjust oral dosage to optimal clinical response as well as desired serum level; clinical effects begin to appear within 4 to 7 days.

Prophylaxis: 300 mg 3 to 4 times/day (serum levels 0.6 mEq/L–1.4 mEq/L) *Note:* blood samples for determination of serum lithium levels should be taken 8 to 12 hours after the previous dose

FATE

Rapidly absorbed orally; peak serum levels in 1 to 2 hours, although optimal clinical response may take a week or more to develop; widely distributed in the body; very little is protein-bound; crosses blood–brain barrier; excreted through the kidneys (half-life about 24 h), the rate being directly proportional to its plasma concentration; excretion is diminished by low sodium levels, for example, those resulting from diminished salt intake or concomitant diuretic therapy

COMMON SIDE EFFECTS

Fine hand tremors, nausea, thirst, polyuria, fatigue, and mild muscle weakness (usually subside with continued therapy)

SIGNIFICANT ADVERSE REACTIONS

(Usually observed at serum levels above 1.5 mEq/L but may occur independent of lithium plasma level)

Neuromuscular: lack of coordination, ataxia, muscle hyperirritability and twitching, choreiform movements, extrapyramidal-like symptoms, coarse hand tremor

CNS: drowsiness, dizziness, restlessness, confusion, slurred speech, tinnitus, incontinence, psychomotor retardation, epileptic-like seizures, stupor, coma

Autonomic: dry mouth, blurred vision

Cardiovascular: hypotension, arrhythmias, bradycardia, edema, circulatory collapse

GI: anorexia, vomiting, diarrhea, abdominal pain

Urinary: albuminuria, glycosuria, oliguria

Dermatologic: rash, pruritus, thinning of hair, folliculitis, topical anesthesia, acneiform eruptions, cutaneous ulceration

Other: hypothyroidism, transient hyperglycemia, excessive weight gain, leucocytosis, scotomas, flattening and inversion of the T wave, worsening of psoriasis

CONTRAINDICATIONS

Severe renal or cardiovascular disease, organic brain syndrome, sodium depletion (low-salt diet, diuretic therapy, dehydration), early pregnancy, and in children under 12. *Cautious use* in elderly, debilitated, or dehydrated persons and in the presence of epilepsy or thyroid disease

INTERACTIONS

Effects of lithium may be decreased by acetazolamide, alkalinizing agents (e.g., sodium bicarbonate, antacids), aminophylline, caffeine, excess sodium chloride, and urea, all substances that increase its excretion

Toxic effects of lithium may be intensified by use of diuretics (sodium loss), methyldopa, antipsychotic drugs, phenytoin, carbamazepine, mazindol, and indomethacin

Combinations of lithium and haloperidol may produce severe encephalopathic symptoms such as parkinsonism, dyskinesias, and dementia

Profound hypothermia may occur with simultaneous use of benzodiazepines (e.g., Valium, Librium) and lithium

Lithium may reduce the pressor effects of sympathomimetic drugs

Lithium may prolong the effects of neuromuscular blocking agents

NURSING CONSIDERATIONS

Nursing Alerts

- Monitor serum levels, which should be obtained at least monthly in stabilized outpatient but as frequently as every other day during initial dosing phase. Toxic effects frequently develop when serum level rises above 1.5 mEq/L.
- Expect dosages to be much higher during the acute phase of treatment. To minimize toxicity, dosage should be reduced proportionately as therapeutic effects become evident.

1. Consult with prescriber if GI irritation occurs. Administration with meals or use of sustained-release forms or smaller, more frequent doses may help. Monitor results of serum level determinations to ensure that they remain consistent.
2. Help to evaluate patient's response to drug. Optimum therapeutic effects usually occur 7 to 14 days after initiation of treatment. Therapy should *not* be continued beyond 4 weeks if no response is evident.
3. Test urine periodically for specific gravity, and note signs of polydipsia and polyuria. These are common in the elderly and do not seem to be dose related; if these symptoms are severe, therapy may need to be discontinued.
4. Observe for signs of developing hypothyroidism (e.g., fatigue, weight gain, cold intolerance, puffy face). Symptoms are reversible upon cessation of therapy but may be controlled by supplemental thyroxine without discontinuing lithium therapy.
5. Provide supplemental fluid and salt in cases of prolonged sweating or diarrhea.

PATIENT EDUCATION

1. Instruct patient to consult physician immediately if signs of toxicity appear, such as diarrhea, vomiting, drowsiness, muscle weakness, ataxia, or tremor.
2. Stress the importance of adequate intake of salt and 2500–3000 mL of fluid per day. Reduced fluid intake can slow lithium excretion, resulting in increased toxicity.
3. Caution person about engaging in activities requiring alertness until reaction to lithium has been established. The drug may cause significant drowsiness and impaired coordination.
4. Teach patient to check for ankle or wrist edema and to record weekly weight. Sudden changes should be reported to drug prescriber.

Pimozide

Orap

Pimozide is a centrally acting dopamine receptor antagonist used to suppress severe motor and phonic tics in patients with Gilles de la Tourette's syndrome. This disorder is characterized by unpredictable and spontaneous outbursts of foul language or barking sounds and by other motor abnormalities. Some cases have been successfully managed by haloperidol, another dopamine antagonist, but pimozide appears to be most effective in treating resistant cases.

Prolonged use of pimozide is associated with a high frequency of tardive dyskinesias (see discussion earlier in the chapter) and dosage must be kept as low as possible to minimize the likelihood of tardive dyskinesias developing. Extrapyramidal reactions occur frequently, often during the first few days of treatment. Their severity and frequency are dose related and are usually reversible with dosage reduction. Many other untoward reactions have occurred in patients receiving pimozide, most of which are also seen with anti-psychotic drug use. Refer to **Significant Adverse Reactions** on p. 213 for a complete listing of potential adverse effects.

Pimozide is *contraindicated* in persons with a history of cardiac arrhythmias or QT interval disturbances, as sudden death has occurred because of ventricular arrhythmias.

The drug must be given *with caution* to patients with impaired renal or hepatic function and during pregnancy and nursing.

Pimozide may lower the convulsive threshold and may therefore interfere with the action of anticonvulsants, and it can potentiate the effects of other CNS depressants.

The initial dose of pimozide (tablets) is 1 mg to 2 mg daily in divided doses. Dosage may be gradually increased every other day until an optimal effect is noted. Usual maintenance doses are 10 mg/day or less. Periodic attempts should be made to reduce the dose to see if the tics persist.

PATIENT EDUCATION

1. Explain that a baseline ECG is usually prescribed prior to initiation of therapy. An ECG should also be obtained periodically throughout therapy, especially during periods of dosage adjustment, because cardiotoxicity can occur.
2. Warn patient to use caution in driving a car or engaging in potentially hazardous activities because hand tremors, drowsiness, and blurred vision may occur.
3. Teach patient and family how to recognize and report symptoms of extrapyramidal reactions. If dosage reduction fails to alleviate symptoms of a reaction, drug should be discontinued.
4. Inform patient that concomitant use of other CNS depressant drugs, including alcohol, will augment CNS depressant effects of pimozide.
5. Discuss interventions to help alleviate dry mouth. See **Plan of Nursing Care 4 (Antihistamines)** in Chapter 14 for specific information.
6. Discuss measures to minimize constipation (e.g., increased intake of fluid and dietary fiber).
7. Instruct patient to report other symptoms of anticholinergic effects (e.g., urinary retention, ataxia, dizziness). These may necessitate dosage reduction.

Droperidol

Inapsine

Droperidol is a butyrophenone producing tranquilization, sedation, and mild peripheral vascular dilation. It has a strong antiemetic effect and can potentiate the action of other CNS depressants. It is principally used in combination with a narcotic analgesic (fentanyl) as Innovar (see Chap. 17) to induce neuroleptanalgesia, which is a state of quietude, reduced motor activity, and indifference to pain. Alone, droperidol is given to provide tranquilization and reduce nausea and vomiting during surgical and diagnostic procedures, and as an adjunct to regional or general anesthesia.

The onset of action with IM or IV use is 3 to 10 minutes, and the duration lasts 2 to 4 hours; although altered consciousness may persist up to 12 hours.

Mild hypotension and tachycardia are common side effects and usually subside spontaneously. Postsurgical drowsiness is also a frequent occurrence with use of droperidol, especially when given as an adjunct to general anesthesia. Extrapyramidal reactions occur in approximately 1% of patients. Other untoward reactions reported include dizziness, shivering, bronchospasm, and postoperative hallucinations. When used in combination with fentanyl, respiratory depression, muscle rigidity, and elevated blood pressure have been noted.

Droperidol should be used *cautiously* in elderly, debilitated, and other poor-risk patients; during pregnancy; in children under 2 years; and in the presence of liver, kidney, or cardiac dysfunction.

Recommended dosage for the indications for droperidol are as follows:

Adults

Premedication: 2.5 mg to 10 mg IM 30 minutes to 60 minutes preoperatively

Adjunct to general anesthesia: 2.5 mg/20 lb to 25 lb IV during induction

Maintenance: 1.25 mg to 2.5 mg IV

Diagnostic procedures: 2.5 mg to 10 mg IM 30 to 60 minutes before procedure, then 1.25 mg to 2.5 mg IV as needed

Children (2–12 yr)

1 mg to 1.5 mg/20 lb to 25 lb for premedication or induction of anesthesia

NURSING CONSIDERATIONS

Nursing Alerts

- Monitor vital signs closely during use. Have fluids, vasopressors, and other necessary measures at hand to manage hypotension should it occur. Do *not* use epinephrine

> because reversal of pressor effect can occur, worsening the hypotension.
> - Observe for additive depressant effects when narcotics or other CNS depressants are used. Dosage of other CNS depressants should be reduced in the presence of droperidol.
> - When used with fentanyl (as Innovar), assess for early signs of respiratory depression such as dyspnea, restlessness, and rigidity, especially if rapid IV injection is given. Be prepared to provide respiratory assistance, and have necessary resuscitative equipment available (e.g., endotracheal tube, oxygen, suction apparatus).

1. Exercise care in moving and positioning patient following administration of droperidol because orthostatic hypotension may develop.
2. Observe for development of extrapyramidal reactions, which may occur up to 1 to 2 days after administration. They can usually be controlled with an antiparkinsonian agent.
3. Postoperatively, assist patient with ambulation and other activities until drowsiness disappears.
4. Carefully evaluate reaction of elderly or debilitated patient to initial dose, which should be small. Incremental doses should be based on response.

Methotrimeprazine

Levoprome
(CAN) Nozinan

A phenothiazine derivative having a profound CNS–depressant effect, methotrimeprazine is characterized by sedation, reduced motor activity, increased pain threshold, and amnesia. Analgesia is comparable to that elicited by morphine but is *not* accompanied by signs of dependence or addiction, even with prolonged use. It rarely produces respiratory depression and does not alter the cough reflex; high incidence of orthostatic hypotension and sedation, but most other phenothiazine-related side effects (e.g., extrapyramidal symptoms, anticholinergic effects) occur less frequently than with other antipsychotic drugs.

The principal indication for use of methotrimeprazine is for relief of moderate to severe pain in nonambulatory patients. Additional uses include obstetrical analgesia when respiratory depression is to be avoided and as a preanesthetic agent to produce somnolence and relief of anxiety and apprehension.

The principal side effect of methotrimeprazine is orthostatic hypotension, accompanied by weakness and fainting. This effect can be avoided by keeping the patient supine for at least 6 hours following the injection. The orthostatic hypotensive effect generally diminishes with continued administration. Other adverse effects include nausea and vomiting, abdominal discomfort, disorientation, weakness, urinary hesitancy, xerostomia, nasal congestion, pain and inflammation at the injection site, and agranulocytosis and jaundice with prolonged high-dose therapy.

Use of methotrimeprazine is *contraindicated* in the presence of severe myocardial, renal, or hepatic disease; significant hypotension; and in patients receiving antihypertensive drugs or CNS depressants, since additive effects can occur. The drug should not be used longer than 30 days, except where narcotics are contraindicated or in terminal illnesses. When used for prolonged periods, regular liver function tests and blood studies should be performed.

Methotrimeprazine is given by deep intramuscular injection into a large muscle mass. Intravenous and subcutaneous administration should be avoided. Usual dosage ranges are as follows:

Analgesia: 10 mg to 20 mg IM every 4 to 6 hours (5 mg–10 mg in elderly patients)
Obstetrical analgesia: 15 mg to 20 mg IM; repeat as needed
Preanesthetic sedation: 10 mg to 20 mg IM 1 to 3 hours before surgery, often with atropine or scopolamine in reduced doses
Postoperative analgesia: 2.5 mg to 7.5 mg IM every 4 to 6 hours as needed

Because methotrimeprazine is a phenothiazine derivative, refer to the discussion of antipsychotic drugs earlier in the chapter for additional information on potential adverse effects as well as drug interactions.

NURSING CONSIDERATIONS

Nursing Alerts
> - Keep patient recumbent for at least 6 hours following administration to avoid orthostatic hypotension. Supervise ambulation and provide assistance as needed.
> - Monitor blood pressure and pulse frequently until response stabilizes. If vasopressors are needed to combat hypotension, methoxamine or phenylephrine should be used. Epinephrine is *contraindicated* because reversal can occur.

1. Administer only by deep IM injection and in a syringe separate from other drugs (except atropine or scopolamine), as incompatibility can result.
2. Clarify appropriateness of long-term administration, as drug should not be used longer than 30 days, except where narcotics are contraindicated or in terminal illness. When used for prolonged periods, liver function tests and blood studies should be performed regularly.

PATIENT EDUCATION
1. Reassure patient receiving drug for prolonged period that hypotensive and sedative effects will diminish.

Selected Bibliography

Cahill C, Arana GW: Navigating neuroleptic malignant syndrome. Am J Nurs 86:671, 1986
Carlsson A: Antipsychotic drugs, neurotransmitters and schizophrenia. Am J Psychiatry 135:164, 1978
Dellefield K, Miller J: Psychotropic drugs and the elderly patient. Nurs Clin North Am 17(6):303, 1982
Diamond R: Drugs and the quality of life: The patient's point of view. J Clin Psychiatry 46:29, 1985
Ehrensing RH: Tardive dyskinesia. Arch Intern Med 138:1261, 1978
Harris E: Antipsychotic medications. Am J Nurs 81:1316, 1981
Harris E: Lithium. Am J Nurs 81:1310, 1981
Jeste DR, Wyatt RJ: Understanding and Treating Tardive Dyskinesia. New York, Gullford Press, 1982
Keltner NL, McIntyre CW: Neuroleptic malignant syndrome. J Neurosurg Nurs 17:363, 1985
Mansch TC: Current concepts in psychiatry: Schizophrenic disorders. N Engl J Med 305:1628, 1981

Rivera-Calimlin L, Hershey L: Neuroleptic concentrations and clinical response. Annu Rev Pharmacol Toxicol 24:361, 1984

Rosel-Greif VL: Drug induced dyskinesias. Am J Nurs 82:66, 1982

Shapiro AK, Shapiro E: Controlled study of pimozide vs placebo in Tourette's syndrome. J Am Acad Child Psychiatry 23:161, 1984

Snyder SH: Dopamine receptors, neuroleptics and schizophrenia. Am J Psychiatry 138:460, 1981

Tosteson DC: Lithium and mania. Sci Am 239:164, 1981

Youssef FA: Compliance with therapeutic regimens: A follow-up study for patients with affective disorders. J Adv Nurs 8:513, 1983

SUMMARY. ANTIPSYCHOTIC DRUGS

Drug	Preparations	Usual Dosage Range
Antipsychotic Agents	See Table 22-3	
Lithium Cibalith-S, Eskalith, Lithane, Lithobid, Lithonate, Lithotabs	Tablets: 300 mg Slow-release tablets: 300 mg, 450 mg Capsules: 300 mg Syrup: 300 mg/5 mL	*Acute mania:* 600 mg 3 times/day; adjust to optimal response *Prophylaxis:* 300 mg 3–4 times/day, or 300-mg slow-release tablets twice a day
Pimozide Orap	Tablets: 2 mg	Initially, 1 mg–2 mg in divided doses; increase dose every other day until optimal effect; maximum 10 mg/day
Droperidol Inapsine	Injection: 2.5 mg/mL	*Adults* Preanesthetic medication: 2.5 mg–10 mg IM Adjunct to general anesthesia: 2.5 mg/20 lb–25 lb IV Maintenance: 1.25 mg–2.5 mg IV Diagnostic procedures: 2.5 mg–10 mg IM initially; repeat with 1.25-mg–2.5-mg increments *Children* (2–12 yr) 1 mg to 1.5 mg/20 lb to 25 lb
Methotrimeprazine Levoprome	Injection: 20 mg/mL	Analgesia: 10 mg–20 mg IM/4–6 h (5 mg–10 mg in elderly) Obstetrical analgesia: 15 mg–20 mg IM, repeated as needed Preanesthetic medication: 10 mg–20 mg IM 1–3 h before surgery Postoperative analgesia: 2.5 mg–7.5 mg IM/4–6 h

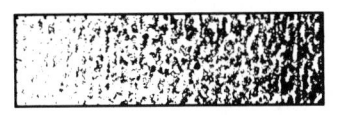

23 ANTIANXIETY DRUGS

Several drugs have the ability to induce mild sedation and reduce anxiety and tension in doses that do not generally impair mental alertness or psychomotor performance. Such drugs have been designated as *antianxiety agents* and have become a widely used and often abused class of drugs.

Pharmacologically, these compounds, especially when given in high doses, resemble the barbiturates in many ways; however, their principal advantage relative to the barbiturates is their significantly higher sedative:hypnotic ratio. In other words, the margin between the calming, tension-relieving dose and the hypnotic, sleep-inducing dose is much greater with the antianxiety agents than with the barbiturates. Likewise, their safety margin—therapeutic/toxic dose levels—is wider than that observed with barbiturates. Their primary use, therefore, is to provide a degree of relief from emotional symptoms (such as agitation, anxiety, muscle tension, and motor hyperactivity) associated with psychoneurotic and psychosomatic disorders. They are rarely satisfactory alone for controlling severely disturbed psychotic patients, although they have been employed in conjunction with antipsychotic drugs in treating acute psychotic episodes.

In contrast to the antipsychotic drugs however, antianxiety agents have a rather low incidence of adverse reactions when administered in normal therapeutic doses. Moreover, their central skeletal muscle−relaxant action may contribute to their effectiveness in treating emotional disorders compounded by excessive muscular tension or spasm. However, their prolonged use is associated with development of tolerance, and a significant potential for habituation and abuse exists with these compounds, whereas it is unlikely with the antipsychotic drugs.

Most antianxiety agents also have clinically significant anticonvulsant activity when administered IV and can effectively control acute convulsive states such as status epilepticus or those associated with acute alcohol withdrawal. Moreover, their use is not accompanied by extrapyramidal or autonomic side effects.

The currently available antianxiety agents can be conveniently classified into one of two groups:

I. *Benzodiazepines*: alprazolam, chlordiazepoxide, clorazepate, diazepam, halazepam, lorazepam, midazolam, oxazepam, prazepam
II. *Miscellaneous*: buspirone, chlormezanone, hydroxyzine, meprobamate

The benzodiazepines are reviewed as a group, followed by individual consideration of the remaining antianxiety agents.

BENZODIAZEPINE ANTIANXIETY AGENTS

Alprazolam	Halazepam
Chlordiazepoxide	Lorazepam
Clorazepate	Oxazepam
Diazepam	Prazepam

The benzodiazepines are the most widely used antianxiety agents. Much of their popularity derives from their demonstrated effectiveness at dosage levels that are not associated with the high risk of untoward reactions or the development of physical dependence that is characteristic of prolonged barbiturate consumption. The drugs in this group that are discussed in this chapter are indicated primarily for the relief of situational anxiety. Other benzodiazepines have somewhat different indications and are found elsewhere in this book. Midazolam is a short-acting drug used IM or IV as an adjunct in minor surgical procedures; it is reviewed following the general discussion of the benzodiazepines. Flurazepam (Dalmane), triazolam (Halcion), and temazepam (Restoril) are effective nonbarbiturate hypnotics used to relieve insomnia and are reviewed in Chapter 21. Clonazepam (Klonopin) is used in certain forms of epilepsy and is discussed in Chapter 25.

The effectiveness of benzodiazepines in relieving symptoms of anxiety over prolonged periods has not been conclusively established; these drugs should not be used for longer than 3 months to 4 months unless careful patient reassessment establishes a definite need for continued treatment.

Although all of the clinically useful benzodiazepines share many common pharmacologic properties (mild sedation, skeletal-muscle relaxation, anticonvulsant action) and differ little in their clinical efficacy, they differ significantly in their duration of action, depending upon whether they are converted to an active metabolite or an inactive conjugate. Table 23-1 lists the usual doses onset of action, metabolic activity, and elimination half-lives of the benzodiazepine drugs. The benzodiazepines are first discussed as a group; characteristics of each individual agent are outlined in Table 23-2.

MECHANISM

Act at several subcortical brain sites such as the limbic system and the reticular formation; higher cortical function is largely unaffected; potentiate the action of gamma-aminobutyric acid (GABA), an inhibitory neurotransmitter in the CNS, possibly by enhancing the binding of GABA to its receptor sites; direct GABA−mimetic action has also been proposed for the benzodiazepines; potentiation of GABA function results in reduced neuronal activity in subcortical brain regions that appear to modulate the level of emotional reactivity; enhancement of GABA activity in the spinal cord decreases activity in motor reflex pathways, resulting in skeletal muscle relaxation; the seizure threshold is elevated, resulting in a clinically significant anticonvulsant action for certain derivatives; even in large amounts, these agents, unlike the barbiturates, do not appear significantly to depress the respiratory or vasomotor centers

USES

Symptomatic relief of anxiety, tension, and irritability associated with neuroses, depression, psychoneuroses, and psychosomatic disorders (short-term use only—maximum 4 months)

Symptomatic relief of the symptoms of acute alcohol withdrawal (chlordiazepoxide, clorazepate, diazepam, oxazepam)

Preoperative sedation

Table 23-1
Benzodiazepine Metabolism

Drug	Usual Daily Dosage Range	Onset of Action: Oral Administration	Activity of Metabolites	Elimination Half-Life
Alprazolam Xanax	0.75–1.5 mg	Moderate	Inactive	10–15 h
Chlordiazepoxide Librium	15–100 mg	Moderate	Active	5–30 h
Clorazepate Tranxene	15–to 60 mg	Fast	Active	30–90 h
Diazepam Valium	4–40 mg	Very fast	Active	20–50 h
Halazepam Paxipam	80–160 mg	Moderate	Active	12–15 h
Lorazepam Ativan	2–8 mg	Moderate	Inactive	10–15 h
Oxazepam Serax	30–120 mg	Slow	Inactive	5–15 h
Prazepam Centrax	20–60 mg	Slow	Active	60–120 h

Relief of muscle hypertonicity associated with anxiety or tension states

Adjunctive therapy in the management of epileptic states (clorazepate, diazepam)

Control of acute (e.g., status epilepticus) or severe recurrent convulsive seizure states (diazepam or lorazepam IV)

Adjunctive treatment prior to cardioversion or endoscopic procedures to lessen anxiety and reduce recall (diazepam or lorazepam IV, IM)

Control of nocturnal enuresis and night terrors (experimental use only)

DOSAGE
See Table 23-2

FATE
Generally well absorbed orally although rates differ widely; IM absorption of lorazepam is rapid and complete, but that of chlordiazepoxide and diazepam is erratic; onset of action ranges from 30 to 60 minutes orally (diazepam has quickest onset of action) and 15 to 30 minutes IM; most drugs have long half-lives, and metabolites may be clinically active as well (see Table 23-1); drugs are lipid soluble and distribute widely throughout the body; protein binding is high (80%–99%); most drugs (except oxazepam and lorazepam) have long elimination half-lives, since their metabolites are also clinically active (see Table 23-1); prazepam and clorazepate are inactive as parent compounds but are metabolized to desmethyldiazepam, an active metabolite; excreted as both unchanged drug and metabolites, largely through the kidneys; elimination may occur in two stages; a rapid (within several hours) phase followed by a slower (within days) phase; danger of accumulation exists with prolonged use

COMMON SIDE EFFECTS
Drowsiness, fatigue, lethargy, and ataxia (most common during early stages of therapy)

SIGNIFICANT ADVERSE REACTIONS
(Not all reactions observed with every drug)

CNS: confusion, disorientation, agitation, slurred speech, headache, syncope, vertigo, depression, hyporeactivity, stupor, tremor; paradoxical excitement (hostility, rage, muscle spasticity, irritability, vivid dreams, euphoria, insomnia, hallucinations) can occur, especially in psychotic patients

Autonomic: dry mouth, constipation, urinary retention, blurred vision, diplopia

Cardiovascular/hematologic: bradycardia, hypotension, edema and weight gain, cardiovascular collapse, agranulocytosis, neutropenia

Hypersensitivity: skin rash, urticaria, fever, angioneurotic edema, bronchial spasm

Other: changes in libido, menstrual irregularities, nasal congestion, salivation, hiccups, difficulty swallowing, hepatic dysfunction (jaundice), pain or thrombophlebitis on IV injection

Overdosage with benzodiazepines alone is seldom fatal; most fatalities result from multiple drug ingestion. Symptoms of overdosage include drowsiness, confusion, ataxia, and hypotension but significant circulatory or respiratory depression is rare

CONTRAINDICATIONS
Severe psychoses, narrow-angle glaucoma, shock, in children under 6 years (except diazepam—children under 6 months). *Cautious use* in addiction-prone persons, in pregnant or nursing women, in elderly or debilitated persons, and in the presence of liver or kidney disease, severe muscle weakness. Injectable benzodiazepines must be given with caution to persons in shock, in acute alcohol intoxication, and those with limited pulmonary reserve

INTERACTIONS
May enhance the CNS-depressant effects of alcohol, barbiturates, antihistamines, phenothiazines, opiates, and other CNS-depressant drugs

The effects of phenytoin may be potentiated by benzodiazepines

An increased muscle-relaxant effect can occur with combinations of benzodiazepines and other centrally and peripherally acting muscle relaxants

The effects of levodopa may be antagonized by benzodiazepines

The effects of benzodiazepines may be lessened in individuals who smoke

Antacids or food may slow oral absorption of some benzodiazepines

The half-life of some benzodiazepines, but *not* lorazepam or oxazepam, can be prolonged by cimetidine

NURSING CONSIDERATIONS

See **Plan of Nursing Care** 7 in this chapter. In addition:
1. Monitor results of blood cell counts and liver function tests, which should be performed periodically during prolonged therapy.
2. Follow proper procedures for handling Schedule IV drugs.

PATIENT EDUCATION

See **Plan of Nursing Care** 7. In addition:
1. Teach patient and family how to identify paradoxical excitatory effects. If they occur, the drug should be discontinued, and appropriate supportive care should be provided.
2. Instruct patient to report early signs of developing jaundice (nausea, diarrhea, abdominal pain, rash) or blood dyscrasias (sore throat, fever, weakness, mucosal ulceration), which are indications for discontinuing the drug.
3. Instruct patient not to abruptly discontinue therapy after long-term treatment because withdrawal symptoms (e.g., vomiting, cramping, sweating, tremor, convulsions) can occur and may persist for several days. If withdrawal symptoms occur, they should be treated symptomatically as needed.
4. Warn woman with childbearing potential that congenital malformations can occur if drug is taken during early pregnancy. Discourage use during this period.

Midazolam
Versed

Midazolam is a short-acting benzodiazepine used parenterally for preoperative and perioperative sedation and as a supplement to nitrous oxide anesthesia for short surgical procedures. Its actions resemble those of the other benzodiazepines, and its onset of sedative action is very rapid following injection. It

---

PLAN OF NURSING CARE 7
PATIENTS TREATED WITH BENZODIAZEPINE ANTIANXIETY DRUGS
Nursing Diagnosis: Potential for Injury related to CNS depression from antianxiety drug therapy
Goal: Patient will not be injured as a result of effects of CNS depression from antianxiety drug therapy.

Intervention	Rationale	Expected Outcome
Assess patient for evidence of excessive CNS depression, such as ataxia, confusion, dizziness, drowsiness, muscle weakness, and slurred speech.	CNS depressant effects are dose-dependent. A dosage reduction usually eliminates excessive CNS depression. Dosage should be carefully regulated in the elderly or debilitated patient because delayed excretion and prolonged half-life usually necessitate smaller, less frequent doses.	Excessive CNS depression will be identified
If CNS effects are pronounced, inform drug prescriber, and discuss potential modifications in drug regimen.		Patient will manifest fewer signs of CNS depression.
Collaborate with patient and health care team to plan optimal dosing schedule.	To minimize daytime drowsiness, a long-acting drug taken once a day at bedtime may promote sleep as well as control anxiety. If necessary, small supplemental doses can be taken during the day.	Patient will verbalize satisfaction with drug regimen.
Protect safety of hospitalized patient: 1. Instruct unsteady patient to seek assistance when getting out of bed. 2. Supervise ambulation. 3. Use siderails for elderly or debilitated patient.	Daytime drowsiness is the most common side effect. As warranted, the patient should be protected from injury. The elderly or debilitated patient is most susceptible to CNS side effects.	Patient will not fall.
With IV administration: 1. Monitor vital signs, have resuscitative equipment available, and observe patient carefully, particularly if patient is elderly, seriously ill, debilitated, or has limited pulmonary reserve. 2. Keep patient supine for several hours following administration, then help patient get out of bed slowly. 3. Assist with ambulation.	IV administration may produce marked muscle weakness, respiratory depression, and hypotension, especially in the presence of narcotics.	Potential adverse consequences of IV administration will either be avoided or recognized and treated promptly.
Warn patient to use caution in engaging in potentially hazardous activities (e.g., driving, operating machinery) during early stages of therapy.	CNS-depressant side effects may be dangerous if mental alertness or motor coordination is required for safety.	Patient will explain hazards of CNS depressant effects in performing potentially dangerous activities.
Explain that sedative effects of antianxiety drugs, alcohol, and other CNS-depressant drugs, both OTC and prescription, are additive.	Excessive CNS depression is most likely to occur with combined usage of CNS depressants.	Patient will state the effect of combined usage of CNS depressants.

Continued

PLAN OF NURSING CARE 7 (continued)
PATIENTS TREATED WITH BENZODIAZEPINE ANTIANXIETY DRUGS

Nursing Diagnosis: Potential Ineffective Individual Coping related to anxiety and the possibility that psychological or physical dependence on antianxiety drugs may develop
Goal: Patient will not become dependent on antianxiety drugs.

Intervention	Rationale	Expected Outcome
Attempt to reduce patient's level of anxiety: 1. Assess contributing factors 2. Alleviate contributing factors as much as possible 3. Provide optimistic, empathic reassurance 4. Decrease sensory stimulation	Reducing the level of anxiety reduces the amount of drug needed to control anxiety.	Patient will manifest fewer physiological signs of anxiety Patient will verbalize feeling calmer
Help patient identify factors contributing to anxiety. Assist patient to recognize and mobilize resources to help resolve issues related to anxiety. Help patient to further develop adaptive coping mechanisms. As needed, refer patient and family to appropriate resources for additional assistance.	It may be possible to help the patient learn to cope more effectively with stressors and anxiety. The more skills the patient has to cope with anxiety, the less likely it is that reliance on drug therapy will develop.	Patient will verbalize increased confidence in ability to cope effectively with anxiety.
Explain that antianxiety drug therapy is intended only for short-term use. Discuss the possibility that psychological or physical dependence may develop. Emphasize the importance of adhering to prescribed regimen.	The effectiveness of antianxiety drug therapy appears to diminish after 3–5 mo. Although abuse liability is low, excessive daily doses or prolonged use (beyond 3–5 mo) can lead to physical dependence. Psychological dependence may also develop.	Patient will express awareness of: 1. The short-term nature of drug therapy 2. The possibility of dependence with long-term use 3. The need to adhere to prescribed regimen
Carefully evaluate requests for higher dosages or shorter dosing intervals.	If higher dosages are needed to maintain similar effects, tolerance, increased anxiety, or both could be factors. Higher dosages, however, increase the likelihood that dependence might develop.	Patient requests for additional medication will be evaluated.

Table 23-2
Benzodiazepines

Drug	Preparations	Usual Dosage Range	Nursing Implications
Alprazolam Xanax	Tablets: 0.25 mg, 0.5 mg, 1.0 mg	Initially, 0.25 mg–0.5 mg 3 times/day; maximum total dose is 4 mg/day Elderly persons: 0.25 mg 2–3 times/day	Metabolized to benzophenone, which is inactive, and alpha hydroxyalprazolam, which is approximately one-half as active as alprazolam; has a short half-life (12–15 h) and relatively brief duration of action; possesses antidepressant activity, particularly at higher doses; drowsiness and light-headedness are common during early stages of therapy (Schedule IV)
Chlordiazepoxide Libritabs, Librium, Lipoxide, Mitran, Reposans-10 (CAN) Apo-Chlordiazepoxide, Medilium, Novopoxide, Solium	Capsules: 5 mg, 10 mg, 25 mg Tablets: 5 mg, 10 mg, 25 mg Powder for injection: 100 mg/5 mL	**Oral** *Adults:* Anxiety—5 mg–10 mg 3–4 times/day up to 25 mg 4 times/day Alcohol withdrawal—50 mg–100 mg up to 300 mg/day	Less potent than diazepam and has less anticonvulsive activity; excreted slowly by the kidneys, so danger of accumulation exists; prepare IM solution immediately before administration and discard unused portion; do not use IM diluent if hazy or opalescent;

Continued

Table 23-2
Benzodiazepines (continued)

Drug	Preparations	Usual Dosage Range	Nursing Implications
		Children (over 6 yr): 5 mg–10 mg 2–4 times/day as needed **Parenteral** Adults: 50 mg–100 mg IM or IV Children (over 12 yr): 25 mg–50 mg IM or IV	IM solution should *not* be given IV because of air bubbles that form in solution; inject slowly and deeply IM; IV solution can be prepared with sterile water or saline; give IV injection slowly over 1 minute; do *not* inject IV solution IM because pain is common; do *not* add to IV infusion because solution is unstable and quickly deteriorates; sterilization by heating should *not* be attempted; available in combination with amitriptyline as Limbitrol for treatment of anxious depressions (Schedule IV)
Clorazepate Gen-Xene, Tranxene (CAN) Novoclopate	Capsules: 3.75 mg, 7.5 mg, 15 mg Tablets: 3.75 mg, 7.5 mg, 15 mg Long-acting tablets: 11.25 mg, 22.5 mg	*Anxiety:* 15 mg–60 mg daily in divided doses *or* 11.25 mg to 22.5 mg once a day; elderly persons: 7.5 mg–15 mg/day *Adjunct to anticonvulsants:* Adults: 7.5 mg 3 times/day initially; increase gradually Children: 7.5 mg twice a day; increase gradually. *Alcohol withdrawal* Day 1: 30 mg initially, then 30 mg–60 mg in divided doses Day 2: 45 mg–90 mg in divided doses Day 3: 22.5 mg–45 mg in divided doses Day 4: 15 mg–30 mg in divided doses	Slow onset (about 60 min) and fairly long duration (up to 24 h) of action: active metabolite is desmethyldiazepam; single daily dose is usually given at bedtime; recommended in children *only* as adjunct to other anticonvulsant drugs; effects parallel those of diazepam (Schedule IV)
Diazepam Valium, Zetran, and several other manufacturers (CAN) E-PAM, Novodipam	Tablets: 2 mg, 5 mg, 10 mg Capsules (sustained-release): 15 mg Injection: 5 mg/mL Oral solution: 1 mg/mL, 5 mg/mL	**Oral** *Adults* Anxiety: 2 mg–10 mg 2–4 times/day *or* 15 mg–30 mg/day sustained-release capsules Alcohol withdrawal: 10 mg 3–4 times/day initially, followed by 5 mg 3–4 times/day Adjunct in muscle spasm and convulsive states: 2 mg–10 mg 2–4 times/day *or* 15 mg–30 mg once daily *Children* (over 6 mo): 1 mg–2.5 mg 3–4 times/day; may increase gradually as required **Parenteral** *Adults* Psychoneuroses: 2 mg–10 mg IM or IV every 3–4 h as necessary depending on severity of symptoms Alcohol withdrawal: 5 mg–10 mg IM or IV; repeat every 3–4 h Preoperative and minor surgical procedures (e.g., endoscopy): 5 mg–10 mg IM *or* 10 mg IV prior to procedure	Effects occur within 20–30 min with oral administration, 15–30 min IM, and immediately IV; when using IV, inject slowly (5 mg/min) and avoid small veins to reduce danger of thrombophlebitis and local swelling and irritation; do *not* mix or dilute with other solutions or add to IV fluids; IM injection should be made deeply and slowly into a large muscle such as the gluteus; when used to control convulsions, be prepared to readminister drug if seizures recur, as duration of action with IV use is rather short; use cautiously in patients with chronic lung disease or unstable cardiovascular status; facilities for respiratory assistance should be present when drug is given parenterally; use of diazepam for endoscopic procedures has been associated with coughing, dyspnea, hyperventilation, laryngospasm, and pain in the throat and chest; use a topical

Continued

Table 23-2
Benzodiazepines (continued)

Drug	Preparations	Usual Dosage Range	Nursing Implications
		Status epilepticus: 5 mg–10 mg IV; repeat at 10–15-min intervals to a maximum of 30 mg Cardioversion: 5 mg–15 mg IV 5–10 min before procedure *Children:* Tetanus: 2 mg–10 mg, IM *or* slow IV every 3–4 h Status epilepticus: Under 5 yr—0.2 mg–0.5 mg by slow IV every 2–5 min; over 5 yr—1 mg every 2–5 min	anesthetic and have countermeasures available (e.g., respiratory assistance); reduce dose of narcotic analgesic by one third when used with diazepam (Schedule IV)
Halazepam Paxipam	Tablets: 20 mg, 40 mg	20 mg–40 mg 3 or 4 times/day; elderly persons—20 mg 1–2 times/day	Long-acting benzodiazepine; maximum plasma levels are attained in 1–3 h; highly protein-bound; do *not* use in children under 18 (Schedule IV)
Lorazepam Alzapam, Ativan, Loraz (CAN) Apo-Lorazepam, Novolorazem	Tablets: 0.5 mg, 1 mg, 2 mg Injection: 2 mg/mL, 4 mg/mL	**Oral** Anxiety: 1 mg–2 mg 2–3 times/day Insomnia: 2 mg–4 mg at bedtime **IM** Preoperative medication: 0.05 mg/kg 2 h before procedure (maximum 4 mg) **IV** Acute anxiety: 2 mg–4 mg	Short-acting drug used for anxiety, preanesthetic medication and temporary relief of insomnia; *not* recommended in children less than 12 yr; dosage must be individually titrated; increase dose gradually to minimize adverse effects; elderly or debilitated persons should receive an initial dose of 1 mg–2 mg/day; less danger of accumulation than with other derivatives because no active metabolites are formed; inject IM deep into muscle mass; dilute in appropriate diluent for IV administration; do not use if discolored (Schedule IV)
Oxazepam Serax, Zaxopam (CAN) Apo-Oxazepam Novoxapam, Ox-Pam, Zapex	Capsules: 10 mg, 15 mg, 30 mg Tablets: 15 mg	Adults: 10 mg–30 mg 3–4 times/day Elderly or debilitated persons: 10 mg 3–4 times/day	Has shorter duration of action than diazepam and produces a lower incidence of side effects; *not* recommended in children under 6 yr of age; paradoxical excitation may occur in first 2 wk of therapy; reduce dosage until symptoms subside (Schedule IV)
Prazepam Centrax	Tablets: 10 mg Capsules: 5 mg, 10 mg, 20 mg	Adults: 20 mg–60 mg/day in divided doses Elderly persons: 10 mg–15 mg/day	Slow onset and prolonged duration of action; not indicated in patients under 18 yr of age; can be used as a single daily dose (20 mg–40 mg) at bedtime; similar to diazepam in actions and toxicity (Schedule IV)

induces a slight to moderate decrease in mean arterial pressure, cardiac output, stroke volume, and systemic vascular resistance.

MECHANISM
See general discussion of the benzodiazepines earlier in the chapter

USES
Preoperative sedation and reduced recall of perioperative events (IM)

Production of sedation prior to short diagnostic or endoscopic procedures (alone or with a narcotic drug; IV)

Induction of general anesthesia, before administration of other anesthetic agents (IV)

Supplementation of nitrous oxide-oxygen anesthesia for short surgical procedures (IV)

DOSAGE
Preoperative/perioperative sedation: 0.07 mg/kg to 0.08 mg/kg IM 1 hour before surgery

Endoscopic or cardiovascular procedures: 0.1 mg/kg to 0.15 mg/kg IV (up to 0.2 mg/kg); dosage should be reduced if narcotic premedication is used or if given to patients over 60 years of age

Induction of general anesthesia: 0.3 mg/kg to 0.35 mg/kg initially (IV); increments of 25% of the initial dose may be given if needed after 2 to 3 minutes. If patient has received narcotic premedication, the recommended dose is 0.15 mg/kg to 0.3 mg/kg IV

FATE
Onset of sedation is within 15 minutes after IM injection and 2 to 3 minutes following IV administration; anesthesia occurs within 2 minutes with IV injection; approximately 97% protein bound; elimination half-life is variable (1–12 h); awakening from general anesthesia usually occurs within 2 hours

COMMON SIDE EFFECTS
Nausea, hiccups, decreased respiratory rate and tidal volume, pain and tenderness on IM injection, headache, muscle stiffness

SIGNIFICANT ADVERSE REACTIONS
CNS: sedation, headache, confusion, dizziness, amnesia, nervousness, agitation, anxiety, delirium, insomnia, nightmares, tremor, involuntary movements, ataxia, paresthesias, slurred speech, blurred vision, and tonic/clonic movements

Cardiovascular: premature ventricular contractions, tachycardia, bigeminy, hematoma at IM injection site

Respiratory: bronchospasm, laryngospasm, dyspnea, hyperventilation, wheezing, tachypnea

Dermatologic: swelling or feeling of burning or warmth at injection site, rash, pruritus, urticaria

Other: salivation, retching, yawning, lethargy, weakness, chills, toothache

Symptoms of overdosage are characteristic of other benzodiazepines and include somnolence, sedation, confusion, impaired coordination, reduced reflexes, and respiratory distress. Treatment is supportive

CONTRAINDICATIONS
Acute narrow-angle glaucoma, acute alcohol intoxication, significantly depressed vital signs, pregnancy. *Cautious use* in persons with respiratory disease, hypotension, congestive heart failure, or renal dysfunction and in elderly or debilitated persons

INTERACTIONS
The duration or degree of respiratory depression may be enhanced by concurrent use of other respiratory depressants, such as barbiturates, narcotics, alcohol, and so on

The dosage of induction or inhalational anesthetics may need to be reduced if midazolam is used preoperatively

The hypnotic effects of midazolam may be accentuated by preanesthetic use of narcotics, barbiturates, or other sedative agents

NURSING CONSIDERATIONS
See benzodiazepines. However, because midazolam use is limited principally to singular occasions, risks associated with ongoing benzodiazepine therapy are negligible.

MISCELLANEOUS ANTIANXIETY AGENTS

Buspirone
BuSpar

Buspirone is a chemically and pharmacologically unique antianxiety agent that appears to be as effective as the benzodiazepines in treating general anxiety but does not possess their muscle-relaxant, anticonvulsant, sedative or alcohol-potentiating actions. In addition, there is no evidence that buspirone use leads to dependence or habituation and it is *not* a controlled substance.

MECHANISM
Interacts with serotonin 1_A receptor sites in several brain regions; may also function as a dopamine agonist; decreases anxiety without producing significant sedation or muscle relaxation; does *not* interact with GABA as do the benzodiazepines; no anticonvulsant activity; drug has not been shown to increase alcohol-induced CNS depression or motor impairment; tolerance and habituation have not been demonstrated upon continual therapy

USES
Short-term management of anxiety disorders (efficacy for longer than 3–4 wk has not been conclusively demonstrated although patients have been given the drug for several months with no obvious untoward effect)

DOSAGE
Initially, 5 mg 3 times a day; increase by 5-mg increments at 2 or 3-day intervals as needed; usual maintenance range is 20 mg/day to 30 mg/day in divided doses

FATE
Oral absorption is rapid and peak plasma levels occur within 45 to 90 minutes; first-pass hepatic metabolism is extensive; approximately 95% of buspirone is protein bound in the plasma; drug is metabolized by the liver, mainly to inactive hydroxylated metabolites, which are excreted largely in the urine (30%–65%) with lesser amounts in the feces (20%–40%); elimination half-life is 2 to 3 hours.

COMMON SIDE EFFECTS
Nausea, headache, dizziness, lightheadedness, nervousness

SIGNIFICANT ADVERSE REACTIONS
CNS: dysphoria, loss of interest, akathisia, fearfulness, hallucinations, seizures, impaired concentration, confusion, depression, paresthesias, tremor, incoordination, slurred speech, cold intolerance, and suicidal ideation

GI: anorexia, dry mouth, diarrhea, salivation, irritable colon, rectal bleeding

Genitourinary: urinary hesitancy, menstrual irregularities, dysuria
Dermatologic: rash, edema, pruritus, flushing, easy bruising, dry skin, hair loss
Musculoskeletal: muscle cramps, arthralgia, muscle spasm
Respiratory: hyperventilation, dyspnea, chest congestion
Neurologic: involuntary movements, slowed reaction time
Other: altered taste or smell sensation, nasal congestion, muscle aching, tinnitus, blurred vision, conjunctivitis, itching of the eyes, altered libido, increased SGOT and SGPT, weight gain, fever

Overdosage can cause vomiting, drowsiness, dizziness, gastric distress, and miosis. No deaths have occurred with doses as high as 375 mg. Treatment is supportive

CONTRAINDICATIONS
No absolute contraindications *Cautious use* in persons with liver or kidney impairment, parkinsonism, in pregnant or nursing women, and in children under 18

INTERACTIONS
Buspirone can displace digoxin from protein binding sites, possibly potentiating its effects and toxicity

Buspirone may have additional CNS-depressive effects when given together with other depressants, such as hypnotics, narcotics, and alcohol, although the likelihood of a clinically significant interaction is minimal

Concurrent use of buspirone and an MAO inhibitor can result in a hypertensive reaction

NURSING CONSIDERATION
1. Advocate use of a different anxiolytic agent if patient needs either immediate relief from anxiety or an intermittent drug regimen for episodic anxiety, because the antianxiety effects of buspirone are not evident until after 1 or 2 weeks of use.

PATIENT EDUCATION
1. Inform patient that anxiolytic effects may not be apparent until after 1 or 2 weeks of use.
2. Warn patient to exercise caution in engaging in potentially hazardous activities until drug effects are known, because dizziness and nervousness may occur. Although significant sedation is unusual with normal therapeutic doses, it may occur at higher doses.
3. Instruct patient to be alert for and to immediately report any abnormal involuntary movements (e.g., dystonias, facial movements), which can occur because of the drug's dopamine-agonistic activity.

Chlormezanone
Trancopal

An infrequently used antianxiety drug for the treatment of mild anxiety and tension states, chlormezanone has a usual dosage range of 100 mg to 200 mg, 3 to 4 times/day for adults, and 50 mg to 100 mg 3 or 4 times/day in children 5 to 12 years of age. Its onset of action is 15 to 30 minutes, and effects persist for up to 6 hours. Adverse reactions can include dizziness, rash, drowsiness, dryness of the mouth, muscle weakness, edema, and depression.

The warnings, precautions, and nursing considerations discussed previously in connection with the benzodiazepines generally pertain to the use of chlormezanone as well. The drug has no particular advantage over the other antianxiety agents and is largely obsolete.

Hydroxyzine
Atarax, Vistaril, and several other manufacturers
(CAN) Apo-Hydroxyzine, Multipax

Hydroxyzine is a diphenylmethane derivative having a mild CNS-depressant action, together with anticholinergic, antihistaminic, local anesthetic, antiemetic, antispasmodic, antisecretory, and skeletal muscle–relaxant effects. It has a good safety margin, and adverse reactions are minimal at recommended doses; it is frequently used in children as a mild sedative.

MECHANISM
Not completely established; may suppress activity in subcortical brain areas but appears to have little effect on the cortex; blocks action of histamine and exerts both a direct and an indirect (through its sedative action) skeletal muscle–relaxant effect

USES
Symptomatic treatment of psychoneurotic states characterized by anxiety, tension, hostility, and motor hyperactivity

Adjunctive preoperative and prepartum therapy to help reduce anxiety and lessen narcotic analgesic requirements

Relief of anxiety symptoms associated with organic disturbances such as digestive disorders, allergic conditions, organic brain syndrome, menopause, alcoholism, and behavioral problems, especially in children

Relief of pruritus associated with urticaria, dermatoses, and other histamine-mediated conditions

Adjunctive treatment of alcohol withdrawal or delirium tremens (IM)

DOSAGE
Oral
  Relief of anxiety: adults—50 mg to 100 mg 4 times/day; children—50 mg to 100 mg/day in divided doses
  Relief of pruritus: adults—25 mg 3 to 4 times/day; children—50 mg to 100 mg/day in divided doses
  Preoperative sedation: adults—50 mg to 100 mg; children—0.6 mg/kg
Intramuscular
  Acute alcoholism: 50 mg to 100 mg every 4 to 6 hours as needed
  Nausea/vomiting: adults—25 mg to 100 mg; children—1.1 mg/kg
  Preoperative/postoperative: adults—25 mg to 100 mg; children—1.1 mg/kg

FATE
Rapidly absorbed orally and parenterally; onset of action within 15 to 30 minutes; effects last for up to 6 hours; metabolized primarily in the liver and largely excreted via the bile in the feces; some drug appears in the urine

COMMON SIDE EFFECTS
Transitory drowsiness, dry mouth

SIGNIFICANT ADVERSE REACTIONS
Involuntary motor activity, dizziness; rarely, hypersensitivity reactions (urticaria, skin eruptions, erythema multiforme)

CONTRAINDICATIONS

Early pregnancy (fetal abnormalities can occur)

INTERACTIONS

May exert additive effects with other CNS depressants (e.g., alcohol, hypnotics, narcotics)

NURSING CONSIDERATION
1. When giving IM, inject deeply into large muscle mass.

PATIENT EDUCATION
1. Caution patient against driving or operating machinery during early stages of therapy because drowsiness can occur.
2. Suggest interventions to relieve mouth dryness. See **Plan of Nursing Care 4 (Antihistamines)** in Chapter 14 for specific information.

Meprobamate

Equanil, Miltown, and several other manufacturers
(CAN) Apo Meprobamate, Meditran, Neotran, Novomepro

Meprobamate is an antianxiety agent that more closely resembles a barbiturate than a benzodiazepine. Its CNS-depressant actions are similar to those of the barbiturates but are generally shorter in duration. Other effects produced by meprobamate include skeletal muscle relaxation and, in large doses, an anticonvulsant action. It also reduces REM sleep time. Prolonged use can result in habituation and dependence, and meprobamate is somewhat more dangerous in this regard than the benzodiazepines.

MECHANISM

Not well established; appears to act at several subcortical loci, including the limbic system and thalamus; no specific depressant effects on the reticular activating system or the autonomic nervous system; suppresses REM sleep and exerts a skeletal muscle–relaxing effect, probably resulting in part from its sedative action

USES

Short-term relief of anxiety and tension associated with various disease states (alternative drug *only* to the benzodiazepines or buspirone)

DOSAGE

Adults: 1200 mg to 1600 mg/day in 3 or 4 divided doses
Children (6–12 yr): 100 mg to 200 mg 2 to 3 times/day

FATE

Well absorbed orally; onset of effect within 1 hour; plasma half-life is 6 to 18 hours but is prolonged with long-term use; uniformly distributed in the body; minimal protein binding; metabolized in the liver and largely excreted in the urine mainly as inactive metabolites; meprobamate induces liver microsomal enzymes and readily crosses placental barrier

COMMON SIDE EFFECTS

Drowsiness, ataxia, rash

SIGNIFICANT ADVERSE REACTIONS

CNS: dizziness, vertigo, slurred speech, weakness, paresthesias, headache, depression, confusion, paradoxical excitation, euphoria, hyperactivity

Hypersensitivity: pruritus, urticaria, fever, edema, petechiae, ecchymoses, adenopathy, bronchospasm, anaphylaxis, exfoliative dermatitis
Hematologic: leukopenia, agranulocytosis, thrombocytopenic purpura, aplastic anemia, pancytopenia
Cardiovascular: hypotension, flushing, syncope, palpitations, tachycardia, arrhythmias
GI: nausea, vomiting, diarrhea, dry mouth, glossitis
Other: exacerbation of porphyria, increased incidence of grand mal attacks, pain at IM injection site

CONTRAINDICATIONS

Acute intermittent porphyria, renal insufficiency (IM use), and children under 6. *Cautious use* in epileptics, persons with liver or kidney impairment, addiction-prone persons, and in elderly or debilitated patients

INTERACTIONS

Additive depressant effects can occur between meprobamate and other CNS depressants (e.g., alcohol, barbiturates, phenothiazines)

Meprobamate may augment the metabolism of oral anticoagulants and steroid hormones, thereby reducing their pharmacologic effects

NURSING CONSIDERATIONS
See **Benzodiazepines.**

PATIENT EDUCATION
See **Benzodiazepines.**

Selected Bibliography

Bellantuono C, Reggi V, Tognoni G, Garatini S: Benzodiazepines: Clinical pharmacology and therapeutic use. Drugs 19:195, 1980

Berger JG (ed): Antianxiety Agents. New York, John Wiley and Sons, 1986

Dement W, Seidel W, Carskadon M: Daytime alertness, insomnia and benzodiazepines. Sleep 5(1):S28, 1982

Goa KL, Ward A: Bispirone: A preliminary review of its pharmacological properties and therapeutic efficacy as an anxiolytic. Drugs 32:114, 1986

Goldberg HL: Benzodiazepine and nonbenzodiazepine anxiolytics. Psychopathology, 17(Suppl 1):45, 1984

Greenblatt DJ, Shader RI, Abernethy DR: Current status of benzodiazepines (2 parts). N Engl J Med 309:354, 410, 1983

Hershey LA, Kim KY: Diagnosis and treatment of anxiety in the elderly. Ration Drug Ther 22(3):1, 1988

Lader M: Clinical pharmacology of benzodiazepines. Annu Rev Med 38:19, 1987

Lader M: Rational use of anxiolytic drugs. Ration Drug Ther 21(9):1, 1987

Lader M, Petursson H: Long-term effects of benzodiazepines. Neuropharmacology 22:527, 1983

Meyer BR: Benzodiazepines in the elderly. Med Clin North Am 66:1017, 1982

Miller CA: PRN drugs . . . to give or not to give. Geriatr Nurs Jan/Feb:37, 1982

Olsen RW: Gaba-benzodiazepine-barbiturate receptor interactions. J Neurochem 37:1, 1981

Owen RT, Tyrer P: Benzodiazepine dependence. Drugs 25:385, 1983

Rosenbaum JF: The drug treatment of anxiety. N Engl J Med 306:401, 1982

Schopf J: Withdrawal phenomena after long-term administration of benzodiazepines: A review of recent investigations. J Pharmacopsychiatry 16:1, 1983

Tallman JF, Paul SM, Skolnick P, Gallager DW: Receptors for the age of anxiety: Pharmacology of the benzodiazepines. Science 207:274, 1980

Taylor DP: Buspirone, a new approach to the treatment of anxiety. FASEB J 2:2445, 1988

Trimble MR (ed): Benzodiazepines Divided: A Multidisciplinary Review. New York, John Wiley & Sons, 1983

Wincor MZ: Insomnia and the new benzodiazepines. Clin Pharm 1:425, 1982

SUMMARY. ANTIANXIETY DRUGS

Drug	Preparations	Usual Dosage Range
Benzodiazepines	See Table 23-2	
Midazolam Versed	Injection: 1 mg/mL, 5 mg/mL	*Sedation:* 0.07–0.08 mg/kg 1 h before surgery. *Endoscopy:* 0.1–0.2 mg/kg IV *Anesthesia:* 0.3–0.35 mg/kg IV; increments of 25% of initial dose every 2–3 min as needed
Buspirone BuSpar	Tablets: 5 mg, 10 mg	Initially: 5 mg 3 times/day *Maintenance dose:* 20 mg–30 mg/day in divided doses
Chlormezanone Trancopal	Tablets: 100 mg, 200 mg	Adults: 100 mg–200 mg 3–4 times/day Children (5–12 yr): 50 mg–100 mg 3–4 times/day
Hydroxyzine Atarax, Vistaril, and several other manufacturers	Tablets: 10 mg, 25 mg, 50 mg, 100 mg Capsules: 25 mg, 50 mg, 100 mg Syrup: 10 mg/5 mL, 25 mg/5 mL Injection: 25 mg/mL, 50 mg/mL Injection: 75 mg/dose, 100 mg/dose	*Oral* Adults: 25 mg–100 mg 3–4 times/day Children over 6 yr: 50 mg–100 mg daily in divided doses Children under 6 yr: 50 mg daily *IM* Adults: 25 mg–100 mg as required Children: 1.1 mg/kg
Meprobamate Equanil, Miltown, and several other manufacturers	Tablets: 200 mg, 400 mg, 600 mg Capsules: 400 mg Sustained-release capsules: 200 mg, 400 mg	*Oral* Adults: 1200 mg–1600 mg/day in divided doses (maximum 2400 mg/day) Children (6–12 yr): 100 mg–200 mg 2–3 times/day

24 ANTIDEPRESSANTS

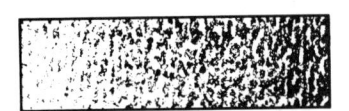

Antidepressants are drugs that can alleviate a variety of symptoms associated with a broad range of psychosomatic disorders collectively known as *depression*. Drug therapy is but one of a number of approaches to depression, however; others may include psychotherapy, counseling, and electroconvulsive therapy.

In some types of depressions, significant therapeutic benefit has been obtained with use of antidepressant drugs. Optimal clinical responses depend mainly upon an accurate diagnosis of the depressive state, and it is here that much controversy still exists. One useful, though not universally accepted, classification of depressions, based primarily upon their etiology, categorizes them as follows:

- Endogenous depressions
- Anxious, neurotic depressions
- Situational, reactive depressions
- Manic–depressive disorders

Endogenous depressions are characterized by absence of pleasure, emotional withdrawal, loss of libido, motor retardation, and sleep disturbances; they do *not* seem to have an external precipitating factor. Central neurohormonal imbalances are likely present in these types of depressions, and they can usually be successfully treated with antidepressant drugs.

Anxious, neurotic depressions are marked by anxiety, tension, "overreactiveness" to disappointment or losses, and signs of irritability, anger, hostility, and even helplessness. Classic antidepressant drugs are usually not very effective in these depressive states, yet they often respond to antianxiety or antipsychotic agents.

The *situational, reactive* types of depression are generally precipitated by stressful or grief-producing external factors, such as death of a loved one, serious illness, or loss of employment, and these comprise most clinical depressions. Because the cause *is* external, the depressive reaction is frequently self-limiting, and remission is often seen in a matter of weeks. Drug therapy is usually not indicated unless the disorder becomes severe or chronic and interferes with normal functioning.

Manic–depressive disorders are characterized by excessive and sometimes violent mood swings that tend to recur regularly. Treatment generally is effected with lithium (see Chap. 22), although antidepressants are sometimes used concurrently.

Severe depressions, in which agitation is a predominant feature or in which risk of suicide is high, are often best treated initially with electroconvulsive therapy (ECT). Rapid and dramatic improvement is frequently noted in severely depressed persons following ECT, making the disorder more amenable to subsequent drug therapy. Concurrent use of antidepressants during ECT may increase the hazards, and such therapy should be avoided. Patients receiving tricyclic antidepressants who are to undergo ECT should have the drugs discontinued for 24 to 48 hours prior to the ECT.

CLASSIFICATION OF ANTIDEPRESSANT DRUGS

The clinically useful antidepressant drugs can be categorized as belonging to one of the following groups:

A. *Tricyclic antidepressants* (e.g., imipramine, amitriptyline)
B. *Second-generation antidepressants* (e.g., fluoxetine, trazodone, bupropion)
C. *Monoamineoxidase inhibitors* (e.g., isocarboxazid, tranylcypromine)
D. *Amphetamines and other CNS stimulants* (e.g., dextroamphetamine, methylphenidate)

The *tricyclic antidepressants* are the most widely used drugs for the treatment of endogenous depression and are reviewed in detail below. Structurally dissimilar but pharmacologically comparable drugs, such as trazodone and fluoxetine are also considered here. They are sometimes referred to as "second-generation" antidepressants because their clinical activity is comparable to that of the tricyclics but their side-effect profile is somewhat different. Monoamine oxidase (MAO) inhibitors display a lower overall clinical effectiveness than the tricyclics but have a greater potential for eliciting untoward reactions, especially hypertensive responses. They are usually reserved for treating severe depressions not managed successfully by the tricyclic drugs. Finally, several central nervous system (CNS) stimulants, most of which are amphetamine derivatives, have been utilized in some instances of mild depressive states, but their lack of potency in more severe depressions and especially their potential for abuse have rendered their use in true depression essentially obsolete. They have other recognized indications, however, and are reviewed in Chapter 27.

TRICYCLIC ANTIDEPRESSANTS

Amitriptyline	Maprotiline (tetracyclic derivative)
Amoxapine	Nortriptyline
Desipramine	Protriptyline
Doxepin	Trimipramine
Imipramine	

Tricyclic antidepressants are so named because of their characteristic three-ring nuclear structure. They are further differentiated into secondary or tertiary amines based upon the configuration of their side chain (see Table 24-1). Some newer compounds (e.g., maprotiline) possess a four-ring nuclear structure. Although similar in most respects to the tricyclic drugs, they may have a lower incidence of some undesirable side effects. The discussion that follows uses the term *tricyclic* as a matter of convention; however, the information refers to the tetracyclic compounds as well. Differences among the several drugs are noted throughout the discussion where appropriate.

The currently available tricyclic antidepressants are structurally analogous to the phenothiazine antipsychotic agents, and there are many similarities in the pharmacologic and toxicologic spectrum of action of these two classes of drugs (e.g., sedation, anticholinergic action, orthostatic hypotension). The tricyclics are characterized by their *specific* blocking action on the uptake of biogenic amines at the nerve ending. Since uptake of these biogenic amines represents the major means by which their synaptic action is terminated, blockade of this reuptake mechanism by tricyclic drugs prolongs and potentiates the action of these amines at the synaptic junction, resulting in a more intense postsynaptic receptor activation.

It is important to realize that blockade of biogenic amine

Table 24-1
Pharmacologic Properties and Side Effects of Antidepressants

	Reuptake Blocking Activity		Side Effects		
	NE	5-HT	Anticholinergic	Sedative	Orthostatic Hypotension
Tricyclics					
Tertiary Amines					
Amitriptyline (Elavil)	+	+++	+++	+++	++
Doxepin (Sinequan, Adapin)	—	+	++	+++	++
Imipramine (Tofranil)	++	+++	++	++	+++
Trimipramine (Surmontil)	+	+	+++	+++	++
Secondary Amines					
Amoxapine (Asendin)	++	++	+	++	+
Desipramine (Norpramin, Pertofrane)	+++	+	+	+	+
Nortriptyline (Aventyl, Pamelor)	++	++	++	++	+
Protriptyline (Vivactil)	—	—	+++	0(+)	++
Tetracyclic					
Maprotiline (Ludiomil)	++	0(+)	+	++	+
Second Generation					
Bupropion (Wellbutrin)	+	+	++	+	0(+)
Trazodone (Desyrel)	0(+)	+++	+	++	++
Fluoxetine (Prozac)	0(+)	+++	++	+	+

+++ = Significant effect
++ = Moderate effect
+ = Slight effect
0(+) = Little or no effect
— = Data inconclusive

uptake into nerve endings is not the sole mechanism of the antidepressant action of the tricyclics. In fact, clinical observations suggest it may be only the initial event in a chain of reactions. It is well known that the therapeutic benefit—the relief of depressive symptoms—of the tricyclics is evident only after several weeks of continual therapy with most of the drugs, whereas the blocking effect of these drugs on amine uptake occurs almost immediately. Therefore, it is difficult to explain the latency of clinical action in view of the immediacy of the biochemical action. Increased synaptic biogenic amine levels subsequent to reuptake inhibition lead to a persistent occupation of postsynaptic receptor sites, which then become fewer in number and *hypo*sensitive. Loss of postsynaptic receptor population, termed *down-regulation,* is slow in developing when a patient is started on a tricyclic antidepressant, and the time course of the postsynaptic receptors' down-regulation closely corresponds to the onset of antidepressant activity in most instances. Therefore, it appears to play a major role in the therapeutic efficacy of the tricyclic antidepressants.

Selective differences exist among the different tricyclic drugs in their relative potency for blocking norepinephrine versus serotonin uptake. These differences, outlined in Table 24-1, may account for the varying degrees of effectiveness among tricyclics observed in different depressed populations, although there appears to be *no* consistent relationship between amine-uptake blocking action and clinical antidepressant efficacy.

Most tricyclic compounds have a sedative action in addition to their antidepressant effect, and all derivatives exert a degree of central and peripheral anticholinergic action and can induce orthostatic hypotension, especially in the elderly. Although these several side effects have been noted with most of the derivatives, the frequency of occurrence and degree of severity vary considerably among the different drugs, as outlined in Table 24-1. Again, however, there appears to be *no consistent relationship* between the differential amine-uptake blocking action of these drugs and the severity of side effects.

It might appear that tricyclics with prominent sedative activity would be most useful in depressive states characterized by anxiety or agitation, whereas a drug such as protriptyline, which is largely nonsedating, might be preferred in retarded or apathetic depressions. However, this differential applicability remains to be proved clinically.

Differences in amine-uptake blockade notwithstanding, the overall pharmacologic profile of the tricyclic antidepressants is quite similar. These drugs consequently are reviewed as a group. A profile of each individual drug is then presented in Table 24-2.

MECHANISM

Inhibit neuronal uptake of biogenic amines (norepinephrine, serotonin) into presynaptic endings, blocking a major mechanism for their inactivation and thereby potentiating their effects; may also exert a blocking effect at presynaptic alpha$_2$ receptor sites to increase release of norepinephrine and possibly serotonin; increased postsynaptic receptor activation cause a gradual decrease in the number and sensitivity of these receptors; the clinical efficacy of these agents is thought to be the result of *down-regulation* of beta-adrenergic and serotonergic receptors; drugs also possess anticholinergic, antihistaminic, and quinidine-like action and produce peripheral vasodilation and mild hypotension

USES

Relief of the symptoms of depression, especially of the endogenous types (see introduction)

Control of anxiety associated with depressive states (especially doxepin or amoxapine)

Treatment of depression in patients with manic–depressive disorders (especially maprotiline or doxepin)

Treatment of childhood enuresis (especially imipramine)

Investigational uses include enhanced control of acute pain (in combination with narcotic analgesics), prevention of migraine and cluster headaches (especially amitriptyline), treatment of obstructive sleep apnea (protriptyline), symptomatic management of peptic ulcer disease (doxepin, trimipramine), and treatment of attention-deficit disorders (desipramine)

DOSAGE

See Table 24-2

Dosage should be tailored to patient's needs: Use lowest effective dose for maintenance therapy, and observe patient carefully for continued clinical progress. Gradually taper dosage after symptoms have been controlled for some time (at least 3 mo), but be alert for possible relapse. Do not use in children under 12 years of age except for treatment of enuresis in children 6 to 12 years; see Table 24-2

FATE

Well absorbed from the GI tract but undergo extensive first-pass hepatic inactivation; peak plasma concentrations attained within 2 to 4 hours; widely distributed in the body and highly bound to plasma proteins (75%–95%); wide individual variation in plasma levels and plasma half-life (e.g., 8–60 h) caused by variability in liver metabolic activity; metabolized in the liver, often to therapeutically active compounds (e.g., imipramine to desipramine; amitriptyline to nortriptyline); hydroxylated metabolites excreted in the urine, along with small amounts of unchanged drug

COMMON SIDE EFFECTS

Sedation, anticholinergic effects (dryness of the mouth, blurred vision, tachycardia, constipation, urinary hesitancy), headache, muscle twitching, and weight gain

In children (*when used for enuresis*): nervousness, insomnia, lethargy, and GI disturbances

SIGNIFICANT ADVERSE REACTIONS

CNS: anxiety, restlessness, agitation, irritability, fever, insomnia, nightmares, disorientation, confusion, delusions, hypomania, hallucinations, dizziness, tinnitus, numbness and tingling in extremities, ataxia, tremors, extrapyramidal symptoms, paresthesias, seizures

Cardiovascular: orthostatic hypotension, arrhythmias, palpitations, congestive heart failure, infarction, heart block, stroke; ECG changes include prolongation of the PR and QT intervals, reduction of the T wave and formation of a prominent U wave (*caution* in persons with cardiovascular disorders)

Allergic: skin rash, pruritus, urticaria, petechiae, photosensitization, edema, fever

GI: nausea, anorexia, vomiting, diarrhea, cramping, epigastric distress, stomatitis

Endocrine: galactorrhea, gynecomastia, testicular and breast swelling, altered libido, delayed ejaculation or impotence, altered blood sugar levels

Hematologic: blood dyscrasias (agranulocytosis, eosinophilia, leukopenia, thrombocytopenia), bone marrow depression

Other: altered liver function (including jaundice), alopecia, parotid gland enlargement, flushing, sweating, chills, nocturia, nasal congestion, lacrimation

Overdosage is characterized by CNS signs, such as confusion, agitation, hyperreflexia, seizures, and hallucinations; autonomic effects such as dilated pupils, flushing, and hyperpyrexia; and cardiovascular complications such as tachycardia, arrhythmias, pulmonary edema, hypotension, and possibly ventricular fibrillation

CONTRAINDICATIONS

Acute recovery phase of myocardial infarction, severe renal or hepatic impairment, concomitant use of MAO inhibitors, narrow-angle glaucoma. *Cautious use* in patients with a history of seizure disorders, cardiovascular disease, urinary dysfunction, or narrow-angle glaucoma. Also in the presence of pregnancy, lactation, hepatic or renal impairment, prostatic hypertrophy, hyperthryoidism, schizophrenia, or other psychoses

INTERACTIONS

Tricyclics may enhance the effects of other CNS depressants (e.g., alcohol, barbiturates, benzodiazepines, hypnotics, phenothiazines); catecholamines; other adrenergic drugs (e.g., ephedrine, amphetamine); anticholinergics; narcotic analgesics; thyroid drugs; disulfiram; anticoagulants; vasodilators; and centrally acting muscle relaxants

Tricyclics may antagonize the action of antihypertensives (e.g., guanethidine, clonidine); beta-blockers; anticonvulsants (increase incidence of seizures); phenylbutazone; and cholinergic drugs

Effects of tricyclics may be potentiated by phenothiazines, methylphenidate, amphetamines, cimetidine, furazolidone, acetazolamide, MAO inhibitors, and urinary alkalinizers (e.g., sodium bicarbonate)

Tricyclics should not be administered within 14 days of MAO inhibitors because hypertension, hyperpyresis, and convulsions can occur

Reserpine and tricyclic antidepressants can result in a stimulating effect, possibly leading to mania

Therapeutic effects of tricyclics may be reduced by barbiturates (enzyme induction), urinary acidifiers such as ammonium chloride and ascorbic acid (decreased renal tubular reabsorption), and oral contraceptives

Increased cardiovascular toxic effects may be seen with thyroid drugs, quinidine, or procainamide in combination with tricyclic antidepressants

NURSING CONSIDERATIONS

Nursing Alerts
- Carefully assess severely depressed patient during initial improvement phase. Suicidal tendency may be increased as depression and psychomotor retardation are lessened.
- Monitor blood pressure and pulse at least twice a day until stable because hypotension, several types of arrhythmias, and other cardiovascular side effects may occur, especially in patients receiving high doses.

1. Provide emotional support during drug therapy. Encourage patient to engage regularly in physical and social activities. Significant others may need to help motivate patient to participate.
2. Ensure that baseline blood and liver function studies and ECG have been completed before initiating drug administration.
3. Assist in evaluating patient's response to drug. The lowest effective dosage should be used for maintenance therapy, and the patient should be carefully observed for continued clinical progress. After symptoms have been controlled for some time (at least 3 mo), dosage should be gradually tapered, but patient should be monitored for possible relapse. If no improvement is observed within 8 weeks, the drug should be discontinued and alternative therapy instituted.

PATIENT EDUCATION

1. Encourage patient to maintain prescribed regimen. Beneficial effects may not become manifest for several weeks, although some newer drugs (e.g., maprotiline) claim a more rapid onset of action (5–7 days).
2. Explain that abrupt discontinuation of therapy could result in nausea, muscle aching, insomnia, and irritability. The drug should be withdrawn gradually under supervision of the prescriber.
3. Reassure patient that many side effects common early in therapy disappear or diminish with continued use; others may remain. The patient should inform prescriber if side effects appear or persist, as dosage adjustment or change to another agent may help minimize them.
4. Warn patient that no other drugs, including OTC preparations, should be taken without consulting the health care provider.
5. Explain that tricyclic antidepressants augment the effects of alcohol and other CNS depressants. Motor coordination may be impaired if they are used in combination.
6. Caution patient not to operate dangerous machinery until response to drug is known because marked sedation is common during early stages of treatment.
7. Teach patient measures that help control orthostatic hypotension. See **Plan of Nursing Care 8 (Antihypertensive Drugs)** for specific information.
8. Teach patient early signs of blood dyscrasia (fever, sore throat, mucosal irritation, fatigue) that need to be reported to physician immediately.
9. Instruct patient to inform physician immediately if fever, nausea, abdominal pain, or rash (early signs of cholestatic jaundice) appear.
10. Suggest interventions to alleviate mouth dryness, which is common in early therapy. See **Plan of Nursing Care 4 (Antihistamines)** for specific information.
11. Teach patient interventions to prevent constipation (increased intake of fluid and dietary roughage), and advise patient to monitor bowel and bladder function because constipation and urinary retention can occur. Dosage adjustment or adjunctive therapy (e.g., stool softener, laxative) may be necessary.
12. Teach diabetic patient how to assess need for adjustment in antidiabetes regimen because both hypoglycemia and hyperglycemia have been reported.
13. Advise patient to avoid excessive exposure to sunlight because photosensitivity reactions may occur.
14. Instruct patient to notify physician or dentist in charge of tricyclic antidepressant use prior to elective surgery. To reduce operative risks (e.g., excessive hypotension or respiratory depression), the drug should be discontinued several days before surgery.

SECOND-GENERATION ANTIDEPRESSANTS

Bupropion
Wellbutrin

Bupropion is an aminoketone antidepressant unrelated to any other antidepressant. It is an alternative to the tricyclics for treating endogenous depression not responding to more conventional therapy.

MECHANISM
Not established. Weakly inhibits norepinephrine and serotonin and may block dopamine reuptake as well; no effect on monoamineoxidase; possesses a CNS stimulating action

USES
Short term treatment of depression (effectiveness longer than 6 wk has not been established

DOSAGE
Initially, 100 mg twice a day; may increase to 100 mg three times/day after 3 days if necessary; maximum 450 mg/day in three divided doses

FATE
Well absorbed orally; peak plasma levels occur within 2 hours; average half-life is 12 to 16 hours; protein binsing is approximately 80%; metabolites are eliminated in both urine and feces

COMMON SIDE EFFECTS
Dry mouth, insomnia, headache, agitation, nausea/vomiting, constipation, tremor

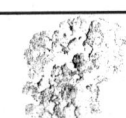

Table 24-2
Tricyclic Antidepressants

Drug	Preparations	Usual Dosage Range	Nursing Implications
Amitriptyline Amitril, Elavil, Emitrip, Endep, Enovil (CAN) Apo-Amitriptyline, Levate, Novotriptyn	Tablets: 10 mg, 25 mg, 50 mg, 75 mg, 100 mg, 150 mg Injection: 10 mg/mL	*Oral* Initially: 75 mg–150 mg/day Maintenance: 50 mg–100 mg/day in divided doses or at bedtime *IM* 20 mg–30 mg 4 times/day initially; replace with oral form as soon as possible	Most effective in endogenous depressions, especially those accompanied by anxiety, or in patients over 50 yr of age; investigational uses include prevention of migraine headaches and control of acute pain, especially in combination with potent narcotics; sedative effect is prominent, especially early in therapy; give drug at bedtime to minimize daytime drowsiness; plasma half-life is 30–40 h
Amoxapine Asendin	Tablets: 25 mg, 50 mg, 100 mg, 150 mg	Initially: 50 mg 2–3 times/day; increase to 100 mg 2–3 times/day on the third day Once effective dose is established, may be given in a single bedtime dose not to exceed 300 mg	Used in a wide range of depressions; exhibits a moderate sedative action; clinical effects are usually observed within 7 days; may be used on a once-daily basis at bedtime; highly bound (90%) to plasma proteins, so interactions with other protein-bound drugs can occur; serum half-life is 8 h, but converted to an active metabolite with a half-life of 30 h; *do not* use in children under 16 yr; most frequent adverse reactions (10%–15%) are sedation, dry mouth, and constipation
Desipramine Norpramin, Pertofrane	Tablets: 10 mg, 25 mg, 50 mg, 75 mg, 100 mg, 150 mg Capsules: 25 mg, 50 mg	Adults: 25 mg–50 mg 3–4 times/day (maximum 300 mg/day) Geriatric patients: 25 mg–100 mg/day	Active metabolite of imipramine, with essentially the same uses and adverse effects; *not* recommended in children; slightly lower incidence of sedation and anticholinergic action than imipramine; increased psychomotor activity may occur in first few weeks of therapy; orthostatic hypotension is common early in treatment—caution against rapid position changes; improvement is usually apparent within 1–2 wks
Doxepin Adapin, Sinequan (CAN) Triadapin	Capsules: 10 mg, 25 mg, 50 mg, 75 mg, 100 mg, 150 mg Oral concentrate: 10 mg/mL	10 mg–50 mg 3 times/day (maximum 300 mg/day) *or* 150 mg once daily at bedtime *Do not* use in children under 12 yr	Indicated for relief of depression and anxiety associated with psychotic or psychoneurotic disorders; antianxiety effects occur within several days, but antidepressant action requires several weeks; sedation is marked during initial stage of treatment; effects of alcohol may be enhanced; dilute oral concentrate with 4 oz of water, juice, or milk prior to administration
Imipramine Janimine, Tipramine, Tofranil (CAN) Apo-Imipramine, Impril, Novopramine	Tablets: 10 mg, 25 mg, 50 mg Long-acting capsules (Tofranil-PM): 75 mg, 100 mg, 125 mg, 150 mg Injection: 25 mg/2 mL	**Depression** *Oral* Initially: 75 mg–150 mg/day in divided doses Maintenance: 50 mg–150 mg/day	Used for relief of symptoms of endogenous depressions and for reducing enuresis in children 6 yr and older; decreases time spent in deep phases of sleep associated with bedwet-

Continued

Table 24-2
Tricyclic Antidepressants

Drug	Preparations	Usual Dosage Range	Nursing Implications
Imipramine (cont'd)		*IM* 100 mg/day in divided doses **Enuresis** Initially: 25 mg–50 mg/night, orally *or* 25 mg in midafternoon and 25 mg at bedtime	ting; may be administered in a single nightly dose (Tofranil-PM) for depression; do *not* use the PM (pamoate salt) dosage form in enuresis; plasma half-life is 10–25 h
Maprotiline Ludiomil	Tablets: 25 mg, 50 mg, 75 mg	Initially: 75 mg/day in single or divided doses; adjust to desired maintenance range, usually 75 mg–225 mg/day (maximum 300 mg/day) Elderly: 50 mg/day–75 mg/day	A *tetracyclic* antidepressant with a slightly lower incidence of cardiovascular reactions and fewer anticholinergic side effects than most tricyclic compounds; may have a rapid response (within 1 wk) in some patients; used in manic–depressive disorders; most common side effects are dry mouth and drowsiness; *not* indicated in children under 18 yr; reduce dosage in elderly patients, and during prolonged maintenance therapy
Nortriptyline Aventyl, Pamelor	Capsules: 10 mg, 25 mg, 50 mg, 75 mg Liquid: 10 mg/5 mL	25 mg 3–4 times/day (maximum 150 mg/day) *Geriatric patients:* 30 mg–50 mg/day	Primarily effective in endogenous depressions; not recommended in children under 12 yr; drug is a metabolite of amitriptyline and is similar to imipramine in most of its pharmacologic effects
Protriptyline Vivactil (CAN) Triptil	Tablets: 5 mg, 10 mg	5 mg–10 mg 3–4 times/day (maximum 60 mg/day) Geriatric patients: 5 mg 3 times/day	Most effective in endogenous depressions in withdrawn and anergic patients; use is associated with less sedation, but drug has more CNS-stimulatory, cardiovascular, and anticholinergic action than other tricyclics; *caution* in cardiac patients or in those with insomnia; *not* recommended in children under 12 yr; last dose should be taken not later than midafternoon to avoid excessive stimulation at bedtime
Trimipramine Surmontil	Capsules: 25 mg, 50 mg, 100 mg	Initially: 75 mg–150 mg/day in divided doses. Maintenance: 50 mg–150 mg/day at bedtime Geriatric patients: 50 mg–100 mg/day	Possesses significant sedative action; similar to amitriptyline in most respects; *not* recommended in children

SIGNIFICANT ADVERSE REACTIONS

WARNING

A risk of seizures is closely associated with use of bupropion. At doses up to 450 mg/day, the risk is about four times that seen with other antidepressants. Seizures incidence increases almost tenfold at doses between 450 mg/day and 600 mg/day. The total daily dose should not exceed 450 mg in three equally divided doses, and the drug should be used with extreme caution in persons with a history of seizures, cranial trauma, or other predisposition toward seizures

CNS: sedation, insomnia, akinesia, confusion, hostility, impaired concentration, decreased libido, anxiety, blurred vision, auditory disturbances
Cardiovascular: dizziness, tachycardia, hypertension, arrhythmias, palpitation
GI: weight loss, anorexia, diarrhea, dyspepsia
Other: menstrual irregularities, impotence, urinary frequency, rash, pruritus, fatigue, arthritic-like symptoms, fever, chills

CONTRAINDICATIONS

Patients with a seizure disorder, anorexia, or bulimia, or those being treated with a MAO inhibitor. *Cautious use* in persons with psychoses, mania, unstable heart disease, impaired liver or kidney function, and in pregnant or nursing women

INTERACTIONS

Bupropion is an enzyme inducer in the liver and may increase the metabolism of other drugs metabolized by the hepatic microsomal enzyme system

Concurrent use of bupropion and levodopa may increase the risk of adverse reactions to levodopa

The toxicity of bupropion may be enhanced by MAO inhibitors

Drugs that lower the seizure threshold increase the risk of seizures with bupropion

NURSING CONSIDERATIONS

See tricyclic antidepressants. In addition:

Nursing Alert
- Use extreme caution when administering bupropion to persons with increased risk of seizures (e.g., alcoholics, epileptics, patients with CNS tumors or trauma). Begin at low doses, make dosage changes gradually, and closely monitor patients. Question patient about any prior seizure episodes and be aware of the danger of seizures in persons with a history of seizure activity.

1. Monitor weight during therapy with bupropion. Weight loss occurs commonly and may be excessive.

PATIENT EDUACTION

See tricyclic antidepressants. In addition:
1. Inform patients that drug may impair the ability to perform tasks requiring judgment or motor skills. Advise caution during early stages of therapy.
2. Impress patients with the importance of adhering to prescribed dosage schedule to minimize the risk of seizures and other adverse reactions.
3. Caution against taking any other medication during therapy with bupropion unless approved by health-care provider.

Fluoxetine
Prozac

Fluoxetine is an antidepressant chemically dissimilar to other available antidepressants but comparable in clinical efficacy. The incidence of anticholinergic, sedative, and hypotensive effects compared to the tricyclics is somewhat reduced, although certain CNS (e.g., headache, nervousness) and GI (e.g., nausea, diarrhea) side effects appear to occur more often with fluoxetine than with other antidepressants

MECHANISM

Inhibits neuronal uptake of serotonin, with minimal effects on norepinephrine uptake; antagonism of cholinergic, histaminergic, and alpha-adrenergic receptors is weak; may slightly reduce heart rate but no ECG changes have occurred; exhibits a weak anorexigenic action and can lead to slight weight loss

USES

Symptomatic treatment of endogenous depression (use in hospitalized depressed patients has *not* been adequately studied)

DOSAGE

Initially, 20 mg once daily in the morning; increase in 20-mg/day increments to a maximum of 80 mg/day. Doses above 20 mg/day should be administered on a twice-daily schedule

FATE

Oral absorption is good and is not appreciably decreased by food; peak plasma levels occur within 6 to 8 hours; plasma protein binding is approximately 95%; extensively metabolized in the liver to norfluoxetine, an equally effective uptake blocker; primarily excreted by the kidneys (elimination half-life of fluoxetine is 2–3 days and of norfluoxetine is 7–9 days); active drug persists in the body for weeks after dosing is terminated

COMMON SIDE EFFECTS

Anxiety, nervousness, insomnia, headache, sweating, mild tremor, lightheadedness, nausea, anorexia

SIGNIFICANT ADVERSE REACTIONS

Listed in order of approximate decreasing frequency within each organ system.

CNS: drowsiness, anxiety, tremor, dizziness, fatigue, decreased libido, abnormal dreams, agitation
GI: diarrhea, dry mouth, constipation, abdominal pain, vomiting, altered taste, flatulence, increased appetite
Dermatologic: rash, pruritus, alopecia, acneiform eruptions, contact dermatitis, urticaria, herpes simplex infection
Respiratory: upper respiratory infection, pharyngitis, flulike syndrome, nasal congestion, sinusitis, cough, dyspnea, rhinitis, bronchitis
Cardiovascular: palpitations, hot flashes, migraine, tachycardia
Musculoskeletal: back, joint, or muscle pain,
Urogenital: frequent urination, painful menstruation, urinary tract infection
Miscellaneous: fever, asthenia, allergic reactions, visual disturbances, weight loss, chest pain, chills

CONTRAINDICATIONS

No absolute contraindications. *Cautious use* in persons with a history of seizures, impaired renal or hepatic function, anorexia, mania or hypomania, in pregnant or nursing women, and in the elderly

INTERACTIONS

Fluoxetine may interact with other highly protein bound drugs, resulting in an increased effect of both drugs

The half-life of diazepam may be prolonged by concomitant administration of fluoxetine

Concurrent use of fluoxetine and an MAO inhibitor may lead to increased adverse effects

NURSING CONSIDERATION

See tricyclic antidepressants. In addition:
1. Carefully evaluate drug effects in patient with liver or kidney disease. Because drug is metabolized primarily in liver, dosage should be lower or another drug should be used if liver function is impaired. Dosage should also be decreased if kidney disease is present.

PATIENT EDUCATION

See tricyclic antidepressants. In addition:
1. Inform patient that antidepressant effect may not be evident until after 4 weeks or longer of use.
2. Emphasize importance of promptly reporting any adverse reactions. Drug withdrawal can be problematic because long half-lives of drug and metabolite cause active drug substance to persist weeks after drug is discontinued.

Trazodone

Desyrel, Trialadine

Trazodone is an effective antidepressant chemically unrelated to tricyclics, tetracyclics, or MAO inhibitors. Its use is associated with minimal anticholinergic and cardiac conductive effects, although arrhythmogenic incidences have occurred with trazodone, particularly at high doses. Symptomatic improvement is often noted within 1 week.

MECHANISM

Selectively inhibits serotonin uptake in the brain; does not elicit CNS stimulation

USES

Treatment of depression, with or without accompanying anxiety

DOSAGE

Initially, 150 mg/day in divided doses; increase by 50-mg/day increments every 3 or 4 days until optimal effect is attained.

Maximum dose is 400 mg/day in outpatients and 600 mg/day in inpatients.

FATE

Well absorbed orally; peak plasma levels occur in 1 hour if taken on an empty stomach and within 2 hours if taken with food. Clinically significant therapeutic response is seen within 2 weeks in 75% of responders; metabolized in the liver; elimination half-life is 4 to 8 hours.

COMMON SIDE EFFECTS

Drowsiness, dizziness, lightheadedness, fatigue, dry mouth, constipation, nasal congestion

SIGNIFICANT ADVERSE REACTIONS

(See also general discussion of tricyclic antidepressants)

Cardiovascular: hypotension, syncope, tachycardia, chest pain
CNS: confusion, headache, insomnia, nervousness, disorientation, reduced concentration, malaise
Autonomic: blurred vision, constipation
GI: nausea, vomiting, salivation
Neurologic: incoordination, paresthesias, tremors
Other: allergic skin conditions; myalgia; sinus congestion; tinnitus; weight gain; tired, itching eyes; sweating; dyspnea; decreased libido; altered menses; anemia, leukopenia

CONTRAINDICATIONS

No absolute contraindications. *Cautious use* in patients with arrhythmias, hypotension, in pregnant or nursing mothers and in persons receiving MAO inhibitors. Drug should not be administered concurrently with ECT or during initial recovery phase following myocardial infarction.

INTERACTIONS

See general discussion of tricyclic antidepressants. In addition:

- Increased serum levels of digoxin and phenytoin have been reported with trazodone therapy
- Increased CNS depression can occur with concurrent use of trazodone and alcohol, barbiturates, and other CNS depressants
- Trazodone may enhance the hypotensive effects of most antihypertensive drugs; however, the effects of clonidine may be inhibited by trazodone

NURSING CONSIDERATIONS

See tricyclic antidepressants.

PATIENT EDUCATION

See tricyclic antidepressants. In addition:
1. Instruct patient to take drug during or shortly following a meal or snack because absorption is enhanced by the presence of food in the stomach.

MONOAMINE OXIDASE INHIBITORS

Isocarboxazid   Tranylcypromine
Phenelzine

Drugs that can form stable complexes with and therefore inhibit the action of the enzyme monoamine oxidase (MAO) have been employed for many years as antidepressants. MAO is an enzyme system that catalyzes the deamination, or inactivation, of several naturally occurring biogenic amines, most notably norepinephrine, epinephrine, and serotonin, in numerous body tissues, especially the liver, kidney, intestines, and nerve endings. It is found within the mitochondria of cells comprising these tissues, and its principal role in neuronal transmission is the regulation of *intra*cellular neurotransmitter levels. Inhibition of MAO in nerve endings increases the amounts of free neurotransmitter available for release after the arrival of a nerve impulse. By blocking a major means for intraneuronal catecholamine (and serotonin) breakdown, MAO inhibitors can increase the synaptic actions of these amine neurohormones, thereby increasing postsynaptic receptor activation. As discussed under tricyclic antidepressants above, continued postsynaptic receptor stimulation ultimately reduces the sensitivity and number of these receptor sites, a process termed *receptor down-regulation*. The amelioration of depressive symptomology is believed to be the result of this down-regulation of central aminergic receptor sites.

Although MAO inhibitors were the first clinically effective antidepressants to be introduced, their relatively high toxicity has restricted their usefulness to serving as alternatives to the more effective and less toxic tricyclic antidepressants. MAO inhibitors are frequently employed in a hospital setting in patients refractive to or intolerant of the tricyclics. Their use in outpatients must be carefully and continually monitored, and necessary precautions must be taken to avoid precipitation of serious adverse reactions and drug interactions.

Since MAO inhibitors interfere with the activity of enzymes responsible for inactivating many endogenous and exogenous amines, the effects of aminergic substances contained in several foods may be markedly enhanced in the presence of an MAO inhibitor. Certain sympathomimetic amines such as tyramine, which is found in many foods, can exert a potent pressor effect. Normally, tyramine is efficiently metabolized by MAO; however, in the presence of an MAO inhibitor, the pressor action of tyramine can be substantially potentiated, and hypertensive crises have occurred with ingestion of tyramine-containing foods (e.g., sausages, aged cheeses, smoked fish, chianti wine, caviar) as well as foods containing other pressor substances normally metabolized by MAO.

MECHANISM

Inhibit the MAO enzyme system by forming an irreversible (stable) complex with the enzyme; consequently, intraneuronal breakdown of catecholamines and serotonin is inhibited, and their concentration rises in several body tissues including the CNS, heart, blood, and intestine. Increased intraneuronal concentrations of these amine neurohormones result in a larger pool of neurohormone available for release and thus an enhanced postsynaptic action. The increased activity of norepinephrine, serotonin, and possibly other neurohormones at postjunctional receptor sites in the CNS is believed to underlie the effectiveness of MAO inhibitors in relieving depression. Likewise, increased neurohormone availability in other body tissues is thought to underlie many of the toxic reactions elicited by these agents. These drugs also inhibit hepatic microsomal drug-metabolizing enzymes, thereby prolonging the action of many other drugs

USES
Management of severe endogenous, exogenous (atypical), or reactive depressions resistant to treatment with tricyclic antidepressants, ECT, or other adjunctive psychotherapy

Control of the depressive phase of manic-depressive psychoses

DOSAGE
See Table 24-3

FATE
Readily absorbed orally; enzyme inhibition occurs rapidly, but clinical effects take several weeks to develop, except with tranylcypromine (10–14 days); termination of drug effect following administration of irreversible inhibitors (isocarboxazid, phenelzine) depends largely on regeneration of MAO enzyme, a process taking several weeks; tranylcypromine effects decline within 3 to 5 days following discontinuation of therapy; drugs are metabolized in the liver and excreted in the urine as metabolites and some unchanged drug

COMMON SIDE EFFECTS
Orthostatic hypotension, dizziness, weakness, fatigue, jitteriness, hyperactivity, insomnia, GI disturbances, headache, disturbances in cardiac rate and rhythm, dry mouth, blurred vision, hyperhidrosis

SIGNIFICANT ADVERSE REACTIONS
CNS: vertigo, tremors, hypomania, euphoria, confusion, memory impairment, drowsiness, ataxia, excessive sweating, delirium, hallucinations, convulsions

Autonomic/cardiovascular: dysuria, incontinence, impotence, palpitations, edema, weight gain

Hematologic/dermatologic: leukopenia, hypochromic anemia, skin rash, hepatocellular jaundice

Other: anorexia, peripheral neuritis, photosensitivity reactions, nystagmus, sodium retention, hypoglycemia, galactorrhea, glaucoma, optic damage

Overdose: restlessness, tachycardia, hypotension, respiratory depression, confusion, incoherence, convulsions, shock

CONTRAINDICATIONS
In children under 16 years of age, congestive heart failure, liver disease, pheochromocytoma, hyperthyroidism, hypertension, cardiovascular or cerebrovascular disease, and elderly or debilitated patients. *Cautious use* in patients with epilepsy, diabetes, depression accompanying drug or alcohol addiction, chronic brain syndromes, history of anginal attacks, impaired renal function, and during pregnancy and lactation

INTERACTIONS
Effects of sympathomimetic drugs (e.g., amphetamines, catecholamines, L-dopa, ephedrine, phenylephrine, methylphenidate) may be potentiated, resulting in severe hypertension, headache, and possibly cerebrovascular hemorrhage

Hypertensive reactions can occur in patients taking MAO inhibitors who ingest foods containing tyramine, a pressor substance (e.g., cheeses, sour cream, beer, red wines, yeasts, yogurt, pickled herring, chicken livers, aged meats, fermented sausages) as well as caffeine, chocolate, and licorice

Concurrent use of MAO inhibitors and tricyclic antidepressants (or within 10 days of each other) can result in severe hypertension, convulsions, fever, sweating, delirium, tremor, circulatory collapse, and coma, although some tricyclic antidepressants have been employed safely in conjunction with MAO inhibitors

MAO inhibitors may increase the toxic effects of barbiturates and phenothiazines by decreasing their metabolism in the liver

Effects of antihypertensive drugs may be potentiated by MAO inhibitors (increased orthostatic *hypo*tension); however, severe *hyper*tension can occur with parenteral use of reserpine or guanethidine, owing to release of large amounts of catecholamines

Hypotension, respiratory arrest, shock, and coma can occur if MAO inhibitors are used in combination with CNS depressants such as alcohol, anesthetics, narcotics (especially meperidine), and sedative–hypnotics

Increased hypoglycemic effects have occurred with combined use of MAO inhibitors and either insulin or oral hypoglycemics

Muscle-relaxing action of succinylcholine may be increased because MAO inhibitors interfere with plasma pseudocholinesterase, the enzyme that inactivates succinylcholine

MAO inhibitors reduce convulsive seizure threshold and may reduce the efficacy of antiepileptic drugs

Effects of anticholinergic, antihistaminic, and antiparkinsonian drugs may be potentiated by MAO inhibitors, which decrease their rate of metabolism

NURSING CONSIDERATIONS
1. Establish baseline blood pressure before therapy is initiated and monitor frequently during therapy.
2. Monitor indicators of fluid retention (intake and output, edema, weight gain) until dosage is stabilized. Advise primary care provider of any changes because renal impairment may result in greatly increased toxicity.
3. Monitor results of liver function studies and blood cell counts, which should be performed prior to initiation of therapy and at regular intervals thereafter.
4. Assist with evaluation of patient's response to therapy. If no significant clinical response occurs within 4 weeks, the patient should be reevaluated, and an alternative form of treatment should be considered.

PATIENT EDUCATION
1. Carefully explain the untoward reactions associated with use of MAO inhibitors, especially the possibility of hypertensive crisis.
2. Emphasize the need to *closely* follow prescribed drug regimen and diet to minimize the danger of untoward reactions.

Table 24-3
MAO Inhibitors

Drug	Preparations	Usual Dosage Range	Nursing Implications
Isocarboxazid Marplan	Tablets: 10 mg	*Initially:* 30 mg/day; reduce to maintenance levels (usually 10 mg–20 mg/day) as soon as possible	Administer with meals to reduce gastric upset; adjust dosage critically, on basis of careful patient observation; note that although therapeutic effects may take several weeks to develop, toxic interactions can occur within hours; may be administered either as a single dose or in divided doses
Phenelzine Nardil	Tablets: 15 mg	*Initially:* 15 mg 3 times/day; reduce slowly to maintenance levels, usually 15 mg every 1–2 days	Effective in moderate to severe depressive states, especially accompanied by anxiety and agitation; do not exceed 75 mg/day
Tranylcypromine Parnate	Tablets: 10 mg	*Initially:* 20 mg–30 mg/day; reduce to 10 mg–20 mg/day as needed *With concurrent ECT:* 10 mg 1–2 times/day	Incidence of hypertensive reactions is higher than with other MAO inhibitors; latency of therapeutic effect is generally shorter (3–5 days) than with other similar drugs; it is a structural analog of amphetamine and probably exerts a direct receptor activation, as well as MAO inhibition

3. Ensure that patient and family have a list of, and fully understand, tyramine-containing foods that should not be eaten. Consumption of such foods could precipitate a hypertensive crisis. Aged cheese, sour cream, imported beer and ale, red wine (especially chianti), yogurt, yeast, pickled herring, aged meat and meat tenderizer, and chicken liver are among the foods that should be avoided. Chocolate and caffeine have also been implicated in blood pressure elevations with MAO inhibitors.
4. Urge patient not to take any other drugs, including OTC preparations, without consulting the health care provider who prescribed the MAO inhibitor because numerous serious drug interactions can occur.
5. Stress the importance of noting and reporting early signs of an impending hypertensive reaction (headache, palpitations, neck stiffness, sweating, nausea, photophobia).
6. Instruct patient not to discontinue drug without supervision. Rapid withdrawal may induce excitability, hallucinations, and possibly severe depression, especially after prolonged use or high dosage.
7. Warn patient to avoid all foods and drugs that may be hazardous for at least several weeks after the last dose of MAO inhibitor has been taken.
8. Teach patient interventions to help minimize orthostatic hypotension. See **Plan of Nursing Care 8 (Antihypertensive Drugs)** for specific information.
9. Advise patient and family to be alert for and to report the development of hypomania, which occurs most often when hyperkinetic symptoms have been masked by concurrent depression. Relief of depression by MAO inhibitors can precipitate agitation, delusion, and exaggeration of feelings. Use of sedatives is indicated.
10. Teach patient how to recognize and report the development of hepatic complications, marked by jaundicelike reactions (e.g., rash, abdominal pain, pruritus, yellowing of skin). If they occur, drug may need to be discontinued.
11. Instruct patient to report immediately any visual disturbances, especially changes in red-green color vision, because these are often the initial signs of drug-induced ocular change.
12. Suggest interventions to relieve mouth dryness. See **Plan of Nursing Care 4 (Antihistamines)** for specific information.
13. Instruct patient to inform physician or dentist of MAO inhibitor use prior to surgery. MAO inhibitors should be discontinued at least 1 week before elective surgery to reduce the danger of interaction with anesthetic agents and postoperative narcotics.
14. Caution patient, especially one with a history of heart disease, to avoid overexertion. MAO inhibitors suppress anginal pain and may, therefore, mask the warning signs of an ischemic attack.
15. Teach diabetic patient how to carefully observe for signs of hypoglycemia, and inform patient that the dosage of antidiabetic agent may need to be adjusted.

Selected Bibliography

Baldessarini RJ: Biochemical Aspects of Depression. Washington, DC, American Psychiatric Press, 1983

Baldessarini RJ: Treatment of depression by altering monoamine metabolism: Precursors and metabolic inhibitors. Psychopharmacol Bull 20:224, 1984

Bloom PE, Baetge G, Deyo S et al: Chemical and physiological aspects of the actions of lithium and antidepressant drugs. Neuropharmacology 22:359, 1983

Cassem N: Cardiovascular effects of antidepressants. J Clin Psychiatry 43:22, 1982

Cavenar JO (ed): Psychiatry. Philadelphia, JB Lippincott, 1985

Davidson J: When and how to use MAO-inhibitors. Drug Ther 13:197, 1983

DeGennaro MD, Hymen R, Crannell AM, Mansky PA: Antidepressant drug therapy. Am J Nurs 81:1304, 1981

Donlon PT: Cardiac effects of antidepressants. Geriatrics 37:53, 1982

Feighner JP: The new generation of antidepressants. J Clin Psychiatry 44(11):49, 1983

Fink M: Convulsive and drug therapies of depression. Annu Rev Med 32:405, 1981

Glassman AH, Bigger JT: Cardiovascular effects of therapeutic doses of tricyclic antidepressants. Arch Gen Psychiatry 38:815, 1981

Goodwin FK: The impact of tricyclic antidepressants and lithium on the course of recurrent affective disorder. McLean Hosp J 8:1, 1983

Harris B: Drugs and depression. Am J Nurs 86:292, 1986

Hollister LE: Second generation antidepressants. Ration Drug Ther 16:1, 1982

Karusu TB: Psychotherapy and pharmacotherapy. Am J Psychiatry 139:67, 1982

Prien RF (ed): Antidepressant drug therapy: The role of the new antidepressants. Psychopharmacol Bull 20:209, 1984

Rawls WN: Trazodone. DNS Intell Clin Pharm 16:7, 1982

Richelson E: Pharmacology of antidepressants in use in the United States. J Clin Psychiatry 43:4, 1982

SUMMARY. ANTIDEPRESSANTS

Drug	Preparations	Usual Dosage Range
Tricyclic–tetracyclic derivatives	See Table 24-2	
Bupropion Wellbutrin	Tablets: 75 mg, 100 mg	Initially, 100 mg twice daily; may increase to 100 mg 3 times/day after 3 days. Maximum dose is 450 mg/day in 3 divided doses
Fluoxetine Prozac	Capsules: 20 mg	Initially, 20-mg once daily; increase in 20-mg increments; maximum 80 mg/day
Trazodone Desyrel, Trialodine	Tablets: 50 mg, 100 mg, 150 mg, 300 mg	Initially, 150 mg/day in divided doses; increase in 50 mg increments; maximum 600 mg/day in patients
MAO inhibitors	See Table 24-3	

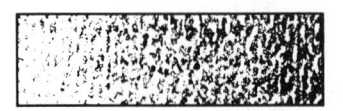

25 ANTICONVULSANTS/ANTIEPILEPTICS

Epilepsy is a chronic CNS disorder estimated to afflict between 0.5% and 1.5% of the population. Attempts have been made to classify the epilepsies according to the type of seizure manifestation (e.g., tonic–clonic convulsions, akinetic–atonic behavior, local muscle hyperactivity), but complete agreement is lacking. However, certain characteristics such as EEG alterations and localized or generalized muscular hyperactivity can aid in distinguishing among the major types of epilepsies, and these are outlined in Table 25-1.

Seizures can be broadly categorized as being *generalized* or *partial* (i.e., localized). Generalized seizures include:

- Tonic–clonic convulsions, frequently referred to as *grand mal epilepsy*
- Simple absence seizures, also known as *petit mal epilepsy*;
- Myoclonic jerking
- Atonic-akinetic seizures
- Infantile spasms.

In contrast, partial seizures may be subdivided according to the degree of total body involvement. Elementary or simple seizures are characterized by minimal spread of the discharge and limited involvement of the extremities. In complex seizures, the discharge becomes more widespread and complex motor or behavioral aberrations are noted. Complex seizures arise primarily in the temporal lobe and are therefore sometimes referred to as *temporal lobe* or *psychomotor* epilepsy.

Anticonvulsant drugs are effective in controlling the various manifestations of the epilepsies, but critical dosage regulation is of paramount importance for optimal seizure control. Drugs and doses must be individualized according to a particular patient's needs. Some antiepileptic drugs are not only ineffective in certain types of seizure disorders but may actually worsen certain aspects of these conditions. Successful therapy, therefore, depends on accurate diagnosis, careful selection of drugs, and critical adjustment of dosage.

Therapy usually is initiated with a single agent, but complete control of most seizure types generally requires addition of a second and often a third drug. Frequent dosage alterations or too-rapid shifting among anticonvulsant drugs should be avoided. The essential requirement of any antiepileptic drug is that it control the seizures without causing undue sedation and with minimal adverse drug effects. While many agents possess significant anticonvulsant activity at doses associated with disabling side effects, the clinically useful antiepileptic drugs provide adequate control of most seizure types without subjecting the patient to frequent and debilitating adverse reactions. Although the drugs do not *cure* the affliction, they do allow the epileptic patient to function productively.

Stabilization of epileptic patients is a difficult task in most cases. Once it is attained, patients should be advised of the dangers inherent in altering the prescribed drug regimen or in subjecting themselves to physical and emotional stresses that might compromise their stable conditions. Patients should be taught to observe their conditions and to report any unusual symptoms that occur during therapy, because these may indicate early manifestations of serious toxicity. Drugs should be discontinued *gradually* whenever necessary, and changes in medication should be accomplished slowly over several weeks. Abrupt discontinuance or alteration in drug therapy can precipitate *status epilepticus*, a series of rapid, repetitive seizures that may be fatal unless terminated quickly (see Table 25-1).

Several agents (including barbiturates and diazepam) that are employed in the emergency control of acute convulsive states resulting from trauma, hyperthermia of infection, or drug overdosage have already been reviewed. The drugs to be considered here are used primarily to treat the various forms of epilepsy and therefore may be regarded, in most cases, as specific antiepileptic agents.

ANTICONVULSANT BARBITURATES

Mephobarbital   Phenobarbital
Metharbital

Although all barbiturates can abolish seizure activity at doses sufficient to produce anesthesia, only three barbiturates—phenobarbital, metharbital and mephobarbital—appear to be particularly suited for long-term treatment of epilepsy. They are effective at nonsedating doses, exert a prolonged action, and tend to be well tolerated during extended drug therapy.

MECHANISM
Reduce excitability of nerve cells by increasing their firing threshold; block the active transport of ions across the neuronal membrane, thereby lowering the firing rate; may also potentiate activity of GABA, an inhibitory neurotransmitter

USES
Generalized tonic–clonic seizures (grand mal); used alone in infants and young children, and most often in combination with phenytoin in adults
Generalized myoclonic jerks
Complex absence seizures with autonomic manifestations
Status epilepticus (phenobarbital IV)
Infantile spasms (effectiveness not conclusively demonstrated)

DOSAGE
See Table 25-2

FATE
Well absorbed orally; onset following oral administration ranges from 30 minutes (phenobarbital) to 2 hours (metharbital); effects are evident in 10 to 15 minutes with IV injection; duration lasts from 8 to 12 hours; partly metabolized in the liver and excreted both as metabolites and unchanged drug in the urine

COMMON SIDE EFFECTS
Lethargy, dizziness, irritability

Table 25-1
Classification and Management of Seizures

Seizure Type	Usual Age at Onset	Characteristics
Generalized		
Tonic–clonic (grand mal)	Any age (usually before 20 yr)	Tonic rigidity of extremities, followed by massive clonic jerking for several minutes; urinary incontinence is common; lassitude and stupor ensue
Simple absence (petit mal)	3–10 yr	Sudden loss of consciousness lasting up to 30 sec but usually of much shorter duration; can occur hundreds of times a day; characteristic 3/sec spike-wave EEG pattern; may be accompanied by some clonic jerking of the eyelids or extremities and autonomic manifestations but frequently no motor activity is evident; rare in the adult
Myoclonic jerking	5–20 yr	Sudden, violent contractions of the extremities, with or without loss of consciousness; occur most often after awakening or before retiring, often in combination with other seizure types
Atonic–akinetic	1–5 yr	Sudden loss of muscle tone, usually lasting 10–60 sec; sagging of head and dropping to ground are noted; EEG shows a slow spike-wave pattern; most often due to an organic brain abnormality
Infantile spasms (hypsarrhythmia)	Under 1 yr	Brief, recurrent myoclonic jerks with abrupt flexion or extension of the limbs or whole body; most patients are mentally retarded; high-voltage, slow waves are predominant in the EEG, but asynchronous spiking can occur.
Status epilepticus	Any age	Repetitive generalized seizure activity in which the patient does *not* regain consciousness during seizure-free intervals; medical emergency; diffuse continuous spiking in EEG waves
Partial		
Elementary (focal) seizures	Any age	Manifestations differ according to site of the lesion; convulsions may be confined to a single limb or muscle group (jacksonian seizures); no impairment of consciousness; sensory disturbances also noted; EEG shows spiking at site of focus
Complex, partial seizures (psychomotor epilepsy)	Any age	Confused behavior, with involuntary, purposeless, repetitive motor activity; usually accompanied by autonomic manifestations and loss of consciousness; seizures last several minutes, but patients have no recall of the attack; bizarre actions are sometimes seen; EEG spiking is present in the temporal lobe; control is difficult

SIGNIFICANT ADVERSE REACTIONS

Nausea, vomiting diarrhea, skin rash (2% of patients), urticaria, angioedema, muscle and joint pain, bradycardia, hypoventilation, laryngospasm, respiratory depression, paradoxical excitation (especially in children and elderly), megaloblastic anemia, insomnia, nightmares, altered behavior, blood dyscrasias (rare)

CONTRAINDICATIONS

Latent or manifest porphyria, respiratory obstruction. *Cautious use* in patients with pulmonary, hepatic, or renal disease, status asthmaticus, hyperthyroidism, diabetes, and in elderly or debilitated patients. Too-rapid IV injection can result in hypotension, laryngospasm, respiratory depression, and apnea

INTERACTIONS

See Chapter 20

NURSING CONSIDERATIONS
See Chapter 20. In addition:

Nursing Alerts
- When administering drugs IV in acute convulsive states, ensure that adequate resuscitative measures are immediately at hand, and monitor vital signs closely. Drugs should be given slowly.
- Drugs may cause neonatal hemorrhage by reducing levels of vitamin K–dependent clotting factors produced in the liver: Be prepared to administer vitamin K prophylactically at birth to infants born to mothers receiving the drug.

1. Follow proper procedures for handling controlled substances. Metharbital is a Schedule III drug. Phenobarbital and mephobarbital are Schedule IV drugs.

PATIENT EDUCATION

See Chapter 20. In addition:
1. Warn patient that drug may impair mental and physical abilities required for performance of many tasks such as driving.
2. Prepare patient and family for the possibility of paradoxical excitatory and other unusual affective reactions, which are particularly likely to occur in the elderly and in young children.
3. Explain that prolonged use, even in rather low doses, can lead to tolerance and habituation. Teach patient to recognize signs of tolerance and inform patient that, if drug must be withdrawn, it should be discontinued *slowly* to avoid possibility of delirium, tremors, and convulsions.
4. Instruct patient to increase intake of vitamin D because drugs may increase vitamin D requirements by stepping up its metabolism, occasionally leading to rickets or osteomalacia with prolonged use.

PRIMIDONE

Myidone, Mysoline
(CAN) Apo-Primidone, Sertan

Although not a true barbiturate, primidone is structurally related to phenobarbital and has a similar profile of action. It is metabolized to phenobarbital and phenylethylmalonamide, both active anticonvulsants.

MECHANISM
Not established, but probably similar to phenobarbital

USES
(May be given alone or with other anticonvulsants)
Grand mal seizures
Psychomotor seizures
Complex partial motor seizures (jacksonian)
Benign familial (essential) tremor (investigational use)

DOSAGE
Adults: Initially, 100 mg to 125 mg daily at bedtime for 3 days; gradually increase to 250 mg 3 or 4 times a day, the usual maintenance dose
Children: Initially, 50 mg a day; increase gradually to 125 mg to 250 mg 3 times a day

FATE
Slowly but well absorbed orally; peak serum levels attained in 3 to 4 hours; prolonged action caused by conversion to active metabolites with half-lives of 2 to 4 days; excreted through kidneys, approximately one fourth as unchanged drug

COMMON SIDE EFFECTS
Lethargy, ataxia, vertigo, irritability

SIGNIFICANT ADVERSE REACTIONS
Nausea, anorexia, vomiting, fatigue, allergic reactions, severe skin rash (macropapular and morbilliform), lymph gland enlargement, megaloblastic anemia (rare), visual disturbances, impotence, personality disorders, drowsiness, blood dyscrasias (leukopenia, thrombocytopenia), and systemic lupus–like reaction

CONTRAINDICATIONS
Latent or manifest porphyria. *Cautious use* in pregnant or nursing women and in persons who must drive or operate heavy machinery

INTERACTIONS
See Anticonvulsant Barbiturates; in addition:

Concurrent administration of phenytoin may increase the toxic effects of primidone by altering its metabolism
Primidone can decrease plasma levels of carbamazepine
Isoniazid may inhibit the metabolism of primidone to active metabolites

NURSING CONSIDERATIONS
See Anticonvulsant Barbiturates. In addition:

Nursing Alerts
- Monitor for early signs of lymph node enlargement, fever, sore throat, bruising, and weakness, possible indications of blood dyscrasias.
- Assess for signs of folic acid deficiency (drug may impair folate absorption), such as anemia, mental dysfunction, neuropathy, and psychiatric disturbances. Use of folic acid (15 mg/day) or vitamin B_6 may be necessary to prevent megaloblastic anemia.
- Before initiating administration, review patient's medication history for evidence of allergy to barbiturates. A patient allergic to barbiturates will probably be allergic to primidone.

1. Observe for early signs of overdosage (e.g., incoordination, slurred speech, blurred vision). If they occur, dosage should be gradually decreased.
2. Expect dosage adjustments to be made gradually and dosage of other antiepileptics to be readjusted if primidone is added to the regimen.

PATIENT EDUCATION
See Anticonvulsant Barbiturates. In addition:
1. With prolonged therapy, inform patient that a complete blood count is recommended at 6-month intervals.

HYDANTOINS

Ethotoin   Phenytoin
Mephenytoin

The hydantoin group of antiepileptic agents generally are the most effective drugs for the treatment of grand mal seizures and can be used in the control of psychomotor epilepsy as well. These drugs, unlike barbiturates, are not CNS depressants and do not interfere with normal sensory function. There are three

Table 25-2
Anticonvulsant Barbiturates

Drug	Preparations	Usual Dosage Range	Nursing Implications
Mephobarbital Mebaral	Tablets: 32 mg, 50 mg, 100 mg	Adults: 400 mg–600 mg/day Children (over 5 yr): 32 mg–64 mg 3–4 times/day; (under 5 yr) 16 mg–32 mg 3–4 times day	Similar to phenobarbital in most respects, producing somewhat less sedation; largely converted to phenobarbital within 24 h; used as a single daily dose at bedtime for nocturnal seizures; withdraw slowly when necessary, and reduce dose of other antiepileptics when added to the regimen (Schedule IV)
Metharbital Gemonil	Tablets: 100 mg	Adults: Initially 100 mg 1–3 times/day; adjust to optimal level Children: 5–15 mg/kg/day	Less effective than phenobarbital, and possesses somewhat greater sedative action; usually used in combination with other antiepileptic drugs for grand mal, petit mal, myoclonic or mixed seizures (Schedule III)
Phenobarbital Various manufacturers	Tablets: 8 mg, 16 mg, 32 mg, 65 mg, 100 mg Capsules: 16 mg Elixir: 15 mg/5 mL, 20 mg/5 mL Injection: 30 mg/mL, 60 mg/mL, 65 mg/mL, 130 mg/mL	*Oral* Adults: 50 mg–100 mg 2–3 times/day Children: Initially, 3 mg/kg–5 mg/kg/day for 7–10 days; adjust to blood level of 10 µg/mL to 15 mcg/mL *IM, IV* Adults: 200 mg–300 mg; repeat in 6 h if needed *or* 300 mg–600 mg initially, then 120 mg–240 mg every 20 min as needed Children (IV): 20 mg/kg initially, then 6 mg/kg every 20 min as needed	Very effective alone for treatment of grand mal (especially in children) and as part of the drug regimen in most other forms of epilepsy; also used IV or IM for status epilepticus and other acute convulsive states; following IV injection, 15 min or more may be required to attain peak CNS concentration; thus, give drug *intermittently,* even though convulsions persist; continuous injection can result in excessive CNS levels of drug after convulsions have ceased, possibly leading to respiratory depression; solutions should be prepared in sterile water for injection and should not be used if not completely clear after 5 min of mixing; inject drug within 30 min after preparation of solution; drowsiness is common in early stages of therapy but diminishes with continued use; frequency of IV administration is determined by patient's response; discontinue drug as soon as desired response is obtained (Schedule IV)

currently marketed hydantoins, of which phenytoin is the most frequently prescribed.

MECHANISM

Inhibit spread of seizure activity to neurons surrounding seizure focus in the motor cortex by raising the threshold of excitability of these neurons; promote sodium efflux from neuronal cells, blocking development of posttetanic potentiation and thereby preventing focal seizure activity from spreading to adjacent cortical areas; may shorten duration of afterdischarges and increase release of GABA, an inhibitory neurotransmitter in the central nervous system

USES

Grand mal seizures (may be combined with primidone or carbamazepine)
Focal, Jacksonian, or psychomotor seizures, either alone or in combination with primidone
Alcohol withdrawal syndrome
Trigeminal neuralgia

Cardiac arrhythmias (especially ventricular arrhythmias due to digitalis intoxication—see Chap. 30)

Status epilepticus and seizures during neurosurgery (IV phenytoin)

DOSAGE
See Table 25-3

FATE
(Discussion applies to phenytoin, the only hydantoin whose pharmacokinetics has been extensively studied)

Generally slowly absorbed orally; rate and extent of phenytoin absorption vary widely among the different available preparations, the sodium salt being the best absorbed; bioavailability also differs markedly (20%–90%) among products of different manufacturers; oral phenytoin sodium *extended* (Dilantin) attains peak plasma levels in 4 to 12 hours; phenytoin sodium *prompt* (other clinically available preparations) achieves peak serum levels in 2 to 3 hours; erratically absorbed following IM injection; peak blood levels occur at varying times up to 24 hours and are significantly lower than blood levels obtained with oral or IV administration; highly bound (85%–95%) to plasma proteins; metabolized in the liver and excreted largely as conjugated metabolites in the urine; elimination half-life ranges from 8 to 60 hours (average 20–30 h)

COMMON SIDE EFFECTS
Sluggishness, ataxia, nystagmus, confusion, slurred speech; less commonly—dizziness, insomnia, nervousness, fatigue, irritability

SIGNIFICANT ADVERSE REACTIONS
GI: nausea, vomiting, diarrhea, abdominal pain, dysphagia
CNS: headache, depression, tremors, behavioral disturbances
Dermatologic: skin rashes (morbilliform, maculopapular, scarlatiniform), urticaria, keratosis, hirsutism, lupus erythematosus, exfoliative dermatitis (rare)
Hematopoietic: blood dyscrasias, anemias, lymphadenopathy, bone marrow depression
Other: gingival hyperplasia (20%–30% incidence, especially children), periodontal infection, polyarthropathy, hepatitis, liver damage, alopecia, hyperglycemia, edema, chest pain, numbness, photophobia, pulmonary fibrosis, osteomalacia
IV administration has resulted in hypotension, cardiac arrhythmias, hyperkinesis, and cardiovascular collapse

CONTRAINDICATIONS
Hematologic disorders, severe hepatic dysfunction, incomplete heart block; IV phenytoin is contraindicated in sinus bradycardia, sinoatrial block, second and third degree AV block, and Adams–Stokes syndrome. *Cautious use* in persons with hypotension, myocardial insufficiency, hyperglycemia, anemia, osteoporosis, or acute intermittent porphyria, and in pregnant or nursing mothers. Abrupt withdrawal of the drug may result in status epilepticus

> **WARNING**
> Consider benefit *versus* risk ratio in pregnant women. Although fetal damage has been reported (cleft palate), discontinuance of therapy may precipitate status epilepticus with resulting hypoxia to the fetus. Carefully weigh all factors when using these drugs during pregnancy

INTERACTIONS
Phenytoin may increase the effects of oral anticoagulants, antihypertensives, thyroid hormones, sedatives and hypnotics, propranolol, and methotrexate

Phenytoin may diminish the effects of corticosteroids, oral contraceptives, disopyramide, quinidine, digitalis glycosides, and tetracyclines (by increasing their liver metabolism)

The effects of phenytoin can be increased by drugs that (1) *inhibit its metabolism* (e.g., allopurinol, cimetidine, diazepam, disulfiram, acute ethanol ingestion, isoniazid, phenacemide, phenylbutazone, succinimides, sulfonamides, trimethoprim, and valproic acid) or (2) *displace the drug from protein-binding sites* (e.g., salicylates and antiinflammatory drugs, valproic acid)

The effects of phenytoin can be reduced by drugs that (1) *increase its metabolism* (e.g., barbiturates, carbamazepine, diazoxide, chronic ethanol ingestion, folic acid, and theophylline), (2) *retard its oral absorption* (e.g., antacids, antineoplastics, calcium, charcoal) and (3) by several other drugs such as influenza virus vaccine, loxapine, nitrofurantoin, and pyridoxine

Tricyclic antidepressants may precipitate seizures, so phenytoin dosage should be adjusted accordingly. Valproic acid and phenytoin may result in breakthrough seizures

Phenytoin can impair the absorption of furosemide.

Concomitant administration of phenytoin and dopamine may lead to hypotension and bradycardia

NURSING CONSIDERATIONS

Nursing Alerts
- When administering drug IV, monitor blood pressure, ECG, and respiration, and ensure that appropriate antidotal measures are on hand (e.g., vasopressors, oxygen, respiratory aids). Hydantoins should be given *slowly* (50 mg/min into running IV) to avoid bradycardia and hypotension, and sterile saline should be injected through the needle or catheter after each injection to avoid local venous irritation caused by alkalinity of the drug solution.
- Monitor patient for early signs of developing blood dyscrasias (e.g., fever, sore throat, mucosal ulceration, malaise) or hepatic dysfunction (dark urine, abdominal cramps, jaundice), and check results of periodic blood counts and urinalyses.
- Assess for nystagmus, confusion, ataxia, dysarthria, and unresponsive pupils, which are signs of overdosage. If these occur, dosage should be carefully readjusted.
- Collaborate with health care team to individually adjust dosage to minimize toxicity. In some patients, peak blood levels after full dosage may be associated with transient signs of CNS toxicity, and these adverse effects may be reduced by using multiple smaller doses.
- Observe for signs of folic acid deficiency (anemia, neuropathy, psychiatric disorders, mental dysfunction) because hydantoins may interfere with folic acid availability. Supplemental folic acid should be given as needed. Additional folic acid can, however, increase phenytoin metabolism and may increase seizure frequency. Dosage should be adjusted accordingly.
- Monitor patient's blood sugar levels because hydantoins may inhibit insulin release, leading to hyperglycemia. Dosage should be carefully adjusted in the diabetic patient.

- Be prepared to administer vitamin K prophylactically during latter stages of pregnancy because hydantoins can reduce levels of vitamin K–dependent clotting factors produced by the liver.

1. Provide emotional support to patient and family.
2. Ensure that brand of phenytoin administered is not changed after therapy is initiated unless serum concentrations are carefully monitored because bioavailability differs significantly among preparations (see Fate). Note that *only Dilantin products* are approved for once-daily use owing to prolonged absorption. All other phenytoin products are classified as *prompt* acting and are used 2 to 4 times a day.
3. Refer patient for dietary consultation to ensure that intake of vitamin D–containing foods is adequate to prevent hypocalcemia; hydantoins can accelerate vitamin D metabolism.
4. Question administration to patient with petit mal seizures because hydantoins may worsen the symptoms. Combined drug therapy is indicated when mixed seizure types are present.
5. Use parenteral solutions immediately after mixing, and do not add to any IV infusion because solubility may be altered by pH differences. Shake suspension thoroughly to obtain correct dosage. Continuous infusions should be avoided.

PATIENT EDUCATION

1. Advise patient to take oral drug with meals, if possible, to minimize gastric irritation; drug is strongly alkaline.
2. Discuss the importance of proper diet, avoidance of fatigue, stress, or illness, and maintenance of prescribed dosage regimen for good seizure control.
3. Warn patient that convulsions may occur if dosage is altered or medication is abruptly discontinued.
4. Advise patient not to take any other drugs, including OTC preparations, unless specifically prescribed because hydantoins interact with many drugs. Excessive use of alcohol or other CNS depressants, for example, may reduce the efficacy of hydantoins.
5. Stress the importance of oral hygiene, regular gum massage, and frequent brushing of the teeth to minimize the severity of gingival hyperplasia, especially in children, in whom the incidence is much higher than in adults.
6. Inform patient that hydantoins may harmlessly color urine pink to reddish-brown.
7. Teach significant others proper methods for dealing with a seizure episode.
8. Urge patient to carry an identification card with pertinent medical information.

OXAZOLIDINEDIONES

Paramethadione   Trimethadione

The oxazolidinediones are effective drugs for the control of simple absence (petit mal) seizures but elicit a rather high incidence of untoward reactions. They are largely reserved for patients intolerant of or unresponsive to other less toxic agents.

The two currently available drugs, trimethadione and paramethadione, differ only slightly in their pharmacologic properties; thus, they are reviewed together and are then listed separately in Table 25-4.

MECHANISM
Complex and incompletely understood; prolong the recovery period of postsynaptic neurons in those CNS systems (primarily thalamocortical) where repetitive discharges produce absence attacks through a negative feedback mechanism; other central effects include elevating the threshold for seizure discharge in the thalamus and interference with the propagation of seizure activity from a cortical focus to the thalamus; possess little sedative or hypnotic action but may exert an analgesic effect

USES
Simple absence (petit mal) seizures refractory to other drugs

DOSAGE
See Table 25-4

FATE
Readily absorbed from GI tract; peak plasma concentrations in 30 minutes to 60 minutes; uniformly distributed and not bound to plasma proteins; metabolized in liver to an active metabolite with an extended half-life; slowly excreted in the urine

COMMON SIDE EFFECTS
Drowsiness, GI distress, hiccups, photophobia

SIGNIFICANT ADVERSE REACTIONS

WARNING
Fetal malformations and other serious side effects have occurred during therapy with oxazolidinediones. Use only where other less toxic drugs are ineffective

GI: nausea, vomiting, abdominal pain, anorexia
CNS: vertigo, irritability, personality changes, headache, paresthesias, precipitation of grand mal seizures
Ocular: diplopia, scotomata, hemeralopia (day blindness), retinal hemorrhage
Hematologic: epistaxis, mucosal bleeding (e.g., gums, vagina), blood dyscrasias (especially neutropenia), changes in blood pressure
Dermatologic: skin rash (acneiform, morbilliform), exfoliative dermatitis, erythema multiforme
Other: albuminuria, alopecia, lymphadenopathy, systemic lupus-like reaction, myasthenia gravis–like reaction, nephrosis, hepatitis

CONTRAINDICATIONS
Hepatic and renal disease, blood dyscrasias, diseases of the retina or optic nerve, myasthenia gravis, pregnancy. *Cautious use* in nursing mothers and in persons with acute intermittent porphyria. Do not use alone in mixed seizure forms because oxazolidinediones can worsen grand mal symptoms

INTERACTIONS
CNS depression induced by oxazolidinediones may be augmented by other depressants, oral anticoagulants, and *p*-aminosalicylic acid

Table 25-3
Hydantoins

Drug	Preparations	Usual Dosage Range	Nursing Implications
Ethotoin Peganone	Tablets: 250 mg, 500 mg	Adults: 250 mg 4 times/day initially; increase to optimal levels (usually 2 g–3 g/day) Children: 750 mg/day initially; maintenance 500 mg–1000 mg/day based on age and weight	Administer with food, and begin therapy at small dose levels; compatible with most other anticonvulsants (dosage must be adjusted) expect phenacemide (danger of paranoid reactions); less effective than phenytoin, but somewhat less toxic as well; *not* used as an antiarrhythmic
Mephenytoin Mesantoin	Tablets: 100 mg	Adults: Initial dose 50 mg–100 mg/day; increase gradually to optimal levels (usual range 200 mg–600 mg/day) Children: 100 mg–400 mg/day based on age, weight, and severity of seizures	Most toxic of the hydantoins; reserved for patients refractory to less toxic anticonvulsants; may be useful in jacksonian seizures; possesses a strong sedative action; blood counts should be performed every 2–4 wk; more rapidly absorbed than other hydantoins with an onset of action in 30 minutes
Phenytoin Dilantin Infatab, Dilantin-30 Pediatric, Dilantin-125 **Phenytoin Sodium, Extended** Dilantin Kapseals **Phenytoin Sodium, Prompt** Diphenylan **Phenytoin Sodium Parenteral** Dilantin	Chewable tablets: 50 mg Suspension: 30 mg, 125 mg/ 5 mL Capsules: 30 mg, 100 mg Capsules: 30 mg, 100 mg Injection: 50 mg/mL	*Oral* Adults: Initially, 100 mg 3 times/day; usual range is 300 mg–400 mg/day Children: Initially 5 mg/kg/day in 2 or 3 divided doses; usual maintenance range is 4–8 mg/kg/day in children under 6 *IV* *Status epilepticus* Adults: 150 mg–250 mg; repeat in 30 min with 100 mg–150 mg if necessary Children: 250 mg/m² body surface area *Arrhythmias* 100 mg every 5 min until arrhythmia is abolished (maximum 1000 mg) *IM* *Neurosurgery* 100 mg–200 mg/4 h during surgery and postoperative period (maximum 1000 mg/day)	Owing to their slower dissolution rate, *extended* phenytoin sodium capsules (Dilantin) can be used on a more convenient once-daily basis when seizure control has been established with divided doses initially; *do not* administer IM in status epilepticus, because erratic absorption prevents attaining sufficient plasma levels; an IM dose 50% greater than the oral dose is necessary to maintain stable plasma levels; margin between the effective and toxic IV dose is very small; administer slowly and carefully monitor vital signs; do *not* exceed IV infusion rate of 50 mg/min and avoid *continuous* infusion; effective against digitalis-induced arrhythmias (see Chap. 30); phenytoin is also available in combination with phenobarbital (Dilantin-Pb capsules)

NURSING CONSIDERATIONS

Nursing Alerts
- Observe closely for early signs of hematologic toxicity (e.g., sore throat, mucosal ulceration, fever, malaise, petechiae). If noted, withhold drug and notify physician.
- Withhold drug and inform physician if skin rash, neutrophil depression (see next item), jaundice, albuminuria, scotomas, lymph node enlargement, or myasthenia symptoms occur because severe toxicity can ensue.
- Monitor results of compete blood counts, liver function tests, and urinalyses, which should be performed prior to and at regular intervals during therapy. Therapy should be discontinued if neutrophil count drops below 2500/mm³.

PATIENT EDUCATION
1. Stress the importance of rigid adherence to prescribed regimen to minimize untoward reactions.
2. Advise patient to report immediately any development of ocular side effects (e.g., glaring, dark spots, blurring), which necessitate dosage reduction. Retinal damage may occur if dosage is too high.
3. Inform patient that the incidence of petit mal attacks may *increase* during first few days of therapy. Reassure patient that clinical benefit will occur within several days.
4. Inform patient that drowsiness will diminish with continued use. A mild stimulant such as caffeine may be employed in early stages of therapy to reduce excessive drowsiness.

Table 25-4
Oxazolidinediones

Drug	Preparations	Usual Dosage Range	Nursing Implications
Paramethadione Paradione	Capsules: 150 mg, 300 mg Solution: 300 mg/mL	Adults: 300 mg–600 mg 3–4 times/day (initial dose 900 mg/day; increase by 300 mg/wk to above range) Children: 300 mg–900 mg/day in 3–4 divided doses	Less effective but slightly less toxic than trimethadione; no myasthenic-like reactions have occurred, but sedation is common; oral solution contains 65% alcohol and should be diluted with water before administration to children
Trimethadione Tridione	Chewable tablets: 150 mg Capsules: 300 mg Solution: 40 mg/mL	Adults: Initially 300 mg 3 times/day; usual maintenance dose 900 mg–2400 mg/day in divided doses Children: 300 mg–900 mg/day in 3–4 divided doses	Plasma level of dimethadione, the active metabolite of trimethadione, may be used as a dosage guide; this level should be maintained about 700 µg/mL for optimal control of petit mal attacks in patients receiving trimethadione; alkalinization of the urine will increase excretion of this metabolite

5. Inform patient that therapy should be discontinued only under the supervision of a health care provider. The drug should be withdrawn gradually to prevent development of simple absence attacks, which can occur with abrupt discontinuation.

SUCCINIMIDES

Ethosuximide   Phensuximide
Methsuximide

Although no more effective than the oxazolidinediones in the treatment of simple absence seizures (petit mal,), the succinimides remain the drugs of choice for these conditions primarily because of their lower toxicity as compared with other drugs used for simple absence seizures. Because they may increase the frequency of grand mal attacks, however, their use in mixed seizure patterns must be accompanied by other antiepileptics capable of controlling tonic–clonic seizures. Three succinimides are currently available, offering little in the way of significant differences among them. They are discussed as a group, then listed individually in Table 25-5.

MECHANISM
Remains to be definitively established; in laboratory tests, drugs' effects generally resemble those of the oxazolidinediones, and they are known to suppress the three-per-second spike-wave EEG pattern characteristic of absence seizures; evidence suggests a depressant effect on the motor cortex and possible elevation of the firing threshold of cortical neurons

USES
Simple absence (petit mal) seizures
Adjunctive treatment of psychomotor and other minor motor seizures (methsuximide *only*)

DOSAGE
See Table 25-5

FATE
Well absorbed orally; peak serum levels in 2 to 4 hours; not bound to plasma proteins; short half-life (2–4 h) except ethosuximide (30–60 h); metabolized by the liver and excreted primarily in the urine as both active and inactive metabolites

COMMON SIDE EFFECTS
GI distress (nausea, upset, cramping, pain, diarrhea), drowsiness, ataxia, dizziness

SIGNIFICANT ADVERSE REACTIONS
CNS: irritability, nervousness, euphoria, aggressiveness, hyperactivity, confusion, lethargy, fatigue, depression, sleep disturbances, night terrors, inability to concentrate, hiccups, insomnia
Ocular: blurred vision, myopia, photophobia, periorbital edema
Hematologic: blood dyscrasias
Dermatologic: urticaria, erythematous rashes, erythema multiforme, systemic lupus erythematosus, Stevens–Johnson syndrome (see Chap. 4)
Genitourinary: urinary frequency, hematuria, albuminuria, renal damage (rare)
Other: alopecia, vaginal bleeding, hyperemia, swelling of the tongue, muscular weakness, hirsutism

CONTRAINDICATIONS
Severe liver or renal damage. *Cautious use* in persons with reduced liver function, mixed seizures, behavioral disturbances, and ulcers

INTERACTIONS
Absorption of ethosuximide may be reduced by amphetamine
Increased libido may result if ethosuximide is combined with other anticonvulsants

PATIENT EDUCATION

1. Caution against engaging in any hazardous activity during initial stages of therapy because drowsiness is common.
2. Explain the significance of adhering to prescribed dosing schedule. Dosage adjustments should always be made gradually because abrupt changes may precipitate increased seizure activity.
3. Stress the importance of carefully noting and reporting the development of untoward reactions. Most adverse effects can be minimized or eliminated by a dosage adjustment if detected early.
4. Instruct patient and family to be alert for and to report development of behavior changes (e.g., depression, aggressiveness). Drug should be withdrawn slowly if these occur.
5. Instruct patient to inform physician if rash, dizziness, fever, blurred vision, joint pain, bruising, or bleeding occur because these may indicate developing toxicity.
6. Encourage patient to obtain all laboratory studies requested. Periodic blood counts should be performed because several blood dyscrasias have been reported.

CARBAMAZEPINE

Carbamazepine

Epitol, Tegretol

(CAN) Apo-Carbamazepine, Mazepine, PMS Carbamazepine

Carbamazepine is structurally related to the tricyclic antidepressants and has a spectrum of action similar to phenytoin. It has been employed successfully to treat the pain of trigeminal neuralgia (tic doloureux). The drug is a fairly toxic agent that is used for the treatment of grand mal and psychomotor seizures in patients not responding satisfactorily to other less toxic drugs.

MECHANISM

Increases latency, decreases responsivity, and suppresses afterdischarges in polysynaptic pathways associated with cortical and limbic function; may reduce posttetanic potentiation; has anticholinergic, antidepressant, and muscle-relaxing action (interferes with neuromuscular transmission)

USES

Psychomotor seizures (alone or with primidone or phenytoin)
Grand mal (with phenytoin)
Adjunctive treatment of mixed seizures or complex partial seizures
Relief of pain associated with trigeminal neuralgia
Experimental uses include treatment of neurogenic diabetes insipidus, alcohol withdrawal syndrome, and certain psychiatric disorders such as bipolar depressive illness and schizoaffective disorders

DOSAGE

A. *Epilepsy*
 1. Adults and children over 12: Initially 200 mg twice a day; increase by 200 mg/day in divided doses until optimal response is achieved; maximum 1200 mg/day; usual maintenance range is 800 mg to 1200 mg/day
 2. Children 6 to 12: Initially, 100 mg twice a day; increase by 100 mg/day until optimal response is achieved; usual maintenance level is 400 mg to 800 mg daily

B. *Trigeminal Neuralgia*
 1. Initially 100 mg twice a day; increase by 100 mg/12 hours; usual maintenance range is 400 mg to 800 mg/day

---

Table 25-5
Succinimides

Drug	Preparations	Usual Dosage Range	Nursing Implications
Ethosuximide Zarontin	Capsules: 250 mg Syrup: 250 mg/5 mL	Adults: Initially 500 mg/day; increase by 250 mg every 4–7 days until control is achieved (maximum 1500 mg/day) Children: 250 mg/day increased slowly to optimal level	Inform patient that drug may color urine pink to reddish-brown; appearance of frequent GI distress, dizziness, ataxia, or other neurologic disorders signifies need for dosage adjustment; administer with meals to reduce GI upset; long half-life, therefore do not exceed recommended dosage as danger of accumulation exists
Methsuximide Celontin	Capsules: 150 mg, 300 mg	Initially 300 mg/day for 1 wk; may increase by 300 mg weekly to a maximum of 1200 mg	Equally effective in petit mal as ethosuximide but somewhat more toxic, especially to the CNS (e.g., severe depression, confusion); may be useful in certain cases of psychomotor epilepsy
Phensuximide Milontin	Capsules: 500 mg	Adults: 500 mg–1000 mg 2–3 times/day (range 1 g–3 g/day) Children: 600 mg–1200 mg 2 or 3 times/day	Slightly less effective and less toxic than other succinimides; may color urine reddish-brown

FATE
Oral absorption is slow but complete; peak plasma levels in 4 hours to 6 hours; widely distributed and highly (75%) protein-bound; serum half-life is 12 to 20 hours on repeated dosing; metabolized in the liver (epoxide metabolite has anticonvulsant activity) and excreted as several metabolites and some unchanged drug through the kidneys

COMMON SIDE EFFECTS
Drowsiness, dizziness, ataxia, nausea, blurred vision, diplopia

SIGNIFICANT ADVERSE REACTIONS

> **WARNING**
> Serious and sometime fatal blood dyscrasias have occurred with carbamazepine. Early detection is vital, because in some patients aplastic anemia is irreversible. See Nursing Alert

CNS: confusion, incoordination, speech disturbances, involuntary movements, dysphasia, visual hallucinations, tinnitus, depression, peripheral neuritis, paresthesias, nystagmus
Dermatologic: rash, sweating, urticaria, photosensitivity reactions, alopecia, exfoliative dermatitis, erythema multiforme, abnormal pigmentation
Hematologic: blood dyscrasias, (aplastic anemia, leukopenia, agranulocytosis, eosinophilia, leukocytosis, thrombocytopenia)
Genitourinary: urinary frequency, albuminuria, glycosuria, urinary retention, oliguria, impotence
GI: diarrhea, vomiting, abdominal pain, anorexia, xerostomia, glossitis
Cardiovascular: hypotension, syncope, arrhythmias, aggravation of coronary artery disease and hypertension, thrombophlebitis, AV block, congestive heart failure
Other: abnormal liver function, osteomalacia, hepatitis, jaundice, muscle aching, fever, chills, lenticular opacities, adenopathy

CONTRAINDICATIONS
History of bone marrow depression, severe hypertension, and concomitant use of MAO inhibitors. *Cautious use* in patients with renal, hepatic, or cardiac disease, hypertension, glaucoma, and in elderly, pregnant, or nursing patients

INTERACTIONS
Carbamazepine may accelerate the metabolism and therefore decrease the effects of other anticonvulsants (phenobarbital, phenytoin, primidone), oral anticoagulants, and tetracyclines
Concurrent use of carbamazepine with MAO inhibitors or tricyclic antidepressants is not recommended because toxicity may be increased
Carbamazepine is highly protein-bound and therefore may potentiate other protein-bound drugs (e.g., salicylates, oral hypoglycemics, anticoagulants, antiinflammatory agents) by displacing them from protein-binding sites
Cimetidine, isoniazid, erythromycin, and propoxyphene can elevate serum levels of carbamazepine, leading to increased toxicity
Carbamazepine can result in breakthrough bleeding in women taking oral contraceptives
Increased CNS toxicity can occur if carbamazepine is used concurrently with lithium

NURSING CONSIDERATIONS

Nursing Alert
- Monitor results of complete blood counts, liver function tests, urinalyses, and BUN tests, which should be performed prior to initiating therapy and at regular intervals thereafter. The drug should be discontinued if findings are abnormal or if any evidence of bone marrow depression develops.

1. Implement interventions to protect elderly patients from injury, as confusion, agitation, and behavioral disturbances occur more commonly in the elderly.

PATIENT EDUCATION
1. Warn patient to avoid hazardous tasks until reaction to drug has been determined. Drowsiness and dizziness are common in initial stages of therapy.
2. Explain the importance of adhering to prescribed dosage schedule. Drug withdrawal or dosage adjustments should be implemented slowly. Abrupt changes may provoke seizures or status epilepticus.
3. Teach patient how to recognize early signs of hematologic toxicity (sore throat, mucosal ulceration, petechiae, bruising, malaise). If any occur, the physician should be notified immediately.
4. Encourage patient to obtain periodic ophthalmologic examinations because drug can cause ocular damage.

VALPROIC ACID DERIVATIVES

Valproic Acid
Depa, Depakene, Deproic
Sodium Valproate
Depakene, Myproic Acid
Divalproex Sodium
Depakote

Although chemically unrelated to other anticonvulsants, valproic acid, its sodium salt, and a stable compound composed of equal parts valproic acid and sodium valproate (i.e., divalproex sodium) generally provide improved seizure control when added to the drug regimen of patients with multiple seizure types whose condition is refractory to treatment. They are most effective against simple and complex absence seizures. Divalproex is an enteric-coated dosage form and has a slightly lower incidence of GI side effects than the other dosage forms

MECHANISM
Elicit a consistent elevation in the functional levels of GABA (an inhibitory neurotransmitter) in the CNS; the contribution of this effect to the antiepileptic efficacy of the drug remains to be established; drug also elicits a metabolic acidosis that may also protect against seizures; inhibits release of prolactin

USES
Simple and complex absence seizures, including petit mal (alone or in combination with other anticonvulsants)
Adjunct in the treatment of multiple-seizure types

Investigational uses include grand mal seizures, myclonic seizures, infantile spasms, complex and elementary partial seizures, and prevention of recurrent febrile seizures

DOSAGE
(Dosage is expressed in valproic acid equivalents)
Initially, 15 mg/kg/day; increase by 5 mg/kg to 10 mg/kg weekly until seizures are controlled (maximum 60 mg/kg/day)

FATE
Valproic acid and sodium valproate are rapidly absorbed orally; divalproex is enteric coated and absorption is delayed but uniform and consistent; peak serum levels occur within 30 to 60 minutes with sodium valproate and within 1 to 4 hours with the other dosage forms; widely distributed and highly (90%) protein-bound; drug is metabolized primarily in the liver and is excreted in the urine, almost entirely as conjugated metabolites

COMMON SIDE EFFECTS
Nausea, vomiting, indigestion, sedation, elevated serum transaminases

SIGNIFICANT ADVERSE REACTIONS

> **WARNING**
> Fatal hepatic failure has occurred in patients receiving valproic acid, usually during the first 6 months of treatment. Frequent liver function tests are required, especially during the initial months of therapy

Diarrhea, abdominal cramps, lenticular opacities, nystagmus, visual disturbances, diplopia, dizziness, incoordination, tremor, dysarthria, skin rash, petechiae, alopecia, depression, aggression, hyperactivity, behavioral disturbances, altered bleeding time (drug inhibits platelet aggregation), muscle weakness, blood dyscrasias (rare), hepatotoxicity

Note: Because the drug has been used in combination with other antiepileptic medication, it is difficult to ascribe the above adverse effects solely to valproic acid

CONTRAINDICATIONS
Hepatic disease or dysfunction. *Cautious use* in persons with bleeding disorders or renal dysfunction and in pregnant or nursing women

INTERACTIONS
Valproic acid may potentiate the depressant effects of other CNS depressant drugs (e.g., barbiturates, narcotics, alcohol)
Serum phenobarbital levels may be elevated by valproic acid
Simultaneous use of valproic acid and clonazepam may *induce* absence seizures
Valproic acid interferes with platelet aggregation and therefore may enhance the action of anticoagulants, dipyridamole, and salicylates
Breakthrough seizures have occurred with use of valproic acid and phenytoin

NURSING CONSIDERATIONS

Nursing Alert
- Monitor results of liver function tests, which should be performed prior to and at frequent intervals during therapy, because hepatic failure has occurred. The drug should be discontinued at the first sign of hepatic dysfunction as indicated by either serum biochemistry or clinical evaluation.

1. Interpret urine tests for ketone bodies cautiously. The drug is excreted in part as a ketone-containing metabolite, which can interfere with these tests.

PATIENT EDUCATION
1. Instruct patient to swallow capsule whole to avoid local mouth and throat irritation and to take with food to minimize GI irritation.
2. Warn patient not to use alcohol or other CNS depressants with valproic acid because additive CNS depression can occur.
3. Advise patient not to engage in hazardous activities because drowsiness and dizziness can occur.
4. Instruct patient to report any visual disturbances immediately because ocular toxicity has been noted.
5. Inform patient that periodic blood counts are advisable during therapy because platelet dysfunction and blood dyscrasias have been reported

CLONAZEPAM

Clonazepam
Klonopin
(CAN) Rivotril

Clonazepam is a benzodiazepine derivative used primarily in absence seizures, especially the akinetic and myoclonic variants. Its use is associated with a significant degree of CNS depression and can result in psychological dependence. As many as 50% of users develop tolerance usually within 3 to 6 months, necessitating a dosage adjustment.

MECHANISM
Not well established; may potentiate inhibitory mechanisms in subcortical brain structures; has been shown to suppress the spike wave discharge characteristic of absence seizures and to decrease the frequency, duration, amplitude, and spread of minor motor seizure discharges

USES
Petit mal variant (Lennox–Gastaut syndrome)
Myoclonic and akinetic seizures
Simple absence seizures refractory to succinimides (may be used alone or as an adjunct; some evidence of benefit in psychomotor and focal seizures in combination with other drugs)

DOSAGE
Adults: Initially 0.5 mg 3 times/day; increase by 0.5 mg to 1.0 mg every 3 days until optimal effect is achieved (maximum 20 mg/day)
Children: Initially 0.01 mg/kg to 0.03 mg/kg/day; increase by 0.25 mg to 0.5 mg every 3 days (usual range 0.1 mg/kg–0.2 mg/kg/day)

FATE
Onset following oral administration in 30 to 60 minutes; maximum plasma levels occur in 1 to 2 hours; duration 6 to 12 hours; half-life varies from 20 to 40 hours; metabolized in the liver and primarily excreted in the urine

COMMON SIDE EFFECTS
Drowsiness, ataxia, abnormal behavior

SIGNIFICANT ADVERSE REACTIONS
CNS: confusion, insomnia, depression, hysteria, headache, hypotonia, involuntary movements, slurred speech, tremor, vertigo, nystagmus, hallucinations, psychosis
GI: anorexia, constipation, dry mouth, gastritis, nausea, sore gums, hepatomegaly, coated tongue
Respiratory: rhinorrhea, shortness of breath, hypersecretion
Dermatologic: rash, ankle edema, hirsutism
Urinary: dysuria, enuresis, nocturia
Other: palpitations, muscle weakness, fever, lymphadenopathy, dehydration, blood dyscrasias (rare), diplopia, abnormal eye movements, increased salivation

CONTRAINDICATIONS
Severe liver disease, narrow-angle glaucoma. *Cautious use* in behaviorally disturbed or drug-addicted persons, persons with renal dysfunction or chronic respiratory diseases, and in pregnant or nursing mothers. Drug should *not* be given alone in the presence of mixed seizures, since it may worsen tonic–clonic seizures

INTERACTIONS
CNS depressive effects may be enhanced by other drugs having a depressant action (e.g., alcohol, narcotics, sedatives, phenothiazines, barbiturates)
Phenytoin and phenobarbital can reduce serum clonazepam levels
Combined use of clonazepam and valproic acid may elicit absence seizures

NURSING CONSIDERATIONS
1. Monitor results of complete blood counts and liver function tests, which should be performed periodically during prolonged therapy.
2. Assist with evaluation of patient response to drug. Dosage should be periodically reviewed and adjusted as necessary. Signs of dependence should be noted and, if drug needs to be discontinued, it should be discontinued slowly to avoid withdrawal symptoms.

PATIENT EDUCATION
1. Caution patient against performing hazardous tasks because incidence of drowsiness is quite high.
2. Inform patient that drug may induce paradoxical increases in seizure activity. If this occurs, the physician should be notified. The drug should not be discontinued abruptly because marked exacerbation of seizures or status epilepticus can result.

DIAZEPAM

Diazepam
Valium, Vazepam
(CAN) Apo Diazepam, Diazemuls, E-Pam, Meval, Novodipam, Rival, Vivol

Diazepam is a benzodiazepine widely used for control of simple anxiety states. It may be useful orally as an adjunct in the management of convulsive disorders, but it rarely is effective alone. Its principal indication is parenterally (IV) for the treatment of status epilepticus and other severe recurrent convulsive seizures. Diazepam may also be used for convulsions accompanying acute alcohol withdrawal. The drug is discussed fully in Chapter 23; thus only those aspects relating to its use as an antiepileptic are reviewed here. Diazepam suppresses polysynaptic neuronal activity in the spinal cord and mesencephalic reticular formation; it also facilitates the action of GABA, an inhibitory neurotransmitter in the CNS.

Oral adult dosage ranges from 2 mg to 10 mg 2 to 4 times a day, whereas children may be given 1 mg to 2.5 mg 3 to 4 times a day. Adult IV doses are 5 mg to 10 mg, to be repeated as needed at 10 to 15-minute intervals to a maximum of 30 mg. Children receive 0.2 mg to 1 mg every 2 to 5 minutes depending on age and body weight.

NURSING CONSIDERATIONS
(*See also* Chapter 23)

Nursing Alerts
- After IV administration to control an acute seizure episode, observe patient carefully. Readministration may be necessary because drug effects are short-lived, and many patients experience recurrent seizure episodes.
- Question IV administration to patient with petit mal or petit mal variants because status epilepticus can be *precipitated* in such a patient.
- To help prevent venous thrombosis, swelling, or phlebitis, inject IV diazepam very slowly (5 mg/min) and do not use small veins (e.g., wrist or dorsum of the hand).

1. When giving IM, inject deep into large muscle mass. Although the IV route is preferred for treating convulsive disorders, the drug may be given IM if severe convulsions preclude IV use.

PHENACEMIDE

Phenacemide
Phenurone

A structural analog of the hydantoins, phenacemide is useful in severe epileptic states, especially mixed forms of psychomotor seizures refractory to other medications. It is generally employed as a last resort, however, because of its extreme toxicity.

The exact mechanism of action of phenacemide is unknown; however, it has been demonstrated to elevate the threshold for experimental electroshock seizures in animals.

Recommended doses in adults are 250 mg to 500 mg orally 3 times a day, initially. The usual maintenance range is 2 g to 3 g a day. Children (5–10 yr) should receive one half of the adult dose.

Phenacemide can produce serious untoward reactions. Most frequently encountered adverse effects are psychic changes (e.g., psychosis, depression), gastrointestinal disturbances, skin rash, drowsiness, dizziness, weakness, and headache. In addition, phenacemide administration has been associated with insomnia, paresthesias, fatigue, fever, muscle pain, palpitations, increased serum creatinine, hepatitis (occasionally fatal), blood dyscrasias (e.g., leukopenia, aplastic anemia), and bone marrow depression. The drug is contraindicated in persons with personality disorders and in pregnant women. *Cautious use* is warranted in patients with a history of allergy or renal dysfunction, and in nursing mothers. Concomitant use of other antiepileptics, especially ethotoin, can increase the incidence of untoward reactions.

NURSING CONSIDERATION

Nursing Alert
- Monitor results of complete blood counts and liver function tests, which should be performed prior to initiating therapy and at regular intervals thereafter. The drug should be discontinued if symptoms of jaundice or hepatitis appear or if blood picture is abnormal.

PATIENT EDUCATION
1. Suggest taking drug with food or milk to minimize GI irritation.
2. Teach patient how to recognize and report early signs of hematologic toxicity (e.g., sore throat, fever, mucosal ulceration, malaise) or liver damage (e.g., pruritus, yellow skin, frothy amber urine, petechiae). If these occur, the drug should be withdrawn slowly.
3. Stress the potential toxicity of the drug and the importance of immediately reporting *any* untoward reaction.

ACETAZOLAMIDE

Acetazolamide
Ak-Zol, Dazamide, Diamox
(CAN) Acetazolam, Apo-Acetazolamide

Acetazolamide is a carbonic anhydrase inhibitor used as an *adjunct* in the control of petit mal and other absence or non-localized seizures, but seldom alone. The drug has also been employed as a mild diuretic, for relief of migraine headaches, and for treatment of chronic open-angle glaucoma (reduces formation of aqueous humor).

Acetazolamide inhibits the enzyme carbonic anhydrase, reducing formation of H^+ and HCO_3^- ions; thus, it appears to retard excessive or abnormal discharges from central neurons, although the mechanism of this effect is not well understood. The beneficial effects may be largely a consequence of the slight acidosis produced by the drug.

The usefulness of acetazolamide in treating epileptic seizures is greatly limited by the rapid onset of tolerance, with return of seizure activity often within a few weeks. The starting dose is 250 mg/day, and the usual maintenance dosage range is 375 mg to 1000 mg a day, generally in combination with another antiepileptic agent.

The most frequently encountered side effects are paresthesias of the face and extremities. Other untoward reactions observed with acetazolamide include polyuria, glycosuria, drowsiness, confusion, myopia, urticaria, rash, hepatic dysfunction, and flaccid paralysis. The drug is contraindicated in patients with sulfonamide allergy, since it is a sulfonamide derivative, and also in the presence of acidosis, hypokalemia, kidney or liver dysfunction, adrenal insufficiency, and early pregnancy. The drug should be used with *caution* in diabetic patients, since it may increase blood glucose levels resulting in the need to alter antidiabetic drug requirements.

NURSING CONSIDERATIONS
1. Assess diabetic patient carefully because acetazolamide may alter antidiabetic drug requirements by increasing blood glucose levels.
2. Use parenteral solution within 24 hours after reconstitution because it contains no preservative.

PATIENT EDUCATION
1. Instruct patient to report signs of hypokalemia (muscle weakness, cramping, cardiac irregularities) and metabolic acidosis (nausea, weakness, malaise, vomiting, abdominal pain, dehydration), which indicate the need for dosage adjustment.

MAGNESIUM SULFATE

Magnesium, in the form of magnesium sulfate, is an effective anticonvulsant in seizures associated with the toxemia of pregnancy and other clinical situations characterized by abnormally low levels of plasma magnesium. The drug may be used IV or IM, depending on the speed of action desired, although IV use is significantly more hazardous. Other clinical applications for magnesium sulfate are its use orally as a cathartic, topically as an antipruritic, and parenterally to control uterine tetany, paroxysmal atrial tachycardia, hypertension, and cerebral edema. It has also been employed as an adjunct in hyperalimentation and for replacement therapy in acute magnesium deficiency.

Magnesium controls convulsions by interfering with neuromuscular transmission, possibly by blocking release of acetylcholine from motor nerve endings. It also exerts a depressant effect on the CNS.

Adult intramuscular doses range from 1 g to 5 g of a 25% to 50% solution, up to 5 times a day as necessary. With intravenous injection, 1 g to 4 g of a 10% to 20% solution may be given at a rate not exceeding 1.5 mL/min; alternately, 4 g in 250 mL of a 5% dextrose solution may be infused at a rate not to exceed 3 mL/min. Pediatric intramuscular doses range from 20 mg to 40 mg/kg in a 20% solution. With repeated administration, knee jerk reflexes should be tested before every dose; if the reflex is absent, magnesium should *not* be administered. The onset of action is immediate with intravenous injection and within 1 hour with intramuscular administration.

Side effects include flushing (common), sweating, hypotension, sedation, confusion, hypothermia, flaccid paralysis, depressed reflexes, cardiac and respiratory depression, and circulatory collapse. Hypocalcemia with tetany has been reported secondary to magnesium sulfate administration. The drug must be given *cautiously* to persons with renal impairment and is *contraindicated* in the presence of heart block and myocardial insufficiency. Additive CNS-depressant effects can occur when magnesium is given together with narcotics, barbiturates, anesthetics, and other sedative–hypnotic drugs. Magnesium may potentiate the muscle-relaxing action of neuromuscular blocking agents.

NURSING CONSIDERATIONS

Nursing Alerts
- When magnesium is administered parenterally, ensure that IV calcium is on hand as an antidote, along with appropriate respiratory equipment.
- Monitor blood pressure and pulse repeatedly during IV therapy.

- Observe patient for appearance of early signs of magnesium toxicity (thirst, feeling of warmth, confusion, depressed tendon reflexes, muscle weakness), which require discontinuation of the drug.
- Monitor intake and output during extended use. The drug should be discontinued if output falls below 100 mL during 4 hours preceding each dose.
- Monitor results of plasma magnesium level determinations during parenteral treatment. Plasma levels above 4 mEq/L are usually associated with untoward reactions.

Selected Bibliography

Bocchese JD, Merker A: Seizure disorders in the neonate. Crit Care Nurs 3:42, 1983

Browne TR, Feldman RG: Epilepsy: Diagnosis and Management. Boston, Little, Brown & Co, 1983

Coulter DL: The treatable epilepsies. N Engl J Med 309:1456, 1983

Dalessio DJ: Current concepts: Seizure disorders and pregnancy. N Engl J Med 312:559, 1985

Delgado-Escueta AV, Treiman DM, Walsh GO: The treatable epilepsies, Parts I and II. N Engl J Med 308:1508, 1576, 1983

Drugs for Epilepsy. Med Lett Drugs Ther 25:81, 1983

Ferrari M et al: Psychologic and behavioral disturbance among epileptic children treated with barbiturate anti-convulsants. Am J Psychiatry 140:112, 1983

Frey HH, Janz D (eds): Antiepileptic drugs. In Handbook of Experimental Pharmacology, Vol. 74. Berlin, Springer-Verlag, 1985

Hachinski V: Management of a first seizure. Arch Neurol 43:1290, 1986

Jobe PC, Dailey JW, Laird HE (eds): Epilepsy: Neurotransmitter abnormalities as determinants of seizure susceptibility and severity. Fed Proc 43:2503, 1984

Norman S, Brown T: Seizure disorders: Nursing management. Am J Nurs 81:990, 1981

Parrish MA: A comparison of behavioral side effects related to commonly used anticonvulsants. Pediatr Nurs 10:149, 1984

Pedley TA, Meldrum BS (eds): Recent Advances in Epilepsy. New York, Churchill Livingstone, 1983

Penry JK, Porter RJ: Epilepsy: Mechanisms and therapy. Med Clin North Am 63:801, 1979

Reynolds EH, Shorvou SD: Single drug or combination therapy for epilepsy. Drugs 21:374, 1981

Sasso SC: Phenytoin for seizure disorders. Matern Child Nurs 9:279, 1984

Solomon GE, Kutt H, Plum F: Clinical Management of Seizures: A Guide for the Physician, 2nd ed. Philadelphia, WB Saunders, 1983

Spero L: Epilepsy. Lancet 2:1319, 1982

Woodbury DM, Penry JK, Pippender CE (eds): Antiepileptic Drugs. New York, Raven Press, 1983

SUMMARY. ANTICONVULSANTS/ANTIEPILEPTICS

Drug	Preparations	Usual Dosage Range
Barbiturates	See Table 25-2	
Primidone (Myidone, Mysoline)	Tablets: 50 mg, 250 mg Suspension: 250 mg/5 mL	*Adults:* Initially 100 mg–125 mg/day for 3 days Usual maintenance range: 250 mg 3–4 times/day *Children:* Initially; 50 mg/day Usual maintenance range: 125 mg–250 mg 3 times/day
Hydantoins	See Table 25-3	
Oxazolidinediones	See Table 25-4	
Succinimides	See Table 25-5	
Carbamazepine (Epitol, Tegretol)	Tablets: 200 mg Chewable tablets: 100 mg Suspension: 100 mg/5 mL	*Epilepsy* *Adults:* 200 mg twice a day, increased by 200 mg/day to optimal response (maximum 1200 mg/day) *Children* (6–12 yr): 100 mg twice a day; increase by 100 mg/day until desired response is achieved; maximum 1000 mg/day *Trigeminal neuralgia* 100 mg twice a day, increased by 100 mg/12 h; usual range 400 mg–800 mg/day
Valproic Acid Derivatives		
Valproic Acid (Depa, Depakene, Deproic)	Capsules: 250 mg	Initially 15 mg/kg/day; increase by 15 mg/kg weekly until optimal effect is noted (maximum 60 mg/kg/day)
Sodium Valproate (Depakene Myproic Acid)	Syrup: 250 mg/5 mL	
Divalproex Sodium (Depakote)	Enteric-coated tablets: 125 mg, 250 mg, 500 mg	

Continued

SUMMARY. ANTICONVULSANTS/ANTIEPILEPTICS (continued)

Drug	Preparations	Usual Dosage Range
Clonazepam Klonopin	Tablets: 0.5 mg, 1 mg, 2 mg	Adults: 0.5 mg 3 times/day increased by 0.5 mg–1 mg every 3 days (maximum 20 mg/day) Children: 0.01 mg/kg–0.03 mg/kg/day; increase to a maintenance range of 0.1 mg/kg–0.2 mg/kg/day
Diazepam Valium, Val-Release, Vazepam	Tablets: 2 mg, 5 mg, 10 mg Sustained-release capsules: 15 mg Solution: 1 mg/mL, 5 mg/mL Injection: 5 mg/mL	*Oral* Adults: 2 mg–10 mg 2–4 times/day Children: 1 mg–2.5 mg 3–4 times/day *IV* Adults: 5 mg–10 mg initially; repeat at 10–15-min intervals to a maximum of 30 mg Children: 0.2 mg–1 mg every 2–5 min based on age and weight
Phenacemide Phenurone	Tablets: 500 mg	Adults: 250 mg–500 mg 3 times/day (usual range is 2 g–3 g/day) Children (5–10 yr): half adult dose
Acetazolamide Ak-Zol, Dazamide, Diamox	Tablets: 125 mg, 250 mg Injection: 500 mg/vial	Initially: 250 mg/day Usual maintenance range: 375 mg–1000 mg/day
Magnesium Sulfate Several manufacturers	Injection: 10%, 12.5%, 25%, 50%	1 g to 2 g IM or IV; IV rate not to exceed 1.5 mL of 10% solution/min

26 ANTIPARKINSONIAN DRUGS

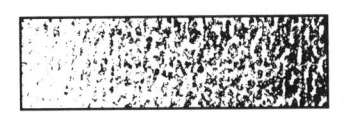

Parkinson's disease, or *paralysis agitans,* is a chronic progressive disorder of the CNS, the etiology of which is largely unknown. The term *parkinsonism* is used to describe the symptom complex that may result either from the normal course of the disease itself or from administration of certain drugs (e.g., phenothiazines) that produce similar symptoms (see Chap. 22). However, the terms are frequently used interchangeably. Although the symptoms vary depending on the stage of the disease—which becomes progressively more disabling—the three cardinal manifestations of Parkinson's disease are the following:

- *Akinesia* (bradykinesia): a lack of or difficulty in initiating voluntary muscle movement; advanced disease states are characterized by "frozen" muscles, resulting in masklike facial expression, impairment of postural reflexes, and inability to adequately care for oneself
- *Rigidity:* usually of the "plastic" or "cogwheel" type; the affected area usually can be moved without great difficulty but often remains fixed once again in its new position
- *Tremor:* coarse (3–7 cycles/sec), repetitive muscle activity, usually worse when the person is at rest; commonly manifested as a "pill-rolling" motion of the hands and a bobbing of the head

Besides the principal symptoms of the disease, affected patients may show disturbances in gait or posture, impaired speech, muscular weakness, and autonomic hyperactivity such as salivation and seborrhea. Advanced stages, however, are frequently characterized by autonomic *insufficiency,* resulting in severe orthostatic hypotension, which may be exacerbated by the anticholinergic drugs used in treatment.

Onset usually occurs in middle age, and during the early stages symptoms frequently are much worse on one side of the body. Diagnosis is largely symptomatic, although definite biochemical changes are present in the CNS. The most characteristic pathologic feature of parkinsonism is a degeneration of dopaminergic neurons having their cell bodies in the substantia nigra. Because motor regulatory areas such as the corpus striatum receive their dopamine supply from the substantia nigra, degeneration of these nigral–striatal neurons decreases the functional amount of dopamine available to the nuclei of the corpus striatum (i.e., caudate nucleus, putamen). This upsets the normal balance between the inhibitory transmitter dopamine and the excitatory transmitter acetylcholine in these brain regions, and therefore allows an excitatory predominance on lower motor centers by the intact cholinergic pathways.

Although striatal dopamine deficiency provides a common basis for the various manifestations of parkinsonism, the only *true* symptom resulting from low striatal dopamine is akinesia. As such, akinesia is the abnormality most benefitted by dopamine-replacement therapy. The other symptoms probably reflect the effects of the abnormal neurotransmitter ratio *triggered* by the dopamine deficit and involve alterations in more complex pathways among central motor regulatory structures. Therefore, tremor and rigidity may be more effectively controlled by both dopamine replacement *and* cholinergic antagonism.

Drug therapy of parkinsonism is directed either toward augmentation of central dopaminergic function or reduction of central cholinergic activity. Drugs effective in the control of Parkinson's disease may be grouped as follows:

I. *Dopaminergic agents*
   A. Dopamine precursor (e.g., levodopa)
   B. Dopamine releasing agent (e.g., amantadine)
   C. Dopamine receptor agonist (e.g., bromocriptine, pergolide)
   D. Inhibitor of dopamine inactivation (e.g., selegiline)
II. *Anticholinergic/antihistaminergic agents* (e.g., benztropine, ethopropazine)

In addition to proper drug treatment, which of course is not curative but simply palliative, adjunctive therapy for parkinsonism should include physical therapy to delay disability and emotional support to help lessen feelings of helplessness and inadequacy as the disease inexorably progresses and limits the patient's activities.

New approaches to the treatment of Parkinson's disease have emerged in recent years, although they are still in the experimental stages. Among the more promising are implantation with adrenal medullary tissue in the brain (providing a source of dopamine) or fetal nigral tissue (which replaces the deficient dopamine-producing cells of the substantia nigra).

A somewhat different type of drug-induced parkinsonism has been reported among drug abusers. Attempts by certain clandestine laboratories to synthesize a meperidine-like narcotic drug have resulted in the formation of certain by-products, one of which is 1-methyl-4-phenyl-1,2,5,6-tetrahydropyridine (MPTP). When this substance was accidentally injected, individuals developed severe parkinsonism within 2 weeks. Subsequent investigation demonstrated that MPTP is a neurotoxin that can selectively destroy dopaminergic neurons in the substantia nigra, leading to the development of classic parkinsonism that is irreversible and requires antiparkinsonian drug therapy. MPTP is now being evaluated in the laboratory as a model for Parkinson's disease.

DOPAMINERGIC AGENTS

Four types of drugs are available that can enhance dopaminergic functioning in the motor regulatory centers of the CNS. *Levodopa* (L-dopa) is the metabolic precursor of dopamine, and its use results in increased concentrations of dopamine in the corpus striatum. It is used rather than dopamine itself because L-dopa readily passes the blood–brain barrier, whereas dopamine does not and therefore does not reach sufficient levels in the CNS following systemic administration. Levodopa is now used almost exclusively in a fixed-ratio combination with carbidopa, the latter being an inhibitor of peripheral dopa decarboxylase, the enzyme responsible for converting dopa to dopamine. (see following discussion of carbidopa/levodopa).

Another drug employed to potentiate the effects of dopamine in the CNS is *amantadine.* Originally developed as an antiviral agent against the Asian (A) influenza strain, amantadine was demonstrated to have a beneficial action in certain parkinsonian patients to whom it was administered. It apparently increases the release of dopamine from presynaptic nerve endings. Therefore, its effectiveness is limited to those patients having functional stores of dopamine present in striatal brain areas.

A third type of dopaminergic drug is typified by *bromocriptine* and *pergolide,* dopamine receptor agonists that find their principal clinical application in cases of parkinsonism refractory to conventional therapy as an adjunct to levodopa/carbidopa treatment. These drugs can provide additional therapeutic benefit in those patients whose condition has begun to deteriorate and may allow a reduction in levodopa dosage, thus reducing the incidence of side effects associated with prolonged levodopa therapy. However, patients whose condition does not respond to levodopa are not likely to benefit from bromocriptine or pergolide.

Finally, *selegiline* is an inhibitor of MAO-B, an enzyme that inactivates dopamine within presynaptic nerve endings. It can also block conversion of environmental toxins into free radicals that may damage nigral neurons and ultimately lead to the development of Parkinson's disease.

Levodopa
Dopar, Larodopa

Carbidopa/levodopa
Sinemet

Although levodopa is the active pharmacologic agent in treating the symptoms of Parkinson's disease, it is seldom used alone, but usually as a fixed ratio (1:4, 1:10) combination of carbidopa and L-dopa. Carbidopa competes for the enzyme dopa decarboxylase, thereby retarding the *peripheral* breakdown of L-dopa. This allows a greater fraction of the administered L-dopa dose to pass the blood–brain barrier, resulting in higher dopamine levels in central motor regulatory centers. Carbidopa itself does not cross the blood–brain barrier and therefore does not interfere with conversion of L-dopa to dopamine in the CNS. Levodopa dosage requirements are reduced approximately 75% by combination with carbidopa, because plasma levels and plasma half-life are increased. Consequently, much less dopamine is formed peripherally than with the use of L-dopa alone, resulting in a lower incidence of many systemic side effects, especially nausea, vomiting, and cardiovascular disturbances. However, adverse *CNS* effects (e.g., dyskinesias) may occur sooner and at lower doses of L-dopa when combined with carbidopa than when given alone, because more levodopa is reaching the brain to be converted there to dopamine.

In addition to being available in two fixed dosage ratios with L-dopa (1:4, 1:10), carbidopa is also marketed alone in 25-mg tablets (Lodosyn) that allow the clinician to more carefully titrate the dosage ratio to obtain better symptom control. Individual dosing of the two drugs allows separate titration of each agent and may provide better control of the symptoms and a lower incidence of side effects than the use of the fixed-dosage combinations. Although most parkinsonian patients can be managed adequately with the carbidopa/levodopa combination (Sinemet), certain patients may require individual titration of each drug, especially when nausea and vomiting are prominent.

The pharmacologic and toxicologic properties of carbidopa/levodopa are similar to those of levodopa in most respects. However, the fixed ratio combinations allow use of lower doses of L-dopa, provide a smoother response, and permit more rapid dosage adjustments than can be obtained with L-dopa alone. Untoward reactions, contraindications, and drug interactions observed with carbidopa/levodopa are essentially the same as those noted with levodopa itself, although blood levels of urea nitrogen, uric acid, and creatinine are lower during carbidopa/levodopa administration than during treatment with levodopa alone.

Levodopa must be discontinued at least 8 hours prior to initiating therapy with carbidopa/levodopa, which should be substituted at a dosage level that will provide approximately 25% of the previous levodopa dose. The combination is *not* recommended in children under 18.

MECHANISM
Levodopa is a precursor of dopamine that readily passes the blood-brain barrier, then is decarboxylated to dopamine. Increased formation of dopamine in motor-regulatory areas of the CNS restores the depleted dopamine levels and improves the symptoms of Parkinson's disease; levodopa is most effective in relieving akinesia and bradykinesia, somewhat less effacacious in controlling rigidity, and seldom of significant benefit in reducing tremor; response to levodopa is greatest at the outset of therapy but diminishes gradually over 2 to 5 years, at which time it is usually necessary to initiate therapy with other antiparkinsonian drugs, such as anticholinergics, amantadine, or bromocriptine

USES
Treatment of parkinsonism, whether idiopathic, postencephalitic, or secondary to injury or cerebral arteriosclerosis
Control of drug-induced extrapyramidal symptoms

DOSAGE
Levodopa Alone
Highly individualized; initially 0.5 g to 1 g/day in 2 or more divided doses; increase gradually in increments of 0.75 g every 3 to 7 days; maximum dose is 8 g/day
Carbidopa/Levodopa
The dosage of carbidopa/levodopa, like that of levodopa itself, is highly individualized. Tablets are available in a fixed ratio of either 10 mg carbidopa/100 mg levodopa, 25 mg carbidopa/100 mg levodopa, or 25 mg carbidopa/250 mg levodopa. Dosage schedules are as follows:

Patients not receiving levodopa: Initially, 1 tablet (10/100 or 25/100) 3 times/day; increase by 1 tablet daily until 6 tablets/day; if more L-dopa is necessary, substitute 1 tablet (25/250) 3 or 4 times/day; increase by ½ to 1 tablet/day to a maximum of 8 tablets (25/250) per day
Patients receiving levodopa: (Discontinue L-dopa for at least 8 hr); initially, 1 tablet (25/250) 3 or 4 times/day in patient previously requiring 1500 mg or more of levodopa alone per day; *otherwise,* 1 tablet (10/100) 3 or 4 times/day; adjust by ½ to 1 tablet a day until control is obtained

FATE
Levodopa is well absorbed from GI tract; peak plasma levels occur in 1 to 2 hours; significant amounts are metabolized to dopamine in the stomach, intestines, and liver; relatively small fraction of administered dose reaches CNS unchanged as levodopa (1%–2%); dopamine metabolites are rapidly and almost completely excreted in the urine. Carbidopa inhibits the decarboxylation of peripheral levodopa but does not cross the blood–brain barrier and therefore does not interfere with the conversion of dopa to dopamine in the CNS. Concurrent use of carbidopa with levodopa reduces the required dose of levodopa by 70% to 80% and increases its plasma half-life

COMMON SIDE EFFECTS

Nausea, vomiting, anorexia, orthostatic hypotension, salivation, dry mouth, dysphagia, ataxia, headache, confusion, dizziness, weakness, fatigue, hand tremor, insomnia, anxiety, euphoria, choreiform and other involuntary movements, nightmares, agitation. Use of carbidopa with levodopa may reduce the incidence of peripheral side effects but can exacerbate the centrally mediated side effects. Dyskinesias occur in a majority of patients receiving long-term therapy and tend to develop with smaller doses as treatment continues.

SIGNIFICANT ADVERSE REACTIONS

GI: diarrhea, GI bleeding, ulceration

Cardiovascular: palpitations, tachycardia, arrhythmias, phlebitis, hemolytic anemia

Neurologic/psychiatric: bradykinetic episodes (on/off phenomena—see Patient Education), muscle twitching, grinding of the teeth, convulsions, paranoid ideation, psychotic reactions, depression, dementia

Ocular: spasmodic winking (blepharospasm), diplopia, blurred vision

Other: urinary retention, bitter taste, skin rash, sweating, hot flashes, edema, alopecia, leukopenia

Drug may elevate BUN, SGOT, SGPT, LDH, bilirubin, alkaline phosphatase, and PBI; may also reduce WBC, hemoglobin, and hematocrit

CONTRAINDICATIONS

Narrow-angle glaucoma, undiagnosed skin lesions or history of melanoma (levodopa can activate malignant melanoma), acute psychoses, and in patients on MAO inhibitor therapy. *Cautious use* in patients with severe cardiovascular, pulmonary, renal, hepatic, or endocrine disease; peptic ulcer; chronic wide-angle glaucoma; diabetes; psychiatric disturbances (including depression); a history of myocardial infarction with residual arrhythmias; and in pregnant or nursing women

INTERACTIONS

Effects of L-dopa may be *decreased* by antipsychotics, phenytoin, papaverine, pyridoxine, reserpine, phenylbutazone, benzodiazepines (e.g., diazepam)

L-dopa may enhance the hypotensive effect of methyldopa, guanethidine, diuretics, and possibly other antihypertensive drugs

Therapeutic effects of L-dopa may be potentiated by propranolol, methyldopa, and anticholinergics

Cardiovascular effects of sympathomimetic drugs such as amphetamines, ephedrine, and epinephrine can be increased by L-dopa

Diabetic control with oral hypoglycemic drugs may be adversely affected by L-dopa

Concurrent use of L-dopa and either tricyclic antidepressants or MAO inhibitors can result in tachycardia and hypertension

NURSING CONSIDERATIONS

1. Carefully evaluate patient's response to and tolerance of L-dopa. Dosage adjustments should be made slowly to minimize adverse effects.
2. Monitor vital signs during early dosage regulation.
3. Check results of tests of hepatic, renal, and cardiovascular function, which should be performed periodically during prolonged therapy.

PATIENT EDUCATION

1. Advise taking drug with food to lessen GI irritation.
2. Instruct patient to promptly report appearance of muscle twitching and blepharospasm (intermittent winking), early signs of overdosage.
3. Teach patient measures to help minimize orthostatic hypotension, which is common during early months of therapy. See **Plan of Nursing Care 8 (Antihypertensive Drugs)** for specific information.
4. Explain that prolonged use often leads to development of abnormal involuntary movements, especially of the face, mouth, tongue, and head, in which case an attempt should be made to reduce the dosage to the lowest effective level to minimize these effects.
5. Prepare patient for the possibility of a *sudden* worsening of symptoms (e.g., extreme weakness, bradykinesia) during prolonged high-dosage therapy, the so-called on/off phenomenon. This condition, which usually lasts several hours, is apparently due to temporarily excessive L-dopa levels, perhaps resulting from altered metabolism.
6. Advise patient to avoid multiple-vitamin preparations containing vitamin B_6 (pyridoxine) because it will reduce the effects of L-dopa by increasing its *peripheral* conversion to dopamine.
7. Inform patient that some improvement generally occurs within 2 to 3 weeks, but in some cases it may be several months before benefits are evident.
8. Advise diabetic patient to monitor condition closely for possible loss of control. Blood sugar should be checked frequently during therapy. Inform patient that drug can cause false negative urine test with Clinistix and false positive with Clinitest.
9. Inform patient that drug may cause urine and sweat to darken.

Amantadine

Symadine, Symmetrel

A synthetic antiviral agent originally used for prophylaxis against the Asian strain of influenza, amantadine can also effectively relieve symptoms of parkinsonism (especially akinesia and rigidity). It is effective in up to 40% of patients but its efficacy tends to diminish within 1 to 2 years. It may be used as initial therapy in milder forms of Parkinson's disease and in conjunction with levodopa in more advanced stages of the disease.

MECHANISM

Not completely understood; may enhance release of dopamine from presynaptic nerve endings, and block presynaptic reuptake of dopamine; effectiveness is greatly reduced in the absence of functional dopamine stores in the corpus striatum; no anticholinergic activity

Antiviral action has been attributed to prevention of the release of viral nucleic acid into host cells; does not interfere with the influenza A viral vaccine (see Chap. 71)

USES

Symptomatic treatment of parkinsonism and drug-induced extrapyramidal reactions

Prophylaxis against Asian influenza virus strains, especially in high-risk patients (see Chap. 71)

Symptomatic management of respiratory disease caused by Asian influenza virus (see Chap. 71)

DOSAGE

Parkinsonism: 100 mg 1 or 2 times/day (maximum 400 mg/day)

Drug-Induced extrapyramidal reactions: 100 mg twice a day (maximum 300 mg/day)

Influenza
Adults: 100 mg twice a day
Children (1–9 yr): 2 mg to 4 mg/lb/day (maximum 150 mg/day)

FATE

Well absorbed orally; peak plasma levels in 2 to 4 hours; long duration of action (half-life 18–24 h); not metabolized to any extent and excreted almost entirely intact through the kidneys; excretion is enhanced in an acid urine

COMMON SIDE EFFECTS

Irritability, anxiety, nausea, dizziness, ataxia, confusion, mild depression, constipation, urinary retention, peripheral edema, livedo reticularis (skin mottling)

SIGNIFICANT ADVERSE REACTIONS

Orthostatic hypotension, vomiting, headache, weakness, fatigue, insomnia, dyspnea, tremors, visual disturbances, skin rash, dermatitis, ankle edema, congestive heart failure, psychotic reactions, leukopenia, and neutropenia

CONTRAINDICATIONS

No absolute contraindications. *Cautious use* in patients with a history or evidence of epilepsy, congestive heart failure, or peripheral edema; also in patients with dermatitis, hypotension, psychotic disturbances, liver or kidney disease, and in elderly patients

INTERACTIONS

Amantadine may worsen the side effects of anticholinergics (e.g., hallucinations, confusion)
Excessive CNS stimulation may occur when given with other stimulants

NURSING CONSIDERATION

1. Carefully evaluate patient's response to drug because therapeutic effectiveness is unpredictable and may decrease abruptly. If drug becomes ineffective, beneficial effects may be regained by increasing the dose or discontinuing the drug briefly, then resuming. Apprise physician of any change in patient's status.

PATIENT EDUCATION

1. Suggest that patient avoid taking last dose close to bedtime because insomnia can result.
2. Inform patient that *abrupt* discontinuation of drug can markedly worsen symptoms. Dosage should be tapered gradually.
3. Warn patient that dizziness, drowsiness, and blurred vision may impair ability to drive a car or operate machinery.
4. Instruct patient to make position changes slowly, especially when arising from bed, because orthostatic hypotension may occur.
5. Explain that livedo reticularis (skin mottling, usually of lower extremities) may occur, particularly if patient is exposed to cold. Effect generally appears early in therapy and will subside once drug is discontinued or possibly when dose is reduced.

Bromocriptine
Parlodel

Bromocriptine is primarily used orally as adjunctive therapy to provide additional therapeutic benefits in patients currently maintained on L-dopa who are beginning to show signs of deterioration in their condition. Because of the progressive degenerative nature of parkinsonism, even persons receiving maximum doses of L-dopa in combination with carbidopa are eventually susceptible to breakthrough effects. These are sometimes referred to as "late L-dopa failures." Examples of such conditions are return of tremor or rigidity, "end-of-dose" failure (appearance of akinesia between dosing), and "on/off" phenomena (abrupt loss of mobility). Bromocriptine may delay the onset of late L-dopa failure and may also ameliorate the symptoms (e.g., dyskinesias) associated with excessive L-dopa levels by allowing a dosage reduction.

MECHANISM

Functions as a direct receptor agonist at dopaminergic sites in the CNS, resulting in increased dopamine receptor activation in the corpus striatum; may provide increased control of parkinsonian symptoms in patients whose condition has begun to deteriorate after prolonged L-dopa therapy; also activates dopamine receptors in the tuberoinfundibular dopaminergic system of the pituitary, resulting in secretion of prolactin inhibitory factor (PIF) from the hypothalamus; secretion of PIF blocks release of prolactin from the anterior pituitary

USES

Adjunctive treatment of Parkinson's disease (usually in combination with levodopa/carbidopa) or drug-induced parkinsonian-like symptoms (may provide increased symptom control and reduce the incidence of levodopa-induced side effects by permitting use of a smaller dose)
Treatment of amenorrhea/galactorrhea associated with hyperprolactinemia (*not* indicated in patients with normal prolactin levels)
Treatment of female infertility associated with hyperprolactinemia
Prevention of postpartum lactation
Reduction of plasma growth hormone levels in patients with acromegaly

DOSAGE

Parkinson's disease: 1.25 mg to 2.5 mg twice daily initially; increase by 2.5-mg increments every 2 to 4 weeks until optimal response occurs

Amenorrhea/galactorrhea: 2.5 mg 2 to 3 times a day; not to exceed 6 months

Prevention of lactation: 2.5 mg 2 to 3 times a day for 14 to 21 days

Treatment of infertility: initially 2.5 mg once daily; increase to 2 or 3 times a day within the first week

Acromegaly: 1.25 mg to 2.5 mg daily for 3 days; increased slowly every 3 to 7 days as tolerated; usual therapeutic range is 20 mg to 30 mg daily to a maximum of 100 mg daily

FATE
Approximately one fourth of an oral dose is absorbed from the gastrointestinal tract; drug is highly protein-bound (90%–95%); metabolized in the liver and excreted almost entirely through the bile into the feces; less than 5% of the dose is eliminated in the urine

COMMON SIDE EFFECTS
Nausea, vomiting, headache, dizziness, drowsiness, lightheadedness, confusion, visual disturbances, nasal congestion, shortness of breath, abdominal discomfort, diarrhea, insomnia, hypotension

SIGNIFICANT ADVERSE REACTIONS
Nightmares, anxiety, anorexia, dysphagia, foot and ankle edema, skin mottling, paresthesia, skin rash, urinary frequency, and epileptiform seizures. In addition, signs and symptoms of ergotism have occurred, such as numbness and tingling in the extremities, cold feet, muscle cramping, and Raynaud's syndrome

Elevations in BUN, SGOT, SGPT, creatine phosphokinase (CPK), alkaline phosphatase, and serum uric acid have been noted but are usually of a transient nature

CONTRAINDICATIONS
Severe ischemic heart disease, peripheral vascular disease, sensitivity to ergot alkaloids, and in pregnant or nursing women. *Cautious use* in the presence of severe hypotension, epilepsy, psychoses, cardiac arrhythmias, and impaired hepatic or renal function; safety and efficacy of bromocriptine in children under 15 years of age have not been established

INTERACTIONS
Bromocriptine can potentiate the hypotensive action of other blood pressure–lowering drugs

Antipsychotic drugs that are dopamine blockers may antagonize the action of bromocriptine

NURSING CONSIDERATIONS

Nursing Alerts
- Carefully evaluate drug effects. The dose effective in parkinsonism (25 mg–100 mg/day) is approximately 10 times that used for amenorrhea/galactorrhea. Consequently, adverse effects are more frequent and often more severe.
- Collaborate with patient, significant others, and health care team to ensure that adequate provision is made for patient's safety in home environment because side effects such as dizziness and hypotension may limit ability to manage self-care, especially early in therapy.

PATIENT EDUCATION
1. Inform amenorrheic woman that treatment with bromocriptine may restore fertility. Encourage use of effective contraceptive measures.
2. Inform woman with childbearing potential that periodic pregnancy tests are recommended during therapy. Treatment should be discontinued immediately if pregnancy occurs.
3. Warn patient to use caution in operating machinery or engaging in other potentially hazardous activities because dizziness and fainting may occur.

Selegiline
Eldepryl

MECHANISM
Irreversibly inhibits MAO-B enzyme in nerve endings in the brain, thereby increasing the intraneuronal levels of dopamine; as a result, more dopamine is available for release. May also interfere with dopamine reuptake into nerve endings and facilitate dopamine release. Does not appear to interfere with activity of MAO-A, the enzyme found in the liver and intestines

USES
Adjunctive treatment of Parkinson's disease in patients being treated with L-dopa when the response begins to deteriorate

Delay need for treatment with L-dopa in Parkinson's disease (investigational use)

DOSAGE
5 mg twice a day, at breakfast and lunch. After 2 or 3 days of treatment, attempt to reduce dose of L-dopa by 10% to 30%. Further reductions may be possible with continued selegiline use

FATE
Rapidly absorbed orally; peak plasma levels are attained in 1 to 2 hours; quickly metabolized to at least three metabolites, which are excreted largely in the urine

COMMON SIDE EFFECTS
Nausea, dizziness, lightheadedness

SIGNIFICANT ADVERSE REACTIONS
CNS: confusion, vivid dreams, headache, anxiety, insomnia, depression, hallucinations, delusions, tremor, involuntary motor movements, personality changes, dyskinesias

Cardiovascular: palpitations, orthostatic hypotension, tachycardia, arrhythmias, sinus bradycardia, peripheral edema

GI: vomiting, diarrhea, anorexia, weight loss, heartburn, dysphagia

Urinary: urinary retention, nocturia, prostatic hypertrophy

Dermatologic: sweating, hair loss, rash, photosensitivity

Other: dry mouth, acne, leg pain, back pain, diplopia, blurred vision, asthma, tinnitus, migraine, chills, altered taste, numbness of fingers and toes

CONTRAINDICATIONS
No absolute contraindications. *Cautious use* in persons in whom dizziness and drowsiness may prove hazardous and in pregnant or nursing women. Doses exceeding 10 mg/day should not be used, since nonselective inhibition of MAO-A may occur, leading to the possibility of hypertensive reactions with tyramine-containing foods (see Chap. 24)

INTERACTIONS
Concurrent used of meperidine and MAO inhibitors may result in severe and sometimes fatal interactions

NURSING CONSIDERATIONS
1. Be aware that the incidence of L-dopa–induced side effects may be increased when selegiline is added to the regimen. A 10% to 30% reduction in L-dopa dosage usually prevents any increase in side effects.

PATIENT EDUCATION

1. Caution patients not to exceed the recommended dose (10 mg/day), because higher doses inhibit MAO-A and may result in a hypertensive reaction to many foods containing tyramine, a potent pressor agent (see Chap. 24)
2. Inform patients of the signs of an MAO-inhibitor hypertensive reaction, such as severe headache, sweating, or flushing.

Pergolide

Permax

Pergolide is a dopamine receptor agonist that directly stimulates dopamine receptors in the nigrostriatal system. It is similar to bromocriptine but is about 100 times more potent on a milligram basis. It is used as adjunctive therapy to L-dopa in Parkinson's disease, allowing for a 5% to 30% reduction in the dose of L-dopa. Most frequently encountered side effects are dyskinesia, nausea, dizziness, hallucinations, rhinitis, somnolence, and confusion. Orthostatic hypotension may also occur frequently, especially during the initial stages of treatment. Cardiac arrhythmias have been reported. The clinical efficacy of pergolide may be decreased by concurrent use of dopamine antagonists such as phenothiazine antipsychotics or metoclopramide. Initial dose is 0.05 mg/day for the first 2 days. Dosage is then increased by 0.1 mg or 0.15 mg/day every third day for 2 weeks, then by 0.25 mg/day until an optimal therapeutic dosage is achieved. The drug is usually administered in three divided doses. The usual daily dose is 3 mg/day; efficacy of doses above 5 mg/day has not been determined.

ANTICHOLINERGIC/ANTIHISTAMINERGIC AGENTS

Benztropine	Orphenadrine
Biperiden	Procyclidine
Diphenhydramine	Trihexyphenidyl
Ethopropazine	

The first drugs used for the treatment of Parkinson's disease were the belladonna alkaloids atropine and scopolamine, and for many years these were the only effective drugs available for this disease. These agents, although still occasionally employed, have been supplanted by a group of synthetic drugs having central anticholinergic (and in some instances antihistaminergic) activity.

These agents are useful on their own in patients with mild symptoms, and the agents appear to be most effective in relieving rigidity and occasional tremor. They are often prescribed in combination with levodopa to obtain more efficient control of the condition than either drug alone is capable of providing. The usefulness of these compounds is mainly limited by their side effects, such as blurred vision, dizziness, and dysuria. Moreover, large doses are frequently associated with development of CNS toxicity, *especially in elderly people,* characterized by confusion, ataxia, delirium, and hallucinations.

In addition to their use in parkinsonism, these drugs are employed to control the extrapyramidal manifestations (akinesia, dystonias, akathisia, tremor) characteristic of treatment with the antipsychotic agents.

The anticholinergic/antihistaminergic drugs used in Parkinson's disease are pharmacologically and toxicologically similar and are reviewed as a group. Most of the individual drugs have been mentioned previously, either in Chapter 11 (anticholinergics) or Chapter 14 (antihistamines). They are listed again here in Table 26-1, where specific information is provided relating to their use in parkinsonism and extrapyramidal disorders.

MECHANISM

Exhibit a blocking effect on central cholinergic excitatory pathways that normally exert increasing effect as a lack of functional dopamine leads to a reduction of dopaminergic inhibition; also retard re-uptake of dopamine into presynaptic nerve endings, thereby blocking its inactivation; some agents may have a direct relaxant effect on smooth muscle

USES

Sole or adjunctive treatment of parkinsonian symptoms, especially rigidity

Prevention and relief of extrapyramidal reactions resulting from antipsychotic drug therapy

DOSAGE

See Table 26-1

FATE

Generally well absorbed orally; onset usually in 30 minutes to 60 minutes; duration of action is variable (average 4–6 h), except for sustained-release preparations (8–12 h); excreted primarily by the kidney, both as metabolites and intact drug

COMMON SIDE EFFECTS

Dryness of mouth, blurred vision, dizziness, nausea, nervousness, drowsiness, urinary hesitancy

SIGNIFICANT ADVERSE REACTIONS

(Usually due to excessive dosage) Confusion, agitation, delirium, hallucinations, depression, memory loss, vomiting, constipation, paralytic ileus, dilatation of the colon, skin rash, flushing, decreased sweating, tachycardia, palpitation, weakness, mild orthostatic hypotension, paresthesias, numbness in extremities, muscle cramping, elevated temperature, mydriasis, diplopia, headache, and increased intraocular pressure

CONTRAINDICATIONS

Acute narrow-angle glaucoma, pyloric or duodenal obstruction, peptic ulcer, prostatic hypertrophy, myasthenia gravis. *Cautious use* in patients with open-angle glaucoma; cardiac, liver, or kidney disorders; and in small children, elderly or debilitated patients; alcoholics, and pregnant or nursing women

INTERACTIONS

Combined use with other drugs having an anticholinergic action (e.g., phenothiazines, tricyclic antidepressants) may result in increased toxicity

May potentiate the sedative action of other CNS depressants (e.g., alcohol, barbiturates, narcotics)

Certain centrally acting anticholinergic drugs can impair the antipsychotic effectiveness of phenothiazines and haloperidol by increasing their rate of gastrointestinal metabolism

Oral absorption of levodopa can be reduced by anticholinergic drugs, since they delay gastric emptying, thus increasing the gastric degradation of levodopa. However, the reduced gastrointestinal motility may increase absorption of slowly dissolving preparations such as digoxin

NURSING CONSIDERATIONS

Nursing Alert
- Be alert for possible early signs of paralytic ileus (e.g., abdominal pain, distention, constipation). Alert physician if these occur.

1. Carefully evaluate patient's response to drug, and assist with decisions to adjust dosage as situation warrants to minimize side effects. Dosage requirements are quite variable and may change as condition deteriorates.
2. Monitor urinary output and bowel function during prolonged therapy.

PATIENT EDUCATION

1. Advise patient to take drug with or following meals to minimize GI irritation.
2. Stress the importance of adhering to prescribed dosage levels. Clinical improvement may not occur for several days or even weeks.
3. Warn patient to exercise caution in driving a car or operating machinery because physical and mental abilities may be impaired, especially during early therapy.
4. Explain that the ability to sweat may be hampered, which may interfere with maintenance of heat equilibrium. If a problem occurs, a dosage reduction should be considered, and patient should be instructed to avoid exertion as much as possible.
5. Suggest interventions to alleviate dry mouth. See **Plan of Nursing Care 4 (Antihistamines)** for specific information.
6. Emphasize the importance of periodic ophthalmic examinations for patient on prolonged therapy.

Table 26-1
Anticholinergic/Antihistaminergic Drugs Used For Parkinsonism

Drug	Preparations	Usual Dosage Range	Nursing Implications
Benztropine Cogentin (CAN) ApoBenzotropine, Bensylate, PMS Benztropine	Tablets: 0.5 mg, 1 mg, 2 mg Injection: 1 mg/mL	*Parkinsonism:* 1 mg–2 mg/day (range 0.5 mg–6 mg) *Extrapyramidal rections:* 1 mg–4 mg 1–2 times/day	IM injection used for rapid response in acute dystonic reactions (onset 15 min); do *not* use in children under 3; effects are cumulative and may take several days to develop; usually not effective against tremors
Biperiden Akineton	Tabelts: 2 mg Injection: 5 mg/mL	*Parkinsonism* 2 mg 3 or 4 times/day *Extrapyramidal reactions* Oral: 2 mg 1–3 times/day IM, IV: 2 mg; may repeat every 30 min to a total of 4 doses	Most effective against akinesia and rigidity; effectively reduces salivation and seborrhea; may produce mood elevation or temporary euphoria, especially parenterally; IV injection can cause hypotension and incoordination
Diphenhydramine Benadryl and others; *see also* Chap. 14	Capsules: 25 mg, 50 mg Tablets: 50 mg Elixir: 12.5 mg/5 mL Syrup: 12.5, 13.3 mg/5 mL Injection: 10, 50 mg/mL	Oral: 25 mg–50 mg 3–4 times/day IV, IM: 10 mg–50 mg (maximum 400/day)	Effective in mild parkinsonism and extrapyramidal reactions (especially dystonias); often combined with other anticholinergics or L-dopa; see Chapter 14 for adverse effects, contraindications, and interactions
Ethopropazine Parsidol (CAN) Parsitan	Tablets: 10 mg, 50 mg	Initially 50 mg 1–2 times/day Increase gradually to a maximum of 600 mg/day in severe cases	A phenothiazine derivative with significant anticholinergic activity; effectively controls most symptoms, including tremor; does *not* potentiate other CNS depressants; high incidence of side effects and poorly tolerated by many older patients; used for treatment of extrapyramidal reactions, even though it is a phenothiazine itself
Orphenadrine HCl Disipal (CAN) Norflex	Tablets: 50 mg	*Parkinsonism:* 50 mg 3 times/day (maximum 250 mg/day)	Antihistamine that is also a centrally acting muscle relaxant; relieves rigidity and controls

Continued

Table 26-1
Anticholinergic/Antihistaminergic Drugs Used For Parkinsonism

Drug	Preparations	Usual Dosage Range	Nursing Implications
Orphenadrine (HCl) (cont'd)			autonomic manifestations as well; minimal drowsiness but high incidence of other atropine-like side effects; use with chlorpromazine has resulted in hypoglycemic coma; may decrease the effects of barbiturates, phenylbutazone, and griseofulvin; also available as the citrate for relief of musculoskeletal disorders (see Chap. 15)
Procyclidine Kemadrin (CAN) PMS Procyclidine, Procyclid	Tablets: 5 mg	*Parkinsonism:* Initially 2.5 mg 3 times/day; increase gradually to a maximum of 20 mg/day *Extrapyramidal reactions:* 2.5 mg 3 times/day (usual range 10 mg–20 mg/day)	Anticholinergic and smooth muscle antispasmodic; most effective against rigidity; controls excessive salivation as well; may temporarily worsen tremor as rigidity is relieved; be alert for confusion, agitation, and behavioral changes, which are common in elderly persons with hypotension; similar to trihexyphenidyl
Trihexyphenidyl Aphen, Artane, Trihexane, Trihexidyl, Trihexy (CAN) Aparkane, Apo-Trihex, Novohexidyl	Tablets: 2 mg, 5 mg Capsules: 5 mg (sustained-release) Elixir: 2 mg/5 mL	*Parkinsonism* Initially 1 mg–2 mg; increase by 2-mg increments every 3–5 days to a maximum of 15 mg/day *Usual range:* 6 mg–10 mg/day, in 3–4 divided doses or 5 mg sustained-release once or twice a day *Extrapyramidal reactions* Initially: 1 mg; increase by 1 mg every few hours until control is obtained Usual range: 5 mg–15 mg/day in divided doses	Anticholinergic and smooth muscle relaxant; do *not* use sustained-release capsules for initial therapy because they do not allow enough flexibility in dosage regulation; major effect is on rigidity, although most symptoms improve to some extent; effects may be potentiated by MAO inhibitors

Selected Bibliography

Calne DB: Progress in Parkinson's disease. N Engl J Med 310:523, 1984

Calne DB, Langston JW: The etiology of Parkinson's disease. Lancet 2:1457, 1983

Campanella G, Roy M, Barbeau A: Drugs affecting movement disorders. Annu Rev Pharmacol Toxicol 27:113, 1987

Fahn S, Calne DB: Considerations in the management of parkinsonism. Neurology 31:371, 1981

Garrett E: Parkinsonism: Forgotten considerations in medical treatment and nursing care. J Neurosurg Nurs 14:13, 1982

Hoehn MM: Bromocriptine and its use in parkinsonism. J Am Geriatr Soc 24:251, 1981

Langston JW, Ballard P, Tetrud JW, Irwin I: Chronic parkinsonism in humans due to a product of meperidine-analog synthesis. Science 219:979, 1983

Leff SE, Creese I: Dopamine receptor re-explained. Trends Pharmacol Sci 4:463, 1983

Nutt JG, Woodward WR, Hammerstad JP et al: The "on-off" phenomenon in Parkinson's disease. N Engl J Med 310:483, 1984

Parkes JD: Adverse effects of antiparkinsonian drugs. Drugs 21:341, 1981

Quinn NP: Antiparkinsonian drugs today. Drugs 28:236, 1984

Riederer P, Przuntek H: MAO-B-inhibitor selegiline: A new therapeutic concept in the treatment of Parkinson's disease. J Neural Trans 25(Suppl):1, 1987

Seeman P: Brain dopamine receptors. Pharmacol Rev 32:229, 1981

Symposium: Current concepts and controversies in Parkinson's disease. Can J Neurol Sci 11(Suppl 1):89, 1984

Todd B: Drugs and the elderly: Therapy for Parkinson's disease. Geriatr Nurs 6(2):117, 1985

Vance ML, Evans WS, Thorner MO: Bromocriptine. Ann Intern Med 100:78, 1984

Young RR: Step therapy for Parkinson's disease. Patient Care 14:24, 1980

SUMMARY. ANTIPARKINSONIAN DRUGS

Drug	Preparations	Usual Dosage Range
Dopaminergic Agents		
Levodopa (L-dopa) Dopar, Larodopa	Tablets: 100 mg, 250 mg, 500 mg Capsules: 100 mg, 250 mg, 500 mg	Initially 0.5 g–1 g/day; increase by 0.75 g every to 7 days to a maximum of 8 g/day
Carbidopa/levodopa Sinemet	Tablets: 10 mg carbidopa and 100 mg levodopa, 25 mg carbidopa and 100 mg levodopa, or 25 mg carbidopa and 250 mg levodopa	Initially 1 tablet (10:100 or 25:100) 3 times/day; increase by 1 tablet daily to 6 tablets/day; *or* 1 tablet (25:250) 3–4 times/day; increase in increments of ½–1–8 tablets/day depending on response
Carbidopa Lodosyn	Tablets: 25 mg	12.5 mg–25 mg as needed with carbidopa/levodopa combination to provide improved symptom control or to reduce side effects
Amantadine Symadine, Symmetrel	Capsules: 100 mg Syrup: 50 mg/5 mL	*Parkinsonism:* 100 mg 1–2 times/day (maximum 400 mg/day) *Extrapyramidal reactions:* 100 mg twice a day (maximum 300 mg/day) *Influenza* Adults: 100 mg twice a day Children (1–9 yr): 2 mg–4 mg/lb/day (maximum 150 mg/day)
Bromocriptine Parlodel	Tablets: 2.5 mg Capsules: 5 mg	Initially, 1.25 mg twice a day; increase by 2.5 mg/day every 2–4 wk until optimal response is achieved
Pergolide Permax	Tablets: 0.05 mg, 0.25 mg, 1 mg	Initially, 0.05 mg/day; increase by 0.1 mg/day to 0.15 mg/day every third day for 2 weeks, then by 0.25 mg/day. Usual daily dose is 3 mg/day
Selegiline Eldepryl	Tablets: 5 mg	5 mg twice a day
Anticholinergic/ Antihistaminergic Agents	See Table 26-1	

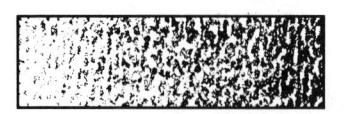

CENTRAL NERVOUS SYSTEM STIMULANTS

27

Although a large number of pharmacologic agents have a stimulating effect on the central nervous system (CNS), the number of drugs actually employed clinically for this purpose is quite small. A useful classification of the therapeutically effective CNS stimulants is as follows:

I. Respiratory stimulants (analeptics; e.g., doxapram)
II. Caffeine
III. Amphetamines (e.g., dextroamphetamine, methamphetamine)
IV. Anorexiants (e.g., phentermine, diethylpropion)
V. Methylphenidate
VI. Pemoline

The *analeptics* are used primarily as physiologic antagonists of respiratory depression due to overdosage with CNS depressants. The only currently available analeptic, doxapram, is discussed below.

Caffeine is the most widely used CNS stimulant, largely because it is consumed in coffee, tea, soda, and many over-the-counter drug combinations. In small amounts it is a relatively weak stimulant that aids in maintaining mental alertness. It can also be employed parenterally as a respiratory stimulant, and it may relieve the pain of vascular headaches by virtue of its constricting action on cerebral blood vessels.

The *amphetamines* are potent CNS stimulants with a high potential for abuse. They have been used to treat obesity, although their usefulness is restricted to a short-term basis (several weeks). A group of amphetamine-related drugs, termed *anorexiants,* are used in the therapy of obesity, with most of the same restrictions and limitations as amphetamine itself. Other approved indications for the amphetamines are the treatment of narcolepsy and attention deficit disorder (ADD).

The remaining drugs listed above (i.e., methylphenidate, pemoline) are primarily indicated as alternatives to amphetamine for the treatment of ADD in children.

RESPIRATORY STIMULANTS (ANALEPTICS)

Drugs having the ability to enhance depressed respiratory function are termed *respiratory stimulants* or *analeptics.* Such agents act at the level of the respiratory center in the brainstem as well as on the peripheral carotid chemoreceptors to increase the depth and, frequently, also the rate of respiration. They are used mainly to overcome respiratory depression due to drug overdosage with the several classes of CNS depressants (e.g., hypnotics, narcotics) or overdosage resulting from general anesthesia. However, their clinical effectiveness in many cases of drug-induced respiratory depression has been questioned, and their potential for eliciting untoward reactions is rather high.

Foremost among their disadvantages is that doses needed to elicit sufficient respiratory stimulation in cases of marked respiratory depression often stimulate other CNS areas as well (e.g., vasomotor center, vomiting center, brainstem reticular formation), causing a variety of undesirable effects ranging from mild cardiovascular stimulation to marked central activation leading to vomiting, hyperreflexia, and convulsions. Since respiratory stimulants have a rather narrow safety margin, they must be administered cautiously by trained personnel and only in conjunction with appropriate resuscitative measures (e.g., oxygen, suction, anticonvulsants, muscle relaxants) as necessary.

Analeptics alone are often insufficient in arousing an individual with severe respiratory depression and should be used only in conjunction with adequate adjunctive measures, such as mechanical assistance, narcotic antagonists, or cholinergic drugs, depending upon the particular drug involved. Obviously, maintenance of an open airway is essential with use of respiratory stimulants.

Doxapram
Dopram

MECHANISM

Enhances depth and rate of respiration by direct stimulation of medullary respiratory center (large doses) and by increasing activation of peripheral carotid chemoreceptors; large doses also stimulate vasomotor center (increase blood pressure and cardiac output) and may cause convulsions; little direct action on cerebral cortex

USES

Reversal of postanesthetic respiratory depression or apnea (except due to muscle relaxants) and facilitation of emergence from anesthesia

Adjunctive treatment of drug-induced CNS and respiratory depression, to hasten arousal and facilitate return of laryngopharyngeal reflexes (*Note:* Respiratory depression due to CNS-depressant overdosage is *best* managed by mechanical ventilation.)

Prevention of elevated arterial carbon dioxide tension during oxygen administration in patients with chronic obstructive pulmonary disease with acute respiratory insufficiency

DOSAGE

Postanesthesia: 0.5 mg to 1 mg/kg IV injection (maximum 2 mg/kg) or 5 mg/min by IV infusion until satisfactory response, then 1 mg to 3 mg/min to maintain respiration

Drug-induced respiratory depression: 2 mg/kg IV injection; repeat in 5 minutes, then at 1- to 2-hour intervals until arousal is sustained (total maximum dose is 3 g); alternatively, 1 mg to 3 mg/min by IV infusion following initial priming dose given above (total maximum dose is 3 g)

Chronic obstructive pulmonary disease: 1 mg to 3 mg/min by IV infusion (2 mg/mL solution) for a maximum of 2 hours

FATE

Onset of action is 20 to 40 seconds and peak effect occurs within 1 to 2 minutes; duration ranges from 5 to 12 minutes

COMMON SIDE EFFECTS

Mild hypertension, variations in heart rate

SIGNIFICANT ADVERSE REACTIONS

CNS/Autonomic: flushing, sweating, pruritus, paresthesias, headache, dizziness, disorientation, mydriasis, tremors, involuntary movements, muscle spasticity, convulsions, increased deep tendon reflexes

Respiratory: cough, dyspnea, bronchospasm, laryngospasm, hiccups, rebound hypoventilation
Cardiovascular: chest pain and tightness, phlebitis, depressed T waves, arrhythmias
GI: nausea, vomiting, diarrhea
Other: urinary retention, incontinence, proteinuria, decreased hemoglobin or hematocrit

CONTRAINDICATIONS

Epilepsy or other convulsive states, airway obstruction, incompetence of the ventilatory mechanism, pneumothorax, extreme dyspnea, acute bronchial asthma, suspected or confirmed pulmonary embolism, respiratory failure due to neuromuscular disorders, pulmonary fibrosis, severe hypertension, head injury, coronary artery disease, and uncompensated heart failure. *Cautious use* in the presence of cerebral edema, severe tachycardia, arrhythmias, cardiac disease, pheochromocytoma, history of bronchial asthma, hyperthyroidism, peptic ulcer, acute agitation; in pregnant women and in children under 12 years

INTERACTIONS

Additive pressor effects may occur if doxapram is combined with sympathomimetics or MAO inhibitors

Doxapram releases epinephrine and thus may increase the incidence of arrhythmias with those general anesthetics that sensitize the myocardium (e.g., halothane, enflurane, cyclopropane)

Doxapram may enhance the CNS effects of amantadine (see Chap. 26)

NURSING CONSIDERATIONS

Nursing Alerts
- Ensure that airway is patent and oxygenation is adequate before drug is administered.
- Use IV infusion control pump to regulate flow rate of infusion, and have proper measures and drugs available (e.g., oxygen, resuscitative equipment, anticonvulsants, antiarrhythmics) to treat possible doxapram overdosage.
- Monitor blood pressure, pulse, and deep tendon reflexes during administration to prevent overdosage. If signs of toxicity (tachycardia, hyperactive reflexes, hypertension) occur, the infusion rate should be reduced or the drug should be discontinued.
- Delay administration of doxapram for 10 to 15 minutes after anesthetics (e.g., halothane, enflurane) have been discontinued because doxapram-induced release of epinephrine may elicit arrhythmias.
- Immediately notify physician if sudden dyspnea or hypotension occurs because the drug should be discontinued.
- Carefully avoid extravasation of solution because thrombophlebitis can result.

1. In patient with obstructive pulmonary disease, ensure that arterial blood gas levels have been determined before doxapram is administered. Blood gases should then be monitored at least every 30 minutes during infusion. Drug should not be infused for more than 2 hours. Supplemental oxygen should be provided as needed.
2. Continue to observe patient closely for at least 1 hour after injection or until patient is fully alert and pharyngeal and laryngeal reflexes are restored.
3. Assist with evaluation of drug effects. Infusion flow rate should be adjusted to sustain desired level of respiratory stimulation with minimal side effects.
4. Expect subsequent doses of doxapram to be readministered only to patient who has responded to initial dose.
5. Do not mix doxapram injection with alkaline solutions because precipitation will result. Injection is compatible with normal saline or dextrose in water.

CAFFEINE

Caffeine
Caffedrine, Dexitac, No Doz, Tirend, Vivarin

Caffeine and Dextrose
Quick-Pep

Caffeine and Sodium Benzoate
Citrated Caffeine

Caffeine is a xanthine derivative possessing relatively weak CNS-stimulant, smooth-muscle relaxant, vasodilatory, diuretic, and myocardial stimulant actions. However, it constricts cerebral arteries and enhances the contraction of skeletal muscles. CNS stimulant effects are exerted mainly on the cortex in small doses, relieving fatigue and improving sensory awareness. Larger doses can further excite lower brain centers (e.g., vasomotor, respiratory, vagal). The drug is used orally alone or in combination with either citric acid or dextrose, and as an injection solution with sodium benzoate.

MECHANISM

Competitively blocks receptors for adenosine, a naturally occurring substance that normally depresses neuronal firing in the CNS, thereby permitting these neurons to fire more readily; also increases the concentration of cyclic AMP in tissues by inhibiting the enzyme phosphodiesterase, which inactivates cyclic AMP; can increase release of calcium from the sarcoplasmic reticulum, improving skeletal muscle tone; stimulates all levels of the CNS when used in sufficient amounts

USES

Allays fatigue and increases sensory awareness (orally)
Treatment of mild to moderate respiratory depression caused by overdosage with CNS depressants such as morphine or alcohol (parenterally)
Relieves pain associated with vascular headaches or spinal puncture (orally or parenterally, often with ergotamine)

DOSAGE

Oral: 100 mg to 200 mg every 4 hours *or* 200 mg to 250 mg sustained-release capsules every 4 to 6 hours. Oral administration of caffeine is not recommended in children
IM: Adults receive 200 mg to 500 mg, repeated as needed every 4 hours. Infants and young children are given 8 mg/kg, with a maximum single dose of 500 mg

FATE

Readily absorbed following injection; well absorbed orally, peak plasma levels occur within 30 to 45 minutes; readily crosses the blood–brain barrier; half-life is 3 to 6 hours; minimally protein-bound; partially demethylated and oxidized in the liver; excreted largely through the kidney, 10% as unchanged drug

COMMON SIDE EFFECTS
Nervousness, insomnia, gastric irritation

SIGNIFICANT ADVERSE REACTIONS
(Usually with large doses) Nausea, vomiting, hematemesis, restlessness, irritability, excitement, tinnitus, scotomas, tremors, flushing, palpitation, tachycardia, extrasystoles, diuresis, hypotension, delirium, and respiratory distress

CONTRAINDICATIONS
No absolute contraindications. *Cautious use* in patients with gastric ulcers, myocardial infarction, respiratory depression, and diabetes

INTERACTIONS
Caffeine may cause hypertensive reactions in combination with MAO inhibitors
Caffeine can increase CNS stimulation due to propoxyphene overdosage, resulting in convulsions
Increased effects of caffeine can occur in combination with oral contraceptives or cimetidine, because these drugs may inhibit caffeine metabolism
Smoking may increase the elimination of caffeine

NURSING CONSIDERATIONS

Nursing Alert
- Administer caffeine and sodium benzoate slowly. Do not exceed 1000 mg per dose because increased respiratory depression may result.

1. Have a short-acting barbiturate on hand when drug is given IM or IV to counteract excessive CNS stimulation.

PATIENT EDUCATION
1. Advise heavy caffeine users that headache, dizziness, palpitations, and nervousness can occur either during use or upon abrupt withdrawal.

AMPHETAMINES

Amphetamine	Dextroamphetamine
Amphetamine complex	Methamphetamine

The amphetamines are synthetic sympathomimetic amines with marked CNS-stimulatory action. They increase alertness and concentration, temporarily elevate mood, and stimulate motor activity. Amphetamines can induce varying degrees of euphoria depending on the dose as well as the personality of the user. Major peripheral effects of these compounds include elevation of blood pressure, relaxation of bronchiolar smooth muscle, contraction of the urinary sphincter, and mydriasis.

Prolonged oral use of amphetamines often leads to irritability, insomnia, and dizziness. The stimulation resulting from amphetamine usage is invariably followed by an equally intense depression, usually accompanied by fatigue and listlessness. The desire to overcome this poststimulatory depression often leads to repetitive amphetamine dosing, and in the susceptible person, this can evolve into a vicious circle culminating in habituation and addiction. Large, repeated doses of amphetamines have brought about a behavioral state that is difficult to distinguish clinically from paranoid schizophrenia. Obviously, the danger is greatly increased when these agents are abused parenterally (IV) as "spree drugs." The acute behavioral changes that ensue with IV injection include extreme disorientation, hallucinations, and paranoid ideation; users are given to violent outbursts that can endanger themselves and others (see Chap. 79 for a discussion of amphetamine abuse).

Approved clinical indications for amphetamines are few; use of these drugs must be undertaken cautiously, and patients closely observed. The amphetamines are discussed as a group, then are listed individually in Table 27-1.

MECHANISM
Promote release of catecholamines from presynaptic nerve terminals and prevent their re-uptake into these nerve endings; net effect is potentiation of endogenous catecholamine activity; may exert a direct-activating effect on adrenergic receptor sites and interfere with the functioning of MAO, an enzyme responsible for intracellular breakdown of monoamines such as norepinephrine, dopamine, and serotonin; stimulant effect thought to be caused by an action on the cerebral cortex and possibly the reticular formation; anorexiant action may be caused by stimulation of a beta receptor–mediated satiety center in lateral hypothalamus; usefulness in attention deficit disorder has been related to potentiation of dopamine action in the CNS and possibly to enhanced stimulus discrimination related to increased activity of the reticular activating system

USES
Short-term (i.e., 4–8 wk) adjunct in the treatment of obesity, as an aid to a total weight control program (potential benefit does *not* outweigh inherent risks—see below)
Treatment of narcolepsy
Treatment of attention deficit disorder (ADD) in children

DOSAGE
See Table 27-1

FATE
Rapidly absorbed from GI tract and widely distributed in the body; high concentrations are found in the brain and cerebrospinal fluid; onset of action is usually in 30 to 60 minutes; plasma half-life is approximately 4 to 6 hours but effects may persist for up to 24 hours; partially metabolized in the liver; metabolites may lead to development of amphetamine psychosis with prolonged use; some unchanged drug is eliminated in the urine

COMMON SIDE EFFECTS
Nervousness, palpitations, insomnia, tachycardia, unpleasant taste

SIGNIFICANT ADVERSE REACTIONS
CNS: dizziness, euphoria or dysphoria, headache, chills, tremor; large doses may cause confusion, hallucinations, panic, aggressiveness, and psychotic episodes
Cardiovascular: hypertension, arrhythmias
GI: nausea, vomiting, diarrhea, anorexia and weight loss, cramping

Other: impotence, urticaria, delayed or difficult urination; large doses can cause dyspnea, anginal pain, syncope, convulsions, and coma
Overdosage: restlessness, irritability, tremor, sweating, hyperreflexia, confusion, hypertension, delirium, arrhythmias, convulsions

CONTRAINDICATIONS
Cardiovascular disease, hypertension, hyperthyroidism, arteriosclerosis, glaucoma, agitated states, severe endogenous depression, history of drug abuse, within 14 days of MAO-inhibitor administration; in children under 3 and in pregnancy. *Cautious use* in emotionally disturbed persons, in the presence of cardiac arrhythmias, and in nursing mothers

INTERACTIONS
Amphetamines may reduce the antihypertensive effects of guanethidine, methyldopa, hydralazine, and possibly other antihypertensive drugs

Effects of amphetamines can be potentiated by acetazolamide, cocaine, furazolidone, propoxyphene, tricyclic antidepressants, MAO inhibitors, and by sodium bicarbonate and other substances that alkalinize the urine

Amphetamines may be antagonized by urinary acidifying agents (ascorbic acid, methenamine, reserpine, glutamic acid, fruit juices), lithium, haloperidol, and phenothiazines

Amphetamines may delay the effects of phenytoin, ethosuximide, and related anticonvulsants by impairing their GI absorption

Concurrent use of amphetamines and general anesthetics may increase the risk of cardiac arrhythmias

NURSING CONSIDERATIONS

Nursing Alerts
- *Note:* The risk of dependence with amphetamines is considerable. Therefore, they should be used for weight control *only* after other programs have failed, and they should be given for no more than a few weeks.
- When administering an amphetamine for weight control, observe patient closely for signs of tolerance. If tolerance develops, the drug should be discontinued rather than increasing the dose.
- Assist with efforts to determine the *lowest* effective dose for each patient to minimize dangers of adverse effects and habituation.

1. When used for attention deficit disorder in children, collaborate with health care team to plan for provision of appropriate educational, psychological, and social interventions along with drug therapy.
2. Follow proper procedures for handling Schedule II substances (see Chap. 8).

PATIENT EDUCATION
1. Suggest taking last dose at least 6 hours before bedtime, if possible, to minimize insomnia.
2. Caution patient that ability to drive or operate machinery may be impaired.
3. Warn patient that poststimulatory depression may occur. Emphasize the need for proper rest and avoidance of hazardous activities during this period.
4. Explain that abrupt discontinuation of drug following prolonged therapy can cause extreme fatigue, depression, and even psychotic behavior.
5. Inform diabetic patient that amphetamines may alter insulin or dietary requirements. Urge patient to report any symptomatic changes.
6. Instruct patient to avoid excessive intake of foods high in tyramine (e.g., aged cheese, beer, red wine, liver, broad beans, soy sauce) because they can cause an excessive rise in blood pressure when amphetamines are being taken.
7. If patient is using drug for weight reduction, stress the importance of adhering to dietary program to obtain maximal benefit.

ANOREXIANTS

Benzphetamine	Phendimetrazine
Diethylpropion	Phenmetrazine
Fenfluramine	Phentermine
Mazindol	Phenylpropanolamine

A group of drugs related structurally to amphetamine have been used in the treatment of exogenous obesity. These agents, termed *anorexiants, anorectics,* or *anorexigenics,* possess essentially the same spectrum of pharmacologic and toxicologic actions as amphetamine. With the exception of fenfluramine, which depresses the CNS, all these drugs evoke varying degrees of stimulation that appear to be a major component of their anorectic action. They are primarily indicated for the temporary, adjunctive management of obesity in conjunction with a carefully supervised program of caloric restriction and proper exercise. Although none of these agents is superior to amphetamine in effectiveness, some do have less potential for habituation than the amphetamines and may be preferable for short-term therapy. It is important to recognize, however, that *all* of these drugs can become habituating with continued use. Since their therapeutic benefit is restricted to a few weeks at best, because of developing tolerance, there is significant danger in their prolonged consumption.

In addition to the prescription-only anorexigenic drugs discussed below, the decongestant *phenylpropanolamine* is available over-the-counter as a diet aid, either alone or in combination with different vitamins or a grapefruit extract. A weak CNS stimulant, phenylpropanolamine has been recommended for the short-term management of obesity, although its efficacy is subject to considerable doubt. Moreover, because it stimulates alpha-adrenergic receptors and releases norepinephrine, it can significantly elevate blood pressure and should not be taken by anyone with even mild hypertension. Severe hypertensive episodes have occurred during concomitant administration of phenylpropanolamine and propranolol or indomethacin. Contraindications to phenylpropanolamine include hypertension, diabetes, kidney disease, arteriosclerosis, symptomatic cardiovascular disease, and hyperthyroidism. Recommended dosages of phenylpropanolamine are 25 mg 3 times/day or 75 mg (sustained-release) once daily. Strict supervision is necessary whenever these nonprescription diet aids are used.

Benzocaine, a local anesthetic (see Chap. 16), is also available

Table 27-1
Amphetamines

Drug	Preparations	Usual Dosage Range	Nursing Implications
Amphetamine Sulfate	Tablets: 5 mg, 10 mg	*Narcolepsy* 5 mg–60 mg/day in divided doses *Attention deficit disorder* 3–5 yr: 2.5 mg/day; increase by 2.5 mg/wk if necessary Over 6 yr: 5 mg 1–2 times/day; increase by 5 mg/wk if necessary *Obesity* 5 mg– 30 mg/day in divided doses 30–60 min before meals	Note development of insomnia or anorexia and reduce dose; give first dose on awakening and last dose 4–6 h before bedtime if possible; attempt to provide drug-free periods in children with attention deficit disorder, especially during periods of reduced stress (e.g., summer vacations, holidays); be aware that response is more variable in children than in adults, and observe more closely (Schedule II)
Amphetamine Complex Biphetamine	Capsules: 12.5 mg, 20 mg (contain 6.25 mg and 10 mg each of dextroamphetamine and amphetamine, respectively)	*Obesity:* 1 capsule daily in the morning	Indicated only for *short-term* adjunctive treatment of exogenous obesity; high potential for abuse; should be prescribed cautiously and patient's consumption monitored carefully (Schedule II)
Dextroamphetamine Sulfate Dexedrine, Ferndex, Oxydess II, Spancap No. 1	Tablets: 5 mg, 10 mg Capsules: 15 mg Capsules: (sustained-release): 5 mg, 10 mg, 15 mg Elixir: 5 mg/5 mL	*Narcolepsy* 5 mg–60 mg/day in divided doses *Obesity* 2.5 mg–10 mg 1–3 times/day *Attention deficit disorder* Over 3 yr: 2.5 mg–5 mg/day; increase gradually to optimal effect (maximum 40 mg/day)	More potent CNS stimulant than amphetamine but less of an effect on the cardiovascular and peripheral nervous systems; give last dose at least 6 h before bedtime; tolerance usually develops within several weeks; possesses the same pharmacologic properties and hazards as amphetamine, and should be used sparingly and cautiously (Schedule II)
Methamphetamine Desoxyn	Tablets: 5 mg, 10 mg Long-acting tablets: 5 mg, 10 mg, 15 mg	*Obesity* 5 mg 3 times/day (long-acting—1 tablet daily) *Attention deficit disorder* Over 6 yr: initially, 5 mg 1 or 2 times/day; increase by 5 mg/week to optimal level (usual range 20 mg–25 mg/day)	CNS effects slightly greater than amphetamine; do *not* use long-acting tablets to initiate dosage; give 30 min before meals and last dose at least 6 h before bedtime; large doses may result in cardiac stimulation; tolerance develops quickly, so drug has high abuse potential; commonly called *speed* among abusers; has caused severe psychotic reactions following repeated injections of dissolved tablets (Schedule II)

as gum and chewable candy as an aid to reducing appetite by deadening taste sensation.

The anorexigenic drugs are discussed as a group, followed by a tabular listing of the agents indicating significant differences in their actions. As with amphetamines, the potential benefit to be derived from these agents does not justify the risks associated with their use.

MECHANISM
Probably similar to amphetamine; exert a CNS-stimulant effect on the cortex and may activate hypothalamic satiety center regulating food intake to decrease appetite; most drugs (except fenfluramine) possess a central excitatory action and can elevate blood pressure

USES
Short-term (8–12 wk) adjunctive management of exogenous obesity in conjunction with caloric restriction
Fenfluramine has been used investigationally in treating autistic children with elevated serotonin levels

DOSAGE
See Table 27-2

FATE
Most drugs are quickly and completely absorbed orally; onset of action occurs within 1 hour, and effects generally persist 4 to 6 hours; sustained-release formulations may have prolonged action (12–18 h). Tolerance develops within several weeks; metabolized by the liver and excreted both as unchanged drug and metabolites by the kidney

COMMON SIDE EFFECTS
Nervousness, irritability, insomnia, tachycardia, palpitations

SIGNIFICANT ADVERSE REACTIONS
Cardiovascular: hypertension, precordial pain, arrhythmias, syncope
CNS: anxiety, dizziness, headache, euphoria, tremors, confusion, incoordination; occasionally depression, (especially fenfluramine), dysphoria, dysarthria; also, drowsiness and impotence with fenfluramine
GI: nausea, vomiting, unpleasant taste, cramping, constipation, glossitis, stomatitis
Genitourinary: dysuria, polyuria, diuresis, cystitis, impotence, menstrual irregularities, changes in libido, gynecomastia
Other: rash, urticaria, erythema, mydriasis, blurred vision, muscle pain, chills, flushing, fever, sweating, alopecia, blood dyscrasias (rare)

CONTRAINDICATIONS
See Amphetamines. *Cautious use* in pregnant or nursing women, and in persons with glaucoma, diabetes, epilepsy, or anxiety neuroses

INTERACTIONS
See Amphetamines. In addition:
Fenfluramine may augment the effects of other CNS depressants (e.g., alcohol, narcotics, barbiturates) and may potentiate the action of antihypertensive drugs
Mazindol may potentiate the pressor effects of exogenous catecholamines and increase the risk of lithium toxicity
Anorexiants may reduce diabetic drug requirements by increasing glucose uptake by skeletal muscle cells, necessitating dosage adjustment

NURSING CONSIDERATIONS

Nursing Alert
- Expect therapy to be discontinued after several weeks to avoid development of tolerance and possible habituation. The recommended dose should not be exceeded in an attempt to increase anorectic effect.

1. Monitor for signs of excessive stimulation (tachycardia, dizziness, restlessness, hypertension), and notify physician immediately if any occur.
2. Follow proper procedures for handling controlled substances. Individual drugs are classified in Schedules II through IV (see Chap. 8).

PATIENT EDUCATION
1. Instruct patient to swallow the delayed or sustained-action dosage forms whole. Chewing or crushing the tablets may release large quantities of medication too quickly.
2. Suggest taking last dose at least 6 hours before bedtime, if possible, to minimize insomnia. Because, however, much overeating occurs at night, advantages and disadvantages of an evening dose should be considered.
3. Caution patient to avoid activities requiring mental alertness and coordination because dizziness and confusion may occur.
4. Explain that extreme fatigue and depression may ensue if drug is abruptly discontinued following use for a prolonged period.
5. Emphasize the importance of careful adherence to the *total* treatment regimen (i.e., drugs, diet, exercise) if weight control is to be successful. Clarify the danger of overreliance on the drug as the answer to an obesity problem.
6. Ensure that patient understands dietary restrictions that must accompany drug therapy to obtain maximal benefit.
7. Advise patient to avoid excessive consumption of foods high in tyramine content (e.g., aged cheese, broad beans, red wine, beer, liver, soy sauce) because they can cause hypertensive reactions in persons taking amphetamine-like drugs.

METHYLPHENIDATE

Methylphenidate
Ritalin

A CNS stimulant with a pharmacologic profile of action similar to that of amphetamine, but having a more marked effect on mental rather than physical or motor activities at normal doses, methylphenidate shares the potential for habituation and psychological addiction possessed by the amphetamines. However, its central excitatory effects are weaker. In usual therapeutic dosage, it does not elevate the blood pressure, heart rate, or respiratory rate; however, with large doses, signs of generalized CNS excitation can occur (e.g., tremors, tachycardia, hyperpyrexia, confusion). It is most widely used as an adjunct in the therapy of attention deficit disorder in children, where its effectiveness equals that of the amphetamines.

MECHANISM
Not definitively established but probably similar to amphetamine; major action appears to be on the cerebral cortex; increases release of catecholamines from presynaptic nerve endings

USES
Adjunctive therapy of attention deficit disorder in children
Treatment of narcolepsy
Relief of mild depression and apathetic or withdrawn senile behavior

DOSAGE
Adults: Initially 10 mg 2 or 3 times/day (maximum 60 mg/day)
Children (over 6 yr): Initially 5 mg 2 times/day; increase by 5 mg to 10 mg/week to optimal dose (maximum 60 mg/day)

During prolonged therapy in children, periodic discontinuation of therapy should be attempted to assess the patient's condition. Drug treatment is not intended to be indefinite

Table 27-2
Anorexiant Drugs

Drug	Preparations	Usual Dose Range	Nursing Implications
Benzphetamine Didrex	Tablets: 25 mg, 50 mg	Initially 25 mg–50 mg/day; increase as necessary (usual range 50 mg–150 mg/day)	Usually given as single daily dose, midmorning or midafternoon (Schedule III)
Diethylpropion Tenuate, Tepanil (CAN) Nobesine, Propion	Tablets: 25 mg Tablets: (sustained-release): 75 mg	25 mg 3 times/day 1 h before meals and in midevening if needed *or* 75 mg daily in the morning	Less effective but somewhat less hazardous than amphetamines; caution in epileptics because drug has been shown to increase convulsions; may alter ECG (T-wave changes) (Schedule IV)
Fenfluramine Pondimin (CAN) Ponderal	Tablets: 20 mg	Initially 20 mg 3 times/day before meals; increase by 20 mg/week to a maximum of 120 mg/day	Differs from other anorexiants because it often produces CNS *depression;* may enhance glucose uptake by skeletal muscles; *use cautiously* in depression and diabetes; diarrhea is often noted early in therapy; reduce dosage or discontinue if severe; do not discontinue abruptly because severe depression can ensue; avoid use in alcoholics, because psychiatric symptoms can develop; may potentiate effects of both CNS stimulants and CNS depressants (Schedule IV)
Mazindol Mazanor, Sanorex	Tablets: 1 mg, 2 mg	1 mg 3 times/day before meals, *or* 2 mg daily before lunch	Take with food if necessary to reduce GI discomfort; may alter diabetic drug requirements by lowering blood glucose levels; elicits CNS and cardiovascular stimulation, and appears to alter mood by an action on the limbic system (Schedule III)
Phendimetrazine Several manufacturers	Tablets: 35 mg Capsules: 35 mg Sustained-release capsules: 105 mg	35 mg 2–3 times/day 1 h before meals *or* 105 mg once a day	Similar to amphetamine in action but somewhat less potent (Schedule III)
Phenmetrazine Preludin	Tablets: 25 mg Tablets (sustained-release): 75 mg	25 mg 2 or 3 times/day 1 h before meals *or* 75 mg daily in the morning	Blood pressure may be elevated by drug; monitor pressure periodically; congenital malformations have occurred but a causal relationship has not been proved; sustained-release forms are no more effective than regular tablets and may be more hazardous if taken in excess; more intense CNS stimulation than most other anorexiants, and greater incidence of abuse (Schedule II)
Phentermine Ionamin and several other manufacturers	Tablets: 8 mg, 15 mg, 30 mg Tablets: (long-acting): 37.5 mg Capsules: 8 mg, 15 mg, 18.75 mg, 30 mg Capsules: (long-acting): 15 mg, 30 mg, 37.5 mg	8 mg 3 times/day before meals *or* 15 mg to 37.5 mg daily in the morning	Less potent stimulant of CNS and cardiovascular activity than amphetamine; available as a resin-complex capsule (15 mg, 30 mg) providing prolonged action (10–15 h); do *not* use resin complex if patient has diarrhea because effectiveness is lost (Schedule IV)

Continued

Table 27-2
Anorexiant Drugs (continued)

Drug	Preparations	Usual Dose Range	Nursing Implications
Phenylpropanolamine Acutrim, Dexatrim, Diadax, Prolamine and several other manufacturers	Tablets: 25 mg Capsules: 37.5 mg Tablets (timed-release): 75 mg Capsules (timed-release): 50 mg, 75 mg	25 mg 3 times/day *or* 50 mg–75 mg once daily in the morning	Over-the-counter diet aid possessing weak central stimulatory action; can activate peripheral alpha and beta receptors, resulting in vasoconstriction and cardiac stimulation; use must be closely supervised as blood pressure elevations have occurred; discontinue drug if tachycardia, dizziness, nervousness, or insomnia occur; do *not* exceed recommended dose

FATE
Absorbed well from GI tract; distributed throughout the body, including CNS; onset of action occurs in 30 to 60 minutes and peak blood levels are achieved in 1 hour to 3 hours; effects persist up to 6 hours with oral administration; excreted through the kidneys, largely as metabolites

COMMON SIDE EFFECTS
Nervousness, insomnia; in children, anorexia, mild weight loss, and tachycardia are also frequent

SIGNIFICANT ADVERSE REACTIONS
CNS: nausea, dizziness, drowsiness, headache, dyskinesia, agitation, toxic psychoses
Cardiovascular: palpitations, blood pressure changes, tachycardia, anginal attacks, arrhythmias
Allergic: skin rash, fever, urticaria, arthralgia, erythema multiforme, necrotizing vasculitis, exfoliative dermatitis
Other: visual disturbances, alopecia, abdominal pain, anemia

CONTRAINDICATIONS
Marked tension, anxiety or agitated states, glaucoma, seizure disorders, and *severe* depression. *Cautious use* in patients with hypertension, in patients with a history of drug dependence or alcoholism, and during pregnancy

INTERACTIONS
Methylphenidate may increase the effects of oral anticoagulants, anticonvulsants, tricyclic antidepressants, and phenylbutazone by inhibiting their metabolism
Hypertensive reactions may occur with vasopressors, MAO inhibitors, and furazolidone
Methylphenidate decreases the antihypertensive action of guanethidine
Effects of methylphenidate can be antagonized by phenothiazines and propoxyphene

NURSING CONSIDERATIONS

Nursing Alert
- Carefully evaluate drug-taking patterns, especially in emotionally unstable person, because chronic abuse can occur.

1. Monitor blood pressure, weight, and results of blood counts, which should be performed periodically during extended periods of treatment.
2. When used for attention deficit disorder in children, collaborate with health care team to plan for provision of appropriate educational, psychological, and social intervention along with drug therapy.
3. Follow proper procedures for handling a Schedule II drug (see Chap. 8).

PATIENT EDUCATION
1. Suggest taking last dose no later than 4 or 5 hours prior to bedtime to minimize insomnia.
2. Advise patient that nervousness and insomnia may occur early in therapy but generally lessen with time. Dosage reduction may, however, be required.
3. Explain that drug should be withdrawn gradually to avoid precipitation of severe depressive episodes or psychotic behavior. The drug should *not* be prescribed for a severely depressed patient.

PEMOLINE

Pemoline
Cylert

A chemically unique CNS stimulant having minimal sympathomimetic effects, pemoline is otherwise pharmacologically comparable to amphetamine and methylphenidate. It appears to have a lower abuse potential than most other CNS stimulants.

MECHANISM
Not established; increases alertness and motor activity and induces a mild euphoria, probably by an action on the cerebral cortex; may increase dopaminergic transmission in CNS structures

USES
Adjunctive therapy of attention deficit disorder in children
Treatment of narcolepsy and excessive sleepiness

DOSAGE
Children (over 6 yr): Initially 37.5 mg/day as single morning dose; increase by 18.75 mg/wk until optimal effects are noted; maximum dose—112.5 mg/day

FATE
Absorbed from GI tract, with peak blood levels in 2 hours to 4 hours; onset of action is gradual over 3 to 4 weeks; plasma half-life approximately 12 hours; metabolized by the liver and excreted in the urine both as unchanged drug (45%) and several conjugated metabolites

COMMON SIDE EFFECTS
Insomnia, anorexia

SIGNIFICANT ADVERSE REACTIONS
Nausea, diarrhea, dizziness, headache, drowsiness, irritability, nystagmus, dyskinesias, abdominal pain, skin rash, jaundice, convulsive movements, and hallucinations

CONTRAINDICATIONS
Children under 6. *Cautious use* in patients with impaired renal or hepatic function, in those with a history of drug abuse, and in pregnant or lactating women

INTERACTIONS
May enhance the effects of other CNS stimulants (e.g., caffeine, amphetamines)

NURSING CONSIDERATIONS

Nursing Alert
- Monitor results of liver function tests, which should be performed periodically during prolonged therapy. Drug should be discontinued if SGOT, SGPT, or serum LDH levels are significantly elevated.

1. Monitor weight of children on prolonged therapy because growth suppression and weight loss can occur.
2. When used for attention deficit disorder in children, collaborate with health care team to plan for provision of appropriate educational, psychological, and social intervention along with drug therapy.
3. Follow proper procedures for handling a Schedule IV drug (see Chapter 8).

PATIENT EDUCATION
1. Suggest that drug be taken once a day in the morning to minimize insomnia.

Selected Bibliography
Brown RT et al: How much stimulant medication is appropriate for hyperactive school children? J Sch Health 54(3):128, 1984

Curatolo PW, Robertson D: Health consequences of caffeine. Ann Intern Med 98:641, 1983

Hallal JC: Caffeine: Is it hazardous to your patient's health? Am J Nurs 86:422, 1986

Huber CJ, Dalldorf, JS: Minimal brain dysfunction syndrome. Nurs Clin North Am 15(1): 51, 1980

Ludwikowski KL: PPA: An innocent over-the-counter drug? Pediatr Nurs 10(6):387, 1984

Soldatos CR, Vales A, Cadieux RJ: Treatment of sleep disorders. II: Narcolepsy. Ration Drug Ther 17(3):1, 1983

Tan TL, Handford HA, Soldatos CR: Current therapy of eating disorders. II: Obesity. Ration Drug Ther 18(2):1, 1984

Tesar GE: The role of stimulants in general medicine. Drug Ther 12:1986, 1982

Weiss G: Controversial issues of the pharmacotherapy of the hyperactive child. Am J Psychiatry 26:385, 1981

SUMMARY. CNS STIMULANTS

Drug	Preparations	Usual Dosage Range
Analeptics		
Doxapram Dopram	Injection: 20 mg/mL	*Postanesthesia:* 0.5 mg–1 mg/kg by IV injection *or* 5 mg/min IV infusion initially, then 1 mg–3 mg/min to sustain respiration *Drug-induced respiratory depression:* 2 mg/kg IV injection at 1–2 h intervals *or* 1 mg–3 mg/min IV infusion after priming dose given above (maximum 3 g/day) *Chronic obstructive pulmonary disease:* 1 mg–3 mg/minute IV infusion for a maximum of 2 h
Caffeine Caffedrine, Dexitac, Nō Dōz, Quick-Pep, Tirend, Vivarin	Tablets: 100 mg, 150 mg (with 300 mg dextrose) 200 mg Timed-release capsules: 200 mg, 250 mg Injection: 250 mg/mL (equal parts caffeine and sodium benzoate)	Oral: 100 mg–200 mg every 3–4 h *or* 200 mg–250 mg timed-release capsules every 4–6 h IM: 200 mg–500 mg; repeat as necessary IV: 500 mg in emergency respiratory failure

Continued

SUMMARY. CNS STIMULANTS (continued)

Drug	Preparations	Usual Dosage Range
Amphetamines	See Table 27-1	
Anorexiants	See Table 27-2	
Methylphenidate Ritalin	Tablets: 5 mg, 10 mg, 20 mg Sustained-release tablets: 20 mg	Adults: 10 mg 2–3 times/day in divided doses (maximum 60 mg/day) Children (over 6 yr): Initially 5 mg 2 times/day; increase by 5 mg–10 mg/week (maximum 60 mg/day)
Pemoline Cylert	Tablets: 18.75 mg 37.5 mg, 75 mg Chewable tablets: 37.5 mg	Initially 37.5 mg/day in the morning; increase by 18.75 mg/wk (maximum 112.5 mg/day)

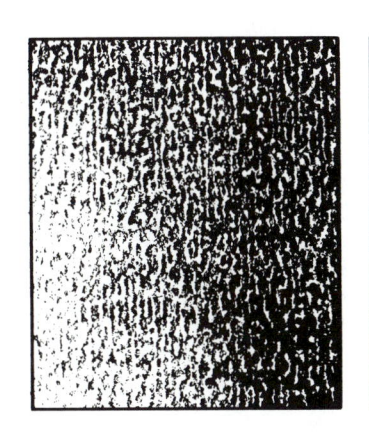

III Drugs Acting on the Cardiovascular System

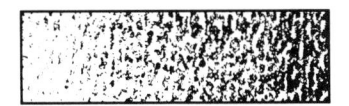

28 CARDIOVASCULAR PHYSIOLOGY: A REVIEW

The cardiovascular system functions as a highly integrated unit to establish and maintain, within a wide range of conditions, the hemodynamic state necessary to meet the moment-to-moment needs of each body tissue.

The rhythmic pumping action of the heart establishes blood flow at an adequate level of pressure. The elastic recoil of the aorta and large arteries transforms the intermittent output of the heart into a relatively steady peripheral flow of blood. Unidirectional flow of blood is maintained by suitable pressure gradients and is aided by strategically placed valves. Blood pressure is maintained by delicate reflex mechanisms, and blood flow to individual body tissues is controlled by local metabolic needs as well as central integrating mechanisms.

THE HEART

The human heart is a four-chambered, highly muscular organ lying within the mediastinum enclosed by a double-layered pericardium (Fig. 28-1). The heart wall is composed of three layers: an outer thin transparent *epicardium* (visceral pericardium); a thick middle muscular *myocardium;* and an inner serous lining, or *endocardium.* In addition to lining the chambers of the heart, the endocardium covers the valves of the heart and is continuous with the endothelium of the blood vessels.

The thin-walled superior chambers, or *atria,* function primarily as reservoirs for blood returning to the heart. The right atrium receives systemic venous blood from the superior and inferior venae cavae and coronary venous blood chiefly through the coronary sinus. The left atrium receives oxygenated blood from the lungs by way of four pulmonary veins. Because no true valves separate the great veins near the heart from the atrial chambers, elevations in right atrial pressure are reflected backward into the systemic venous circulation, whereas elevations in left atrial pressure lead to pulmonary congestion.

The inferior chambers or *ventricles* are thick walled, being formed by three indistinct layers of muscle arranged in a complex spiral fashion. During contraction, the myocardium of each ventricle generates a force sufficient to overcome the existing pressure in the receiving artery. The right ventricle ejects its contents into the pulmonary artery, while the left ventricle pumps oxygenated blood into the aorta. Because the pulmonary circulation is maintained at a considerably lower pressure than the systemic circulation, the thickness of the right ventricular wall is approximately one third that of the left, reflecting the lighter workload of the right ventricle.

Unidirectional blood flow through the heart is maintained by two types of valves: the *atrioventricular* (AV) valves and the *semilunar* valves. The AV valves separate the atria from the ventricles. Each valve is composed of leaflets or cusps that attach to the papillary muscles of the ventricles by way of chordae tendinae. A *tricuspid* valve separates the right atrium from the right ventricle, while a *bicuspid* or mitral valve is found between the left atrium and left ventricle.

The semilunar valves consist of three symmetrical cuplike cusps secured onto a fibrous ring. The *pulmonic* valve is situated between the right ventricle and the pulmonary artery, while the *aortic* valve is located between the left ventricle and the aorta. Immediately above the free margins of the aortic valve are the sinuses of Valsalva and the openings of the coronary arteries.

THE CORONARY CIRCULATION

The myocardium is richly vascularized, its blood supply coming by way of the coronary circulation. The coronary vessels course around the heart in two external anatomic grooves: the atrioventricular groove and the interventricular groove.

The coronary arteries arise from the ascending aorta immediately above the free margins of the aortic semilunar valve. They form a crown around the heart and provide branches to supply the atrial and ventricular myocardium.

The right coronary artery, with its marginal and posterior interventricular branches, supplies the right atrium, right ventricle, and a portion of the left ventricle. The left coronary artery and its major branches, the circumflex and anterior interventricular arteries, supply the left atrium, left ventricle, and part of the right ventricle. Anastomoses between arterial branches exist and serve as potential routes for collateral circulation if gradual occlusion of a vessel occurs. Coronary veins accompany the coronary arteries. The most significant myocardial venous return occurs by way of the coronary sinus, which opens into the right atrium near the orifice of the inferior vena cava.

Blood flow through the coronary arteries occurs primarily during ventricular relaxation (*diastole*) because ventricular contraction (*systole*) compresses the arteries and impedes arterial flow. The reduced time in diastole that occurs at rapid heart rates can markedly decrease coronary arterial perfusion, a potentially critical situation in patients with coronary artery or cardiac disease.

Coronary perfusion is primarily controlled by local metabolites and is minimally affected by autonomic nervous system activity. Coronary vessels dilate in response to increased acidity (reduced pH), increased carbon dioxide, and diminished oxygen availability in the blood.

If a coronary artery is partially occluded by a plaque or embolus, the vasodilation that automatically occurs distal to the block may provide sufficient blood flow to meet the needs of a resting heart. During exercise or emotional stress, however, such vasodilation may not be sufficient to meet the increased demand on the heart, and ischemia may result. Moderate inadequacy of coronary perfusion is associated with a characteristic substernal thoracic pain that occasionally radiates along the medial aspect of the left arm and is termed *angina pectoris.* Angina pectoris is usually relieved by rest and vasodilators such as nitroglycerin. Severe and prolonged ischemia of the myocardium causes irreversible damage to the heart. This state, termed *myocardial infarction,* is characterized by severe substernal oppression and may lead to shock, arrhythmias, cardiac dysfunction, or sudden death.

THE CONDUCTION SYSTEM

The heart muscle, or *myocardium,* exhibits the physiologic properties of excitability, conductivity, contractility, and auto-

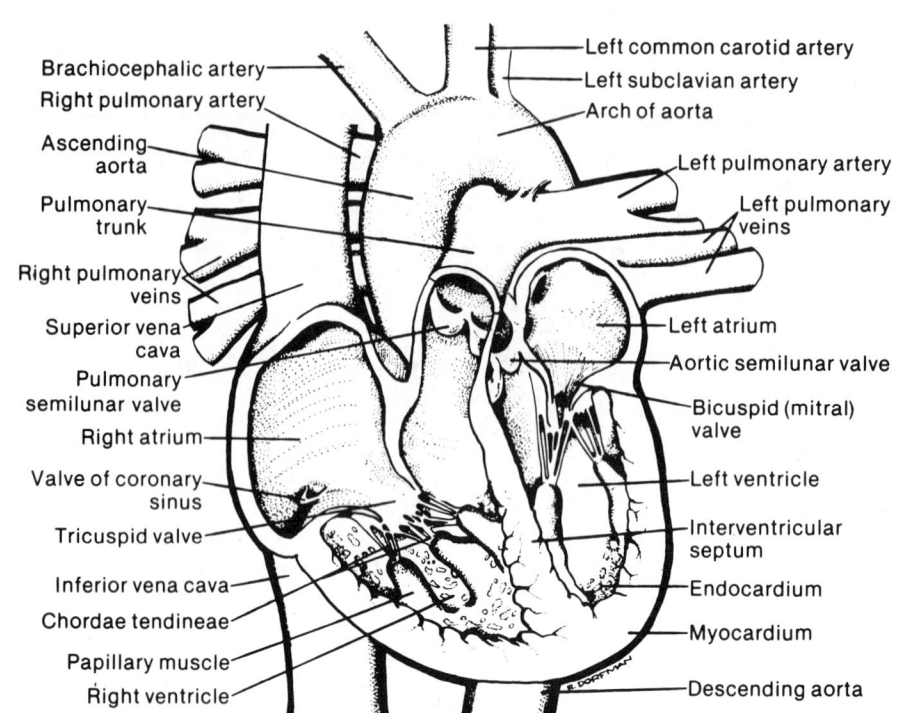

Figure 28-1 The human heart contains four chambers and is enclosed by a double-layered pericardium.

rhythmicity. The heart spontaneously and rhythmically generates electrical impulses (action potentials) that are distributed along specialized conduction pathways to all parts of the myocardium, permitting synchronous contraction of the ventricular myocardium. Like all excitable tissues, the myocardium exhibits refractory periods. During such times of decreased reactivity, the myocardium is unresponsive to a second stimulus.

The rhythmic synchronized activity of the heart is maintained by a spontaneously active, highly specialized conduction system illustrated in Figure 28-2.

The cardiac impulse normally originates in the *sinoatrial (SA) node*, a small mass of modified myocardial tissue located in the posterior wall of the right atrium, below the opening of the superior vena cava.

A second specialized mass of conduction tissue, the *AV node*, lies in the posterior right side of the interatrial septum near the opening of the coronary sinus. The AV node is continuous with a tract of conducting tissue termed the *AV bundle* or the *bundle of His*. Descending along the interventricular septum, the AV bundle divides into right and left bundle branches that descend along opposite sides of the interventricular septum and ultimately terminate in an extensive network of fine branches known as *Purkinje fibers.*

The spread of the cardiac impulse over the Purkinje fibers is extremely rapid, thereby ensuring virtually simultaneous excitation of the entire ventricular myocardium. Adjacent myocardial cells approximate at specialized junctions of low resistance, called *intercalated disks.* These intercalated disks facilitate the rapid spread of excitation from cell to cell, thereby allowing the heart to function as a *syncytium.*

The SA node initiates a wave of depolarization that spreads rapidly throughout the atria. Upon reaching the AV node, the impulse is delayed briefly (0.08–0.12 sec) to allow completion of atrial contraction. Excessive delay or failure of impulse conduction at the AV node results in heart block. Following the normally brief delay at the AV node, the cardiac impulse then proceeds along the bundle of His and its right and left bundle branches to the rapidly depolarizing fibers of the Purkinje network. The impulse sweeps through the ventricular myocardium from the endocardial (inner) to the epicardial (outer) surface.

Although all parts of the conduction system can rhythmically discharge cardiac action potentials, the cells of the SA node intrinsically depolarize at the highest frequency (60–100 times/min), thereby setting the pace or rhythm of the heart. Hence the SA node is commonly termed the cardiac *pacemaker.* The discharge rate of the SA node may be affected extrinsically by the autonomic nervous system, as well as by certain hormones, drugs, and even temperature changes. If the SA node fails to generate rhythmic cardiac impulses, other sites, such as the AV node or AV bundle, may assume a pacemaker role.

Disturbances of normal cardiac rhythm, or *arrhythmias,* are caused by altered myocardial electrophysiology. Cardiac arrhythmias may result from abnormal sites of impulse formation (ectopic foci), abnormal rates of impulse formation, or abnormal rates or routes of impulse conduction (see Chap. 30). A shortened myocardial refractory period may also contribute to the development of cardiac arrhythmias. Other predisposing factors include cardiac ischemia, electrolyte imbalance, excessive autonomic stimulation, and drug toxicity.

THE ELECTROCARDIOGRAM

The *electrocardiogram* (ECG or EKG) is a graphic record of the electrical activity of the heart. A typical ECG (lead II tracing) is shown in Figure 28-3. The *P wave* depicts atrial depolarization, the *QRS complex* depicts ventricular depolarization, and the *T wave* depicts ventricular repolarization.

The PR interval (normally 0.12–0.20 sec) indicates conduction time through the atria and includes the delay at the AV node. Abnormal prolongation of the PR interval indicates first-degree heart block.

The QT interval encompasses both ventricular depolariza-

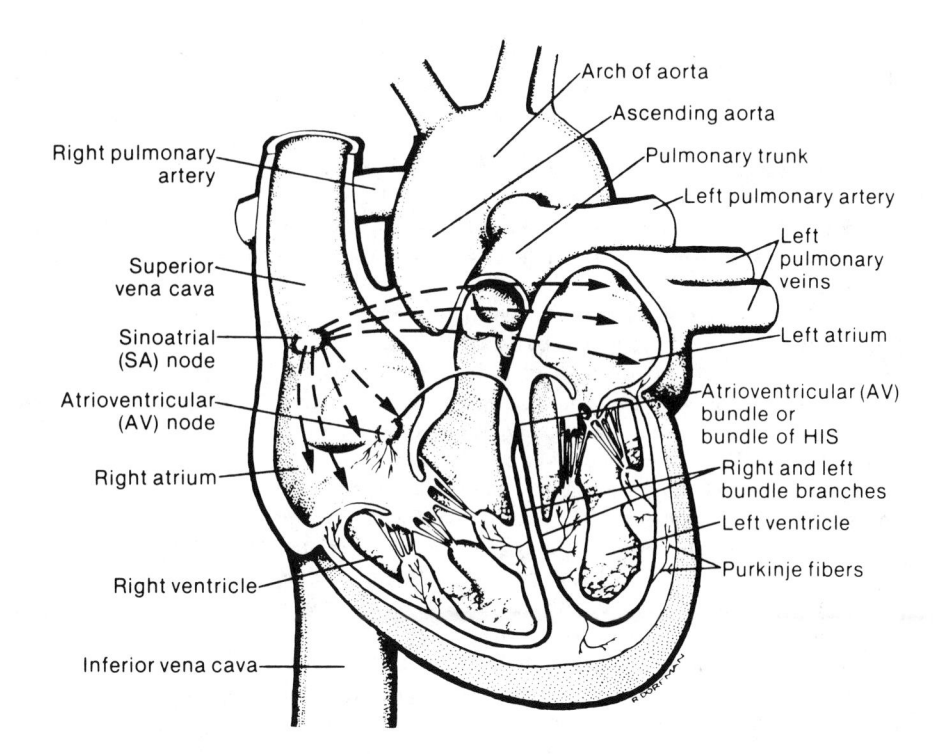

Figure 28-2 A highly specialized conduction system maintains the rhythmic synchronized activity of the heart.

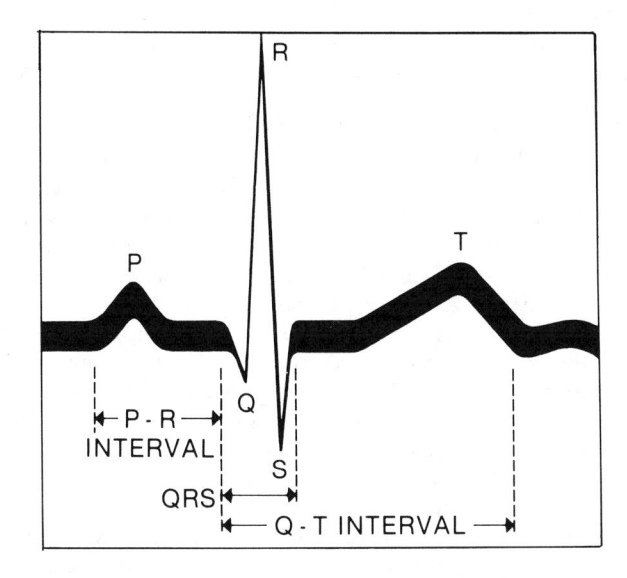

Figure 28-3 A typical electrocardiogram includes the following features: the P wave (depicting atrial depolarization), the QRS complex (depicting ventricular depolarization), and the T wave (depicting ventricular repolarization).

tion and repolarization. The QT interval may be prolonged by some antiarrhythmic drugs such as quinidine.

The T wave may be flattened or inverted by digitalis overdosage. Hyperkalemia causes peaking and elevation of the T wave. To a skilled reader, the ECG offers valuable information about cardiac rhythm (atrial and ventricular rates), conduction rate, chamber hypertrophy, presence of infarction, ionic imbalance, and drug effects.

THE CARDIAC CYCLE

The *cardiac cycle* consists of an orderly sequence of interdependent electrical and mechanical events associated with one complete cycle of contraction (systole) and relaxation (diastole) of the heart. Electrical excitation of the heart precedes contraction.

During diastole, the atrial and ventricular chambers are relaxed and the semilunar valves are closed. Blood that has entered the atria through the great veins flows passively from the atria to the ventricles through the open AV valves. The period of slow ventricular filling is termed *diastasis,* and it occurs in mid-diastole. During late diastole, a wave of depolarization (P wave) sweeps through the atria, leading to contraction of the atrial musculature. Atrial contraction (atrial systole) contributes approximately 30% to the ventricular blood volume.

Ventricular contraction follows the wave of depolarization through the ventricular conduction system and myocardium (QRS complex). When the ventricular pressures exceed the atrial pressures, the AV valves close, generating the first heart sound. During this phase of ventricular systole, the arterial pressures within the aorta and pulmonary artery exceed the ventricular pressures, thereby keeping the semilunar valves closed and maintaining the ventricular volumes constant (period of isovolumetric contraction). Eventually the sustained ventricular contraction generates sufficient ventricular pressure to exceed the arterial pressure. At this point the semilunar valves open, and the ventricles eject the blood into the pulmonary artery and aorta.

A wave of repolarization (T wave) sweeps through the ventricles, causing the ventricular myocardium to relax. As the ventricles relax, the ventricular pressures drop below the arterial pressures of the pulmonary artery and aorta, causing the semilunar valves to close and generating the second heart sound.

With continued ventricular relaxation, the ventricular pressures fall below the atrial pressures, causing the AV valves to open. The venous blood that has been accumulating in the atria during ventricular systole now rapidly flows through the open AV valves into the ventricles. At rest, approximately 70% of ventricular filling takes place during this period of early diastole.

CARDIAC OUTPUT

The work of the heart may be expressed in terms of *cardiac output*, that is, the volume of blood ejected from each ventricle in 1 minute. Cardiac output is the product of stroke volume multiplied by heart rate. The cardiac output of a resting adult falls in the range of 4.5 to 5 liters/min; however, during exercise an average adult may achieve a cardiac output of 15 to 20 liters/min.

Multiple factors contribute to the control of cardiac output. The *stroke volume* (the volume of blood ejected from a ventricle during a single contraction) is equal to the difference between the end-diastolic and end-systolic volumes. The end-diastolic volume represents the degree of ventricular filling, and it is determined by factors such as ventricular filling time, atrial contraction, myocardial distensibility, and the effective filling pressure. Normally, the bulk of ventricular filling occurs during early diastole, so that ventricular filling time is inversely related to the heart rate. At very rapid heart rates, the ventricular filling time is substantially reduced. In this case, atrial contraction may contribute significantly to the ventricular volume.

The effective filling pressure is directly related to the venous return, which is determined largely by the circulating blood volume and venous tone. Venous return to the heart is enhanced by the thoracicoabdominal pump and by skeletal muscle contraction. The pressure within the thorax is negative with respect to atmospheric pressure, whereas the pressure within the abdominal cavity is slightly positive. The pressure gradient, which becomes even greater during inspiration, favors the return of blood from the abdomen to the thorax. According to *Starling's Law of the Heart,* there is, within physiologic limits, a direct relationship between myocardial fiber length and the force of ventricular contraction. The degree of stretch of myocardial fibers before contraction is termed *preload*, and it is determined largely by the end-diastolic ventricular volume.

Increased preload will, within physiologic limits, increase the force of ventricular contraction and thereby increase the stroke volume. *Excessive* stretching of myocardial fibers will, however, ultimately lead to cardiac failure.

The end-systolic volume is primarily determined by the afterload and the contractility of the myocardium. The term *afterload* refers to the amount of tension that a ventricle must develop during systole in order to open the semilunar valve and to eject blood into the receiving artery. Afterload is a function of arterial pressure and ventricular size. As the size of a ventricle increases, the ventricle must develop a greater tension in order to generate a given pressure. Therefore, a dilated ventricle would have to develop a greater tension than a normal ventricle to generate the same systolic pressure.

Elevations in arterial pressure will also increase resistance to the outflow of blood from a ventricle, thereby necessitating an increase in ventricular tension. Chronic or excessive increases in afterload will adversely affect the cardiac output by elevating end-systolic volume, thereby reducing stroke volume.

The contractility of the myocardium is affected by a multitude of factors, including the metabolic state of the myocardium, physical and mechanical factors (Starling's Law of the Heart), nervous activity, hormones, and pharmacologic agents.

Factors that enhance the contractility of the myocardium are said to have a positive inotropic effect on the heart. Sympathetic stimulation, epinephrine, and isoproterenol, for example, enhance the contractile force of the myocardium and thereby increase the stroke volume and cardiac output. Cardiac output may also be altered by changes in heart rate.

Heart rate is responsive to extrinsic control by the autonomic nervous system. The SA and AV nodes are richly innervated by sympathetic and parasympathetic nerve fibers. The atria receive some innervation from each division of the autonomic nervous system, while the ventricles are innervated principally by sympathetic fibers. Sympathetic stimulation, through the release of norepinephrine from adrenergic nerve terminals, accelerates the heart rate and the speed of cardiac impulse conduction. Sympathetic activation also can markedly enhance the force of myocardial contractility.

Parasympathetic nerves to the heart are anatomically vagal and functionally cardioinhibitory. Vagal stimulation, through mediation of the neurotransmitter acetylcholine, produces a notable decrease in the heart rate and the speed of impulse conduction and a slight reduction of cardiac contractility.

BLOOD FLOW: HEMODYNAMICS

The cardiovascular system forms a continuous closed circuit for the distribution of blood to all body tissues. With each contraction, the left ventricle ejects the blood with a force sufficient to propel it through the entire systemic circuit. The elasticity of the aorta and large arteries transforms the intermittent output of the heart into a relatively steady peripheral blood flow. Blood flows through the arteries, arterioles, capillaries, venules, and veins according to existing pressure gradients, the progressive drop in pressure across the systemic circuit promoting undirectional forward flow.

According to Poiseuille's law, blood flow is directly proportional to the driving pressure and inversely proportional to the resistance. Resistance to blood flow is directly related to the viscosity of blood and is inversely related to the vascular radius. The viscosity of blood depends upon the hematocrit, the rate of flow, and the diameter of the vessel. With a constant hematocrit, the viscosity changes over normal ranges of flow are insignificant. The variable resistance to blood flow is determined largely by the radius of the blood vessels, notably the small muscular arteries and arterioles (resistance vessels). Because the vascular resistance to flow varies inversely as the fourth power of the vascular radius, even a small change in the caliber of a blood vessel can produce a pronounced change in blood flow.

Blood flow varies widely among the different organs and tissues of the body. The brain and kidneys, which represent only a small fraction of the total body mass, receive a generous blood supply; skeletal muscle, despite its large mass, receives only a small percentage of the cardiac output at rest.

Distribution of the cardiac output among the organs and tissues is determined by individual metabolic requirements of the tissue as well as by neural and humoral factors. Because the needs of individual body tissues are continually changing, blood flow must continually be adjusted. Blood flow to a given organ may be enhanced by increasing the cardiac output or by shunting blood from other body tissues. Distribution of the cardiac output is controlled by intrinsic as well as extrinsic mechanisms, which will now be examined in greater detail.

Intrinsic Control of Blood Flow

Local metabolic conditions and individual tissue requirements play an important role in the regulation of regional blood flow. Factors involved in the intrinsic control of blood flow include tissue oxygen requirements and availability, rate of tissue metabolism, and presence of certain tissue metabolites. The vascular smooth muscle of the microcirculation (arterioles, precapillaries, and precapillary sphincters) is highly sensitive to lack of oxygen. The vessels respond to tissue ischemia by vasodilation. Local increases in carbon dioxide and hydrogen ions also produce vasodilation and increased blood flow independently of nervous reflexes. Local control of perfusion is particularly evident in the heart and brain.

In addition to changes in pH and gas tension, endogenous vasodilators such as bradykinin, histamine, adenosine, and potassium ions may act locally to increase blood flow, especially during times of tissue injury or inflammation. The precise role and importance of these vasodilators and of other vasoactive substances such as prostaglandins, angiotensin, serotonin, and acetylcholine in the regulation of regional blood flow probably vary from tissue to tissue and remain to be clarified.

Autoregulation of blood flow assumes the inherent ability of a vascular bed to maintain a constant flow rate despite fluctuations in arterial pressure. Central to the mechanism of autoregulation is the ability of vascular smooth muscle to respond to distention caused by increased intraluminal pressure with appropriately graded contraction. Chemical influences have also been implicated in the mechanism of autoregulation.

Extrinsic Control of Blood Flow

The walls of small arteries and arterioles are abundantly innervated by autonomic vasomotor fibers, most of which are sympathetic. Sympathetic vasoconstrictor nerves are important in the regulation of peripheral resistance. Arteriolar vasomotor tone changes in accordance with the level of sympathetic activity. Increased sympathetic discharge of vasoconstrictor fibers leads to a reduction in vascular caliber and thereby to an increase in peripheral resistance to blood flow. All vasoconstrictor fibers are adrenergic.

Vasodilator nerves are of minor functional significance in most vascular beds, with the exception of skeletal muscle. In addition to possessing sympathetic adrenergic vasoconstrictor fibers, the vasculature of skeletal muscle is uniquely equipped with sympathetic cholinergic vasodilator nerves that elicit vasodilation in response to stress or exercise. Parasympathetic vasodilator nerves (also cholinergic) innervate only certain organs such as the salivary glands, bladder, and external genitalia. These vasodilator fibers do not significantly influence peripheral vascular resistance. Rather, their specific and limited distribution suggests a more specialized physiologic role.

In addition to neural regulation, humoral agents such as epinephrine and angiotensin extrinsically influence peripheral vascular resistance and blood flow.

ARTERIAL BLOOD PRESSURE

The arterial blood pressure serves as the driving force for blood flow through the vascular system. The magnitude of arterial blood pressure changes throughout the cardiac cycle. The maximum pressure (*systolic pressure*) occurs at the peak of ventricular contraction or systole. The magnitude of systolic pressure may be altered by changes in cardiac output or arterial distensibility. An increase in stroke volume, and hence cardiac output, will elevate systolic pressure, as will a reduction in arterial distensibility such as that occurring in arteriosclerosis.

The lowest pressure (*diastolic pressure*) occurs during diastole, just before ventricular contraction. Changes in peripheral resistance alter the level of diastolic pressure.

The difference between the systolic and diastolic pressures is termed *pulse pressure*. Pulse pressure is directly related to stroke volume and is inversely related to heart rate and peripheral resistance.

The mean arterial pressure is generally assumed to equal the diastolic pressure plus one third of the pulse pressure. At rapid heart rates, the times spent in systole and diastole are more nearly equal, and mean arterial pressure equals approximately one half of the sum of systolic and diastolic pressures.

The mean arterial pressure equals the product of cardiac output and peripheral resistance. Any factor or condition that alters either or both of these variables will therefore affect the blood pressure.

The arterial blood pressure must be constantly and carefully regulated to provide a driving force sufficient to distribute blood to all body tissues without imposing an excessive load upon the heart and blood vessels. Several control mechanisms exist for the continuous and precise regulation and integration of cardiovascular functions.

Within the medulla of the brainstem are cardiovascular (cardiac and vasomotor) control centers that receive and integrate input from numerous sensory receptors. Homeostatically, the most important of these are the pressure-sensitive baroreceptors located in the carotid sinus and aortic arch. Associated with the baroreceptors are branches of the glossopharyngeal (IX) and vagus (X) nerves, which serve as "buffer" nerves for the physiologic regulation and maintenance of systemic arterial pressure.

In response to blood pressure changes detected by the baroreceptors, afferent (sensory) impulses travel along the glossopharyngeal (sinus) and vagus (aortic) nerves to the cardiovascular integrating centers of the medulla. Activation of autonomic sympathetic and parasympathetic efferent nerves to the heart and blood vessels produces appropriate changes in cardiac output and peripheral resistance for the homeostatic restoration of blood pressure.

Efferent responses to an elevated blood pressure include the following: (1) a slowing of the heart (bradycardia) induced by increased parasympathetic and decreased sympathetic activity, (2) reduced myocardial contractility caused by decreased sympathetic discharge, and (3) vasodilation resulting from decreased sympathetic tone. The reduction in cardiac output (resulting from a decreased heart rate and stroke volume) and the decreased peripheral vascular resistance restore the blood pressure toward normal.

The activity of the medullary cardiovascular integrating centers may also be influenced by afferent impulses from higher brain centers such as the hypothalamus and cerebral cortex. It is through such afferent input that emotional responses, for example, fear or rage, alter blood pressure.

A peripheral mechanism operative in the control of blood pressure is the renin–angiotensin–aldosterone system, which is outlined in Figure 28-4. Renin is released from renal juxtaglomerular cells (see Fig. 36-3) in response to a number of stimuli, including hypotension, reduced renal perfusion pressure, and beta-adrenergic stimulation. Renin acts upon the plasma protein angiotensinogen to form the decapeptide angiotensin I, which is then converted by endothelial cell and plasma enzymes into the physiologically active angiotensin II. Angiotensin II is a potent vasopressor that acts through several mechanisms, but primarily by direct stimulation of vascular smooth muscle, to produce intense vasoconstriction and in-

```
↑Renal           ↓Blood         Beta-adrenergic
perfusion        pressure       innervation
       \            |            /
        →  Juxtaglomerular cells ←
                    |
                    ↓
                  Renin
Angiotensinogen ─────────────→ Angiotensin I
                                     |  converting
                                     |  enzyme
                                     ↓
Peripheral  ←──────────────── Angiotensin II
vasoconstriction                     |
      |                              ↓
      |                        Adrenal cortex
      |                              |
      ↓                              ↓
↑Peripheral                      Aldosterone
resistance                           |
      |                              ↓
      |                        ↑Na⁺ Reabsorption
      |                              |
      |                              ↓
      |                        ↑H₂O Reabsorption
      |                              |
      ↓                              ↓
  ↑Blood   ←──────────────── ↑Plasma volume
  pressure
```

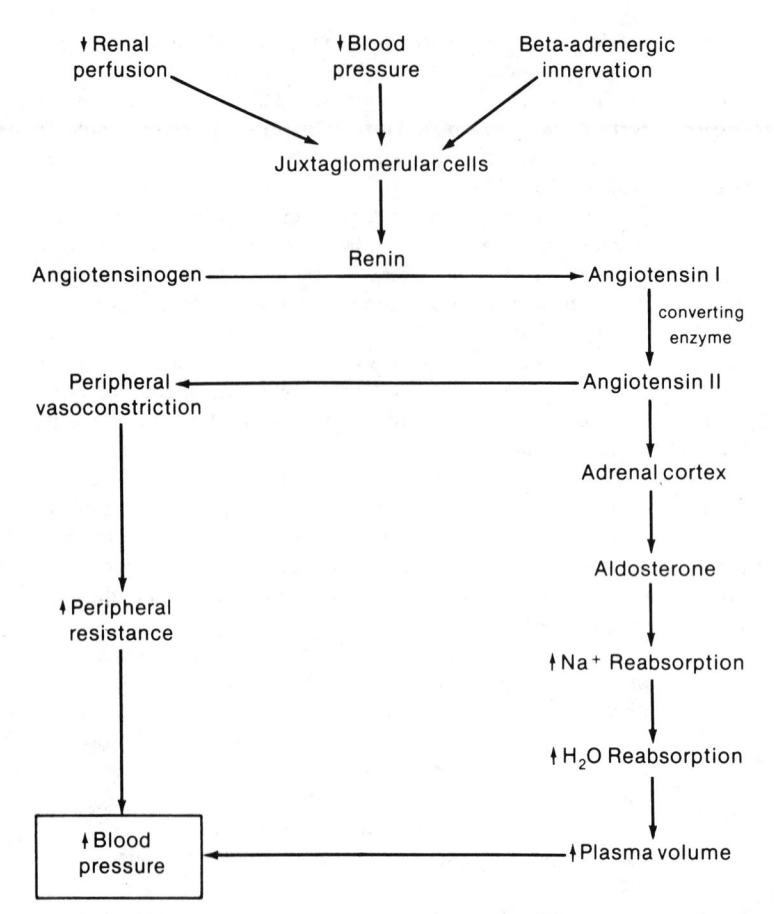

Figure 28-4 Renin-angiotensin-aldosterone mechanism for blood pressure regulation.

creased peripheral resistance. Angiotensin II also stimulates release of aldosterone from the adrenal cortex. Aldosterone stimulates renal tubular reabsorption of sodium, thereby promoting water reabsorption and increasing blood volume. The increased blood volume and the increased peripheral resistance both contribute to the elevation of blood pressure.

The contribution of the renin–angiotensin–aldosterone system to hypertension, other than those cases resulting from renal dysfunction or renovascular stenosis, has yet to be definitively established. Although it does not appear that abnormalities of this system are a *consistent* factor in the development of most forms of hypertension, several compounds that interfere with conversion of angiotensin I to angiotensin II are being used successfully in treating many forms of hypertension (see Chap. 31). In addition, other currently used antihypertensives reduce the release of renin, presumably because of a beta-blocking action, and this action may contribute to their efficacy in reducing blood pressure.

29 CARDIOTONIC DRUGS

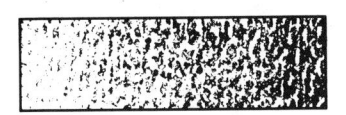

Drugs that have a cardiotonic action are capable of increasing the force of contraction of cardiac muscle, thus improving its functional capability. The term has traditionally been applied to a group of drugs known as the digitalis glycosides, although newer drugs that exhibit similar properties are now available and are termed positive inotropic agents. Cardiotonic drugs are primarily indicated for the treatment of congestive heart failure because of their ability to improve the force of contraction of the failing heart. In addition to the digitalis glycosides and the positive inotropic agents to be discussed in this chapter, other drugs are also used in managing the symptoms of congestive heart failure. Thus, diuretics (see Chap. 37) and vasodilators (see Chaps. 31 and 32) are also of great usefulness in treating certain types of congestive heart failure. Optimal therapy often includes two or more of the above-mentioned drugs

CARDIOACTIVE GLYCOSIDES

The cardioactive glycosides encompass a group of three semisynthetic steroidal compounds having qualitatively similar effects on cardiac function. These drugs are derived from the leaves of either *Digitalis purpurea* or *Digitalis lanata*, both species of the foxglove plant. Because digitalis is the name of the principal botanical source of these agents, they may also be referred to collectively as the digitalis glycosides.

Digitalis Glycosides

Deslanoside   Digoxin
Digitoxin

Although all the digitalis glycosides have similar pharmacologic effects on the heart, they differ with respect to onset and duration of action (owing to differences in absorption, biotransformation, and extent of protein binding) as well as mode of administration. The drugs can be divided arbitrarily into three groups according to their routes of administration: oral only, parenteral only, and both oral and parenteral. The major characteristics of the currently available cardioactive glycosides, grouped according to their methods of administration, are listed in Table 29-1.

The digitalis glycosides increase myocardial contractility in both normal and failing hearts. Consequently, there is significant improvement in cardiovascular performance and an associated decrease in the size of the ventricles. Although there is some increase in oxygen demand because of increased contractility, this is more than compensated for by the reduced oxygen demand that occurs as ventricular size is reduced. Therefore, in the failing heart, there is an overall increase in efficiency (work performed: energy required).

The overall cardiodynamic effects of the digitalis agents are quite complex, being a combination of direct actions on the myocardium as well as indirect actions that alter the normal electrophysiologic properties of the heart (automaticity, conductivity, refractoriness). Moreover, the benefits of the digitalis drugs, are significantly greater in the failing heart than in the normal heart, a further indication that the drugs are acting to correct the hemodynamic imbalances associated with heart failure.

The direct action of the digitalis glycosides on the myocardium is largely responsible for the increased force of contraction (positive inotropic effect) noted with these drugs. Conversely, their effects on the heart's electrical properties play an essential role in their ability to alter the rate and rhythm of the heartbeat. This latter action is responsible for both the therapeutic effect of the drugs in managing certain supraventricular arrhythmias, and their toxic effects on the heart, namely the development of other types of arrhythmias. A review of the major cardiovascular actions of the digitalis glycosides is found in Table 29-2.

The progressive atrioventricular (AV) block seen with increasing dosage can lead to a major manifestation of digitalis toxicity—disturbances in cardiac rhythm. The arrhythmias that develop following administration of these drugs also are attributable to a shortened AV refractory period, suppression of normal pacemaker activity, and increased ventricular automaticity. Many factors can predispose the heart to digitalis toxicity, the most important being hypokalemia (reduced serum potassium levels), hypercalcemia (elevated serum calcium levels), catecholamine depletion, concurrent use of quinidine, systemic alkalosis, and renal or hepatic impairment. These drugs display a rather narrow safety margin and between 10% and 20% of patients receiving them will develop signs of toxicity.

Following administration, digitalis glycosides are distributed widely in the body, into both inactive reservoir (binding) sites and active receptor sites in the myocardium. Therefore, to achieve the desired effect at the active myocardial receptor sites, it is necessary to administer sufficient drug to saturate the reservoir of nonspecific binding sites. In *acute* congestive failure, large loading doses of drug may be administered rapidly to achieve the desired effect quickly. This process, termed *digitalization*, carries the risk of serious toxicity if the loading dose is excessive. Therefore, in less acute conditions, the patient should be loaded (digitalized) more slowly to reduce the risk of potential toxicity. Such slow loading can often be effectively accomplished simply by administering the small recommended maintenance doses from the beginning of therapy.

The *maintenance* dose is the amount of drug sufficient to replace the amount of drug eliminated between dosings, and thereby to maintain a steady-state plasma level of the drug. Maintenance doses therefore are smaller than rapid loading doses and must be individually adjusted according to the patient's condition and the type of digitalis preparation used (long- or short-acting). Periodic clinical assessment is necessary to ensure that the optimal maintenance dose of the cardiac glycoside is being used and that adverse reactions are kept at a minimum. Because there is a substantial difference between the digitalizing and maintenance doses of some agents, both dosage ranges will be given for each drug throughout the chapter.

The digitalis glycosides are reviewed as a group because they have similar pharmacologic properties; characteristics of individual drugs are then given in Table 29-3.

MECHANISM
Inhibit sodium–potassium (Na^+–K^+) membrane ATPase, the enzyme responsible for breakdown of ATP to supply energy for

Table 29-1
Characteristics of Digitalis Glycosides

	Onset IV	Onset PO	Maximum Effect IV	Maximum Effect PO	Plasma Half-life	Extent of GI Absorption	Protein Binding
Parenteral							
Deslanoside	10–30 min		60–90 min		30–36 h		20%–30%
Oral/Parenteral							
Digoxin	10–30 min	1–2 h	2–4 h	4–8 h	32–40 h	60%–90%	20%–30%
Oral							
Digitoxin		2–3 h		6–12 h	5–7 days	95%–97%	90%–100%

Table 29-2
Cardiovascular Actions: Digitalis Glycosides

Excitability of myocardium
   Small doses 0 (↑)
   Large doses ↓
Conduction velocity
   AV conduction system ↓ (dose-dependent)
   Cardiac muscle 0 (↑)
Refractory period
   AV conduction system ↑ (dose-dependent)
   Cardiac muscle ↓
Heart rate ↓
Force of contraction ↑
Cardiac output ↑
Blood pressure
   Venous ↓
   Systolic slight ↑
   Diastolic slight ↓
ECG
   P–R interval prolonged
   Q–T interval shortened
   S–T segment depressed
   T wave decreased *or* inverted
Diuretic action
   Renal blood flow and glomerular filtration ↑
   Aldosterone release (deactivation of renin–angiotensin mechanism) ↓
   Sodium reabsorption in renal tubules ↓

0 no effect; ↑, increased or prolonged; ↓, decreased or shortened.

---

the cellular Na^+–K^+ pump; therefore, electrical properties of the myocardium are altered, and intracellular sodium and extracellular potassium concentrations are elevated; subsequently, increased sodium–calcium exchange occurs across the sarcolemmal membrane and additional calcium is liberated from binding sites on the sarcoplasmic reticulum; elevated free intracellular calcium levels facilitate the interaction of actin and myosin by removing the inhibitory effect of the troponin–tropomyosin complex; therefore cardiac contraction is enhanced and cardiac output is increased. Heart rate is slowed by both vagal and extravagal mechanisms. Vagally, the drugs stimulate medullary vagal nuclei and increase sensitivity of pacemaker cells to the action of acetylcholine; extravagally, the drugs decrease AV conduction and increase the AV refractory period. Diuretic effect is primarily caused by increases in renal blood flow and glomerular filtration rate secondary to higher cardiac output but may also involve a reduction in aldosterone release and possibly direct interference with sodium reabsorption in renal tubules

USES

Treatment of congestive heart failure, especially low-output failure associated with depressed left ventricular function
Note: Drugs are of little value in "high output"congestive heart failure or in patients with mitral stenosis and normal sinus rhythm
Treatment of certain cardiac arrhythmias, including atrial fibrillation, atrial flutter, and paroxysmal atrial tachycardia, where ventricular rate is elevated
Treatment of cardiogenic shock accompanied by pulmonary edema

DOSAGE
See Table 29-3

FATE
Variable rates of absorption, onset of action, and duration of effect are observed among the different digitalis glycosides (see Table 29-1). Digitoxin is highly lipid soluble and extensively absorbed orally. Digoxin is somewhat less well absorbed (60%–90%). The digitalis glycosides are widely distributed in peripheral tissues; preparations are bound to varying degrees by plasma proteins (see Table 29-1) and are excreted through the kidneys, either as unchanged drug (e.g., digoxin, deslanoside) or as hepatic metabolites (e.g., digitoxin)

COMMON SIDE EFFECTS
Anorexia, nausea, slow or irregular pulse, altered color perception (yellow or green vision)

SIGNIFICANT ADVERSE REACTIONS
(More common at large doses)

GI: vomiting, diarrhea, abdominal pain
CNS: weakness, lethargy, disorientation, headache, confusion, depression, paresthesias, amblyopia, diplopia, visual disturbances (e.g., flashes, halos, white dots, "snowflakes"), neuralgia-like pain, delirium
Cardiac: arrhythmias (all types are possible); most common are

ventricular premature beats and paroxysmal atrial tachycardia

Other: thromboembolism, pruritus, urticaria, fever, facial edema, joint pain, gynecomastia

CONTRAINDICATIONS
Ventricular tachycardia or fibrillation, severe myocarditis. *Cautious use* in patients with Adams–Stokes syndrome, acute myocardial infarction, severe pulmonary disease, advanced heart failure, myxedema, incomplete AV block, chronic constrictive pericarditis, or hypertrophic subaortic stenosis; also in the presence of hypoxia, hypomagnesemia, hypokalemia, hypercalcemia, renal or hepatic insufficiency, and in elderly, debilitated, pregnant, or nursing patients

INTERACTIONS
Absorption of digitalis drugs may be reduced by antacids, anticholinergics, cholestyramine resin, laxatives, metoclopramide, neomycin and possibly other aminoglycosides

Effects of digitalis drugs can be reduced by agents that increase their metabolism, such as anticonvulsants, antihistamines, barbiturates, oral hypoglycemics, and pyrazolones

Toxic effects of cardiac glycosides (especially arrhythmias) may be *increased* by adrenergics, amphotericin, calcium salts, corticosteroids, diuretics (except potassium-sparing drugs), glucose, insulin, magnesium, pancuronium, reserpine, succinylcholine, and thyroid preparations

Marked bradycardia may develop if digitalis drugs are given in combination with carbamazepine, guanethidine, phenytoin, propranolol, and reserpine.

Digitalis drugs may decrease the effects of oral anticoagulants and heparin

Quinidine, nifedipine, and verapamil can increase serum levels of digoxin, possibly by displacement from tissue binding sites or reduced renal clearance

Increased plasma levels of digitalis drugs can result from combined use with potassium-sparing diuretics or propantheline

NURSING CONSIDERATIONS

Nursing Alerts
- Because the margin between the therapeutic and toxic dose of cardiac glycosides is extremely narrow, closely monitor patient for early symptoms of impending toxicity (weakness, nausea, vomiting, diarrhea, blurred vision, diplopia, halo vision, dizziness, precordial pain, palpitations, anxiety, and facial pain). Many symptoms of digitalis intoxication are, however, the same as those associated with conditions for which digitalis is used (e.g., nausea and vomiting due to heart failure, arrhythmias). Careful determination of cause (i.e., disease versus digitalis overdose) is essential to proper management.
- Because hypokalemia greatly increases the incidence of digitalis toxicity, monitor for early indications of potassium deficiency (e.g., drowsiness, paresthesias, muscle weakness, anorexia, depressed reflexes, orthostatic hypotension, polyuria), especially if patient is receiving potassium-wasting diuretics. Potassium supplementation (KCl liquid, orange juice, bananas) should be considered.
- Monitor for changes in pulse rate (e.g., sudden increase above 120 when rate has been slowing or a fall below 60/min) or rhythm, possible signs of overdosage. Ventricular arrhythmias may, in fact, occur even when other signs of digitalis toxicity are absent, especially in the patient with advanced heart failure, severe pulmonary disease, rheumatic carditis, or Wolff–Parkinson–White syndrome.
- If the patient is a child, carefully assess for presence of atrial arrhythmias. Because nausea, vomiting, and neurologic and visual disturbances rarely occur in children, atrial arrhythmias are often the most reliable indication of developing toxicity. Premature, immature, and newborn infants are particularly sensitive to digitalis drugs and should be digitalized very cautiously. Arrhythmias also occur very frequently in children with rheumatic carditis.

1. Ensure that baseline data (i.e., clinical symptoms, serum electrolytes, vital signs) have been obtained before initiating administration.
2. Expect to give drug parenterally only when oral administration is not feasible (e.g., need for *rapid* digitalization, severe vomiting, unconsciousness).
3. Take apical pulse for 1 minute immediately before giving drug. In patient with atrial fibrillation, determine pulse deficit (apical minus radial pulse). Check with physician to determine limits (both high and low) for withholding drug.
4. Monitor intake–output and body weight, and check for edema. Dosage adjustments may be necessary to improve renal function if fluid retention occurs.
5. Monitor results of renal and liver function tests and ECG and serum electrolyte determinations, which should be performed periodically.

PATIENT EDUCATION
1. Instruct patient to take drug after meals if nausea and vomiting are present. If symptoms do not subside, they may reflect digitalis toxicity through central emetic action. The physician should be notified immediately.
2. Emphasize importance of adhering to prescribed dosage regimen and recommended diet in order to obtain maximal benefit with minimal toxicity.
3. Instruct patient not to take an "extra" dose of medication to compensate for a missed dose. The possibility of toxicity is increased if doses are taken too close together because of the danger of accumulation.
4. Teach patient how to monitor pulse rate, urinary output, and weight to determine if therapy is appropriate.
5. Instruct patient to report untoward reactions immediately because toxicity can develop rapidly.
6. Instruct patient to notify physician at once if protracted diarrhea or vomiting occurs because these conditions can alter electrolyte balance and possibly lead to toxicity.
7. Advise patient to avoid using OTC drugs high in sodium (e.g., Alka Seltzer, Bromo Seltzer, Bisodol).
8. Refer patient to dietician for instruction regarding reduction of overall salt intake. High-salt foods as well as addition of table salt to foods should generally be avoided.
9. If patient is overweight, refer to appropriate resource for assistance with a weight reduction program to lessen demands on cardiovascular system.
10. Inform patient that consumption of large quantities of licorice, which contains glycyrrhizic acid, may cause salt and water retention, hypokalemia, and other symptoms of congestive heart failure.

Table 29-3
Cardioactive Glycosides

Drug	Preparations	Usual Dosage Range — Digitalizing	Maintenance	Nursing Implications
Deslanoside Cedilanid-D	Injection: 0.2 mg/mL	IV: 1.6 mg as 1 injection *or* in 0.8-mg portions IM: 0.8 mg at each of 2 sites		Rapid-acting glycoside used for emergency treatment of acute pulmonary edema and supraventricular arrhythmias; maintenance therapy with an oral glycoside may be instituted within 12 h after deslanoside; give injection slowly over 5 min
Digitoxin Crystodigin	Tablets: 0.05 mg, 0.1 mg, 0.15 mg, 0.2 mg	*Rapid:* 0.6 mg initially, followed by 0.4 mg, then 0.2 mg at intervals of 4–6 h *Slow:* 0.2 mg twice a day for 4 days	Adults: 0.05 mg–0.3 mg/day (usual—0.1 mg/day) Children: one tenth of digitalizing dose	Long-acting, potent glycoside mainly employed for maintenance rather than digitalizing therapy; slow onset and extremely long half-life makes digitalization difficult; danger of accumulation toxicity is high with this drug; do *not* give full digitalizing doses to patients receiving other digitalis glycosides within the preceding 3 wk
Digoxin Lanoxin, Lanoxicaps (CAN) Novodigoxin	Tablets: 0.125 mg, 0.25 mg, 0.5 mg Capsules: 0.05 mg, 0.1 mg, 0.2 mg Elixir (pediatric): 0.05 mg/mL Injection: 0.1, 0.25 mg/mL	**Oral** *Adults* Rapid: 0.5 mg–0.75 mg initially, followed by 0.25 mg–0.5 mg every 6–8 h to a total of 1 mg–1.5 mg Slow: 0.125 mg–0.25 mg daily for 7 days *Children* Newborn: 40 µg/kg–60 µg/kg 1 mo–2 yr: 60 µg/kg–80 µg/kg 2–10 yr: 40 µg/kg–60 µg/kg **IV** *Adults:* 0.25 mg–0.5 mg initially, then 0.25 mg every 4–6 h to a total of 1 mg *Children:* 25 µg/kg–50 µg/kg in divided doses	**Oral/IV** *Adults:* 0.125 mg–0.5 mg/day (average 0.25 mg/day) *Children:* 20%–30% of the total digitalizing dose daily	Widely used for both rapid digitalization and maintenance therapy; little danger of accumulation because drug is rapidly excreted; capsules have greater bioavailability than tablets; therefore 0.2-mg capsule is equivalent to 0.25-mg tablet and 0.1-mg capsule is equivalent to 0.125-mg tablet; drug can be given IM but absorption is erratic; do *not* give full digitalizing dose if patient has received a more slowly excreted cardiac glycoside within the preceding 2 wk; administration with food slows rate of absorption but does not affect the total amount absorbed; closely monitor patients with renal insufficiency because drug is primarily excreted unchanged through the kidney; dosage may need to be decreased in patients receiving quinidine (see Interactions)

Digoxin Immune Fab—Ovine
Digibind

Digoxin immune Fab consists of antigen-binding fragments (Fab) derived from antidigoxin antibodies produced in immunized sheep. The antibodies are papain-digested, and digoxin-specific Fab fragments are then isolated and purified. The preparation contains 40 mg/vial of lyophilized powder for reconstitution. Each vial binds approximately 0.6 mg of digoxin (or digitoxin).

Digoxin immune Fab is used to treat potentially life-threatening digoxin (or digitoxin) intoxication. In most instances, amelioration of signs and symptoms of intoxication is noted within 1 hour. The drug is administered IV over 30 minutes but may be given as a bolus injection if cardiac arrest is imminent. Dosage guidelines are provided with the drug packaging and differ according to the amount of digoxin (or digitoxin) to be neutralized. If this value is not readily obtainable, administration of 20 vials (800 mg) is usually adequate to treat most life-threatening intoxications in adults and children. Larger doses have a more rapid onset of action than smaller doses but are associated with a greater likelihood of febrile or allergic reactions. Hypokalemia may also occur, and withdrawal from the effects of digoxin may result in reduced cardiac output and worsening of congestive heart failure.

POSITIVE INOTROPIC AGENTS

Amrinone
Inocor

Amrinone is the first of a new class of positive inotropic agents that are structurally and mechanistically unlike the digitalis glycosides. Amrinone and its close structural analog milrinone increase myocardial contractility and exert a peripheral vasodilatory action. They can provide additional symptomatic relief of congestive heart failure in patients whose condition is not satisfactorily controlled by conventional therapy (i.e., digitalis drugs, diuretics, vasodilators). The drug is administered IV only in an acute setting; prolonged use increases the likelihood of thrombocytopenia and should be avoided.

MECHANISM
Drug appears to inhibit myocardial cell phosphodiesterase (the enzyme responsible for inactivating cyclic AMP), thus increasing cellular levels of cyclic AMP which facilitate the contractions of myocardial muscle cells; also exhibits a relaxant effect on vascular smooth muscle, thereby reducing both preload and afterload (see review of cardiac physiology in Chap. 28); drug is *not* a beta-adrenergic agonist, nor does it inhibit the activity of Na^+-K^+ ATPase, as do the digitalis glycosides; increased inward calcium flux during the action potential has also been postulated as a contributory mechanism; effects noted following amrinone administration include enhanced myocardial contractility *even after full doses of digitalis,* increased cardiac output, reduced ventricular filling pressure and pulmonary capillary wedge pressure, increased left ventricular ejection fraction, and improved exercise capacity; there is little change in heart rate or arterial pressure

USES
Short-term management of congestive heart failure in patients who have not responded adequately to digitalis drugs, diuretics, and vasodilators

DOSAGE
Initially, 0.75 mg/kg by IV bolus over 2 to 3 minutes, followed by a maintenance infusion of 5 μg/kg/min to 10 μg/kg/min to a total daily dose of 10 mg/kg (including bolus). An additional bolus injection may be given 30 minutes after the initial bolus, if needed

FATE
Peak effect occurs within 10 minutes; duration of action is dose-dependent (range 30 min–2 h); protein binding is variable (10%–50%); metabolized in the liver; elimination half-life is 3 to 4 hours, although it can range from 3 to 15 hours depending on status of heart function

SIGNIFICANT ADVERSE REACTIONS
Arrhythmias (3%) and thrombocytopenia (2.5%) can occur, especially with prolonged therapy; other adverse effects associated with amrinone therapy are nausea, vomiting, anorexia, abdominal pain, hepatotoxicity, hypotension, fever, chest pain, burning at injection site; asymptomatic platelet count reductions (less than 150,000/mm^3) may be noted and are usually reversed within 1 week of dosage reduction

CONTRAINDICATIONS
No absolute contraindications. *Cautious use* in patients with aortic or pulmonic valvular disease, hypertrophic subaortic stenosis, arrhythmias, thrombocytopenia, hypotension, and following an acute myocardial infarction or vigorous diuretic therapy. Safety for use in pregnant or nursing women and in children has not been established

Note: If liver enzymes are elevated or platelet count is reduced *together* with clinical symptoms, the drug should be discontinued. If these changes occur in the *absence* of clinical symptoms, consider the benefit: risk ratio in deciding whether to discontinue therapy

INTERACTIONS
Additive hypotensive effects may occur with concurrent use of disopyramide.

NURSING CONSIDERATIONS

Nursing Alerts
- If given as a bolus in a peripheral IV, dilute with normal saline because drug is extremely irritating. Irritation is not a problem with a central line.
- Assess patient for evidence of unusual bleeding, such as petechiae, purpura, hematuria, or melena.
- Monitor results of platelet counts, which should be obtained regularly. Levels below 150,000/mm^3 represent thrombocytopenia.
- Assess patient for signs and symptoms of hepatotoxicity.
- Monitor results of liver enzyme determinations, which should be performed periodically.
- Check results of ECGs, which should be performed periodically to detect arrhythmias.

1. Assess patient for presence of GI symptoms (e.g., anorexia, nausea, vomiting, abdominal pain). Symptoms can be ameliorated by reducing drug dosage.
2. Do not dilute drug with solutions containing dextrose because a chemical interaction occurs with prolonged contact.
3. Do not administer through an IV line with other drugs because physical incompatabilities are highly likely.

Selected Bibliography
Aronow WS: Treatment of congestive heart failure, Parts I and II. Ration Drug Ther 16(9) and 16(10):1982
Bristol JA, Evans DB: Agents for the treatment of heart failure. Med Res Rev 3:259, 1983

Colucci WS, Wright MD, Braunwald E: New positive inotropic agents in the treatment of congestive heart failure. N Engl J Med 314(6):349, 1986

Farah AF, Alousi AA, Schwarz RP: Positive inotropic agents. Ann Rev Pharmacol Toxicol 24:275, 1984

Franciosa JA: Intravenous amrinonc: An advance or a wrong step? Ann Intern Med 102:399, 1985

Hoffman BF: The pharmacology of cardiac glycosides. In Rosen MR, Hoffman BF (eds): Cardiac Therapy, p 387. Boston, Martinus Nighoff, 1983

Jafri SM, Levine TB, Kloner RA: Congestive heart failure: Recent advances in medical management. Mod Med 56(12):50, 1988

McCall D, O'Rourke RA: Congestive heart failure. I. Biochemistry, pathophysiology, and neurohumoral mechanisms. Mod Concepts Cardiovasc Dis 54:55, 1985

McCauley K, Burke KG: Your detailed guide to drugs for C.H.F. Nursing '84 14(5):47, 1984

Parmley WW: Pathophysiology of congestive heart failure. Am J Cardiol 55:9A, 1985

Potempa K, Roberts KV: Cardiovascular drugs and the older adult. Nurs Clin North Am 17:263, 1982

Smith TW: Digitalis: Mechanisms of action and clinical use. N Engl J Med 318(6):358, 1988

Ward A, Brogden RN, Heel RC: Amrinone: A preliminary review of its pharmacologic properties and therapeutic use. Drugs 26:468, 1983

Willerson JT: What is wrong with the failing heart? N Engl J Med 307:243, 1982

SUMMARY. CARDIOTONIC DRUGS

Drug	Preparations	Usual Dosage Range
Digitalis Glycosides	*See* Table 29-3	
Digoxin Immune Fab Digibind	Injection: 40 mg/vial with 75 mg sorbitol	Depends on amount of digoxin or digitoxin to be neutralized; see package instructions
Amrinone Inocor	Injection: 5 mg/mL	Initially, 0.75 mg/kg by IV bolus; maintenance infusion of 5–10 µg/kg/min up to a total daily dose of 10 mg/kg

ANTIARRHYTHMIC DRUGS

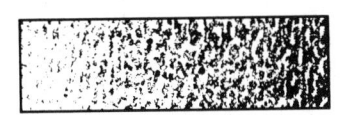

30

Cardiac arrhythmias can be regarded as any deviation from the normal rate and rhythm of contractions of the heart. Depending on the type of arrhythmia present, a number of hemodynamic complications can ensue, cardiac output may be reduced, and serious rhythm alterations may be lethal.

The conductile system of the heart is discussed in detail in Chapter 28 and outlined schematically in Figure 28-2. Deviations from the orderly propagation and conduction of impulses through this cardiac conductile system result in a decrement in cardiac function and reduced flow of oxygenated blood to the body organs. Irregularities in rate and rhythm of the heart markedly impair its ability to function and are a cause of eventual development of cardiac failure.

Cardiac arrhythmias arise from electrophysiologic disturbances of cardiac function. The two principal alterations are:

- *Disorders of impulse formation:* impulses arise in areas of the heart other than the normal SA node; these are often termed *ectopic beats.*
- *Disorders of impulse conduction:* impulses spread throughout the heart by abnormal pathways; examples include delayed AV conduction (AV block), bundle branch block, and reentry excitation, a complex phenomenon in which impulses reenter an area of the myocardium from a direction opposite to normal flow, reactivating the fibers.

While certainly serious, *atrial arrhythmias* are usually not life-threatening if normal ventricular function is maintained. Conversely, disturbances in *ventricular* rhythm of even a few minutes' duration can be fatal, and therefore require immediate and vigorous therapy. The purposes of antiarrhythmic drug treatment, therefore, are twofold: to restore normal cardiac rhythm, and to prevent recurrence or extension of an existing arrhythmia.

Although the electrophysiologic properties of antiarrhythmic drugs are quite complex, attempts have been made to classify these drugs based on their primary mechanisms of action. Table 30-1 outlines the different groups of antiarrhythmic drugs categorized according to their principal actions on the heart. Drugs within a particular group (e.g., group IA) generally share similar electrophysiological effects but can differ significantly in other respects such as oral versus parenteral availability and frequency and type of side effects.

Selection of an appropriate antiarrhythmic agent depends on the type of arrhythmia present as well as the characteristics of the drugs themselves—their onset, duration, type, and incidence of side effects, in addition to other factors.

The major pharmacokinetic properties as well as the electrophysiological effects of the principal antiarrhythmic drugs are listed in Table 30-2.

Drugs used in treating arrhythmias alter the heart's basic electrical properties, including excitability, conduction velocity, refractory period, and automaticity. These, then, are potentially dangerous drugs. Because not all arrhythmias require drug therapy, careful diagnosis of the type of disordered rhythm present is essential for effective and safe management of these conditions. Since the overall pharmacology and toxicology of the different drugs vary to a significant degree, they are discussed individually in this chapter.

GROUP IA DRUGS

Quinidine

Cardioquin, Cin-Quin, Duraquin, Quinaglute Dura-Tabs, Quinatime, Quinidex Extentabs, Quinora, Quin-Release
(CAN) Apo-Quinidine, Biquin Durules, Novoquinidin, Quinate

MECHANISM
Complexes with lipoproteins in myocardial cell membrane, thereby decreasing sodium influx during depolarization and potassium efflux during repolarization; depresses cardiac excitability (elevates firing threshold to screen out weak ectopic impulses), slows conduction velocity and prolongs effective refractory period of the myocardium; slows phase 0 (depolarization) and prolongs phase 4 (diastolic depolarization) of the ventricular action potential; exerts anticholinergic action (decreases vagal tone and prevents cardiac slowing due to vagal activation)

USES
Treatment of the following arrhythmias:
    Paroxysmal supraventricular tachycardia
    Atrial flutter and fibrillation (following digoxin to control AV conduction)
    Premature atrial and ventricular contractions
    Paroxysmal AV junctional rhythm
    Paroxysmal ventricular tachycardia not associated with complete heart block
Maintenance therapy after electrical conversion of atrial flutter or fibrillation

DOSAGE
Oral
    Usual: 10 mg/kg to 20 mg/kg/day in 4 to 6 divided doses (200 mg–300 mg 4 times/day) individually adjusted to patient's response
    Paroxysmal supraventricular tachycardia: 400 mg to 600 mg every 2 hours to 3 hours until paroxysm is terminated
    Premature atrial and ventricular contractions: 200 mg to 300 mg 3 to 4 times/day
    Atrial fibrillation: 200 mg every 2 hours to 3 hours for 5 to 8 doses; increase gradually until sinus rhythm is restored (maximal daily dose is 3 g–4 g)
    Maintenance: 200 mg to 300 mg 3 to 4 times/day (sustained-release forms—1 to 2 tablets 2 to 3 times/day)
IM
600 mg gluconate salt initially, then 400 mg every 2 hours as needed
IV
200 mg to 750 mg gluconate salt or equivalent by slow IV infusion of a dilute (800 mg gluconate/50 mL 5% glucose) solution at a rate of 1 mL (16 mg) per minute
Note: Use prolonged-acting forms of quinidine (i.e., Quinaglute Dura-Tabs, Quinidex Extentabs) only for maintenance therapy. Make appropriate dosage adjustments when changing preparations (Quinaglute Dura-Tabs are 62% base; quinidine sulfate is 82% base).

Table 30-1
Classification of Antiarrhythmic Drugs

Group	Drugs	Principal Cardiac Actions	Major Indications
IA	Quinidine Procainamide Disopyramide	Slow conduction velocity Prolong myocardial refractory period Prolong action potential duration	Prophylaxis of atrial fibrillation Premature atrial contractions Premature ventricular contractions Ventricular tachycardia
IB	Lidocaine Tocainide Phenytoin[a] Mexiletine	Enhance conduction Shorten repolarization	Premature ventricular contractions Ventricular tachycardia Digitalis-induced arrhythmias
IC	Flecainide Encainide	Decrease conduction (especially His–Purkinje) Prolong ventricular refractory period	Life-threatening ventricular arrhythmias
II	Propranolol Acebutolol	Slow AV conduction Prolong AV nodal refractory period Decrease automaticity of SA node	Atrial tachycardia or flutter Supraventricular tachycardia Exercise-induced arrhythmias
III	Bretylium Amiodarone	Prolong refractory period Increase action potential duration	Life-threatening ventricular arrhythmias (not responding to other treatment)
IV	Verapamil	Prolong AV nodal refractory period Decrease sinus node automaticity	Supraventricular tachyarrhythmias Control of rapid ventricular rate in atrial fibrillation

[a]Phenytoin is not approved for treatment of arrhythmias but is used for digitalis-induced arrhythmias.

Table 30-2
Pharmacokinetic and Electrophysiologic Properties of Antiarrhythmic Drugs

Drugs	Onset (min)	Duration (h)	Plasma Half-life (h)	Protein Binding (%)	Automaticity SA Node	Automaticity Ectopic Pacemakers	Conduction Velocity AV Node	Conduction Velocity Purkinje Fibers	Refractory Period AV	Refractory Period Purkinje	Refractory Period Ventricle	Heart rate
Quinidine	30	6–10	6–7	70–90	↑↓	↓	↑↓	↓	↑	↑	↑	↑↓
Procainamide	30	3–5	3–5	15–25	↑↓	↓	↑↓	↓	↑	↑	↑	↑↓
Disopyramide	30	5–7	4–8	30–60	↑↓	↓	↑	↓	↑	↑	↑	↑↓
Lidocaine	1–3[a]	0.2	1–2	40–80	0	↓	↑	↑	↑↓	↑↓	↑↓	0
Phenytoin	30–60	24	24–36	90–95	↑↓	↓	↑	↑	↑↓	↑↓	↑↓	↑↓
Tocainide	30–60	4–8	10–15	10–20	↑↓	↓	0	0	↓	↑↓	↓	0
Mexiletine	30–60	4–8	10–12	50–60	↓	↓	0	0	↑↓	↑	↑	—
Flecainide	30–60	8–12	12–24	40–50	↓	↓	↓	↓	0	↑	↑	0
Encainide	30–60	8–12	1–2	75–85	↑↓	↓	↓	↓	↑	↑	↑	0
Propranolol	30	3–6	2–4	90–95	↓	↓	↓	↓	↑	↑	↑	↓
Acebutolol	30	12–16	3–4	25–30	↓	↓	↓	↓	↑	0	0	↑
Bretylium	1–3[a]	6–8	6–10	10	↑	↑	0	↑	↑↓	↑	↑	0
Amiodarone	b	b	1–4 days	95	↓	↓	↓	↓	↑	↑	↑	—
Verapamil	30	6–8	4–8	90	↓	↓	↓	0	↑	0	0	↓

↑, increase; ↓, decrease; 0, no significant effect; ↑↓, variable effect.
[a]Onset reflects time after IV administration.
[b]Onset may take several weeks and effects persist from weeks to months, even after drug is discontinued.

FATE
Completely absorbed orally; maximum effects occur in 1 to 3 hours, and action persists for at least 6 to 8 hours (8 h–12 h with sustained-release forms); widely distributed in the body and significantly bound (70%–90%) to plasma proteins; metabolized in the liver and excreted through the kidneys both as metabolites (80%) and unchanged (20%); elimination half-life is 6 hours.

COMMON SIDE EFFECTS
Nausea, diarrhea, abdominal distress; large doses can result in *cinchonism*, characterized by headache, tinnitus, dizziness, blurred vision and mild tremor

SIGNIFICANT ADVERSE REACTIONS
GI: vomiting, cramping
CNS: fever, vertigo, impaired hearing, altered color perception, photophobia, diplopia, scotomas, excitement, confusion, delirium, syncope
Cardiovascular: ventricular ectopic beats, cardiac asystole, hypotension, severe bradycardia, atrial or ventricular flutter and fibrillation, arterial embolism
Hematologic/dermatologic: acute hemolytic anemia, thrombocytopenic purpura, leukopenia, agranulocytosis (rare), flushing, urticaria, angioedema, pruritus, sweating
Other: arthralgia, dyspnea, respiratory depression, asthmatic episodes
IV use: sweating, nervousness, vomiting, cramping, urge to urinate or defecate

CONTRAINDICATIONS
AV conduction defects or complete AV block, ectopic impulses and rhythms due to escape mechanisms, thrombocytopenic purpura, acute rheumatic fever, myasthenia gravis, cardiac enlargement due to congestive heart failure, renal dysfunction with azotemia. *Cautious use* in the presence of incomplete heart block, digitalis intoxication, congestive heart failure, hypotension, respiratory disorders, potassium imbalance (e.g., diuretic therapy), and impaired renal or hepatic function

INTERACTIONS
Quinidine may increase the effects of oral anticoagulants, antihypertensives, neuromuscular blocking agents, anticholinergics, digitalis, and other antiarrhythmics

Blood levels of quinidine can be elevated by substances that alkalinize the urine (e.g., sodium bicarbonate, antacids, carbonic anhydrase inhibitors), thereby retarding quinidine excretion

Effects of cholinergic drugs (e.g., neostigmine, edrophonium) may be antagonized by quinidine

Additive cardiac depressant effects may occur with use of propranolol or phenothiazines with quinidine

Administration of phenytoin, rifampin, or barbiturates may reduce the serum half-life of quinidine because of enzyme induction

Quinidine may elevate blood levels of digoxin by reducing its tissue binding or by retarding its renal clearance

Cimetidine may enhance the effects of quinidine by slowing its hepatic metabolism

Concurrent use of nifedipine and quinidine may result in lowered plasma levels of quinidine

NURSING CONSIDERATIONS

Nursing Alerts
- In treatment of atrial flutter or fibrillation, ensure that patient has been pretreated with digitalis prior to administering quinidine to retard AV conduction and to reduce the danger of ventricular tachycardia resulting from a progressive reduction in the degree of AV block to a 1:1 ratio.
- Closely monitor patient receiving quinidine (especially parenterally or in large oral doses), and note evidence of developing cardiotoxicity (widening of QRS complex greater than 25%, ventricular extrasystoles, abolition of P waves). Advise physician immediately if signs of toxicity appear, as the drug should be discontinued.
- During parenteral therapy, monitor ECG, pulse rate and rhythm, and blood pressure. Have sodium lactate, vasopressors, and cardiopulmonary resuscitative equipment on hand.
- Keep patient supine during IV administration, and monitor blood pressure for development of severe hypotension. Monitor results of serum quinidine levels, which should be determined frequently to prevent the cardiac toxicity that often occurs at levels greater than 8 mg/liter.

1. If time permits, be prepared to assist with administration of a preliminary test dose (200 mg PO or IM) to determine if hypersensitivity exists.

PATIENT EDUCATION
1. Suggest taking drug with food to minimize GI distress.
2. Inform patient that diarrhea is common early in therapy but should disappear. Advise consulting physician if diarrhea persists because dosage adjustment may be required.
3. Instruct patient to be alert for signs of quinidine overdosage, collectively termed *cinchonism*. If tinnitus, impaired vision, dyspnea, palpitations, nausea, headache, or chest tightness appear, the physician should be informed, and the dosage should be reduced.
4. Instruct patient to report immediately feelings of dizziness or faintness, possible indications of ventricular arrhythmias and depressed cardiac output.
5. Encourage patient on prolonged therapy to obtain the periodic blood counts, serum electrolyte determinations, and liver and kidney function tests that should be performed.
6. Advise patient to use moderation in the consumption of caffeine or alcohol and in smoking, which can alter the irritability of the heart.
7. Instruct patient to avoid consumption of large amounts of citrus fruits because they can alkalinize the urine and reduce excretion of quinidine.

Procainamide
Procan SR, Promine, Pronestyl, Pronestyl-SR, Procamide SR, Rhythmin

MECHANISM
Essentially identical to quinidine in pharmacologic actions; decreases cardiac excitability (screening out weaker ectopic impulses), slows conduction in the atria, ventricles, and bundle of His, and prolongs the refractory period of the atria; little effect

on contractility or cardiac output; may elicit tachycardia because of its anticholinergic (i.e., vagal blocking) action; produces peripheral vasodilation (especially IV) and hypotension; large doses can result in progressive AV block and ventricular extrasystoles

USES

Treatment of premature ventricular contractions (PVCs), ventricular tachycardia, paroxysmal atrial tachycardia, and atrial fibrillation

Treatment of arrhythmias associated with surgery, general anesthesia, or myocardial infarction (IV administration)

DOSAGE

Oral

Ventricular tachycardia: initially, 1-g loading dose, then 50 mg/kg/day in divided doses every 3 hours (every 6 h with sustained-release tablets); *atrial fibrillation and paroxysmal atrial tachycardia:* initially, 1.25 g, followed in 1 hour by 0.75 g; then, 0.5 g to 1 g every 2 hours until arrhythmia is interrupted; maintenance dose 0.5 g to 1 g every 4 hours to 6 hours

IM

Initially, 50 mg/kg/day in divided doses every 3 to 6 hours; switch to oral therapy as soon as possible (for arrhythmias during anesthesia or surgery, 0.1 g–0.5 g IM). *Deep* IM injection is recommended

IV

Injection: 100 mg every 5 minutes by slow IV injection (25 mg–50 mg/min) to a maximum of 500 mg; usual serum level is 4 µg/mL to 8 µg/mL; continuous ECG monitoring must be performed

Infusion (extreme emergencies only): 20 mg to 25 mg/min of a diluted solution over 30 minutes to a maximum of 600 mg with continual ECG monitoring; if necessary, change to a second infusion (2 mg–6 mg/min) for maintenance

Therapeutic plasma levels are 3 µg/mL to 10 µg/mL

FATE

Well absorbed orally, except in patients with severely compromised cardiovascular function; onset is 30 minutes with oral use and duration is 3 to 4 hours (up to 6 h with sustained-release preparations); onset following IM or IV administration is immediate; maximum plasma levels in 15 to 30 minutes; minimal protein binding (15%–25%); slowly hydrolyzed by liver esterases, approximately one fourth converted to *n*-acetylprocainamide, an active metabolite with a 6-hour half-life; primarily (60%–70%) excreted by the kidneys, at least half as the unchanged drug; half-lives of procainamide and metabolites are prolonged in patients with congestive heart failure

COMMON SIDE EFFECTS

Anorexia, nausea (orally); hypotension (IV)

SIGNIFICANT ADVERSE REACTIONS

Orally: vomiting, diarrhea, urticaria, angioedema, maculopapular rash, weakness, depression, psychotic behavior, agranulocytosis, systemic lupus–like reaction (fever, rashes, muscle and joint pain, pericarditis, skin lesions seen with prolonged use) pleural effusion, hepatomegaly, hemolytic anemia, thrombocytopenia

IV: flushing, ventricular asystole, ventricular fibrillation

CONTRAINDICTIONS

Myasthenia gravis, second-or-third-degree AV block, and hypersensitivity to local anesthetics (drug is a derivative of procaine). *Cautious use* in patients with liver or kidney disease because accumulation can occur; advise patient to report possible signs of renal dysfunction (e.g., dysuria, oliguria)

INTERACTIONS

Procainamide may potentiate the muscle-relaxing action of neuromuscular blocking agents and those antibiotics (especially aminoglycosides) having a skeletal muscle–relaxant effect

Additive effects on the heart may occur with combinations of procainamide and other antiarrhythmic or digitalis-like drugs

Procainamide may increase the hypotensive effects of antihypertensives and diuretics

Effects of procainamide can be potentiated by agents that alkalinize the urine and reduce urinary excretion, such as acetazolamide, sodium lactate, and sodium bicarbonate

The action of cholinesterase inhibitors in treating myasthenia gravis can be antagonized by procainamide

Cimetidine can reduce the renal clearance of procainamide and its metabolite

NURSING CONSIDERATIONS

Nursing Alerts

- During IV infusion, keep patient supine, and monitor ECG and blood pressure continually. If blood pressure falls more than 15 mm Hg or if ventricular rate slows significantly without development of regular AV conduction, infusion should be discontinued. Have pressor agent (e.g., levarterenol or dopamine) available to combat extreme hypotension.
- Be prepared to stop infusion when arrhythmia is terminated or if excessive widening of QRS complex or prolongation of PR interval occurs. Arrhythmias are usually abolished within minutes following IV infusion.
- In treatment of atrial arrhythmias, be alert for sudden development of ventricular tachycardia when rapid atrial rate is slowed during drug infusion, allowing 1:1 AV conduction. Prior digitalization reduces this danger.
- In patient receiving large oral doses over prolonged periods, observe carefully for signs of possible lupus-like reaction (e.g., fever, arthralgia, skin lesions, pericarditis, chest pain, coughing, pleural effusion). Review results of antinuclear antibody titers, which should be measured periodically. The drug should be discontinued if clinical signs of lupus appear or if titer rises (quinidine may be substituted). Steroid therapy should be initiated if symptoms persist or worsen.
- Watch for indications of developing agranulocytosis (fever, sore throat, mucosal ulceration, respiratory tract infection), and check results of leukocyte counts. Medication should be discontinued if values are abnormal.

1. Monitor results of ECG determinations and blood counts, which should be performed periodically in patients on prolonged therapy.
2. For patient simultaneously taking oral anticoagulant, expect dosage of oral anticoagulant to remain unchanged. Procainamide does not appear to increase effects of oral anticoagulants as does quinidine.

PATIENT EDUCATION

1. Suggest taking drug with meals or milk to reduce GI upset.
2. Inform patient that drug may cause lightheadedness and dizziness owing to hypotensive effect. Advise caution in driving a car or operating machinery.
3. Advise patient to avoid using other medications, including OTC preparations, that can alter cardiac stability (e.g., sympathomimetics, anticholinergics) during long-term therapy with procainamide.

Disopyramide

Napamide, Norpace, Norpace CR
(CAN) Rythmodan

MECHANISM

Decreases the rate of diastolic depolarization (phase 4) in myocardial cells, and decreases upstroke velocity of the action potential (phase 0); prolongs action potential duration and effective refractory period of the atria and ventricles, thereby decreasing automaticity and conduction velocity; minimal effect on AV conduction or AV nodal refractory period; possesses some anticholinergic activity and exerts a negative inotropic effect (decreased force of contraction), especially in persons with reduced left ventricular function

USES

Suppression and prevention of recurrence of the following arrhythmias:
  Unifocal premature (ectopic) ventricular contractions
  Premature (ectopic) ventricular contractions of multifocal origin
  Paired premature ventricular contractions
  Episodes of ventricular tachycardia

DOSAGE

Note: Patients with atrial flutter or fibrillation should be digitalized prior to administering disopyramide to ensure that the drug-induced increase in AV conduction does not result in unacceptably rapid ventricular rates

Initially, 200 mg to 300 mg loading dose, followed by 150 mg every 6 hours; controlled-release capsules (Norpace CR) may be given every 8 hours; usual dose is 400 mg to 800 mg/day

In patients weighing less than 50 kg, or in those with hepatic or mild renal insufficiency: 200 mg loading dose followed by 100 mg every 6 hours

In patients with cardiomyopathy or cardiac decompensation: 100 mg every 6 hours with *no* loading dose

Pediatric dosage (divided doses every 6 h):
1 to 4 yr: 10 mg/kg to 20 mg/kg/day
4 to 12 yr: 10 mg/kg to 15 mg/kg/day
12 to 18 yr: 6 mg/kg to 15 mg/kg/day

FATE

Rapidly and almost completely absorbed; onset within 30 minutes; peak serum levels occur within 2 to 3 hours; duration approximately 4 to 6 hours; plasma half-life 4 to 10 hours; approximately 25% to 30% protein-bound; excreted mainly in the urine, one half as unchanged drug; remainder is excreted as metabolites, either through the kidney or in the feces; renal excretion is independent of urinary pH

COMMON SIDE EFFECTS

Dry mouth, urinary hesitancy, nausea, bloating, GI pain, constipation, blurred vision, fatigue, headache, malaise

SIGNIFICANT ADVERSE REACTIONS

Cardiovascular: Hypotension, congestive heart failure, (due to decreased force of contraction), edema, cardiac conduction disturbances, QRS widening, AV block, chest pain, dyspnea
CNS: Dizziness, nervousness, insomnia, depression
Dermatologic/hematologic: Rash, pruritus, dermatoses, decreased hemoglobin, thrombocytopenia, agranulocytosis (rare)
Other: Urinary retention; anorexia; diarrhea; vomiting; elevated liver enzymes; impotence; elevated creatinine; reversible cholestatic jaundice; elevated cholesterol, triglycerides, and blood urea nitrogen; hypokalemia; hypoglycemia; anaphylactoid reaction

CONTRAINDICATIONS

Cardiogenic shock, second- or third-degree AV block, uncompensated congestive heart failure or hypotension, and in nursing mothers. *Cautious use* in patients with glaucoma, urinary retention, prostatic hypertrophy, sick sinus syndrome, Wolff–Parkinson–White syndrome, bundle branch block, renal impairment, hepatic dysfunction, and in children and pregnant women

INTERACTIONS

Effects of disopyramide may be enhanced by concurrent use of other antiarrhythmic drugs, beta-adrenergic blockers and calcium channel blockers

Plasma levels can be increased by the presence of other protein-bound drugs (e.g., sulfonamides, antiinflammatory agents, oral anticoagulants, oral hypoglycemics)

Therapeutic effects may be reduced by the presence of hypokalemia (e.g., diuretic therapy)

Effects of cholinesterase inhibitors in relieving myasthenia gravis may be impaired by disopyramide

Plasma levels of disopyramide may be lowered by the presence of enzyme inducers, such as phenytoin, barbiturates, glutethimide, or primidone

NURSING CONSIDERATIONS

Nursing Alerts

- Monitor blood pressure and cardiac function closely. Be alert for signs of developing toxicity, such as excessive widening of QRS complex, hypotension, conduction disturbances, bradycardia, and worsening of congestive heart failure. Progressive congestive failure should be treated with cardiac glycosides and diuretics.
- Expect dosage to be reduced if first-degree heart block occurs. If block persists, benefits of continuing therapy should be weighed against risk of causing higher degrees of heart block.

1. Monitor intake and output because urinary retention can occur.

PATIENT EDUCATION

1. Warn patient not to drive a car until effects of drug are known because lightheadedness and dizziness can occur.

2. Advise patient to avoid using all drugs, including OTC preparations, that have sympathomimetic effects (e.g., cough or cold preparations, nasal decongestants) because they may alter cardiac stability.
3. Suggest interventions to relieve the mouth dryness that often occurs. See **Plan of Nursing Care 4 (Antihistamines)** for specific information.

GROUP IB DRUGS

Lidocaine

Lidopen, Xylocaine
(CAN) Xylocard

MECHANISM
Increases the electrical stimulation threshold of the ventricle during diastole; suppresses automaticity of ectopic pacemaker, shortens the refractory period, and decreases the duration of the action potential in Purkinje fibers, thereby slowing spontaneously firing ectopic ventricular rhythms; little effect on atrial muscle, AV conduction, systolic arterial pressure, myocardial contractility, and cardiac output, also has a local anesthetic action (see Chap. 16)

USES
Management of acute ventricular arrhythmias such as those resulting from myocardial infarction, cardiac surgery or catheterization, and digitalis intoxication

Emergency control of arrhythmias where IV administration is impractical, such as in a mobile emergency unit (IM administration)

DOSAGE
(Loading dose is given initially, followed by a maintenance infusion to maintain a therapeutic plasma level of 2 µg/mL–5/µg/mL)

IV injection: 1 mg/kg at a rate of 25 mg to 50 mg/min; may repeat at one-third to one-half initial dose in 5 minutes if necessary; maximum is 300 mg/h

IV infusion: 20 µg/kg to 50 µg/kg/min (1 mg–4 mg/min) of a 0.1% to 0.2% solution (1 g–2 g lidocaine in 1 liter 5% dextrose in water)

IM: 300 mg in an average 70-kg individual (approximately 4.3 mg/kg); may repeat in 60 to 90 minutes; use only 10% solution, or LidoPen Auto-Injector (300 mg/3 mL)

FATE
Onset with IV injection is immediate and duration is 10 minutes to 20 minutes; following IM injection, onset is 5 to 15 minutes and duration is approximately 60 to 120 minutes. Plasma half-life is 1 to 2 hours; although the initial distribution half-life from the plasma is 5 to 10 minutes; widely distributed in the body and significantly bound to plasma proteins (40%–80%); largely (90%) metabolized in the liver and excreted in the urine

COMMON SIDE EFFECTS
Drowsiness; lightheadedness; slurred speech; sensations of heat, cold, or numbness; paresthesias; mild tremor

SIGNIFICANT ADVERSE REACTIONS
CNS: dizziness, impaired hearing or vision, anxiety, apprehension, euphoria, vomiting, muscle twitching, tremors, convulsions, respiratory depression

Cardiovascular: hypotension, bradycardia, cardiovascular collapse, cardiac arrest (overdosage)

Dermatologic: urticaria, peripheral edema, cutaneous lesions

Other: pain at IM injection site, excessive perspiration, local thrombophlebitis (IV infusion); *rarely,* malignant hyperthermia

CONTRAINDICATIONS
Adams-Stokes syndrome; Wolff-Parkinson-White syndrome; severe SA, AV, or intraventricular block; hypersensitivity to local anesthetics. *Cautious use* in the presence of liver or kidney disease, congestive heart failure, severe respiratory depression, hypovolemia, shock, or myasthenia gravis

Note: In patients with sinus bradycardia or incomplete heart block, acceleration of the heartbeat with isoproterenol or electric pacing should be accomplished prior to administering lidocaine to avoid precipitation of more frequent or serious ventricular arrhythmias or complete heart block.

INTERACTIONS
Cardiac depression may increase if lidocaine is used along with other antiarrhythmic drugs, especially phenytoin or propranolol

Concurrent administration of procainamide may result in additive neurologic effects

Muscle-relaxant effects of neuromuscular blocking agents (e.g., succinylcholine, aminoglycosides) may be increased by lidocaine

Lidocaine inhibits the antibacterial action of sulfonamides

Barbiturates may decrease the action of lidocaine through enzyme induction

Serum levels of lidocaine can be elevated by concurrent use of cimetidine or beta blockers

NURSING CONSIDERATIONS

Nursing Alerts
- Have resuscitative equipment (e.g., respiratory aids) and drugs (e.g., IV fluids, vasopressors, muscle relaxants) on hand to treat adverse reactions involving the CNS or the cardiovascular or respiratory systems.
- Use a microdrip infusion set and an infusion control pump to ensure close regulation of IV flow rate. Adequate plasma levels must be maintained because lidocaine has a short duration of action.
- Monitor cardiac function and blood pressure closely. Infusion should be discontinued if signs of cardiac depression (e.g., prolonged PR interval, widened QRS complex) or increased arrhythmias develop.
- Observe patient carefully for indications of CNS toxicity (e.g., confusion, paresthesias, excitement, tremors), particularly during IV infusion. CNS effects are especially problematic in patient with congestive heart failure. Be prepared to terminate IV infusion as soon as cardiac rhythm is stable (or signs of toxicity develop). Patient should be changed to oral antiarrhythmic for maintenance as soon as possible, usually within 24 hours.
- Do *not* add lidocaine to transfusion assemblies.

1. For treatment of arrhythmias, do not use lidocaine solutions containing either preservatives or epinephrine.
2. Give IM injections into deltoid muscle because therapeutic blood levels occur sooner, and peak blood level is higher than with other IM injection sites.
3. If IM route is used often, interpret serum creatine phosphokinase (CPK) levels cautiously because levels may be increased. This can interfere with diagnosis of myocardial infarction.

Tocainide

Tonocard

MECHANISM
Similar to that of lidocaine but effective orally; decreases myocardial cell excitability, reduces automaticity, and decreases the effective refractory period of the Purkinje fibers and ventricular muscle cells; sinus node function is largely unaltered and conduction times are not changed appreciably. No significant changes in heart rate, blood pressure, or myocardial contractility, although a slight degree of depression of left ventricular function is noted, usually without appreciable change in the cardiac output in well-compensated patients; a slight increase in vascular resistance and pulmonary arterial pressure may occur

USES
Treatment of symptomatic ventricular arrhythmias such as premature ventricular contractions, ventricular tachycardia, and unifocal or multifocal couplets

DOSAGE
Initially, 400 mg orally every 8 hours; usual maintenance range is 1200 mg to 1800 mg/day in divided doses; maximum dose is 2400 mg/day

FATE
Oral absorption is rapid and complete; peak serum levels are attained in 30 minutes to 3 hours; food delays the rate but not the extent of absorption; only 10% to 20% of a dose is protein-bound; drug is inactivated in the liver and is excreted in the urine as metabolites as well as unchanged drug (30%–50%); elimination half-life is approximately 12 to 15 hours and is increased in the presence of severe renal dysfunction; pharmacokinetics of the drug are not appreciably altered in patients with a myocardial infarction

COMMON SIDE EFFECTS
Lightheadedness, dizziness, nausea, paresthesias, numbness, mild tremor, giddiness

SIGNIFICANT ADVERSE REACTIONS
CNS: nervousness, visual disturbances, tinnitus, headache, drowsiness, nystagmus, ataxia, anxiety, incoordination, confusion, disorientation, altered mood, hallucinations
Cardiovascular: bradycardia, hypotension, palpitations, chest pain, ventricular arrhythmias, congestive heart failure, AV or bundle branch block, cardiomegaly
GI: Anorexia, loose stools, diarrhea, vomiting, abdominal pain, dysphagia
Other: Sweating, rash, skin lesions, arthralgia; rarely, blood dyscrasias, lupus-like syndrome, pulmonary fibrosis and edema, pneumonia

CONTRAINDICATIONS
Second- and third-degree heart block, hypersensitivity to amide-type local anesthetics. *Cautious use* in persons with heart failure, reduced cardiac reserve, conduction disturbances, atrial arrhythmias (ventricular rate may increase), pulmonary dysfunction, hypokalemia, severe liver or kidney disease, and in pregnant or nursing women

INTERACTIONS
Concurrent use of tocainide with other drugs having a negative inotropic action (e.g., beta blockers, verapamil, disopyramide) may further depress left ventricular function

NURSING CONSIDERATIONS

Nursing Alerts
- Carefully review patient's past medication history for evidence of allergy to amide-type local anesthetics, a contraindication to tocainide use.
- Assess patient carefully for indications of CNS toxicity (e.g., drowsiness, dizziness, lightheadedness, confusion, headache, visual disturbances, tinnitus, mood alterations, hallucinations). Neurologic side effects are usually early warning signs of toxicity.
- Monitor ECG results for manifestations of prodysrhythmic effect (incidence estimated at approximately 1%–2% for tocainide).

1. Assess patient for evidence of GI symptoms (e.g., nausea, vomiting, anorexia, diarrhea). The patient who develops GI or CNS side effects on divided doses every 12 hours may tolerate therapy better if drug is given every 8 hours instead and is taken with a meal.

PATIENT EDUCATION
1. Recommend that bedtime doses be taken with snacks.
2. Inform patient that most side effects are transient. If symptoms persist, however, the physician should be notified.
3. Instruct patient to report any unusual bleeding (e.g., petechiae, bruising, hematuria) because thrombocytopenia has occurred in rare instances.
4. Instruct patient to report signs of infection (e.g., sore throat, fever, chills) because leukopenia and agranulocytosis have occurred, although infrequently.
5. Advise patient to report respiratory problems (e.g., exertional dyspnea, cough, wheezing) because pulmonary reactions such as fibrosis, pneumonitis, pneumonia, and edema have occurred on rare occasions.

Phenytoin

Dilantin, Diphenylan
(Although this is not an approved indication, phenytoin has been employed in treating certain arrhythmias, particularly those resulting from digitalis toxicity.)

MECHANISM
Depresses ectopic pacemaker activity and shortens action potential duration in isolated Purkinje tissue; improves AV and intraventricular conduction in the digitalis-depressed heart; increases membrane responsiveness in Purkinje fibers; slightly impairs force of contraction and has little effect on arterial pressure; exerts an anticonvulsant activity (see Chap. 25), and is widely used in grand mal seizures

USES

Treatment of paroxysmal atrial tachycardia, particularly if associated with digitalis intoxication

Treatment of ventricular ectopic rhythms, especially those resulting from digitalis overdosage

DOSAGE

IV injection: 100 mg every 5 to 10 minutes until arrhythmia is abolished or toxicity appears (maximum dose is 1000 mg/24 h)

Oral: Initially 1000 mg first day in divided doses, then 500 mg to 600 mg on second and third days; maintenance is 100 mg 2 to 4 times/day; usual serum level is 10 µg/mL to 20 µg/mL

FATE

(*See also* Chap. 25)

Onset of action orally is 30 to 60 minutes; plasma half-life is 24 to 36 hours; highly protein-bound (85%–95%); metabolized by the liver and excreted largely by the kidneys as conjugated metabolites

COMMON SIDE EFFECTS

Nystagmus, diplopia, nausea, GI upset (see also Chap. 25)

SIGNIFICANT ADVERSE REACTIONS

(*See also* Chap. 25)

Cardiovascular: bradycardia, hypotension, cardiac arrest
CNS: confusion, nervousness, ataxia, drowsiness, tremors, visual disturbances

CONTRAINDICATIONS

(*See also* Chap. 25)

Severe bradycardia, second-degree or complete heart block

INTERACTIONS

See Chapter 25

NURSING CONSIDERATIONS

See Chapter 25. In addition:

Nursing Alert

- During IV administration, have atropine available to reverse bradycardia or heart block. Inform patient that infusion may be quite painful, and check infusion site frequently for signs of phlebitis. Infusion may be accomplished with a dilute solution (1 g/L of dextrose in water) given over 2 to 4 hours.

1. Expect to administer large initial doses in some cases. It takes 6 to 12 days to attain steady-state plasma levels with oral administration because of long half-life. This time can be shortened by administration of loading doses.
2. Refer to Chapter 25 for discussion of potential adverse effects when drug is given orally for prolonged periods. Because of these, therapy should be limited to the shortest feasible period of time. However, because most arrhythmias respond to phenytoin at plasma concentrations below toxic levels, cautious therapy should eliminate most short-term adverse effects.

PATIENT EDUCATION

See Chapter 25.

Mexiletine

Mexitil

MECHANISM

Similar to lidocaine and tocainide in its actions; reduces the rate of rise of phase 0 of the action potential, decreases the effective refractory period in Purkinje fibers, and shortens the action potential duration; mexiletine has minimal effects on impulse generation or propagation, cardiac output, force of contraction, pulse rate, blood pressure, and peripheral vascular resistance

USES

Management of symptomatic ventricular arrhythmias (e.g., premature ventricular contractions, ventricular tachycardia)

DOSAGE

Initially, 200 mg orally every 8 hours (up to 400 mg initially may be given for rapid control of ventricular arrhythmias); adjust dosage in 50-mg increments to optimal response

FATE

Oral absorption is good; peak serum levels occur in 2 hours to 3 hours; the effective plasma range of 0.5 µg/mL to 2 µg/mL can be maintained with 2- to 3-times-daily dosing; 50% to 60% protein-bound, drug is metabolized in the liver and metabolites are excreted in the urine together with approximately 10% unchanged drug; elimination half-life is 10 to 12 hours with normal liver function but may be prolonged up to 25 to 30 hours in patients with liver impairment

COMMON SIDE EFFECTS

GI distress, lightheadedness, dizziness, impaired coordination, palpitations, nervousness, headache, mild tremor

SIGNIFICANT ADVERSE REACTIONS

GI: diarrhea, loss of appetite, abdominal pain, dysphagia, GI bleeding, peptic ulcer, altered taste, oral mucosal ulceration
CNS: confusion, short-term memory loss, depression, hallucinations, convulsions, psychotic behavior
Cardiovascular: angina-like pain, premature ventricular contractions, bradycardia, hypotension, syncope, edema, conduction disturbances, atrial arrhythmias
Other: rash, arthralgia, fever, urinary hesitancy, hiccups, dyspnea, sweating, hair loss, decreased libido, impotence, systemic lupus–like syndrome, blood dyscrasias, abnormal liver function tests, positive ANA titer

Note: Mexiletine can worsen arrhythmias, especially in more seriously ill patients

CONTRAINDICATIONS

Cardiogenic shock, second- and third-degree heart block. *Cautious use* in patients with sinus node dysfunction, conduction abnormalities, hypotension, congestive heart failure, liver or kidney disease, or history of convulsive disorders and in pregnant or nursing women

INTERACTIONS

Phenytoin, phenobarbital, rifampin, and other hepatic enzyme inducers may lower mexiletine plasma levels

Cimetidine can reduce mexiletine clearance and increase its plasma levels

Drugs that alkalinize the urine may slow mexiletine excretion, whereas acidifying agents can enhance its rate of excretion

NURSING CONSIDERATIONS

See tocainide. In addition:
1. Monitor results of liver function studies, which should be performed periodically to detect hepatotoxicity.

PATIENT EDUCATION

1. Recommend that drug be taken with food or antacid to slow absorption time, which may help to reduce side effects. CNS and GI side effects may be quite disabling, can occur with normal doses, and may necessitate dosage reduction.
2. Warn patient to limit driving or operation of hazardous equipment until response to drug is known because dizziness and drowsiness may occur.
3. Teach patient interventions to help minimize orthostatic hypotension (see **Plan of Nursing Care 8, Chap. 31**) related to drug's hypotensive effects.

GROUP IC DRUGS

Flecainide
Tambocor

MECHANISM
Possesses membrane-stabilizing activity and has local anesthetic-like properties; decreases conduction in all parts of the heart, with the greatest effect noted in the His–Purkinje system; ventricular refractory period is prolonged; suppresses single and multiple premature ventricular contractions and can decrease the recurrence of ventricular tachycardia; alterations in heart rate and blood pressure are minimal; drug can cause new arrhythmias or worsen existing ones, and its use is associated with a wide range of untoward reactions.

USES
Treatment of documented life-threatening ventricular arrhythmias (e.g., sustained ventricular tachycardia)—*only approved indication:* see *Warning* below

DOSAGE
Initially, 100 mg every 12 hours; increase in 50-mg increments twice a day every 4 days *only;* most patients are controlled at 300 mg/day; maximum dose 400 mg/day.

FATE
Oral absorption is complete and peak plasma levels are attained in about 3 hours; steady-state plasma levels occur within 3 to 5 days, and the plasma half-life ranges from 12 to 24 hours; cumulation rarely occurs during prolonged therapy; plasma protein binding is approximately 40%; about one third of an oral dose is eliminated unchanged in the urine; the remainder is metabolized in the liver and conjugated metabolites are excreted in the urine; renal impairment lengthens the drug's half-life

COMMON SIDE EFFECTS
Lightheadedness, faintness, visual disturbances, headache, nausea, dizziness, palpitations, dyspnea, constipation

SIGNIFICANT ADVERSE REACTIONS

> **WARNING**
>
> Flecainide can initiate or worsen arrhythmias. The likelihood of this effect is related to the dose and the degree of underlying cardiac disease. Therapy with flecainide should be initiated in the hospital and patients monitored closely since fatalities have occurred. The drug also exhibits a negative inotropic effect and may cause or worsen congestive heart failure, particularly in patients with cardiomyopathy, preexisting heart failure, or low ejection fractions

Cardiovascular: sinus bradycardia, sinus arrest, second-degree or third-degree heart block, anginal-like symptoms, hypotension
CNS: flushing, sweating, tinnitus, paresthesias, ataxia, somnolence, anxiety, depression, weakness, speech disorders, stupor, amnesia, euphoria, convulsions, morbid dreams
GI: diarrhea, vomiting, anorexia, dyspepsia, dry mouth, altered taste
Ocular: blurred vision, diplopia, photophobia, eye pain, nystagmus
Other: decreased libido, impotence, polyuria, skin rash, urticaria, pruritus, exfoliative dermatitis, fever, swollen lips or tongue, bronchospasm, arthralgia, myalgia, leukopenia, thrombocytopenia

Large doses may significantly lengthen the PR interval; increase the QRS duration, QT interval, and amplitude of the T wave; and reduce heart rate and contractile force. Conduction disturbances, hypotension, respiratory failure, and asystole have resulted from overdosage

CONTRAINDICATIONS
Second- or third-degree heart block, bundle branch block, cardiogenic shock. *Cautious use* in persons with congestive heart failure, myocardial dysfunction, sick sinus syndrome, renal impairment, electrolyte imbalances, liver disease, or implanted pacemakers, and in pregnant or nursing women

INTERACTIONS
Concurrent use of flecainide with propranolol (and probably other beta blockers), verapamil, or disopyramide can cause additive negative inotropic effects
Acidification of the urine can increase the renal elimination of flecainide, whereas alkalinization reduces the rate of excretion
Plasma levels of flecainide and propranolol may both be increased when the two drugs are given together

NURSING CONSIDERATIONS

Nursing Alerts
- Carefully review patient's medication history for evidence of allergy to amide-type local anesthetics, a contraindication to drug use.
- Ensure that baseline assessment of ECG and cardiovascular function is obtained before therapy is initiated because many cardiovascular side effects can occur.
- Assess patient for signs of developing congestive heart failure. Most side effects develop within 1 to 2 weeks after initiation of therapy.

- Monitor ECG results for manifestations of prodysrhythmic effects (incidence is approximately 7% for flecainide, 10% for encainide—see below).
- Monitor results of serum drug level determinations, which should be obtained periodically. Drug should be administered every 12 hours because effectiveness is enhanced by maintenance of consistent blood levels.
- Assess patient for indications of CNS toxicity (e.g., drowsiness, dizziness, lightheadedness, confusion, headache, visual disturbances, tinnitus, mood alterations, hallucinations). Neurologic side effects are usually the early warning signs of toxicity.

1. Assess patient for evidence of GI symptoms (e.g., nausea, vomiting, anorexia, diarrhea).

PATIENT EDUCATION
1. Instruct patient to report immediately any rapid weight gain, swelling of hands or feet, or difficulty in breathing, possible signs of congestive heart failure.
2. Instruct patient to report any unusual bleeding (e.g., petechiae, bruising, hematuria) because thrombocytopenia has occurred in rare instances.

Encainide
Enkaid

MECHANISM
Similar to flecainide; blocks sodium channel of Purkinje fibers and myocardium and slows phase 0 depolarization; increases the ratio of the effective refractory period to action potential duration; decreases intracardiac conduction in all parts of the heart; blood pressure is unchanged

USES
Treatment of documented life-threatening arrhythmias, such as sustained ventricular arrhythmia—*only approved indication:* see *Warning* below

DOSAGE
Initially, 25 mg orally every 8 hours; increase to 35 mg every 8 hours after 3 to 5 days, and, if necessary, to 50 mg every 8 hours; maximum dose for life-threatening arrhythmias is 75 mg 4 times daily

FATE
Oral absorption is complete; peak plasma levels occur within 30 to 90 minutes; plasma protein binding is 75% to 85%; steady-state plasma levels are attained within 3 to 5 days; drug has two active metabolites which are eliminated more slowly than the parent compound (4–8 h versus 1–2 h); major route of elimination is via the kidneys

COMMON SIDE EFFECTS
Dizziness, blurred vision, headache

SIGNIFICANT ADVERSE REACTIONS
WARNING
Encainide can initiate or worsen an existing ventricular arrhythmia in approximately 10% of patients and some fatalities have occurred; these proarrhythmic events occur most often during the first week of therapy and are more common when doses exceed 200 mg/day

Cardiovascular: palpitations, tachycardia, syncope, peripheral edema, prolonged QRS interval, congestive heart failure
CNS: nervousness, somnolence, tremor, anorexia, insomnia
GI: abdominal pain, constipation, nausea, vomiting, dry mouth
Other: dyspnea, cough, skin rash, tinnitus, altered taste, paresthesia, lower-extremity pain, chest pain

CONTRAINDICATIONS
Preexisting second- or third-degree heart block, right bundle branch block (unless a pacemaker is present), cardiogenic shock. *Cautious use* in patients with congestive heart failure, electrolyte disturbances, sick sinus syndrome, or renal or hepatic impairment, and in pregnant or nursing women

INTERACTIONS
Concurrent use of cimetidine may increase the plasma levels of encainide

NURSING CONSIDERATIONS
See flecainide.

GROUP II DRUGS

Propranolol
Inderal
(CAN) Apo-Propranol, Detensol, Novopranol, PMS Propranolol

Acebutolol
Sectral

Propranolol and acebutolol are beta-adrenergic blocking agents that have been employed in treating a variety of arrhythmias, particularly exercise-induced arrhythmias or those associated with excessive sympathetic stimulation or circulating catecholamine levels. The beta blockers are used for a number of pathologic conditions, and they are reviewed in detail as a group in Chapter 13. The following discussion is limited to their usefulness in treating arrhythmias.

MECHANISM
Competitively antagonize the action of adrenergic agents at beta receptor sites; specifically, on the heart, reduce rate, force of contraction, irritability, AV conduction, and automaticity of the SA node and ectopic pacemakers; large doses exert a direct quinidine-like depressant effect on the myocardium, suppressing overall cardiac functioning

USES
Treatment of the following arrhythmias:
  Exercise-induced ventricular tachycardia
  Supraventricular tachyarrhythmias
  Digitalis-induced arrhythmias
  Tachycardia due to thyrotoxicosis or excessive catecholamine activity
  Persistent premature ventricular extrasystoles

DOSAGE
Propranolol
Oral: 10 mg to 30 mg 3 to 4 times/day
IV (life-threatening arrhythmias *only*): 1 mg to 3 mg at a rate of 1 mg/minute
Acebutolol

Oral: initially, 200 mg twice a day; increase gradually until desired response is achieved; usual range 600 mg to 1200 mg daily

FATE

(Orally—see Chap. 13.) With IV administration, onset is 1 to 2 minutes and duration lasts 3 to 6 hours

NURSING CONSIDERATIONS

See Chapter 13 and **Plan of Nursing Care 3.** In addition:

Nursing Alerts
- Be alert for development of severe bradycardia and hypotension when propranolol is administered IV, especially in patient with digitalis intoxication. Keep patient supine, closely monitor ECG and blood pressure, and have atropine injection available.
- Closely monitor patient on propranolol and digitalis therapy because their effects are additive in depressing AV conduction. Use of propranolol in digitalis overdosage may further depress myocardial contractility and can lead to cardiac failure. Propranolol should be withdrawn if signs of cardiac failure persist.

PATIENT EDUCATION

See Chapter 13 and **Plan of Nursing Care 3.**

GROUP III DRUGS

Bretylium

Bretylol
(CAN) Bretylate

MECHANISM

Complex and incompletely understood; prolongs the effective refractory period of Purkinje fibers and ventricular muscle fibers; increases ventricular fibrillation threshold and action potential duration; initially releases norepinephrine from adrenergic nerve endings, which may result in tachycardia, increased blood pressure, and a transient worsening of arrhythmias; subsequently, release of norepinephrine is reduced in response to nerve stimulation, although stores in the nerve ending are not depleted

USES

Treatment of *life-threatening* ventricular arrhythmias that have not responded to lidocaine or procainamide (use is restricted to intensive- or coronary-care units with appropriate facilities for continuous monitoring of cardiac function)

DOSAGE

Acute ventricular fibrillation IV: 5 mg/kg (undiluted) by rapid injection; may repeat at 10 mg/kg every 15 to 30 minutes to a total dose of 30 mg/kg

Other ventricular arrhythmias IV: 5 mg/kg to 10 mg/kg of a diluted solution by IV infusion over 10 to 30 minutes; repeat at 1- to 2-hour intervals

Dilution—10 mL (500 mg) diluted to a minimum of 50 mL with dextrose or sodium chloride injection

IM (do *not* dilute): 5 mg/kg to 10 mg/kg; may repeat in 1 to 2 hours, then every 6 to 8 hours thereafter (maximum injection volume is 5 mL)

Maintenance Dosage
5 mg/kg to 10 mg/kg of diluted solution infused over 8 to 10 minutes every 6 hours *or* 1 mg/kg to 2 mg/kg of diluted solution by constant infusion

FATE

Adequately absorbed IM; peak plasma concentrations in 60 to 90 minutes; however, maximum antiarrhythmic effects are not seen for 6 to 9 hours; effects of a single dose persist for 6 to 8 hours; onset following IV injection within minutes; excreted largely unchanged by the kidneys, approximately 70% to 80% of a dose within 24 hours

COMMON SIDE EFFECTS

Hypotension, nausea and vomiting (especially with rapid IV injection), lightheadedness

SIGNIFICANT ADVERSE REACTIONS

Vertigo, syncope, bradycardia, transitory hypertension, increased arrhythmias (initially), anginal attacks, substernal pressure and pain

Other (cause–effect relationship has not been definitively established): diarrhea, flushing, hyperthermia, dyspnea, anxiety, abdominal pain, erythematous rash, diaphoresis, confusion, nasal congestion, renal dysfunction

CONTRAINDICATIONS

There are no absolute contraindications to use in treating life-threatening ventricular arrhythmias; use in less serious arrhythmias is contraindicated in severe pulmonary hypertension or in aortic stenosis and in patients with fixed cardiac output. *Cautious use* in pregnant women, in children, and in persons with reduced renal function

INTERACTIONS

May increase digitalis toxicity by releasing norepinephrine
Peripheral vasodilation occurring in patients already receiving procainamide or quinidine may be increased by bretylium

NURSING CONSIDERATIONS

Nursing Alerts
- Keep patient supine until tolerance to hypotensive action of the drug has developed, which often does not occur for several days. Assist with ambulation as needed.
- Monitor cardiac function closely during therapy, and have appropriate equipment and drugs (e.g., dopamine) on hand to treat adverse effects such as hypotension.
- Expect dosage to be reduced in patient with impaired renal function to prevent accumulation toxicity because drug is excreted primarily through the kidneys.

1. Because transient hypertension and arrhythmias can develop during *early* stages of therapy because of initial release of catecholamines, monitor patient closely and inform physician if effects are severe or prolonged.

Amiodarone
Cordarone

MECHANISM
Prolongs myocardial cell action potential duration (APD) and refractory period; possesses both an alpha-adrenergic and a beta-adrenergic blocking action; vascular smooth muscle is relaxed and peripheral vascular resistance is reduced; automaticity of cardiac cells is decreased, but amiodarone can cause marked sinus bradycardia and has resulted in heart block and sinus arrest; electrocardiographic changes include increased PR and QT intervals, appearance of U waves, and altered T wave contour

USES
Treatment of life-threatening recurrent ventricular arrhythmias (ventricular fibrillation, hemodynamically unstable ventricular tachycardia) that do not respond to other antiarrhythmics

DOSAGE
Initially, loading doses of 800 mg to 1600 mg daily in divided doses; when arrhythmia is controlled, reduce dosage to 600 mg to 800 mg daily for 1 month, then to 400 mg daily

FATE
Oral absorption is slow and variable; peak plasma levels occur in 3 to 7 hours, but clinical effects often take days to weeks to become manifest; widely distributed in the body and accumulates in fatty tissue; protein binding is approximately 95%; eliminated largely via the bile following hepatic metabolism; plasma half-life is extremely variable (20–120 days)

COMMON SIDE EFFECTS
Nausea, vomiting, corneal microdeposits, photosensitivity, fatigue, tremor, incoordination, paresthesias

SIGNIFICANT ADVERSE REACTIONS

> **WARNING**
> Amiodarone is a highly toxic drug. Fatalities have occurred as a result of pulmonary toxicity (e.g., interstitial pneumonitis/alveolitis), liver disease, arrhythmias, heart block, and sinus bradycardia. Owing to its slow onset and very prolonged duration of action, even after drug discontinuation, patients must be monitored very closely during therapy and for several months following termination of therapy. Drug treatment should be initiated in a hospital setting and prolonged hospitalization may be required in unstable patients

CNS: insomnia, headache, dizziness, ataxia, anorexia, sleep disturbances, decreased libido, visual disturbances, photophobia
Cardiovascular: bradycardia, congestive heart failure, SA node dysfunction, hypotension, conduction abnormalities, arrhythmias (most often exacerbation of existing arrhythmias)
Dermatologic: Solar dermatitis, blue skin discoloration, rash, alopecia, spontaneous ecchymoses
Other: Abdominal pain, dryness of the eyes, peripheral neuropathy, hepatic disease, hepatitis, abnormal taste and smell, salivation, edema, altered thyroid function, coagulation abnormalities, pulmonary inflammation

CONTRAINDICATIONS
Marked sinus bradycardia, second- or third-degree heart block, syncope due to bradycardia. *Cautious use* in patients with reduced hepatic function, thyroid abnormalities (drug increases levels of T_4 and reduces levels of T_3), electrolyte disturbances, coagulation difficulties, pulmonary disease, and in pregnant or nursing women

Drug should be discontinued if patients develop pulmonary infiltrates or fibrosis, paroxysmal ventricular tachycardia, congestive heart failure, or symptoms of hepatic dysfunction

INTERACTIONS
Amiodarone can increase serum levels of digoxin, quinidine, procainamide, and phenytoin if given concurrently. Dosage reductions of one third to one half may be necessary for these drugs

Beta blockers and calcium channel blockers (especially verapamil) may result in potentiation of bradycardia and increase the risk of AV block or sinus arrest when given together with amiodarone

Amiodarone may increase the hypoprothrombinemic effects of warfarin, leading to serious bleeding

NURSING CONSIDERATIONS

Nursing Alerts
- Monitor patient closely because a wide range of debilitating side effects can occur. The drug is usually used only as a last resort when other drugs have failed. Unfortunately, side effects may not resolve for days to weeks even after cessation of therapy because the drug has a long half-life.
- Assess patient for evidence of developing congestive heart failure (e.g., dyspnea, rales, edema, lip cyanosis, neck vein distention) or pulmonary fibrosis.
- Weight patient daily to monitor early development of congestive heart failure.
- Measure intake and output to monitor possible fluid retention.
- Review results of baseline and periodic determinations of arterial blood gases and hepatic function (hepatotoxicity may also occur).
- Instill artificial tears 4 to 6 times daily to facilitate excretion of small crystals deposited as some of drug is excreted through lacrimal ducts. Because corneal deposits may develop, complete ocular examinations should be performed when therapy is initiated and periodically thereafter during therapy.
- Assess patient's neurologic status periodically because headaches and peripheral neuropathies, especially in hands and feet, can occur.
- Monitor results of thyroid function studies (T_3, T_4), which should be obtained periodically, because either hyperthyroidism or hypothyroidism (more likely) may occur.

1. Administer with food if GI disturbances occur. However, because absorption is slow, food may merely prolong symptoms.
2. Implement interventions to prevent constipation (e.g., increased intake of fluid and dietary fiber). Laxatives should be avoided if possible because they may impair drug absorption.

PATIENT EDUCATION

1. Warn patient that photophobia is likely to occur. Dark glasses may afford sufficient protection, but some patients are unable to go outdoors at all in the daytime.
2. Instruct patient to report development of blurred vision, halos around lights, especially at night, or altered visual acuity.
3. Advise patient to use sunscreens and protective clothing and to limit exposure to direct sunlight because photosensitivity reactions may occur.
4. Inform patient that a reversible blue-gray skin discoloration may occur, particularly in fair-skinned females.
5. Instruct patient to report development of symptoms of hyperthyroidism (e.g., rapid heart rate, increased perspiration, increased appetite with weight loss, and insomnia) or hypothyroidism (e.g., lethargy, puffy hands and feet, periorbital edema, cool skin, vertigo, constipation).

GROUP IV DRUGS

Verapamil

Calan, Isoptin

Verapamil is a calcium channel blocker that together with other calcium channel blockers is used orally for the treatment of angina (see Chap. 32). The drug is also used orally for the control of mild to moderate hypertension (see Chap. 31). In addition, verapamil is indicated for the treatment of supraventricular tachyarrhythmias because it has a much greater effect on SA and AV nodal function than do the other calcium blockers. Its use as an antiarrhythmic is discussed below.

MECHANISM

Inhibits influx of calcium ions through slow channels into cells of the cardiac conductile system; AV conduction is slowed and the effective refractory period of the AV node is prolonged, thus reducing elevated ventricular rate, interrupting AV nodal impulse reentry, and restoring normal sinus rhythm in supraventricular tachycardias; decreases myocardial contractility and reduces aortic impedance to left ventricular ejection (i.e., afterload); may transiently lower systemic arterial pressure, and raise left ventricular filling pressure

USES

Treatment of supraventricular tachyarrhythmias, such as paroxysmal atrial tachycardia

Control of excessive ventricular rate in patients with atrial flutter or atrial fibrillation

Long-term management of angina (see Chap. 32)

Treatment of mild to moderate hypertension (see Chap. 31)

DOSAGE

(Given by slow IV injection)

Adults: initially, 5 mg to 10 mg over 2 to 3 minutes; repeat with 10 mg 30 minutes after first dose if initial response is inadequate

Children: 0 to 1 yr—0.75 mg to 2 mg over 2 minutes; 1 to 15 yr—2 mg to 5 mg over 2 minutes; may repeat initial dose in 30 minutes, if necessary

FATE

Effects are usually noted within 2 to 5 minutes of injection. Duration of action of a single injection is 30 to 45 minutes. Elimination half-life is 3 to 8 hours. Verapamil is rapidly metabolized in the liver, and metabolites are excreted in the urine (70%) and feces (15%–20%). It is highly protein-bound (90%).

COMMON SIDE EFFECTS

Transient hypotension and dizziness, bradycardia

SIGNIFICANT ADVERSE REACTIONS

(Infrequent)

Cardiovascular: tachycardia, marked hypotension, asystole, AV block, congestive heart failure
CNS: headache, depression, vertigo, fatigue, nystagmus
GI: nausea, abdominal discomfort
Other: diaphoresis, muscle weakness

CONTRAINDICATIONS

Severe hypotension, cardiogenic shock, second-or third-degree AV block, severe congestive heart failure, sick sinus syndrome, concurrent administration of IV beta blocker or disopyramide. *Cautious use* in patients with hypertrophic cardiomyopathy and renal or hepatic dysfunction

INTERACTIONS

Verapamil may be potentiated by other strongly protein-bound drugs, such as oral anticoagulants, anti-inflammatory drugs, and sulfonamides

The desired effects of verapamil may be reduced by administration of supplemental calcium

The depressant action of verapamil on the myocardium and AV node can be enhanced by simultaneous use of an IV beta-blocking drug or disopyramide

Excessive bradycardia or AV block can occur if verapamil is given together with a digitalis drug. Prolonged verapamil therapy increases serum digoxin levels

Verapamil can enhance the blood pressure–lowering action of antihypertensive drugs

NURSING CONSIDERATIONS

Nursing Alerts

- Ensure that complete monitoring and proper resuscitative equipment is available when verapamil is first administered because patient may respond with rapid ventricular rate or, conversely, with marked hypotension and extreme bradycardia. Cardioversion, lidocaine, or procainamide are effective in treating rapid ventricular rate. Norepinephrine or metaraminol may be used to treat hypotension, and isoproterenol or atropine is indicated to reverse bradycardia or AV block.
- Administer IV injection over at least 3 minutes in older patient to minimize possibility of adverse reactions. Keep patient recumbent for 1 hour after injection to minimize hypotension. Closely monitor patient receiving verapamil along with digitalis drugs, beta blockers, or other antiarrhythmic drugs because adverse effects can be increased.

1. Monitor urinary output because impaired renal function can prolong duration of action.

2. Be prepared for possible occurrence of complexes resembling premature ventricular contractions during conversion to normal sinus rhythm. These events have no clinical significance.

PATIENT EDUCATION
1. Explain to patient on prolonged therapy that OTC products containing calcium may impair effectiveness of verapamil.

Selected Bibliography

Advances in antiarrhythmic drug therapy—Changing concepts (Proceedings of a symposium). Fed Proc 45(8):2184, 1986

Anderson JL: Criteria for selection of oral drug therapy in chronic ventricular arrhythmia. Mod Med 55:48, 1987

Garfein OB (ed): Clinical pharmacology of cardiac antiarrhythmic agents. Ann NY Acad Sci 432:1, 1984

Greenspon AJ, Vlasses PH, Ferguson RK: Amiodarone: A new drug for the treatment of cardiac arrhythmias. Ration Drug Ther 18(81):1, 1984

Hoffman BF, Rosen MR: Cellular mechanisms of cardiac arrhythmias. Circ Res 49:1, 1981

Kienzle MG et al: Antiarrhythmic drug therapy for sustained ventricular tachycardia. Heart Lung 13(6):614, 1984

Mason JW: Amiodarone. N Engl J Med 316:455, 1987

Morganroth J: New antarrhythmic agents: Mexiletine, tocainide, encainide, flecainide and amiodarone. Ration Drug Ther 21(4):1, 1987

Pratt CM, Delclos G, Wierman AM et al: The changing baseline of complex ventricular arrhythmias: A new consideration in assessing long-term antiarrhythmic drug therapy. N Engl J Med 313:1444, 1985

Roberts WC: Symposium on the management of ventricular dysrhythmias. Am J Cardiol 54:1A, 1984

Rosen MR, Wit AL: Electropharmacology of antiarrhythmic drugs. Am Heart J 106:829, 1983

Rossi L: Nursing care for survivors of sudden cardiac death. Nurs Clin North Am 19(3):411, 1984

Ruskin JN: Arrhythmias: Are you selecting the right drug. Mod Med 54(11):54, 1986

Scherer P: New drugs of 1985 in theory and in practice. Am J Nurs 86:406, 1986

Sjogren ER: Tonocard. Crit Care Nurs 3(6):12, Nov/Dec, 1983

Smith A: Amiodarone: Clinical considerations. Focus Crit Care 11(5):30, 1984

Stone KS, Scordo KA: Understanding the calcium channel blockers. Heart Lung 13(5):563, 1984

Tocainide for arrhythmias. Med Lett Drugs Ther 27:9, 1985

Treatment of cardiac arrhythmias. Med Lett Drugs Ther 25:21, 1983

Wilson H: Drug therapy for cardiac arrhythmias. American Druggist, April 1985:137

Woosley RL, Echt DS, Roden DM: Treatment of ventricular arrhythmias in the failing heart: Pharmacologic and clinical considerations. Ration Drug Ther 19(10):1, 1985

Woosley RL: Mexiletine and tocainide: A profile of two lidocaine analogs. Ration Drug Therap 21(3):1, 1987

SUMMARY. ANTIARRHYTHMIC AGENTS

Drug	Preparations	Usual Dosage Range
Group IA		
Quinidine Cardioquin, Cin-Quin, Duraquin, Quinaglute Dura-Tabs, Quinatime, Quinidex Extentabs, Quinora, Quin-Release	Tablets: 100 mg, 200 mg, 300 mg Sustained-release tablets: 300 mg, 324 mg, 330 mg Capsules: 200 mg, 300 mg Injection: 80 mg, 200 mg/mL	*Oral* Usually: 200 mg–600 mg 4 times/day individualized to patient's response Maximal daily dose: 3 g–4 g Maintenance: 200 mg–300 mg 3–4 times/day or 1–2 sustained-acting tablets 2–3 times/day *IM (gluconate):* Initially: 600 mg; *then* 400 mg every 2 h as needed *IV (gluconate or sulfate):* 200 mg–750 mg by slow IV infusion (800 mg/50 mL 5% glucose at a rate of 1 mL/min or 16 mg/min)
Procainamide Procamide SR, Procan SR, Promine, Pronestyl, Pronestyl SR, Rhythmin	Capsules: 250 mg, 375 mg, 500 mg Tablets: 250 mg, 375 mg, 500 mg Sustained-release tablets: 250 mg, 500 mg, 750 mg, 1000 mg Injection: 100 mg, 500 mg/mL	*Oral* Initially: 1 g; then 50 mg/kg/day in divided doses every 3 h *IM:* 50 mg/kg/day in divided doses every 3–6 h For arrhythmias during surgery or anesthesia: 0.1 g–0.5 g IM *IV infusion* 20 mg–25 mg/min to a maximum of 600 mg
Disopyramide Norpace, Norpace CR, Napamide	Capsules: 100 mg, 150 mg Sustained-release capsules: 100 mg, 150 mg	*Adults:* initially 200 mg–300 mg, then 150 mg every 6 h (every 8 h with sustained-release capsules); usual dosage range 400 mg–800 mg/day *Children:* 6 mg/kg–20 mg/kg/day in divided doses every 6 h depending on age

Continued

SUMMARY. ANTIARRHYTHMIC AGENTS (continued)

Drug	Preparations	Usual Dosage Range
Group IB		
Lidocaine LidoPen, Xylocaine	Injection: 10 mg, 20 mg, 40 mg, 100 mg, 200 mg/mL IV infusion: 2 mg, 4 mg, 8 mg/mL in 5% Dextrose	*IV injection:* 1 mg/kg at a rate of 25 mg–50 mg/min; may repeat in 5 min at one half dose *IV infusion:* 20 μg/kg–50 μg/kg/min (1 mg–4 mg/min) of a 0.1% solution *IM:* 300 mg in a average-size patient (4.3 mg/kg); may repeat in 60–90 min
Tocainide Tonocard	Tablets: 400 mg, 600 mg	Initially, 400 mg every 8 h; usual dosage range 1200 mg–1800 mg daily in divided doses
Phenytoin Dilantin, Diphenylan, Ditan	Chewable tablets: 50 mg Capsules: 30 mg, 100 mg, 250 mg Suspension: 30 mg, 125 mg/5 mL Injection: 50 mg/mL	*IV injection:* 100 mg every 5–10 min until arrhythmia is abolished or toxicity appears *Oral:* initially 1000 mg first day, then 500 mg–600 mg 2nd and 3rd days; maintenance dose 100 mg 2–4 times/day
Mexiletine Mexitil	Capsules: 150 mg, 200 mg, 250 mg	Initially, 200 mg every 8 h; adjust in 50-mg increments to optimal dosage
Group IC		
Flecainide Tambocor	Tablets: 50 mg, 100 mg, 150 mg	Initially, 100 mg every 12 h; increase in 50-mg increments every 4 days; usual dose range 300 mg–400 mg daily
Encainide Enkaid	Capsules: 25 mg, 35 mg, 50 mg	Initially, 25 mg every 8 h; increase gradually as needed; maximum 75 mg 4 times/day
Group II		
Propranolol Inderal	Tablets: 10 mg, 20 mg, 40 mg, 60 mg, 80 mg, 90 mg Sustained-release capsules: 80 mg, 120 mg, 160 mg Injection: 1 mg/mL	*Oral:* 10 mg–30 mg 3–4 times/day *IV:* 1 mg–3 mg at a rate of 1 mg/min
Acebutolol Sectral	Capsules: 200 mg, 400 mg	Initially, 200 mg twice daily; usual dose range 600 mg–1200 mg/day
Group III		
Bretylium Bretylol	Injection: 50 mg/mL	*IV injection:* 5 mg/kg undiluted solution by rapid IV injection; may repeat at 10 mg/kg to a total dose of 30 mg/kg *IV infusion:* 5 mg/kg–10 mg/kg of a diluted solution over at least 8 min–10 min *IM:* 5 mg/kg–10 mg/kg undiluted solution; repeat in 1–2 h, then every 6–8 h thereafter
Amiodarone Cordarone	Tablets: 200 mg	Initially, loading dose of 800 mg–1600 mg daily in divided doses; reduce to 400 mg–800 mg daily as arrhythmias are controlled
Group IV		
Verapamil Calan, Isoptin	Tablets: 40 mg, 80 mg, 120 mg Sustained-release tablets: 240 mg Injection: 2.5 mg/mL	*Adults:* 5 mg–10 mg IV over 2–3 min; repeat with 10 mg 30 min after the first dose *Children:* 0.75 mg–5 mg IV over 2–3 min depending on age; repeat in 30 min if necessary

ANTIHYPERTENSIVE DRUGS

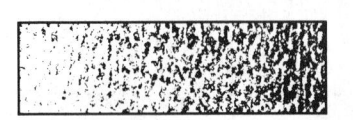

31

Drug therapy of hypertension is directed toward reducing elevated arterial pressure, which is believed to be the primary cause of vascular degeneration and other complications that impair health and reduce life expectancy. The etiology of most cases of hypertension is unknown, thus treatment is essentially palliative—that is, directed at lowering the elevated systolic and diastolic pressures.

Nevertheless, judicious use of one or more of the available antihypertensive agents can provide excellent control of blood pressure for extended periods. The agents can also markedly delay the onset of vascular damage and can significantly prolong the life of the hypertensive patient. Drug therapy, however, is only one aspect of a complete therapeutic regimen that should also include proper diet, exercise, and reduced salt intake.

The wide range of antihypertensive medications in clinical use today allows the physician to carefully tailor drug therapy to the needs of each hypertensive patient. Milder forms of hypertension frequently can be controlled by single-drug therapy, whereas more elevated pressures may require one or more additional antihypertensive agents in the regimen. Combination drug therapy enhances the pharmacologic effects of each drug so that smaller individual doses can be used and the incidence and severity of untoward reactions thereby reduced. Control of all degrees of blood pressure can therefore be attained, in most instances, with minimal untoward effects on the patient. Controversy exists about the necessity for drug treatment of mild or labile hypertension (diastolic pressure 90 mm Hg to 100 mm Hg), especially where other risk factors are absent (e.g., if there is lack of tissue or organ damage, no familial history of hypertension, and the patient is not young, male, or black). Elimination of certain contributory factors (e.g., stress, overweight, smoking, dietary salt) is often sufficient to adequately control the arterial pressure in this labile hypertensive population. On the other hand, there is clear indication for the use of antihypertensive medications in patients who exhibit sustained diastolic pressures above 100 mm Hg, or in high-risk patients (e.g., presence of diabetes or hypercholesterolemia, young black males, genetic predisposition toward hypertension) whose diastolic pressures are consistently above 90 mm Hg.

Clinically effective antihypertensive drugs act at many sites in the body and through numerous mechanisms. They have a wide range of potencies, side effects, and potential interactions. Choice of a suitable antihypertensive drug depends on many factors, such as the degree of hypertension being treated, the presence of other disease states (e.g., reserpine is contraindicated in active hepatic disease), the presence of other drugs (e.g., antidepressants reduce guanethidine's effectiveness), and a patient's acceptance of the mild yet often inescapable side effects of many agents. Although many antihypertensive drugs have more than one site or mechanism of action, they can be conveniently grouped according to their *principal sites* of action, recognizing, however, that these may not be the only active sites for many of the compounds. Such a grouping is presented in Table 31-1.

Another means of classifying the many available antihypertensive drugs is based on a suggested progressive drug regimen that treats all stages of hypertension, from mild to severe. This so-called stepped-care approach is widely followed, and despite some minor disagreements on the placement of certain drugs, is generally regarded as the preferred approach for managing the hypertensive patient. A typical stepped-care classification is presented in Table 31-2. Mild hypertension is usually treated initially with a diuretic or a beta blocker, the latter drugs being of use especially in younger patients with a high pulse pressure (i.e., systolic minus diastolic) and rapid heartbeat, and in patients with arrhythmias, angina, or hyperuricemia. Small doses of angiotensin-converting enzyme (ACE) inhibitors have also been advocated for use in managing mild hypertension.

Adrenergic inhibitors (e.g., clonidine, guanabenz, guanfacine, prazosin, terazosin, methyldopa) are added next (step 2), when maximally tolerated doses of step 1 drugs fail to provide sufficient control; however, a diuretic is often continued in lower doses. Significant differences in mechanisms and side effects among the antiadrenergic drugs, however, mandate that careful drug selection be made to optimize the therapeutic benefit. Several different step 2 drugs should be tried before adding a third drug. Calcium channel blockers (see Chap. 32) are also now being used successfully in the control of mild hypertension and represent alternatives in the management of mild to moderate hypertension.

Direct-acting vasodilators, such as hydralazine, are considered step 3 drugs and may provide additional therapeutic benefit in moderate degrees of hypertension refractive to combinations of step 1 and step 2 drugs. ACE inhibitors in somewhat larger doses than employed for mild hypertension can be useful in controlling more severe forms of hypertension; however, the risk of serious adverse effects is increased at higher doses.

Severe hypertension may not be controlled by combination antihypertensive regimens. In these instances, the extremely potent step 4 drugs, guanethidine or minoxidil, may be substituted for the other drugs or added to the existing regimen. However, these latter agents are associated with severe side effects and many drug interactions, and patients must be carefully monitored.

Hypertensive emergencies are best managed by IV sodium nitroprusside or diazoxide, both vascular smooth muscle relaxants, or by trimethaphan, a ganglionic blocking agent. Pheochromocytoma, a catecholamine-secreting tumor of chromaffin tissue (e.g., adrenal medulla), leads to marked elevations in blood pressure. Metyrosine or possibly phentolamine can be used to reduce the excessively high blood pressure seen in pheochromocytoma.

Several classes of antihypertensive agents have been discussed in previous chapters (e.g., alpha- and beta-adrenergic blocking agents, ganglionic blocking agents); only those aspects relating to their antihypertensive action will be mentioned here. Likewise, diuretics are reviewed in detail in Chapter 37 and are not considered in this chapter. Calcium channel blockers are are also useful antihypertensive agents because of their peripheral vasodilating action; their antihypertensive action is discussed below, while their other uses are considered in Chapters 30 and 32.

Table 31-1
Antihypertensive Drugs: Principal Sites of Action

CNS

Cortex
  reserpine and rauwolfia derivatives
Cardiovascular centers (hypothalamus, medulla)
  clonidine/guanabenz/guanfacine
  methyldopa
  beta-adrenergic blockers

Sympathetic Ganglia

  ganglionic blocking agents

Adrenergic Nerve Endings

  alpha-adrenergic blockers
  beta-adrenergic blockers
  reserpine and rauwolfia derivatives
  guanethidine/guanadrel
  metyrosine
  pargyline

Vascular Smooth Muscle

  hydralazine
  diazoxide
  minoxidil
  nitroprusside
  diuretics
  calcium channel blockers

Kidney and Afferent Arteriole

  diuretics
  beta-adrenergic blockers

Renin-Angiotensin System

  angiotensin–converting enzyme inhibitors

Table 31-2
Stepped-Care Approach to the Treatment of Hypertension

Step 1 (mild hypertension)

diuretics (thiazides, ? high-ceiling diuretics)
beta-blockers
angiotensin–converting enzyme inhibitors (captopril, enalapril, lisinopril)—low doses

Step 2 (mild to moderate hypertension)

beta blockers/labetalol
angiotensin–converting enzyme inhibitors
clonidine/guanabenz/guanfacine
methyldopa
prazosin/terazosin
calcium channel blockers (verapamil)
reserpine (rarely used)

Step 3 (moderate to severe hypertension)

hydralazine
angiotensin–converting enzyme inhibitors (large doses)

Step 4 (severe hypertension)

guanethidine/guanadrel
minoxidil

Hypertensive Emergencies

nitroprusside
diazoxide
trimethaphan
labetalol (IV)

STEP 1 DRUGS

Diuretics
See Chapter 37.

Beta-Adrenergic Blocking Agents

Acebutolol	Penbutolol
Atenolol	Pindolol
Carteolol	Propranolol
Metoprolol	Timolol
Nadolol	

Diuretics are still recognized as initial drugs of choice for mild hypertension *in the majority of patients,* and their overall safety record is quite good, especially when electrolyte levels are controlled. However, serious untoward reactions such as arrhythmias (some fatal), and increases in serum triglycerides, blood viscosity, and platelet aggregation have been associated with use of diuretics, particularly in large doses or in patients with cardiac abnormalities. These have prompted a reevaluation of the relative role of diuretics versus beta blockers as initial therapy in treating mild uncomplicated hypertension, and have also suggested a possible role for the ACE inhibitors as drugs for treating mild hypertension.

Owing to the concerns about diuretics, there is increasing support for the use of beta blockers in the initial pharmacologic treatment of mild hypertension, although it must be recognized that these drugs are capable of causing untoward reactions as well, such as bradycardia, congestive heart failure, and bronchoconstriction. Although the choice of a diuretic versus a beta blocker as a step 1 antihypertensive drug is still largely a matter of physician preference, there are definite cautions that must be observed when making this choice. Diuretics are generally preferred in patients with congestive heart failure, sinus bradycardia, and asthma, whereas beta blockers are a logical choice in patients with cardiac arrhythmias, tachycardia, angina, hyperuricemia, and coagulation disorders.

Beta blockers have numerous clinical indications and are considered in detail in Chapter 13. Most of the available beta blockers are approved for use in treating hypertension, and that particular indication is discussed below.

MECHANISM
Not completely established; these agents can decrease cardiac output, reduce release of renin from the juxtoglomerular cells of the kidney (thus decreasing production of angiotensin and secretion of aldosterone), and impede outflow of sympathetic (i.e., vasoconstrictor and cardioaccelerator) impulses from brainstem vasomotor control centers to peripheral organs; in addition, beta blockers may retard release of norepinephrine from adrenergic nerve endings by blockade of presynaptic beta receptors, thereby reducing the vasoconstrictive action of endogenous norepinephrine

DOSAGE
(for hypertension only)

Acebutolol (Sectral)

Initially, 400 mg in a single or twice-daily dose; usual dosage—range is 400 mg to 800 mg daily to a maximum of 1200 mg/day

Atenolol (Tenormin)

Initially, 50 mg as a single daily dose; increase to 100 mg as a single dose if an optimal response is not achieved within 2 weeks; further dosage increases are unlikely to provide additional benefit; available in combination with chlorthalidone (25 mg) as Tenoretic

Carteolol (Cartrol)

Initially, 2.5 mg as a single daily dose; may increase up to 10 mg once daily if necessary; usual dosage range 2.5 mg to 5 mg once daily

Metoprolol (Lopressor)

(CAN) Apo-Metoprolol, Betaloc, Novometoprol

Initially 100 mg/day in a single dose or 2 divided doses; increase at weekly intervals until optimal blood pressure reduction is attained; usual maintenance range is 100 mg to 450 mg/day; once-daily administration may not provide 24-hour control, especially with lower doses; larger or more frequent doses may be necessary; available in combination with hydrochlorothiazide as Lopressor HCT

Nadolol (Corgard)

Initially, 40 mg once daily; increase gradually in 40-mg to 80-mg increments until optimal effect is noted; usual maintenance range is 80 mg to 320 mg/day in a single dose; also available in fixed combination with bendroflumethiazide (5 mg) as Corzide

Penbutolol (Levatol)

20 mg once daily; may increase to 40 mg once daily if necessary

Pindolol (Visken)

Initially, 10 mg twice a day (or 5 mg 3 times/day); adjust dosage in increments of 10 mg/day at 2- to 3-week intervals; maximum dose is 60 mg/day

Propranolol (Inderal)

(CAN) Apo-Propranolol, Detensol, Noropranol, PMS Propranolol

Initially, 40 mg twice a day or 80 mg (sustained-release) once daily; adjust gradually to optimal effect; usual dosage ranges are 120 mg to 240 mg/day in 2 to 3 divided doses or 120 mg to 160 mg once daily as sustained-release dosage forms; maximum daily dose is 640 mg; available in combination with hydrochlorothiazide as Inderide

Timolol (Blocadren)

Initially, 10 mg twice a day; usual maintenance range is 20 mg to 40 mg/day in 1 or 2 divided doses; maximum dose is 60 mg/day in 2 divided doses; available in combination with hydrochlorothiazide as Timolide

Angiotensin–Converting Enzyme Inhibitors

Captopril   Lisinopril
Enalapril

These drugs are orally effective antihypertensive drugs which are used either alone or in combination with other antihypertensive agents in treating mild to moderate hypertension. These drugs (especially captopril) may also be used at higher doses for controlling more severe resistant forms of hypertension, although at these elevated dose levels serious toxicity such as blood dyscrasias or renal damage can occur with captropril.

They are discussed as a group, then listed individually in Table 31-3.

MECHANISM

Drugs inhibit an enzyme (angiotensin-converting enzyme; ACE) that hydrolyzes inactive angiotensin I to active angiotensin II in the plasma and lungs. (See Fig. 28-4). Inhibition of ACE reduces the formation of the pressor substance angiotensin II and decreases the angiotensin-mediated secretion of aldosterone from the adrenal cortex. Peripheral vascular resistance is lowered, and salt and water retention is reduced. Plasma renin activity increases owing to loss of negative feedback, and serum potassium may rise owing to absence of aldosterone activity. No significant change in cardiac output occurs, but renal blood flow is increased. Both supine and standing blood pressure are lowered to approximately the same extent. Orthostatic hypotension is rare, and reflex tachycardia seldom occurs.

Inhibition of the converting enzyme by these drugs also appears to *decrease* the inactivation of bradykinin, a potent endogenous vasodilator, an action that may also contribute to the blood pressure–lowering effect. An increased synthesis of prostaglandin E, which may result in peripheral vasodilation, has been proposed as an additional action, possibly resulting from the increased levels of bradykinin.

In patients with congestive heart failure, these agents decrease systemic vascular resistance (i.e., afterload) and pulmonary capillary wedge pressure and increase cardiac output

USES

A. Treatment of all degrees of hypertension, either alone or combined with other drugs, especially diuretics, as blood pressure–lowering effects are additive
   1. *Small doses* may be used in mild hypertension in patients with normal renal function, especially where other step 1 or step 2 drugs are inappropriate or ineffective
   2. *Large doses* may be used in moderate to severe forms of hypertension in patients who fail to respond to or cannot tolerate other multiple drug regimens (risk of toxicity is significantly increased)
B. Treatment of refractive congestive heart failure, sometimes combined with digoxin and/or a diuretic
C. Symptomatic treatment of rheumatoid arthritis (investigational use for captopril)

DOSAGE
See Table 31-3

FATE

Drugs are adequately absorbed orally, although the presence of food can reduce absorption of captopril by 30% to 40%; maximal blood pressure–lowering effect is achieved within 60 to 90 minutes with captopril and within 4 to 6 hours with enalapril and lisinopril; however, optimal clinical antihypertensive effects may require several weeks to develop. Following absorption, enalapril is converted to enalaprilat, a more potent ACE inhibitor. The elimination half-life of captopril is less than 2 hours but may be up to 12 hours for lisinopril and up to 36 hours for enalaprilat. Approximately 95% of a dose of each drug is eliminated within 24 hours, in both the urine and the feces

COMMON SIDE EFFECTS
Captopril

Loss of taste sensation, rash, pruritus

Enalapril
Headache, dizziness, fatigue
Lisinopril
GI upset, lightheadedness, anergia

SIGNIFICANT ADVERSE REACTIONS

> **WARNING**
> Excessive hypotension has occurred following ACE-inhibitor administration, especially in severely salt- or volume-depleted patients, such as those with severe congestive heart failure who are receiving diuretics. Excessive perspiration, vomiting, diarrhea, or dehydration may increase the likelihood of extreme hypotension. Caution must be used when initiating therapy with these agents in patients who are receiving other blood pressure–lowering drugs such as diuretics or adrenergic inhibitors

Note: Not all of the following adverse reactions have been noted with each drug

Cardiovascular: tachycardia, chest pain, palpitations, flushing, hypotension, angina, congestive heart failure, myocardial infarction (rare)
GI: nausea, gastric irritation, abdominal pain, diarrhea, vomiting, peptic ulcer
CNS: dizziness, malaise, insomnia, headache
Hematologic: neutropenia, agranulocytosis, eosinophilia, hemolytic anemia
Dermatologic: photosensitivity, angioedema, paresthesias, flushing, pallor, alopecia, hyperhidrosis
Renal: proteinuria, oliguria, polyuria, urinary frequency, renal insufficiency
Other: dry mouth, dyspnea, lymphadenopathy, Raynaud's disease, laryngeal edema, elevated liver enzymes

CONTRAINDICATIONS

No absolute contraindications. *Cautious use* in patients with severe renal dysfunction, systemic lupus–like syndrome, reduced white cell counts, valvular stenosis, or diabetes mellitus and in pregnant or nursing women

INTERACTIONS

The hypotensive effects of ACE inhibitors may be increased by diuretics, adrenergic blocking agents, other antihypertensive drugs, nifedipine, and by severe salt or fluid restriction (see *Warning* under Significant Adverse Reactions)
Serum potassium levels can be elevated by concurrent use of ACE inhibitors and potassium-sparing diuretics or potassium supplements
Vasodilators (e.g., nitrites) may be potentiated by these agents and should be discontinued before beginning therapy with ACE inhibitors
The antihypertensive efficacy of captopril can be reduced by indomethacin and possibly by aspirin and other salicylates

NURSING CONSIDERATIONS

See **Plan of Nursing Care 8** in this chapter. In addition:

> **Nursing Alerts**
> - Monitor results of urinary protein estimates, which should be performed prior to therapy and at monthly intervals thereafter. If proteinuria exceeds 1 g/day, drug should be discontinued unless benefits clearly outweigh risks.
> - Review results of white blood cell and differential counts, which should be obtained prior to therapy and at 2-week intervals during early months of treatment.

PATIENT EDUCATION

See **Plan of Nursing Care 8** in this chapter. In addition:
1. Explain that several weeks of careful monitoring may be required to gradually titrate the dosage to achieve full therapeutic benefit.
2. Instruct patient to take drug with water either 1 hour before or 2 hours after a meal (to enhance absorption).
3. Advise patient that drug may alter taste perception during therapy.
4. Stress importance of reporting any signs of infection (fever, sore throat), possible signs of neutropenia, which are indications for withdrawing drug if white cell count is abnormal.
5. Instruct patient to notify physician if mouth sores, swelling of hands or feet, irregular heartbeat, or chest pains occur.
6. Recommend that patient maintain the same salt intake as prior to therapy because salt restriction can lead to a precipitous drop in blood pressure with initial doses of these drugs.
7. Warn patient that excessive perspiration and dehydration (e.g., due to diarrhea, vomiting) may lead to drastic reduction in blood pressure.

STEP 2 DRUGS

Labetalol
Normodyne, Trandate

MECHANISM

A unique adrenergic blocking agent that combines an alpha$_1$ blocking action with a nonspecific beta-blocking action at both beta$_1$ and beta$_2$ receptor sites; ratio of alpha to beta blockade with oral administration is approximately 1:3; blood pressure is lowered by labetalol, standing pressure more so than supine (owing to the alpha$_1$ blocking action), but changes in heart rate are minimal; exercise-induced increases in heart rate and blood pressure are blunted, and elevated plasma renin levels are reduced; cardiac output and renal function are relatively unaffected, as are AV conduction time and refractory period; also appears to possess some intrinsic beta$_2$ agonistic activity, although the clinical significance of this action is not known; postural hypotension can occur

USES

Treatment of mild to moderate hypertension, either alone or combined with other antihypertensive agents, especially diuretics
Emergency control of blood pressure in severe hypertension (IV administration)

DOSAGE

Oral: 100 mg twice a day as an initial dose; increased in increments of 100 mg twice a day every 2 to 3 days until the desired effect is obtained; usual oral maintenance dose is 200 mg to 400 mg twice a day, although up to 2400 mg/day has been used in severe hypertension.

(*Text continued on page 310*)

PLAN OF NURSING CARE 8
PATIENTS TREATED WITH NONDIURETIC ANTIHYPERTENSIVE DRUGS

Nursing Diagnosis: Potential Noncompliance with Antihypertensive Drug Therapy related to inadequate understanding of hypertension or nature of side effects of antihypertensive drugs

Goal: Patient will comply with prescribed antihypertensive drug regimen.

Intervention	Rationale	Expected Outcome
See also **Plan of Nursing Care 2 (Compliance)**. Teach patient about hypertension: 1. Asymptomatic nature 2. Long-term risks of cardiovascular damage (stroke, heart attack, kidney damage) if not controlled	It may be difficult to accept the need to take medication, probably for the remainder of patient's life, to treat an asymptomatic condition. Awareness of long-term risks of uncontrolled hypertension may improve motivation to comply with antihypertensive drug therapy.	Patient will verbalize understanding of: 1. The nature of hypertension 2. The rationale for drug treatment
Reassure patient that many drug side effects are transient or diminish over time.	Awareness that many side effects diminish or disappear over time is likely to enhance compliance.	3. The transience of many drug side effects
Inform patient that it may be possible to alter drug regimen if side effects are intolerable. Explain that it often takes several weeks for maximum antihypertensive drug action to develop.	Compliance may be jeopardized if patient becomes unduly discouraged by continuing side effects or lack of evidence of antihypertensive effectiveness.	Patient will express awareness of: 1. The possibility of altering drug regimen 2. The length of time required for maximum drug action to develop
As appropriate for specific drugs (e.g., clonidine, hydralazine), warn patient that sudden discontinuation may cause serious symptoms.	Sudden termination of certain drugs may cause symptoms of sympathetic rebound (e.g., rapid rise in blood pressure, headache, insomnia, restlessness, tachycardia, tremors) to appear within several days.	3. The hazards of sudden discontinuation of drug

Nursing Diagnosis: Potential Knowledge Deficit related to antihypertensive drug therapy

Goal: Patient will possess knowledge and skills needed to implement antihypertensive drug regimen and related actions.

Intervention	Rationale	Expected Outcome
See also **Plan of Nursing Care 1 (Knowledge Deficit)**. As supportively as possible, discuss side effects commonly experienced with specific drugs and interventions patient can implement to minimize them.	With potential drug side effects so numerous and compliance a major problem, patient should fully understand the drug regimen and related actions. Mental depression and sexual dysfunction are two particularly troublesome potential side effects with certain drugs. Mental depression occurs most often with drugs that have central antiadrenergic effects. Sexual dysfunction occurs with other antiadrenergic drugs. Headache and palpitations are particularly likely to occur with direct-acting vasodilators, as their marked hypotensive effect may activate baroreceptors that function to increase heart rate (reflex tachycardia) and cardiac output.	Patient will discuss potential side effects of specific drugs and measures that help minimize them.
Emphasize the need to check with drug prescriber or pharmacist before using any OTC drug.	Many OTC allergy, cough, and cold preparations contain vasoconstrictors or CNS depressants that may interfere with blood pressure control or enhance sedation or orthostatic hypotension.	Patient will voice awareness of the need to seek consultation before using OTC drugs.
Teach patient, if indicated, how to monitor blood pressure at home: 1. Technique 2. Record keeping 3. Amount of change to be reported	The dosage schedule and type of medication needed for control can be more closely regulated when blood pressure is monitored frequently.	Patient will demonstrate: 1. Accurate blood pressure measurement 2. Recording of results Patient will state normal blood pressure for self and amount of change that should be reported.

Continued

PLAN OF NURSING CARE 8 (continued)
PATIENTS TREATED WITH NONDIURETIC ANTIHYPERTENSIVE DRUGS

Nursing Diagnosis: Potential Knowledge Deficit related to antihypertensive drug therapy
Goal: Patient will possess knowledge and skills needed to implement antihypertensive drug regimen and related actions.

Intervention	Rationale	Expected Outcome
Encourage patient, as appropriate, to implement adjunctive measures to help control hypertension: 1. Reduce dietary salt intake 2. Lose excess body weight 3. Decrease or eliminate caffeine intake 4. Stop smoking 5. Reduce stress (e.g., biofeedback, lifestyle modification)	Measures that decrease blood volume, peripheral resistance, vasoconstriction, adrenergic activity, or cardiac output help lower blood pressure.	Patient will discuss adjunctive measures that help lower blood pressure and the rationale for their effectiveness.
Refer patient to dietitian or other resources as appropriate.		Patient will be taught how to implement appropriate adjunctive measures.
Suggest that patient wear bracelet or tag indicating the drug regimen taken for hypertension. Provide information on how to obtain one.	In an emergency, it is important for care providers to be aware of patient's hypertension and drugs taken for it.	Patient will explain how to obtain a medical alert tag.

Nursing Diagnosis: Potential Alteration in Tissue (Cerebral) Perfusion: Decrease related to postural (orthostatic) hypotension from antihypertensive drug therapy
Goal: Patient will maintain adequate cerebral circulation to avoid injury.

Intervention	Rationale	Expected Outcome
If patient is hospitalized, take supine and standing blood pressures at least every 4 h when drug therapy is initiated, dosage is adjusted, another drug is added, or patient reports symptoms of hypotension (dizziness, lightheadedness, weakness, or syncope upon standing).	Hypotension occurs most often when drug therapy is started, new drugs are added, or dosages are altered. For some drugs, the effective maintenance dose is determined by monitoring blood pressure with patient in the upright position at times of maximal drug effect and titrating dose to a level just below that which produces signs of orthostatic hypotension.	Patient's blood pressure will be maintained within safe limits.
Use precautions for postural hypotension with hospitalized patient: 1. Instruct patient not to get out of bed without help. 2. Assist patient to rise slowly from recumbent to sitting to erect positions. 3. Supervise patient's ambulation. 4. Use utmost caution with elderly patient.	Hypotension occurs most often when moving rapidly from a supine to an upright position, especially in the morning. Slow movement gives homeostatic mechanisms more time to adjust. The elderly are particularly vulnerable to postural hypotension.	Patient will not fall when getting out of bed.
Reassure patient that symptoms of orthostatic hypotension usually wane over time.	Adaptation gradually occurs over a period of time.	Patient will explain that symptoms of orthostatic hypotension are usually transient.
If orthostatic effect is strong, discuss feasibility of bedtime administration with drug prescriber.	Depending on drug characteristics, it may be possible to administer drug at bedtime so that peak effects occur during sleep.	Patient will state that symptoms of orthostatic hypotension have lessened.
Explain to patient the relationship between blood pressure in recumbent versus upright position and resulting effect on cerebral blood flow.	Normally, blood pressure drops with sudden movement from a reclining to an upright position as blood drains from the head and remains in the periphery. Most antihypertensive drugs decrease either peripheral resistance or cardiac output (beta blockers) and thus inhibit the vascular or cardiac mechanisms that adjust for position changes. Until adaptation occurs, blood pressure may be low enough to induce symptoms of diminished blood flow and oxygen to the brain.	Patient will discuss dynamics of hypotension.

Continued

PLAN OF NURSING CARE 8 (continued)
PATIENTS TREATED WITH NONDIURETIC ANTIHYPERTENSIVE DRUGS

Nursing Diagnosis: Potential Alteration in Tissue (Cerebral) Perfusion: Decrease related to postural (orthostatic) hypotension from antihypertensive drug therapy

Goal: Patient will maintain adequate cerebral circulation to avoid injury.

Intervention	Rationale	Expected Outcome
Teach patient interventions that help control postural hypotension and provide written guidelines: 1. If symptoms of hypotension occur, lie down immediately and elevate legs or sit down and lower head until symptoms pass. 2. When arising from a recumbent position, sit on edge of bed with feet dangling for 1 or 2 min. 3. When arising from a sitting position, rise slowly and hold on to a sturdy object. 4. Wear waist-high support hose. 5. Apply support garment while lying flat before getting out of bed. 6. If standing a long time is unavoidable, perform isometric foot and leg exercises. 7. Avoid straining (e.g., lifting, during bowel movement). 8. Be particularly cautious in the morning; in very hot weather; during hot showers, hot baths, exercise, or squatting; and after ingestion of a large meal or alcohol. 9. If symptoms continue or worsen, contact health care provider.	Actions that improve venous return or prevent vasodilation or venous pooling help control postural hypotension, as enhanced venous return increases cardiac output, blood pressure, and cerebral circulation.	Patient will describe measures that help control postural hypotension and will possess written guidelines.

Nursing Diagnosis: Potential Alteration in Fluid Volume: Excess: Edema related to fluid retention from antihypertensive drug therapy

Goal: Patient will receive treatment for fluid overload.

Intervention	Rationale	Expected Outcome
With hospitalized patient, monitor fluid balance: 1. Measure intake and output. 2. Weigh daily. 3. Check extremities for pitting edema. Teach outpatient how to detect fluid retention: 1. Obtain daily comparable body weights (same scale, same time, same amount of clothing). 2. Record results. 3. Report gain of 2 or more pounds within 1 day to appropriate person.	Antihypertensive drugs lower blood pressure, renal perfusion, and glomerular filtration rate. As a result, sodium and water are retained, urinary output diminishes, and increased fluid volume adds to body weight.	Patient will receive treatment for fluid overload. Patient will verbalize procedure for monitoring fluid retention at home.

Nursing Diagnosis: Potential for Injury related to sedation from antihypertensive drug therapy

Goal: Patient will not be injured as a result of sedation.

Intervention	Rationale	Expected Outcome
Advise patient that any activity that requires alertness (e.g., driving a car, operating heavy machinery) should be avoided or at least performed very cautiously until the effects of newly initiated drugs or increased dosages of drugs have been ascertained.	Drowsiness may occur when drug therapy is initiated or when dosages are increased. Many antihypertensive drugs induce sedation by interfering with central adrenergic functions.	Patient will express awareness of precautions for sedation.

Continued

PLAN OF NURSING CARE 8 (continued)
PATIENTS TREATED WITH NONDIURETIC ANTIHYPERTENSIVE DRUGS
Nursing Diagnosis: Potential for Injury related to sedation from antihypertensive drug therapy
Goal: Patient will not be injured as a result of sedation.

Intervention	Rationale	Expected Outcome
Warn patient that alcohol and other CNS depressant drugs, including those in OTC preparations, will enhance drug-induced sedation.	CNS depressants have an additive effect on drug-induced sedation.	Patient will explain interaction between antihypertensive drug and CNS-depressant drugs.
Reassure patient that sedative effects are usually transient.	Sedation diminishes as adaptation occurs.	
If sedation becomes problematic, collaborate with pharmacist and drug prescriber to determine if drug dosing schedule can be altered to minimize sedative effects.	Once-daily doses at bedtime minimize sedative effects. Even with divided doses, a bedtime dose may reduce late-day sedation. The dosage schedule may depend, however, on half-life and other drug characteristics.	Patient will state that sedation has abated.

See also **Plan of Nursing Care 3** for additional considerations related to **Beta-adrenergic blockers**.
See **Plan of Nursing Care 9** for **Diuretics**.

Table 31-3
Angiotensin Converting–Enzyme Inhibitors

Drug	Preparations	Usual Dosage Range	Nursing Implications
Captopril Capoten	Tablets: 12.5 mg, 25 mg, 37.5 mg, 50 mg, 100 mg	*Mild hypertension:* 12.5 mg–25 mg 2–3 times/day; increase gradually as needed *Moderate-severe hypertension:* initially 25 mg 3 times/day; usual dosage range 50 mg–150 mg 2–3 times/day	Used alone for mild hypertension and most often together with a diuretic and other antihypertensives for severe hypertension; also used as adjunctive therapy in congestive heart failure (see Chap. 29), as it reduces preload and afterload; rash is a common occurrence; proteinuria and neutropenia can occur at high doses
Enalapril Vasotec	Tablets: 5 mg, 10 mg, 20 mg Injection: 1.25 mg enalaprilat/mL	*Oral:* initially 5 mg once daily; usual dosage range 10 mg–40 mg daily in a single or 2 divided doses *IV:* 1.25 mg every 6 h given over 5 min; in persons receiving diuretics, 0.625 mg IV over 5 min	Following absorption, drug is hydrolyzed to enalaprilat, a more potent ACE inhibitor; also used in congestive heart failure; headache and dizziness are most common side effects; may elevate serum potassium; also available for IV injection as enalaprilat; peak effects may not occur for 4 h, however; has been used up to 7 days IV
Lisinopril Prinivil, Zestril	Tablets: 5 mg, 10 mg, 20 mg	Initially 10 mg once daily; usual dosage range 20 mg–40 mg/day	Long-acting ACE inhibitor; a diuretic may be added if control with lisinopril alone is inadequate; reduce initial dose in elderly and in persons with impaired renal function

IV (hypertensive emergency): 20 mg injected over 2 minutes; additional injections of 40 mg to 80 mg can be given every 10 minutes thereafter until the desired supine blood pressure is attained or a total of 300 mg has been administered; alternatively, 2 mg/min (2 mL/min of diluted injection solution) can be infused IV until the desired blood pressure response has been attained; usual IV dosage range is 50 mg to 200 mg. Labetalol is compatible with and stable in 5% dextrose, 0.9% sodium chloride, dextrose and sodium chloride mixtures, Ringer's solution, and lactated Ringer's solution. It is *not* compatible with 5% sodium bicarbonate injection

FATE
Completely absorbed orally; peak plasma levels occur within 1 to 2 hours; maximum effects with a single dose are noted within 2 to 4 hours, and effects persist 8 hours to 12 hours; undergoes extensive first-pass hepatic metabolism; drug is approximately 50% protein-bound

Maximum effect following IV injection occurs within 5 minutes and persists for up to 12 to 15 hours following discontinuation; drug is partially metabolized in the liver and excreted both in the urine and feces and by way of the bile as conjugated metabolites as well as unchanged drug; elimination half-life following oral and IV administration is 6 hours and 5.5 hours, respectively

COMMON SIDE EFFECTS
Nausea, fatigue, dizziness, rash, tingling of skin and scalp

SIGNIFICANT ADVERSE REACTIONS
Systemic lupus–like reaction; in addition, refer to Chapter 13 for the adverse reactions associated with alpha- and beta-adrenergic blockers, which may also occur with labetalol

CONTRAINDICATIONS
Bronchial asthma, severe bradycardia, second- or third-degree heart block, cardiac failure, cardiogenic shock. *Cautious use* in persons with bronchitis, emphysema, diabetes mellitus, or hepatic dysfunction and in pregnant or nursing women

INTERACTIONS
Labetalol can reduce the bronchodilator effects of beta-adrenergic agonists

The incidence of tremor with combined use of labetalol and tricyclic antidepressants is significantly higher than with use of labetalol alone

Cimetidine can increase the plasma levels of labetalol

Labetalol reduces the reflex tachycardia seen with direct-acting vasodilators

In addition, see Chapter 13 for a list of other potential interactions for alpha$_1$ antagonists and beta-adrenergic antagonists.

NURSING CONSIDERATIONS
See **Plan of Nursing Care 8** in this chapter. In addition:

Nursing Alerts
- Take lying and standing blood pressures 1 to 3 hours after an initial oral dose or dose increment to detect postural hypotension.
- Prior to IV administration, prepare patient for prolonged supine positioning. During and for up to 3 hours following IV administration, maintain patient in supine position to avoid postural hypotension (high incidence).
- Immediately before IV injection and at 5 and 10 minutes after each injection, take patient's supine blood pressure (maximum effect usually occurs within 5 minutes after injection).
- During IV infusion, monitor blood pressure every 15 to 30 minutes. For IV infusion, a pump is recommended to maintain accurate flow rate.
- For patient on long-term therapy, review results of antinuclear antibody titers, which should be performed periodically to detect a systemic lupus–like reaction.

1. Recognize that drug has both alpha- and beta-antiadrenergic effects. Unlike drugs with only beta-antiadrenergic effects, labetalol does not require routine monitoring of heart rate and cardiac output.

PATIENT EDUCATION
See **Plan of Nursing Care 8** in this chapter. In addition:
1. Recommend that patient take drug with food if nausea occurs. Nausea is an early, but usually transient, side effect.
2. Instruct patient on long-term therapy to report any symptoms of a systemic lupus–like reaction, such as joint pain, stiffness, or dyspnea.

Clonidine
Catapres
(CAN) Dixarit
Guanabenz
Wytensin
Guanfacine
Tenex

Clonidine, guanabenz, and guanfacine are similar, orally active antiadrenergic agents that are indicated in the treatment of mild to moderate hypertension. In addition, clonidine is available as a transdermal patch (Clonidine-TTS). They are centrally acting antihypertensive drugs with a very low incidence of serious toxicity; principal side effects are drowsiness and dry mouth.

MECHANISM
Activation of presynaptic adrenergic alpha$_2$ receptors in cardiovascular integrating centers in the brainstem, resulting in a decreased outflow of sympathetic vasoconstrictor and cardioaccelerator impulses; moderate reduction in pulse rate and cardiac output; decrease plasma renin activity; initially, may stimulate peripheral alpha-adrenergic receptors, causing transient vasoconstriction

USES
Treatment of mild to moderate degrees of hypertension, either alone or with a diuretic or another antihypertensive drug

Investigational uses for *clonidine* include prophylaxis of migraine, treatment of episodes of menopausal flushing, symptomatic management of opiate detoxification, and treatment of Gilles de la Tourette's disease

DOSAGE
Clonidine
Hypertension: Initially 0.1 mg twice a day; increase by 0.1 mg to 0.2 mg/day to desired response; usual range is 0.2 mg to 0.8 mg/day in divided doses; maximum 2.4 mg/day; may be effective as a single daily dose; transdermal patch—apply 1 patch every 7 days; begin with 0.1 mg system and increase in 0.1-mg increments as needed

Opiate withdrawal: 10 µg/kg to 17 µg/kg/day in divided doses (experimental use only)

Gilles de la Tourette's disease: 0.05 mg to 0.6 mg/day

Guanabenz

Initially, 4 mg twice a day; increase in increments of 4 mg to 8 mg/day every 1 to 2 weeks; maximum dose is 32 mg a day in divided doses

Guanfacine

Initially, 1 mg daily at bedtime (usually with a diuretic); may increase up to 3 mg/day if necessary

FATE

Onset for all drugs is 30 to 60 minutes following oral administration; maximum effect in 2 to 4 hours; duration 6 to 8 hours; plasma half-life is 12 to 16 hours for clonidine and guanfacine and 6 to 8 hours for guanabenz; metabolized by the liver and excreted mainly in the urine both as unchanged drug and as metabolites

COMMON SIDE EFFECTS

Dry mouth, drowsiness, sedation, constipation, dizziness, headache, fatigue

SIGNIFICANT ADVERSE REACTIONS

(Not all reactions observed with all drugs)

GI: anorexia, nausea, vomiting, parotid pain, liver function test abnormalities

CNS: insomnia, nervousness, anxiety, depression, vivid dreams or nightmares

Dermatologic: rash, angioedema, urticaria, hives, hair loss, pruritus

Cardiovascular: Raynaud's phenomenon (pallor, cyanosis, pain in extremities), palpitation, flushing, congestive heart failure (rare)

Other: weight gain, hyperglycemia, gynecomastia, urinary retention, impotence, itching or burning of eyes, pallor, dryness of nasal mucosa

CONTRAINDICATIONS

No absolute contraindications. *Cautious use* in patients with coronary insufficiency, cerebrovascular disease, chronic renal failure, thromboangiitis obliterans, history of depression, or recent myocardial infarction, and in pregnant women

INTERACTIONS

Clonidine, guanabenz, and guanfacine may intensify the CNS-depressant effects of alcohol, barbiturates, narcotics, and other depressants

Effects of clonidine, guanabenz, and guanfacine may be antagonized by tricyclic antidepressants (except doxepin) and tolazoline

Excessive bradycardia can occur when clonidine, guanabenz, and guanfacine used in combination with digitalis agents, propranolol, or guanethidine

NURSING CONSIDERATIONS

See **Plan of Nursing Care 8** in this chapter. In addition:

Nursing Alert
- Do not discontinue therapy abruptly because agitation, tachycardia, and rebound hypertension can occur. Discontinue therapy gradually over 3 to 4 days. If symptoms occur, be prepared to reinstitute drug or to administer both an alpha- and a beta-adrenergic blocker.

PATIENT EDUCATION

See **Plan of Nursing Care 8** in this chapter. In addition:

1. Suggest that significant others closely observe patient with a prior history of mental depression because these drugs can evoke depressive episodes.
2. Instruct patient to report any changes in pattern of urination because urinary hesitancy can occur.
3. Instruct patient to undergo periodic eye examinations during prolonged therapy because retinal degeneration may occur.
4. Inform patient that tolerance to drug effects can develop. If tolerance occurs, therapy should be reevaluated, and addition of other antihypertensive medications should be considered.
5. Inform patient that sensitivity to alcohol may be increased.

Methyldopa

Aldomet, Amodopa

(CAN) Apo-Methyldopa, Dopamet, Novomedopa, PMS Dopazide

MECHANISM

Inhibits the enzyme aromatic-amino-acid-decarboxylase by competitive antagonism, and is itself converted to alpha-methyl norepinephrine, which functions as an activator of central alpha-2 adrenergic receptors. Stimulation of brainstem alpha receptors results in a decreased outflow of sympathetic vasoconstrictor and cardioaccelerator impulses, thereby producing vasodilation and bradycardia; may reduce plasma renin activity but does not significantly affect renal blood flow; cardiac output is usually decreased; diurnal blood pressure variations occur rarely; has a sedative action and promotes sodium and water retention

USES

Treatment of sustained moderate to moderately severe hypertension, either alone or more commonly with other antihypertensive agents

Treatment of acute hypertensive crises (methyldop*ate* ester, IV); infrequently used owing to slow onset of action

DOSAGE

Oral

Adults: Initially 250 mg 2 to 3 times/day; adjust dosage by increments at intervals of not less than 2 days until desired response occurs; usual maintenance dosage 500 mg to 2000 mg/day in 2 to 4 divided doses (maximum 3 g/day)

Children: 10 mg/kg/day in 2 to 4 divided doses adjusted to desired level; maximum dose 65 mg/kg or 3 g daily

IV Infusion

Adults: 250 mg to 500 mg at 6-hour intervals (dose is added to 100 mL 5% dextrose injection and infused over 30 to 60 min); maximum dose 1 g every 6 hours

Children: 20 mg to 40 mg/kg in divided doses every 6 hours; maximum dose 3 g/day

FATE

Oral absorption is variable (range 10%–60%); peak plasma levels occur in 2 to 4 hours, but maximal antihypertensive effect may not occur for several days; duration may persist for 24 hours even though elimination half-life is 2 to 3 hours; following IV infusion, maximal effects are seen in 4 to 8 hours and last 12 to 16 hours; appears rapidly in the urine, predominantly in unaltered form

COMMON SIDE EFFECTS
Sedation, headache, weakness, dry mouth, nasal stuffiness, weight gain, and positive direct Coombs' test (see below)

SIGNIFICANT ADVERSE REACTIONS
Cardiovascular: bradycardia, anginal pain, orthostatic hypotension, edema, myocarditis, paradoxical pressor response with IV use
CNS: dizziness, paresthesias, parkinsonian-like symptoms, choreoathetoid movements, psychoses, depression, nightmares, memory impairment
GI: nausea, vomiting, constipation, "black" tongue, abdominal distention, pancreatitis, sialadenitis
Hematologic: hemolytic anemia, leukopenia, thrombocytopenia, granulocytopenia
Hepatic: jaundice, liver dysfunction
Other: fever, myalgia, arthralgia, dermatoses, rash, nasal congestion, breast enlargement, gynecomastia, lactation, impotence, decreased libido
Laboratory test variations: abnormal liver function tests; positive tests for antinuclear antibody, lupus erythematosus cells, and rheumatoid factor; rise in BUN; falsely high urinary catecholamines

CONTRAINDICATIONS
Active hepatic disease, blood dyscrasias. *Cautious use* in patients with chronic liver dysfunction, angina, renal impairment, pheochromocytoma, endocrine disorders, or anemia and in pregnant or nursing women

INTERACTIONS
Additive hypotensive effects can occur with methyldopa and anesthetics, alcohol, diuretics and other antihypertensive drugs, fenfluramine, narcotics, methotrimeprazine, levodopa, quinidine, vasodilators, verapamil
Hypotensive action of methyldopa can be antagonized by amphetamines, catecholamines (except levodopa), tricyclic antidepressants, MAO inhibitors, phenothiazines, sympathomimetics, and vasopressors
Methyldopa can potentiate the hypoglycemic action of tolbutamide
Elevated serum lithium levels can occur with methyldopa
Psychiatric disturbances can result from combined use of methyldopa and haloperidol
Phenoxybenzamine and methyldopa together have resulted in reversible urinary incontinence
Combinations of methyldopa and propranolol have occasionally resulted in paradoxical hypertension

NURSING CONSIDERATIONS
See **Plan of Nursing Care 8** in this chapter. In addition:

Nursing Alerts
- Monitor results of complete blood counts and direct Coombs' tests, which should be performed prior to initiating therapy and periodically during drug treatment because a positive Coombs' test, as well as hemolytic anemia and liver disorders, can occur and can lead to potentially fatal complications. A positive Coombs' test is observed in approximately 20% of patients on chronic therapy. It is dose-dependent and may persist for 3 to 18 months after drug is withdrawn. In most cases, it is *not* clinically significant in the absence of other complications (e.g., anemia, hepatitis). If a positive test develops, hemolytic anemia needs to be ruled out. Although a positive test is not in itself an indication for stopping therapy, if Coombs'-positive hemolytic anemia, non-dose-dependent drug fever, or hepatitis occur, the drug should be discontinued immediately.
- During IV administration, check blood pressure repeatedly until stabilized, and monitor urinary output.
- Be alert for development of paradoxical pressor response with IV use of methyldopate ester.

PATIENT EDUCATION
See **Plan of Nursing Care 8** in this chapter. In addition:
1. Teach patient to be alert for development of fever, chills, headache, pruritus, rash, arthralgia, and enlarged liver because reversible methyldopa hepatotoxicity occasionally occurs, especially during the first few months of therapy. Patient should notify physician if these occur so that liver function tests can be performed. If fever, jaundice, or liver function abnormalities appear, the drug should be discontinued.
2. Instruct patient to watch for appearance of involuntary movements and to advise physician if these occur because the drug should be discontinued.
3. Inform patient that a breakdown product of drug may harmlessly darken urine.

Prazosin
Minipress
Terazosin
Hytrin

MECHANISM
Selectively block postsynaptic alpha$_1$ receptor sites and dilate both resistance (i.e., arterioles) and capacitance (i.e., veins) vessels; therefore, little change in cardiac output, heart rate, renal blood flow, or glomerular filtration rate; blood pressure is lowered in both supine and standing positions, and effects are most pronounced on the diastolic pressure; reduce venous return (preload) and aortic impedance to left ventricular ejection (afterload); sodium and water retention can occur

USES
Treatment of mild to moderate hypertension, either alone or with a diuretic or other antihypertensive agent
Adjunctive treatment of severe, refractive congestive heart failure

DOSAGE
Prazosin
Initially 1 mg 2 to 3 times/day; increase slowly to optimal response, up to 20 mg/day; usual maintenance range is 6 mg to 15 mg/day in 2 or 3 divided doses
Terazosin
Initially, 1 mg at bedtime; increase slowly to optimal response; usual dose range is 1 mg to 5 mg daily; maximum dose 20 mg/day

FATE
Oral absorption is good and is not affected by food; peak plasma levels occur within 1 to 3 hours; protein binding is 90% to 95%; elimination half-life is 2 to 3 hours for prazosin and 9 to 12 hours for terazosin; drugs are excreted both in the urine and the bile

COMMON SIDE EFFECTS

Dizziness, headache, malaise, drowsiness, weakness, palpitations, nausea, nasal congestion

SIGNIFICANT ADVERSE REACTIONS

(Causal relationships not established in all cases)

GI: vomiting, constipation, abdominal pain
Cardiovascular: tachycardia, angina, syncope (see Nursing Alert regarding first-dose phenomenon) edema, orthostatic hypotension
CNS: nervousness, paresthesias, vertigo, depression
Other: urinary frequency or incontinence, impotence, rash, pruritus, dyspnea, blurred vision, tinnitus, dry mouth, epistaxis, diaphoresis, arthralgia, leukopenia, drug-induced lupus-like syndrome (rare)

CONTRAINDICATIONS

No absolute contraindications. *Cautious use* in persons who must drive or operate heavy machinery during early stages of therapy

INTERACTIONS

Enhanced hypotensive effects can occur in combination with other antihypertensive drugs, especially propranolol

Effects of prazosin may be potentiated by other highly protein-bound drugs

NURSING CONSIDERATIONS

See **Plan of Nursing Care 8** in this chapter. In addition:

Nursing Alert
- Monitor blood pressure frequently during changes in drug regimen. The initial dose of prazosin should be limited to 1 mg, dosage adjustments should be made gradually, and other antihypertensive medications should be added cautiously to avoid excessive hypotensive reactions.

PATIENT EDUCATION

See **Plan of Nursing Care 8** in this chapter. In addition:
1. Warn patient that fainting caused by excessive orthostatic hypotension can occur shortly after small, initial doses of prazosin. This is called the *first-dose phenomenon.*
2. Explain that tolerance may develop with continued use and that drug may lose effectiveness within a few months.

Calcium Channel Blockers

Diltiazem (Cardizem)
Nicardipine (Cardene)
Verapamil (Calan, Isoptin)

In addition to their use in treating arrhythmias (see Chap. 30) and for the prophylaxis of angina (see Chap. 32), several calcium channel blockers have been employed for the control of mild to moderate hypertension. The drugs relax vascular smooth muscle and elicit peripheral vasodilation, thereby lowering blood pressure. They are well tolerated by most patients, the most frequent side effects being headache, nausea, dizziness, and mild peripheral edema. Adverse effects such as impotence, depression, and elevated serum lipids that have occurred with other agents used in mild hypertension do not seem to occur with calcium channel blockers.

DOSAGE

Diltiazem
(sustained-release tablets)
60 mg to 120 mg twice daily; adjust dosage when maximum effect is achieved (usually within 14 days); usual dosage range is 240 to 300 mg/day

Nicardipine
Initially, 20 mg 3 times/day; usual range is 20 mg to 40 mg 3 times/day

Verapamil
Initially, 80 mg 3 times/day; increase gradually as necessary up to 360 mg/day.

CONTRAINDICATIONS

Diltiazem
Second- or third-degree heart block, systolic hypotension (<90 mm Hg), sick-sinus syndrome acute pulmonary congestion

Nicardipine
Advanced aortic stenosis

Verapamil
Second- or third-degree heart block, systolic hypotension, sick-sinus syndrome, left ventricular dysfunction, cardiogenic shock, severe congestive heart failure

NURSING CONSIDERATIONS

See Chapters 30 and 32 and **Plan of Nursing Care 8** in this chapter.

PATIENT EDUCATION

See Chapters 30 and 32 and **Plan of Nursing Care 8** in this chapter.

Rauwolfia Alkaloids

Alseroxylon	Rescinnamine
Deserpidine	Reserpine
Rauwolfia whole root	

The rauwolfia derivatives are a group of products derived from the Rauwolfia family of plants, comprising whole root rauwolfia, an extraction of alkaloids (alseroxylon), and the refined alkaloids deserpidine, rescinnamine, and reserpine. These agents are infrequently used today, since they are no more effective than most other available antihypertensive medications and have the potential to elicit a wide range of troublesome side effects. Their pharmacology is reviewed briefly, and individual drugs are listed in Table 31-4.

MECHANISM

Deplete central and peripheral neuronal stores of biogenic amines (i.e., norepinephrine, serotonin) by blocking amine uptake into vesicular storage sites within the nerve ending; decrease blood pressure, heart rate, and cardiac output; exert a CNS-depressant (sedating) action; do not markedly affect renal blood flow

USES

Treatment of mild to moderate essential hypertension, usually in combination with other antihypertensive medications

Management of psychotic behavior, primarily in patients incapable of tolerating other antipsychotic drugs (except alseroxylon and rescinnamine)

DOSAGE

See Table 31-4

FATE

Onset of action following oral administration is generally slow (several days); maximum antihypertensive effect requires several weeks to develop; effects persist for weeks following discontinuation of therapy; primarily excreted in the urine, mainly as metabolites; following IM injection, reserpine has an onset in approximately 1 to 2 hours with maximum effects occurring within 4 to 6 hours

COMMON SIDE EFFECTS

Drowsiness, nasal congestion, diarrhea, bradycardia

SIGNIFICANT ADVERSE REACTIONS

GI: nausea, vomiting, abdominal pain, hypersecretion, bleeding

CNS: nervousness, anxiety, nightmares, depression, extrapyramidal symptoms (large doses)

Cardiovascular: palpitations, arrhythmias, angina-like symptoms, orthostatic hypotension, syncope, cutaneous vasodilation and flushing

Other: rash, pruritus, uveitis, blurred vision, dryness of mouth, epistaxis, headache, dysuria, impotence, breast engorgement, pseudolactation, gynecomastia, asthma, dyspnea, muscle aching, weight gain, menstrual irregularities

CONTRAINDICATIONS

Mental depression, active peptic ulcer, ulcerative colitis, pheochromocytoma, in patients receiving ECT, therapy with MAO inhibitors. *Cautious use* in patients with arrhythmias, obesity, epilepsy, bronchitis, gallstones, renal or hepatic dysfunction, and in pregnant women or nursing mothers

INTERACTIONS

Enhanced hypotensive effects may be seen when rauwolfia derivatives are combined with anesthetics, barbiturates, diuretics and other antihypertensive drugs, methotrimeprazine, phenothiazines, quinidine, propranolol, and vasodilators

Cardiac arrhythmias can occur if reserpine is given with digitalis, quinidine, or theophylline

CNS-depressant effects of other agents (e.g., alcohol, barbiturates, narcotics, antihistamines, phenothiazines) may be enhanced by reserpine

Rauwolfia derivatives may decrease the effects of anticholinergics (antisecretory action), anticonvulsants, indirect-acting sympathomimetics (e.g., ephedrine, amphetamine), levodopa, morphine, salicylates, vasopressors (e.g., metaraminol, mephentermine)

If used with tricyclic antidepressants, rauwolfia derivatives may cause excitation and mania

Excitation and hypertension can initially result from combined use of rauwolfia drugs and MAO inhibitors, but prolonged therapy can lead to severe depression and markedly increased GI activity

NURSING CONSIDERATIONS

See **Plan of Nursing Care 8** in this chapter.

PATIENT EDUCATION

See **Plan of Nursing Care 8** in this chapter. In addition:

1. Recommend that drug be taken with food or milk to minimize GI distress.
2. Teach patient and significant others to report the first signs of drug-induced depression (despondency, insomnia, anorexia, impotence). Depressive effects of drug can, however, persist for months after withdrawal.
3. Inform patient that, although orthostatic hypotension is uncommon, dizziness and fainting may occur.
4. Inform patient that alcohol may increase both the hypotensive and CNS-depressant effects of the drug.
5. Explain that therapeutic effects may persist for up to 1 month following termination of therapy.
6. Inform patient that, after prolonged use of rauwolfia alkaloids, ingestion of agents containing sympathomimetic amines, such as decongestants, cold preparations, or adrenergic bronchodilators, can result in excessive elevation of blood pressure because the receptivity of postsynaptic adrenergic receptors may be increased when presynaptic neurohormonal stores are depleted.
7. Instruct patient to inform surgeon or dentist of drug use prior to elective surgery because the drug should be discontinued several weeks earlier to avoid severe hypotension during anesthesia.

STEP 3 DRUGS

Hydralazine

Alazine, Apresoline

MECHANISM

Direct relaxation of vascular smooth muscle, primarily arteriolar, leading to decreased peripheral resistance; little effect on venous capacitance vessels; diastolic pressure is usually lowered more than systolic; no change or possibly an increase in renal and cerebral blood flow; reflex increase in heart rate, stroke volume, and cardiac output. In congestive heart failure, drug lowers peripheral arteriolar resistance, thereby improving cardiac output

USES

Management of moderate forms of hypertension, sometimes alone but more commonly in combination with other antihypertensive medications

Short-term treatment of severe essential hypertension (IV or IM)

Adjunctive treatment of congestive heart failure and severe aortic insufficiency and following valve replacement

DOSAGE

Oral: initially 10 mg 4 times/day for 2 to 4 days; increase to 25 mg 4 times/day for balance of week; for second and subsequent weeks, increase to 50 mg 4 times/day; adjust to lowest effective levels for maintenance; twice daily dosage may be adequate

Table 31-4
Rauwolfia Alkaloids

Drug	Preparations	Usual Dosage Range	Nursing Implications
Alseroxylon Rauwiloid	Tablets: 2 mg	Initially 2 mg–4 mg/day Usual maintenance dose is 2 mg/day	Used for treatment of mild essential hypertension; be alert for serious mental depression that can occur at high doses; instruct patients to limit alcohol intake, as CNS depression can be enhanced
Deserpidine Harmonyl	Tablets: 0.25 mg	Hypertension: Initially 0.75 mg–1 mg/day; maintenance dose 0.25 mg/day Psychoses: Initially 0.5 mg/day; usual range is 0.125 mg–1 mg/day	Used for treatment of mild essential hypertension and for relief of symptoms in agitated psychotic states; do *not* make dosage adjustments more frequently than every 10 to 14 days because effects of the drug are slow to develop
Rauwolfia whole root Raudixin and several other manufacturers	Tablets: 50 mg, 100 mg	Usual starting dose is 200 mg–400 mg/day in divided doses Maintenance dose is 50 mg–300 mg/day in a single or 2 divided doses	Used in mild essential hypertension and for relief of symptoms in agitated psychotic states; administer with food or milk to minimize GI upset; rarely used today
Rescinnamine Moderil	Tablets: 0.25 mg, 0.5 mg	Initially 0.5 mg twice a day Usual maintenance dose is 0.25 mg–0.5 mg daily	Used in mild essential hypertension and may be effective as an adjunct to other antihypertensive medications in more severe forms of hypertension; lower incidence of sedation and bradycardia reported with rescinnamine than with reserpine
Reserpine Serpasil and several other manufacturers (CAN) Novoreserpine, Reserfia	Tablets: 0.1 mg, 0.25 mg, 1 mg	Hypertension: initially 0.5 mg/day; reduce slowly to 0.1 mg–0.25 mg/day Psychiatric disorders: 0.1 mg to 1 mg/day adjusted to patient's response	Used for treating mild hypertension and for relief of symptoms of agitated psychotic states; doses higher than 0.25 mg/day may cause severe depression; combined with other antihypertensive drugs (e.g., diuretics, hydralazine) for treatment of more severe forms of hypertension

IM, IV: initially, 5 mg to 10 mg; titrate upward slowly as needed and give at 30-minute intervals

Children—0.1 mg/kg to 0.2 mg/kg every 4 to 6 hours

FATE
Well absorbed orally; peak plasma levels occur within 1 hour; half-life is 2 to 8 hours; effects last for 6 to 8 hours; highly protein bound (85%–90%); onset following IM injection is 10 to 15 minutes and duration lasts 3 to 4 hours; IV administration results in immediate onset, with maximal response in 1 hour; metabolized by the liver and rapidly excreted, largely in the feces

COMMON SIDE EFFECTS
Headache, nausea, vomiting, diarrhea, sweating, palpitations, tachycardia

SIGNIFICANT ADVERSE REACTIONS
Paresthesias, numbness and tingling in extremities, anginal pain, tremors, disorientation, anxiety, depression, flushing, lacrimation, conjunctivitis, urticaria, pruritus, fever, chills, nasal congestion, muscle cramping, arthralgia, eosinophilia, constipation, difficulty in micturition, dyspnea, and paralytic ileus

Reduced hemoglobin, leukopenia, agranulocytosis, and purpura

Systemic lupus–like syndrome (doses greater than 400 mg/day) marked by fever, dermatoses, myalgia, arthralgia, anemia, splenomegaly, edema, and lymphadenopathy

CONTRAINDICATIONS
Rheumatic heart disease, coronary artery disease, and systemic lupus erythematosus. *Cautious use* in persons with renal impairment, cerebral vascular disease, or peripheral neuritis and in pregnant or nursing women

INTERACTIONS
Hypotensive action of hydralazine can be antagonized by amphetamines, ephedrine, and other sympathomimetic agents, and the incidence of tachycardia and anginal pain increased

Additive hypotensive effects can occur with combined use of hydralazine and anesthetics, antidepressants, other antihypertensives, diuretics, quinidine, and procainamide

NURSING CONSIDERATIONS
See **Plan of Nursing Care 8** in this chapter. In addition:

Nursing Alert
- Closely observe patient receiving large amounts (dosage should not exceed 400 mg/day) for signs of developing lupus-like reaction (e.g., fever, myalgia, dermatoses, arthralgia, anemia, skin lesions). Drug should be discontinued and alternative antihypertensive medication used if signs develop. Most symptoms regress when drug is withdrawn, but residual effects may persist for years.

1. Note that hydralazine is available in three strengths in fixed combination with hydrochlorothiazide as Apresazide and others.

PATIENT EDUCATION
See **Plan of Nursing Care 8** in this chapter. In addition:
1. Suggest taking drug with meals because bioavailability is reportedly *enhanced* by concurrent ingestion of food, which may decrease first-pass hepatic metabolism.
2. Inform patient that headache and palpitations may occur during early stages of therapy, but usually disappear.
3. Teach significant others how to recognize changes in patient's mental acuity because these may indicate cerebral ischemia. The physician should be notified if these occur.
4. Instruct patient to report signs of hydralazine-induced peripheral neuritis (paresthesias, numbness, tingling) to physician. Pyridoxine (vitamin B_6) may be used to alleviate these symptoms.
5. Explain to patient that periodic blood counts, lupus erythematosus cell preparations, and antinuclear antibody titer determinations should be performed during prolonged therapy.

STEP 4 DRUGS

Guanadrel
Hylorel
Guanethidine
Ismelin

(CAN) Apo-Guanethidine

Guanadrel and guanethidine are two antihypertensive drugs with similar pharmacologic and toxicologic properties. Yet, guanadrel is generally classified as a step 2 drug, whereas guanethidine is largely viewed as a step 4 drug. Although both drugs are effective in the treatment of severe, refractory hypertension, guanadrel has been employed successfully in treating mild to moderate hypertension. It should, however, be reserved for patients who have not responded to other step 2 drugs.

MECHANISM
Accumulate in peripheral adrenergic nerve endings, where they inhibit norepinephrine release in response to nerve stimulation; a gradual depletion of norepinephrine stores in the nerve endings ensues, resulting in a prolonged reduction in heart rate and peripheral vascular resistance; venous return is diminished, cardiac output is reduced, and plasma renin activity is decreased; blood pressure reduction is greater in the standing than prone position, and orthostatic effects are common and can result in significant dizziness and weakness; renal blood flow is reduced relative to blood flow to the heart and brain, thus sodium and water retention is significant; sensitivity of adrenergic receptors to circulating norepinephrine is enhanced due to impaired neuronal uptake

USES
Treatment of moderate to severe hypertension not adequately controlled by other antihypertensive drugs. (Although guanadrel has been used for milder degrees of hypertension, it should be viewed as an alternative drug, at best, to other step 2 antihypertensive drugs)

Treatment of renal hypertension, including that secondary to renal artery stenosis and pyelonephritis

DOSAGE
Guanadrel

Initially, 10 mg/day; increase gradually until optimal effect is seen; usual dosage range is 20 mg to 75 mg in twice daily doses

Guanethidine

Ambulatory patients: initially 10 mg/day; increase gradually every 5 to 7 days to achieve optimal response; usual dose is 25 mg to 50 mg/day in a single dose

Hospitalized patients: initially 10 mg to 50 mg, depending on other antihypertensive drugs being used; increase by 10 mg to 25 mg every 2 to 4 days until desired response is obtained

Children: initially 0.2 mg/kg/day as a single oral dose; increase by 0.2 mg/kg/day increments every 7 to 10 days; maximum dose is 3 mg/kg/day

FATE
Guanethidine is poorly but consistently absorbed orally; peak effect occurs within 8 hours of a single dose; half-life is 5 days, so drug accumulates slowly; partially metabolized by the liver and excreted as active drug and inactive metabolites primarily by the kidneys

Guanadrel is rapidly absorbed orally and attains peak plasma concentration in 1.5 to 2 hours; effects are noted within 2 hours and maximal blood pressure decreases occur within 4 to 6 hours; excreted primarily in the urine, approximately 40% as unchanged drug

COMMON SIDE EFFECTS
Fatigue, headache, faintness, drowsiness, nocturia, urinary urgency, increased bowel movements, diarrhea, shortness of breath on exertion, palpitations, bradycardia, fluid retention, ejaculation disturbances

SIGNIFICANT ADVERSE REACTIONS
Nausea, vomiting, paresthesias, incontinence, dermatitis, anorexia, constipation, leg cramps, hair loss, nasal congestion, blurred vision, asthma, chest pains, myalgia, tremor, depression, and cardiac irregularities

CONTRAINDICATIONS
Pheochromocytoma, congestive heart failure not caused by hypertension, and concurrent use with MAO inhibitors. *Cautious use* in patients with fever, bronchial asthma, renal disease, coronary insufficiency, recent myocardial infarction, cerebral vascular disease, colitis, or peptic ulcer, and during pregnancy

INTERACTIONS

The antihypertensive effects of guanethidine and guanadrel may be antagonized by amphetamines, antidepressants, antihistamines, antipsychotics (e.g., phenothiazines, thioxanthenes, haloperidol), cocaine, diethylpropion, ephedrine, MAO inhibitors, methylphenidate, oral contraceptives, and sympathomimetic agents

Enhanced hypotensive effects may be observed when guanethidine or guanadrel is given in combination with alcohol, diuretics, hydralazine, levodopa, methotrimeprazine, propranolol, quinidine, reserpine, or vasodilator drugs

Excessive bradycardia can occur if guanethidine or guanadrel is used in combination with digitalis drugs

Guanethidine or guanadrel may impair the hyposecretory effect of anticholinergics

Guanethidine or guanadrel may exert an additive hypoglycemic effect with insulin or oral antidiabetic drugs

Increased responses to adrenergic agents (e.g., catecholamines, phenylephrine, metaraminol) may occur with guanethidine or guanadrel

NURSING CONSIDERATIONS

See **Plan of Nursing Care 8** in this chapter. In addition:
1. Assess patient's sexual health throughout therapy by providing supportive, nonthreatening opportunities to discuss concerns. Drug-related sexual dysfunctions may not be reported but may be responsible for noncompliance.

PATIENT EDUCATION

See **Plan of Nursing Care 8** in this chapter. In addition:
1. Instruct patient to inform physician of development of persistent diarrhea or sudden weight gain or edema. Dosage adjustment or additional medication may be required.
2. Instruct patient to be alert for development of adverse reactions such as urinary hesitancy or retention, weakness, and bradycardia, and to report these effects promptly.
3. Inform patient that periodic blood counts and liver and kidney function tests are advisable when therapy is prolonged.
4. Explain that physician or dentist in charge should be informed of drug use prior to surgery. If possible, drug should be withdrawn 48 to 72 hours before the use of general anesthetics to reduce the possibility of vascular collapse and cardiac arrest.
5. Explain that drug has prolonged duration of action. Dosage adjustments should be made carefully, and sufficient time should be allowed between dosage changes (e.g., 3–5 days) for effects to become manifest.
6. Inform patient that a diuretic is often given concurrently to minimize sodium and water retention as well as to enhance hypotensive response.
7. Encourage patient on antihyperglycemic medication to monitor blood sugar carefully because guanadrel or guanethidine may have additive hypoglycemic effects.
8. Warn patient that alcohol may intensify the hypotensive reaction.

Minoxidil

Loniten

MECHANISM

Direct relaxation of arteriolar smooth muscle, possibly due to blockade of calcium uptake *via* the cell membrane, thus decreasing peripheral vascular resistance—little effect on venous tone; microcirculatory blood flow is maintained in all systemic vascular beds; does not enter CNS or interfere with vasomotor reflexes; therefore does not elicit orthostatic hypotension; reflexly increases heart rate and cardiac output, renin secretion, and salt and water retention; topical application (as Rogaine) may increase hair growth in balding areas but effect lasts only as long as drug is applied

USES

Treatment of severe hypertension not manageable by maximum doses of a diuretic plus two other antihypertensive drugs; usually given together with a diuretic or a beta blocker, or both; methyldopa and clonidine have also been used concurrently

Treatment of male pattern baldness (alopecia areata, androgenic alopecia) based on drug's ability to increase growth of fine body hair (see Common Side Effects)

DOSAGE

(Oral)

Adults: initially 5 mg/day as a single dose; increase stepwise to 40 mg/day in divided doses, or until optimal control is attained; usual range is 10 mg to 40 mg/day (maximum is 100 mg/day)

Usually given with a diuretic to minimize fluid retention and with a beta blocker to reduce reflex bradycardia.

Children (under 12): initially, 0.2 mg/kg/day as a single dose; increase in 50% to 100% increments until optimal control is attained; usual range is 0.25 mg/kg to 1.0 mg/kg/day (maximum is 50 mg/day)

FATE

Well absorbed from the GI tract; maximum plasma levels occur within 60 minutes, effects are maximal in 2 to 3 hours and persist up to 24 hours; half-life is approximately 4 hours; almost completely metabolized in the liver and excreted principally in the urine; does not bind to plasma proteins

COMMON SIDE EFFECTS

Hypertrichosis (elongation, thickening, and enhanced pigmentation of fine body hair—80% of patients within 3–6 wk), temporary edema, ECG (i.e., T wave) changes *not* associated with other symptoms, sweating, headache, temporary edema

SIGNIFICANT ADVERSE REACTIONS

> **WARNING**
> Use only in severe hypertension because serious adverse reactions have occurred. Pericardial effusion, occasionally progressing to tamponade, has been reported, and anginal symptoms may be exacerbated

Nausea; vomiting; fatigue; pericardial effusion; tamponade; reflex tachycardia; breast tenderness; temporary decreases in hemoglobin, hematocrit, and erythrocytes; increases in alkaline phosphatase and serum creatinine; hypersensitivity reactions

CONTRAINDICATIONS

Pheochromocytoma, acute myocardial infarction, dissecting aortic aneurysm. *Cautious use* in patients with cardiac disease, renal or hepatic insufficiency, in edematous states, and in pregnant or nursing women

INTERACTIONS

Minoxidil may markedly worsen the degree of orthostatic hypotension caused by guanethidine

NURSING CONSIDERATIONS

See **Plan of Nursing Care 8** in this chapter. In addition:

Nursing Alerts

- Closely monitor patient for development of adverse reactions. Minoxidil should be administered only under close supervision to patient with severe hypertension who has not responded to maximum doses of a diuretic plus two other antihypertensive drugs.
- Carefully assess patient for evidence of a pericardial disorder; if one is suspected, echocardiographic studies should be performed. Pericardial effusion occurs in about 3% of treated patients not on dialysis, especially those with impaired renal function.
- When minoxidil is used in patient already receiving guanethidine, continually monitor blood pressure following minoxidil administration to detect a too-large or too-rapid drop. The patient should be hospitalized.

1. Monitor fluid and electrolyte balance, intake–output ratio, and body weight.
2. Help to evaluate patient's response to drug. At least 3 days should elapse between dosage adjustments to permit the full response to a given dose to become manifest.

PATIENT EDUCATION

See **Plan of Nursing Care 8** in this chapter. In addition:
1. Stress the importance of taking other antihypertensive medications exactly as prescribed along with minoxidil to increase drug's effectiveness and to reduce untoward reactions. Patient should not discontinue any other drugs without consulting drug prescriber.
2. Teach patient how to detect and report increased pulse rate (20 or more beats/min over normal), rapid weight gain, swelling in the extremities, dyspnea, or chest pain. If these occur, a dosage adjustment is indicated.
3. Inform patient that fine body hair will probably increase and darken within 3 to 6 weeks (80% incidence). While bothersome, this is not associated with hormonal changes and is probably not dangerous. It is first noticeable in eyebrows, sideburns, and temple area, later extending to back, arms, and legs. This condition regresses and eventually disappears within 2 to 6 months after treatment is discontinued.

DRUGS FOR HYPERTENSIVE EMERGENCIES

Hypertensive emergencies, or marked elevations in blood pressure, require immediate treatment to avoid serious and often life-threatening complications. A number of drugs are available to rapidly lower blood pressure, and they are commonly administered IV, frequently with or following a diuretic. Among the drugs indicated for hypertensive emergencies that have been discussed previously are trimethaphan, a ganglionic blocking agent (reviewed in Chap. 11), and methyldopa, hydralazine, and labetalol, three orally effective antihypertensive drugs, discussed in this chapter, that can be given IV in acute hypertension. The other drugs frequently used in acute hypertensive emergencies are diazoxide parenteral and nitroprusside; these are considered in detail below.

Diazoxide, Parenteral

Hyperstat IV

MECHANISM

Direct relaxation of arteriolar smooth muscle, resulting in vasodilation; reflexly increases heart rate, stroke volume and cardiac output; renal blood flow is increased; causes sodium and water retention and inhibits tubular secretion of uric acid; elicits hyperglycemia by inhibiting insulin secretion from the pancreas; elevates serum free fatty acids

USES

Acute treatment (IV) of hypertensive emergencies and severe hypertension
Production of controlled hypotension during surgery
Management of hypoglycemia caused by hyperinsulinism (e.g., islet cell carcinoma); available in *oral* form as Proglycem—see Chapter 42

DOSAGE

(IV)
1 mg/kg to 3 mg/kg (maximum 150 mg per injection) by IV push within 30 seconds or less; repeat at intervals of 5 to 15 minutes until a satisfactory response is attained, then at 4- to 24-hour intervals until a regimen of oral antihypertensive drug becomes effective

Note: Do not give for longer than 10 days or by IV infusion

FATE

Onset usually within 1 to 2 minutes, with maximal blood pressure decrease in 5 minutes; pressure then slowly increases over 2 to 12 hours; extensively bound to serum proteins (90%); excreted slowly through the kidneys; plasma half-life is 20 to 36 hours

COMMON SIDE EFFECTS

Nausea, hypotension, dizziness, weakness (most often seen with large doses); repeated injections can result in fluid retention and hyperglycemia

SIGNIFICANT ADVERSE REACTIONS

Cardiovascular: myocardial and cerebral ischemia, palpitations, arrhythmias, sweating, flushing, supraventricular tachycardia
CNS: (secondary to blood flow changes in the brain) confusion, headache, lightheadedness, somnolence, hearing impairment, euphoria, convulsions, paralysis
GI: abdominal pain, vomiting, anorexia, parotid swelling, salivation, dry mouth, constipation or diarrhea, ileus
Dermatologic/hypersensitivity: rash, fever, leukopenia
Respiratory: cough, dyspnea, choking sensation
Other: pancreatitis, weakness, lacrimation, cellulitis, pain along injected vein, back pain, nocturia, hyperuricemia

CONTRAINDICATIONS

Hypersensitivity to thiazide diuretics, coronary artery disease, compensatory hypertension (e.g., aortic coarctation, arteriovenous shunt), and dissecting aortic aneurysm. *Cautious use* in the presence of impaired cerebral or coronary circulation, hyperglycemia, or congestive heart failure and in pregnant or nursing women

INTERACTIONS

Combined use of diuretics with diazoxide may intensify its hyperglycemic, hyperuricemic, and antihypertensive effects

Diazoxide may potentiate the action of other highly protein-bound drugs (e.g., oral anticoagulants, antiinflammatory agents, sulfonamides, phenytoin, quinidine, propranolol) by displacing them from binding sites

Chlorpromazine and furosemide may potentiate the hyperglycemic effect of diazoxide

An increased hypotensive response can occur when diazoxide is used along with other antihypertensive drugs such as vasodilators (e.g., nitrites, hydralazine), catecholamine-depleting drugs (e.g., reserpine), beta blockers, or centrally acting agents

Diazoxide can accelerate the hepatic metabolism of phenytoin

Diazoxide may blunt the effectiveness of oral hypoglycemic agents by impairing insulin secretion

NURSING CONSIDERATIONS

See **Plan of Nursing Care 8** in this chapter. In addition:

Nursing Alerts

- When drug is administered, have vasopressors (e.g., metaraminol) on hand to treat marked hypotension. Smaller than recommended doses can be given by IV injection with less danger of sharp drop in blood pressure. IV infusion may be effective if patient is receiving other antihypertensive drugs concurrently.
- Assist with drug administration as needed. Drug should be given only in a peripheral vein, and extravasation should be avoided because solution is alkaline and very irritating.
- Keep patient recumbent during, and for at least 30 minutes after, injection. Monitor blood pressure closely until stabilized, then hourly during expected duration of effect. Check blood pressure with patient in upright position before ending surveillance.
- With repeated injections, assess patient for, and inform physician of, signs of developing congestive heart failure (cough, dyspnea, edema, distended neck veins, rales) and renal or bowel dysfunction (urinary hesitancy, decreased urine output, constipation, abdominal distention).

1. Ensure that appropriate blood glucose and electrolyte determinations are obtained (usually at start of therapy and frequently during repeated dosing).
2. When diuretics are used in conjunction with diazoxide, keep patient supine for 8 to 10 hours because of added hypotensive effect. Concomitant diuretic use prevents sodium and water retention elicited by diazoxide and increases the antihypertensive effect.
3. Monitor diabetic patient for signs of hyperglycemia. Diazoxide-induced hyperglycemia is usually transient, reversible, and clinically insignificant in the nondiabetic patient, but the dosage of antidiabetic drugs may need to be adjusted in the diabetic patient.
4. Be prepared to administer a beta blocker (e.g., propranolol) if reflex tachycardia and increased cardiac output become clinically significant.

Nitroprusside

Nipride, Nitropress

MECHANISM

Direct relaxation of arteriolar and venular smooth muscle, resulting in marked reduction of arterial pressure, slight reflex increase in heart rate, and a small decrease in cardiac output; renin activity is markedly increased

In the presence of left ventricular failure, reduces both afterload (aortic resistance) and preload (ventricular filling pressure), improves cardiac output, and reduces pulmonary capillary wedge pressure. Heart rate is essentially unchanged

USES

Emergency treatment of hypertensive crises (*Note:* Oral antihypertensive medication should be initiated while blood pressure is being controlled by IV nitroprusside)

Production of controlled hypotension during surgery or anesthesia

Adjunctive therapy of severe, refractory congestive heart failure, treatment of lactic acidosis due to reduced peripheral perfusion, and attenuation of the vasoconstrictor effects of norepinephrine and dopamine

DOSAGE

Adults and children: used only by IV infusion; 3 μg/kg/minute (range 0.5 μg/kg–10/μg/kg/min) of a 50 mg in 250 mL to 1000 mL of 5% dextrose in water dilution

FATE

Immediate onset of action (30–60 seconds); effects are maximum within 1 to 2 minutes; upon termination of the infusion, blood pressure can return to pretreatment levels within several minutes; decomposes to cyanide in the blood which either reacts with methemoglobin to form cyanmethemoglobin or is converted in the liver and kidneys to thiocyanate, which is slowly cleared by the kidneys and has a half-life of 4 days in patients with normal renal function; in patients with impaired renal function, prolonged infusion or excessive doses can cause cyanide toxicity

COMMON SIDE EFFECTS

(Usually result of too-rapid infusion) Nausea, sweating, headache, restlessness, muscle twitching, palpitations, dizziness, substernal discomfort

SIGNIFICANT ADVERSE REACTIONS

(Usually due to thiocyanate accumulation [see Fate] especially in patients with impaired renal function) Blurred vision, tinnitus, dyspnea, ataxia, diminished reflexes, mydriasis, delirium, and convulsions; also, hypothyroidism, methemoglobinemia

CONTRAINDICATIONS

Compensatory hypertension (arteriovenous shunt, aortic coarctation), and inadequate cerebral circulation. *Cautious use* in patients with hypothyroidism, renal or hepatic impairment, anemia, hypovolemia, and in elderly or poor surgical risk patients

INTERACTIONS

Enhanced hypotension can occur if nitroprusside is given to patients receiving other antihypertensive medications, circulatory depressants, and volatile liquid anesthetics

Tolbutamide may decrease the effects of nitroprusside

NURSING CONSIDERATIONS

See **Plan of Nursing Care 8** in this Chapter. In addition:

Nursing Alerts

- Administer *only* by slow IV infusion. Determine blood pressure frequently, and adjust rate of flow to achieve desired response. Do not allow systolic pressure to go below 70 mm Hg.
- Do not exceed infusion rate of 10 μg/kg/min. If blood pressure is not reduced within 10 minutes at this dose, drug should be discontinued. Dosage should be reduced in patient already receiving antihypertensive medication.
- Have drugs on hand to treat cyanide intoxication in case of overdose because nitroprusside is metabolized to cyanide, then to thiocyanate. If treatment is continued longer than 2 to 3 days, thiocyanate blood levels should be determined; drug should be discontinued if levels exceed 10 mg/100 mL. To treat overdosage, 2.5 mL to 5 mL/minute of 3% sodium nitrite is injected to a total of 15 mL, followed by sodium thiosulfate 12.5 g/50 mL of 5% dextrose over 10 minutes by IV infusion. Treatment is repeated at one half of these doses if signs of overdose reappear.

1. Discard any solution that is strongly colored (freshly prepared solutions have a faint brownish tinge), and use solutions within 4 hours after preparation. Cover infusion container with opaque material to exclude light, which can increase rate of decomposition to cyanide ion.
2. Do *not* add other drugs or preservatives to infusion solution.
3. Check infusion site for indications of extravasation (e.g., swelling, pain) because irritation may occur.
4. When drug is used to produce controlled hypotension during surgery, ensure that preexisting anemia or hypovolemia has been corrected prior to nitroprusside administration.
5. Expect patient to be started on oral antihypertensive medication as soon as possible. Oral drug may be started while blood pressure is being brought under control by nitroprusside.

Trimethaphan

Arfonad

Trimethaphan is a ganglionic blocking agent used parenterally for rapid blood pressure reduction. In addition to blocking ganglionic receptor sites, it may also exert a direct relaxant effect on peripheral vascular smooth muscle. Onset of action is rapid, and the effects persist for only a short time after the infusion is terminated. Trimethaphan is discussed in Chapter 11.

USES

Production of controlled hypotension during surgery
Short-term management of hypertensive emergencies, (e.g., dissection of the aorta)
Emergency treatment of pulmonary edema in patients with pulmonary hypertension

DOSAGE

Dilute 10 mL of drug to 500 mL 5% dextrose injection; infuse initially at a rate of 3 mL to 4 mL/min and adjust to desired blood pressure control; range is 0.3 mL to 6 mL/min

MISCELLANEOUS ANTIHYPERTENSIVE DRUGS

Mecamylamine

Inversine

Mecamylamine is a potent, orally effective ganglionic blocking agent that exerts a considerable orthostatic hypotensive effect. Owing primarily to its many side effects, it is used only for the control of severe hypertension in patients not responding to a combination of other antihypertensive drugs. The drug is reviewed further in Chapter 11

DOSAGE

Initially 2.5 mg twice a day; increase by 2.5 mg every 2 days until desired response is attained; average dose is 25 mg/day in 2 to 4 divided doses; usually given after meals, with the larger fraction of the dose administered later in the day

Metyrosine

Demser

MECHANISM

Inhibits tyrosine hydroxylase, the enzyme that catalyzes the conversion of tyrosine to dopa, which is the initial reaction in the biosynthesis of the catecholamines dopamine, norepinephrine, and epinephrine. Therefore, catecholamine production is reduced.

USES

Symptomatic treatment of patients with pheochromocytoma (a tumor of the sympathetic nervous system, usually of the adrenal medulla)

Preoperative preparation
Management of patients when surgery is contraindicated
Chronic therapy of malignant pheochromocytoma

DOSAGE

Initially 250 mg 4 times/day; increase by 250 mg to 500 mg every day as needed to a maximum of 4 g/day in divided doses

COMMON SIDE EFFECTS

Sedation, extrapyramidal symptoms (drooling, fine tremor, speech difficulties), diarrhea

SIGNIFICANT ADVERSE REACTIONS

Anxiety, depression, hallucinations, confusion, headache, nasal congestion, decreased salivation, vomiting, dry mouth, abdominal pain, impotence, galactorrhea, breast swelling, crystalluria, dysuria, hematuria, hypersensitivity reactions (urticaria, rash, pharyngeal edema)

INTERACTIONS

Extrapyramidal effects may be intensified by concurrent use of phenothiazines or other antipsychotic drugs
Metyrosine may have additive effects with alcohol or other CNS depressants

NURSING CONSIDERATIONS

See **Plan of Nursing Care 8** in this chapter. In addition:

Nursing Alerts
- Ensure that patient receiving metyrosine maintains adequate intravascular fluid volume postoperatively to avoid hypotension and reduced perfusion of vital organs.
- Continually monitor blood pressure and ECG during surgery because arrhythmias can occur. Have lidocaine and a beta-adrenergic blocking agent on hand.
- Observe for, and inform physician of, first signs of drooling, speech difficulty, fine tremors, diarrhea, disorientation, or jaw stiffness.

1. Encourage patient to maintain fluid intake sufficient to achieve daily urine volume of 2000 mL or more to minimize danger of drug crystallization in urine.
2. Interpret results of urinary catecholamine measurements cautiously because the drug can interfere with them.
3. If patient's blood pressure is not adequately controlled with metyrosine, be prepared to add an alpha-adrenergic blocking agent to drug regimen.

Pargyline
Eutonyl

Pargyline is an infrequently used oral antihypertensive drug that exerts predominantly an orthostatic effect. It is an MAO inhibitor (see Chap. 24), but the exact mechanism of its hypotensive action is unknown. Pargyline has been used in the treatment of moderate to severe hypertension, usually in combination with diuretics or other antihypertensives.

Commonly noted side effects are dry mouth, insomnia, nervousness, weakness, palpitations, dizziness, sweating, muscle twitching, blurred vision, fluid retention, and mild constipation. Because pargyline is an MAO inhibitor, all of the adverse reactions listed for the other MAO inhibitors in Chapter 24 are theoretically possible with this drug.

DOSAGE
Initially 25 mg/day in a single dose; increase by 10-mg increments weekly until desired response; usual dosage range is 25 mg to 50 mg daily

NURSING CONSIDERATIONS

See MAO inhibitors (Chap. 24) and **Plan of Nursing Care 8** in this chapter. In addition:

Nursing Alerts
- Do not administer pargyline to patient receiving methyldopa or guanethidine because severe CNS stimulation and hypertension can occur.
- Closely observe patient because risk of severe untoward reactions is considerable. Pargyline should be used only when all other less toxic antihypertensive agents have proved ineffective or intolerable.

1. Monitor blood pressure with patient in standing position to determine need for dosage adjustment because drug exerts a strong orthostatic effect.

PATIENT EDUCATION

See MAO inhibitors (Chap. 24) and **Plan of Nursing Care 8** in this chapter. In addition:

1. Instruct patient to notify physician immediately if faintness, dizziness, palpitations, or weakness occur; dosage adjustment is indicated to alleviate orthostatic hypotension.

Phenoxybenzamine
Dibenzyline

An orally effective, long-acting, nonselective alpha-adrenergic blocking agent indicated for the control of episodes of hypertension and sweating associated with pheochromocytoma. Phenoxybenzamine produces a chemical sympathectomy, interrupting impulse transmission through alpha-adrenergic receptor sites, thereby reducing blood pressure and increasing blood flow to the skin, mucosa, and abdominal organs. In addition to its use in pheochromocytoma, it has been shown effective in disorders of the bladder that cause impaired urination.

Principal adverse reactions with phenoxybenzamine are nasal congestion, orthostatic hypotension, miosis, tachycardia, and impaired ejaculation. These effects are due to adrenergic blockade and generally disappear with time. Phenoxybenzamine should be used with *caution* in patients with coronary or cerebral vascular insufficiency or renal damage. Phenoxybenzamine is discussed in detail in Chapter 13.

DOSAGE
Initially 10 mg/day orally; increase by 10 mg every 4 days until desired response is achieved; usual dosage range is 20 mg to 60 mg/day

Note: At least 2 weeks generally are required to attain significant improvement, and possibly several more weeks are required for full benefits

Phentolamine
Regitine
(CAN) Rogitine

Phentolamine is a nonselective alpha-adrenergic blocking agent used by injection to control hypertensive episodes that might occur in patients with pheochromocytoma during surgery for removal of the chromaffin tumor. The drug has also been employed to prevent the dermal necrosis and sloughing that can occur upon extravasation during IV infusion of epinephrine, norepinephrine, or dopamine solutions. Treatment of rebound hypertension during withdrawal of antihypertensive medications has also been accomplished by injection of phentolamine. In addition to its alpha-blocking action, the drug has a direct relaxant effect on vascular smooth muscle.

Tachycardia and cardiac arrhythmias may occur with use of phentolamine. Other adverse effects include weakness, dizziness, flushing, orthostatic hypotension, nasal stuffiness, vomiting, and diarrhea.

DOSAGE
Hypertension: IV, IM, 5 mg (adults); 1 mg (children)
Necrosis/sloughing: 10 mg/L of IV infusion solution, or 5 mg to 10 mg/10 mL saline injected into area of extravasation

Selected Bibliography

Alexander JK: Managing the elderly patient with hypertension. Mod Med 55(1):58, 1987

Caris TN: Hypertension in older patients: What drugs to use and when. Geriatrics 37:38, 1982

Dollery CT: Hypertension and new antihypertensive drugs: Clinical perspectives. Fed Prod 42:207, 1983

Drayer JI, Weber MA: The impact of antihypertensives on cardiovascular risks. Drug Ther 13(4):116, 1983

Drugs for hypertension. Med Lett Drugs Ther 29:1, 1987

Ferguson RK, Vlasses PH, Riley LJ: Captopril and enalapril: Angiotensin converting enzyme (ACE) inhibitors. Ration Drug Ther 18:1, 1984

Finnerty FA: Step-down treatment of mild systemic hypertension. Am J Cardiol 53:1304, 1984

Freis ED: Should mild hypertension be treated? N Engl J Med 307:306, 1982

Frishman WH, Stroh JA, Greenberg S et al: Calcium channel blockers in systemic hypertension. Med Clin North Am 72:449, 1988

Frolich ED, Cooper RA, Lewis RJ: Review of the overall experience of captopril in hypertension. Arch Intern Med 144:1441, 1984

Hypertension Detection and Follow-up Program Cooperative Group: The effect of treatment on mortality in mild hypertension. N Engl J Med 307:1976, 1982

Johnson BE: Choices in antihypertensive therapy: Beta blockers or calcium channel antagonists. Mod Med 57(7):56, 1989

Johnson CI, Arnolda L, Hiwatari M: Angiotensin-converting enzyme inhibitors in the treatment of hypertension. Drugs 27:271, 1984

Kaplan NM: New approaches to the therapy of mild hypertension. Am J Cardiol 51:621, 1983

Kelley M, Mongiello R: Hypertension in pregnancy: Labor, delivery and postpartum. Am J Nurs 83:813, 1983

Kirschenbaum HL, Rosenberg JM: Emergency antihypertensives. RN 46:53, 1983

Lees KR: Angiotensin-converting enzyme inhibitors. Ration Drug Ther 22(9):1, 1988

Reichgott M et al: The nurse practitioner's role in complex patient management: Hypertension. J Natl Med Assoc 75:1197, 1983

Spivack C, Ocken S, Frishman WH: Calcium antagonists: Clinical use in the treatment of systemic hypertension. Drugs 25:154, 1983

Westfall TC, Meldrum MJ: Alterations in the release of norepinephrine at the vascular neuroeffector junction in hypertension. Annu Rev Pharmacol Toxicol 25:621, 1985

SUMMARY. ANTIHYPERTENSIVE DRUGS

Drug	Preparations	Usual Dosage Range
Step 1 Drugs		
Diuretics	See Chapter 37	
Beta Blockers		
Acebutolol Sectral	Capsules: 200 mg, 400 mg	Initially 400 mg in a single or 2 divided doses; usual dosage range 400 mg–800 mg/day
Atenolol Tenormin	Tablets: 50 mg, 100 mg	Initially 50 mg/day in a single dose; increase to 100 mg/day in 2 wk if response is inadequate
Carteolol Cartrol	Tablets: 2.5 mg, 5 mg	Initially, 2.5 mg/day in a single dose; may increase up to 10 mg/day if needed
Metoprolol Lopressor	Tablets: 50 mg, 100 mg Injection: 1 mg/mL	Initially 100 mg/day in a single or divided doses; increase at weekly intervals; usual maintenance range 100 mg–450 mg/day
Nadolol Corgard	Tablets: 40 mg, 80 mg, 120 mg, 160 mg	Initially 40 mg once daily; increase in 40-mg–80-mg increments; usual dose is 80 mg–320 mg/day
Penbutolol Levatol	Tablets: 20 mg	20 mg–40 mg once daily
Pindolol Visken	Tablets: 5 mg, 10 mg	Initially 10 mg twice a day or 5 mg 3 times a day; adjust in increments of 10 mg/day at 2–3-wk intervals
Propranolol Inderal, Inderal LA	Tablets: 10 mg, 20 mg, 40 mg, 60 mg, 80 mg, 90 mg Long-acting capsules: 60 mg, 80 mg, 120 mg, 160 mg Injection: 1 mg/mL	Initially 40 mg twice a day or 80 mg once daily; increase gradually until optimal response is achieved; usual maintenance range is 160 mg–480 mg/day in 2–3 divided doses, or once daily with long-acting capsule
Timolol Blocadren	Tablets: 5 mg, 10 mg, 20 mg	Initially 10 mg twice a day; increase gradually; usual maintenance range is 20 mg–40 mg/day
Angiotensin-Converting Enzyme Inhibitors	See Table 31-3	

Continued

SUMMARY. ANTIHYPERTENSIVE DRUGS (continued)

Drug	Preparations	Usual Dosage Range
Step 2 Drugs		
Labetalol Normodyne, Trandate	Tablets: 100 mg, 200 mg, 300 mg Injection: 5 mg/mL	*Oral:* initially 100 mg twice a day; usual maintenance dose 200 mg–400 mg twice a day *IV:* 20 mg given over 2 min *or* 2 mg/min by IV infusion
Clonidine Catapres	Tablets: 0.1 mg, 0.2 mg, 0.3 mg Transdermal patch: release 0.1 mg, 0.2 mg, or 0.3 mg/24 h	*Oral:* initially 0.1 mg twice a day; increase by 0.1 mg–0.2 mg/day to desired response (maximum 2.4 mg/day) *Topical:* apply 1 patch every 7 days; begin with 0.1 mg patch and increase as necessary
Guanabenz Wytensin	Tablets: 4 mg, 8 mg	Initially 4 mg twice a day; increase in increments of 4 mg–8 mg every 1–2 wk; maximum dosage is 32 mg/day
Guanfacine Tenex	Tablets: 1 mg	Initially 1 mg/day; may increase up to 3 mg/day if necessary
Methyldopa Aldomet, Amodopa	Tablets: 125 mg, 250 mg, 500 mg Oral suspension: 250 mg/5 mL Injection: 250 mg methyldopate HCl/5 mL	*Oral:* Adults: 250 mg 3–4 times/day; adjust to desired response; usual dosage range is 500–2000 mg/day in 2–4 divided doses Children: 10 mg/kg/day in 2–4 divided doses (maximum 65 mg/kg/day or 3 g) *IV infusion:* Adults: 250 mg–500 mg at 6-h intervals infused over 30–60 min; maximum dose 1 g every 6 h Children: 20 mg–40 mg/kg in divided doses every 6 h; maximum dose 3 g/day
Prazosin Minipress	Capsules: 1 mg, 2 mg, 5 mg	Initially 1 mg 2–3 times/day; increase *slowly* to desired level, up to 20 mg/day
Terazosin Hytrin	Tablets: 1 mg, 2 mg, 5 mg	Initially 1 mg at bedtime; usual dosage range 1 mg–5 mg daily; maximum 20 mg/day
Calcium Channel Blockers		
Diltiazem Cardizem	Tablets: 30 mg, 60 mg, 90 mg, 120 mg Capsules (sustained-release): 60 mg, 90 mg, 120 mg	60 mg–120 mg sustained-release capsule twice daily; increase as necessary; usual dosage range is 240 mg–360 mg daily
Nicardipine Cardene	Capsules: 20 mg, 30 mg	Initially 20 mg 3 times/day; usual range is 20 mg–40 mg 3 times/day
Verapamil Calan, Isoptin	Tablets: 40 mg, 80 mg, 120 mg Tablets (sustained-release): 240 mg Injection: 5 mg/2 ml	Initially, 80 mg 3 times/day; increase gradually as needed up to 360 mg/day
Rauwolfia Alkaloids	*See* Table 31-4	
Step 3 Drugs		
Hydralazine Alazine, Apresoline	Tablets: 10 mg, 25 mg, 50 mg, 100 mg Injection: 20 mg/mL	Oral: initially 10 mg 4 times/day for 2–4 days; increase to 25 mg 4 times/day for balance of first week, then to 50 mg 4 times/day if necessary IM, IV: initially, 5 mg–10 mg; titrate upward slowly as needed; *Children*— 0.1 mg/kg to 0.2 mg/kg every 4 h–6 h

Continued

SUMMARY. ANTIHYPERTENSIVE DRUGS (continued)

Drug	Preparations	Usual Dosage Range
Step 4 Drugs		
Guanethidine Ismelin	Tablets: 10 mg, 25 mg	Ambulatory: 10 mg/day initially; increase slowly every 5–7 days; usual dose is 25 mg–50 mg/day Hospital: 10 mg–50 mg initially; increase by 10 mg–25 mg every 2–4 days
Guanadrel Hylorel	Tablets: 10 mg, 25 mg	Initially 10 mg/day; increase gradually until optimal effect is reached; usual dosage range is 20 mg–75 mg daily in 2 divided doses
Minoxidil Loniten	Tablets: 2.5 mg, 10 mg	Adults: initially 5 mg/day; increase gradually until optimal control is attained (usual range 10 mg–40 mg/day) Children (under 12): initially 0.2 mg/kg/day; increase in 50% to 100% increments (usual range is 0.25 mg/kg–1 mg/kg/day)
Drugs for Hypertensive Emergencies		
Diazoxide Parenteral Hyperstat IV	Injection: 300 mg/20 mL	1 mg/kg to 3 mg/kg (maximum 150 mg) by IV push within 30 sec; repeat at 5–15-min intervals
Nitroprusside Nipride, Nitropress	Injection: 50 mg/vial	IV infusion *only*: 3 µg/kg/min (range 0.5 µg/kg–10 µg/kg/min) of a 50 mg in 250 mL–1000 mL 5% dextrose in water dilution
Trimethaphan Arfonad	Injection: 50 mg/mL	Dilute 10 mL of drug solution to 500 mL with 5% dextrose injection; infuse at a rate of 3 mL–4 mL/min (range is 0.3 mL–6 mL/min)
Miscellaneous Antihypertensive Drugs		
Mecamylamine Inversine	Tablets: 2.5 mg	Initially 2.5 mg twice a day; increase by 2.5 mg every 2 days until desired response; average dose is 25 mg/day in 3–4 divided doses
Metyrosine Demser	Capsules: 250 mg	Initially 250 mg 4 times/day; increase by 250 mg–500 mg every day to a maximum of 4 g/day
Pargyline Eutonyl	Tablets: 10 mg, 25 mg	Initially 25 mg/day in a single dose; increase by 10 mg/wk until desired response is achieved; usual range is 25 mg–50 mg/day
Phenoxybenzamine Dibenzyline	Capsules: 10 mg	Initially 10 mg/day, increase by 10 mg/4 days until optimal effects are noted; usual range is 20 mg–60 mg/day
Phentolamine Regitine	Injection: 5 mg/ampule	*Hypertension* IV, IM: 5 mg (adults); 1 mg (children) Prevent necrosis: 10 mg/L of infusion solution Treat necrosis: 5 mg–10 mg/10 mL saline injected into area

32 ANTIANGINAL AGENTS/VASODILATORS

Drugs that can improve blood flow through circulatory vessels by increasing their diameter are termed *vasodilators*. These agents are usually effective in reducing the incidence and severity of exertional pain in patients with coronary artery disease (e.g., angina) but are generally of limited clinical usefulness for improving circulation in peripheral vascular diseases. The drugs discussed in this chapter are therefore divided into those principally used for the treatment of angina pectoris and those usually indicated for the treatment of peripheral and cerebrovascular insufficiency.

ANTIANGINAL AGENTS

Angina pectoris is a condition characterized by intermittent substernal (chest) pain, often of a "crushing" nature, which may remain localized in the sternal region or may radiate to other areas of the body (e.g., the left shoulder or left arm). The pain is the result of ischemia (reduced blood supply) in an area of the myocardium, leading to decreased cardiac oxygenation, especially during periods of exertion or stress.

Angina may be classified on the basis of the etiology of the myocardial ischemia as:

- *Classic, stable angina:* increased oxygen demand resulting from exercise, stress, physical exertion
- *Unstable angina:* pain occurs even at rest; probably owing to significantly compromised coronary blood flow
- *Vasospastic (Prinzmetal's) angina:* ischemia results from coronary vasospasm; death can occur from attendant arrhythmias

Acute anginal attacks are triggered when the oxygen demand of the heart exceeds the capacity of the coronary circulation to supply the needed oxygen. However, merely increasing myocardial blood flow via coronary artery dilation is not usually beneficial unless the workload on the heart is also reduced. Effective management of the anginal condition requires the use of drugs that can increase *overall* myocardial oxygenation. In fact, the primary effect of the vasodilators such as the nitrates used in the treatment of angina is reduction of *total* peripheral vascular resistance rather than selective dilation of coronary arteries. The resultant decrease in venous return to the heart and in systemic vascular resistance reduces the oxygen requirement of the myocardium and the workload on the anginal heart.

Drug therapy of angina is twofold: namely, to provide relief of pain during an acute anginal attack, and to decrease the overall frequency and severity of attacks by improving the oxygen supply:demand ratio. Treatment of an acute anginal attack is usually accomplished by sublingual administration of one of the rapid-acting nitrites or nitrates (e.g., nitroglycerin, isosorbide dinitrate), drugs that have a quick onset and a relatively short duration of action. Prophylaxis against anginal episodes can be conferred by use of longer-acting, orally effective nitrates (e.g., pentaerythritol, erythrityl), topical nitroglycerin, beta-adrenergic blockers, and calcium channel blockers.

While the efficacy of the rapid-acting agents in aborting an acute anginal attack is unquestioned, controversy surrounds the use of the long-acting nitrates as prophylactic drugs. Although clinical evidence suggests that these long-acting agents may improve exercise tolerance in some anginal patients, there are conflicting data on their efficacy in reducing the incidence and severity of anginal attacks when used repeatedly. Tolerance to the effects of nitrates develops rapidly with continued usage, and attempts to maintain stable plasma levels of these drugs with a *regular* dosing schedule invariably lead to loss of effectiveness, sometimes within a matter of days. Similarly, use of nitrates as transdermal patches or topical ointment quickly leads to a loss of improvement in exercise tolerance due to rapid development of tolerance to the drug. Many clinicians are now advocating "pulse" dosing of nitrates, in which the drugs are given for a portion of each day but the patient remains drug free for a given period each day, such as overnight. This dosing method reportedly results in much less tolerance and increased effectiveness.

A chemically unique type of compound, the calcium channel blocker, is also indicated for *prophylaxis* of anginal attacks. The calcium channel blockers act by reducing the influx of calcium through the so-called slow membrane channels, thus reducing the contractile activity of smooth muscle and cardiac muscle. They are effective in alleviating pain and improving exercise tolerance in many anginal patients while exhibiting a fairly low incidence of side effects. The calcium channel blockers are employed orally in chronic, stable angina as well as in the vasospastic (Prinzmetal's) variant form. In addition, verapamil reduces AV conduction and SA nodal automaticity and prevents abnormal impulse reentry at the AV node; it is also used IV in the management of supraventricular tachyarrhythmias, a condition in which the drug is now considered by many to be the drug of choice. This latter indication is reviewed in detail in Chapter 30. Calcium channel blockers are also useful in treating hypertension, and this aspect of their pharmacology in considered in Chapter 31.

The nitrites and nitrates are discussed as a group because they exhibit qualitatively similar actions; individual drugs are then listed in Table 32-1. The calcium channel blockers are likewise considered together; the individual drugs are then detailed in Table 32-2 and 32-3. Beta blockers useful in the prophylaxis of angina are also reviewed briefly.

Nitrites/Nitrates

Amyl nitrite	Nitroglycerin
Erythrityl tetranitrate	Pentaerythritol tetranitrate
Isosorbide dinitrate	

MECHANISM
Direct relaxing effect on vascular smooth muscle (probably due to increased synthesis of cyclic guanosine monophosphate—GMP), resulting in generalized vasodilation, venous effects predominate, resulting in pooling of blood in the great veins and reduced venous return, which lowers the left ventricular end-diastolic pressure (LVEDP), also known as the *preload*. Decreased venous return also leads to reduced cardiac output and lowered myocardial oxygen demand. Decline in LVEDP results

in improved blood flow to deeper (subendocardial) layers of the myocardium, which may be oxygen starved.

Relaxation of arteriolar smooth muscle occurs to a lesser extent, which lowers systemic vascular resistance and aortic impedance to left ventricular ejection (*afterload*), also reducing the workload on the heart. Pulmonary vascular pressures are reduced, and heart size is decreased.

Total coronary blood flow is probably not significantly increased by nitrites/nitrates; however, the drugs may cause a shunting or redistribution of flow to ischemic areas by dilation of collateral channels; most nonvascular smooth muscle is transiently relaxed, and reflex tachycardia due to a drop in blood pressure can occur

USES

Relief of pain of acute anginal attacks (rapid-acting drugs dosage forms [e.g., sublingual, translingual spray])

Prevention of anginal episodes and reduction in frequency and severity of acute attacks (long-acting or sustained-release forms of nitrates; transdermal nitroglycerin)

Reduction of cardiac work load in patients with myocardial infarction or congestive heart failure

Production of controlled hypotension or control of blood pressure during surgery (IV nitroglycerin)

DOSAGE

See Table 32-1

FATE

Onset with sublingual administration is 1 to 2 minutes; duration ranges from 30 to 45 minutes (nitroglycerin) to 2 hours (isosorbide); onset following oral ingestion is 20 to 30 minutes, with a duration of 4 to 6 hours for regular tablets or capsules, and perhaps up to 12 hours with sustained-release dosage forms. Topical administration (ointment, transdermal patch) produces effects within 30 to 60 minutes; initial duration of action is 4 to 6 hours with ointment, and up to 24 hours with transdermal patch; however, rapid tolerance occurs, and duration of action declines quickly with continued use; drugs are rapidly metabolized in the liver. Following oral administration, there is extensive first-pass hepatic metabolism, although hepatic enzyme activity can be saturated by large oral doses of these drugs; two metabolites have some vasodilator activity and longer plasma half-life than the parent compounds; metabolites are excreted in the urine

COMMON SIDE EFFECTS

(Most frequent with rapid-acting drugs) Headache, flushing, dizziness, palpitation, burning sensation in sublingual area

Topical application causes localized irritation

SIGNIFICANT ADVERSE REACTIONS

Orthostatic hypotension, tachycardia, vertigo, confusion, weakness, skin rash, and exfoliative dermatitis (rare)

Occasional hypersensitivity reaction marked by vomiting, profound weakness, restlessness, tachycardia, incontinence, syncope, perspiration, pallor, pronounced hypotension, and collapse

CONTRAINDICATIONS

Severe anemia, marked hypotension, increased intracranial pressure, cerebral hemorrhage, and acute stages of myocardial infarction. *Cautious use* in patients with hypotension, glaucoma, severe hepatic or renal disease and in pregnant or nursing women

INTERACTIONS

Hypotensive effects of nitrites and nitrates may be enhanced by alcohol, beta blockers, antihypertensives, narcotics, tricyclic antidepressants

Nitrates can potentiate the effects of antihistamines, tricyclic antidepressants, and other anticholinergic drugs

Cross-tolerance can occur between all nitrites and nitrates

Nitrites and nitrates can antagonize the pressor actions of sympathomimetic drugs

PATIENT EDUCATION

1. Encourage patient to avoid situations that might precipitate angina (e.g., stress, heavy exercise, smoking, overeating). Recommend, as appropriate, reduction in caloric intake and development of a program of regular exercise.
2. Recommend using sublingual nitroglycerin in anticipation of situations in which acute anginal episodes have predictably occurred.
3. Instruct patient to place sublingual tablets under the tongue. Long-acting tablets or capsules should be swallowed whole.
4. Advise patient to sit or lie down to take medication and to rest for 10 to 15 minutes afterward taking drug because dizziness, weakness, syncope, and other signs of orthostatic hypotension can occur following administration, especially sublingual.
5. Instruct patient to take additional sublingual tablets (up to 3) at 5-minute intervals if necessary. If pain is not relieved after 15 minutes, either a physician should be contacted immediately or patient should report to a hospital.
6. Reassure patient that headaches which may occur following drug administration usually disappear within 20 to 30 minutes. Prolonged headache can be relieved with analgesics.
7. Discuss danger associated with alcohol consumption in conjunction with nitroglycerin therapy: A shocklike syndrome (flushing, pallor, weakness, hypotension, syncope) can occur.
8. Instruct patient to inform physician if skin rash, visual disturbances, dry mouth, or severe or persistent headaches occur because the medication may need to be adjusted.
9. Warn patient to be alert for development of tolerance to rapid-acting drug (inadequate pain relief following several tablets). Temporary discontinuation (several days) is usually sufficient to restore sensitivity. Tolerance can be minimized by using smallest effective dose.
10. Assist patient to develop a system for recording frequency of anginal attacks, number of tablets required for relief, and development of side effects.
11. Instruct patient to store drug (especially sublingual nitroglycerin) in original container. Tablets may rapidly lose potency in metal, plastic, or cardboard containers.
12. Suggest that patient discard unused sublingual tablets 6 months after original container is opened because potency is probably reduced. A burning or stinging sensation under the tongue following administration is a good indication that potency is adequate.

Table 32-1
Nitrites and Nitrates

Drug	Preparations	Usual Dosage Range	Nursing Implications
Amyl nitrite Aspirols, Vaporole	Inhalation ampules: 0.18 mL, 0.3 mL	0.18 mL–0.3 mL inhaled as required	Available as thin ampules in a woven fabric cover; ampule is wrapped in gauze or cloth, crushed between fingers, and contents inhaled; drug has a strong, fruity odor; volatile and highly flammable; tachycardia often occurs for a brief period following inhalation; has been employed to relieve renal and gallbladder colic but infrequently used now because of odor, cost, and inconvenience; excessive doses may cause methemoglobinemia, an impaired oxygen-carrying capacity of red blood cells
Erythrityl tetranitrate Cardilate	*Tablets* Oral: 5 mg, 10 mg Sublingual: 5 mg, 10 mg	Sublingual: 5 mg–10 mg 3 times/day or prior to stressful episodes Oral: 10 mg 3–4 times/day	Comparable onset but longer duration (4 h) of action than nitroglycerin; used mainly for prophylaxis in patients with frequent, recurrent anginal pain and reduced exercise tolerance; vascular headaches are common early in therapy—less frequent with oral than sublingual administration; GI disturbances are noted with high oral doses
Isosorbide dinitrate Isordil, Sorbitrate, and several other manufacturers (CAN) Apo-ISDN, Coronex, Novosorbide	*Tablets* Sublingual: 2.5 mg, 5 mg, 10 mg Oral: 5 mg, 10 mg, 20 mg, 30 mg, 40 mg Sustained-release: 40 mg Chewable: 5 mg, 10 mg *Capsules* Oral: 40 mg Sustained-release: 40 mg	Sublingual: 2.5 mg–10 mg as needed for relief of pain *or* every 2–3 h for prophylaxis Chewable: 5 mg–10 mg every 2–3 h for prophylaxis Tablets: 10 mg–40 mg 3 times a day for prophylaxis Sustained-release: 40 mg–80 mg every 8–12 h	Sublingual and chewable forms rated "probably effective" for treatment of acute anginal attacks and to prevent attacks in high-risk situations (e.g., stress); oral dosage forms rated "possibly effective" for prevention of anginal episodes; should be taken on an empty stomach unless vascular headaches are severe—then drug may be taken with meals; duration following sublingual administration is 1–3 h, and up to 6 h with oral administration (8 h with sustained-release forms)
Nitroglycerin, sublingual Nitrostat and several other manufacturers	Tablets: 0.15 mg, 0.3 mg, 0.4 mg, 0.6 mg	0.15 mg–0.6 mg under the tongue or in the buccal pouch at first indication of acute anginal attack; repeat as needed up to 3 tablets within 15 min	Very effective in relieving pain of acute anginal episodes and for preventing attacks when taken immediately prior to a stressful event; onset is almost immediate, and effects persist 30–45 min; keep bottles tightly capped, store in cool and dry place, and, if possible, only a week's supply of tablets should be carried at any one time—remainder should be kept in stock bottle
Nitroglycerin, translingual Nitrolingual	Oral spray: 0.4 mg per metered dose (200 doses/cannister)	1–2 sprays onto oral mucosa; no more than 3 sprays within 15 min	Oral spray used for relief of an acute attack of angina *or* prophylactically immediately

Continued

Table 32-1
Nitrites and Nitrates (continued)

Drug	Preparations	Usual Dosage Range	Nursing Implications
			before engaging in strenuous activities; if chest pain persists after three sprays, prompt medical attention is needed; spray should not be inhaled
Nitroglycerin, transmucosal Nitrogard	Controlled-release buccal tablets: 1 mg, 2 mg, 3 mg	1 tablet placed in buccal pouch every 3–5 h while awake	Tablets are placed between lip and gum above incisors or between cheek and gum and adhere to mucosa; drug is slowly absorbed over several hours; used for long-term management of angina; caution must be exercised in drinking and eating; if tablet is accidently swallowed, insert a new tablet as most of the drug that is swallowed is metabolized upon first pass through the liver
Nitroglycerin, topical ointment Nitro-Bid, Nitrol, Nitrong, Nitrostat	Ointment: 2%	Initially, half-inch strip of ointment every 4–8 h; apply by spreading a thin, uniform layer on skin; do *not* rub in; increase by half-inch increments until optimal response is obtained; usual dose is 1–2 in/8 h, although up to 4–5 in have been used every 4 h	Effective prevention of anginal attacks, especially at night; begin with half-inch of ointment/dose, and increase by half-inch every succeeding dose until vascular headache occurs, then decrease slightly; ointment is measured by squeezing a ribbon onto calibrated measuring tapes provided; rotate sites of application to prevent dermal inflammation and sensitization; area may be covered with plastic wrap to protect clothing; equally effective when applied to any skin area; *gradually* reduce dosage and frequency of application upon termination of drug to prevent sudden withdrawal reaction; one inch ointment equals approximately 15 mg nitroglycerin
Nitroglycerin, sustained release Nitro-Bid, Nitrospan, Nitrostat SR, and several other manufacturers	Sustained-release tablets: 2.6 mg, 6.5 mg, 9.0 mg Sustained-release capsules: 2.5 mg, 6.5 mg, 9.0 mg	Initially 2.5 mg every 6–8 h; increase in 2.5-mg increments 2–4 times/day until side effects limit the dose	Rated "possibly effective" for prophylaxis of anginal attacks; drug should be taken on an empty stomach, and tablets or capsules should be swallowed whole; monitor blood pressure closely
Nitroglycerin, injection Nitrostat IV, Nitro-Bid IV, Tridil	Injection: 0.5 mg/mL, 0.8 mg/mL, 5 mg/mL, 10 mg/mL	Initially 5 µg/min by IV infusion; increase gradually in 5-µg/min increments every 3–5 min up to 20 µg/min; if no response, further increases should be made in increments of 10 µg/min, then 20 µg/min until an effect is noted	Used to reduce the incidence of myocardial ischemic injury resulting from an acute myocardial infarction, to control hypertension associated with certain surgical procedures, to provide "controlled hypotension" during surgery, and to treat acute angina pectoris in patients not responding to other means of therapy; dilute and store solutions only in glass containers because nitroglycerin can be absorbed

Continued

Table 32-1
Nitrites and Nitrates (continued)

Drug	Preparations	Usual Dosage Range	Nursing Implications
			by plastic; some preparations contain alcohol; use caution with intracoronary injections; to discontinue, gradually decrease dose 5 μg/min every 5 min and monitor blood pressure
Nitroglycerin transdermal systems Deponit, Nitrocine, Nitrodisc, Nitro-Dur, Transderm-Nitro	*Adhesive pads providing stated release rates* Deponit: 5 mg/24 h, 10 mg/24 h Nitrocine: 5 mg/24 h; 10 mg/24 h; 15 mg/24 h Nitrodisc: 5 mg/24 h; 7.5 mg/24 h; 10 mg/24 h Nitro-Dur: 2.5 mg/24 h; 5 mg/24 h; 7.5 mg/24 h; 10 mg/24 h; 15 mg/24 h Transderm-Nitro: 2.5 mg/24 h; 5 mg/24 h; 10 mg/24 h; 15 mg/24 h	Apply one patch to a nonhairy skin area once every 16–18 h (remove patch for 6–8 h overnight)	Transdermal patch system provides for continuous drug absorption over approximately 24 h although absorption rates and hence nitroglycerin plasma levels can vary significantly; tolerance develops rapidly if patches are left on 24 h/day; dosage is stated in amount of drug absorbed over 24 h; patch must be in complete contact with skin to be effective; any tears or breaks in the patch system will change the rate of absorption; rotate application sites to minimize undue skin irritation; dosage is individualized and titrated to clinical response and tolerance of side effects (e.g., headache, hypotension); terminate usage gradually over 4–6 wk to prevent sudden withdrawal reactions; *not* intended for treatment of acute anginal attacks
Pentaerythritol tetranitrate P.E.T.N., Peritrate, and other manufacturers	Tablets: 10 mg, 20 mg, 40 mg, 80 mg Sustained-release tablets: 80 mg Sustained-release capsules: 30 mg, 45 mg, 60 mg, 80 mg	Initially 10 mg–20 mg 3 times/day; increase gradually to a maximum 40 mg 3 times/day; maintenance 30 mg–80 mg sustained-release forms every 12 h	Rated "possibly effective" for prophylactic treatment of angina; observe for development of skin rash or persistent headaches and caution patient that prolonged use may reduce effectiveness of rapid-acting drugs

13. Explain that topical nitroglycerin dosage forms are *not* intended for relief of acute anginal attacks because their onset of action is slower.
14. Advise patient to check patch to ensure that it is intact following showering, swimming, or heavy perspiration, which may affect drug response.
15. Explain that increased anginal episodes can result from excessive consumption of caffeine (in coffee, tea, and other foods).

Calcium Channel Blockers

Diltiazem   Nimodipine
Nicardipine Verapamil
Nifedipine

Most types of smooth muscle and cardiac muscle cells are dependent on transmembrane calcium influx for maintenance of normal resting tone and for activation. This influx occurs subsequent to the rapid influx of sodium noted during the initial depolarization phase and proceeds at a much slower rate by way of membrane channels that are relatively selective for calcium. These so-called *slow membrance channels* are blocked by a group of drugs known as calcium channel blockers. The entry of extracellular calcium into smooth muscle cells and myocardial cells is inhibited by these agents, resulting in vasodilation, bradycardia, decreased force of contraction, and reduced AV nodal conduction. Some of these agents are useful in treating angina, mild hypertension, and certain types of arrhythmias. In addition, nimodipine is indicated as an adjunctive agent in subarachnoid hemorrhage (see Uses). The following discussion pertains to the oral use of these agents in angina. While *all* of the calcium blockers except nimodipine are effective in treatment of angina pectoris, significant differences exist among the drugs with regard to their pharmacologic effects on cardiovascular function. Table 32-2 outlines some of the more important differences in the actions of the calcium channel blockers, while Table 32-3 presents dosage ranges and additional information.

MECHANISM

Calcium channel blockers inhibit the influx of extracellular calcium ions into cardiac muscle and smooth muscle cells through specific slow calcium channels. Antianginal effects include dilation of coronary arteries and arterioles and prevention of coronary artery spasm. Dilation of peripheral arterioles also occurs, reducing total resistance against which the heart must work; thus, there is a corresponding reduction in myocardial energy consumption and oxygen demand. Verapamil also markedly decreases calcium influx into cardiac contractile and conductile cells of the SA node and AV node. This latter action slows AV conduction, prolongs effective AV refractory period, and interrupts reentry of impulses at the AV node, thus restoring normal sinus rhythm. Nimodipine appears to have a greater effect on cerebral rather than peripheral arteries and may prevent arterial spasm subsequent to subarachnoid hemorrhage

USES

Management of all forms of angina (chronic stable, unstable, or vasospastic); the combination of a calcium channel blocker with a beta blocker appears to be more effective than either drug alone (all drugs except nimodipine)

Treatment of supraventricular tachyarrhythmias and control of rapid ventricular rate in atrial flutter or atrial fibrillation (IV verapamil—see Chap. 30)

Control of mild to moderate hypertension—diltiazem, nicardipine, nifedipine, and verapamil only (see Chap. 31)

Improvement of neurological deficits resulting from cerebral arterial spasm following subarachnoid hemorrhage

Investigational uses include treatment of bronchial asthma and Raynaud's phenomenon, and migraine prophylaxis

DOSAGE

See Table 32-3

FATE

(See Table 32-2.) All drugs are well absorbed orally, but diltiazem and verapamil undergo extensive first-pass hepatic metabolism; onset of action is within 30 minutes and effects persist for 4 to 6 hours (up to 12 h with sustained release dosage forms). All drugs are highly protein bound. Hepatic metabolism is extensive and excretion proceeds largely via the kidneys, except for diltiazem, which is eliminated primarily in the feces

COMMON SIDE-EFFECTS

(Most frequent with nifedipine.) Flushing, headache, weakness, dizziness, nausea, lightheadedness, peripheral edema; also, constipation with verapamil and giddiness with nifedipine

SIGNIFICANT ADVERSE REACTIONS

Cardiovascular: palpitations, hypotension, bradycardia, myocardial infarction, heart failure; in addition, third-degree AV block with verapamil

Respiratory: dyspnea, cough, wheezing, chest congestion, pulmonary edema

GI: heartburn, diarrhea, cramping, flatulence, sore throat

CNS: fatigue, tremor, nervousness, confusion, mood changes, blurred vision, insomnia

Musculoskeletal: muscle cramping, joint stiffness, inflammation

Other: hair loss, menstrual irregularities, claudication, dermatitis, urticaria, fever, sweating, chills, impotence

CONTRAINDICATIONS

(Verapamil and diltiazem) Severe left ventricular dysfunction, sick sinus syndrome, second- or third-degree heart block, cardiogenic shock, systolic pressure less than 90 mm Hg; diltiazem is also contraindicated in acute myocardial infarction and pulmonary congestion; nicardipine is contraindicated in advanced aortic stenosis. In addition, do not give IV verapamil and IV beta blockers concurrently—severe myocardial depression may occur; nifedipine has no absolute contraindications. *Cautious use* in patients with impaired hepatic or renal function, hypotension, reduced left ventricular function, or pulmonary edema, and in pregnant women and nursing mothers

INTERACTIONS

Calcium blockers and beta blockers together may be beneficial in some patients with chronic, stable angina but can also increase the likelihood of congestive heart failure or severe hypotension and may worsen existing angina, especially when given IV in patients with left ventricular dysfunction or conduction defects

Verapamil and nifedipine can elevate serum levels of digoxin if used concurrently, possibly leading to digitalis toxicity

Calcium blockers may have an additive antihypertensive effect if administered together with other antihypertensive drugs

Actions of calcium blockers may be enhanced by concomitant use of other highly protein-bound drugs (e.g., anticoagulants, antiinflammatory agents, sulfonamides, barbiturates)

The effectiveness of verapamil may be reduced by combined use with calcium and vitamin D

Nifedipine may decrease serum quinidine levels in patients with diminished left ventricular function

Cimetidine may augment the effects of calcium channel blockers by decreasing their hepatic metabolic rate

Lithium plasma levels may be decreased by verapamil

The effects of theophylline can be augmented by concurrent use of calcium channel blockers

Cyclosporine plasma levels can be increased by diltiazem, nicardipine, and verapamil

NURSING CONSIDERATIONS

See Table 32-3 for additional information.

Nursing Alerts

- Carefully monitor blood pressure during initial stages of therapy and whenever dosages are altered because excessive hypotension can occur, especially in patient already receiving beta blocker or other antihypertensive drug.
- Monitor ECG for development of bradycardia, sometimes accompanied by nodal escape rhythms, because verapamil and, to a lesser extent, diltiazem have significant negative inotropic effects and markedly slow AV conduction (see Table 32-2). First-degree AV block may also occur during peak serum concentrations. If such changes persist or worsen, the dose should be reduced, and preparations should be made to institute appropriate antidotal therapy if necessary.
- Assess for signs of developing congestive heart failure, especially if patient is also receiving a beta blocker. Mild peripheral edema can occur, usually in the legs, especially with nifedipine, and may be treated with diuretics. This

must be differentiated from the edema that results from heart failure. If heart failure develops, the drug should be discontinued.

1. Monitor results of liver enzyme determinations, which should be obtained periodically because occasional elevations of transaminase and alkaline phosphatase have been reported. Although elevations are usually not associated with clinical symptoms, and their significance is unclear, the potential for hepatic injury exists.

PATIENT EDUCATION
1. Inform patient that sublingual nitroglycerin may be used as needed to control acute anginal attacks while taking a calcium channel blocker.

Beta Blockers

The beta-adrenergic blocking agents approved for use in the treatment of angina include atenolol, metoprolol, propranolol, and nadolol. They are particularly suited for patients who experience frequent or severe acute attacks at rest because they can markedly reduce the myocardial oxygen demand. The principal hemodynamic actions of the beta blockers responsible for this effect include a decreased heart rate, blood pressure, and myocardial contractility, all of which reduce cardiac workload. Decreased heart rate may also result in lengthened diastolic perfusion time, leading to increased coronary blood flow. Although beta blockers may cause a slight increase in the end-diastolic pressure owing to the slowed heart rate, this potentially undesirable action can readily be offset by concurrent use of one of the nitrates. Conversely, the reflex tachycardia frequently seen with nitrates is attenuated by beta blockers. Therefore, combined nitrate-beta blocker therapy is frequently more advantageous than use of either drug alone.

The beta blockers are discussed in detail in Chapter 13, and only those aspects of the use of propranolol, metoprolol, nadolol, and atenolol in angina is considered here.

Propranolol
Inderal, Inderal LA, Ipran
(CAN) Apo-Propranolol, Detensol, Novopranol, PMS Propranolol
A nonselective beta blocker used for management of moderate to severe angina, frequently in combination with nitrates

DOSAGE
Initially 10 mg to 20 mg 3 to 4 times/day; increase gradually at weekly intervals until optimal response is obtained; usual maintenance dosage range is 80 mg to 160 mg/day in a single (sustained-release) or divided doses

Metoprolol
Lopressor
(CAN) Apo-Metoprolol, Betaloc, Novometoprol
A beta-selective blocker that is well absorbed orally and displays moderate lipid solubility. It is useful for treating angina as well as hypertension and for preventing reinfarction following a myocardial infarction

DOSAGE
Initially, 50 mg twice a day, increase gradually at weekly intervals as necessary; usual dosage range is 100 mg to 400 mg daily in two divided doses

Nadolol
Corgard
A nonspecific beta-adrenergic blocking agent indicated for the long-term management of patients with angina, its actions resemble those of propranolol. Unlike propranolol, however, nadolol does not appear to exert a direct depressant action on the myocardium. The long half-life of nadolol (20–24 h) permits once-daily dosing.

DOSAGE
Initially 40 mg once daily; increase by 40 mg to 80 mg at 3- to 7-day intervals until optimal clinical response is observed, or

Table 32-2
Pharmacokinetic and Pharmacologic Properties of Calcium Channel Blockers

	Diltiazem	Nifedipine	Verapamil	Nicardipine	Nimodipine
Pharmacokinetics					
Onset of action (min)	15–30	20	30 (2–5 IV)	20	—
Peak effect (h)	0.5–1	1–2	2–4 (0.2 IV)	1–2	0.5–1
Half-life (h)	3–6	2–4	4–8	2–4	1–2
Protein binding (%)	70–80	90–95	85–90	95–98	95–98
Pharmacologic effects					
Coronary vasodilation	↑↑↑	↑↑↑	↑↑↑	↑↑↑	—
Peripheral vasodilation	↑	↑↑↑	↑↑	↑↑↑	—
Heart rate	↓	↑ (reflex)	↑ or ↓	↑	—
Contractility	0 (↓)	↑ (reflex)	↓↓	0	—
AV nodal conduction	↓↓	0 (↓)	↓↓↓	0(↑)	—
SA nodal automaticity	↓	0	↓↓	0	—

↑↑↑ or ↓↓↓, marked effect; ↑↑ or ↓↓, moderate effect; ↑ or ↓, minimal effect; 0 (↑) or 0 (↓), variable effect; 0, no effect; —, no data.

Table 32-3
Calcium Channel Blockers

Drug	Preparations	Usual Dosage Range	Remarks
Diltiazem Cardizem	Tablets: 30 mg, 60 mg, 90 mg, 120 mg Capsules (sustained-release): 60 mg, 90 mg, 120 mg	*Angina:* Initially 30 mg 4 times/day; increase gradually at 1–2-day intervals to achieve optimal response; maximum dose is 360 mg/day in divided doses *Hypertension:* 60 mg to 120 mg sustained release twice a day; usual dosage range is 240 mg/day to 360 mg/day	Potent coronary vasodilator with little or no negative inotropic effect; also used in treating mild–moderate hypertension; heart rate is slightly reduced; slows AV conduction and may have additive bradycardic effects with beta blockers or digitalis; incidence of adverse reactions is very low; nausea, headache and peripheral edema are occasionally reported; elevated serum transaminases and hyperbilirubinemia have occurred but are reversible upon cessation of therapy; *not* recommended for children
Nicardipine Cardene	Capsules: 20 mg, 30 mg	*Angina/Hypertension:* Initially 20 mg 3 times/day; usual range is 20 mg–40 mg 3 times/day	Potent peripheral vasodilator used for treating angina and mild–moderate hypertension; significantly increases cardiac output; may also be useful in adjunctive treatment of congestive heart failure; decrease dosage in patients with hepatic impairment
Nifedipine Adalat, Procardia	Capsules: 10 mg, 20 mg	Initially 10 mg 3 times/day; increase slowly until optimal effect is noted; usual dosage range is 10 mg–20 mg 3 times/day; maximum recommended dose is 180 mg/day	Orally effective calcium blocker used in chronic, stable angina as well as vasospastic angina; does not alter conduction system of the heart as does verapamil, thus is of no use in arrhythmias; marked reduction in peripheral resistance coupled with minimal increase in heart rate suggests possible use as an antihypertensive; discontinue drug gradually if necessary
Nimodipine Nimotop	Capsules: 30 mg	60 mg every 4 h for 21 consecutive days	Orally effective drug used to improve neurological deficit due to cerebral arterial spasm subsequent to subarachnoid hemorrhage; treatment should be initiated within 96 h of the onset of hemorrhage; may also be effective in treating migraine and cluster headaches.
Verapamil Calan, Isoptin	Tablets: 40 mg, 80 mg, 120 mg Sustained-release tablets: 240 mg Injection: 5 mg/2 mL	Oral *Angina:* Initially 80 mg 3–4 times/day; increase at daily or weekly intervals until optimal effect is attained; usual dosage range is 300 mg–480 mg daily *Hypertension:* Initially, 40 mg–80 mg 3 times/day; usual dose is 240 mg as a single dose IV See Chapter 30	Orally effective calcium blocker used in angina and for relief of mild to moderate hypertension; also administered IV for treatment of supraventricular tachyarrhythmias (see Chap. 30); significantly reduces SA nodal automaticity and AV conduction and decreases force of contraction; high oral doses are necessary owing to extensive first-pass metabolism; use with *caution* in patients with left ventricular dysfunction

until there is pronounced slowing of heart rate; usually maintenance dose is 80 mg to 240 mg/day

Atenolol

Tenormin

A beta$_1$ selective blocker with a long half-life (once-daily dosing) and low lipid solubility, which decreases the incidence of central side effects such as drowsiness

DOSAGE

50 mg once daily; may increase to 100 mg once daily

NURSING CONSIDERATIONS

See Chapter 13 and **Plan of Nursing Care 3.** In addition:
1. Assist with ongoing evaluation of patient's response to drug because dosage requirements may change as condition stabilizes or deteriorates.

PATIENT EDUCATION

See Chapter 13 and **Plan of Nursing Care 3.**

Dipyridamole

Dipyridamole

Persantine, Pyridamole
(CAN) Apo-Dipyridamole

Dipyridamole is an orally effective coronary vasodilator and inhibitor of platelet aggregation. It has been employed to prevent reinfarction and to decrease the incidence of transient ischemic attacks due to platelet hyperaggregation, although these above indications are viewed solely as investigational. The drug has been extensively used as an anginal prophylactic agent although this is no longer an FDA-approved indication.

MECHANISM

Inhibits the activity on adenosine deaminase, thereby increasing functional levels of adenosine and other vasodilatory nucleotides; also appears to block the action of phosphodiesterase, resulting in elevated levels of cyclic AMP, another coronary vasodilator; increased cyclic AMP also reduces platelet aggregation; synthesis of prostacyclin is increased by dipyridamole, resulting in further vasodilation and impaired platelet aggregation; blood pressure is relatively unchanged, and systemic blood flow is largely unaffected; a mild positive inotropic action has also been reported

USES

Adjunct to coumarin anticoagulants in preventing postoperative thromboembolic complications of cardiac valve replacement

Investigational uses include prevention of thrombotic complications associated with cerebrovascular or ischemic heart diseases, prevention of myocardial reinfarction and mortality following infarction, and prevention of coronary bypass graft occlusion

DOSAGE

75 mg 4 times a day as an adjunct to the usual anticoagulant dose
(The average for most other nonapproved uses is 50 mg 3 times a day, 1 h before meals; clinical effects may take several months to become evident)

FATE

Oral absorption is good, although bioavailability is variable (25%–75%). Peak plasma concentrations occur within 2 to 3 hours, although, as noted above, therapeutic effects may not be evident for weeks to months. Protein binding is extensive (90%–97%). The drug is metabolized in the liver and excreted in the feces by enterohepatic recirculation

SIGNIFICANT ADVERSE REACTIONS
(Infrequent)

Headache, nausea, GI distress, weakness, dizziness, syncope, skin rash; occasionally, aggravation of angina pectoris

CONTRAINDICATIONS

No absolute contraindications. *Cautious use* in the presence of hypotension

INTERACTIONS

Dipyridamole can enhance the effects of oral anticoagulants and heparin

PATIENT EDUCATION

1. Instruct patient to take drug 1 hour before meals.
2. Inform patient that headache or dizziness may occur, but that they are usually transient.

PERIPHERAL VASODILATORS

Vasodilator drugs may increase blood flow through circulatory vessels by either a direct action (smooth-muscle relaxation) or an indirect action (interference with sympathetic nerve supply). Although these agents may improve blood flow to limbs and body organs in the *normal* person, their efficacy in relieving the ischemia of peripheral vascular disease is severely limited. It is unlikely that any peripheral vasodilator can markedly increase blood flow distal to an occlusion. Moreover, regulatory mechanisms in cerebral and skeletal vascular beds elicit compensatory vasodilation in response to ischemia; thus vasodilator drugs probably increase blood flow primarily to nonischemic areas. Therefore, minimal therapeutic benefit should be expected from the treatment of peripheral vascular disease with the peripheral vasodilators. Despite this fact, they continue to be frequently prescribed for symptomatic treatment of chronic occlusive vascular disease, at a significant cost to the public. Their use in treating cerebrovascular insufficiency in the elderly patient is particularly hazardous, inasmuch as these drugs can elicit a significant degree of hypotension, which can actually result in *reduced* cerebral perfusion, negating any potential benefit derived from dilation of cerebral vessels. Peripheral circulation should be closely monitored when any of these drugs is used. In addition, reflex tachycardia can occur with use of these peripheral vasodilators, which may prove dangerous in the patient with cardiac disease. Lastly, increased intraocular pressure may occur. Patients taking these drugs should be warned to immediately report any vision change or eye pain.

Cyclandelate

Cyclan, Cyclospasmol

Cyclandelate is a direct-acting vascular smooth muscle relaxant with no significant sympathomimetic or adrenergic blocking action. It is rated only "possibly effective" for treatment of ischemic peripheral and cerebrovascular disease (e.g., intermittent claudication, arteriosclerosis obliterans, Raynaud's phenomenon, thrombophlebitis, nocturnal leg cramps)

Initial oral dosage is 400 mg 3 to 4 times a day, which is gradually reduced to the usual maintenance dosage of 400 mg/day to 800 mg/day in 2 to 4 divided doses. Side effects include flushing, headache, weakness, sweating, dizziness, tachycardia, and GI distress. Most of these are transient; GI distress can be minimized by taking the drug with meals. The drug must be used cautiously in patients with glaucoma, severe coronary artery or cerebral vascular disease, and bleeding tendencies (prolonged bleeding time has been noted at high doses). Clinical benefit, if any, is slow to develop.

Ergoloid Mesylates

Gerimal, Hydergine, Hydroloid-G, Niloric

Ergoloid mesylates contain equal parts of three dihydrogenated ergotoxine alkaloids, namely dihydroergocornine, dihydroergocristine, and dihydroergocryptine. The compound is used to provide symptomatic relief of those signs and symptoms associated with a decline in mental acuity and capacity in the elderly, such as confusion and forgetfulness and lessened self-care, sociability, and appetite. A degree of improvement in these conditions is observed within 8 to 12 weeks and may be related to improved cerebral circulation. Although the precise mechanism by which ergoloid mesylates are able to improve mentation is not known, it is believed the drug can increase metabolic activity of the brain, thereby improving cerebral blood flow. Vasodilation of cerebral vessels may also play a role, albeit minor, in the action of the drug. Blood pressure may decline, reducing cerebral perfusion, and orthostatic effects have been noted.

The drug is erratically absorbed orally when administered as a tablet, capsule or liquid, and undergoes extensive first-pass hepatic metabolism. Thus, the preferred route of administration is sublingual, although this may be difficult in elderly or senile patients. Recommended starting dosage is 1 mg 3 times a day. Onset of clinical response is gradual, and results may not be evident for 3 to 4 weeks. Doses up to 12 mg/day have been used for extended periods.

Side effects are generally mild and include GI upset, nausea, sublingual irritation, lightheadedness, nasal stuffiness, blurred vision, skin rash, and orthostatic hypotension. Ergoloid mesylates should not be used in persons with acute or chronic psychosis, or in persons with a history of acute intermittent porphyria.

Isoxsuprine

Vasodilan, Voxsuprine

Isoxsuprine is a peripheral vasodilator that can increase resting blood flow in skeletal muscle. The drug possesses a beta-adrenergic agonistic, alpha-adrenergic antagonistic, and direct vascular smooth muscle relaxant effect. Because its vasodilatory actions are *not* blocked by beta-blocking agents, it is doubtful whether its beta-agonistic properties contribute to its vasodilatory action. Isoxsuprine can also increase heart rate, myocardial contractility, and cardiac output, and can relax uterine smooth muscle, probably by means of a beta-activating action. High doses may inhibit platelet aggregation. It is rated only "possibly effective" for the relief of symptoms associated with cerebral and peripheral vascular insufficiency. In addition, isoxsuprine has been employed IM to inhibit premature labor and to prevent threatened abortion, although these latter indications are considered experimental.

Oral dosage is 10 mg to 20 mg 3 to 4 times a day. When given IM, 5 mg to 10 mg may be administered 2 to 3 times a day. The drug should not be given IV because the likelihood of side effects is greatly increased. Flushing, palpitations, nausea, dizziness, skin rash, tachycardia, abdominal distress, hypotension, and nervousness have been reported with the use of isoxsuprine. The drug is discussed further in Chapter 12.

Nylidrin

Adrin, Arlidin
(CAN) PMS Nylidrin

The vasodilatory action of nylidrin appears to be the result of both a beta-adrenergic agonistic action and a direct relaxant effect on vascular smooth muscle. Heart rate and cardiac output are increased, and blood pressure may be lowered. Nylidrin is rated "possibly effective" in treating peripheral vascular diseases such as arteriosclerosis obliterans, diabetic vascular disease, Raynaud's disease, or acroparesthesia. It has also been used in treating circulatory disturbances of the inner ear, such as cochlear cell, macular or ampullar ischemia, or labyrinthine artery spasm. Oral dosage is 3 mg to 12 mg 3 to 4 times a day. Side effects include nausea, nervousness, weakness, dizziness, tremor, palpitations, and postural hypotension. Nylidrin is contraindicated in myocardial infarction, paroxysmal tachycardia, progressive angina pectoris, and thyrotoxicosis. Additional information on nylidrin is found in Chapter 12.

Papaverine

Cerespan, Pavabid, Paverolan, and others
Ethaverine

Ethaquin, Ethatab, Ethavex-100, Isovex

Papaverine and its closely related analog ethaverine exert a direct, nonspecific relaxant effect on smooth muscle. Vasodilatory effects are noted on the coronary, cerebral, pulmonary, and systemic blood vessels. The drugs may elevate the levels of cyclic AMP in vascular smooth muscle. Cerebral blood flow may be increased by means of decreased cerebral vascular resistance; however, blood pressure may decline, offsetting the beneficial effect of reduced cerebral vascular resistance. Papaverine and ethaverine have been used orally for relieving cerebral, myocardial, and peripheral ischemia resulting from vascular spasm, although their clinical effectiveness has not been conclusively demonstrated. They have also been employed as smooth muscle spasmolytics for treatment of a number of spastic states of GI, urinary, ureteral, or biliary smooth muscles.

Oral dosage of *papaverine* is 100 mg to 300 mg 3 to 5 times a day or 150 mg sustained-release preparation every 12 hours. IV or IM dosage ranges from 30 mg to 120 mg every 3 hours. For immediate effect, the IV route is recommended, and administration may be by *slow* injection or intermittent infusion. Absorption from sustained-release preparations is highly variable, and plasma levels may be very low following this mode of administration. Recommended dosage for *ethaverine* is 100 mg to 200 mg 3 times a day.

Side effects associated with these drugs include nausea, abdominal distress, flushing, sweating, headache, fatigue, skin rash, diarrhea, dizziness, tachycardia, and anorexia. Hepatic hypersensitivity can also occur and may be manifested as eosinophilia, jaundice, and elevated serum transaminases and alkaline phosphatase. IV administration of papaverine can lead to increased blood pressure, respiratory rate, and heart rate, and to profound sedation. Large doses of these agents can suppress AV nodal conduction and may lead to arrhythmias. The drugs are contraindicated in severe liver disease, complete AV block, and serious arrhythmias, and they must be used with caution in patients with glaucoma (increase intraocular pressure), myocardial depression, or impaired liver function.

Intraocular pressure may increase during drug use. The patient should be told to immediately report any change in vision, eye pain, or scleral redness.

PATIENT EDUCATION

1. Recommend that patient exercise caution in driving and performing other hazardous tasks until effects of drug have been determined because dizziness and drowsiness may occur.
2. Teach patient interventions to minimize orthostatic hypotension. See **Plan of Nursing Care 8**, Chapter 31, for specific information.
3. Teach patient how to monitor heart rate because abnormalities can occur. Dosage should be reduced or drug should be discontinued if heart rate is significantly altered.
4. Inform patient that flushing, a sensation of warmth, and headache can occur during initial stages of therapy, but that they usually disappear with slight dosage reduction.
5. Explain that beneficial effects may occur gradually and that adherence to dosage schedule is important to obtain maximal therapeutic benefit.
6. Stress the importance of good health practices (e.g., proper diet, rest, exercise, cessation of smoking) in the successful management of peripheral vascular disease.

Selected Bibliography

Anders Vedin J, Wilhelmsson CF: Beta receptor blocking agents with secondary prevention of coronary heart disease. Annu Rev Pharmacol Toxicol 23:29, 1983

Baumwald E: Mechanism of action of calcium-channel blocking agents. N Engl J Med 307:1618, 1982

Butler JD, Harrison L: Keeping pace with calcium channel blockers. Nursing 83 13(7):38, 1983

Cauvin C, Loutzenhiser R, Van Breeman C: Mechanisms of calcium antagonist-induced vasodilation. Annu Rev Pharmacol Toxicol 23:373, 1983

Herlihy B et al: A nursing care plan for the patient receiving calcium antagonists. Crit Care Nurs 4(1):38, 1984

Mar DD: New topical nitroglycerin preparations. Am J Nurs 82:462, 1982

McGourty JC, Silas JH, Solomon SA: Tolerability of combined treatment with verapamil and beta-blockers in angina resistant to monotherapy. Postgrad Med J 61:229, 1985

Meyer JS: Calcium channel blockers in the prophylactic treatment of vascular headache. Ann Intern Med 102:395, 1985

Opie LH (ed): Calcium Antagonists and Cardiovascular Disease, Vol. 6: Perspectives in Cardiovascular Research. New York, Raven Press, 1984

Parker JO: Nitrate therapy in stable angina pectoris. N Engl J Med 316:1635, 1987

Piepho RW: The calcium antagonists: Mechanisms of action and pharmacologic effects. Drug Ther 13:69, 1983

Purcell JA, Holder CK: Intravenous nitroglycerin. Am J Nurs 82:254, 1982

Roberts R: Intravenous nitroglycerin in acute myocardial infarction. Am J Med 74 (Suppl):45, 1983

Roberts R (ed): Second North American Conference on Nitroglycerin Therapy: Perspectives and mechanisms. Am J Med 76:1, 1984

Rossi LP, Antman EM: Calcium channel blockers: New treatment for cardiovascular disease. Am J Nurs 83:382, 1983

Schneck DW: Calcium-entry blockers: A review of their basic and clinical pharmacology and therapeutic applications. Ration Drug Ther 19(5):1, 1985

Schroeder JS: Calcium and beta blockers in ischemic heart disease: When to use which. Mod Med 26:94, 1982

Scriabine A: Current and potential indications for calcium antagonists. Ration Drug Ther 21(11):1, 1987

Shub C, Ulietstra RE, McGoon MD: Selection of optimal drug therapy for the patient with angina pectoris. Mayo Clin Prac 60:539, 1985

Snyder SH, Reynolds IJ: Calcium-antagonist drugs: Receptor interactions that clarify therapeutic effects. N Engl J Med 313:995, 1985

Strauss WE, Parisi AF: Superiority of combined diltiazem and propranolol therapy for angina pectoris. Circulation 71(5):951, 1985

Thadani U, Whitsett TL: Nitrate therapy: Continuous or pulse dosing. Ration Drug Therap 21(7):1, 1987

Zelis R, Flaim SF: Calcium blocking drugs for angina pectoris. Annu Rev Med 33:465, 1982

SUMMARY. ANTIANGINAL DRUGS—VASODILATORS

Drug	Preparations	Usual Dosage Range
Antianginal Drugs		
Nitrites/nitrates	See Table 32-1	
Calcium channel blockers	See Table 32-3	
Beta blockers		
Propranolol Inderal, Ipran	Tablets: 10 mg, 20 mg, 40 mg, 60 mg, 80 mg, 90 mg Long-acting capsules: 60 mg, 80 mg, 120 mg, 160 mg Oral solutions: 20 mg/5 mL, 40 mg/5 mL, 80 mg/mL Injection: 1 mg/mL	10 mg–20 mg 3 to 4 times/day; increase gradually at 3–7-day intervals; usual range is 80 mg–160 mg/day

Continued

SUMMARY. ANTIANGINAL DRUGS—VASODILATORS (continued)

Drug	Preparations	Usual Dosage Range
Metoprolol Lopressor	Tablets: 50 mg, 100 mg Injection: 1 mg/mL	Initially, 50 mg twice a day; increase gradually at weekly intervals; usual range is 100 mg–400 mg daily
Nadolol Corgard	Tablets: 20 mg, 40 mg, 80 mg, 120 mg, 160 mg	Initially 40 mg once daily; increase by 40 mg–80 mg every 3–5 days; usual range is 80 mg–240 mg/day
Atenolol Tenormin	Tablets: 50 mg, 100 mg	50 mg once a day; may increase to 100 mg once day
Dipyridamole **Persantine, Pyridamole**	Tablets: 25 mg, 50 mg, 75 mg	75 mg 4 times/day
Peripheral Vasodilators		
Cyclandelate Cyclan, Cyclospasmol	Tablets: 200 mg, 400 mg Capsules: 200 mg, 400 mg	Initially 400 mg 3–4 times/day; usual maintenance dose is 400 mg–800 mg/day in divided doses
Ergoloid mesylates Hydergine and several other manufacturers	Tablets (oral): 1 mg Tablets (sublingual): 0.5 mg, 1 mg Liquid: 1 mg/mL Capsules: 1 mg	Initially 1 mg 3 times/day; adjust upward gradually, depending upon response
Ethaverine Ethaquin, Ethatabs, Ethavex-100, Isovex	Tablets: 100 mg Capsules: 100 mg	100 mg–200 mg 3 times/day
Isoxsuprine Vasodilan, Voxsuprine	Tablets: 10 mg, 20 mg Injection: 5 mg/mL	Oral: 10 mg–20 mg 3–4 times/day IM: 5 mg–10 mg 2–3 times/day
Nylidrin Adrin, Arlidin	Tablets: 6 mg, 12 mg	3 mg–12 mg 3–4 times/day
Papaverine Cerespan, Pavabid, Paverolan, and several other manufacturers	Tablets: 30 mg, 60 mg, 100 mg, 200 mg, 300 mg Tablets (timed-release): 200 mg Capsules (timed-release): 150 mg, 300 mg Injection: 30 mg/mL	Oral: 100 mg–300 mg 3–5 times/day Oral (timed-release): 150 mg every 8–12 h IM, IV: 30 mg–120 mg every 3 h as required

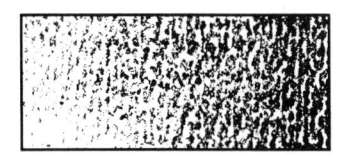

33 PROPHYLAXIS OF ATHEROSCLEROSIS: HYPOLIPEMIC DRUGS

Atherosclerosis is a condition characterized by deposition of lipid (fatty) material within the walls of the arterial system, resulting in a gradual occlusion of blood flow. Clinical consequences of this lipid deposition include the development of ischemic heart disease, cerebrovascular disease (including stroke), peripheral ischemia, and renovascular hypertension. The presence of generalized atherosclerosis greatly increases the risk of mortality from one or more of these conditions.

Although the basic mechanism involved in the development of the atherosclerotic process is still somewhat uncertain, there appears to be a metabolic disturbance in the synthesis, transport, and utilization of lipids; this, in combination with damage to the vascular endothelial lining, results in the adherence and eventual buildup of fatty deposits within the lining of the vessel walls.

Lipids do not circulate freely in the bloodstream, but rather are bound to plasma proteins (albumin, globulins). These complexes are termed *lipoproteins* and contain varying proportions of high-density proteins and low-density lipids. The four major types of lipoproteins, and a brief description of their characteristics, are listed below.

- *Chylomicrons:* largest and lightest of the lipoproteins, formed in the intestine during absorption of dietary fat; composed mainly (80%–90%) of triglycerides and impart a cloudiness to plasma; normally cleared rapidly from the blood; their presence in plasma taken from a fasting patient suggests an inability to handle dietary fats
- *Very low density lipoproteins (VLDL):* prebeta lipoproteins containing large amounts (50%–60%) of triglycerides that were synthesized in the liver; major means by which endogenous triglycerides are carried from the liver to the plasma
- *Low-density lipoproteins (LDL):* beta lipoproteins derived partly from breakdown of VLDL, containing about 50% to 60% cholesterol, 25% protein, and very few triglycerides; most of the circulating serum cholesterol is transported in this form, and elevated plasma levels of LDL indicate excessive cholesterol levels and suggest that the patient is at high risk for developing atherosclerosis
- *High-density lipoproteins (HDL):* alpha lipoproteins, the smallest and most dense (heaviest) of the lipoproteins, containing approximately 50% protein, 25% cholesterol, and very small amounts of triglycerides; believed to play an important role in clearing cholesterol from body tissues and may protect against development of atherosclerosis by blocking uptake of LDL cholesterol by vascular smooth muscle cells

Approximately one fourth of all adults have elevated levels of one or more of the plasma lipids or lipoproteins, which may reflect improper diet, excessive alcohol consumption, secondary disease (such as hypothyroidism or diabetes), or an inherited trait. Measurements of serum cholesterol and triglycerides can easily be done and are a common component of laboratory blood studies. However, a more accurate and useful classification of patients having defects in lipid metabolism or transport is based on the types of lipoproteins that are elevated in the plasma. This grouping allows precise diagnosis and treatment of each patient's condition. The term *hyperlipoproteinemia* is used to indicate an increase in one or more of the classes of lipoproteins. Table 33-1 lists the types of hyperlipoproteinemias that are currently recognized, with a brief description of each type and the most effective treatment of each subgroup.

There is increasing evidence that lowering serum levels of cholesterol and other lipids reduces the risk of atherosclerosis. It appears that elevated plasma cholesterol or LDL is a major risk factor for development of atherosclerosis, and results of a recent multicenter, randomized clinical study strongly suggest that reductions in plasma concentrations of LDL cholesterol can significantly reduce the risk of coronary artery disease.

Several therapeutic strategies may be employed in the treatment of hyperlipoproteinemias. The cornerstone of therapy remains diet modification and weight reduction. Reduced consumption of cholesterol and saturated animal fats is recommended for all types of hyperlipoproteinemias. Protein intake is either maintained or increased in most instances. Other risk factors should be eliminated as well: such as cessation of smoking, curtailment or abstinence from alcohol, treatment of elevated blood pressure, and maintenance of an adequate program of exercise and physical fitness.

Drug therapy of hyperlipoproteinemia involves the use of agents that can lower plasma concentrations of lipoproteins, either by blocking their production or by enhancing their removal from the plasma. These drugs, termed *hypolipemic* or *hypolipidemic* agents, are employed in a significant percentage of the population with hyperlipoproteinemia. However, in view of the potential for many hypolipemic drugs to cause untoward reactions, dietary changes are usually undertaken initially before drug therapy is instituted. If diet alone is ineffective in controlling plasma lipids, drug therapy is then warranted but only upon careful diagnosis of the type of hyperlipoproteinemia present. Drug therapy is entirely prophylactic—that is, hypolipemic agents can reduce the rate and extent of fatty deposition within arterial walls by lowering plasma lipid concentrations, but they do *not* dissolve or remove existing lipid deposits.

Bile Acid Sequestering Resins

Cholestyramine   Colestipol

These two bile acid sequestering agents are anion-exchange resins that combine with bile acids in the intestines, preventing their reabsorption and therefore increasing their excretion in the feces. They are effective plasma cholesterol–lowering drugs, and cholestyramine is also used for relieving pruritus associated with partial biliary obstruction. They are discussed together here, then listed individually in Table 33-2.

MECHANISM
Form an insoluble complex with bile acids in the intestine, increasing their fecal excretion; this leads to increased oxidation of cholesterol to bile acids, decreased serum cholesterol

Table 33-1
Classification of Hyperlipoproteinemias

Type	Descriptive Name	Characteristic Features	Treatment Diet	Treatment Drugs
I	Fat-induced (exogenous)	Relatively rare; increase in plasma chylomicrons containing large amounts of triglycerides of dietary origin; frequently seen in infancy and marked by abdominal pain; does not lead to atherosclerosis	Low fat; no alcohol; no restrictions on proteins, carbohydrates, or cholesterol	None effective
IIa	Familial hypercholesterolemia	High levels of LDL; normal VLDL; slight elevation of triglycerides; fairly common, and a definite risk for development of atherosclerosis and coronary artery disease	Low cholesterol; low saturated fats; increased intake of polyunsaturated fats	cholestyramine colestipol dextrothyroxine lovastatin probucol
IIb	Combined hyperlipoproteinemia	Elevated LDL and VLDL; presence of hypercholesterolemia and hypertriglyceridemia; lipid deposits occur on feet, elbows, knees	See IIa	cholestyramine colestipol dextrothyroxine lovastatin nicotinic acid probucol
III	Broad beta lipoproteinemia	Elevated LDL and VLDL; cholesterol and triglycerides are elevated; relatively uncommon but associated with atherosclerosis; recessively inherited disorder	Weight reduction; low cholesterol; low saturated fats; maintain high protein	clofibrate dextrothyroxine nicotinic acid
IV	Carbohydrate-induced (endogenous)	Marked elevation of VLDL; triglycerides are increased but LDL and cholesterol are normal or slightly elevated; most common type; definite risk for atherosclerosis and coronary artery disease	Weight reduction; low carbohydrate; low cholesterol; low alcohol; maintain protein intake	clofibrate (?) gemfibrozil nicotinic acid
V	Mixed hyperlipemia	Elevated VLDL and triglycerides; chylomicrons are increased; relatively uncommon type not generally associated with atherosclerosis or heart disease; xanthomas, hyperuricemia and pancreatitis can occur	Low fat; high protein, low carbohydrate; low alcohol	clofibrate (?) gemfibrozil (?) nicotinic acid

levels, and reduced beta lipoprotein (LDL) levels; little effect on serum triglyceride levels; may interfere with absorption of calcium, fats, fat-soluble vitamins (A, D, E, K), and many other drugs (see Interactions)

USES
Adjunctive treatment of primary type II hyperlipoproteinemia
Relief of pruritus associated with partial biliary obstruction (cholestyramine only)
Investigational uses for cholestyramine include treatment of antibiotic-induced pseudomembranous colitis and treatment of poisoning with the pesticide chlordecone (Kepone)

DOSAGE
See Table 33-2

FATE
Not absorbed from the GI tract nor hydrolyzed by digestive enzymes; excreted in feces as insoluble bile acid complex

COMMON SIDE EFFECTS
Constipation (occasionally severe), abdominal discomfort, flatulence, belching, nausea, anorexia

SIGNIFICANT ADVERSE REACTIONS
Vomiting; steatorrhea; fecal impaction; vitamin-K deficiency with bleeding tendencies; vitamin A, D, and E deficiencies; rash and irritation of the skin, tongue, and perianal region; and osteoporosis

A wide variety of other adverse reactions has been reported in persons taking these drugs, but their relationship to the drugs themselves is unclear

CONTRAINDICATIONS
Complete biliary obstruction. *Cautious use* in patients with constipation, anemia, bleeding tendencies, systemic acidosis, or hypothyroidism and in pregnant or nursing women

INTERACTIONS
May interfere with oral absorption of anticoagulants, cephalexin, clindamycin, digitalis drugs, iron preparations, phenobarbital, phenylbutazone, thiazide diuretics, thyroid drugs, tetracyclines, trimethoprim, and vitamins A, D, E, and K

NURSING CONSIDERATIONS

Nursing Alerts
- Monitor bowel function for development of constipation, especially when dose is high or patient is elderly. If bowel function is problematic, dosage may be lowered, or a stool softener or laxative may be used.
- Observe patient for early symptoms of hypoprothrombinemia related to vitamin K deficiency, such as pe-

techiae, mucosal bleeding, and tarry stools. Parenteral vitamin K₁ is indicated if this occurs. Recurrences can be prevented by oral administration of vitamin K (2.5 mg–10 mg).
- Advocate supplemental therapy with parenteral or water-miscible forms of vitamins A, D, and E in patient on prolonged therapy because deficiencies can occur.
- Carefully observe infant or child because hypochloremic acidosis has occurred in these patients. Therapy should be initiated with small doses because a dosage schedule has not been established for infants or children.

1. Monitor results of serum cholesterol and triglyceride levels, which should be determined at start of therapy and at regular intervals thereafter.
2. Prepare drug as instructed before giving orally (see Table 33-2). Dissolve powder in an appropriate vehicle (e.g., flavored liquid, thin soup, juice) to disguise disagreeable taste. Ingestion of powder alone is very irritating and may cause esophageal impaction.

PATIENT EDUCATION

1. Instruct patient to take other oral medications at least 1 hour before or 4 hours following resin administration, if possible, to avoid interference with their absorption.
2. Instruct patient to eat foods high in bulk (fruit, raw vegetables) and to maintain liberal fluid intake to minimize constipation.
3. Inform patient that GI side effects usually subside with continued therapy.

Clofibrate

Atromid-S

(CAN) Claripex, Novofibrate

MECHANISM

Not definitively established; lowers elevated triglyceride and VLDL levels, possibly by increasing breakdown of free fatty acids in the liver via action of lipoprotein lipase; also, decreases release of VLDL from liver to plasma and interferes with binding of free fatty acids to albumin; may slightly reduce plasma cholesterol and LDL, presumably by inhibiting cholesterol biosynthesis and increasing biliary and fecal excretion of cholesterol; reduces serum fibrinogen levels and platelet adhesiveness

USES

Adjunctive treatment of type III hyperlipoproteinemia that does not respond adequately to diet

Adjunctive treatment of types IV and V hyperlipoproteinemia characterized by very high serum triglyceride levels and a risk of pancreatitis

DOSAGE

Adults: Initially 2 g/day in divided doses; adjust to desired response

Note: Drug should be discontinued after 3 months if response is inadequate

FATE

Following administration, drug is hydrolyzed to *p*-chlorophenoxyisobutyric acid (CPIB), the active form of the drug, which is slowly but completely absorbed; peak CPIB plasma levels occur in 3 to 6 hours; plasma half-life ranges from 6 to 24 hours; much longer (up to 100 h) in patients with renal impairment; CPIB is highly protein bound (90%–95%) and is largely metabolized in the liver and excreted in the urine

COMMON SIDE EFFECTS

Nausea, dyspepsia, abdominal distress, flatulence

SIGNIFICANT ADVERSE REACTIONS

WARNING

Clofibrate has produced benign and malignant tumors in rats at 5 to 8 times the human dose. The drug has the potential to elicit hepatic tumors in humans, produce cholelithiasis (twice the risk of nonusers), and evoke a wide range of other untoward reactions. Because of these characteristics, coupled with the lack of substantial evidence for a beneficial effect for clofibrate on cardiovascular mortality, it should be reserved for those patients with *significant hyperlipidemia* and a high risk of coronary artery disease who have not responded adequately to diet, weight loss, and other less toxic drugs

GI: diarrhea, vomiting, gastritis, stomatitis, increased gallstones, hepatomegaly

Cardiovascular: arrhythmias, swelling, and phlebitis at site of xanthoma, angina, thromboembolic complications

Table 33-2
Bile Acid Sequestering Resins

Drug	Preparations	Usual Dosage Range	Nursing Implications
Cholestyramine Questran	Powder: 4 g resin/9 g powder	Initially 4 g resin 2–3 times/day before meals, adjust to patient's needs (range 16 g–24 g/day)	Place drug on surface of 4–6 oz liquid; allow to stand 1–2 min without stirring, then gently twirl container or stir slowly to obtain a uniform suspension; rinse glass with fluid to assure taking entire dose; may also be mixed with soups or pulpy fruits (e.g., applesauce); relief of pruritus may take 1–2 wk to become evident; decline in serum cholesterol is usually apparent by 1 mo
Colestipol Colestid	Water-insoluble beads: 5-g packets or 500-g bottles	15 g–30 g/day in divided doses 2–4 times/day	Add prescribed amount of drug to at least 3 oz of liquid and stir until completely mixed (does *not* dissolve); may also be added to cereals, soups, or pulpy fruits; does not have the disagreeable odor or taste of cholestyramine

Dermatologic: rash, urticaria, pruritus, alopecia, dry skin, dry hair
Hematologic: leukopenia, anemia, eosinophilia
Neurologic: drowsiness, weakness, dizziness, headache
Other: myalgia and flulike symptoms, arthralgia, impotence, decreased libido, dysuria, hematuria, decreased urinary output, weight gain, polyphagia, abnormal liver function tests, hepatic tumors

CONTRAINDICATIONS

Hepatic or renal dysfunction, primary biliary cirrhosis, and in pregnant and nursing women. *Cautious use* in the presence of peptic ulcer, cardiac arrhythmias, or gout and in persons receiving oral anticoagulants or oral hypoglycemic drugs (see Interactions)

INTERACTIONS

Clofibrate may enhance the effects of oral anticoagulants, hypoglycemic agents, cholinesterase inhibitors, furosemide, and thyroxine

Oral contraceptives, other estrogens, and rifampin can antagonize the action of clofibrate

The effects of clofibrate may be enhanced by acidifying agents, neomycin, probenecid, and thyroxine

NURSING CONSIDERATIONS

Nursing Alert
- Monitor results of liver function tests and blood counts, which should be performed frequently during therapy. Drug should be withdrawn if results are abnormal.

1. Monitor results of serum cholesterol and triglyceride analyses, which should be performed before initiating therapy and at 2- to 4-week intervals during treatment. A *rebound rise* in lipid levels may occur after 2 to 3 months of therapy, but further decreases will then ensue.

PATIENT EDUCATION

1. Instruct patient to notify physician immediately if chest pain, dyspnea, irregular heartbeat, stomach pain, vomiting, fever, chills, sore throat, hematuria, oliguria, or swelling of the extremities occurs.
2. Instruct patient to report development of flulike symptoms (muscle aching, weakness, soreness, cramping) because these may indicate a need for dosage reduction.
3. Encourage woman with childbearing potential to use effective birth-control measures because fetal damage can occur. Drug should be withdrawn several months prior to attempted conception.
4. Stress the importance of adhering to recommended diet.

Dextrothyroxine
Choloxin

MECHANISM

Synthetic *d*-isomer of thyroxine, possessing much less metabolic stimulating action than the naturally occurring *l*-isomer (*l*-thyroxine); reduces serum cholesterol and LDL levels but has no *consistent* effect on triglycerides or VLDL; accelerates breakdown of cholesterol in the liver resulting in increased biliary excretion; may also increase number of LDL receptors on all membranes

USES

Adjunctive treatment for reduction of elevated cholesterol and LDL levels in type II (and possibly type III) euthyroid patients with no evidence of organic heart disease

Treatment of hypothyroidism in patients with cardiac disease who cannot tolerate other thyroid drugs

DOSAGE

Hypercholesterolemia
Adults: initially 1 mg to 2 mg/day; increase by 1-mg to 2-mg increments at monthly intervals to a maintenance range of 4 mg to 8 mg/day
Children: initially 0.05 mg/kg/day; increase by 0.05-mg/kg/month increments to desired level (usually 0.1 mg/kg/day)
Hypothyroidism
Initially 1 mg; increase in 1-mg/mo increments to optimal level (usually 4 mg/day)

FATE

Adequately absorbed from GI tract; minimal protein binding metabolized by the liver and rapidly excreted in the urine

COMMON SIDE EFFECTS

Nervousness, sweating, flushing, palpitations, dyspepsia

SIGNIFICANT ADVERSE REACTIONS

(Most common in hypothyroid patients or patients with organic heart disease)

Cardiovascular: angina, arrhythmias, myocardial damage, increased heart size
CNS: insomnia, tremors, headache, hyperthermia, dizziness, visual disturbances, tinnitus, paresthesias, psychic changes
GI: vomiting, diarrhea, anorexia
Other: hair loss, weight loss, diuresis, menstrual irregularities, altered libido, hoarseness, muscle pain, skin rash, gallstones, hyperglycemia, elevated protein-bound iodine levels, worsening of peripheral vascular disease

CONTRAINDICATIONS

Organic heart disease (angina, arrhythmias, myocardial infarction, congestive heart failure, rheumatic heart disease), hypertension (other than mild, labile forms), liver or kidney disease, pregnancy, and lactation. *Cautious use* in persons with diabetes mellitus

INTERACTIONS

Dextrothyroxine may potentiate the effects of oral anticoagulants

Toxic actions of digitalis preparations may be enhanced by dextrothyroxine

Dextrothyroxine can antagonize the effects of oral hypoglycemics and insulin by increasing blood sugar levels

Increased response to injections of epinephrine or norepinephrine (e.g., episodes of coronary insufficiency) may occur in the presence of dextrothyroxine

Concurrent use of dextrothyroxine and other CNS stimulants (tricyclic antidepressants, amphetamines, caffeine) may result in increased CNS excitation and tachycardia

NURSING CONSIDERATIONS

Nursing Alerts
- Carefully assess patient with known or suspected cardiac disease for signs of increasing cardiac decompensation (e.g., dyspnea, nocturnal coughing, pain on exertion, palpitations, edema). If signs appear, inform physician immediately; dosage reduction or discontinuation of drug is warranted.
- In patient with organic heart disease, question prescription of more than 4 mg dextrothyroxine/day because myocardial oxygen requirements may be dangerously elevated.

1. Interpret results of serum protein-bound iodine (PBI) levels appropriately. Increased levels occur in patient taking dextrothyroxine, but they indicate drug absorption and transport drug rather than a hypermetabolic state. Levels in the range of 10 to 25 µg/dL are common and do not necessitate dosage adjustment.

PATIENT EDUCATION
1. Advise patient to promptly report symptoms of iodism (excessive use of iodine-containing compounds), such as acneiform rash, itching, coryza, conjunctivitis. Drug may have to be withdrawn if these occur.
2. Encourage woman of childbearing potential to use effective birth-control measures because fetal damage can occur.
3. Teach diabetic patient to carefully assess blood glucose control. Loss of control (e.g., glycosuria, polyuria, polydipsia) may require dosage adjustments (increase antidiabetic drugs or decrease dextrothyroxine).
4. Encourage patient to obtain all blood tests requested. Serum lipids should be determined prior to therapy and monthly during therapy.
5. Inform patient that decreased cholesterol levels may not occur for several weeks after initiation of therapy and that maximal response may require 2 to 3 months.

Gemfibrozil
Lopid

MECHANISM
Not completely established; lowers elevated serum triglycerides, primarily the VLDL fraction and less frequently the LDL fraction; may also increase the high-density lipoprotein fraction, an action also considered to be beneficial in atherosclerosis; biochemical mechanisms of action may include inhibition of peripheral lipolysis, reduction of liver triglyceride production, and impairment in the synthesis of VLDL carrier apoprotein; may also reduce incorporation of long-chain fatty acids into newly formed triglycerides and accelerate removal of cholesterol from the liver

USES
Treatment of type IV and V hyperlipoproteinemia associated with high serum triglyceride levels and a definite risk of pancreatitis in patients who do not respond adequately to dietary therapy

DOSAGE
600 mg twice a day, 30 minutes before the morning and evening meal

FATE
Well absorbed from the GI tract; peak serum levels occur in 1 to 2 hours; plasma half-life is 1 to 2 hours but elimination half-life is considerably longer owing to enterohepatic circulation; excreted in the urine largely as unchanged drug (70%) and some metabolites; small amounts are also eliminated in the feces

COMMON SIDE-EFFECTS
Abdominal pain, diarrhea, nausea

SIGNIFICANT ADVERSE REACTIONS
WARNING
Due to pharmacologic similarities between gemfibrozil and clofibrate, the serious adverse effects reported in patients receiving clofibrate must be considered a possibility in patients receiving gemfibrozil as well. Refer to the discussion of clofibrate for details

GI: vomiting, constipation, dry mouth, gas pain, anorexia
CNS: headache, dizziness, blurred vision, vertigo, insomnia, tinnitus, paresthesias
Musculoskeletal: arthralgia, back pain, myalgia, muscle cramping, swollen joints
Dermatologic: rash, dermatitis, pruritus, urticaria
Hepatic: liver function abnormalities (increased SGOT, SGPT, LDH, CPK, alkaline phosphatase)
Other: anemia, eosinophilia, leukopenia, malaise, syncope, cholelithiasis

CONTRAINDICATIONS
Hepatic or severe renal dysfunction, gallbladder disease, biliary cirrhosis. *Cautious use* in patients with diabetes mellitus, cardiac arrhythmias, or altered liver function values and in pregnant or nursing women

INTERACTIONS
Gemfibrozil may potentiate the effects of oral anticoagulants

NURSING CONSIDERATIONS

Nursing Alert
- Monitor results of liver function tests and blood counts, which should be performed periodically during therapy. Drug should be discontinued if abnormalities persist for any length of time or worsen.

1. Assist with evaluation of patient's response to drug. If lipid response is still inadequate after 3 months as determined by serum lipid levels, drug should be withdrawn.

PATIENT EDUCATION
1. Urge caution in performing hazardous tasks, especially in early stages of therapy, because dizziness or blurred vision may occur.
2. Inform patient to inform physician if GI symptoms (abdominal pain, nausea, vomiting, diarrhea) persist or worsen. Dosage may have to be reduced or drug discontinued.
3. Instruct patient to notify physician if symptoms of gallbladder disease occur (e.g., upper abdominal discomfort, bloating, belching, fried-food intolerance). Appropriate diagnostic studies should be performed. Drug should be discontinued if gallstones are found.

4. Carefully explain that adherence to prescribed diet and restricted intake of sugars, cholesterol, saturated fats, and alcohol are very important to successful control of hyperlipidemia.

Lovastatin
Mevacor

MECHANISM

Hydrolyzed to a beta-hydroxy acid form, which is a potent inhibitor of HMG-CoA reductase, an enzyme that catalyzes the conversion of HMG-CoA to mevalonate, an early and *rate-limiting* step in the biosynthesis of cholesterol: lowers both normal and elevated LDL cholesterol levels; reduces the concentration of circulating LDL particles, increases HDL cholesterol levels, and reduces VLDL cholesterol and plasma triglycerides; does not appear to affect steroidogenesis adversely

USES

Adjunct to diet for reducing elevated total and LDL cholesterol levels in patients with primary hypercholesterolemia (types IIa and IIb)

Reduction of elevated LDL cholesterol levels in patients with combined hypercholesterolemia and hypertriglyceridemia

DOSAGE

Initially, 20 mg once daily. Usual dosage range 20 mg to 80 mg daily in a single or divided doses

FATE

Less than one third of an oral dose is absorbed, and the drug undergoes extensive first-pass hepatic metabolism such that less than 5% of an oral dose reaches the systemic circulation as active drug or metabolite; maximum therapeutic response occurs within 4 to 6 weeks and is maintained by single daily dosing in the evening; both lovastatin and its beta-hydroxy acid metabolite are highly protein-bound in the plasma (95%); excretion is largely in the feces by way of the bile (about 85%) with some drug and metabolite (10% to 15%) appearing in the urine

COMMON SIDE EFFECTS

Headache, abdominal discomfort, flatulence, diarrhea, nausea, rash, pruritus, elevated creatine phosphokinase

SIGNIFICANT ADVERSE REACTIONS

Dizziness, blurred vision, peripheral neuropathy, increased serum transaminases with prolonged therapy, myalgia, muscle tenderness

CONTRAINDICATIONS

Acute liver disease, persistent elevation of serum transaminases, pregnancy, or lactation. *Cautious use* in patients at risk for developing renal failure (such as those with severe acute infections, hypotension, trauma, or severe metabolic, endocrine, or electrolyte disturbances), and in those with uncontrolled seizures, chronic liver dysfunction, or skeletal muscle disorders

NURSING CONSIDERATIONS
1. Monitor results of serum cholesterol determinations, which should be obtained periodically throughout therapy to guide dosage adjustments.
2. Monitor results of liver function tests, which the manufacturer recommends be obtained every 4 to 6 weeks for the first 15 months of therapy and periodically thereafter, because unexplained elevations of serum transaminases may occur. The patient who consumes large amounts of alcohol or has a history of liver disease should be monitored especially carefully.

PATIENT EDUCATION
1. Emphasize that drug acts in conjunction with reductions in dietary fat and cholesterol.
2. Refer patient to dietitian for instruction regarding low fat, low cholesterol diet.
3. Instruct patient to take once daily with evening meal because drug is absorbed much better when taken with food, and evening doses appear to be more effective than morning doses.
4. Advise patient to use caution in performing hazardous activities until drug effects have been determined because dizziness and blurred vision may occur.

Nicotinic acid—Niacin
Several manufacturers

Nicotinic acid (vitamin B_3) is a water-soluble vitamin that is discussed in Chapter 73. In large doses, it can lower elevated plasma lipid levels and has been used as adjunctive therapy in certain types of hyperlipoproteinemias.

MECHANISM

Not completely established; reduces lipolysis and release of free fatty acids from adipose tissue and decreases hepatic synthesis of VLDL and triglycerides; LDL formation is also reduced; increases activity of lipoprotein lipase and accelerates removal of chylomicron triglycerides; hepatic cholesterol synthesis may also be inhibited

USES

Adjunctive therapy in patients with elevated cholesterol or triglycerides who do not respond adequately to diet and weight loss

DOSAGE

1 g to 2 g one to three times/day; increase slowly, first to 4.5 g then to 6 g/day after several weeks if necessary

FATE

Readily absorbed orally; peak serum levels occur within 1 hour; elimination half-life is 45 to 60 minutes; partially metabolized by the liver and excreted as both metabolites and unchanged drug by the kidneys

COMMON SIDE EFFECTS

GI distress, flushing, feeling of warmth, pruritus, paresthesias

SIGNIFICANT ADVERSE REACTIONS

Headache, dizziness, palpitations, diarrhea, hypotension, hyperuricemia, gouty arthritis, skin rash, dermatoses, epigastric pain, jaundice, decreased glucose tolerance, activation of peptic ulcer, increased sebaceous gland activity, toxic amblyopia, and impaired liver function

CONTRAINDICATIONS

Hepatic dysfunction, active peptic ulcer, severe hypotension, hemorrhaging, and gastritis. *Cautious use* in patients with allergic disorders, glaucoma, jaundice, gallbladder disease, diabetes, or gout, and in pregnant or lactating women

INTERACTIONS
Nicotinic acid may enhance the blood pressure–lowering effects of antihypertensive medications

Nicotinic acid may antagonize the effects of hypoglycemic agents by elevating blood glucose levels

PATIENT EDUCATION
1. Instruct patient to take drug with food to minimize GI distress and with cold water, not hot beverages, to facilitate swallowing. Reduction in serum lipids may be enhanced if tablets are chewed, rather than swallowed whole, and ingested with large amounts of water.
2. Inform patient that liver function tests and blood glucose determinations are usually performed frequently during early stages of therapy to determine if adverse effects are occurring.
3. Warn patient that hypotension with accompanying dizziness or weakness can occur following ingestion of nicotinic acid. If this occurs, physician should be informed because dosage may need to be reduced.

Probucol
Lorelco

MECHANISM
Not determined; may inhibit hepatic synthesis of cholesterol at an early stage; does not affect later stages; increased excretion of fecal bile acids occurs, and absorption of dietary cholesterol may be impaired

USES
Treatment of elevated serum cholesterol in patients with primary hypercholesterolemia (type II hyperlipoproteinemia) who have not responded to diet and weight reduction (*not* indicated where hypertriglyceridemia is the predominant factor)

DOSAGE
500 mg twice a day with meals

FATE
Variable GI absorption; peak blood levels are higher and less variable when taken with food; accumulates in fatty tissues and is very slowly eliminated in the feces via the bile

COMMON SIDE EFFECTS
Diarrhea, flatulence, abdominal pain, nausea

SIGNIFICANT ADVERSE REACTIONS
Headache, dizziness, paresthesias, vomiting, decreased hemoglobin, rash, pruritus, insomnia, impotence, blurred vision, tinnitus, impaired taste, anorexia, indigestion, GI bleeding, petechiae, nocturia, angioedema, palpitations, syncope, chest pain, eosinophilia, thrombocytopenia, peripheral neuritis, and elevated levels of serum transaminases, bilirubin, alkaline phosphatase, uric acid, glucose, and creatine phosphokinase

CONTRAINDICATIONS
Patients with cardiac arrhythmias or prolongation of the QT interval, pregnant or nursing women. *Cautious use* in persons with gout, impaired hepatic function, anemia, peptic ulcer, arrhythmias

NURSING CONSIDERATION
1. Monitor results of serum triglyceride analyses, which should be performed during therapy. If levels are elevated and remain so, probucol therapy should be discontinued, and another drug that reduces both cholesterol and triglycerides should be prescribed.

PATIENT EDUCATION
1. Instruct patient to take drug with food to minimize GI upset and to provide more consistent blood levels.
2. Inform patient that serum cholesterol levels are usually determined prior to initiation of therapy and frequently during initial months of therapy. Reductions should occur within first 2 months of therapy. Drug may be continued as long as favorable trend continues.
3. Encourage woman with childbearing potential to use effective birth-control measures during therapy and for several months thereafter because drug may induce fetal damage.

Several other drugs have the capacity to lower elevated serum lipid levels, but are largely unsuitable for the treatment of hyperlipoproteinemia, primarily because of their high incidence of untoward reactions and the availability of more effective and less toxic agents. *Neomycin sulfate* reduces plasma cholesterol by blocking its gastric absorption and lowers LDL levels as well, especially when given in combination with cholestyramine resin. However, neomycin is highly toxic (GI distress, ototoxicity, kidney damage) and is employed only in type II disease that is resistant to other forms of therapy.

Estrogens effectively lower cholesterol and LDL levels but may elevate triglycerides and VLDL. They are obviously unsuited for use in males because of their feminizing action, and they can cause thromboembolic disorders, abdominal pain, and pancreatitis in women. Administration of *norethindrone acetate,* a progestin, has decreased VLDL levels in some women with type V hyperlipoproteinemia. However, this agent has significant estrogenic activity and is therefore associated with many of the same adverse effects as the estrogens themselves.

Finally, although *heparin* can increase the conversion of triglycerides to free fatty acids, resulting in degradation of chylomicrons to soluble, dispersible complexes, heparin is of no clinical use as a hypolipemic drug because of its potential to cause hemorrhage and its need to be administered parenterally.

Selected Bibliography

Alexander S: Diet and drug therapy in the treatment of lipid disorders. Mod Med 56:68, 1988

Connor WE, Connor SL: The dietary treatment of hyperlipidemia. Med Clin North Am 66:485, 1982

Dujovne CA, Block JE: Drug treatment of hyperlipidemia. Ration Drug Ther 18(6):1, 1984

Dujovne CA, Harris WS: The pharmacological treatment of dyslipidemia. Annu Rev Pharmacol Toxicol 29:265, 1989

Feldman EB, Kuske TT: Lipid disorders: Diet and drug therapy. Mod Med 56(9):60, 1988

Gwynne JT, Lawrence MK: Hypercholesterolemia: Current concepts in evaluation and treatment. Mod Med 57(3):126, 1989

Heel RC, Brogden RN, Pakes GE, Speight TM, Avery GS: Colestipol: A review of its pharmacological properties and therapeutic efficacy in patients with hypercholesterolemia. Drugs 19:161, 1980

Kane JP, Malloy HJ: Treatment of hypercholesterolemia. Med Clin North Am 66:537, 1982

Krauss R: Regulation of HDL levels. Med Clin North Am 66:417, 1982

Lipid Research Clinic's Coronary Primary Prevention Trial. The relationship of reduction and incidence of coronary heart disease to cholesterol lowering. JAMA 251:365, 1985

Samuel P: Effects of gemfibrozil on serum lipids. Am J Med 74:23, 1983

SUMMARY. HYPOLIPEMIC DRUGS

Drug	Preparations	Usual Dosage Range
Bile Acid Sequestering Resins	See Table 33-2	
Clofibrate Atromid-S	Capsules: 500 mg	2 g/day in divided doses; adjust to desired response
Dextrothyroxine Choloxin	Tablets: 1 mg, 2 mg, 4 mg, 6 mg	Initially: 1 mg–2 mg/day; increase by 1-mg–2-mg/mo increments to desired response (usual range is 4 mg–8 mg/day) Children: 0.05 mg/kg/day increased by 0.05-mg/kg/mo increments to desired level (usual dose is 0.1 mg/kg/day)
Gemfibrozil Lopid	Capsules: 300 mg	600 mg twice a day, 30 min before the morning and evening meals
Lovastatin Mevacor	Tablets: 20 mg	Initially, 20 mg once a day; increase gradually at 4-wk intervals; usual dosage range is 20 mg–80 mg/day
Nicotinic Acid Niacin	Tablets: 25 mg, 50 mg, 100 mg, 250 mg, 500 mg Timed-release capsules: 125 mg, 250 mg, 300 mg, 400 mg, 500 mg Timed-release tablets: 150 mg Elixir: 50 mg/5 mL Injection: 100 mg/mL	1 g–2 g 3 times/day, with or following meals; increase slowly to a maximum of 6 g/day
Probucol Lorelco	Tablets: 250 mg	500 mg twice a day

34 ANTIANEMIC DRUGS

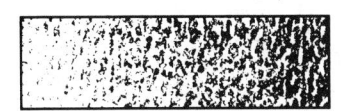

The term *anemia* describes a group of clinical conditions characterized by a reduction in the number of erythrocytes or in the hemoglobin concentration within erythrocytes, or both. Because oxygen is transported in the bloodstream primarily in combination with hemoglobin contained within the red blood cell, either condition will impair the oxygen-carrying capacity of the blood and thereby lead to inadequate tissue oxygenation.

Red cells are formed continually in the bone marrow, their synthesis requiring many nutrients, of which the most important are iron, folic acid, and vitamin B_{12} (cyanocobalamin). These substances are usually present in sufficient amounts in the diet; if they are adequately absorbed from the GI tract, erythrocyte formation and hemoglobin synthesis proceed normally. However, if the diet is deficient in any of these nutrients, or if their GI absorption is impaired, symptoms of anemia develop. Anemia may also result from extreme loss or destruction of red blood cells (e.g., trauma, hemorrhage, excessive menstruation), thereby increasing the nutritional requirements above the level that can be supplied by diet alone.

Although anemias can occur in a number of ways (e.g., deficiency or impaired availability of dietary factors, excessive destruction or loss of red blood cells, loss of bone marrow cells), most anemias are the result of inadequate amounts of iron, folic acid, or vitamin B_{12}, and so they are considered *deficiency* anemias. Correction of the deficiency has proved highly successful in treating these conditions, if an accurate diagnosis of the type of anemia as well as any underlying causative factor (e.g., ulcers, malignancy) has been made.

Of the deficiency anemias, those that result from lack of iron are characterized by fewer than normal erythrocytes, which are frequently smaller (microcytic) and paler (hypochromic) than usual, because they contain less hemoglobin. These anemias are referred to as *microcytic* or *hypochromic*. Other hypochromic microcytic anemias result from failure to incorporate adequate iron into the developing cells, although an actual nutritional deficiency may not be present.

Anemias that occur because of insufficient levels of folic acid or vitamin B_{12} (i.e., dietary deficiency, reduced absorption) are characterized by the presence of large, immature red cells (megaloblasts) in the bone marrow and blood, as well as enlarged erythrocytes (macrocytes) that may contain abnormally high levels of hemoglobin. These anemias are labeled *megaloblastic, macrocytic,* or *hyperchromic.*

Other types of anemias include *acute hemorrhagic anemia; aplastic anemia,* which is due to bone marrow damage; and *hemolytic anemia,* which is due to destruction of circulating red cells. The latter two anemias are usually the result of drug toxicity and are discussed in Chapter 4.

Since hypochromic and hyperchromic anemias seldom occur together, the importance of accurate diagnosis for proper replacement therapy is obvious. Likewise, carefully differentiating those anemias caused by nutritional iron deficiency from those caused by failure of iron incorporation into red blood cells is essential, because supplemental iron in the latter case is not only ineffective but can result in iron overload (hemochromatosis) and subsequent toxicity. The "shotgun" approach of combining many factors (e.g., iron, B_{12}, folic acid) in treating anemias has no place in clinical medicine and should never be used in lieu of careful diagnosis and *selective* replacement of the deficient factor, as well as correction of any underlying pathologic disorder.

The antianemic drugs to be discussed in this chapter include the iron preparations, folic acid, and vitamin B_{12}. In addition to these agents, therapy may also include other drugs and measures to correct any underlying abnormality that may be responsible for the anemia. Self-medication with any of the antianemic drugs should be strongly discouraged, because the apparent beneficial effects gained by treating oneself often may mask the symptoms of a more serious underlying disorder (e.g., internal bleeding, neurologic dysfunction).

ORAL IRON PREPARATIONS

Ferrous fumarate   Polysaccharide–iron complex
Ferrous gluconate
Ferrous sulfate

The primary use of supplemental iron is the prevention or treatment of iron-deficiency anemia. The most common cause of iron deficiency in adults is blood loss, which can result from heavy or frequent menstruation, as well as from GI bleeding, especially if it goes unrecognized for extended periods. GI bleeding must always be considered as a cause of unexplained iron-deficiency anemia, and careful evaluation is necessary to rule out a more serious underlying disorder, such as GI carcinoma or peptic ulcers.

Iron-deficiency states can also occur in infants (especially premature infants), in young children during periods of rapid growth, and in pregnant and lactating women. Supplemental iron is frequently given during these periods in the growth and reproductive cycle to meet the increased need.

Several types of preparations containing iron (capsules, tablets, liquids, injections) are used as replacement therapy in iron-deficiency anemias. The oral forms of therapy are preferred; parenteral administration of iron is largely restricted to those persons who cannot tolerate oral iron because of its gastric irritative action, those who do not absorb sufficient iron from the GI tract, or those who are unable to comply with an oral regimen. Oral iron is available in either the bivalent (ferrous) or trivalent (ferric) forms; bivalent iron is more widely used because it is better absorbed and somewhat less irritating than the trivalent form. An acid environment favors reduction of trivalent to bivalent iron, which increases absorption. GI distress can be reduced by using one of the iron complexes or sustained-release forms, but the absorption of elemental iron may be retarded with use of these specialized dosage forms, because much of their iron content may be released beyond the major iron absorptive sites in the duodenum and jejunum.

The oral iron preparations are essentially alike in terms of their pharmacologic action, because they all release elemental iron, and therefore they are reviewed as a group. Individual salts and dosage forms are then listed in Table 34-1. The parenteral iron preparation, iron dextran, is then discussed in detail.

MECHANISM

Provide replacement for insufficient iron, thereby correcting the hemoglobin and tissue iron deficiency; iron is an essential component of hemoglobin because transport of oxygen by hemoglobin requires molecular iron in the bivalent state; corrects the abnormal red blood cell condition

USES

Prevention and treatment of iron-deficiency anemias
Prophylactic therapy during periods of increased iron requirements, e.g., pregnancy, rapid growth, and sustained hemorrhaging

DOSAGE

See Table 34-1

FATE

Absorption occurs primarily from the duodenum and jejunum; only 5% to 10% of dose is absorbed in normal persons and up to 20% in iron-deficient patients. Ferrous iron (i.e., Fe^{+2}) is much more efficiently absorbed than ferric iron (i.e., Fe^{+3}). Bivalent iron is then converted to trivalent iron in gastric mucosal cells and then either combined with transferrin for transport to bone marrow cells or converted to ferritin or hemosiderin and stored either in gastric mucosal cells, liver, spleen, or bone marrow. Excretion of iron is minimal (generally less than 1 mg/day) and occurs mainly in feces through sloughing of iron-containing intestinal mucosal cells. Very small amounts of iron may also be eliminated in the urine and sweat

COMMON SIDE EFFECTS

GI irritation, nausea, constipation, darkened stools

SIGNIFICANT ADVERSE REACTIONS

(Usually occur with large doses) Vomiting, diarrhea, allergic reactions, drowsiness, abdominal pain, stomach and intestinal erosion, hypotension, weak pulse, shock, convulsions

CONTRAINDICATIONS

Peptic ulcer, ulcerative colitis, regional enteritis, hemochromatosis, hemosiderosis, hemolytic anemia. *Cautious use* in hepatic cirrhosis

INTERACTIONS

Absorption of iron may be impaired by antacids (especially those containing magnesium trisilicate), cholestyramine, and pancreatic extracts, as well as by ingestion of eggs or milk
Oral iron retards absorption of tetracyclines and penicillamine
Effectiveness of iron may be impaired by vitamin E, hydroxyurea, and oral contraceptives
Vitamin C may facilitate iron absorption by maintaining it in the ferrous state
Chloramphenicol can delay clearance of iron from the plasma and its incorporation into red blood cells
Allopurinol may interfere with the action of an enzyme that controls iron absorption, leading to excessive absorption

NURSING CONSIDERATIONS

1. Refer patient to dietitian for assessment of dietary iron intake, if possible, and note other drugs patient is taking that may contribute to anemia (e.g., quinidine, antiinflammatory drugs, sulfonamides). Blood counts and hemoglobin values should be obtained before iron is prescribed.
2. Note that oral iron preparations are available in combination with many other drugs (e.g., B and C vitamins, folic acid, dessicated liver, antacids, stool softeners).

PATIENT EDUCATION

1. Warn patient that self-medication with iron preparations may mask symptoms of a more severe underlying disease.
2. Inform patient that GI disturbances (irritation, cramping, constipation) are common in initial stages of therapy but can usually be minimized by reducing the dose, taking the drug with food, or changing the type of preparation taken.
3. Suggest taking drug with food if GI irritation occurs, although this may reduce absorption. Milk or antacids should be avoided because they may further impair absorption.
4. Instruct patient using liquid form to take drug through a straw and to rinse mouth immediately after ingestion because preparation can stain teeth.
5. Inform patient that oral iron preparations can cause black or dark green stools, which are *not* usually a sign of GI bleeding.
6. Inform patient that hemoglobin and reticulocyte values will probably be checked periodically during therapy. Improvement should be noted within 2 to 4 weeks. If not, reassessment is warranted.

PARENTERAL IRON PREPARATION

Iron Dextran

Imferon and other manufacturers

Iron dextran is a complex of ferric hydroxide with dextran in physiologic saline used either IV or IM for treating iron-deficiency anemias in patients intolerant of or resistant to oral iron preparations.

MECHANISM

Hydrolysis of the iron–dextran complex by reticuloendothelial cells of liver, spleen, and bone marrow releases ferric iron, which combines with transferrin and is transported to the bone marrow to be used in the synthesis of hemoglobin, as it is gradually converted to a utilizable form of iron

USES

Treatment of iron-deficiency anemias in patients where oral iron administration is ineffective or poorly tolerated

DOSAGE

(1 mL iron dextran complex equals 50 mg elemental iron) To determine quantity of iron needed, the following formula may be used:

$$0.3 \times wt\ (lb) \times \left(100 - \frac{Hb\ in\ g\% \times 100}{14.8}\right) = mg\ iron$$

A more practical rule is 250 mg iron for each gram of hemoglobin below normal.
Recommended dosing procedures are:

IM: test dose of 25 mg (i.e., 0.5 mL) on first day to test for allergic reactions—if no evidence of hypersensitivity within 1 to 2 hours, the remainder of the first day's dose can be

Table 34-1
Oral Iron Preparations

Drug	Preparations	Usual Dosage Range	Nursing Implications
Ferrous Fumarate Femiron, Feostat, Fumasorb, Fumerin, Hemocyte, Ircon, Palmiron, Span-FF, (CAN) Neo-Fer-50, Novofumar, Palafer	Tablets: 63 mg, 195 mg, 200 mg, 300 mg, 324 mg, 325 mg Chewable tablets: 100 mg Suspension: 100 mg/5 mL Drops: 45 mg/0.6 mL Controlled-release capsules: 325 mg	Adults: 200 mg–300 mg 1–3 times/day Children (under 6): 100 mg–300 mg/day in divided doses	Contains 33% elemental iron; essentially similar to ferrous sulfate in most respects, with slightly lower incidence of some GI side effects; available in combination with docusate as timed-release capsules (Ferocyl, Ferro-Sequels)
Ferrous Gluconate Fergon, Ferralet, Simron, (CAN) Fertinic, Novoferrogluc	Tablets: 300 mg, 320 mg, 325 mg Capsules: 86 mg, 325 mg, 435 mg Elixir: 300 mg/5 mL	Adults: 300 mg–650 mg 3 times/day Children (6–12 yr): 300 mg 1–3 times/day Children (under 6 yr): 100 mg–300 mg/day in divided doses	Contains 11.6% elemental iron; somewhat better tolerated and better utilized than other forms of iron; lower incidence of GI distress
Ferrous Sulfate Feosol, Fer-In-Sol, Fer-Iron, Ferralyn, Fero-Gradumet, Ferospace, Mol-Iron, Slow FE, (CAN) Fesofor, Novoferrosulfa	Tablets: 195 mg, 200 mg, 300 mg, 325 mg Timed-release capsules: 150 mg, 160 mg, 250 mg Timed-release tablets: 160 mg, 525 mg Syrup: 90 mg/5 mL Elixir: 220 mg/5 mL Drops: 75 mg/0.6 mL, 125 mg/mL	Adults: 300 mg–1200 mg/day in divided doses Children (6–12 yr): 120 mg–600 mg/day in divided doses Children (under 6 yr): 300 mg/day in divided doses	Contains 20% elemental iron; most widely used form of oral iron; best absorbed and least expensive; high degree of GI irritation that can be minimized by using sustained-release forms; available in combination with magnesium–aluminum hydroxide as Fermalox
Polysaccharide–Iron Complex Hytinic, Niferex, Nu-Iron	Tablets: 50 mg iron Capsules: 150 mg iron Elixir: 100 mg iron/5 mL	Adults: 50 mg–300 mg/day in divided doses as required Children: 50 mg–100 mg/day	Water-soluble complex of elemental iron and a low-molecular-weight polysaccharide; fewer GI side effects than with other forms of iron, no teeth staining, and no metallic aftertaste; fairly expensive

given; each day's dose should not exceed 25 mg iron for infants under 10 lb, 50 mg iron for children under 20 lb, 100 mg iron for patients under 110 lb, and 250 mg iron for other patients until the calculated total dose has been given

IV infusion: Dilute the calculated iron dose in 200 mL to 250 mL of normal saline; administer a test dose of 25 mg over 5 minutes; if no adverse effects occur, infuse the rest of the dose over 1 to 2 hours

Note: IV infusion of iron dextran is not a labeled indication, but it is widely used because it eliminates the need for multiple IM injections, pain and skin staining at the IM injection site, danger of abscess formation, and the possibility of poor absorption from muscle. It is used in patients who have poor IM absorptive capacity or uncontrolled bleeding, or where prolonged therapy is indicated

FATE
Slowly but well absorbed from IM injection sites (60% within 2–3 days and 90% within 1–2 wk); distributed through the reticuloendothelial system; excreted in urine, bile, and feces

COMMON SIDE EFFECTS
Flushing, dizziness (especially with too-rapid IV administration)

SIGNIFICANT ADVERSE REACTIONS
Anaphylactic reactions, other hypersensitivity reactions (rash, pruritus, urticaria, dyspnea, arthralgia, fever, chills, sweating, myalgia), soreness and inflammation at injection site, brown discoloration and sterile abscesses at IM injection sites, headache, vomiting, shivering, hypotension, lymphadenopathy, local phlebitis (IV injection), chest pain, tachycardia, arrhythmias, and convulsions

CONTRAINDICATIONS
Anemias other than iron-deficiency anemias, marked liver impairment, and pregnancy. *Cautious use* in patients with asthma or a history of allergies, rheumatoid arthritis, liver impairment, or ankylosing spondylitis, and in women of childbearing potential

NURSING CONSIDERATIONS

Nursing Alerts
- Have epinephrine (1:1000) solution available to treat acute hypersensitivity because fatal anaphylactic-type reactions have occurred. A small initial test dose should always be administered to determine patient's sensitivity,

and patient should be carefully observed for signs of hypersensitivity.
- Keep patient recumbent for 30 to 60 minutes following IV administration to minimize orthostatic hypotension. Drug should be used IV only in patient with insufficient muscle mass, impaired IM absorptive capacity (e.g., edema), or uncontrolled bleeding, or for whom massive or prolonged therapy is indicated.

1. Administer IM injections into upper, outer quadrant of buttock using a large (19 or 20 gauge, 2–3 in) needle. Use Z-track technique to avoid leakage into and staining of overlying subcutaneous tissue (see Chap. 1).
2. When giving IM to patient who is standing, have patient bear weight on leg opposite injection site. Place supine patient in lateral position with injection site uppermost.
3. Monitor results of hemoglobin, hematocrit, and reticulocyte analyses, which should be obtained periodically during therapy. *Oral* iron therapy should be initiated as soon as feasible.
4. Periodically assess degree of pain and swelling experienced by patient with rheumatoid arthritis because iron dextran may cause an increase.
5. Do not use multiple-dose vials for IV administration because they contain a preservative (phenol).
6. Do not mix other drugs in solution with iron dextran.

VITAMIN B$_{12}$ AND FOLIC ACID

Vitamin B$_{12}$ and folic acid are two vitamins essential for normal deoxyribonucleic acid (DNA) synthesis. A deficiency of either can result in impaired DNA synthesis, inhibition of normal cell division, and anemia.

Cyanocobalamin, Crystalline

Betalin 12, Redisol, Rubramin PC and other manufacturers
(CAN) Anacobin, Rubion and other manufacturers

Cyanocobalamin (vitamin B$_{12}$) is a cobalt-containing substance essential for normal growth, cell reproduction, hematopoiesis, and nucleoprotein synthesis. It is a biologically potent compound, so only minute amounts (1 µg–2 µg) are necessary in the daily diet to supply the normal body needs. The most common cause of vitamin B$_{12}$ deficiency is insufficient GI absorption, due primarily to reduced availability of the *intrinsic factor*, a glycoprotein secreted by the gastric mucosal cells that is necessary for adequate absorption of B$_{12}$. This condition is referred to as *pernicious anemia* and is characterized hematologically by megaloblasts in the bone marrow and macrocytes in the plasma. The patient feels fatigued, and frequently there are GI and neurologic complications. Symptoms are usually readily reversed by supplemental injections of cyanocobalamin crystalline.

Cyanocobalamin is available over-the-counter for oral use as tablets and by prescription for IM or SC injection. Tablets containing less than 500 µg are *not* intended for treatment of pernicious anemia but should only be used as nutritional supplements (see Chap. 73).

MECHANISM

Activate folic acid coenzymes necessary for the synthesis of red blood cells, and facilitate the maturation of megaloblasts into normal erythrocytes; in vitamin B$_{12}$ deficiency states, cyanocobalamin improves GI function; relieves neurologic symptoms such as numbness, tingling, and incoordination; and arrests further neurologic damage

USES

Treatment of vitamin B$_{12}$ deficiency states caused by impaired GI absorption (e.g., pernicious anemia, GI dysfunction or surgery, tapeworm infestation, sprue)
Prevention of vitamin B$_{12}$ deficiency resulting from increased requirements (e.g., pregnancy; hemorrhage; malignancy; thyroid, liver or renal disease) or inadequate dietary intake (e.g., poverty, famine, alcoholism, vegetarian diet)
Performance of the Vitamin B$_{12}$ absorption test (Schilling test)
Treatment of nutritional vitamin B$_{12}$ deficiency (see Chap. 73)

DOSAGE

(Dependent on extent of vitamin B$_{12}$ deficiency)

Initially: 30 µg to 100 µg IM or SC daily for 5 to 10 days, then on alternate days for 2 weeks, then every third or fourth day for 2 to 3 weeks, then 100 µg to 200 µg once a month. (Up to 1000 µg/day has been used in seriously ill patients.) May be given orally if GI absorptive mechanisms are *not* impaired.
Children: 100 µg/dose to a total of 1 mg to 5 mg over 2 weeks, then 30 µg to 60 µg monthly.
Schilling test: 1000 µg IM 2 hours after an oral dose of radioactive cobalt—B$_{12}$ (0.5 µg–1 µg); urine is collected for 24 hours and radioactivity is measured; impaired absorption indicated by less than 5% urinary excretion of vitamin B$_{12}$ (normal is 10%–30%)

FATE

Intestinal absorption is dependent on the availability of sufficient intrinsic factor and calcium; vitamin B$_{12}$–intrinsic factor complex is transported through cells of the distal ileum by a specific receptor-mediated transport system; absorption from intramuscular or subcutaneous sites is rapid and the plasma level peaks within 1 hour; stored mainly in the liver and slowly released as needed for cellular metabolism; deficiency states only develop after considerable time in the absence of supplemental B$_{12}$; trace amounts (2 µg–5 µg) are normally lost in the urine and feces; however, when administered in large doses, 50% to 98% of the dose appears in the urine within 48 hours, mostly within the first 8 hours

COMMON SIDE EFFECTS

(Usually with parenteral therapy) Transient diarrhea, itching, flushing

SIGNIFICANT ADVERSE REACTIONS

Urticaria, pain at injection site, hypokalemia, peripheral vascular thrombosis, pulmonary edema, congestive heart failure, polycythemia vera, optic nerve atrophy, and anaphylactic shock

CONTRAINDICATIONS

Cobalt hypersensitivity, optic nerve damage. *Cautious use* in persons with infections, uremia, bone marrow depression, pulmonary edema, hypokalemia, neurologic disorders

INTERACTIONS

GI absorption of cyanocobalamin may be impaired by alcohol, *p*-aminosalicylic acid, colchicine, neomycin, and potassium chloride

Chloramphenicol may antagonize the beneficial therapeutic response to vitamin B_{12}

NURSING CONSIDERATIONS

Nursing Alerts
- Expect to administer vitamin B_{12} parenterally in cases of pernicious anemia because oral administration is unreliable, and prolonged oral therapy may therefore result in permanent neurologic complications.
- Monitor results of serum potassium tests, which should be performed prior to treatment and regularly during initial days of therapy. Improvement of condition increases erythrocyte potassium requirements and may result in severe hypokalemia, with a possibly fatal outcome.
- Assess patient for indications of pulmonary edema (e.g., dyspnea, night cough), which can occur early in therapy.

1. Refer patient to dietitian for a dietary history. If possible, dietary deficiencies should be corrected. Strict vegetarian diets can lead to vitamin B_{12} deficiency. Good sources of vitamin B_{12} are red meats, liver, egg yolk, dairy products, clams, oysters, and sardines. Because single vitamin B_{12} deficiency is rare, multiple vitamin supplementation is often indicated.
2. Interpret results of vitamin B_{12} or folic acid blood assays cautiously if patient is taking an antibiotic or methotrexate.
3. Assist with evaluation of drug therapy. Therapeutic response is usually rapid (within 48 h), as measured by improved hematologic status, lessened GI and neurologic symptoms, and decreased fatigue. Reticulocyte counts rise in 3 to 4 days, peak in 7 to 8 days, than gradually decline as erythrocyte counts and hemoglobin rise.

PATIENT EDUCATION
1. Instruct patient to take oral vitamin B_{12} with meals to increase absorption (food stimulates production of intrinsic factor) and to avoid mixing drug with citrus juices because ascorbic acid may adversely affect its stability.
2. Stress the importance of *continual* vitamin B_{12} therapy in patient with pernicious anemia. Interruption of treatment can result in progressive neurologic damage.
3. Explain that excessive consumption of alcohol may cause malabsorption of vitamin B_{12}.
4. Instruct patient to report the development of an infection because decreased vitamin B_{12} effectiveness can result. Dosage may have to be temporarily increased.
5. Instruct patient to check with physician before using multiple B vitamin preparations because doses of vitamin B_{12} greater than 10 μg/day may mask symptoms of folate deficiency.

Hydroxocobalamin, Crystalline

AlphaRedisol and several other manufacturers
(CAN) Acti-B_{12}

Hydroxocobalamin is a source of vitamin B_{12} similar in actions, indications, and untoward reactions to cyanocobalamin. It is more slowly absorbed than cyanocobalamin, resulting in a more sustained rise in serum cobalamin levels and less urinary excretion of cobalamin following each injection, and may be taken up by the liver in larger quantities than cyanocobalamin.

Hydroxocobalamin is used for the same indications as cyanocobalamin and is preferred by some because it remains in the circulation longer. In addition, hydroxocobalamin has been used to treat cyanide toxicity, such as that associated with excessive doses of sodium nitroprusside (see Chap. 31). It can combine with cyanide to yield cyanocobalamin, which is nontoxic and readily excreted in the urine. IM dosage is 30 μg/day for 5 to 10 days, then 100 μg/mo to 200 μg/mo as maintenance. Mild pain and irritation at injection site has been reported.

Folic Acid

Folvite
(CAN) Apo-Folic, Novofolacid

Folic acid, also known as folate or vitamin B_9 is a member of the B complex vitamin group essential for synthesis of nucleoproteins and maintenance of normal erythrocyte production. Folic acid stimulates production of red and white blood cells as well as platelets in megaloblastic anemias. Dietary folate is ultimately converted in the body to tetrahydrofolic acid, which functions as a coenzyme in may reactions, especially the synthesis of purine and pyrimidine precursors of nucleic acids. Folate is available in many different foods (e.g., vegetables, milk, eggs, liver), so deficiencies rarely occur. Most likely causes are malnutrition, greatly increased demands (e.g., repeated pregnancy), and malabsorption syndromes such as sprue or celiac disease. Patients lacking sufficient folic acid usually develop a megaloblastic anemia similar to that observed in pernicious anemia, although the incidence of neurologic damage is much less than the damage observed in cases of vitamin B_{12} deficiency. Oral or parenteral administration of folic acid readily corrects the anemia, both symptomatically and hematologically, and improvement can be maintained by very small daily doses of folic acid.

MECHANISM
Converted to tetrahydrofolic acid, which is essential for proper synthesis of purines and pyrimidines, and ultimately nucleic acids; deficiency of folic acid impairs production of bone marrow blood cell precursors

USES
Treatment of megaloblastic anemias caused by deficiency of folic acid, as seen in malnutrition, alcoholism, pregnancy, infancy, sprue or celiac disease

DOSAGE
Initially up to 1.0 mg daily until clinical symptoms have subsided; maintenance is 0.1 mg to 0.4 mg daily depending on age; 0.8 mg daily for pregnant or lactating women

FATE
Well absorbed from GI tract and widely distributed; highly bound to plasma proteins; in the liver; excreted in the urine, feces, and breast milk

COMMON SIDE EFFECTS
(Rare) Flushing following IV injection

SIGNIFICANT ADVERSE REACTIONS
(Rare) Allergic reactions (rash, itching, bronchospasm), GI distress, irritability, confusion, and depression

CONTRAINDICATIONS
Pernicious, aplastic, and normocytic anemias

INTERACTIONS

Effects of folic acid may be decreased by barbiturates, chloramphenicol, oral contraceptives, phenytoin, and primidone

Folic acid may reduce phenytoin blood levels, requiring an increase in dosage

Trimethoprim, triamterene, and pyrimethamine may interfere with utilization of folic acid

NURSING CONSIDERATIONS

1. Expect to administer drug orally, although it can be given IM, IV, or SC in severe diseases or if GI absorption is impaired, and to use higher than normal dosages in the presence of alcoholism, hemolytic anemia, chronic infection, and anticonvulsant therapy (especially with hydantoins).
2. Assist with evaluation of drug therapy. Beneficial effects may appear within 24 hours (decreased malaise, improved outlook), although it may take 3 to 5 days for hematologic studies to improve.

PATIENT EDUCATION

1. Caution patient against self-medication with folic acid because this may delay recognition of other types of anemia.
2. Inform patient that foods high in folates include green vegetables, fruits, liver, and yeasts and that much of the folate content is destroyed by prolonged cooking or canning.

Leucovorin Calcium—Folinic Acid

Wellcovorin

Leucovorin is a metabolite of folic acid that is used IM to treat folate-deficient megaloblastic anemia when oral folic acid therapy is not feasible. The drug is also indicated for "leucovorin rescue," that is, to minimize the cellular toxicity resulting from large doses of methotrexate used in certain neoplastic diseases. Leucovorin prevents severe methotrexate-induced toxicity by preferentially protecting or "rescuing" normal cells from the action of folic-acid antagonists such as methotrexate without interfering with the desired oncolytic action of the drug. This cellular protective function is considered further in Chapter 72.

In treating megaloblastic anemia, leucovorin is administered IM in a dose of 1 mg/day. It should not be used in anemias secondary to a vitamin B_{12} deficiency, because the hematologic picture may improve while the neurologic deficit continues to accrue. Allergic reactions represent the principal group of adverse reactions.

Selected Bibliography

Callender ST: Treatment of iron deficiency. Clin Haematol 11:327, 1982

Cook JD: Clinical evaluation of iron deficiency. Semin Hematol 19(1):6, 1982

Cooper BA: Megaloblastic anemia. Drug Ther 14(4):65, 1984

Hallberg L: Bioavailability of dietary iron in man. Annu Rev Nutr 1:123, 1981

Hoffbrand AV, Wickremasinghe RG: Megaloblastic anemia. In Hoffbrand AV (ed): Recent Advances in Hematology, p 25. Edinburgh, Churchill-Livingstone, 1982

Huebers H, Huebers E, Csiba E et al: The significance of transferrin for intestinal iron absorption. Blood 61:283, 1983

Lee GR: The anemia of chronic disease. Semin Hematol 20:61, 1983

Pollit E, Leibel RL (eds): Iron Deficiency: Brain Biochemistry and Behavior. New York, Raven Press, 1982

Siegel RS, Lessin LS: The hemolytic anemias: Guidelines to rational management. Drug Ther 14(4):87, 1984

SUMMARY. ANTIANEMIC DRUGS

Drug	Preparations	Usual Dosage Range
Oral Iron Preparations	See Table 34-1	
Iron Dextran Imferon and other manufacturers	Injection: ferric hydroxide and dextran equivalent to 50 mg iron/mL	See text
Cyanocobalamin, Crystalline Betalin 12, Redisol, Rubramin PC, and other manufacturers	Tablets: 500 µg, 1000 µg Injection: 30 µg, 100 µg, 1000 µg/mL (See also Chap. 73)	*Adults* SC, IM: 30 µg/day to 100 µg/day for 5–10 days, then 100 µg–200 µg/mo *Children* 100 µg/dose to a total of 1 mg–5 mg over 2 wk, then 30 µg–60 µg/mo
Hydroxocobalamin, Crystalline AlphaRedisol and other manufacturers	Injection: 1000 µg/mL	IM: 30 µg/day for 5–10 days, then 100 µg–200 µg/mo
Folic Acid Folvite	Tablets: 0.1 mg, 0.4 mg, 0.8 mg, 1.0 mg Injection: 5 mg/mL, 10 mg/mL	Initially up to 1.0 mg/day Maintenance is 0.1 mg–0.4 mg/day depending on age; 0.8 mg/day for pregnant women
Leucovorin Calcium Wellcovorin	Tablets: 5 mg, 25 mg Injection: 3 mg/mL, 5 mg/mL, 10 mg/mL Powder for oral solution: 1 mg/mL after reconstitution	Megaloblastic anemia: 1 mg/day, IM, leucovorin rescue—see Chap. 72

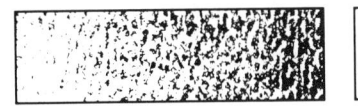

35 ANTICOAGULANT, THROMBOLYTIC, AND HEMOSTATIC DRUGS

The process of blood clot formation, and subsequent clot resolution, or lysis, is characterized by a chemically complex series of events that involves the interaction of a large number of substances (coagulation factors) present in blood plasma, blood cells (especially platelets), and, to a lesser extent, in body tissues.

The *coagulation factors*, which are listed in Table 35-1, function in either of two distinct pathways, the intrinsic clotting pathway and the extrinsic clotting pathway. The *intrinsic pathway* is so named because all of the coagulation proteins are present in the blood itself. The reactions are relatively slow, and several minutes are required to produce a clot. The *extrinsic pathway* is triggered by clotting factors derived from injured cells in tissues. It is a much more rapidly acting system: It can cause a blood clot to form within seconds. The interaction of the intrinsic and extrinsic pathways to produce a fibrin clot is shown schematically in Figure 35-1.

Drugs capable of affecting the coagulation process generally act on one or more of the stages shown in Figure 35-1. Agents preventing the formation of new clots are termed *anticoagulants*. Drugs increasing the rate of resolution (or lysis) of preformed clots are referred to as *thrombolytic agents*. Compounds enhancing blood clot formation, thereby reducing bleeding, are characterized as *hemostatic drugs*.

ANTICOAGULANT DRUGS

Therapy with anticoagulant drugs is directed primarily toward preventing development of intravascular thromboses, a major cause of death in thromboembolic disorders. Although these compounds are widely used, therapy with them is often empirical, (i.e., based on clinical experience), and their efficacy in treating some conditions for which they are used has been questioned. Moreover, they are potentially dangerous drugs, capable of causing severe, possibly fatal hemorrhaging, and therefore must be carefully prescribed and closely monitored. *Long-term* therapy with anticoagulant drugs remains a controversial area; nevertheless, when judiciously selected and properly employed, the several anticoagulant agents have an important place in clinical therapy and can markedly reduce the likelihood of vascular clotting, thus improving the quality of life and preventing mortality.

There are two classes of therapeutically useful anticoagulant drugs, the parenteral and oral agents. Heparin is the sole representative of the parenteral class, while the oral anticoagulant group encompasses several drugs characterized as either coumarin or indandione derivatives. Following a separate discussion of heparin, the oral anticoagulants are discussed as a group, followed by a listing of individual drugs. Mention is also made under this heading of both protamine sulfate, a heparin antagonist, and vitamin K and its derivatives, which are antagonists of the oral anticoagulant drugs. Finally, pentoxifylline, a drug that decreases blood viscosity and improves vascular flow, is considered under anticoagulants in this chapter.

Parenteral Anticoagulant

Heparin Sodium
Liquaemin
Heparin Calcium
Calciparine
(CAN) Calcilean, Hepalean, Minihep

Heparin is a mucopolysaccharide extracted from bovine lung or porcine intestinal tissue. Its potency is standardized by a biological assay and is expressed in units. The compound is a strong organic acid, possessing an electronegative charge that is essential for its anticoagulant activity. Blood clotting is inhibited in vivo as well as in vitro, and the effects of heparin are noted immediately upon administration. Heparin is usually given as the sodium salt but is also available as heparin calcium, which is equally effective.

MECHANISM
Accelerates the rate at which antithrombin III, an alpha-2-globulin produced by the liver, inactivates factors IX, X, XI and XII, as well as thrombin; thus, conversion of fibrinogen to fibrin is blocked, and activation of the fibrin-stabilizing factor (XIII) is also impaired; the rate-limiting step in the coagulation cascade is activation of factor X, which is inhibited by lower doses of heparin than those needed to neutralize thrombin, thus prophylactic therapy is accomplished with much lower doses than those necessary once the coagulation process has begun; may also reduce platelet adhesiveness; no fibrinolytic activity but may exert a diuretic and hypolipemic action, although the latter two actions are of no clinical value

USES
Prophylaxis and treatment of venous thromboses, pulmonary embolism, and atrial fibrillation with embolization
Prevention of postoperative deep venous thrombosis and pulmonary embolism in patients undergoing major (abdominothoracic, cardiac, arterial) surgery (low-dose regimen)
Prevention of cerebral thrombosis in evolving stroke
Diagnosis and treatment of acute and chronic consumption coagulopathies (disseminated intravascular coagulation)
Prevention of peripheral venous thrombosis following acute myocardial infarction
Anticoagulant in blood transfusion, dialysis procedures, blood samples for laboratory procedures, and extracorporeal circulation

DOSAGE
The dosage depends upon the patient's coagulation tests. Dosage is adequate when whole blood clotting time is 2.5 to 3 times the control value *or* the partial thromboplastin time (PTT) is 1.5 to 2 times the control value. *Recommended dosage guidelines for average size patients are:*

Table 35-1
Blood Coagulation Factors

Factor	Name	Function
I	Fibrinogen	Precursor of fibrin
II	Prothrombin	Precursor of thrombin
III	Thromboplastin	Triggers extrinsic coagulation pathway
IV	Calcium	Essential for several reactions in coagulation pathways
V	Proaccelerin	Accelerates conversion of prothrombin to thrombin
VII	Proconvertin	Accelerates the extrinsic coagulation pathway
VIII	Antihemophilic factor	Accelerates activation of factor X
IX	Christmas factor (plasma thromboplastin component; PTC)	Accelerates activation of factor X
X	Stuart-Prower factor	Accelerates conversion of prothrombin to thrombin
XI	Plasma thromboplastin antecedent (PTA)	Accelerates activation of factor IX
XII	Hageman factor	Triggers intrinsic coagulation pathway—activates factor XI
XIII	Fibrin stabilizing factor	Strengthens fibrin clot when activated by thrombin and calcium

Anticoagulation
SC: 10,000 to 20,000 units initially, then 8000 to 20,000 units every 8 to 12 hours
IV injection: 10,000 units initially, then 5000 to 10,000 units every 4 to 6 hours
IV infusion: 20,000 to 40,000 units/day in 1000 ml of isotonic sodium chloride solution, preceded by a 5000-unit IV loading dose
Children: 50 units/kg IV drip initially, followed by 100 units/kg IV every 4 hours *or* 20,000/m^2/24 hours by continuous infusion.

Postoperative prophylaxis
SC: 5000 units 2 hours before surgery and 5000 units every 8 to 12 hours for 7 days following surgery

Heart/blood vessel surgery
IV: 150 units/kg to 400 units/kg depending on length of surgery

Blood transfusion
7500 units/100 mL sterile sodium chloride injection; 6 mL to 8 mL of dilution is added per 100 mL whole blood

Laboratory samples
70 to 150 units/10 mL to 20 mL whole blood sample

FATE
Not active orally; immediate onset IV, with peak effect in 5 to 10 minutes and duration of 2 to 6 hours; gradually absorbed SC, with onset of 30 to 60 minutes and duration of 8 to 12 hours; highly bound to plasma proteins; plasma half-life averages 60 to 90 minutes but is prolonged at high doses; partially metabolized by the liver, and excreted in the urine as metabolites and unchanged drug; not found in appreciable amounts in the fetus or in breast milk

COMMON SIDE EFFECTS
Spontaneous bleeding, local irritation at SC and IM injection sites

Note: Thrombocytopenia may occur in up to one third of patients receiving heparin and is of two types. *Early* thrombocytopenia develops within 2 to 3 days after initiating therapy, is usually mild, and is seldom of clinical consequence. It appears to be due to a direct action of heparin on platelets and may remain stable or even reverse even if heparin is continued. *Delayed* thrombocytopenia occurs 6 to 12 days after initiation of therapy, probably reflects the presence of an immunoglobulin that induces platelet aggregation, and may be associated with hemorrhage and paradoxical thromboembolic episodes due to irreversible aggregation of platelets, the so-called white-clot syndrome. This condition may lead to skin necrosis, gangrene, pulmonary embolism, myocardial infarction, or stroke. If significant thrombocytopenia develops during heparin therapy, the drug should be discontinued and oral anticoagulants substituted. Most instances of delayed thrombocytopenia are attributable to heparin prepared from bovine lung rather than porcine intestine

SIGNIFICANT ADVERSE REACTIONS
Hemorrhaging, hypersensitivity (chills, urticaria, fever, rhinitis, asthmatic-like reaction, lacrimation, diarrhea, anaphylactic reaction), vasospastic reaction, increased serum transaminases, elevated blood pressure, chest pain, alopecia, osteoporosis, and impaired renal function

CONTRAINDICATIONS
Active bleeding or significant bleeding tendencies (e.g., hemophilia, purpura, thrombocytopenia), presence of a drainage tube, and threatened abortion. *Cautious use* in patients with a history of allergy (heparin is derived from animal tissue), renal or hepatic disease or alcoholism; during menstruation, pregnancy, or the immediate postpartum period; when administer-

Anticoagulant, Thrombolytic, and Hemostatic Drugs

INTRINSIC PATHWAY

Blood Vessel Damage → Exposure of subendothelial collagen

XII (Hageman factor) → XII$_a$

XI (Plasma thromboplastin antecedent) → XI$_a$ (Ca^{2+})

Liver cells, Vitamin K → IX (Christmas factor) → IX$_a$

Liver cells → X (Stuart Prower factor)

EXTRINSIC PATHWAY

Tissue Damage → III (Tissue thromboplastin)

VII (Proconvertin) ← Vitamin K ← Liver cells

VII → VII$_a$ (Ca^{2+})

FINAL COMMON PATHWAY

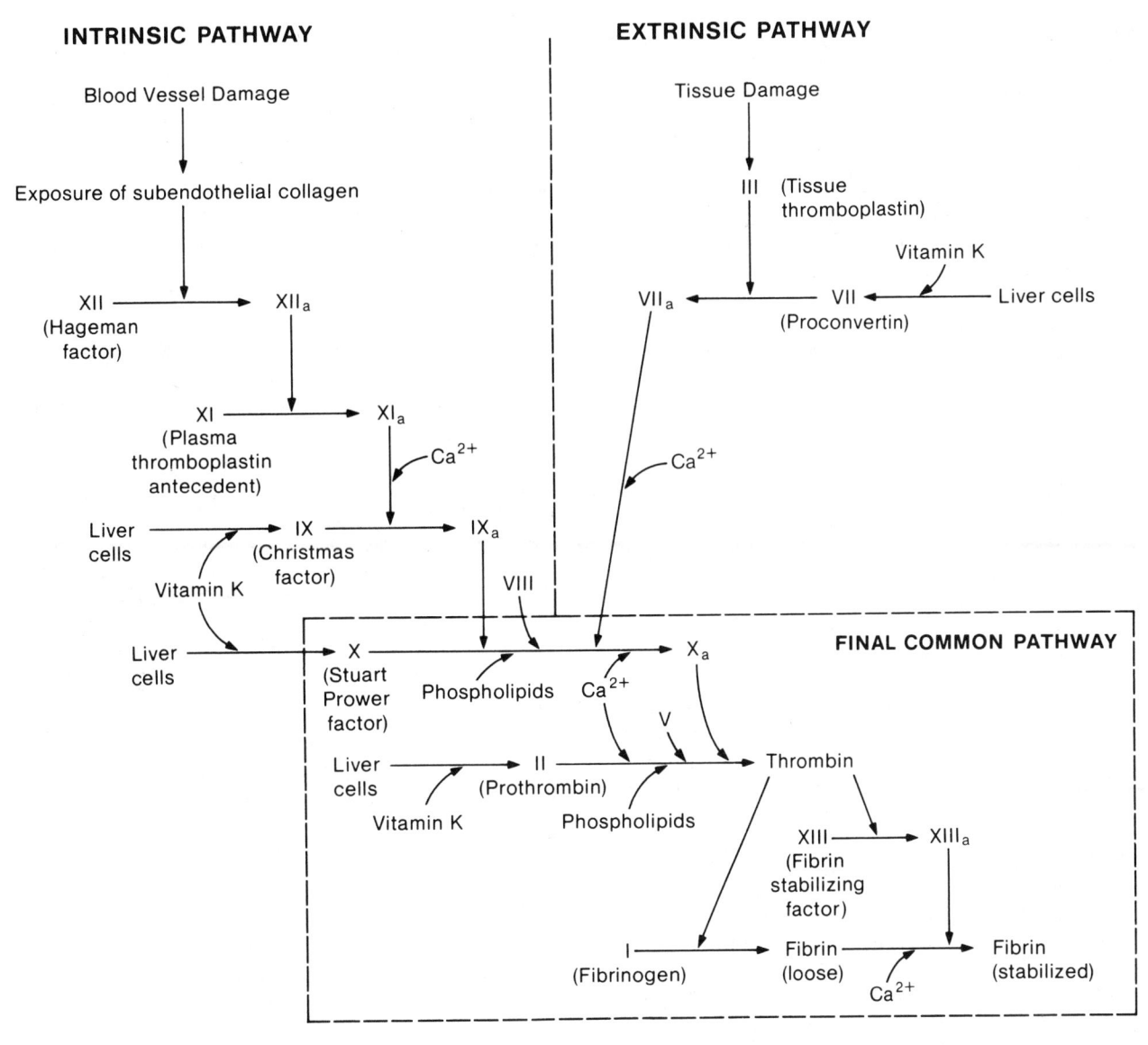

X + VIII + Phospholipids + Ca^{2+} → X$_a$

Liver cells, Vitamin K → II (Prothrombin) + V + Phospholipids → Thrombin

XIII (Fibrin stabilizing factor) → XIII$_a$

I (Fibrinogen) → Fibrin (loose) → Fibrin (stabilized) (Ca^{2+})

Figure 35–1 Coagulation pathways involved in hemostasis.

---

ing acid citrate dextrose (ACD)–converted blood, because heparin activity persists for several weeks following conversion of such blood; and in any condition in which there is increased risk of hemorrhage (e.g., following surgery of the brain, eye, or spinal cord); shock; severe hypertension; jaundice; ulcerative lesions; and in patients with indwelling catheters

INTERACTIONS

An increased risk of bleeding is present when heparin is used in combination with other drugs that can interfere with platelet aggregation, such as salicylates; phenylbutazone, nonsteroidal anti-inflammatory drugs, dipyridamole, valproic acid, dextran, and hydroxychloroquine

Heparin can antagonize the action of ACTH, insulin, and corticosteroids

The action of heparin may be partially reduced by antihistamines, hydroxyzine, digitalis, tetracyclines, and phenothiazines, although the mechanism of this interaction is not established

Heparin may elevate the plasma levels of diazepam

NURSING CONSIDERATIONS

Nursing Alerts
- Have available protamine sulfate, a specific heparin antagonist (see below), as well as whole blood or plasma, in case of heparin overdosage. Monitor vital signs during therapy.
- Check results of most recent clotting test, such as activated partial thromboplastin time (APTT), prior to each SC or IV injection. During early stages of IV infusion, tests should be performed every 4 hours. Careful titration of dosage based on test results is critical for safe, effective therapy. Heparin should not be administered to any patient who cannot be kept under careful observation with periodic coagulation tests.
- Monitor results of platelet counts, which should be performed prior to initiating therapy and regularly thereafter to detect thrombocytopenia (see Common Side Effects, above).

- Assess patient frequently for signs of unusual bleeding (e.g., discoloration of urine or feces, bruising, petechiae, or low back pain, which may indicate abdominal bleeding).
- Observe for early signs of an allergic reaction (chills, fever, itching, dyspnea).
- Inform physician if fever or other symptoms of infection develop because the patient with an infection, as well as the postoperative patient or one with thrombophlebitis, thrombosis, myocardial infarction, or cancer, may be resistant to heparin.

1. Administer SC or IV only because hematoma can occur with IM administration.
2. Give SC injection deep into fatty layers of abdomen or above iliac crest to minimize local irritation. Alternate injection sites, and observe for hematoma. Do not aspirate syringe. Use "bunching" technique or Z-track method (see Chap. 1).
3. When administering heparin with oral anticoagulants, ensure that at least 5 hours elapse after the last IV dose and 24 hours after the last SC dose before blood is drawn for a prothrombin time. Heparin may be withdrawn when prothrombin activity is in the desired range. Oral anticoagulant and heparin therapy usually overlap for 3 to 5 days.
4. Note that solutions of heparin diluted in saline (10 units or 100 units/mL) are available for use as an IV flush (Heparin Sodium Lock Flush Solution) to maintain the patency of indwelling IV catheters. These solutions are *not* intended for therapeutic use.

PATIENT EDUCATION

1. Inform patient that diuresis can occur following heparin therapy. During prolonged treatment, suggest potassium supplementation (e.g., orange juice, bananas).
2. Warn patient that indiscriminate use of alcohol or OTC preparations containing aspirin or the cough suppressant guaifenesin may alter response to heparin.
3. Reassure patient that alopecia, if it occurs, is temporary.

Heparin Antagonist

Protamine Sulfate

Protamine sulfate is a mixture of proteins exhibiting a strongly positive charge that is capable of chemically combining with heparin, producing a stable salt and thereby neutralizing the anticoagulant action of heparin. However, it may exert an anticoagulant effect when administered alone or when dosage exceeds that required to neutralize heparin.

USES

Treatment of heparin overdosage

DOSAGE

Each mg of protamine sulfate neutralizes approximately 90 units of heparin activity derived from lung tissue and 115 units of heparin activity derived from intestinal mucosa

Administer slowly IV over 1 to 3 minutes, not to exceed 50 mg in a 10-minute period

FATE

Onset of action within 5 minutes; duration lasts 1 to 2 hours

COMMON SIDE EFFECTS

Flushing, feeling of warmth

SIGNIFICANT ADVERSE REACTIONS

(Especially with too-rapid injection)
Sudden hypotension, bradycardia, dyspnea, and allergic reactions

CONTRAINDICATIONS

No absolute contraindications. *Cautious use* in patients with cardiovascular disease or fish allergies (protamine is derived from fish sources); have facilities available to treat shock

NURSING CONSIDERATIONS

Nursing Alerts

- Monitor vital signs during administration and for at least 3 to 4 hours afterwards.
- Observe patient for signs of increased bleeding if very large doses are used because protamine itself has weak anticoagulant properties. It should not be used to treat hemorrhage resulting from any condition other than heparin overdosage.

1. Monitor results of blood coagulation studies (e.g., heparin titration test, plasma thrombin time), which should be performed to determine the need for repeat doses.

Oral Anticoagulants

Coumarin derivatives Indandione
Dicumarol   Anisindione
Warfarin

MECHANISM

Depress the hepatic synthesis of vitamin K–dependent clotting factors II, VII, IX, and X by inhibiting vitamin K_2, 3-epoxide reductase enzymes; factor VII is the first to be depleted, (since it has the shortest half-life), followed sequentially by factors IX, X, and II, which have longer half-lives. Thus, initial prolongation of prothrombin time occurs within 8 to 12 hours, but maximal anticoagulant activity requires several days to develop. These drugs exert no effect on established thrombus but may prevent further extension of the formed clot, thereby preventing secondary thromboembolic complications

USES

Prophylaxis and treatment of venous thrombosis and its extension
Treatment of atrial fibrillation with embolism
Prophylaxis and treatment of pulmonary embolism
Adjunctive treatment of coronary occlusion
Prophylaxis in patients with prosthetic valves
Investigational uses include prevention of recurrent transient ischemic attacks and reduction of risk of recurrence following myocardial infarction

DOSAGE

See Table 35-2

FATE

(See Table 35-2 for individual drug properties.) Most are almost completely absorbed orally, although absorption rates vary widely; peak activity usually occurs within 2 to 4 days; effects persist 2 to 5 days with warfarin, 2 to 10 days with dicumarol, and 1 to 3 days with anisindione; all drugs are highly but weakly bound to plasma proteins; metabolized by hepatic microsomal enzymes, and excreted primarily in the urine as inactive metabolites

COMMON SIDE EFFECTS

Hemorrhagic episodes (nosebleed, petechiae, bleeding gums, hematuria, bleeding from wounds)

SIGNIFICANT ADVERSE REACTIONS

Coumarins: nausea, anorexia, severe bleeding, adrenal hemorrhage, vomiting, abdominal cramping, diarrhea, urticaria, dermatitis, alopecia, fever, agranulocytosis, leukopenia, mucosal ulceration, nephropathy

Indandione: dermatitis, urticaria, fever, diarrhea, jaundice, nephropathy, agranulocytosis

CONTRAINDICATIONS

Hemorrhagic tendencies; hemophilia; thrombocytopenic purpura; recent or contemplated surgery (especially eye or CNS surgery); active bleeding; ulcerative, traumatic, or surgical wounds; visceral carcinoma; diverticulitis; colitis; aneurysm; acute nephritis; suspicion of cerebrovascular hemorrhage; eclampsia or preeclampsia; threatened abortion; uncontrolled hypertension; hepatic insufficiency; polyarthritis; polycythemia vera; subacute bacterial endocarditis; ascorbic acid (vitamin C) deficiency; spinal puncture; continuous GI drainage; and regional block anesthesia. *Cautious use* in the presence of congestive heart failure, mild liver or kidney dysfunction, alcoholism, tuberculosis, history of ulcerative disease, diabetes, allergic disorders, poor nutritional states, collagen disease, pancreatic disorders, vitamin K deficiency, hypothyroidism, x-ray therapy, edema, and hyperlipidemia

INTERACTIONS

The hypoprothrombinemic effect of oral anticoagulants may be enhanced by drugs that decrease vitamin K levels (antibiotics, cholestyramine, mineral oil); drugs that displace the anticoagulants from their protein binding sites (clofibrate, chloral hydrate, diazoxide, miconazole, nalidixic acid, phenylbutazone, salicylates, sulfonamides, oral hypoglycemics); drugs that inhibit the metabolism of anticoagulants (alcohol, allopurinol, amiodarone, chloramphenicol, cimetidine, cotrimoxazole, disulfiram, methylphenidate, metronidazole, phenylbutazone, propoxyphene, sulfinpyrazone, tricyclic antidepressants); and also by anabolic steroids, erythromycin, gemfibrozil, glucagon, sulindac, danazol, ketoconazole, propranolol, and thyroid drugs

Increased incidence of hemorrhage can occur with combined use of oral anticoagulants and inhibitors of platelet aggregation (cephalosporins, dipyridamole, indomethacin, pyrazolones, salicylates), inhibitors of procoagulant factors (antimetabolites, alkylating agents, quinidine, salicylates), or ulcerogenic drugs (corticosteroids, indomethacin, pyrazolones, potassium salts, salicylates).

A decreased anticoagulant effect may be observed if oral anticoagulants are used in the presence of enzyme inducers (barbiturates, carbamazepine, ethchlorvynol, glutethimide, griseofulvin, phenytoin, rifampin); activators of procoagulant factors (estrogens, oral contraceptives, vitamin K); and drugs that can decrease GI absorption (cholestyramine, colestipol)

Oral anticoagulants may potentiate the action of phenytoin and the oral hypoglycemic drugs by inhibiting their liver metabolism

Concurrent use of oral anticoagulants with thrombolytic agents (see discussion later in this chapter) can increase the risk of bleeding

NURSING CONSIDERATIONS

Nursing Alerts

- Obtain careful drug history prior to initiation of therapy.
- Monitor results of prothrombin determinations, which should be obtained daily during initial stages of therapy and during periods of dosage adjustment or addition of other drugs. Prothrombin time should be maintained at 1.5 to 2 times the control value.
- Expect dosages to be prescribed daily after results of prothrombin times are available. Initial doses are based on anticipated maintenance levels. Excessive loading doses have been associated with increased bleeding complications. Heparin is preferred if rapid anticoagulation is desired.
- Observe for signs of overdosage during early stages of therapy because onset of clinical effects is delayed several days, during which time the drug may accumulate.

1. During maintenance therapy, ensure that prothrombin time is determined at 1- to 4-week intervals depending upon drug response. Periodic blood counts, urinalyses, and liver function tests should also be obtained.
2. Expect therapy to be withdrawn gradually over 3 to 4 weeks. It should not be terminated abruptly. Prothrombin activity returns to normal within 2 to 10 days following cessation of therapy.

PATIENT EDUCATION

1. Stress the importance of strict compliance with the prescribed dosage schedule (see **Plan of Nursing Care 2, Chap. 7**). Compliance is poorest in elderly, alcoholic, and emotionally unstable persons. Their drug-taking practices should be closely monitored.
2. Caution patient to avoid starting or discontinuing any other medications without professional guidance.
3. Ensure that patient understands the need to observe for signs of abnormal bleeding (e.g., hematuria, tarry stools, hematemesis, petechiae, ecchymoses, bleeding gums, nosebleed, excessive menses). Bleeding should be immediately reported to health care provider because dosage adjustment is indicated.
4. Inform patient that minor overdosage, which is characterized by petechiae, oozing from cuts, or bleeding of gums after brushing, can be treated by omitting one or more doses until prothrombin time returns to therapeutic range. More severe bleeding can be treated with oral (1 mg–10 mg) or parenteral (20 mg–40 mg) vitamin K, depending on severity. Occasionally, transfusion with fresh whole blood or fresh-frozen plasma may be required.

Table 35-2
Oral Anticoagulants

Drug	Preparations	Usual Dosage Range	Nursing Implications
Coumarins			
Dicumarol Dicumarol	Tablets: 25 mg, 50 mg	200 mg–300 mg first day; 25 mg–200 mg/day thereafter, depending on prothrombin time	Slowly and incompletely absorbed orally; peak effect in 3–5 days; be alert for accumulation toxicity (especially bleeding), because drug is long acting; poorly water soluble; half-life increases with increasing dose
Warfarin Sodium Carfin, Coumadin, Panwarfin, Sofarin, (CAN) Warfilone	Tablets: 2 mg, 2.5 mg, 5 mg, 7.5 mg, 10 mg Injection: 50 mg/vial with 2-mL diluent	Initially 10 mg–15 mg/day (up to 60 mg/day) orally; thereafter, adjust based on prothrombin time Usual maintenance—2 mg–15 mg/day (may be given IM or IV for 1 dose if necessary)	Well absorbed orally; peak effect in 1–3 days, and duration of 3–5 days; most widely used oral anticoagulant, giving most uniform response; reduce dose by half in elderly or debilitated patients; do not use injectable solution if precipitate is present
Indandione			
Anisindione Miradon	Tablets: 50 mg	300 mg first day, 200 mg second day, 100 mg third day; then 25 mg–250 mg daily for maintenance	Indandione derivative infrequently used as oral anticoagulant; peak effects occur with 2–3 days and persist for 1–3 days; dermatitis is the most common side-effect; may turn urine red-orange

5. Warn patient to note development of early signs of agranulocytosis (fever, chills, sore throat, malaise, mucosal ulceration) or hepatitis (itching, dark urine, jaundice) and report at once. Discontinuation of medication is advisable.
6. Advise patient that many factors may affect anticoagulant response, including maintenance of a well-balanced diet and avoidance of excessive alcohol consumption.
7. Encourage patient to carry some form of identification at all times stating the type of medication taken and health care provider's name.
8. Instruct patient to restrict intake of foods rich in vitamin K (see Table 74-1) because they may reduce the effectiveness of oral anticoagulants.

Oral Anticoagulant Antagonist

Vitamin K is effective as an antidote to overdosage with the oral anticoagulant drugs. Two forms of vitamin K are available; (1) phytonadione (vitamin K_1), a fat-soluble derivative resembling naturally occurring vitamin K; and (2) menadiol (vitamin K_4), a synthetic water-soluble analog which is converted to menadione (vitamin K_3) in vivo. Phytonadione is the preferred drug for treatment of anticoagulant-induced prothrombin deficiency because menadiol is less potent, less dependable, less rapid acting, and shorter acting than K_1.

The complete pharmacology of the vitamin K preparations is reviewed in detail in Chapter 74. The present discussion is limited to the use of phytonadione (vitamin K_1), the preferred antidote, for the treatment of oral anticoagulant overdosage.

Phytonadione (K_1)

AquaMEPHYTON, Konakion, Mephyton

MECHANISM

Promotes hepatic synthesis of blood clotting factors II, VII, IX, and X, thereby reversing oral anticoagulant–induced prothrombin depression; no antidotal effects against heparin

USES

Treatment of anticoagulant-induced prothrombin deficiency (oral or parenteral K_1)
Treatment of hypoprothrombinemia secondary to antibacterial therapy, obstructive jaundice, biliary fistulas, or salicylate administration (oral or parenteral K_1)
Prophylaxis and therapy of newborn hemorrhagic disease (parenteral K_1)
Treatment of hypoprothrombinemia secondary to malabsorption or impaired synthesis of vitamin K such as can occur in ulcerative colitis, obstructive jaundice, celiac disease, intestinal resection, or regional enteritis (parenteral K_1)

DOSAGE

(Use smallest effective dose)
Anticoagulant overdosage:
Oral: 2.5 mg to 10 mg (maximum 50 mg) initially; repeat in 12 to 24 hours as needed
SC, IM: 0.5 mg to 10 mg (maximum 25 mg) initially; repeat in 6 to 8 hours as needed

IV (emergency only—see Significant Adverse Reactions): 0.5 mg to 10 mg at a rate of 1 mg/min

FATE
Effects appear in 6 to 10 hours with oral use and 1 to 2 hours with parenteral use (15 min following IV injection); oral absorption requires presence of bile in the GI tract; normal prothrombin level usually is obtained within 12 to 16 hours

COMMON SIDE EFFECTS
Flushing, GI upset

SIGNIFICANT ADVERSE REACTIONS

> **WARNING**
> Severe anaphylactic reactions have occurred following IV injection of AquaMEPHYTON (an aqueous colloidal solution of K_1), resulting in shock, cardiac arrest, and respiratory arrest. Therefore, the IV route should be used *only* when other routes are not feasible and with full consideration of all risks.

Pain, swelling, and tenderness at injection site, allergic reactions (bronchospasm, dyspnea, anaphylaxis), cramping, chills, fever, weakness, dizziness, chest constriction, profuse sweating, erythema, cyanosis

CONTRAINDICATIONS
No absolute contraindications. *Cautious use* during pregnancy and in the presence of severe liver disease

INTERACTIONS
Concurrent administration of phytonadione with mineral oil or cholestyramine may result in impaired vitamin K absorption

When large doses of phytonadione are used, temporary resistance to oral anticoagulants may be encountered; if anticoagulant therapy becomes necessary, heparin may be required

Oral antibiotics, quinidine, and salicylates may interfere with vitamin K activity

NURSING CONSIDERATIONS

Nursing Alerts
- In cases of severe hemorrhage, be prepared to administer whole blood or plasma transfusions because it takes several hours for vitamin K to enhance prothrombin synthesis.
- Dilute IV injection with sodium chloride or dextrose solution, and administer very slowly. Severe reactions, including fatal anaphylaxis, have occurred following IV injection (see Significant Adverse Reactions).
- Expect to administer the smallest dose that is effective in restoring normal prothrombin time. Overzealous use may promote return of thromboembolic complications and can interfere with action of oral anticoagulants for an extended period (2–3 wk). If patient who has received large doses of phytonadione exhibits resistance to subsequent oral anticoagulant therapy, larger than normal doses of the oral drugs or use of heparin may be required.

1. Monitor results of prothrombin times, which should be performed frequently during therapy to aid in determining dosage and frequency of administration.
2. Question the use of drugs that can interfere with vitamin K activity (e.g., oral antibiotics, quinidine, salicylates) during phytonadione therapy.
3. Use IV dilution immediately, and discard unused portion. Protect from light by wrapping container during use.

PATIENT EDUCATION
1. Instruct patient to restrict intake of foods rich in vitamin K (see Table 74-1) during therapy.

Hemorheologic Agent

Pentoxifylline
Trental

Pentoxifylline is a xanthine derivative, structurally related to caffeine and theophylline. It is termed a hemorheologic agent, inasmuch as it lowers blood viscosity and improves the flexibility of red blood cells. Therefore, in patients with impaired blood flow in microcirculatory areas, pentoxifylline can increase oxygenation of tissues supplied by these occluded vessels by improving microcirculatory blood flow. It is used principally in the treatment of intermittent claudication resulting from chronic occlusive arterial disease of the limbs.

MECHANISM
Improves regional blood flow by reducing blood viscosity and improving red blood cell flexibility; increases cellular ATP content, thereby decreasing tendency of red cells to aggregate; may also stimulate release of prostacyclin and impair formation of thromboxane A_2, which also decreases likelihood of platelet aggregation and promotes vasodilation

USES
Symptomatic treatment of intermittent claudication due to chronic occlusive arterial disease
Symptomatic treatment of cerebrovascular insufficiency (investigational use)

DOSAGE
400 mg three times daily with meals for at least 8 weeks. If gastrointestinal or central nervous system side effects are bothersome, dosage may be decreased to 400 mg twice a day

FATE
Following oral administration, peak plasma levels occur within 2 to 4 hours and remain constant thereafter; plasma half-life ranges from 30 to 90 minutes, but therapeutic effects generally are not seen for 4 to 8 weeks; the drug is metabolized in the liver and excreted primarily in the urine

COMMON SIDE EFFECTS
Nausea, dyspepsia, dizziness

SIGNIFICANT ADVERSE REACTIONS
Vomiting, dry mouth, anorexia, constipation, headache, anxiety, mild tremor, nasal congestion, epistaxis, flulike symptoms, pruritus, rash, urticaria, brittle fingernails, blurred vision, conjunctivitis, scotomata, bad taste in mouth, earache, salivation, malaise, sore throat, dyspnea, hypotension, edema, swollen glands, and leukopenia

CONTRAINDICATIONS

Sensitivity to methylxanthines, such as caffeine. *Cautious use* in patients with angina, arrhythmias, or severe hypotension and in pregnant or nursing women

PATIENT EDUCATION

1. Instruct patient to take drug with meals to minimize GI side effects.
2. Caution patient to notify drug prescriber if persistent nausea, dyspepsia, dizziness, or headache occur because dosage reduction may be indicated.
3. Explain that beneficial effects of drug may not be apparent for 2 to 4 weeks. Results are often manifested by gradual increase in ability to walk longer distances without experiencing pain (claudication).
4. Inform patient that treatment will probably continue for at least 8 weeks.

THROMBOLYTIC DRUGS

Alteplase, recombinant   Streptokinase
Urokinase

Thrombolytic (or fibrinolytic) drugs facilitate the dissolution of blood clots by activating the fibrinolytic enzyme plasmin (fibrinolysin). They are used in the treatment of several thromboembolic disorders and have become widely used in the early stages of a myocardial infarction to effect recannalization of an occluded coronary artery. Most evidence indicates that thrombolytic drugs are most effective when administered within 4 hours to 6 hours of the *onset* of symptoms of a myocardial infarction; more delayed administration is much less successful in promoting reperfusion of occluded vessels.

The currently available thrombolytic drugs are enzymes, one derived from beta-hemolytic streptococci (streptokinase), another from human kidney cells (urokinase), and a third produced in tissue culture by recombinant DNA techniques (alteplase). These drugs are associated with a definite risk of bleeding, especially from sites of invasive procedures; such procedures should be limited within the first 48 hours following administration. Streptokinase and urokinase can produce a *generalized* lytic state, in which normally protective hemostatic thrombi are lysed as well as the intracoronary thrombi. This condition can lead to internal bleeding and represents a potentially serious complication of thrombolytic therapy. Alteplase appears to be more *clot-specific*, inasmuch as it produces only limited amounts of plasmin in the absence of fibrin. The reduced systemic lytic potential of alteplase brought about its increasing use in myocardial infarction.

Since these three drugs are quite similar in their actions, they are reviewed as a group; individual agents are then listed in Table 35-3.

MECHANISM

Convert plasminogen (profibrinolysin), an inactive plasma protein, to plasmin (fibrinolysin), an active fibrinolytic enzyme, which degrades fibrin clots, fibrinogen, and other plasma proteins. Streptokinase first combines with plasminogen to form an activator complex, resulting in cleavage of peptide bonds on plasminogen to form plasmin; *urokinase* activates plasminogen directly; *alteplase* binds to fibrin and converts the enmeshed plasminogen to plasmin, with only limited conversion to plasmin in the systemic circulation. Increased formation of fibrin degradation products (FDPs) provides for additional anticoagulant activity.

USES

Lysis of coronary artery thrombi associated with an evolving myocardial infarction, as an aid to reperfusion of the blocked vessel (most effective if given within 4 hours of onset of symptoms)
Lysis of acute, massive pulmonary emboli
Lysis of acute, extensive deep vein thromboses (streptokinase)
Clearance of occluded arteriovenous cannulae (streptokinase)
Restoration of patency of IV and central venous catheters obstructed by clotted blood (urokinase)

DOSAGE

See Table 35-3

FATE

Plasminogen is activated almost immediately upon IV infusion of these drugs; their metabolism is poorly understood; plasma half-life of streptokinase is 15 to 20 minutes initially, while antistreptokinase antibodies are present; following saturation of antibodies with a loading dose, half-life is prolonged up to 90 minutes; serum half-life of urokinase is less than 20 minutes but it is prolonged in the presence of impaired liver function; alteplase is cleared quickly from the plasma, more than one-half the dose within 5 minutes; excretion is by way of the urine and bile

COMMON SIDE EFFECTS

Minor bleeding episodes (especially at sites of invasive procedures), bruising. Mild allergic reactions, fever, headache and muscle pain are common with *streptokinase*.

SIGNIFICANT ADVERSE REACTIONS

Severe hemorrhage (cerebral, GI, retroperitoneal); allergic reactions (dyspnea, angioedema, periorbital swelling, bronchospasm, anaphylactic reaction); blood pressure alterations, and phlebitis at site of IV injection

CONTRAINDICATIONS

Active internal bleeding, intracranial or intraspinal surgery, intracranial neoplasm, and recent cerebrovascular accident. *Cautious use* in the following situations: recent or imminent surgery, ulcerative wounds, trauma with internal injuries, malignancies, urinary or GI lesions (e.g., colitis, diverticulitis), severe hypertension, diabetic retinopathy, hepatic or renal disease, hemorrhagic disorders, chronic lung disease, rheumatic heart disease, subacute bacterial endocarditis, history of allergic reactions, pregnancy, immediate postpartum period, and in children

INTERACTIONS

Drugs that alter platelet function (e.g., salicylates, dipyridamole, indomethacin, phenylbutazone) or coagulation (e.g., heparin, warfarin) may increase the risk of hemorrhage with streptokinase

NURSING CONSIDERATIONS

Nursing Alerts

- Avoid unnecessary delays in initiating thrombolytic therapy for myocardial infarction. The sooner a thrombolytic drug is given after symptoms of myocardial infarction are first noted, the more likely it is that the drug will limit damage to the heart muscle. Treatment should begin within 4 to 6 hours of the onset of symptoms.
- Observe patient for signs of potentially serious internal or external bleeding (hematuria, ecchymoses, epistaxis, bleeding from sites of recent invasive procedures).
- Discontinue infusion if serious bleeding occurs and cannot be controlled adequately by local application of pressure or if thrombin time is less than half normal. Whole fresh blood, packed red cells, or fresh-frozen plasma may be administered. Aminocaproic acid may be given if hemorrhage is unresponsive to blood replacement. Therapy should be reinstituted only if signs of bleeding cease.
- Avoid arterial invasive procedures before and during treatment. If an arterial puncture is performed, apply manual pressure to the site for 30 minutes, then apply a pressure dressing. Perform venipuncture as carefully and infrequently as possible, and apply prolonged manual pressure to site afterwards. Avoid IM injections because hematomas are likely to form.
- Monitor patient very carefully during first few hours of infusion for signs of serious allergic reactions (e.g., wheezing, hypotension). Discontinue infusion, and prepare to assist with symptomatic treatment (e.g., epinephrine, antihistamines, corticosteroids) if allergic manifestations occur.
- When streptokinase is used, check results of streptokinase resistance levels, which should be measured prior to instituting therapy. Although recent streptococcal infection may require use of higher loading doses, streptokinase should not be given if resistance levels exceed 1,000,000 units.

1. If streptokinase or urokinase is administered directly into coronary arteries (intracoronary) rather than IV, prepare patient for cardiac catheterization procedure.
2. Prior to initiating therapy, ensure that a blood sample is drawn to determine thrombin time.
3. Maintain patient on bed rest during entire course of therapy and avoid handling patient unnecessarily because bruising occurs readily.
4. Following completion of therapy with streptokinase or urokinase, or concurrent with initiation of therapy with alteplase, begin continuous IV heparin infusion. Heparin therapy is followed by oral anticoagulant therapy. Heparin should be discontinued when prothrombin time reaches 2 to 3 times the normal control value.

HEMOSTATIC DRUGS

Hemostatic drugs may be used to control bleeding in a variety of situations. Systemically administered agents are employed to elevate or replenish one or more coagulation factors that may be deficient because of a hereditary or acquired defect, and to treat excessive systemic bleeding resulting from surgical complications, hematologic disorders, or neoplastic disease. Topically applied hemostatics are primarily used to control continual oozing or mild bleeding from capillaries and other small blood vessels (e.g., following surgery), or in the treatment of decubitus or chronic leg ulcers.

Systemic Hemostatics

Aminocaproic Acid
Amicar

MECHANISM

Inhibits plasminogen activators and interferes with binding of plasmin to fibrin, thereby retarding clot breakdown

USES

Treatment of severe bleeding resulting from systemic hyperfibrinolysis, such as that associated with heart surgery, hematologic disorders, abruptio placentae, cirrhosis of the liver, or neoplastic disorders

Treatment of urinary hyperfibrinolysis, such as that associated with severe trauma, shock, prostatectomy, nephrectomy, or renal malignancies

Treatment of overdosage with fibrinolytic drugs (e.g., alteplase, streptokinase, urokinase)

Preventing recurrence of subarachnoid hemorrhage, aborting or preventing attacks of hereditary angioneurotic edema, and decreasing need for platelet transfusion in cases of amegokaryocytic thrombocytopenia (investigational uses only)

DOSAGE

Oral: 5 g initially, followed by 1 g to 1.25 g/h for 8 hours or until bleeding has ceased; maximum dose 30 g/day

IV infusion: 4 g to 5 g in 250 mL diluent during first hour, followed by continuous infusion at a rate of 1 g/h in 50 mL diluent for 8 hours or until bleeding ceases

FATE

Rapidly absorbed orally; peak plasma levels occur in 1 to 2 hours; widely distributed; rapidly excreted, largely in the form of unmetabolized drug

COMMON SIDE EFFECTS

Nausea, cramping, diarrhea, malaise

SIGNIFICANT ADVERSE REACTIONS

Dizziness, tinnitus, weakness, fatigue, pruritus, headache, hypotension, delirium, nasal congestion, skin rash, menstrual cramping, reversible acute renal failure, thrombophlebitis, and auditory and visual hallucinations

CONTRAINDICATIONS

Active intravascular clotting, hematuria of upper urinary tract origin. *Cautious use* in persons with cardiac, renal, or hepatic disease, in pregnant women and in children

INTERACTIONS

Oral contraceptives may increase the danger of increased coagulation

Serum potassium levels can be elevated by aminocaproic acid

Table 35-3
Thrombolytic Agents

Drug	Preparations	Usual Dosage Range	Nursing Implications
Alteplase, recombinant *Activase*	Powder for injection: 20 mg (11.6 million units), 50 mg (29 million units)/vial	100 mg, given as 60 mg, the first hour (6 mg–10 mg as a bolus the first 1–2 min); 20 mg over the second hour; 20 mg over the third hour	Thrombolytic prepared by recombinant DNA technique using a human melanoma cell line; relatively clot specific—requires fibrin as a cofactor, therefore is less likely to produce systemic lysis than other thrombolytics; heparin is given concurrently for at least 48 h; aspirin may be given either during or following heparin; doses of 150 mg have been associated with increased intracranial bleeding; reconstitute *only* with sterile water for injection and use within 8 h; do *not* add other medications to infusion solution
Streptokinase *Kabikinase, Streptase*	Powder for injection: 250,000; 600,000; 750,000; 1,500,000 U/vial	*Myocardial infarction* IV: 250,000 U initially, followed by 100,000 U/h for 24 h; *or* 1,500,000 U in a single IV infusion over 1 h *Intracoronary:* 20,000 U by bolus initially, followed by 2000 U/min for 1 h *Venous thrombosis and pulmonary or arterial embolism* Initially: 250,000 U IV over 30 min, *then:* 100,000 U/h over 72 h for venous thrombosis *or* 100,000 U/h over 24–72 h for pulmonary embolism or arterial thrombosis *Arteriovenous cannula occlusion* Infuse by pump at a constant rate, 250,000 U/2 mL IV solution, into each occluded limb of cannula over 30 min, then clamp off for 2 h; aspirate contents of infusion cannula, flush with saline, and reconnect cannula	Used by either IV (preferred) or intracoronary route of administration; fever is common and is treated symptomatically; may not be effective if given between 5 days and 6 months of prior streptokinase injection or streptococcal infections owing to the presence of antistreptokinase antibodies; reconstitute contents of each vial with 5 mL sodium chloride injection or 5% dextrose injection directed to the side of the vial rather than directly into the solution; vial is rolled or tilted gently to reconstitute the drug but should *not* be shaken; contents are then diluted further to total volume as recommended for the specific indication; refer to package instructions for additional diluting information
Urokinase *Abbokinase*	Powder for injection: 250,000 U/vial, 500 U/mL	Initial priming dose of 4400 U/kg is given over 10 min at a rate of 1.5 mL/min, followed by continuous infusion of 4400 U/kg/h at rate of 15 mL/h for 12 h; tubing is then flushed with normal saline injection or 5% dextrose injection at same rate; approximately 3–4 h following urokinase therapy, a continuous heparin IV infusion should be initiated *Lysis of coronary artery thrombi:* Following a bolus dose of heparin (2500 U–10,000 U), urokinase infused into occluded artery at rate of 4 mL/min (6000 U/min) for up to 2 h; therapy should be continued until artery is maximally opened	Used for treating coronary artery thrombosis and pulmonary emboli and for restoring patency to IV catheters; does not result in antibody formation as does streptokinase; powder is reconstituted by adding 5.2 mL of sterile water for injection to the vial, rolling it gently to aid mixing (*do not shake*), then diluting with either normal saline or 5% dextrose injection to the desired concentration before infusing; drug should be mixed immediately before infusing since the solution contains no preservatives; do *not* add other medications to the solution

NURSING CONSIDERATIONS

Nursing Alerts
- In life-threatening bleeding situations, be prepared to administer emergency treatment, such as fresh whole blood transfusions or fibrinogen infusions.
- Be alert for signs of possible thromboembolic complications (e.g., chest or leg pain, dyspnea).

1. Monitor results of plasma levels, which should be 0.13 mg/mL or higher to inhibit systemic hyperfibrinolysis.

Tranexamic Acid

Cyklokapron

MECHANISM
Competitively inhibits plasminogen activation; may also directly interfere with action of plasmin at high concentrations; prolongs thrombin time but does not alter platelet aggregation or coagulation time

USES
Reduction or prevention of hemorrhage during and following tooth extraction in patients with hemophilia (short-term use, 3–8 days)

DOSAGE
Oral: 25 mg/kg 3–4 times/day 1 day prior to dental surgery, then 25 mg/kg 3–4 times/day for up to 8 days following surgery
IV: 25 mg/kg the day before surgery *or* 10 mg/kg immediately prior to surgery

FATE
Oral absorption is 25% to 50% of administered dose; peak plasma levels occur in 2 to 3 hours; plasma protein binding is minimal; effective plasma concentrations persist for up to 8 hours; more than 95% of a dose is eliminated unchanged in the urine

COMMON SIDE EFFECTS
Nausea, diarrhea with oral use
Hypotension with too-rapid IV injection

SIGNIFICANT ADVERSE REACTIONS
Vomiting, visual disturbances (e.g., altered color vision)

CONTRAINDICATIONS
Subarachnoid hemorrhage, acquired defective color vision. *Cautious use* in persons with renal insufficiency and in pregnant or nursing women

NURSING CONSIDERATIONS

Nursing Alerts
- Monitor patient taking drug for more than several days for changes in visual acuity, color vision, visual fields, or visual fundus. If changes are found, drug should be discontinued.
- With IV injection, administer solution at rate of 1 mL/min. If drug is injected too rapidly, hypotension may occur.

1. Do not mix solution with blood or with solutions that contain penicillin.

PATIENT EDUCATION
1. Instruct patient to report persistent nausea, vomiting, or diarrhea. Dosage reduction usually alleviates these.

Antihemophilic Factor, Human (AHF)

H.T. Factorate, Hemofil T, Koate-HS, Koate-HT, Monoclate
(CAN) Kryobulin VH

MECHANISM
A plasma protein (factor VIII) that is essential for the conversion of prothrombin to thrombin; replaces deficient endogenous factor VIII in cases of classic hemophilia, thereby decreasing bleeding tendency

USES
Treatment of classic hemophilia A, in which there is a demonstrated deficiency of clotting factor VIII, to control bleeding episodes or perform surgical procedures

DOSAGE
(Administered IV) Dosage expressed in AHF units; one AHF unit (U) equals the activity present in 1 mL of human plasma pooled from at least 10 donors and tested within 1 hour of collection

Dose is individually adjusted on the basis of patient's weight, severity of bleeding, presence of factor VIII inhibitors, and the desired level of factor VIII. Therapy should be based on factor VIII level assays. The following average doses are recommended:

Prophylaxis of spontaneous hemorrhage: 10 U/kg as a single dose; do not repeat in mild cases unless further bleeding occurs
Moderate hemorrhage/minor surgery: 15 U/kg to 25 U/kg initially, followed by 10 U/kg to 15 U/kg every 8 to 12 hours as needed
Severe hemorrhage: 40 U/kg to 50 U/kg initially, followed by 20 U/kg every 8 to 12 hours

Doses less than 34 U/mL may be given at a rate of 10 mL to 20 mL over 3 minutes; doses greater than 34 U/mL should be given at a maximum rate of 2 mL/min. If a significant increase in pulse rate occurs, the rate of administration should be decreased

FATE
Coagulant levels rise rapidly following administration, then quickly decrease. Plasma half-life following the initial dose ranges from 8 to 24 hours and increases with subsequent doses

COMMON SIDE EFFECTS
Mild allergic reactions, headache, flushing

SIGNIFICANT ADVERSE REACTIONS
Nausea, vomiting, chills, erythema, hives, fever, tachycardia, hypotension, backache, visual disturbances, clouded consciousness; massive doses may cause hemolytic anemia, increased bleeding tendency, and hyperfibrinogenemia

Note: Since this product is prepared from human plasma, the risk of transmitting viral hepatitis and the AIDS virus exists, and while minimal, must be recognized

CONTRAINDICATIONS
Approximately 5% to 10% of hemophilia A patients have inhibitors to factor VIII. In these patients, the response to AHF may be markedly reduced or absent; such patients may be candidates

for antiinhibitor coagulant complex (see following section). Large or frequent doses of AHF in patients with blood types A, B, or AB may result in intravascular hemolysis and anemia; appropriate blood monitoring is necessary during extended or high-dosage therapy

NURSING CONSIDERATIONS

Nursing Alerts
- Question administration if diagnosis of factor VIII deficiency has not been made. Drug is of no benefit in other bleeding disorders.
- Administer at a rate no greater than 10 mL/min because vasomotor reactions can occur.
- Be prepared to administer much larger than normal doses of antihemophilic factor or antiinhibitor coagulation complex (see following discussion) to the patient who is one of a small percentage who develop inhibitors to factor VIII (incidence is about 10%).

1. Store drug vials between 2° and 8°C until reconstituted. Warm concentrate and diluent to room temperature before mixing.
2. During reconstitution, rotate vial gently but do not shake. Do not use if gel formation occurs.
3. Do *not* refrigerate after reconstitution because precipitation can occur.
4. Administer within 3 hours after reconstitution to avoid possible untoward effects caused by bacterial contamination during mixing. Use plastic syringe because solution may adhere to surface of glass syringes.

Antiinhibitor Coagulant Complex
Autoplex, Feibo VH Immuno

MECHANISM
Concentrate of activated and precursor clotting factors and factors of the kinin-generating system prepared from pooled human plasma; reduces level of factor VIII inhibitory activity in hemophilic patients, thus decreasing bleeding episodes

USES
Treatment of symptoms of hemophilia in patients with significant levels of factor VIII inhibitors who are bleeding or about to undergo surgery

DOSAGE
(IV only) 25 to 100 factor VIII correctional units/kg depending on severity of bleeding at a rate of 2 mL to 10 mL infusion solution/minute; repeat in 6 hours if necessary (1 unit [U] of factor VIII correctional activity is that amount of activated prothrombin complex which, upon addition to an equal amount of factor VIII–deficient plasma, will correct the clotting time to 35 sec)

SIGNIFICANT ADVERSE REACTIONS
Hypersensitivity reactions (fever, chills, alterations in blood pressure); headache, flushing, tachycardia, hypercoagulability (dyspnea, chest pain, cough, changes in pulse rate)

CONTRAINDICATIONS
Fibrinolysis, disseminated intravascular coagulation (DIC). *Cautious use* in patients with liver disease or a history of allergies, and in small children

Note: This product is prepared from large pools of human plasma and the risk of transmission of viral diseases such as hepatitis or AIDS exists and, while minimal, must be recognized

INTERACTIONS
The possibility of hypercoagulability states is increased with concomitant use of antiinhibitor coagulant complex and aminocaproic acid

NURSING CONSIDERATIONS

Nursing Alerts
- Provide patient with appropriate reassurance and emotional support with regard to the risk of contracting viral hepatitis and possibly other diseases (e.g., AIDS) with administration of product.
- Observe closely for indications of intravascular coagulation (e.g., dyspnea, coughing, chest or leg pain). Infusion should be terminated if these occur.
- Ensure that appropriate medications (e.g., epinephrine, corticosteroids, antihistamines) are available to manage any hypersensitivity reactions that may develop.
- Avoid rapid infusion rates (e.g., 5 mL–10 mL/min) because incidence of side effects is much higher.

1. Monitor results of prothrombin times. Drug should not be reinfused unless *post*infusion prothrombin time is at least two thirds of the *pre*infusion value.
2. Store unreconstituted product under refrigeration. Use diluent provided to prepare infusion solution according to package directions. Each bottle is labeled with units of factor VIII correctional activity that it contains.

Factor IX Complex, Human
Konyne, Profilnine, Proplex

MECHANISM
Concentrate of dried plasma fractions of human coagulation factors II, VII, IX, and X with small amounts of other plasma proteins; provides replacement therapy for a congenital or acquired deficiency of one or more factors that can result in increased bleeding tendencies

USES
Treatment of factor IX deficiency (hemophilia B or Christmas disease) to prevent or control bleeding episodes (not a substitute for fresh-frozen plasma in patients with *mild* factor IX deficiency)
Control of bleeding episodes in patients with factor VIII inhibitors (Proplex)
Reversal of oral anticoagulant–induced hemorrhaging

DOSAGE
Highly individual, depending on patient status, severity of bleeding, and degree of factor deficiency as determined by coagulation assays prior to treatment; dosage measured in units (1 unit [U] is the activity present in 1 mL of normal plasma less than 1 h old). Potency is adjusted based on factor IX, because the other factors (II, VII, X) are present in approximately the same amount.
Recommended IV dosage guidelines are as follows:
Treatment of bleeding in hemophilia A patients with inhibitors to factor VIII: 75 U/kg; repeat in 12 hours if needed

Anticoagulant, Thrombolytic, and Hemostatic Drugs   363

Reversal of Coumarin effect: 15 U/kg

Hemarthroses in hemophiliacs with factor VIII inhibitors: 75 U/kg; repeat in 12 hours if necessary

Prophylaxis in patients with congenital deficiency of procoagulant factors: 10 U to 20 U/kg once or twice a week to prevent spontaneous bleeding

The infusion rate should not exceed 10 mL/min

COMMON SIDE EFFECTS

Flushing, tingling (especially with too-rapid infusion)

SIGNIFICANT ADVERSE REACTIONS

Chills, fever, headache, tachycardia, hypotension, viral hepatitis, and intravascular hemolysis

CONTRAINDICATIONS

Liver disease with signs of intravascular coagulation or fibrinolysis, and in patients undergoing elective surgery

Note: This product is obtained from pooled human plasma and therefore is associated with the risk of transmission of viral diseases such as hepatitis or AIDS; while minimal, this risk must be recognized

NURSING CONSIDERATIONS

Nursing Alerts

- Provide patient with appropriate reassurance and emotional support with regard to the risk that the preparation may contain the causative agent of viral hepatitis or other diseases such as AIDS.
- Monitor infusion rate constantly, and note development of symptoms (e.g., cough, chest pain, respiratory distress, altered pulse and blood pressure) that signify increased intravascular coagulation. If these occur, infusion should be stopped immediately. To minimize risk of intravascular coagulation, no attempt should be made to raise factor IX level to more than 50% of normal.
- Infuse *slowly* IV. Rapid infusion (greater than 10 mL/min) can produce vasomotor symptoms (e.g., tachycardia, hypotension). If chills, fever, tingling, flushing, or headache occurs during infusion, dosage reduction (slower infusion rate) is indicated.

1. Monitor results of coagulation assays, which should be performed prior to initiation of treatment and regularly thereafter. Dosage is adjusted on the basis of assay results.
2. Monitor levels of coagulation factors, which should be checked repeatedly during infusion because excessive levels increase the risk of intravascular coagulation.
3. Store product under normal refrigeration until reconstituted, but do not freeze. Warm to room temperature just before mixing. Do *not* use if gel forms.
4. Administer within 3 hours following reconstitution, and do *not* refrigerate reconstituted soution because precipitation can occur.

Topical Hemostatics

A variety of substances are applied topically to control minor bleeding episodes and to reduce oozing and leakage from small blood vessels that may occur as a result of trauma or surgery. These topical hemostatics are rarely effective in controlling extensive hemorrhaging. Many of these products are employed during or following surgery to retard blood loss through capillary and small vessel leakage. Most of the products are slowly absorbable and therefore provide a temporary framework on which platelets can adhere. Others are of a gelatin composition, which can absorb many times its weight in blood and which adheres to the damaged site, slowing further blood loss. The clinically available topical hemostatic products are discussed briefly below.

Gelatin Film, Absorbable

Gelfilm

MECHANISM

Nonantigenic, absorbable gelatin film with the consistency of cellophane; moistened and cut to desired size and shape, and applied to tissue to reduce bleeding; absorbed completely within 2 weeks to 3 months

USES

Reduce local bleeding in thoracic, ocular, or neurosurgery

DOSAGE

Immerse in sterile saline, and allow to soak until pliable; fit to desired size and shape, and apply to surface of tissue

NURSING CONSIDERATIONS

1. Do not use in grossly contaminated or infected surgical wounds, because rate of absorption is markedly increased.
2. Use immediately after opening package envelope to minimize contamination.

Gelatin Sponge, Absorbable

Gelfoam

MECHANISM

A pliable, nonantigenic sponge capable of absorbing many times its weight in whole blood; prepared from specially treated, purified gelatin solution; completely absorbed in 4 to 6 weeks when implanted into tissues; presence of anticoagulants does not interfere with its effectiveness; liquefies within several days when applied to actively bleeding areas

USES

Providing control of capillary and small blood vessel bleeding in many forms of surgery

Enhancing wound healing by providing a framework for granulation tissue

DOSAGE

(Use sterile technique) Cut to desired size, and apply either dry or saturated with sodium chloride injection or thrombin solution to desired area. Hold in place with moderate pressure for 10 to 15 seconds, then allow to remain in contact with bleeding site. Wound may be closed over sponge.

Decubitus ulcers may be packed with sponge and a dressing applied

CONTRAINDICATIONS

Presence of infection, postpartum bleeding, menorrhagia, bleeding due to blood dyscrasias, and closure of skin incisions

NURSING CONSIDERATIONS

1. Compress sponge before inserting into cavities or closed tissue spaces to reduce expansion and possible disturbances of surrounding structures. Do *not* overpack a particular area, because sponge may expand excessively, interfering with function of surrounding structures.
2. Note that effectiveness can be enhanced by soaking in a thrombin solution.
3. Use sponges as soon as possible after opening package to minimize bacterial contamination.
4. Do not resterilize by heating (changes absorption time) or with ethylene oxide (irritating to tissues).

Gelatin powder, absorbable

Gelfoam

MECHANISM
Acts as a hemostatic when applied locally; promotes growth of granulation tissue and facilitates healing of ulcerated areas

USES
Control of bleeding from cancellous bone when other conventional procedures are ineffective or impractical
Stimulation of granulation tissue in treating leg ulcers, decubitus ulcers, and other oozing lesions (unlabeled use)

DOSAGE
Contents of jar (1 g) are poured into a beaker and 3 mL to 4 mL of sterile saline is added to prepare a paste, which is smeared onto cut surface of bone. Excess is removed when bleeding stops

CONTRAINDICATIONS
Closure of skin incisions, postpartum bleeding or menorrhagia, presence of infection or use as the sole hemostatic agent in persons with blood dyscrasias

Microfibrillar Collagen Hemostat

Avitene

MECHANISM
A dry, fibrous, water-insoluble preparation of purified bovine corium collagen; when applied to the source of bleeding, it attracts platelets, which adhere to the fibrils of the preparation, triggering further platelet aggregation into thrombi; stimulates a mild, chronic inflammatory response; response is not inhibited by heparin; does not interfere with bone regeneration or healing

USES
Adjunct to hemostasis in surgical procedures when control of bleeding by conventional procedures (e.g., ligation) is ineffective or impractical

DOSAGE
Compress surface to be treated with a dry sponge prior to applying dry hemostat preparation, then apply pressure over the hemostat for several minutes. The amount of product required depends on size of area and severity of bleeding. Remove excess material after several minutes. Do *not* handle with wet instruments or gloves

SIGNIFICANT ADVERSE REACTIONS
Potentiation of infection, hematomas (sealing over of exit site for deeper hemorrhage), adhesion formation, and allergic reactions

CONTRAINDICATIONS
Closure of skin incisions, use on bone surfaces to which prosthetic materials are to be attached

NURSING CONSIDERATIONS

Nursing Alerts
- Do not sterilize product because it is inactivated by autoclaving. Avoid wetting product because its hemostatic efficacy is impaired.
- Avoid spilling product on nonbleeding surfaces (especially abdominal or thoracic viscera) because it will adhere to any moist surface, possibly resulting in adhesions.

1. Remove excess material after several minutes by gentle teasing or irrigation. If breakthrough bleeding occurs, apply additional hemostat.
2. Do not use gloved fingers to apply pressure; a dry sponge is preferred.

Negatol

Negatan

MECHANISM
Highly acidic compound that coagulates protein substances and possesses a germicidal action

USES
Astringent and hemostatic on skin and mucous membranes (e.g., vagina, cervix, vulva)

DOSAGE
Cleanse and dry area to be treated; apply either full strength (45%) or as a 1:10 dilution.

Vaginal: soak gauze in 1:10 dilution and use as a pack; remove within 24 hours and douche
Cervical: soak gauze in full strength solution and insert into cervical canal

SIGNIFICANT ADVERSE REACTIONS
Skin irritation, burning, erythema, and superficial desquamation

NURSING CONSIDERATIONS
1. Make initial application in vagina with 1:10 dilution, and observe for signs of hypersensitivity. Concentration can be increased if no untoward reactions are noted.
2. Advise patient to wear perineal pads to avoid soiling clothing.

Oxidized Cellulose

Novocell, Oxycel, Surgicel

MECHANISM
Upon saturation with blood, cellulose material swells into a gelatinous tenacious mass that serves as a clot nucleus; slowly absorbed from sites of implantation with minimal tissue reaction; does not alter normal blood clotting mechanism

USES
Adjunctive control of minor hemorrhage (capillary, venous, small arterial) in cases in which conventional methods (e.g., ligation) are inappropriate

Production of hemostasis in oral and dental surgery

DOSAGE
Place desired size pad, strip, or pellet of material on bleeding site; usually removed following development of hemostasis by irrigation with sterile water or saline

SIGNIFICANT ADVERSE REACTIONS
Stinging, burning, headache, sneezing (nasal application), foreign body reactions, encapsulation of fluid, obstruction (e.g., urinary, intestinal) caused by adhesion formation, necrosis of nasal membranes

CONTRAINDICATIONS
Implantation in bone defects (e.g., fractures), use as packing or wadding (must be removed following hemostasis), hemorrhage from large arteries, and control of nonhemorrhagic oozing

NURSING CONSIDERATIONS

Nursing Alerts
- Do not enclose oxidized cellulose in contaminated wounds without drainage.
- *Always* remove following development of hemostasis in laminectomy procedures (may cause nerve damage), from foramina of bone, and from large open wounds.
- Do not apply silver nitrate or other similar materials before using oxidized cellulose because absorption may be impaired.
- Avoid wadding or packing the cellulose material, especially within rigid cavities, because swelling may cause obstruction or necrosis.
- Ensure that none of the material is aspirated by the patient, as when it is used to control bleeding following tonsillectomy or to reduce epistaxis.

1. Avoid adding anti-infective agents, buffers, or other hemostatics to oxidized cellulose. The low pH of the product destroys these other additives.
2. Always irrigate before removal of oxidized cellulose to avoid tearing tissues and reinstituting bleeding.
3. Do not moisten prior to application because hemostatic effect is greater when dry.
4. Do not resterilize because autoclaving causes physical breakdown. Discard opened, unused product.
5. Use least amount necessary to produce hemostasis. Remove any excess before surgical closure.

Thrombin, Topical
Thrombinar, Thrombostat

MECHANISM
Catalyzes the conversion of fibrinogen to fibrin

USES
Reduce oozing and minor bleeding from capillaries and small venules (e.g., laryngeal or nasal surgery, plastic surgery, bleeding from cancellous bone, dental extractions)

DOSAGE
Prepare solutions in sterile distilled water or saline; intended use determines concentration of solution, which may range from 100 unit to 2000 units/mL depending on extent and severity of bleeding.

Spray or flood area (using syringe and fine-gauge needle) with solution; alternatively, dried powder from vial may be placed directly on area *or* absorbable gelatin sponge may be soaked in thrombin solution and then placed on area of bleeding

SIGNIFICANT ADVERSE REACTIONS
Allergic reactions, fever

NURSING CONSIDERATIONS

Nursing Alert
- Never administer thrombin parenterally or allow it to enter large blood vessels because extensive intravascular clotting and death can result.

1. Use solutions the day they are prepared. Refrigerate solutions if several hours are to elapse between preparation and use.
2. Be aware that acids, alkalies, heat, and heavy metal salts reduce thrombin activity.
3. Do not sponge treated surfaces because clot may be dislodged.
4. Ensure that wound is relatively free from blood before application of drug.

Selected Bibliography
Anderson JL et al: A randomized trial of intracoronary streptokinase in the treatment of acute myocardial infarction. N Engl J Med 308:1312, 1983

Arnesen H, Hoiseth A, Ly B: Streptokinase or heparin in the treatment of deep vein thrombosis. Acta Med Scand 211:65, 1982

Baker DE, Campbell RK: Pentoxifylline: A new agent for intermittent claudication. Drug Intell Clin Pharm 19:345, May, 1984

Bjork I, Lindahl U: Mechanism of the anticoagulant action of heparin. Mol Cell Biochem 48:161, 1982

Bouchier-Hayes D: Drugs in the treatment of thromboembolic diseases. Ir Med J 76:101, 155, 1983

Bouman CC: Intracoronary thrombolysis and percutaneous transluminal coronary angioplasty. Nurs Clin North Am 19(3):397, 1984

Buckler P, Douglas AS: Antithrombotic treatment. Br Med J 287:196, 1983

Cipolle RJ, Rodrold RA, Seifert R et al: Heparin-associated thrombocytopenia: A prospective evaluation of 211 patients. Ther Drug Monit 5:205, 1983

Gever LN: Stopping bleeding with aminocaproic acid. Nursing 84 14(9):8, 1984

Jacques LB: Heparin: A unique misunderstood drug. Trends in Pharmacological Science 3:289, 1982

Laffel GL, Braunwald E: Thrombolytic therapy: A new strategy for the treatment of acute myocardial infarction. N Engl J Med 311:710 and 770, 1984

Loscalzo J, Braunwald E: Tissue plasminogen activator. N Engl J Med 319(14):925, 1988

Marder VJ, Sherry S: Thrombolytic therapy: Current status (2 parts). N Engl J Med 318(23):1512, 318(24):1585, 1988

Miller P, Yardley S: White clot syndrome: A complication of heparin therapy. Am J Nurs 85:1051, 1985

Nelson PH, Moser KM, Stoner C, Moser KS: Risk of complications during intravenous heparin therapy. West J Med 136:189, 1982

Nissen MB: Streptokinase therapy in acute myocardial infarction. Heart Lung 13:223, 1984

Pepper G: New drug for intermittent claudication. Nurse Pract 10(5):54, May, 1985

Serlin MJ, Breckenridge AM: Drug interactions with warfarin. Drugs 25:610, 1983

Sherry S: Tissue plasminogen activator (t-PA): Will it fulfill its promise? N Engl J Med 313:1014, 1985

Sherry S: Thrombolytic agents for acute evolving myocardial infarction: Comparative effects. Ration Drug Ther 21(1):1, 1987

Sherry S: Appraisal of various thrombolytic agents in the treatment of acute myocardial infarction. Am J Med 83(Suppl 2A):31, 1988

Sherry S, Gustafson E: The current and future use of thrombolytic therapy. Annu Rev Pharmacol Toxicol 25:413, 1985

Spann JF et al: High-dose, brief intravenous streptokinase early in acute myocardial infarction. Am Heart J 104:939, 1982

Taylor GJ et al: Intravenous versus intracoronary streptokinase therapy for acute myocardial infarction in community hospitals. Am J Cardiol 54:256, 1984

TIMI Study Group: The thrombolysis in myocardial infarction (TIMI Trial): Phase I findings. N Engl J Med 321:932, 1985

Totly WG et al: Low-dose intravascular fibrinolytic therapy. Radiology 143:59, 1982

Vanbree NS, Hollerback AD, Brooks GP: Clinical evaluation of three techniques for administering low-dose heparin. Nurs Res 33(1):15, 1984

Van de Werf F et al: Coronary thrombolysis with tissue-type plasminogen activator in patients with evolving myocardial infarction. N Engl J Med 310:609, 1984

SUMMARY. ANTICOAGULANT, THROMBOLYTIC, AND HEMOSTATIC DRUGS

Drug	Preparations	Usual Dosage Range
Anticoagulants		
Parenteral Anticoagulant		
Heparin sodium Liquaemin	Injection: 1000; 2500; 5000; 7500; 10,000; 15,000; 20,000; 40,000 U/mL or unit dose	*Anticoagulant* SC: 10,000 units–20,000 units initially, 8000–20,000 U/8–12 h
Heparin calcium Calciparine	Injection: 5000; 12,500; 20,000 U/dose	IV: 10,000 units initially, then 5000–10,000 units every 4–6 h IV infusion: 20,000–40,000 U/day *Perioperative* SC: 5000 U 2 h before surgery, then 5000 U every 8–12 h for 7 days
Heparin sodium lock flush solution Hep-Lock, Hep-Lock U/P	Injection: 10 U, 100 U/mL	Use as IV flush in indwelling IV catheters
Heparin Antagonist		
Protamine sulfate	Injection: 10 mg/mL	1 mg neutralizes 90 units–120 units of heparin; administer slowly IV over 1–3 min; maximum dosage is 50 mg within 10-min period
Oral Anticoagulants	See Table 35-2	
Oral Anticoagulant Antagonist		
Phytonadione AquaMEPHYTON, Konakion, Mephyton	Tablets: 5 mg Injection: 2 mg, 10 mg/mL (Konakion for IM use only)	Oral: 2.5 mg–25 mg initially; may repeat in 12–24 h SC, IM: 0.5 mg–10 mg initially; may repeat up to 25 mg in 6–8 h IV: 0.5 mg–10 mg at a rate of 1 mg/min
Hemorrheologic Agent		
Pentoxifylline Trental	Tablets (controlled-release): 400 mg	400 mg 3 times/day with meals

Continued

SUMMARY. ANTICOAGULANT, THROMBOLYTIC AND HEMOSTATIC DRUGS (continued)

Drug	Preparations	Usual Dosage Range
Thrombolytics	*See* Table 35-3	
Hemostatics		
Systemic Hemostatics		
Aminocaproic acid Amicar	Tablets: 500 mg Syrup: 250 mg/mL Injection: 250 mg/mL	Oral: 5 g initially then 1 g–1.25 g/h until bleeding stops (maximum is 30 g/day) IV infusion: 4 g–5 g initially, during first hour, then 1 g/h thereafter
Tranexamic acid Cyklokapron	Tablets: 500 mg Injection: 100 mg/mL	Oral: 25 mg/kg 3–4 times/day 1 day before dental surgery, then for up to 8 days following surgery IV: 25 mg/kg day before surgery *or* 10 mg/kg immediately prior to surgery
Antihemophilic factor, human Hemofil M, Koate-HS, Koate-HT, Monoclate	Vials: 10 mL, 20 mL, 25 mL, 30 mL, 40 mL, 50 mL and single dose containing a dried preparation of human antihemophilic factor (units indicated on vial) with diluent	Individually adjusted to patient's weight, severity of bleeding, presence of factor VIII inhibitors Average dose range is 10 units–20 units/kg every 6–12 h; prior to surgery 30 units–40 units/kg; prophylaxis 250 units–500 units/day, in the morning
Antiinhibitor coagulant complex Autoplex T, Feiba VH Immuno	Vials: 30 mL containing a dried autoinhibitor coagulant complex obtained from pooled human plasma (units of factor VIII correctional activity indicated on each vial) with diluent	25–100 factor VIII correctional units/kg at a rate of 2 mL–10 mL infusion solution/min; repeat in 6 h if necessary
Factor IX complex, human Konyne, Profilnine, Proplex	Dried plasma fraction of factors II, VII, IX, and X in vials with diluent	Highly individualized; coagulation assays should be performed prior to treatment and at regular intervals during treatment, and dosage should be based upon assay results
Topical Hemostatics		
Gelatin film, absorbable Gelfilm	Strips: 100 mm × 125 mm, and 25 mm × 50 mm	Soak in sterile saline until pliable, cut to desired size, and apply to tissue surface
Gelatin sponge, absorbable Gelfoam	Sponges, dental packs, and prostatectomy cones of several dimensions	Apply dry or saturated with saline injections or thrombin solution
Microfibrillar collagen hemostat Avitene	Jars: 1 g, 5 g (fibrous form) Strips: 70 mm × 70 mm and 70 mm × 35 mm	Place on affected area and apply pressure for several minutes; remove excess material after several minutes
Negatol Negatan	Solution: 45%	Apply either full strength *or* as a 1:10 dilution; also used as a soak for gauze packing
Oxidized cellulose Oxycel, Surgicel	Pads, strips, and pledgets of several sizes Pellets for dental application	Place desired size pad, strip, or pellet onto bleeding area; remove by irrigation following the development of hemostasis
Thrombin, topical Thrombinar, Thrombostat	Powder: 1000-; 5000-; 10,000-; 20,000-unit vials	Topical: spray or flood area of bleeding with solution of thrombin in sterile water or saline; *or* dry powder from vial may be placed on bleeding site

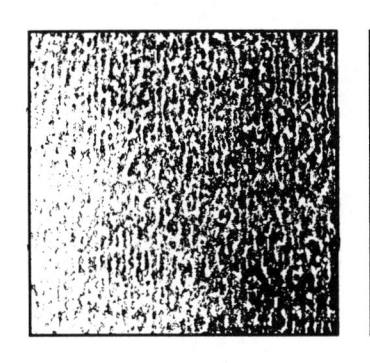

IV Drugs Acting on the Renal System

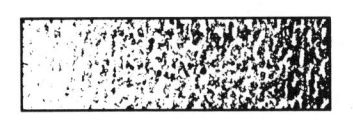

36 RENAL PHYSIOLOGY: A REVIEW

The kidneys play a major role in the maintenance of homeostasis by regulating the volume and composition of the extracellular fluid that serves as the internal environment for each cell. In addition to controlling the water, electrolyte, and solute concentrations of the extracellular fluid, the kidneys selectively excrete drugs, hormones, and byproducts of metabolism. The kidneys also participate in the maintenance of acid–base balance, renin and angiotensin production, and vitamin D metabolism.

GROSS ANATOMY OF THE KIDNEY

The kidneys are paired, bean-shaped organs located retroperitoneally on each side of the vertebral column at the level of the 12th thoracic to the third lumbar vertebrae. The right kidney is slightly lower than the left because of displacement by the liver.

Each kidney is invested by a fibrous capsule that is interrupted medially at the *hilus* for passage of blood vessels, lymphatics, nerves, and a ureter.

A frontal section of the kidney reveals an outer granular *cortex* located deep to the capsule and an inner *medulla* composed of several striated *pyramids* (Fig. 36-1). Interspersed among the pyramids are columns of cortical tissues known as the renal columns of Bertin.

The apex of each renal pyramid forms a *papilla*, which projects into a cuplike minor *calyx*. Several minor calyces unite to form major calyces, and the latter merge to form the *renal pelvis*. The renal pelvis is continuous with the *ureter*, which drains its contents into the *urinary bladder*.

Renal Blood Supply

Paired *renal arteries* arise from the abdominal aorta, branching as they enter the hilus. These branches divide into *interlobar arteries*, which pass between the medullary pyramids. At the corticomedullary junction the vessels form the *arcuate arteries*, which arch over the bases of the pyramids. Branching from the arcuate arteries are numerous *interlobular arteries*, which penetrate the cortical substance and give rise to *afferent arterioles* supplying individual nephron units.

Each afferent arteriole terminates in a tuft of capillaries, the *glomerulus*; these capillaries rejoin to form the *efferent arteriole*. Efferent arterioles terminate in *peritubular capillaries*, which surround the renal tubules. The peritubular capillaries eventually converge into venules that carry the blood into a series of veins corresponding in name and in course to the arteries described above.

A series of long, straight peritubular capillaries termed *vasa recta* course through the medulla, turning sharply at various levels. The vasa recta participate in countercurrent exchange of substances between the renal tubules and vascular bed as detailed later in this chapter.

MICROSCOPIC ANATOMY OF THE KIDNEY

The basic anatomical and functional unit of the kidney is the *nephron* (Fig. 36-2). There are approximately 1 million nephrons in each human kidney. A nephron consists of a renal corpuscle and a long, often tortuously coiled renal tubule composed of the following anatomically modified and functionally distinct segments: the proximal convoluted tubule, the loop of Henle, and the distal convoluted tubule, which empties into a confluent collecting tubule.

Each nephron originates as a double-walled cup, the *Bowman's capsule*, which encloses the glomerular capillaries. Collectively, the Bowman's capsule and the glomerulus are termed the *renal (malpighian) corpuscle*. The epithelium of the Bowman's capsule is of the simple squamous type, with the inner (visceral) layer containing modified cells called *podocytes*. The podocytes exhibit numerous footlike extensions called *pedicels*, which contact the basement membrane of the glomerular capillaries.

The podocyte layer (visceral epithelium) of the Bowman's capsule together with the basement membrane and fenestrated endothelium of the glomerulus forms a functional filtration membrane.

The outer (parietal) layer of the Bowman's capsule becomes continuous with the epithelium of the *proximal convoluted tubule*. The proximal convoluted tubule then straightens and plunges toward the medulla, forming the thick descending segment (pars recta) of the *loop of Henle*.

The loop of Henle is a U-shaped structure composed of a thick descending segment (pars recta), a thin segment, and a thick ascending segment. The thick ascending segment becomes continuous with the *distal convoluted tubule* at a modified site, the *macula densa*, where the tubular cells and their prominent nuclei are densely crowded.

The distal tubule coils in the area of the renal cortex before joining a collecting tubule. The latter descends into the medulla as part of a renal pyramid and empties through the papilla into a minor calyx.

Histologically, the proximal and distal segments of the tubule differ somewhat, reflecting differences in function.

The epithelium of the proximal segments (proximal convoluted tubule and pars recta) is characterized by a luminal "brush border" of extensive microvilli that greatly increase the free surface area available for reabsorption of filtered substances.

By contrast, the epithelia of the thick ascending limb of Henle's loop and the distal tubule are flatter with few microvilli. The epithelium of the thin segment of Henle's loop is simple squamous and lacks microvilli.

Juxtaglomerular Apparatus

At its origin the distal convoluted tubule lies close to the afferent and efferent arterioles. Here the distal tubular epithelium cells with their prominent nuclei are densely crowded, forming a discrete area termed the *macula densa*. Adjacent to the macula densa are modified afferent arteriolar cells called *juxtaglomerular cells*, which contain granules of the proteolytic enzyme *renin*. Collectively the juxtaglomerular cells and the macula densa are termed the *juxtaglomerular apparatus* (Fig. 36-3).

The juxtaglomerular cells secrete renin in response to reduced renal perfusion (renal ischemia), hypotension hypo-

372   Drugs Acting on the Renal System

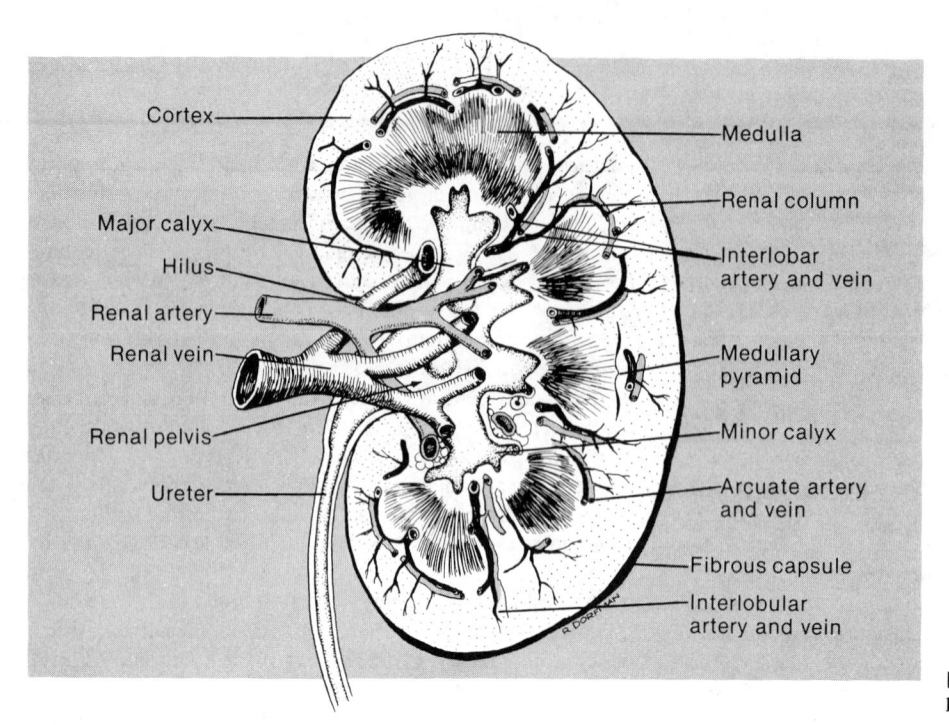

Figure 36-1 Frontal section of a human kidney.

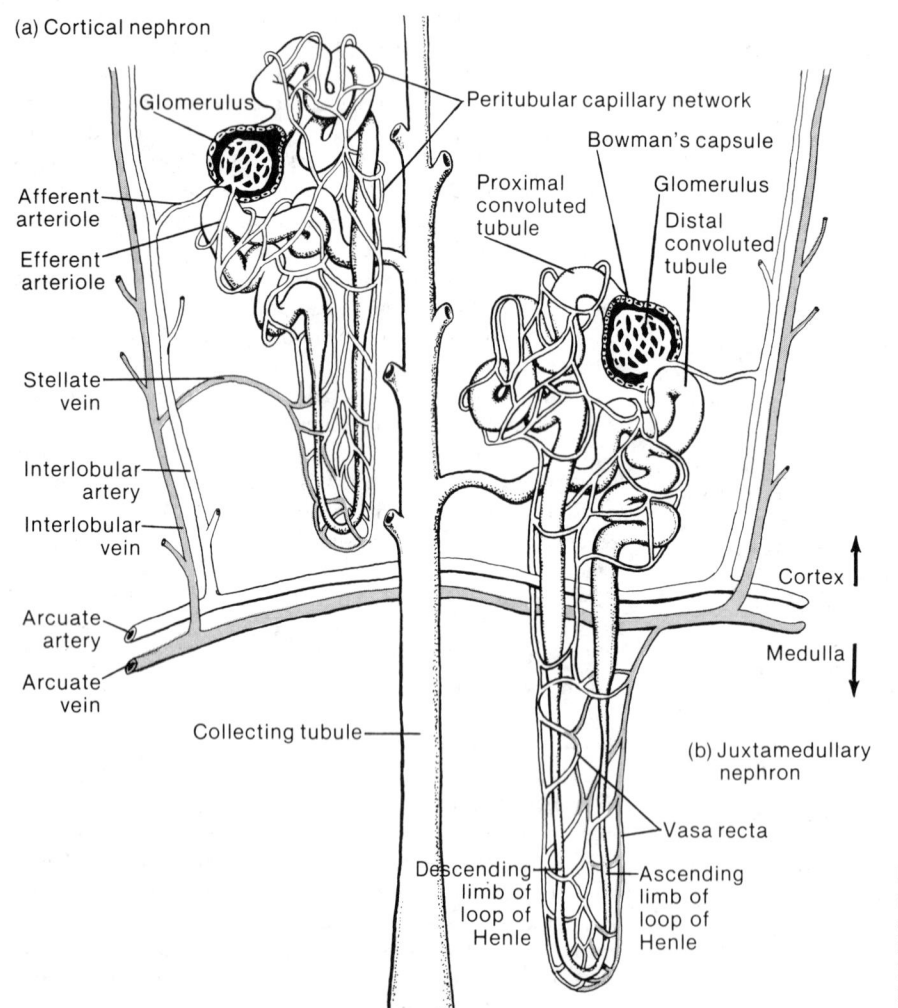

Figure 36-2 Diagram of two nephrons and their blood supply. One nephron (*left*) has a short loop of Henle; the other nephron (*right*) has a long loop of Henle and a more extensive blood supply. (After Chaffee EE, Lytle IM: Basic Physiology and Anatomy, 4th ed. Philadelphia, JB Lippincott, 1980)

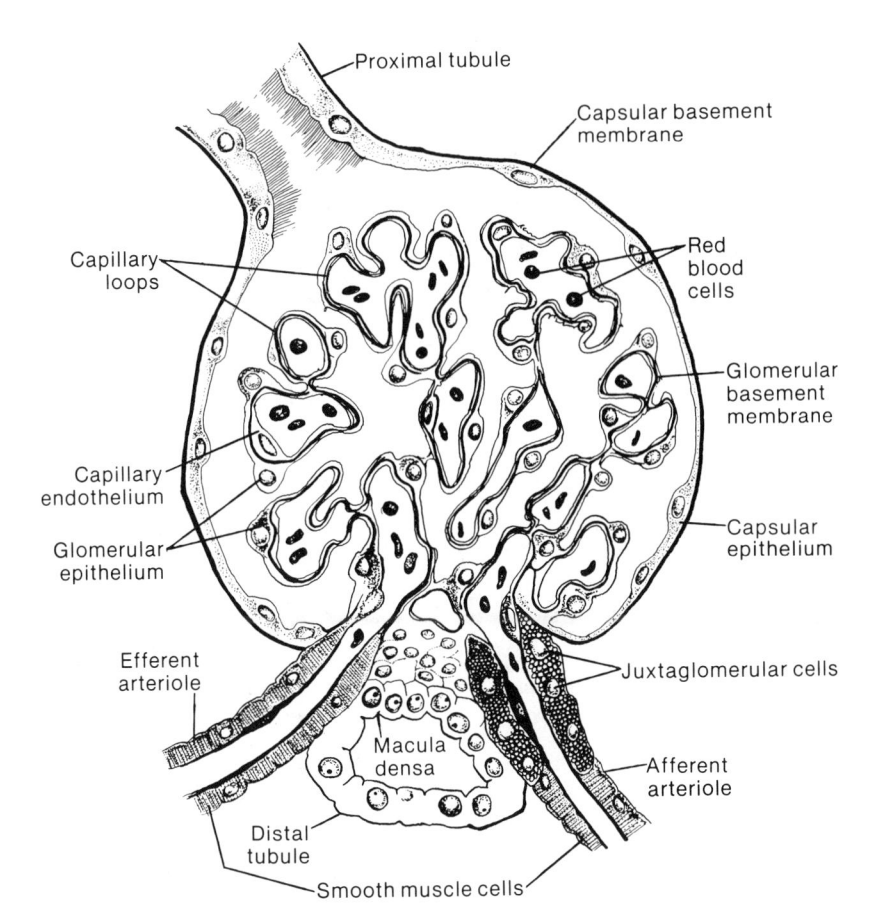

Figure 36-3 Semidiagrammatic drawing of a renal corpuscle. Note that the distal tubule appears to be attached to the afferent arteriole. Also depicted are the macula densa and the juxtaglomerular cells. The combined structure at the point of attachment is called the juxtaglomerular apparatus.

natremia, hyperkalemia, and beta-adrenergic receptor stimulation.

By way of the macula densa, the nature of the tubular fluid in the distal tubule can also influence secretion of renin by the juxtaglomerular cells.

Upon entering the blood, renin converts the plasma protein angiotensinogen into the decapeptide *angiotensin I*. Converting enzymes found largely in the lungs split a dipeptide from angiotensin I to form the physiologically active *angiotensin II*. Angiotensin II is a potent vasopressor substance that elevates blood pressure by promoting intense peripheral vasoconstriction and by stimulating secretion of the sodium-retaining hormone aldosterone, as outlined in Figure 28-4 in Chapter 28.

CONTROL OF RENAL BLOOD FLOW

Sympathetic vasoconstrictor nerve fibers arising from thoracolumbar segments of the spinal cord innervate the kidneys. In an average adult at rest the kidneys receive 20% to 25% of the cardiac output. Pain, cold, fright, strenuous exercise, hemorrhage, deep anesthesia, and other stressors reduce renal blood flow by activating sympathetic mechanisms for constriction of renal blood vessels.

RENAL PHYSIOLOGY

The formation of urine by the nephrons involves three basic processes: glomerular filtration, renal tubular reabsorption, and renal tubular secretion.

Glomerular Filtration

Glomerular filtration is a process whereby approximately one fifth of the plasma flowing through each glomerulus is passively transferred into the Bowman's capsule. The glomerular filtration membrane acts as a sieve, allowing passage of small molecules while restricting transfer of high molecular weight substances such as proteins.

The driving force for filtration is the hydrostatic pressure within the glomerular capillaries, which is ultimately derived from the work of the heart. The hydrostatic pressure in the glomerular capillaries is notably higher than that in other capillaries because each glomerulus is interposed between two arterioles.

Forces opposing filtration include the colloidal osmotic pressure of the plasma and the hydrostatic pressure of the Bowman's capsule. The colloidal osmotic pressure of the Bowman's capsule is close to zero because the glomerular filtrate is essentially protein-free.

Net filtration pressure (NFP) is equal to glomerular capillary hydrostatic pressure (GCHP) *minus* the plasma colloidal osmotic pressure (PCOP) *plus* the capsular hydrostatic pressure (CHP). This rule can be expressed as a formula:

$$NFP = GCHP - [PCOP + CHP]$$

For example, with a glomerular capillary hydrostatic pressure of 50 mm Hg, a plasma colloidal osmotic pressure of 30 mm Hg, and a capsular hydrostatic pressure of 10 mm Hg:

$$(50 \text{ mm Hg}) - (30 \text{ mm Hg} + 10 \text{ mm Hg}) = 10 \text{ mm Hg } NFP$$

Approximately 125 mL of filtrate are formed each minute. An intrinsic mechanism of autoregulation keeps the glomerular filtration rate (GFR) remarkably stable within a rather wide range of blood pressure variation. Glomerular filtration may be affected by changes in plasma colloidal osmotic pressure, a force that opposes glomerular filtration. Decreases in plasma colloidal osmotic pressure will enhance filtration and vice versa.

The high rate of glomerular filtration (125 mL/min) yields a total of 180 liters of plasma filtered in 1 day. Yet the average volume of urine excreted in 1 day is less than 2 liters. Hence, over 99% of the glomerular filtrate is reabsorbed during passage through the renal tubules.

Renal Tubular Reabsorption and Secretion

Renal tubular reabsorption involves the transport of filtered substances across the renal tubular epithelium from the tubular lumen to the blood of the peritubular capillaries.

In contrast, renal tubular secretion involves transtubular movement of substances from the blood of the peritubular capillaries to the tubular lumen.

Substances may be reabsorbed or secreted passively by diffusion along existing chemical, electrical, or osmotic gradients. They may also be actively transported against electrical or chemical gradients into or out of the tubular lumen by selective, carrier-mediated and energy-requiring transport systems. Each active renal transport system exhibits a *transport maximum* (T_m), which is the maximal rate at which a given substance can be carried across the renal tubular epithelium. For actively reabsorbed substances such as glucose, the plasma concentration of the substance that causes its transport maximum to be exceeded is termed the *renal threshold*.

Nutrients such as glucose and amino acids, and vitamins such as ascorbic acid (vitamin C) are actively reabsorbed in the proximal tubule. Uric acid, an end product of purine metabolism, is actively reabsorbed and actively secreted in the proximal tubule. Urea, the major end product of nitrogen metabolism, is formed chiefly in the liver in accordance with the rate of protein catabolism. Filtered urea is passively reabsorbed by the renal tubules to an extent determined by the rate of urine flow and degree of water reabsorption.

Creatinine, a product of muscle metabolism, and histamine are actively secreted in the proximal tubule.

Many organic compounds of medical importance are also actively secreted in the proximal tubule. Among these are the drugs and diagnostic agents listed in Table 36-1. Because renal tubular secretion supplements glomerular filtration and enhances the removal of substances from the blood, impaired renal function may interfere with the excretion of therapeutic agents and may therefore require an adjustment (reduction) in drug dosage.

Renal Handling of Ions and Water

The amount of sodium excreted is normally equivalent to the amount ingested, over a wide range of dietary sodium intake. Renal handling of sodium is of singular importance to the maintenance of extracellular fluid volume, because renal tubular reabsorption of sodium is the major driving force for the passive reabsorption of water. Also linked to the active reabsorption of sodium are the secretion of hydrogen and potassium and the reabsorption of chloride and bicarbonate in certain tubular segments. Chloride and bicarbonate reabsorption are reciprocally related. If chloride reabsorption increases, bicarbonate reabsorption decreases, and vice versa, so that total anion concentration of the plasma remains constant.

Sodium reabsorption begins in the proximal tubule, where it is actively reabsorbed. Bicarbonate and chloride are also reabsorbed there and are accompanied by an osmotically equivalent volume of water, so that tubular fluid osmolarity in this segment equals that of the plasma. The reabsorption of water in this segment is termed *obligatory*.

In the thick ascending limb of Henle, chloride together with sodium and potassium are transported across the tubular cell membrane by way of a complex energy-dependent carrier. Sodium and chloride are avidly reabsorbed in this section of the tubule; however, this segment is water impermeable, and the result is a net loss of sodium and chloride from tubular fluid leading to *hypo*-osmolarity of the fluid entering the distal tubule.

Active reabsorption of sodium resumes in the distal tubule and is coupled to chloride reabsorption along a rather small length of the distal tubule. Upon entering the cortical collecting tubule, sodium is absorbed through the tubular cells by way of conductive channels while, at the same time, potassium is extruded into the tubular fluid. Aldosterone is able to facilitate potassium excretion and sodium reabsorption in this segment through several mechanisms.

The passive reabsorption of water from the distal and collecting tubules is under the control of antidiuretic hormone (ADH). In the absence of ADH the epithelium of the distal and collecting tubules is essentially impermeable to water. The tubular fluid remains hypotonic and urinary volume is high. In the presence of ADH the epithelium of these tubular segments becomes highly permeable to water, permitting the *facultative* reabsorption of water according to osmotic gradients established in the loop of Henle through the countercurrent mechanism.

Table 36-1
Organic Compounds of Medical Importance Actively Secreted by the Proximal Tubule

Compound	Medical Use
Drugs	
Acetazolamide Diamox	Carbonic anhydrase (CA) inhibitor
Chlorothiazide Diuril	Diuretic
Penicillin	Antibiotic
Probenecid Benemid	Uricosuric agent
Salicylates	Analgesic and antiinflammatory agents
Tolazoline Priscoline	Alpha-adrenergic blocking agent
Diagnostic Agents	
Iodopyract Diodrast	Urologic contrast medium
Para-aminohippuric acid PAH	Measurement of renal plasma flow and tubular secretion
Phenolsulfonphthalein Phenol red or PSP	Measurement of renal plasma flow

Countercurrent Mechanism

The conservation of water and concentration of urine by the kidneys is made possible by the operation of a countercurrent mechanism. Within this mechanism the loops of Henle act as countercurrent multipliers that establish an osmotic gradient in the renal medulla, whereas the vasa recta serve as countercurrent exchangers to maintain this gradient.

In the water-impermeable thick ascending limb of Henle's loop, chloride is actively transported out of the tubular fluid, followed passively by sodium, thus creating a *hyper*osmolarity in the medullary interstitium. The permeability of the epithelium in the descending limb of Henle's loop permits diffusion of water from the tubular fluid into the hyperosmolar medullary interstitium and diffusion of sodium chloride and urea into the tubular fluid. Thus, a gradually increasing osmolarity of the tubular fluid and medullary interstitium is created as the turn in the loop of Henle is approached. ADH controls the final volume of urine available for excretion by promoting the facultative reabsorption of water from the collecting tubules passing through the medullary pyramids according to the osmotic gradient established by the countercurrent mechanism.

Renal Function in Acid–Base Regulation

The renal tubular epithelium participates in acid–base regulation by reabsorbing sodium bicarbonate and secreting hydrogen ions and ammonia. The hydrogen ions are derived from the dissociation of carbonic acid (H_2CO_3), which forms when carbon dioxide and water combine in the presence of the enzyme catalyst *carbonic anhydrase*. Hydrogen ions thus secreted into the tubular lumen combine chemically with phosphate buffers present in the tubular fluid to form monosodium phosphate (NaH_2PO_4).

Secreted hydrogen ions may also combine with the ammonia produced by the renal tubular epithelium from the deamination of amino acids such as glutamine. The secreted hydrogen ions and ammonia combine to form the ammonium ion (NH_4^+), which is excreted together with tubular anions such as chloride (Cl^-).

37 DIURETICS

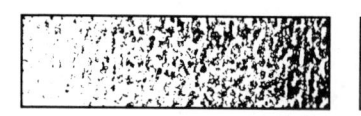

A *diuretic* is an agent capable of increasing the volume of urine and promoting a net loss of body water. The retention of excess fluid by the body depends in large measure on the retention of sodium. Therefore, the effectiveness of a diuretic is primarily related to its ability to increase the excretion of sodium, which is accomplished in most cases by interfering with the reabsorption of sodium ions in the tubules of the kidney. Loss of sodium is accompanied by excretion of an osmotically equivalent quantity of water, which is derived from body fluids removed from the tissues.

The handling of electrolytes by the kidney involves a complex series of interrelated mechanisms. Drugs such as diuretics that affect the handling of one electrolyte (e.g., sodium) almost invariably alter the handling of other electrolytes as well (such as chloride, potassium, hydrogen, bicarbonate). Depending on the mechanism of action of the individual diuretic drugs, therefore, electrolyte or acid–base balance disturbances, or both, can develop during diuretic therapy. These electrolyte imbalances are responsible for many of the disturbing and occasionally serious side effects resulting from diuretic administration, and an understanding of the sites and mechanisms of action of the diuretics can aid in predicting the types of electrolyte changes expected with any one drug. The overall drug regimen can then be tailored to produce an optimal diuretic action with a minimal degree of electrolyte-induced side effects (e.g., combining a drug that produces potassium loss with a potassium-sparing drug).

The effectiveness and safety of diuretics are greatly compromised in the presence of kidney disease. Most diuretics are of little value in patients with significantly impaired renal function, and in many instances they can be quite hazardous. These drugs should be prescribed to patients with known or suspected kidney impairment only after consideration of the potential risks.

A large number of chemically dissimilar compounds have a diuretic action, and the diuretic drugs are usually classified on the basis of their predominant sites and mechanisms of action. The major categories of diuretics reviewed in this chapter are listed in Table 37-1, along with their principal sites of action in the kidney and the major electrolyte disturbances associated with each group. Refer to Chapter 36 for a discussion of the renal handling of water and ions; reference to Chapter 36 will also aid in understanding the sites and mechanisms outlined for each class of diuretics in the subsequent discussion.

CARBONIC ANHYDRASE INHIBITORS

Acetazolamide   Methazolamide
Dichlorphenamide

Compounds in the group of carbonic anhydrase inhibitors are sulfonamide derivatives that interfere with the activity of the enzyme carbonic anhydrase (CA), thus blocking the hydration of carbon dioxide (CO_2) to carbonic acid (H_2CO_3) and subsequent ionization to yield hydrogen (H^+) and bicarbonate (HCO_3^-) ions. In addition to their mild diuretic action, these agents reduce aqueous humor production and are often used adjunctively in the treatment of glaucoma. They are also used in treating some forms of epilepsy (see Chap. 25). The CA inhibitors are reviewed as a group, followed by a listing of individual drugs in Table 37-2.

MECHANISM
Decrease production of H^+ and HCO_3^- in renal tubules, thereby reducing HCO_3^- absorption in proximal tubule; increased distal delivery of HCO_3^- exceeds absorptive capacity of distal nephron, resulting in excretion of HCO_3^-, K^+, and water; sodium loss is minimal; diuretic effect of carbonic anhydrase inhibitors is transient, because tolerance develops as serum bicarbonate levels decline.

In the eye, carbonic anhydrase inhibitors reduce the rate of aqueous humor formation, thereby lowering intraocular pressure. These drugs may also reduce the frequency of seizures (especially petit mal), possible by lowering the pH of brain tissue

USES
Adjunctive treatment of drug-induced edema or edema due to congestive heart failure refractory to single drug therapy (not indicated alone in edema)

Adjunctive treatment of glaucoma (open-angle, secondary glaucoma, preoperative in narrow-angle) to lower intraocular pressure

Adjunctive treatment of certain forms of epilepsy, especially petit mal

Prophylaxis of acute mountain sickness (e.g., weakness, dizziness, nausea) at high altitudes (acetazolamide)

DOSAGE
See Table 37-2

FATE
Readily absorbed from GI tract; onset of action following oral administration is 1 to 2 hours (longer with methazolamide); peak plasma levels occur in 2 to 4 hours (except sustained-release forms, which peak in 8–12 h); largely excreted within 24 hours, either as unchanged drug or *N*-dealkylated metabolites, some of which are active

COMMON SIDE EFFECTS
Paresthesias, drowsiness

SIGNIFICANT ADVERSE REACTIONS
CNS: confusion, myopia, tinnitus, malaise, vertigo, headache, xerostomia, depression, nervousness, weakness, flaccid paralysis, convulsions, tremor, ataxia

Dermatologic/hypersensitivity: skin eruptions, urticaria, pruritus, melena, photosensitivity

Hepatic/renal: hepatic insufficiency, pancreatitis, polyuria, dysuria, glycosuria, hematuria, urinary frequency, ureteral colic

Electrolyte: hypokalemia, hyponatremia

Other: aplastic anemia, diarrhea, vomiting, anorexia, loss of taste and smell

Table 37-1
Diuretic Drugs: Sites of Action and Electrolyte Disturbances

Classes of Diuretics	Major Sites of Action	Electrolyte Disturbances
Carbonic anhydrase inhibitors (e.g., **acetazolamide**)	Proximal tubule	Hyponatremic acidosis Hyperchloremic acidosis Hypokalemia
Loop (high-ceiling) diuretics (e.g., **furosemide**)	Thick ascending loop of Henle and possibly proximal and distal tubules	Hypokalemia Hypochloremic alkalosis Hyponatremia (excessive diuresis) Hypocalcemia
Osmotics (e.g., **mannitol**)	Proximal tubule, descending loop of Henle, and collecting tubule	Minimal
Potassium-sparing diuretics (e.g., **triamterene**)	Distal tubule	Hyperkalemia
Thiazides/sulfonamides (e.g., **hydrochlorothiazide, chlorthalidone, indapamide**)	Distal convoluted tubule and cortical thick ascending loop of Henle	Hypokalemia Hypochloremic alkalosis Hyponatremia Hypercalcemia

Note: Drugs are sulfonamide derivatives. See Chapter 57 for other potential adverse reactions

CONTRAINDICATIONS
Severe liver or kidney disease, chronic pulmonary disease, adrenocortical insufficiency, hyperchloremic acidosis, electrolyte imbalances, sensitivity to sulfonamides, pregnancy, and chronic noncongestive angle-closure glaucoma. *Cautious use* in patients with impaired hepatic function, respiratory disease, diabetes, and gout

INTERACTIONS
CA inhibitors make the urine alkaline and thus may enhance the action of amphetamines, catecholamines, procainamide, quinidine, tricyclic antidepressants, and any other basic drug by increasing their reabsorption

CA inhibitors can decrease the effects of lithium, barbiturates, nitrofurantoin, salicylates, and other acidic substances by reducing their renal tubular reabsorption

A reduced response to insulin and oral hypoglycemics has been reported with CA inhibitors

Increased hypokalemia can result with combinations of CA inhibitors and other diuretics, corticosteroids, and amphotericin B

CA-induced hypokalemia may augment digitalis toxicity

Metabolic acidosis can occur if CA inhibitors are given together with salicylates

NURSING CONSIDERATIONS
See **Plan of Nursing Care** 9 in this chapter. In addition:
1. Ensure that same brand of CA inhibitor is used consistently in each patient because different products are not always therapeutically equivalent.

PATIENT EDUCATION
See **Plan of Nursing Care** 9 in this chapter. In addition:
1. As appropriate, explain that an alternate-day regimen (see Usual Dosage Range, Table 37-2) is used to minimize development of tolerance and loss of diuretic potency. If diuretic effect decreases, *reducing* dose or frequency of administration often restores effectiveness.
2. Teach patient to recognize and report symptoms of metabolic acidosis (nausea, vomiting, malaise, abdominal pain, hyperpnea, tinnitus, disorientation, dysuria, numbness in extremities). If signs occur, drug should be temporarily discontinued, and dosage should be reduced upon resumption.
3. Instruct patient to inform physician immediately if signs of hypersensitivity (rash, fever) or possible blood dyscrasias (sore throat, bruising, mucosal ulceration) occur because CA inhibitors are sulfonamide derivatives. Periodic (4–6 mo) blood cell counts are recommended during prolonged therapy.
4. Warn patient that prolonged exposure to sunlight may cause photosensitivity.
5. Inform diabetic patient that dosage of hypoglycemic drugs may need to be increased because CA inhibitors may raise blood glucose.

LOOP (HIGH-CEILING) DIURETICS

Bumetanide   Furosemide
Ethacrynic acid

Several diuretic drugs are classified as "high-ceiling" agents, inasmuch as their peak diuretic effect is much greater than that observed with other clinically available oral diuretic drugs. Moreover, they exhibit a prompt onset of action when given orally, their action is independent of acid–base disturbances, and they are effective in patients with impaired renal function, whereas most other diuretics are not. The term *loop* derives from their site of action, the thick ascending loop of Henle, where a significant fraction of the filtered sodium load is reabsorbed. They are potent diuretics, and can lead to significant electrolyte disturbances. Careful medical supervision is therefore essential whenever these drugs are employed, and the

Table 37-2
Carbonic Anhydrase Inhibitors

Drug	Preparations	Usual Dosage Range	Nursing Implications
Acetazolamide Ak-Zol, Dazamide, Diamox (CAN) Acetazolam, Apo-Acetazolamide	Tablets: 125 mg, 250 mg Sustained-release capsules: 500 mg Injection: 500 mg/vial (sodium salt)	*Glaucoma:* 250 mg orally, 1–4 times/day depending on response; children—10 mg–15 mg/kg/day in divided doses every 6–8 h *Edema:* 250 mg–375 mg orally, once daily in the morning for 1–2 days; then skip a day; children—5 mg/kg once daily in the morning; IV, 500 mg initially; then 125 mg–250 mg every 4 h as needed in acute situation (500 mg/5 mL sterile water for injection) *Epilepsy:* Adults and children—8 mg–30 mg/kg/day in divided doses *Acute mountain sickness:* 500 mg–1000 mg daily in divided doses; initiate 24–48 h before ascent and continue as long as needed to control symptoms	Used for edema of congestive heart failure, certain forms of epilepsy, chronic open-angle glaucoma, and preoperatively in narrow-angle glaucoma; doses in excess of 1000 mg do not usually produce an increased effect. Sustained-release form may be used on a twice-daily basis; reconstituted injection solution should be used within 24 h; *avoid* IM administration if possible because alkaline solution is painful when injected
Dichlorphenamide Daranide	Tablets: 50 mg	100 mg–200 mg initially, followed by 100 mg/12 h until desired response is achieved; maintenance 25 mg–50 mg 1–3 times/day	Indicated as adjunctive treatment for open-angle glaucoma and preoperatively in narrow-angle glaucoma, together with miotics and osmotic diuretics
Methazolamide Neptazane	Tablets: 25 mg, 50 mg	50 mg–100 mg 2–3 times/day	Adjunctive therapy for both open-angle and narrow-angle glaucoma, with miotics and osmotic diuretics; contraindicated in severe or absolute glaucoma, hemorrhagic glaucoma, or that due to peripheral anterior synechiae; higher incidence of drowsiness than with other CA inhibitors

dosage must be critically adjusted for each patient. The drugs in this category are reviewed together; information pertaining to each individual drug is then presented in Table 37-3.

MECHANISM
Inhibit active tubular reabsorption of sodium and chloride by blocking the sodium–potassium–chloride cotransport system in the thick ascending loop of Henle, resulting in excretion of large quantities of urine high in sodium chloride; magnesium and calcium excretion is increased secondarily, and prolonged use of loop diuretics can lead to hypomagnesemia and hypocalcemia; renal blood flow is increased (perhaps owing to increased production of vasodilatory prostaglandins), and left ventricular filling pressure is lowered; no effect on carbonic anhydrase or aldosterone

USES
Treatment of severe edema associated with congestive heart failure, hepatic cirrhosis, and renal disease
Relief of acute pulmonary edema (IV administration)
Adjunctive treatment of hypertension (furosemide)
Management of ascites due to malignancy, idiopathic edema, and lymphedema (ethacrynic acid)
Short-term management of pediatric patients with congenital heart disease or the nephrotic syndrome (ethacrynic acid)
Treatment of acute hypercalcemia (IV furosemide with normal saline infusion)

DOSAGE
See Table 37-3

(Text continued on page 382)

PLAN OF NURSING CARE 9
PATIENTS TREATED WITH DIURETIC DRUGS

Nursing Diagnosis: Potential Alteration in Pattern of Urinary Elimination related to increased frequency of voiding from diuretic drug therapy

Goal: Patient will adapt to increased frequency of voiding.

Intervention	Rationale	Expected Outcome
See also **Plan of Nursing Care 2 (Noncompliance)**, Chapter 7.		
Inform patient that amount and frequency of urine output will increase, as this is the desired effect of diuretic drug.	Diuretics reduce body fluid by increasing urine output. The patient who is prepared for anticipated effects is less anxious, better able to cope with results, and more compliant.	Patient will express awareness that urine output will increase.
Collaborate with patient and health care team to plan dosing schedule that, to the extent possible, coordinates peak drug action with patient's daily routine and availability of bathroom facilities. Also consider the following: 1. It is usually best to take once-daily doses in the morning 2. It is usually best to take twice-daily doses around 8 a.m. and 2 p.m. 3. The last dose should be taken no later than 6 p.m.	Inconvenience jeopardizes compliance. Poor compliance may result from annoyance with frequent and excessive urination. If drug is taken too near bedtime, nocturia may disturb sleep and may pose a safety hazard with patient getting out of bed at night to void.	Patient will report that inconvenience of dosing schedule is minimal. Patient will report that diuretic has not caused nocturia.
Reassure patient that, once regimen is stabilized, duration of diuresis will be predictable.	The patient can plan activities around diuresis when its duration is known.	Patient will verbalize ability to predict length of diuresis.
For bedfast patient, ensure that urinal or bedpan is within reach.	Frustration is minimized when patient is able to use urinal or bedpan quickly and easily without waiting for someone to get it.	Patient will not manifest frustration due to delayed access to urinal or bedpan.
For ambulatory hospitalized patient, assist patient to bathroom according to needs.	Care must be taken to avoid injury from falls because the patient usually needs to go to the bathroom frequently, and orthostatic hypotension may occur with diuretic therapy, particularly during initial stages of therapy and in the elderly patient.	Patient will not fall getting out of bed to go to bathroom.

Nursing Diagnosis: Potential Fluid Volume Deficit related to diuresis from diuretic drug therapy

Goal: Patient will maintain or quickly regain normal fluid and electrolyte balance during diuretic drug therapy.

Intervention	Rationale	Expected Outcome
Assess patient's predisposition to develop fluid and electrolyte imbalance, which includes the following factors:	The greater the patient's predisposition to fluid and electrolyte disturbances, the more intensely the patient should be monitored.	Intensity of monitoring for fluid and electrolyte imbalance will be based on patient's degree of risk.
1. Type of diuretic prescribed	*Loop (high-ceiling) diuretics* are extremely potent and affect fluid and electrolyte balance much more profoundly than other classes of diuretics.	
2. Route of administration	Effects are more pronounced when a loop diuretic is administered IV than when it is given orally.	
3. Stage of diuretic therapy	Fluid and electrolyte disturbances occur more frequently during initial stages of therapy when diuretic effects are most potent.	
4. Age and condition of patient	The elderly and debilitated are particularly sensitive to effects of diuretics.	

Continued

PLAN OF NURSING CARE 9
PATIENTS TREATED WITH DIURETIC DRUGS (continued)

Nursing Diagnosis: Potential Fluid Volume Deficit related to diuresis from diuretic drug therapy
Goal: Patient will maintain or quickly regain normal fluid and electrolyte balance during diuretic drug therapy.

Intervention	Rationale	Expected Outcome
5. Presence or absence of vomiting or diarrhea	Vomiting or diarrhea contribute to fluid and electrolyte deficits, especially hypokalemia.	
6. Nature and amount of intake	Inadequate intake of appropriate types or amounts of food, fluids, or dietary supplements may precipitate fluid and electrolyte imbalance in the patient on diuretic therapy.	
Inform patient that weight loss is an expected result of diuretic therapy	Patient must be prepared for the weight loss that occurs.	Patient will express awareness that weight loss will occur.
Advise patient to avoid excessive intake of water.	Diuresis may induce thirst, but excessive water intake may lead to hyponatremia.	Patient will not develop hyponatremia.
Obtain baseline and daily weights. Weigh at the same time, preferably early morning before patient has eaten but after bladder has been emptied, under standard conditions.	Weight fluctuation is the best indication of body water changes. Rapid fluid loss, as reflected by excessive weight reduction, predisposes to fluid volume deficit.	Excessive weight loss will be detected promptly.
Teach patient to weigh self and to keep a record of results.		Patient will explain proper procedures for obtaining and recording weight.
Monitor intake and output.	Output greater than intake may reflect excessive fluid loss. Normal urine output is 1500 mL/day. Normal fluid intake is 2000–3000 mL/day.	Fluid volume deficit will be detected promptly.
Observe degree of urine concentration or measure urine specific gravity.	Highly dilute urine may reflect potential for fluid and electrolyte imbalance from rapid diuresis. Highly concentrated urine may reflect dehydration.	
Assess patient for signs and symptoms of dehydration: dry skin and mucous membranes; thirst; decreased skin turgor; nausea; anorexia; lightheadedness; weakness; decreased level of consciousness; increased temperature, pulse, and respirations; decreased blood pressure; oliguria.	Excessive fluid loss may lead to dehydration.	Dehydration will be detected promptly.
Teach patient to recognize and report signs and symptoms of dehydration.		Patient will state signs and symptoms of dehydration.
Check hematocrit results.	Elevation above 45% reflects hemoconcentration from dehydration.	
Notify, or instruct patient to notify, primary health care provider if a weight loss of greater than 3 lb/day occurs or other indications of excessive fluid loss appear.	Discontinuation, dosage reduction, or other alterations in medication regimen may be indicated.	Fluid volume deficit will be corrected.
Instruct patient to promptly report pain in chest, calves, or pelvis to appropriate person.	Excessive fluid loss (dehydration) can reduce blood volume (hypovolemia) and cause decreased cardiac output, hypotension, circulatory collapse (rarely), and thromboembolism (from hemoconcentration).	Thromboembolism will be detected promptly.
Assess patient with pain in chest, calves, or pelvis for possible thromboembolism.		
Implement appropriate interventions for orthostatic hypotension (see **Plan of Nursing Care 8** in Chap. 31).	Symptoms of orthostatic hypotension may occur, particularly during early stages of therapy. Although thiazide diuretics do not appear to exert a direct antihypertensive effect on normal blood pressure, other diuretics may, especially with rapid diuresis.	See **Plan of Nursing Care 8,** Chapter 31, for Expected Outcomes for interventions related to orthostatic hypotension.
Warn patient that hazardous activities should be performed very cautiously until effects of drug are known.	In addition to hypotension, fatigue and other commonly occurring side effects may render hazardous activities unsafe for the patient.	Patient will verbalize awareness of safety risks posed by drug.

Continued

PLAN OF NURSING CARE 9
PATIENTS TREATED WITH DIURETIC DRUGS (continued)
Nursing Diagnosis: Potential Fluid Volume Deficit related to diuresis from diuretic drug therapy
Goal: Patient will maintain or quickly regain normal fluid and electrolyte balance during diuretic drug therapy.

Intervention	Rationale	Expected Outcome
Advise patient to moderate consumption of alcohol, caffeine, and sugars.	These mild diuretics may add to the effect of diuretic therapy, and alcohol can produce severe hypotension when taken in conjunction with diuretics.	Patient will state effects of consumption of mild diuretic substances.
Emphasize the importance of adhering to prescribed drug and dietary regimen and of maintaining regular health care supervision.	Consequences of deviating from prescribed regimen can be quite serious. Drug effects must be monitored so that dosage and regimen can be adjusted accordingly.	Patient will explain significance of compliance with diuretic therapy regimen.
Monitor results of serum electrolyte determinations.	Electrolytes, particularly sodium and potassium, are lost in urine. Diuretics increase urine production by enhancing urinary excretion of sodium and water either directly or indirectly by impairing sodium reabsorption in the renal tubules. Excessive diuresis may result in serum electrolyte deficiencies.	Serum electrolyte abnormalities will be detected.
If patient is receiving a **non-potassium-sparing diuretic,** *implement interventions to monitor and prevent the development of* **hypokalemia,** as follows:	Most diuretics except those in the potassium-sparing group *enhance* renal excretion of potassium. Potassium is exchanged for sodium in the renal tubules.	
Assess patient for signs and symptoms of hypokalemia: weak or irregular pulse, palpitations, hypotension, shallow respirations, dyspnea, dry mouth, thirst, anorexia, nausea, vomiting, fatigue, lethargy, drowsiness, confusion, restlessness, hypoactive reflexes, decreased peristalsis or paralytic ileus, abdominal distention, paresthesias, and skeletal muscle weakness, tremors, pain or cramps.	Potassium is the major intracellular electrolyte. It affects acid-base balance and cellular hydration. High or low levels interfere with conduction of nerve impulses through skeletal, smooth, and cardiac muscle.	Hypokalemia will be detected promptly.
Teach patient to recognize and report signs and symptoms of hypokalemia.		Patient will state signs and symptoms of hypokalemia.
Monitor results of serum potassium determinations.	Levels below 3.5 mEq/liter reflect hypokalemia.	
Check ECG pattern.	Low voltage, flattened T wave, and depressed ST segment are characteristic of hypokalemia. Cardiac arrhythmias and enhanced cardiac-glycoside cardiotoxicity, such as bradycardia and ventricular irritability, may also occur.	
Discuss potential prevention or treatment with patient, such as the following:	Hypokalemia can be prevented or treated by increasing potassium intake.	Patient will express awareness of measures used to prevent hypokalemia.
1. A potassium supplement may be prescribed		
2. A potassium-sparing diuretic may be added to the regimen		
3. Potassium in diet may be increased:		
a. review and give patient list of foods high in potassium content (dates, raisins, prunes, apricots, bananas, fruit juices, oranges, raw carrots, potatoes, tomatoes, beef, chicken, fresh fish, liver, whole grain cereals, Gatorade, Pepsi-Cola, skim milk)		
b. refer patient to dietician for instruction regarding dietary potassium		

Continued

PLAN OF NURSING CARE 9
PATIENTS TREATED WITH DIURETIC DRUGS (continued)
Nursing Diagnosis: Potential Fluid Volume Deficit related to diuresis from diuretic drug therapy
Goal: Patient will maintain or quickly regain normal fluid and electrolyte balance during diuretic drug therapy.

Intervention	Rationale	Expected Outcome
Instruct patient to avoid eating licorice.	Licorice contains glycyrrhizic acid, which can cause severe hypokalemia if ingested in large amounts.	Patient will state that large amounts of licorice should not be eaten.
If evidence of hypokalemia is present, notify, or instruct patient to notify, primary health care provider.	Drug dosage should be adjusted or potassium replacement therapy should be instituted.	Patient will be treated for hypokalemia. Patient's serum potassium will return to normal.
If patient is receiving a **potassium-sparing diuretic,** *implement interventions to monitor and prevent the development of* **hyperkalemia,** *such as follows:*	Potassium-sparing diuretics *block* renal excretion of potassium by inhibiting active tubular reabsorption of sodium and chloride, which results in excretion of sodium, potassium, and other electrolytes.	
Assess patient for signs and symptoms of hyperkalemia: confusion, fatigue, weakness, malaise, nausea, diarrhea, intestinal cramps, paresthesias, hypotension, bradycardia, irregular pulse.	Potassium is the major intracellular electrolyte. It affects acid-base balance and cellular hydration. High or low levels interfere with conduction of nerve impulses through skeletal, smooth, and cardiac muscle.	Hyperkalemia will be detected promptly.
Monitor results of serum potassium determinations.	Levels above 5 mEq/L reflect hyperkalemia.	
Check ECG pattern.	Prolonged PR interval; wide QRS complex; tall, peaked T wave; and depressed ST segment are characteristic of hyperkalemia. Cardiac arrhythmias that progress to ventricular fibrillation and asystole may also occur.	
Teach patient to recognize and report signs and symptoms of hyperkalemia.		Patient will state signs and symptoms of hyperkalemia.
Instruct patient to limit intake of substances high in potassium content, including salt substitutes.	With renal potassium excretion reduced, serum potassium can build to toxic levels. This risk can be minimized by limiting oral potassium intake. Salt substitutes contain potassium.	Patient will express awareness of need to limit oral potassium intake.
If evidence of hyperkalemia is present, notify, or instruct patient to notify, primary health care provider immediately.	Appropriate treatment should be promptly instituted.	Patient will be treated for hyperkalemia. Patient's serum potassium will return to normal.

FATE
Onset of diuresis following oral administration is 30 to 60 minutes; peak effect occurs in 1 to 2 hours, and duration is 6 to 8 hours, except for bumetanide (3–6 h). IV injection produces a diuretic response within 5 to 10 minutes, which then peaks within 15 to 30 minutes and persists for 2 hours. Drugs are highly bound to plasma proteins (94%–98%) and are rapidly excreted in the urine, both as metabolites and unchanged drug. Approximately one third of the dose is eliminated by way of the bile in the feces.

COMMON SIDE EFFECTS
Bumetanide: abdominal discomfort, orthostatic hypotension
Ethacrynic acid: anorexia, abdominal discomfort
Furosemide: orthostatic hypotension (initial period of therapy)

SIGNIFICANT ADVERSE REACTIONS
All Drugs
GI: vomiting, diarrhea, dysphagia, acute pancreatitis, jaundice
CNS: headache, blurred vision, tinnitus, hearing loss, weakness, vertigo
Electrolyte: hypokalemia, hyponatremia, hypochloremic alkalosis, hypomagnesemia, hypocalcemia
Other: rash, pruritus, hyperglycemia, hyperuricemia, azotemia, increased serum creatinine, agranulocytosis, thrombocytopenia

Bumetanide
Dry mouth, arthritic pain, muscle cramping, hives, premature ejaculation, ECG changes, chest pain, hyperventilation, breast tenderness

Ethacrynic Acid
GI bleeding, *profuse* watery diarrhea, fever, chills, hematuria, neutropenia, confusion, fatigue, hypovolemia, hypocalcemia, orthostatic hypotension, muscle cramping, and nystagmus

Furosemide
GI irritation, constipation, paresthesias, leukopenia, anemia, urticaria, photosensitivity, erythema multiforme, exfoliative dermatitis, necrotizing angiitis, weakness, urinary frequency, urinary bladder spasm, and thrombophlebitis

WARNING
A dose-related *reversible* ototoxic effect, manifested as tinnitus, hearing impairment, and rarely deafness, can occur. This effect is usually associated with overzealous therapy (e.g., rapid IV injection of large doses) in patients with reduced renal function

CONTRAINDICATIONS
Anuria, hepatic coma, dehydration, severe electrolyte depletion, early pregnancy, and in infants (especially ethacrynic acid). *Cautious use* in patients with hepatic cirrhosis, hearing impairment, orthostatic hypotension, diabetes, gout, or cardiogenic shock; in persons receiving digitalis drugs or potassium-depleting steroids, and in elderly patients, and pregnant or nursing women

INTERACTIONS
Loop diuretics may potentiate the action of antihypertensive medications

Loop diuretics may increase the toxicity of aminoglycoside antibiotics (ototoxicity), cisplatin (ototoxicity), cephalosporins (nephrotoxicity), salicylates, lithium, and cardiac glycosides

Increased orthostatic hypotension can occur with combinations of loop diuretics and alcohol, narcotics, or barbiturates

Increased potassium loss may occur when corticosteroids are given with loop diuretics

Loop diuretics may reduce the effectiveness of uricosuric drugs by elevating serum uric acid levels

Probenecid may reduce the diuretic effectiveness of bumetanide and furosemide

Indomethacin, and possibly other nonsteroidal anti-inflammatory drugs may impair the action of loop diuretics by decreasing prostaglandin synthesis

Loop diuretics can potentiate the muscle-relaxing effects of the antidepolarizing neuromuscular-blocking drugs (e.g., tubocurare, gallamine) but may enhance the muscle-relaxing action of succinylcholine

Increased requirements for oral hypoglycemic drugs or insulin may occur in persons taking loop diuretics, which can elevate blood glucose levels

Furosemide (and possibly bumetanide) can potentiate the pharmacologic effects of theophylline

Ethacrynic acid may displace oral anticoagulants from their protein-binding sites

Concurrent use of furosemide and metolazone may result in profound diuresis and excessive electrolyte loss

NURSING CONSIDERATIONS
See **Plan of Nursing Care 9** in this chapter. In addition:

Nursing Alerts
- Expect therapy to be initiated with small doses. Dosage should be adjusted carefully on the basis of serum electrolyte levels and clinical response.
- When giving IV, check blood pressure frequently, and monitor infusion rate, which should not exceed 4 mg/minute. Check for signs of extravasation, which commonly causes pain and irritation.
- Assess for signs of joint swelling, tenderness, or pain, which may signify onset of gout. If these occur, advise physician.

1. Monitor results of CO_2, BUN, WBC, and liver function studies, which should be performed periodically during prolonged therapy.
2. Assess adequacy of glucose control in known and suspected diabetics. Advise physician of increased blood glucose or altered glucose tolerance.
3. Seek clarification if diuretic is prescribed for patient in hepatic coma or a state of electrolyte deficiency. These underlying conditions should be corrected before diuretic therapy is initiated.

PATIENT EDUCATION
See **Plan of Nursing Care 9** in this chapter. In addition:
1. Instruct patient to take drug with meals or food if GI irritation occurs.
2. Explain that an intermittent dosage schedule (e.g., 3–4 days/wk interspersed with a rest period) is used when possible to allow electrolyte and acid–base balance to stabilize.
3. Instruct patient to report immediately any indication of impaired hearing (often preceded by vertigo and tinnitus). Dosage should be reevaluated because danger of permanent hearing loss exists with prolonged high-dose therapy.
4. Instruct patient to report any *weight gain*.
5. Inform patient that GI side effects occur most frequently after 1 to 2 months of therapy. Diarrhea or abdominal pain should be reported because dosage adjustment may be warranted.

OSMOTIC DIURETICS

The term *osmotic diuretic* refers to any solute that is readily filtered by the kidney but poorly reabsorbed in the renal tubules. When these agents are taken, the large amount of nonreabsorbed material increases the osmotic pressure of the tubular fluid, causing an osmotically equivalent amount of water to be carried through the tubule with it, eventually to be excreted. Sodium excretion is not significantly increased, however, by normal therapeutic doses of the osmotic diuretics. For this reason, and because most of these diuretics must be administered IV in large doses, they are infrequently used for routine treatment of edema and are primarily indicated for the prevention of acute renal failure associated with a sharply reduced glomerular filtration rate.

Their osmotic effects are not confined to the kidney but extend to the bloodstream as well, where the presence of the drug in the circulation draws fluid from tissue spaces *into* the blood. This effect underlies their application in reducing elevated intraocular and intracranial pressures, actions important in treating cranial injuries and acute congestive glaucoma, and as an aid to neurosurgery.

Glycerin
Glyrol, Osmoglyn

MECHANISM
Elevates plasma osmotic pressure, thus drawing fluid from extravascular spaces; decreases intraocular and intracranial pressure

Table 37-3
Loop (High-Ceiling) Diuretics

Drug	Preparations	Usual Dosage Range	Nursing Implications
Bumetanide Bumex	Tablets: 0.5 mg, 1 mg, 2 mg Injection: 0.25 mg/mL	Oral: 0.5 mg–2 mg/day, as a single dose; maximum oral dose is 10 mg/day IV, IM: 0.5 mg–1 mg; repeat at 2–3-h intervals to a maximum of 10 mg as needed	Drug is more chloruretic than natriuretic; may have an additional action in the proximal tubule; hypokalemia may be less severe than with furosemide; cross-sensitivity with furosemide is rare; use an intermittent dosage schedule for prolonged therapy; use parenteral solutions within 24 h; safety and efficacy in children under 18 has not been established
Ethacrynic acid Edecrin	Tablets: 25 mg, 50 mg Injection: 50 mg/vial (sodium salt)	*Oral* Adults: initially 50 mg–100 mg daily; maintenance dose 50 mg–200 mg/day on an intermittent schedule Children: initially 25 mg/day; adjust dosage in 25-mg increments to achieve optimal response *IV* 0.5 mg/kg–1 mg/kg (usual adult dose 50 mg); a second dose of 50 mg at a different site may be required (maximum 100 mg/dose)	Reconstitute IV solution by adding 50 mL 5% dextrose injection or sodium chloride injection to vial; do *not* inject SC or IM, because pain and irritation may occur; direct IV injection should be made over several minutes; do not use solution if cloudy; discard within 24 h after preparation; when used IV, be alert for presence of pain in calf, chest, or pelvic area, possible signs of thromboembolic complications; safety and efficacy of ethacrynic acid in treating hypertension has not been established; hypoproteinemia may reduce response to ethacrynic acid; discontinue drug if diarrhea occurs
Furosemide Fumide, Furomide M.D., Lasix, Luramide (CAN) Apo-Furosemide, Furoside, Novosemide, Uritol	Tablets: 20 mg, 40 mg, 80 mg Oral solution: 10 mg/mL, 40 mg/5 mL Injection: 10 mg/mL	ORAL *Adults* Diuresis: 20 mg–80 mg as a single dose; may increase by 20-mg–40-mg increments to a maximum of 600 mg/day Hypertension: 40 mg twice a day; adjust according to response; usual maintenance dose 40 mg–80 mg/day in 1 or 2 divided doses *Children* Initially 2 mg/kg as a single dose; may increase by 1-mg/kg–2-mg/kg increments to a maximum of 6 mg/kg/day PARENTERAL *Adults* 20 mg–40 mg IV or IM as a single dose; may increase by 20-mg increments every 2–3 h until desired response is obtained Acute pulmonary edema: 40 mg IV over 1–2 min; may increase to 80 mg IV after 1 h *Children* 1 mg/kg IV or IM; may increase by 1 mg/kg no sooner than 2 h after previous dose; maximum 6 mg/kg	Oral doses should be given on an intermittent schedule (e.g., 2–4 days/wk); parenteral therapy is indicated for emergency situations only and should be replaced by oral therapy as soon as possible; do *not* mix parenteral solutions with highly acidic preparations; use mixture within 24 h of preparation and do *not* use if solution is yellow; use *cautiously* in patients allergic to sulfonamides, because cross-reactions can occur; when adding drug to an existing antihypertensive regimen, reduce dose of other drugs by half to avoid excessive drop in blood pressure and titrate furosemide dosage to obtain optimal hypotensive effect; in patients with impaired renal function, use controlled IV infusion (4 mg/min) to minimize danger of azotemia or oliguria; drug can stimulate renal synthesis of prostaglandin E_2, which can complicate the neonatal respiratory distress syndrome

USES
Interruption of an acute attack of glaucoma
Preoperative reduction in intraocular pressure as an aid to ophthalmic surgery (e.g., for glaucoma, cataracts)
Reduction of intracranial or intraocular pressure (investigational use for IV administration)

DOSAGE
Orally 1 g/kg to 1.5 g/kg of a 50% or 75% solution 1 to 1.5 hours before surgery

FATE
Rapidly absorbed when taken orally; intraocular pressure is reduced within 15 minutes, maximal effect occurring in 1 hour; action persists 4 to 6 hours; metabolized in the liver

SIGNIFICANT ADVERSE REACTIONS
Nausea, vomiting, diarrhea, headache, disorientation, confusion. Rarely, arrhythmias, dehydration, hyperglycemia

Diuretics

CONTRAINDICATIONS
Anuria, severe dehydration, acute pulmonary edema, severe cardiac decompensation. *Cautious use* in persons with hypervolemia, confusion, diabetes, or congestive heart disease, and in elderly or senile individuals

NURSING CONSIDERATION
1. Do not inject glycerin. It is for oral administration *only*. The 50% solution is lime-flavored. The palatability of unflavored solutions may be improved by addition of lemon juice or other flavoring agents.

Isosorbide
Ismotic

MECHANISM
Increases plasma osmotic pressure, thereby reducing elevated intraocular pressure by promoting redistribution of fluid toward the circulatory vessels

USES
Short-term reduction of elevated intraocular pressure prior to and following surgery for glaucoma or cataract to interrupt an acute attack of glaucoma

DOSAGE
Initially, 1.5 g/kg orally 2 to 4 times a day; usual range is 1 g/kg to 3 g/kg 2 to 4 times a day

FATE
Rapidly absorbed orally; onset of action is within 30 minutes; peak effect occurs in 1 to 1.5 hours and duration is 5 to 6 hours

SIGNIFICANT ADVERSE REACTIONS
Nausea, vomiting, diarrhea, thirst, headache, dizziness, lightheadedness, lethargy, irritability, rash, hiccups, hypernatremia

CONTRAINDICATIONS
Anuria due to severe renal disease, severe dehydration, acute pulmonary edema, and hemorrhagic glaucoma. *Cautious use* in patients with hypertension, congestive heart failure

NURSING CONSIDERATIONS

Nursing Alerts
- Maintain proper fluid and electrolyte balance during prolonged administration.
- Monitor urinary output. Drug should be discontinued if output continues to decrease because extracellular fluid overload can occur.

1. Pour medication over cracked ice and instruct patient to sip it to improve palatability.

Mannitol
Osmitrol

MECHANISM
Not appreciably metabolized following IV injection, rapidly excreted by the kidneys; not reabsorbed in the renal tubules, hence raises the osmotic pressure of tubular fluid, thereby reducing reabsorption of water and increasing urine flow; may increase electrolyte excretion when used in large doses; decreases elevated intracranial and intraocular pressure by raising plasma osmotic pressure

USES
Prevention and treatment of the oliguric phase of acute renal failure before irreversible renal failure occurs
Treatment of cerebral edema and elevated intracranial pressure (e.g., resulting from head injury or surgery)
Reduction of elevated intraocular pressure in acute congestive glaucoma
Treatment of acute chemical poisoning, by enhancing renal excretion of toxic substances
Measurement of glomerular filtration rate (GFR)

DOSAGE

> NOTE
> Use by IV infusion only: Carefully evaluate patient's cardiovascular status before administering mannitol solution IV, because sudden expansion of extracellular fluid volume may aggravate or precipitate congestive heart failure

Acute renal failure: 50 g to 100 g as a 5% to 25% solution
Reduction of intracranial pressure: 1.5 g/kg to 2 g/kg as a 15% to 25% solution over 30 to 60 minutes
Reduction of intraocular pressure: 1.5 g/kg to 2 g/kg as a 15% to 25% solution over 30 to 60 minutes.
Acute chemical poisoning: 100 g to 200 g depending on fluid requirement and urinary output
Measurement of glomerular filtration rate: 100 mL of 20% solution diluted with 180 mL of sodium chloride injection infused at a rate of 20 mL/min
Test dose (patients with marked oliguria to determine drug's effectiveness): 0.2 g/kg infused over 3 to 5 minutes to produce a urine flow of at least 30 mL to 50 mL/h

FATE
Confined to extracellular space; only slightly metabolized and rapidly excreted by the kidneys (80% of a dose appears in the urine within 3 h); less than 10% is reabsorbed by the kidneys; diuresis occurs in 1 to 2 hours, and elevated cranial and ocular pressures are reduced within 30 minutes

SIGNIFICANT ADVERSE REACTIONS
(Infrequent) Dry mouth, thirst, headache, blurred vision, nausea, vomiting, rhinitis, diarrhea, marked diuresis, electrolyte imbalance, acidosis, fever, chills, dizziness, hypotension, dehydration, tachycardia, angina-like pain

CONTRAINDICATIONS
Anuria, severe pulmonary edema or congestive heart failure, intracranial bleeding, severe dehydration, progressive renal disease after initiating mannitol therapy, and in children under 12 years of age. *Cautious use* in patients with marked cardiopulmonary or renal dysfunction and in pregnant women

NURSING CONSIDERATIONS

Nursing Alerts
- Carefully assess patient's cardiovascular status prior to and during administration because congestive heart failure may occur.
- During infusion, monitor urine output continually. Infusion should be terminated if output declines because

> accumulation of mannitol can result in expanded extracellular fluid volume, which may aggravate or precipitate congestive heart failure.
> - Monitor results of plasma electrolyte measurements, which should be performed if administration is prolonged. Infusion should be adjusted to prevent electrolyte imbalance.
> - Administer concurrently with whole blood only if at least 20 mEq/L of sodium chloride is added to mannitol solution to prevent pseudoagglutination.
> - In patient with severe renal impairment, be prepared to administer test dose (see Dosage above). A second test dose may be given if response to first is inadequate (urine flow less than 30 mL/h).

1. Adjust infusion rate to maintain urine flow of at least 30 mL to 50 mL/h.
2. Consult physician regarding allowable fluid intake.
3. If solution is crystallized (exposed to low temperatures), warm in hot water bath, then cool to body temperature before injecting. Do not administer if crystals are present.

Urea
Ureaphil

MECHANISM
Filtered but not reabsorbed by the kidney; increased osmotic pressure in tubular fluid prevents water reabsorption and increases rate and volume of urine flow; elevates osmotic pressure of blood, thus increasing movement of fluid from body tissues to bloodstream

USES
Reduction of intracranial and intraocular pressure (alternative drug *only*)
Induction of abortion (intraamniotic injection)—*investigational use*

DOSAGE
(IV infusion *only* as a 30% solution)
Maximum infusion rate 4 mL/min; maximum dose 120 g/day

Adults: 1 g/kg to 1.5 g/kg
Children: 0.5 g/kg to 1.5 g/kg
Infants: 0.1 g/kg to 0.5 g/kg

FATE
Onset of diuretic effect is 4 to 8 hours; intracranial–intraocular pressure is reduced within 1 to 2 hours; widely distributed by the bloodstream and excreted by the kidney essentially unchanged

COMMON SIDE EFFECTS
Headache, nausea

SIGNIFICANT ADVERSE REACTIONS
Syncope, disorientation, confusion, agitation, pain, irritation, phlebitis and thrombosis at site of infusion, electrolyte imbalances, tachycardia, and hypotension

CONTRAINDICATIONS
Severely impaired renal function, marked dehydration, intracranial bleeding, and frank liver failure. *Cautious use* in patients with liver impairment or kidney disease, and in pregnant or lactating women

INTERACTIONS
Urea may potentiate the action of anticoagulants
Urea can reduce the effectiveness of lithium by increasing its excretion

NURSING CONSIDERATIONS

Nursing Alerts
- Closely monitor intake and output during infusion. Comatose patient should have an indwelling bladder catheter. If diuresis does not occur within 6 to 12 hours after injection, or if BUN exceeds 75 mg/dL, drug should be discontinued, and renal function should be reevaluated.
- Use extreme care to avoid extravasation of solution because irritation, thrombosis, and tissue necrosis can occur.
- Do not infuse into veins of lower extremities in elderly patients because thrombosis and phlebitis of deep veins may result.

1. Do not infuse through the administration set used for blood infusion.
2. Keep infusion rate below 4 mL/min to avoid hemolysis.
3. Prepare solution by reconstituting it with 5% or 10% dextrose injection or 10% invert sugar in water. Use within a few hours if stored at room temperature (within 48 h if stored at 2° to 8°C).
4. Discard unused portion.

POTASSIUM-SPARING DIURETICS

Unlike most other major classes of diuretic drugs, the potassium-sparing diuretics do *not* cause a loss of potassium by way of the kidney but rather act to conserve potassium by reducing its distal tubular secretion in conjunction with sodium reabsorption. These agents are not potent diuretic drugs when used alone, and their use as single agents can result in significant hyperkalemia. Their principal application, therefore, is in combination with other oral diuretics (e.g., thiazides, high-ceiling drugs) both to increase the excretion of sodium and water and, more important, to minimize the potassium loss normally induced by the more potent drugs. Because several important differences exist among the available potassium-sparing diuretics, they are reviewed individually.

Amiloride
Midamor

MECHANISM
Acts principally on the distal tubule to inhibit active sodium reabsorption and potassium secretion across tubular membranes; inhibition of Na^+-K^+-ATPase enzyme may play a role in blocking transtubular transport of these ions; also decreases magnesium excretion which occurs with thiazide and loop diuretics; possesses weak diuretic and blood pressure–lowering activity and does not significantly alter renal blood flow or GFR.

USES
Adjunctive treatment with potassium-depleting diuretics (e.g., thiazides, loop diuretics) to minimize potassium loss or restore normal serum potassium levels (rarely used alone)

DOSAGE

Initially 5 mg/day orally as a single dose added to the diuretic regimen; increase if necessary in 5-mg increments. Maximum recommended dose is 20 mg/day for severe, persistent hypokalemia

FATE

Onset of action with oral administration is 2 hours; peak effects occur between 6 and 10 hours; duration is 24 hours; plasma half-life is 6 to 9 hours; not metabolized, but excreted largely unchanged in both urine and feces in approximately equivalent amounts

COMMON SIDE EFFECTS

Nausea, anorexia, diarrhea, headache, vomiting, hyperkalemia (paresthesias, muscle weakness, fatigue, bradycardia)

SIGNIFICANT ADVERSE REACTIONS

GI: abdominal pain, dyspepsia, constipation, flatulence, GI bleeding
CNS: dizziness, encephalopathy, confusion, insomnia, tremors, depression
Respiratory: dyspnea, coughing
Musculoskeletal: muscle cramping; weakness; pain in joints, back, neck, shoulders
Other: impotence, polyuria, dysuria, arrhythmias, photosensitivity, skin rash, pruritus, alopecia, visual disturbances, nasal congestion, tinnitus, increased intraocular pressure

CONTRAINDICATIONS

Hyperkalemia, impaired renal function, and concomitant use with other potassium-sparing diuretics or potassium supplements. *Cautious use* in patients with diabetes, renal impairment, cardiopulmonary disease; in pregnant women or nursing mothers; in children; and in elderly, debilitated, or severely ill patients

INTERACTIONS

Amiloride may increase lithium toxicity by reducing its renal clearance
Hyperkalemia may be augmented by concomitant use of other potassium-sparing drugs (e.g., spironolactone, triamterene) or potassium supplements
Amiloride can reduce the clinical effectiveness of digitalis drugs but also reduces the risk of toxicity resulting from hypokalemia

NURSING CONSIDERATIONS

See **Plan of Nursing Care** 9 in this chapter. In addition:
1. Monitor results of BUN determinations, which should be performed frequently during extended therapy, and inform primary health care provider of change in renal function.
2. Note that amiloride (5 mg) is available in fixed combination with hydrochlorothiazide (50 mg) as Moduretic.

PATIENT EDUCATION

See **Plan of Nursing Care** 9 in this chapter. In addition:
1. Suggest drug be taken with food to minimize GI upset.

Spironolactone

Alatone Aldactone

(CAN) Novospiroton, Sincomen

MECHANISM

Competitive antagonist of the naturally occurring hormone aldosterone at distal tubular sites involved in sodium reabsorption and potassium excretion; aldosterone normally stimulates enzymes that supply energy for active sodium and potassium transport in the distal tubule; inhibition of aldosterone results in excretion of sodium and retention of potassium; does not appear to elevate serum uric acid or alter carbohydrate metabolism but can interfere with testosterone synthesis, leading to increased estrogenic:androgenic activity ratio

USES

Management of edema associated with congestive heart failure, primary hyperaldosteronism, cirrhosis of the liver, and nephrotic syndrome
Treatment of essential hypertension, usually combined with other diuretics or antihypertensive drugs
Adjunctive therapy with other potent diuretics to minimize potassium loss
Diagnosis and treatment of primary hyperaldosteronism
Investigational uses include treatment of hirsutism and relief of symptoms of premenstrual syndrome (PMS)

DOSAGE

(Oral administration *only*)

Edema: Adults, 25 mg to 200 mg/day in a single dose or divided doses; Children, 3.3 mg/kg in a single dose or divided doses
Hypertension: 50 mg to 100 mg daily in a single dose or divided doses; maximum 200 mg/day
Diagnosis of hyperaldosteronism: 400 mg/day for 4 days; if serum potassium increases during this time, then falls when drug is stopped, a presumptive diagnosis of primary hyperaldosteronism may be considered
Treatment of hyperaldosteronism: 100 mg to 400 mg/day
Hypokalemia: 25 mg to 100 mg/day to prevent diuretic-induced potassium loss

FATE

Peak plasma levels occur in 3 to 4 hours following a single dose; maximal diuretic action is seen in 2 to 3 days and may persist for several days after therapy is discontinued; highly bound to plasma proteins; rapidly and extensively metabolized and excreted primarily in the urine, with small amounts in the bile

COMMON SIDE EFFECTS

Gynecomastia and breast tenderness (in men and women), GI upset, lethargy

SIGNIFICANT ADVERSE REACTIONS

> **WARNING**
> Spironolactone has been shown to be a tumorigen in chronic toxicity studies in rats at significantly higher than recommended doses. Its use should be restricted to those indications outlined above for which other diuretic drugs are ineffective or inappropriate

Cramping, diarrhea, vomiting, cutaneous eruptions, urticaria, fever, ataxia, drowsiness, confusion, impotence, hirsutism, irregular menses, voice deepening, postmenopausal bleeding, fluid and electrolyte disturbances (especially hyperkalemia and hyponatremia), mild acidosis, and elevated BUN

CONTRAINDICATIONS

Anuria, acute renal insufficiency or significantly impaired renal function, and hyperkalemia. *Cautious use* in decreased renal function and in pregnant or nursing women

INTERACTIONS

Spironolactone may potentiate the effects of other diuretics and antihypertensive drugs

Salicylates may reverse the effects of spironolactone

Spironolactone may reduce the clinical effectiveness of digitalis drugs but also reduces the likelihood of digitalis-induced arrhythmias occurring as a result of hypokalemia

The renal clearance of lithium may be reduced by spironolactone

The effects of oral anticoagulants may be reduced owing to hemoconcentration of clotting factors resulting from diuretic action

Ammonium chloride and other acidifying agents can induce systemic acidosis when given in combination with spironolactone

Hyperkalemia may result if potassium supplements are used together with spironolactone, or if patients consume a potassium-rich diet

NURSING CONSIDERATION

See **Plan of Nursing Care** 9 in this chapter. In addition:
1. Note that spironolactone is available in two fixed dosage combinations with hydrochlorothiazide as Alazide, Aldactazide, Spironazide, and Spirozide.

PATIENT EDUCATION

See **Plan of Nursing Care** 9 in this chapter. In addition:
1. Inform patient that swelling and tenderness of breasts may occur, most often with prolonged therapy, but that this effect is usually reversible when therapy is discontinued.

Triamterene
Dyrenium

MECHANISM

Inhibits active reabsorption of sodium and secretion of potassium by distal tubular cells; does not appear to interfere with aldosterone but acts directly on the renal tubule

USES

Treatment of edema associated with congestive heart failure, cirrhosis of the liver, or the nephrotic syndrome, and in steroid-induced or idiopathic edema

Adjunctive therapy of hypertension, in combination with other diuretics, for its added diuretic effect as well as its potassium-conserving effect

DOSAGE

When used alone, 100 mg twice a day (maximum 300 mg/day); dosage should be reduced when given in combination with other diuretics

FATE

Well absorbed from the GI tract; onset of action is 2 to 4 hours; maximal diuretic effect occurs within 6 to 8 hours; duration of action is approximately 16 hours after a single dose; 50% to 70% bound to plasma proteins; metabolized primarily in the liver and excreted by the kidneys

COMMON SIDE EFFECTS

GI upset, nausea, leg cramps

SIGNIFICANT ADVERSE REACTIONS

Headache, weakness, metallic taste, dryness of the mouth, skin rash, photosensitivity, elevated BUN, hyperuricemia, hyperkalemia, hypotension, and blood dyscrasias (rare)

CONTRAINDICATIONS

Anuria, severe hepatic disease, hyperkalemia, and severe or progressive kidney dysfunction (except nephrosis). *Cautious use* in persons with gout or gouty arthritis, reduced renal function, or hepatic cirrhosis and in pregnant or nursing women

INTERACTIONS

See spironolactone. In addition:

Serum levels of digitalis glycosides may be increased by triamterene

Acute renal failure has been reported when indomethacin was given with triamterene

NURSING CONSIDERATIONS

See **Plan of Nursing Care** 9 in this chapter. In addition:

Nursing Alert
- Monitor results of BUN and serum creatinine determinations, which should be performed periodically during extended therapy, especially in patients with kidney dysfunction as well as in elderly or diabetic patients. Note possible early signs of renal insufficiency (e.g., fatigue, vomiting, stomatitis, confusion, bad taste in mouth).

1. Monitor diabetic patient for hyperglycemia because drug can elevate blood glucose.
2. Expect drug to be withdrawn *gradually* over several days to prevent excessive rebound potassium excretion.
3. Note that triamterene is available in combination with hydrochlorothiazide in several dose ratios as Dyazide and Maxzide.

PATIENT EDUCATION

See **Plan of Nursing Care** 9 in this chapter. In addition:
1. Suggest drug be taken with meals to minimize nausea.
2. Instruct patient to report immediately the development of fever, sore throat, mucosal ulceration, extreme fatigue, or weakness, possible symptoms of a blood dyscrasia. If symptoms occur, blood counts should be performed.

THIAZIDES/SULFONAMIDES

Bendroflumethiazide	Indapamide*
Benzthiazide	Methyclothiazide
Chlorothiazide	Metolazone*
Chlorthalidone*	Polythiazide
Cyclothiazide	Quinethazone*
Hydrochlorothiazide	Trichlormethiazide
Hydroflumethiazide	

*sulfonamide derivative

The largest group of orally effective diuretic drugs, thiazides/sulfonamides are structurally related to the sulfonamide antibacterial drugs; however, they possess no anti-infective properties. Most of these sulfonamide diuretics are derived from a benzothiadiazine nucleus and hence are commonly referred to as *thiazide diuretics*. A few other sulfonamide diuretics differ slightly in their chemical structure from the thiazides, although their pharmacologic and toxicologic properties are essentially similar, and these compounds are referred to as *sulfonamide-* or *thiazide-like* diuretics. Structural differences notwithstanding, all of these drugs possess parallel dose-response curves; that is, there is essentially no difference among them in their clinical efficacy, and all drugs in this category possess similar sites and mechanisms of diuretic action.

The thiazide/sulfonamide diuretics are the most widely used drugs for the treatment of edematous states and for the control of mild to moderate hypertension. Because of the similarity of action among the drugs in this class, they are reviewed as a group. Individual drugs are then listed in Table 37-4.

MECHANISM
Diuretic
Impair active sodium and chloride reabsorption in the early portion of the distal segment of the renal tubule and also in the cortical thick ascending loop of Henle, resulting in excretion of these ions with an osmotically equivalent volume of water; possess weak carbonic anhydrase inhibitory activity, although the importance of this action to their diuretic effect is probably minimal; bicarbonate excretion is slightly increased, whereas calcium excretion is reduced; potassium is lost in conjunction with sodium reabsorption in the distal tubule

Antihypertensive
May be due to (1) reduction of plasma volume and sodium levels, (2) direct relaxation of arteriolar smooth muscle, and (3) decreased reactivity of vascular smooth muscle to endogenous pressor substances, possibly the result of alterations in sodium content within the muscle fibers

Other
Interfere with insulin release, possibly a result of hypokalemia, and compete with uric acid for renal tubular secretory sites, thus elevating serum uric acid levels; exert a paradoxical *antidiuretic* effect in diabetes insipidus, possibly by enhancing the action of antidiuretic hormone (ADH) as a consequence of sodium depletion

USES
Treatment of edema associated with congestive heart failure, hepatic cirrhosis, renal dysfunction, and steroid or estrogen therapy

Management of all forms of hypertension, either alone (mild cases) or in combination with other antihypertensive drugs (moderate to severe cases)

Symptomatic treatment of diabetes insipidus to reduce polyuria

Prevention of formation and recurrence of calcium stones in hypercalciuria, either alone or with amiloride or allopurinol (investigational use)

DOSAGE
See Table 37-4

FATE
Well absorbed orally; onset of diuresis is usually 1 to 2 hours after oral administration (except cyclothiazide 4–6 h); peak diuretic effect generally occurs in 4 to 6 hours, and duration ranges from 6 to 72 hours (average duration is 12–18 h); several days are necessary for development of the antihypertensive action, and peak antihypertensive effects generally occur after 2 to 4 weeks; many drugs are highly bound to plasma proteins; excreted in the urine, both as unchanged drug and metabolites

COMMON SIDE EFFECTS
Lightheadedness, hypokalemia (muscle weakness, dizziness, paresthesias, cramping), especially if potassium supplements are not employed

SIGNIFICANT ADVERSE REACTIONS
GI: nausea, GI irritation, vomiting, anorexia, dry mouth, diarrhea, cramping, bloating, jaundice, pancreatitis, sialadenitis, hepatitis

Cardiovascular: orthostatic hypotension, palpitation, irregular heartbeat, premature ventricular contractions, angina-like pain, hemoconcentration

CNS: headache, vertigo, blurred vision, syncope, fatigue, drowsiness, restlessness, depression

Hypersensitivity: rash, photosensitivity, fever, purpura, urticaria, vasculitis, Stevens–Johnson syndrome, dyspnea, pneumonitis, anaphylactic reactions

Hematologic: blood dyscrasias (rare)

Other: muscle spasm, chills, impotence, hyperglycemia, hyperuricemia, elevated BUN, hypercalcemia

CONTRAINDICATIONS
Sulfonamide hypersensitivity, anuria, renal decompensation, IV administration in infants and children; metolazone is also contraindicated in patients with hepatic coma or precoma. *Cautious use* in patients with renal or hepatic disease, bronchial asthma, diabetes mellitus, gout, history of allergies or cardiac arrhythmias, lupus erythematosus, advanced arteriosclerosis, or advanced heart disease, and in elderly or debilitated persons, patients receiving digitalis drugs, and pregnant women or nursing mothers

INTERACTIONS
Thiazides potentiate the hypotensive action of other antihypertensive drugs and may increase the incidence of orthostatic hypotension associated with use of alcohol, narcotics, barbiturates and other CNS depressants, phenothiazines, and tricyclic antidepressants

The effects of oral anticoagulants, vasopressors, hypouricemic drugs, and oral hypoglycemics may be antagonized by thiazide diuretics

Hypokalemia may be intensified if thiazides are combined with corticosteroids

Thiazide-induced hypokalemia may increase digitalis toxicity

Indomethacin and the pyrazolones may reduce the diuretic efficacy of the thiazides owing to excessive fluid retention

Hypercalcemia can occur if thiazides are given with calcium carbonate or other calcium-containing products

Thiazides can potentiate amphetamines, quinidine, and lithium by decreasing their excretion

Prolonged relaxation of skeletal muscle (including respiratory) may occur if thiazides are given together with nondepolarizing muscle relaxants (e.g., curare, gallamine, pancuronium, atracurium)

Oral absorption of thiazides may be impaired by cholestyramine and colestipol

Table 37-4
Thiazide/Sulfonamide Diuretics

Drug	Preparations	Usual Dosage Range	Nursing Implications
Bendroflumethiazide Naturetin	Tablets: 5 mg, 10 mg	*Edema:* initially 5 mg–20 mg/day; maintenance 2.5 mg–5 mg/day *Hypertension:* initially, 5 mg–20 mg/day; maintenance 2.5 mg–15 mg/day	Short-acting preparation (6–12 h); low doses do not appreciably alter serum electrolyte levels; available in fixed combinations with rauwolfia (Rauzide) and nadolol (Corzide)
Benzthiazide Aquatag, Exna, Hydrex, Marazide, Proaqua	Tablets: 50 mg	*Edema:* initially 50 mg–200 mg/day; maintenance 50 mg–150 mg/day *Hypertension:* initially 50 mg–100 mg/day; maintenance 50 mg 2–4 times/day	Maximal effect in 4–6 h, with a duration of 12–18 h
Chlorothiazide Diachlor, Diurigen, Diuril	Tablets: 250 mg, 500 mg Suspension: 250 mg/5 mL Injection: 500 mg/20 mL	*Edema* Adults: 0.5 g–1 g 1 to 2 times a day, 3 to 5 days/wk Children: 22 mg/kg/day in 2 doses *Hypertension:* 0.5–1 g/day, adjusted to optimal response	Following oral administration, onset within 2 h and duration of 6–12 h; IV solution prepared by adding 18 mL sterile water to vial; do *not* administer with plasma or whole blood nor give SC or IM; use IV *only* in emergency situations and avoid extravasation—IV injections are not recommended in children; solutions may be stored up to 24 h at room temperature; available with reserpine (Diupres) and methyldopa (Aldoclor) in oral form
Chlorthalidone Hygroton, Hylidone, Thalitone, (CAN) Apo-Chlorthalidone, Novothalidone, Uridon	Tablets: 25 mg, 50 mg, 100 mg	*Edema:* 50 mg–100 mg/day *or* 100 mg/day 3 times/wk on alternate days *Hypertension:* initially 25 mg–50 mg; adjust to optimal response; maximum 100 mg/day; children—3 mg/kg/day, 3 times/wk	Sulfonamide diuretic; onset 2–3 h and duration 24–48 h; given by single daily dosage in the morning; effective hypotensive agent, often used as initial therapy in mild hypertension; doses above 25 mg/day offer little additional antihypertensive action but increase potassium loss; may elevate plasma levels of cholesterol, triglycerides, and LDL; available with clonidine (Combipres), reserpine (Regroton, Demi-Regroton) and atenolol (Tenoretic)
Cyclothiazide Anhydron	Tablets: 2 mg	*Edema:* 1 mg–2 mg/day; reduce to 1 mg–2 mg 2–3 times/wk as necessary *Hypertension:* 2 mg once a day (maximum 6 mg once a day)	Slow onset (4–6 h) and prolonged duration of action (18–24 h); given in early morning to minimize sleep disturbance
Hydrochlorothiazide Esidrix, Hydrodiuril, and several other manufacturers (CAN) Apo-Hydro, Novohydrazide, and other manufacturers	Tablets: 25 mg, 50 mg, 100 mg Solution: 50 mg/5 mL Intensol solution: 100 mg/mL	*Edema:* initially 25 mg–200 mg/day; maintenance 25 mg–100 mg/day, usually on an intermittent schedule *Hypertension:* initially 50 mg–100 mg/day; adjust to desired response; usual range 25 mg–100 mg/day; children—2.2 mg/kg/day	Most widely used thiazide diuretic; onset 1–2 h and duration 6–12 h; available in fixed combination with many other antihypertensive drugs; oral absorption may be improved if taken with food
Hydroflumethiazide Diucardin, Saluron	Tablets: 50 mg	*Edema:* initially 50 mg–100 mg/day; usual maintenance dose 25 mg–200 mg/day on an intermittent schedule	Rapid onset (1–2 h) and short duration (6–12 h); do not exceed 200 mg/day; available with reserpine (Salutensin)

Continued

Table 37-4
Thiazide/Sulfonamide Diuretics (continued)

Drug	Preparations	Usual Dosage Range	Nursing Implications
Indapamide Lozol (CAN) Lozide	Tablets: 2.5 mg	*Hypertension:* 50 mg twice a day; adjusted to desired response Initially, 2.5 mg/day as a single daily dose; may increase to 5 mg/day after 1–4 wk if necessary	Indoline derivative used for hypertension and edema of congestive heart failure; increases serum uric acid an average of 1 mg/dL; doses greater than 5 mg/day do not provide additional therapeutic benefit but are associated with a greater degree of hypokalemia than smaller doses
Methyclothiazide Aquatensen, Enduron, Ethon (CAN) Duretic	Tablets: 2.5 mg, 5 mg	*Edema:* 2.5 mg–10 mg daily *Hypertension:* 2.5 mg–5 mg daily	Onset in 2 h and duration lasts about 24 h; do not exceed 10 mg/day; available with reserpine (Diutensen-R), deserpidine (Enduronyl), pargyline (Eutron), and cryptenamine (Diutensen)
Metolazone Diulo, Microx, Zaroxolyn	Tablets: 2.5 mg, 5 mg, 10 mg	*Edema:* 5 mg to 20 mg once daily *Hypertension:* 2.5 mg–5 mg once daily	Sulfonamide derivative with rapid onset (1 h) and moderate duration (12–24 h) of action; dosage should be in upper end of range in patients with congestive heart failure to ensure diuretic effect for full 24 h; *not* recommended in children; profound volume and electrolyte depletion can occur in combination with furosemide
Polythiazide Renese	Tablets: 1 mg, 2 mg, 4 mg	*Edema:* 1 mg–4 mg/day *Hypertension:* 2 mg–4 mg/day	Onset 1–2 h and duration 24–36 h; available with reserpine (Renese-R) and prazosin (Minizide)
Quinethazone Hydromox (CAN) Aquamox	Tablets: 50 mg	50 mg–100 mg in a single daily morning dose; maximum 200 mg/day	Sulfonamide diuretic with an onset of 2 h and a duration of 18–24 h; available with reserpine (Hydromox-R)
Trichlormethiazide Diurese, Metahydrin, Naqua, Niazide, Trichlorex	Tablets: 2 mg, 4 mg	*Edema:* 1 mg–4 mg/day *Hypertension:* 2 mg–4 mg/day; children—0.07 mg/kg/day	Onset 2 h and duration 24 h or longer; available with reserpine (Metatensin, Naquival)

Concurrent use of thiazides and diazoxide can increase the likelihood of hyperglycemia, hyperuricemia, and hypotension

NURSING CONSIDERATIONS
See **Plan of Nursing Care** 9 in this chapter. In addition:

Nursing Alerts
- Monitor results of baseline and periodic determinations of BUN, CO_2, uric acid, blood glucose, and blood counts.
- If patient is taking a digitalis, hypouricemic, or oral hypoglycemic preparation, carefully monitor for loss of drug effectiveness or development of toxic reactions. Dosage adjustments may be necessary.

1. When a thiazide is added to an existing antihypertensive regime, expect dose of each drug to be reduced by one-half to avoid excessive hypotension. Dosage may then be slowly titrated to obtain maximal benefit.
2. Ensure that drug is discontinued for several days before parathyroid function tests because it may decrease calcium excretion.

PATIENT EDUCATION
See **Plan of Nursing Care** 9 in this chapter. In addition:
1. Suggest drug be taken with food to minimize gastric irritation.
2. Inform patient that physician or dentist in charge should be notified of thiazide use prior to surgery. Drug should be discontinued 48 hours before surgery be-

cause it may enhance action of muscle relaxants and reduce effectiveness of pressor amines.
3. Encourage patient to avoid high-sodium foods and to refrain from adding table salt to other foods.

Selected Bibliography

Brater DC: Pharmacodynamic considerations with use of diuretics. Annu Rev Pharmacol Toxicol 23:45, 1983

Cragoe EJ (ed): Diuretics: Chemistry, Pharmacology and Medicine. New York, John Wiley & Sons, 1983

Flamenbaum W, Friedman R: Pharmacology, therapeutic efficacy and adverse effects of bumetanide, a new "loop" diuretic. Pharmacotherapeutics 2:213, 1982

Francisco LL, Ferris TF: The use and abuse of diuretics. Arch Intern Med 142:28, 1982

Greenberg A: What's new in diuretic therapy? Pract Ther 33(5):200, 1986

Jacobson HR: Diuretics: Mechanisms of action and uses. Hosp Pract, Dec 1987, 120

Lamy P: Side effects of diuretics a danger for the aged. J Geront Nurs 11(6):44, June 1985

Lant A: Diuretic drugs: Progress in clinical pharmacology. Drugs 31(Suppl 4):40, 1986

Madias NE, Zelman SJ: What are the metabolic complications of diuretic treatment? Geriatrics 37(2):93, 1983

Perez-Stable E, Carolis PV: Thiazide-induced disturbances in carbohydrate, lipid and potassium metabolism. Am Heart J 106:245, 1983

Shoback DM, Williams GH: Potassium-sparing diuretics: Clinical pharmacology and therapeutic uses. Drug Ther 12(2):113, 1982

Symposium—Indapamide: A new indoline diuretic agent. Am Heart J 106:183, 1983

Warren SE, Blantz RC: Mannitol. Arch Intern Med 141:493, 1981

SUMMARY. DIURETICS

Drug	Preparations	Usual Dosage Range
Carbonic Anhydrase (CA) Inhibitors	See Table 37-2	
Loop (High-Ceiling) Diuretics	See Table 37-3	
Osmotic Diuretics		
Glycerin Glyrol, Osmoglyn	Oral solution: 50%, 75%	1 g/kg–1.5 g/kg, 1–1.5 hour before ocular surgery
Isosorbide Ismotic	Oral solution: 45%	1 g/kg–3 g/kg 2–4 times a day
Mannitol Osmitrol	Injection: 5%, 10%, 15%, 20%, 25%	50 g to 200 g/24 h by IV infusion Rate adjusted to maintain a urine flow of 30 mL–50 mL/h
Urea Ureaphil	Injection: 40 g/vial	Adults: 1 g/kg–1.5 g/kg (Maximum dose 120 g/day) Children: 0.5 g/kg–1.5 g/kg Infants: 0.1 g/kg–0.5 g/kg
Potassium-Sparing Diuretics		
Amiloride Midamor	Tablets: 5 mg	5 mg–10 mg/day added to the diuretic regimen; maximum dose is 20 mg/day
Spironolactone Alatone, Aldactone	Tablets: 25 mg, 50 mg, 100 mg	Edema: 25 mg–200 mg/day in divided doses Children: 3.3 mg/kg/day in divided doses Hypertension: 50 mg–100 mg/day in divided doses Hyperaldosteronism: 100 mg–400 mg/day prior to surgery
Triamterene Dyrenium	Capsules: 50 mg, 100 mg	100 mg twice a day (maximum 300 mg/day)
Thiazides/Sulfonamides	See Table 37-4	

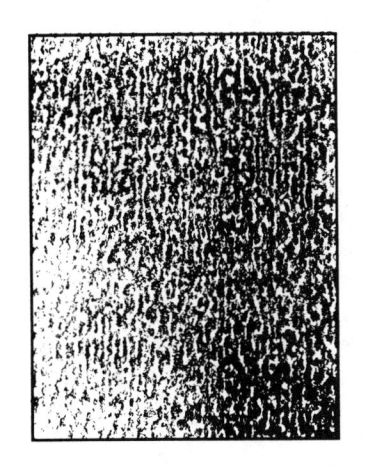

V Drugs Acting on the Endocrine Glands

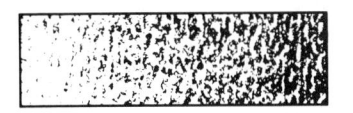

38 THE ENDOCRINE GLANDS: A REVIEW

The endocrine system functions in close harmony with the nervous system in regulating, coordinating, and integrating the wide range of metabolic and physiologic activities essential to the maintenance of homeostasis in an ever-changing environment.

The anatomically distinct and functionally diverse organs of the endocrine system participate in the regulation of the following basic activities: (1) energy metabolism, (2) electrolyte and water metabolism, (3) reproduction, (4) growth and development, and (5) response to stress.

The products of endocrine glands, the *hormones*, are characteristically produced in small amounts by specialized glandular cells and are secreted directly into the bloodstream, whereby they are transported to specific target tissues upon which they exert regulatory control.

Chemically, hormones may be

- Polypeptides or proteins (e.g., insulin and growth hormone)
- Steroids (e.g., aldosterone and cortisol)
- Amines (e.g., epinephrine and thyroxine)

TRANSPORT AND METABOLISM OF HORMONES

Most hormones are transported through the blood bound to plasma proteins. Because only free (unbound) hormone is physiologically active and subject to biodegradation (metabolic transformation), protein binding affords a mechanism by which reserve hormones are readily available. Hormones may be inactivated by the liver or kidneys, or, more rarely, by the target tissues. Because of the great importance of the liver and kidneys in the metabolism and excretion of hormones, the state of hepatic and renal function should be established during the course of diagnosing specific endocrine dysfunction.

MECHANISMS OF HORMONE ACTION

The mechanisms whereby hormones exert their specific effects on target tissues vary. Steroid hormones such as aldosterone bind to intracellular receptors and affect DNA transcription, ultimately modifying protein synthesis. Several hormones, including epinephrine and glucagon, act through a second messenger to activate specific enzymes, whereas others, such as insulin and antidiuretic hormone (ADH), alter the permeability of selected cell membranes to certain substrates.

Second Messenger Mechanism

Several hormones have been shown to exert their effects by way of a "second messenger." The hormone, acting as the first messenger, binds to specific receptors at the outer surface of a target cell membrane. The hormone–receptor interaction leads to the activation of the enzyme *adenyl cyclase,* which then converts cytoplasmic adenosine triphosphate (ATP) into cyclic adenosine monophosphate (cyclic AMP).

Before being inactivated by phosphodiesterase enzymes, the cyclic AMP acts as the second messenger to bring about a specific cellular action (e.g., enzyme activation or change in membrane permeability to a given substrate).

REGULATION OF HORMONE SECRETION

Secretion of certain hormones is under the direct control of the nervous system. Other hormones are controlled by the blood level of an electrolyte (e.g., calcium) or a metabolite (e.g., glucose). Most, however, are controlled by a negative feedback mechanism (Fig. 38-1) whereby an elevation in the plasma concentration of a given hormone inhibits its production by the endocrine gland.

PITUITARY GLAND

The pituitary gland, sometimes called the "master gland," secretes several polypeptide hormones that directly or indirectly regulate a wide variety of metabolic and physiologic processes essential to normal growth and development as well as to the maintenance of homeostasis. Many of the hormones secreted by the pituitary gland are critical to the activity of target glands, including the thyroid, adrenals, and gonads.

Anatomy

The pituitary gland (*hypophysis cerebri*) is located at the base of the brain, resting within the sella turcica of the sphenoid bone. The pituitary gland maintains elaborate neural and vascular connections with the hypothalamus of the brain, which plays a central role in the integration of neuroendocrine activity (Fig. 38-2).

The pituitary gland has two major divisions: the neurohypophysis and the adenohypophysis.

NEUROHYPOPHYSIS

The *neurohypophysis*, which is connected directly to the hypothalamus by the *infundibular* (pituitary) *stalk*, is rich in nerve fibers of hypothalamic origin (the *hypothalamohypophyseal tract*).

Neurosecretory cells in the *supraoptic* and *paraventricular nuclei* of the hypothalamus produce two hormones: *antidiuretic hormone* (ADH or vasopressin) and *oxytocin*. These hormones are then transported along the axons of the hypothalamohypophyseal tract to the *pars nervosa* (posterior lobe) of the pituitary gland for storage and ultimate release.

ADENOHYPOPHYSIS

The *adenohypophysis* is served by an elaborate vascular system, including the *hypothalamohypophyseal portal system,* which transports hypothalamic regulating hormones (factors) to the glandular cells of the adenohypophysis. The classification of cells in the adenohypophysis is based on specific immunohistochemical techniques. Accordingly, there are five recognized cell types:

1. *Somatotrophs,* which secrete growth hormone or somatotropin.
2. *Lactotrophs,* which secrete prolactin.
3. *Corticotrophs,* which produce corticotropin (ACTH) by splitting a large peptide called proopiomelanocortin.
4. *Thyrotrophs,* which secrete thyrotropin (TSH).
5. *Gonadotrophs,* which produce folliculotropin (FSH) and luteotropin (LH).

HORMONES OF THE NEUROHYPOPHYSIS

Antidiuretic Hormone (ADH; Vasopressin)

CONTROL OF SECRETION

Antidiuretic hormone (ADH) is a polypeptide hormone of hypothalamic origin (supraoptic nuclei) that is stored in and released from the neurohypophysis in response to a variety of stimuli. Included among these are increased plasma osmolality, reduced extracellular fluid (ECF) volume, pain, emotional stress, and pharmacologic agents such as morphine, nicotine, ether, and the barbiturates.

Decreased plasma osmolality, increased ECF volume, and alcohol inhibit ADH secretion.

Osmoreceptors found in the anterior hypothalamus monitor changes in plasma osmolality, whereas ECF volume changes are detected by volume ("stretch") receptors located in the wall of the left atrium. The osmoreceptors and volume receptors work in concert to exert precise control over ADH secretion, thus forming a delicate homeostatic feedback mechanism for the regulation of ECF volume and concentration.

ACTIONS

The principal physiological role of ADH is to regulate extracellular fluid volume and osmolality by controlling the final volume and concentration of urine.

ADH, acting through the second messenger cyclic AMP, increases the permeability of the distal nephron (distal convoluted tubules and collecting tubules) to water. The enhanced reabsorption of water from the renal tubules results in the production of a concentrated urine that is reduced in volume.

Pharmacologic amounts of ADH produce a *pressor* (hypertensive) effect that results from a direct constrictor action of the hormone on vascular smooth muscle.

The early observations that posterior pituitary extracts produce a marked elevation of arterial blood pressure led to the initial naming of this hormone as *vasopressin.*

Clinical States

DIABETES INSIPIDUS

Inadequate ADH secretion leads to the excretion of large volumes of dilute urine (polyuria). Intense thirst and consumption of large amounts of liquid (polydipsia) are also characteristic of diabetes insipidus.

This disorder may be idiopathic, or it may follow trauma or cranial injury, central nervous system disease, infection, or emotional shock. The deficit may be related to the supraoptic nuclei, the hypothalamohypophyseal tract, or the neurohypophysis.

A rare ADH-resistant or *nephrogenic* diabetes also exists. In this inherited disorder, ADH secretion is normal, but the renal tubules are unresponsive to the hormone. Treatment of diabetes insipidus is discussed in Chapter 39.

INAPPROPRIATE ADH SYNDROME

The inappropriate ADH syndrome, a clinical state characterized by hypersecretion of ADH, may result from generalized infec-

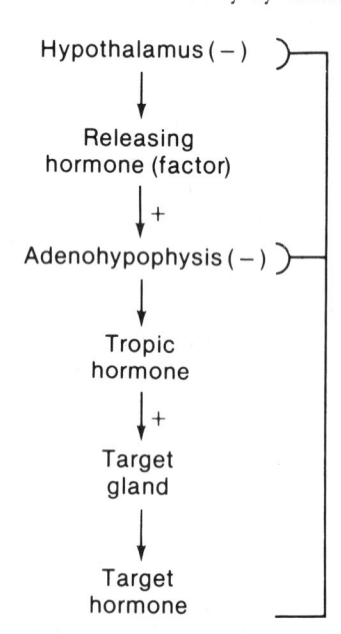

Figure 38–1 Negative feedback mechanism regulating endocrine hormone secretion.

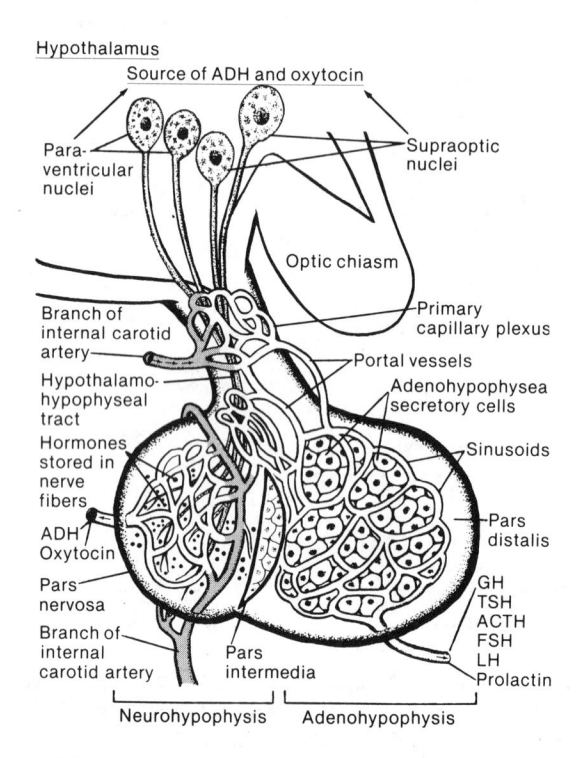

Figure 38–2 The pituitary gland (hypophysis) and its relationship with the hypothalamus.

tion, mediastinal tumors, metastatic tumors to the brain, pathologic CNS changes, or intracranial surgery.

Abnormal fluid retention leads to dilution of plasma sodium (dilutional hyponatremia), and urine becomes inappropriately concentrated. Fluid intake must be stringently restricted to minimize water intoxication.

Oxytocin

CONTROL OF SECRETION AND ACTIONS

The two major physiologic actions of oxytocin are exerted upon female reproductive structures.

Galactokinetic Action

The ejection of milk from a primed, lactating mammary gland follows a neuroendocrine reflex in which oxytocin serves as the efferent limb. The reflex is normally initiated by suckling, which stimulates cutaneous receptors in the areola of the breast. Afferent nerve impulses travel to the paraventricular nuclei of the hypothalamus to effect the release of oxytocin from the neurohypophysis. Oxytocin is carried by the blood to the mammary gland, where it causes contraction of *myoepithelial cells* surrounding the alveoli and lactiferous ducts to bring about the ejection of milk (milk letdown).

In lactating women, tactile stimulation of the breast areola, emotional stimuli, and genital stimulation may also lead to oxytocin release.

Oxytocic Action

Oxytocin acts directly upon uterine smooth muscle to elicit strong, rhythmic contractions of the myometrium. Uterine sensitivity to oxytocin varies with its physiological state and with hormonal balance. The gravid (pregnant) uterus is highly sensitive to oxytocin, particularly in the late stages of gestation. Uterine sensitivity to oxytocin is greatly enhanced by estrogen and inhibited by progesterone.

Oxytocin release appears to follow a neuroendocrine reflex initiated by genital stimulation.

There is some evidence that oxytocin may affect sperm transport through the female genital tract.

HORMONES OF THE ADENOHYPOPHYSIS

The secretion of hormones by the adenohypophysis (pars distalis and pars intermedia) is controlled by hypothalamic regulatory hormones (factors) that are transported to the pituitary gland by the hypothalamohypophyseal portal system illustrated in Figure 38-2.

There appear to be 10 such regulatory (hypophysiotropic) hormones produced by the hypothalamus:

- Growth hormone release–inhibiting hormone (somatostatin; GRIH; SRIH)
- Growth hormone–releasing factor (somatocrinin; GRF; SRF)
- Prolactin release–inhibiting hormone (dopamine; PIH)
- Prolactin-releasing factor (prolactoliberin; PRF)
- Adrenocorticotrophic hormone–releasing hormone (corticoliberin; CRH)
- Thyroid stimulating hormone–releasing hormone (thyroliberin, TRH)
- Luteinizing hormone–releasing hormone (gonadoliberin; GnRH; LHRH)
- Follicle-stimulating hormone–releasing hormone (gonadoliberin; GnRH; FSHRH)
- Melanocyte-stimulating hormone release–inhibiting factor (melanostatin; MRIF)
- Melanocyte-stimulating hormone–releasing factor (melanoliberin; MRF)

Growth Hormone (GH); Somatotropin (STH)

CONTROL OF SECRETION

Factors Promoting GH Secretion

GRF (Somatocrinin)
Hypoglycemia and fasting
Elevated plasma levels of amino acids (e.g., arginine)
Stress
Exercise
Levodopa
Glucagon

Factors Inhibiting GH Secretion

GRIH (Somatostatin)
Hyperglycemia
Elevated plasma levels of free fatty acids
Cortisol
Alpha-adrenergic blocking agents
GH (negative feedback mechanism): GH secretion in response to hypoglycemia, fasting, and exercise appears to be reduced by obesity.

ACTIONS

Effects on Growth

GH accelerates overall body growth by increasing the mass of both skeletal and soft body tissues through hyperplasia (increased cell number) and hypertrophy (increased cell size).

The effects of GH are particularly evident in hard tissues where chondrogenesis (cartilage formation) and osteogenesis (bone formation) are enhanced, leading to an increase in linear growth and stature before epiphyseal closure and in bone thickness following closure of the epiphyses.

GH stimulates certain tissues, notably hepatic, to produce *somatomedins* (formerly termed *sulfation factor*). Somatomedins are low molecular weight peptides that mediate certain effects of GH, including the stimulation of collagen synthesis, chondrogenesis, and incorporation of sulfate into cartilage.

Metabolic Effects

- *Protein metabolism:* GH increases protein synthesis and nitrogen retention by enhancing the incorporation of amino acids into protein. The protein anabolic action results from (1) accelerated entry of amino acids into cells and (2) increased ribonucleic acid (RNA) synthesis.
- *Lipid metabolism:* GH stimulates the mobilization and utilization of fats, enabling the body to use stored fats as an energy source. The elevation of plasma levels of free fatty acids resulting from the hydrolysis of triglycerides (stored neutral fats) is potentially ketogenic.

- *Carbohydrate metabolism:* GH causes hyperglycemia by increasing the hepatic output of glucose and impairing glucose transport into muscle ("anti-insulin" action on muscle). Excessive secretion of GH may precipitate or increase the severity of clinical diabetes mellitus ("diabetogenic" effect).
- *Electrolyte metabolism:* GH enhanced gastrointestinal absorption of calcium and phosphorus and reduces renal excretion of sodium and potassium.

Prolactin (PRL)

CONTROL OF SECRETION

Prolactin secretion is controlled by the hypothalamus, with prolactin release–inhibiting hormone (dopamine; PIH) normally dominating. Tactile stimulation of the breast may initiate neuronal activity leading to the release of prolactin-releasing factor (prolactoliberin; PRF) from the hypothalamus, thus promoting prolactin secretion from the lactotrophs of the adenohypophysis. Prolactin secretion is normally suppressed, however, by liberation of PIF from the hypothalamus.

ACTIONS

Prolactin initiates and maintains milk secretion from breasts primed for lactation by other hormones such as estrogens, progesterone, and insulin.

Prolactin also appears to act synergistically with estrogen to stimulate growth of the mammary glands.

Prolactin and growth hormone are very closely related structurally and may therefore exert some overlapping functions.

Follicle Stimulating Hormone (Folliculotropin; FSH)

CONTROL OF SECRETION

FSH secretion is controlled by the hypothalamus by way of the releasing hormone GnRH or FSHRH. Circulating levels of androgens (testosterone), inhibin, and estrogens participate in this control by inhibiting GnRH or FSHRH secretion by the hypothalamus. Surgical stress usually inhibits FSH secretion. The pineal gland has also been implicated in the control of gonadotropin secretion.

ACTIONS

FSH directly stimulates the germinal epithelium of testicular seminiferous tubules, thereby promoting spermatogenesis in the male. In the female, FSH stimulates follicular growth and development within the ovaries.

Luteinizing Hormone (Luteotropin—LH; Interstitial Cell Stimulating Hormone—ICSH)

CONTROL OF SECRETION

LH secretion is controlled by the hypothalamus through GnRH or LHRH.

The release of LH is inhibited by testosterone and by estrogens, except for a brief priming effect exerted by estrogen to allow a surge of LH needed to effect ovulation.

ACTIONS

In the male, this hormone stimulates testosterone production by testicular interstitial cells (of Leydig); hence the name, interstitial cell stimulating hormone (ICSH).

In the female, LH stimulates ripening of the ovarian follicles, controls ovulation, and promotes the formation and maintenance of the corpus luteum.

In many animals, LH elicits the behavioral manifestations of estrus (heat).

Thyroid Stimulating Hormone (Thyrotropin; TSH)

CONTROL OF SECRETION

Thyroid stimulating hormone–releasing hormone (TRH) and cold promote secretion of TSH by the thyrotrophs of the adenohypophysis. Elevated plasma levels of free thyroid hormones inhibit thyrotropin secretion as outlined in Figure 38-3.

ACTIONS

TSH stimulates growth (hypertrophy) of the thyroid gland and promotes the synthesis and release of thyroid hormones thyroxine and triiodothyronine. The actions of TSH on the thyroid gland are mediated by cyclic AMP, and they are detailed in the section on the thyroid gland.

TSH may also act directly on the ocular orbital tissue to cause exophthalmos (protrusion of the eyeballs).

Adrenocorticotropic Hormone (Corticotropin; ACTH)

CONTROL OF SECRETION

ACTH secretion is regulated by neural factors and a hormonal negative feedback mechanism. ACTH is secreted in response to adrenocorticotropic hormone releasing–hormone (CRH) and to several forms of stress, including fear, pain, cold, trauma, and hypoglycemia.

Elevated plasma glucocorticoid (cortisol) levels inhibit CRH and ACTH secretion.

ACTIONS

ACTH exerts its tropic effects upon the adrenal glands, promoting growth and steroidogenesis in the adrenal cortex. The stimulation of corticosteroid production (steroidogenesis) in response to ACTH is mediated by the second messenger, cyclic AMP.

Melanocyte-Stimulating Hormone (MSH)

CONTROL OF SECRETION

MSH secretion by the pars intermedia is controlled by hypothalamic inhibiting (i.e., MRIF) and releasing (i.e., MRF) hormones.

ACTIONS

MSH acts upon the skin of fish, reptiles, and amphibians to disperse melanophore granules leading to changes in skin coloration.

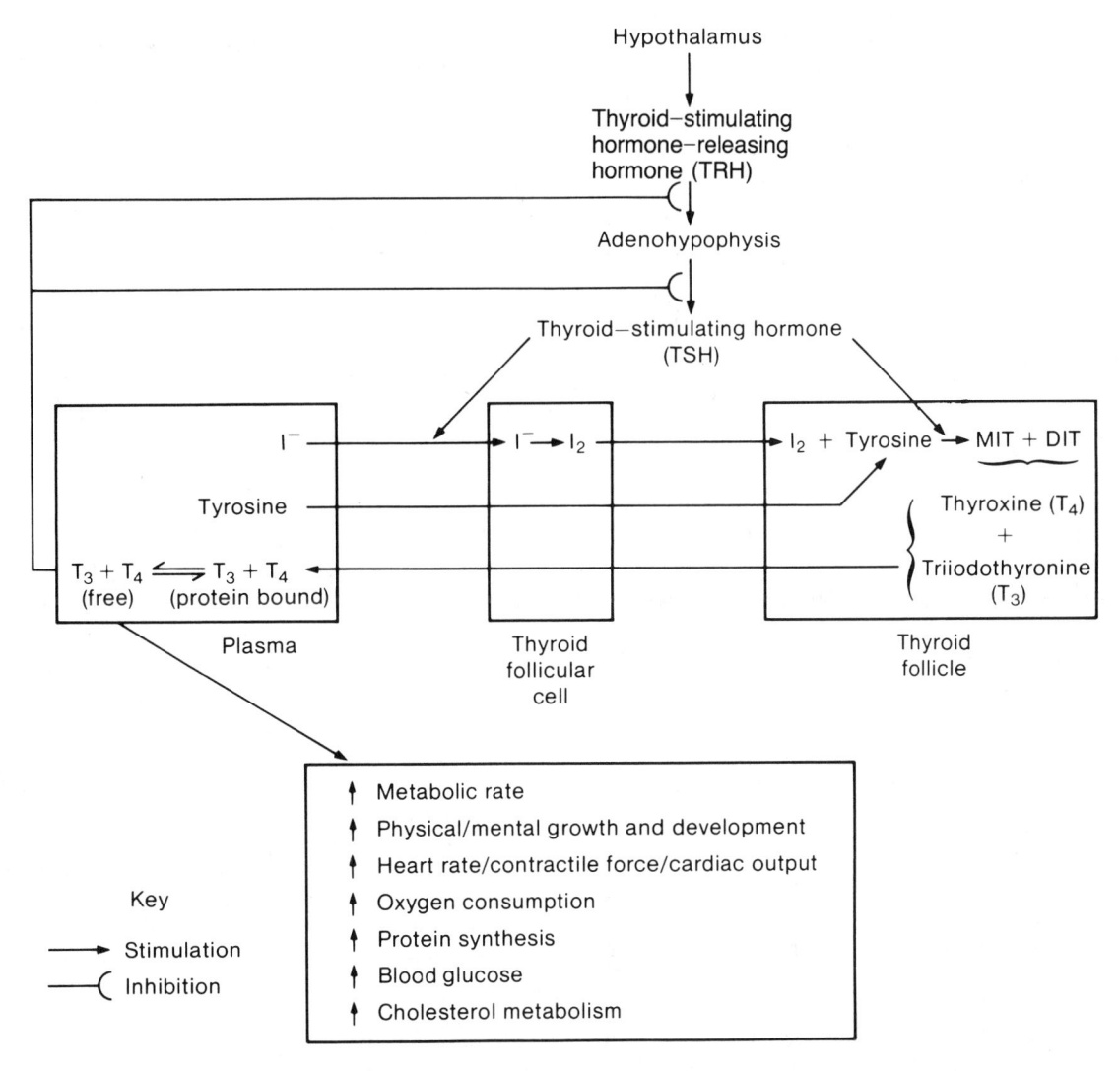

Figure 38-3 Synthesis, storage, release, and actions of thyroid hormones.

Mammals, including humans, do not possess melanophores, but rather melanin-containing cells called *melanocytes*. Thus there appears to be no major physiological role for MSH in humans. Some neurotropic effects of MSH have been observed; however, the physiological significance of these remains unclear.

Abnormally large amounts of MSH (such as with functional pituitary tumors) may produce hyperpigmentation of skin in humans.

ACTH and MSH are structurally similar, and both are derived from the same precursor peptide proopiomelanocortin so that hyperpigmentation associated with certain pathologic states may result from ACTH or MSH hypersecretion, or both.

Disorders of the Adenohypophysis

HYPOFUNCTIONAL STATES

Hypopituitarism (Pituitary Insufficiency)

In the adult, hypopituitarism may be manifested in a variety of forms, such as panhypopituitarism, Simmond's disease (pituitary cachexia), or Sheehan syndrome.

Pituitary insufficiency may be related to hypothalamic lesions, cysts or tumors affecting the pituitary, surgical hypophysectomy, infiltrative granulomatous disease, vascular collapse, or thrombosis.

The deficiency in the production of tropic hormones leads to functional deficiency and atrophy of target glands such as the adrenal cortex, thyroid, and gonads. Symptoms of pituitary insufficiency may include weakness; decreased resistance to stress, cold, and infection; sexual dysfunction (e.g., infertility, amenorrhea, decreased secondary sex characteristics); sallow, dry, wrinkled skin; and hypotension.

Pituitary Dwarfism

The hallmark of hypopituitarism in children is growth retardation or dwarfism. Despite the small stature, the pituitary dwarf has normal body proportions. Hypoglycemia, hypogonadism, and hypothyroidism may also occur.

HYPERFUNCTIONAL STATES

Gigantism and Acromegaly

Excessive secretion of growth hormone (GH) is usually caused by acidophilic adenomas. Hypersecretion of GH occurring before closure of the epiphyses leads to proportional but immense growth. An individual may grow to 7 or 8 feet in height; hence the term *gigantism*.

Excessive secretion of GH following epiphyseal closure results in *acromegaly*. Because the bones can no longer increase in length, overall height (stature) is not affected. However, the bones thicken considerably, an effect particularly noticeable in the face, hands, and feet. Overgrowth of the mandible results in prognathism (jaw protrusion) and separation of the lower teeth. The skeletal changes predispose to joint disorders such as osteoarthritis.

Increased sweating, thickening of the skin, and increased body hair (in women) are common. Hyperglycemia and glucose intolerance may be noted. Headaches and visual disturbances may result from pressure by the tumor.

THYROID GLAND

The hormones of the thyroid gland exert a wide spectrum of metabolic and physiologic actions that affect virtually every tissue in the body.

Anatomy

The thyroid gland is a bi-lobed organ overlying the trachea anteriorly. The thyroid gland is composed of numerous closely packed spheres or follicles.

Each follicle consists of a simple cuboidal epithelium (*follicular cells*) enclosing a lumen or cavity containing a viscous hyaline substance termed *colloid*. The chief constituent of the colloid is the iodinated glycoprotein *thyroglobulin*.

Interspersed among the follicles are small clusters of *parafollicular* (C) cells, which secrete *calcitonin* (thyrocalcitonin), a hormone affecting calcium metabolism.

Thyroid Hormones

The follicular cells of the thyroid gland secrete two hormones, thyroxine (3,3′, 5,5′-tetraiodothyronine or T_4) and 3,3′, 5-triiodothyronine (T_3). The plasma levels of these hormones are regulated by the hypothalamopituitary axis as outlined in Figure 38-3. Intrinsic (intrathyroidal) mechanisms, as well as bioavailability of iodine, influence thyroid hormone production.

BIOSYNTHESIS OF THYROID HORMONES

1. *Iodide uptake:* Ingested iodine is readily absorbed from the GI tract in the reduced iodide state. Iodide ions are actively transported from the blood into the thyroid follicles by an energy-requiring "trapping" mechanism often called the *iodide pump*. The normal thyroid: serum ratio of iodide is 25:1. The uptake of iodide is enhanced by TSH and may be blocked by anions such as perchlorate and thiocyanate.
2. *Oxidation to iodine:* Upon entering the colloid, iodide is rapidly oxidized to iodine in the presence of peroxidase enzymes. Thiouracil appears to inhibit peroxidase activity.
3. *Iodination of tyrosine:* Free molecular iodine spontaneously combines with tyrosine residues on the thyroglobulin to form 3-monoiodotyrosine (MIT) and 3,5-diiodotyrosine (DIT). This organic iodination is enhanced by TSH and blocked by agents such as propylthiouracil and methimazole. Goitrogens found in cabbage, kale, and turnips, as well as cobalt and phenylbutazone, also block organification of iodine.
4. *Coupling reaction:* Two iodinated tyrosines combine to form either T_3 or T_4. The coupling occurs within the thyroglobulin molecule, and the reaction appears to be promoted by TSH.
5. *Storage and release of thyroid hormones:* T_3 and T_4 remain stored within the colloid bound to thyroglobulin until released by protease enzymes that free the hormones, allowing them to diffuse out of the colloid, through the follicular cells into the plasma.

TSH, acting through cyclic AMP, increases the production of thyroid hormones by promoting several steps in the biosynthetic mechanism, including the release of the hormones from storage in thyroglobulin.

TRANSPORT

Circulating thyroid hormones bind specifically with *thyroxine-binding globulin* and *thyroxine-binding prealbumin*, and nonspecifically with serum albumin. The extent of plasma protein binding can be measured as protein-bound iodine (PBI).

Only a small fraction of circulating thyroid hormones is in the free (unbound), biologically active form.

Several drugs, including phenytoin and the salicylates, compete for plasma protein binding sites, thus lowering the PBI and increasing the percentage of free, active hormones. High levels of estrogen, such as those occurring in pregnancy or during oral contraceptive therapy, elevate plasma protein levels, thereby increasing PBI levels.

FATE

Thyroid hormones are inactivated by deiodination, deamination, decarboxylation, or conjugation with glucuronic acid or sulfate. Much of the iodine released during biodegradation is recycled and reutilized for synthesis of new hormones. The remainder is excreted in the urine. Metabolism occurs chiefly in the liver, and excretion is mainly through the kidneys. The conjugated hormones are excreted through the bile and eliminated in the feces.

ACTIONS

The thyroid hormones increase the rate of metabolism, total heat production, and oxygen consumption in most body tissues. They also promote normal physical and mental development and growth, and they potentiate the cardiovascular and metabolic actions of the catecholamines (epinephrine and norepinephrine).

At the cellular level, the thyroid hormones increase mitochondrial permeability, accelerate protein synthesis, and uncouple oxidative phosphorylation. Although T_4 is quantitatively the major hormone produced by the thyroid follicles, it appears that T_3 is biologically more potent. It is likely that T_4 is converted peripherally into the more active T_3 form.

The pharmacologic uses of the thyroid hormones are discussed in Chapter 40.

Disorders of the Thyroid

SIMPLE GOITER

Goiter, an enlargement of the thyroid gland, most commonly results from an insufficient dietary intake of iodine. The gland becomes hyperplastic and filled with colloid lacking in iodine. TSH levels are usually high because plasma levels of free thyroid hormones are insufficient to suppress TSH production by the adenohypophysis. More rarely, goiter may result from excessive intake of goitrogens (such as cabbage) or may be due to congenital lack of biosynthetic enzymes.

Transient simple goiter may occur during pregnancy or at the onset of puberty, when the demand for thyroid hormones increases.

HYPOTHYROIDISM

Hypothyroidism may result from primary disease of the thyroid gland itself, or it may be secondary to a deficiency of pituitary TSH or hypothalamic TRH.

Because thyroid hormones affect a wide range of physiologic and metabolic processes including growth and development, the time of onset of a deficiency state is most important.

Cretinism (Congenital or Neonatal Hypothyroidism)

Cretinism results from fetal or neonatal thyroid hormone deficiency, which may be due to anatomical dysgenesis of the thyroid, iodine deficiency, or inborn errors of iodine metabolism.

Cretinism is characterized by mental retardation and dwarfism due to delayed skeletal maturation. Other signs of this disorder include the presence of thick, dry skin, large protruding tongue, and umbilical hernia. The child appears apathetic or lethargic and has a low body temperature. TSH and serum cholesterol levels are elevated.

Myxedema (Adult Hypothyroidism)

Primary myxedema may follow thyroidectomy, eradication of the thyroid by radioactive iodine, ingestion of goitrogens, or chronic thyroiditis. Idiopathic atrophy, possibly involving autoimmune mechanisms, may also lead to hypothyroidism.

Early symptoms of myxedema include cold intolerance, weakness, fatigue, dryness of the skin, thinning hair, and thin brittle nails. Among later signs are weight gain, pallor, dyspnea, peripheral edema, anginal pain, bradycardia, and slow speech. Cardiac enlargement may result from pericardial effusion, and macrocytic anemia may occur.

The low turnover of protein leads to the accumulation of a protein-rich fluid under the skin, lending a puffiness and thickness to the skin.

Manifestations of personality changes and organic psychoses ("myxedema madness") may occur.

It is noteworthy that myxedematous patients are unusually sensitive to opiates and may die from average doses of these agents.

HYPERTHYROIDISM (THYROTOXICOSIS)

Hyperthyroid states are characterized by some degree of glandular hyperplasia and excessive thyroid hormone production. Nervousness, excessive sweating, heat intolerance, warm moist skin, weight loss despite increased appetite, restlessness, and tremor are common signs of hyperthyroidism. Tachycardia, high pulse pressure, and systolic hypertension frequently occur.

When associated with toxic diffuse goiter, elevated metabolic rate and exophthalmos, hyperthyroidism is termed *Graves disease*. Long-acting thyroid stimulator (LATS) is an immunoglobulin (antibody) with TSH-like activity that has been isolated from the serum of patients with Graves disease.

The treatment of thyroid disorders is detailed in Chapter 40.

Calcitonin

Calcitonin (thyrocalcitonin) is a polypeptide hormone secreted by the cells of the thyroid gland in response to *hypercalcemia* (elevated blood calcium).

Calcitonin lowers serum calcium principally by inhibiting the rate of calcium release from bone.

In addition to inhibiting bone resorption, calcitonin appears to accelerate bone formation and mineral deposition. Calcitonin may also inhibit the renal calcium reabsorptive action of *parathyroid hormone* (PTH)

In addition to secretion by the parafollicular cells of the thyroid, calcitonin may also be secreted by cells found in the parathyroid and thymus glands. Because calcitonin is not the principal calcium-regulating hormone, no clinical syndromes are associated with abnormal rates of calcitonin secretion.

PARATHYROID GLANDS

The parathyroid glands, usually four in number, are embedded in the dorsal surface of the thyroid gland.

In response to *hypocalcemia* (low serum calcium), the chief cells of the parathyroid glands secrete a single polypeptide hormone known as *parathyroid hormone* (PTH).

PTH regulates serum calcium levels by exerting its effects on the following three target tissues:

- *Bone:* PTH stimulates bone resorption by activating the bone-destroying osteoclasts. The demineralization of bone elevates serum calcium and phosphate levels.
- *Kidneys:* PTH promotes renal tubular reabsorption of calcium and increases renal excretion of phosphate by blocking its reabsorption.
- *GI tract:* PTH enhances calcium and phosphate absorption from the small intestine in the presence of adequate amounts of vitamin D.

The major actions of PTH are mediated by cyclic AMP. Calcium metabolism and the clinical uses of PTH and calcitonin are discussed in Chapter 41.

Disorders of the Parathyroid Glands

HYPOPARATHYROIDISM

Hypoparathyroidism is not common. When it occurs, usually following accidental removal of or damage to the parathyroid glands during thyroidectomy, signs of *hypo*calcemia ensue. Among these are neuromuscular hyperexcitability (related in severity to the degree of hypocalcemia), tetany, and mental disturbances. Respiratory difficulties mimicking asthma may occur.

HYPERPARATHYROIDISM

Primary hyperparathyroidism may result from adenoma, carcinoma, or primary hyperplasia of the parathyroid glands. It may also be associated with ectopic production of PTH by carcinomas elsewhere in the body.

Signs and symptoms characteristic of hyperparathyroidism include *hyper*calcemia, anorexia, vomiting, thirst, polyuria, and renal calculi (kidney stones). Skeletal manifestations may range from simple joint or back pain to pathologic fractures and cystic bone lesions throughout the skeleton (osteitis fibrosa cystica). The skeletal abnormalities result from the excessive demineralization of bone, while the occurrence of kidney stones is related to excessive renal excretion of minerals (calcium and phosphate).

PANCREAS

The endocrine functions of the pancreas are performed by the *islets of Langerhans* (also called pancreatic islets)—small, highly vascularized masses of cells scattered throughout the pancreas and representing only 1% to 3% of the entire organ.

The islets of Langerhans contain four types of secretory cells, as follows:

Alpha (A) cells, which secrete *glucagon*
Beta (B) cells, which secrete *insulin*
Delta (D) cells, which secrete *somatostatin*
PP (F) cells, which secrete *pancreatic polypeptide*

Insulin-secreting beta cells are the most numerous, making up 70% to 80% of the islet cell population. The A cells containing glucagon comprise approximately 20% of islet cell mass, whereas the somatostatin-containing D cells account for 3% to 5% of pancreatic islet cells. The F cells make up less than 2% of islet cells and contain a polypeptide that is believed to assist in digestion in a yet undetermined manner.

The physiologic roles of glucagon and insulin in the regulation of intermediary metabolism are well established. The exact physiologic role of pancreatic somatostatin remains unclear. Because somatostatin inhibits the release of both glucagon and insulin from the pancreatic islets, it may function, at least in part, as a hormone regulating pancreatic secretion.

Glucagon

Glucagon is a 29 amino-acid polypeptide hormone secreted by the alpha cells of the pancreatic islets primarily in response to *hypoglycemia* (low blood sugar). Glucagon is essentially a catabolic hormone that decreases carbohydrate and lipid energy stores and increases the amount of glucose and fatty acids available for oxidation.

Extrapancreatic glucagon ("gut glucagon") is secreted by certain cells of the stomach and duodenum. Both pancreatic glucagon and gut glucagon stimulate secretion of insulin from the beta cells of the pancreatic islets.

CONTROL OF SECRETION
The plasma glucose concentration is the major physiologic regulator of glucagon secretion. In addition to hypoglycemia and fasting, the following factors promote glucagon secretion: ingestion of a high protein meal (amino acids), exercise, stress, gastrin, pancreozymin, and beta-adrenergic stimulation. The rate of glucagon secretion is inhibited by elevated blood levels of glucose and free fatty acids, and by somatostatin, phenytoin, and alpha-adrenergic stimulation.

MAJOR ACTIONS
- *Carbohydrate metabolism:* Glucagon stimulates hepatic glycogenolysis, thereby promoting the release of glucose from liver glycogen stores. This action is mediated by cyclic AMP, which stimulates protein kinase activity leading to the activation of phosphorylase, the glycogenolytic enzyme. In addition to stimulating hepatic glycogenolysis, glucagon inhibits glycogenesis and raises the rate of hepatic gluconeogenesis. The net effect is an elevation of blood glucose (*hyperglycemia*).
- *Lipid metabolism:* Glucagon stimulates lipolysis, thereby increasing the release of free fatty acids and glycerol from adipose tissue. Glucagon also promotes the uptake and oxidation of fatty acids by liver and muscle.
- *Protein metabolism:* Glucagon exerts a catabolic action on proteins and inhibits the incorporation of amino acids into hepatic protein.
- *Cardiac effects:* Large amounts of exogenous glucagon produce a positive inotropic effect on the heart by increasing myocardial levels of cyclic AMP. A direct chronotropic effect has also been reported. The net effect is an increase in cardiac output resulting from an increased force of myocardial contraction and increased heart rate.

All the major actions of glucagon—hepatic glycogenolysis, lipolysis, stimulation of insulin release, and the inotropic effect on the heart—are mediated by cyclic AMP.

Insulin

STRUCTURE, BIOSYNTHESIS, AND SECRETION
Insulin is a polypeptide hormone composed of 51 amino acids arranged in two chains (A and B), linked by disulfide bridges.

Insulin is derived from a large polypeptide precursor—*proinsulin*—which is synthesized in the endoplasmic reticulum of beta cells and packaged into membrane-bounded granules within the Golgi complex.

A connecting (C) peptide is removed from the proinsulin molecule by proteolytic cleavage before the secretion of insulin in its biologically active form.

Insulin secretion occurs through exocytosis (emiocytosis), a calcium-dependent process that is enhanced by cyclic AMP and potassium. Upon entering the circulation, insulin is transported largely in free molecular form, not bound to plasma proteins.

CONTROL OF SECRETION
The secretion of insulin is regulated primarily by the blood glucose level, with an elevation of blood glucose (hyperglycemia) increasing both production and release of insulin. Ingested glucose effects a far greater secretion of insulin than an equivalent amount of intravenously administered glucose because several gastrointestinal hormones, including gastrin, secretin, pancreozymin, and glucagon, stimulate insulin secretion.

Insulin secretion is also increased by mannose, fructose, certain amino acids, vagal stimulation (acetylcholine), cyclic AMP, potassium, and oral hypoglycemic drugs such as tolbutamide. Hyperglycemia, somatostatin, alpha-adrenergic stimulation, thiazide diuretics, phenytoin, and diazoxide inhibit insulin secretion.

MAJOR ACTIONS
- *Cellular membrane permeability:* Insulin facilitates the transport of glucose across selected cell membranes, thereby accelerating the entry of glucose into muscle, adipose tissue, fibroblasts, leukocytes, mammary glands, and the anterior pituitary. The transport of glucose into the liver, brain, renal tubules, intestinal mucosa, and erythrocytes is *independent* of insulin. Exercise and hypoxia mimic the effect of insulin upon cellular permeability to glucose in skeletal muscle. The insulin requirements of diabetics engaging in strenuous exercise may be reduced substantially and therefore must be monitored carefully to avoid hypoglycemia. Insulin also increases cellular permeability to amino acids, fatty acids, and potassium, particularly in muscle and adipose tissue.
- *Carbohydrate metabolism:* Insulin effectively lowers the level of blood glucose by enhancing the transport and peripheral utilization of glucose. Insulin increases muscle and liver glycogen stores by activating enzymes involved in glycogen-

esis while inhibiting those that produce glycogenolysis. Glycolytic enzymes are also activated by insulin, whereas several enzymes involved in gluconeogenesis are inhibited.

- *Protein metabolism:* Insulin is strongly anabolic, increasing protein synthesis and inhibiting protein catabolism. Insulin increases the incorporation of amino acids into protein by accelerating the entry of amino acids into the cell and possibly by increasing RNA synthesis.
- *Lipid metabolism:* Insulin stimulates formation of triglycerides (*lipogenesis*) and inhibits their breakdown (*lipolysis*). Insulin accelerates synthesis of fatty acid and glycerol phosphate and enhances cellular permeability to fatty acids, leading to increased deposition of triglycerides in adipose tissue.

Somatostatin (Growth Hormone Release–Inhibiting Hormone; GRIH; SRIH)

Somatostatin is a tetradecapeptide that has been isolated from the hypothalamus, the pancreas, and the upper gastrointestinal tract. Within the pancreatic islets, the somatostatin-secreting delta (D) cells are located between the glucagon-secreting alpha (A) cells and the central mass of insulin-secreting beta (B) cells. Such an arrangement could permit the product of the D cells—somatostatin—to directly influence the secretion of glucagon and insulin by the A and B cells, respectively.

ACTIONS

Although the precise role or roles of somatostatin remain unclear, several endocrine and nonendocrine activities have been attributed to this hormone. These biological actions include the following:

Endocrine

Inhibition of secretion of:

Growth hormone (GH)
Thyroid stimulating hormone (TSH)
Glucagon
Insulin
Gastrin
Secretin
Renin

Nonendocrine

Inhibition of:

Gastric acid secretion and gastric emptying
Pancreatic bicarbonate and enzyme release
Gallbladder contraction
Xylose absorption
Splanchnic blood flow
Platelet aggregation
Electrical activity of CNS neurons
Acetylcholine release from peripheral nerves

Disorders of Glucose Metabolism

HYPOGLYCEMIA

Hypoglycemic states are characterized by the presence of an abnormally low blood glucose level. This represents a threat to the brain, which depends upon glucose as its source of energy.

Normally, when the blood glucose falls below a critical level, insulin secretion is inhibited and release of glucagon, epinephrine, GH, and glucocorticoids is increased. Only the release of the catecholamine epinephrine leads to observable symptoms, such as sweating, palpitation, anxiety, and weakness.

Impairment of brain function, confusion, amnesia, bizarre behavior, or blurred vision may occur if the blood glucose falls below a level of 40 mg/dL. Severe hypoglycemia may ultimately lead to hypothermia, convulsions, and coma. Hypoglycemic disorders may be divided into two types: *fasting* (food-deprived) and *postprandial* (food-stimulated or reactive).

Possible causes of fasting hypoglycemia are:

- *Hyperinsulinism:* insulinomas (insulin-secreting tumors of the pancreas), overdosage with exogenous insulin or sulfonylurea drugs (oral hypoglycemic agents)
- *Endocrine disorders:* Addison's disease (adrenocortical insufficiency), hypopituitarism (e.g., Simmond's disease), myxedema
- *Liver disease:* hepatic necrosis, malignancy, or advanced cirrhosis, which may lead to impairment of glycogenesis and gluconeogenesis, thereby reducing liver glycogen stores and hepatic output of glucose
- *Acute alcoholism*
- *Extrapancreatic tumors*

The possible causes of *postprandial (reactive) hypoglycemia* include early or alimentary hypoglycemia, which may follow gastric intestinal surgery or result from increased vagal tone, and late hypoglycemia (early or occult diabetes mellitus).

DIABETES MELLITUS

Diabetes mellitus is a chronic disorder of metabolism characterized by carbohydrate intolerance and inappropriate hyperglycemia resulting from a deficiency of insulin secretion or a reduction in its biological efficacy ("relative" insulin deficiency).

The insulin deficiency, be it absolute or relative, triggers a series of biochemical changes in the metabolism of carbohydrates, lipids, and proteins, as outlined in Figure 38-4. These metabolic abnormalities lead to the classic symptoms of diabetes mellitus—*polyuria* (frequent urination), *polydipsia* (excessive thirst), *polyphagia* (hunger), and fatigue.

Long-term, serious complications of diabetes mellitus include gangrene, visual impairment resulting from proliferative retinopathy, myocardial infarction, polyneuropathy, and uremia. Pathologic changes in the blood vessels, particularly in the microcirculation (microangiopathy), appear to underlie the majority of these complications.

Diabetes mellitus is a disorder of heterogenous etiology. Predisposition to diabetes is inherited, although the genetic factors are complex. There are two generally recognized types of diabetes mellitus: (1) *insulin dependent* (type I or *juvenile onset*) and (2) *noninsulin dependent* (type II or *maturity onset*).

Insulin-Dependent (Type I) Diabetes

Generally occurs in nonobese persons before the age of 30, most commonly in adolescence. Circulating insulin is virtually absent, and the beta pancreatic cells fail to respond to all normal stimuli for insulin secretion. The islet beta cell reserve is markedly reduced or totally absent, and ketosis usually develops in the course of the disease. Patients respond to exogenous insulin, which is required to reverse the hyperglycemia and the general catabolic state and to prevent ketosis.

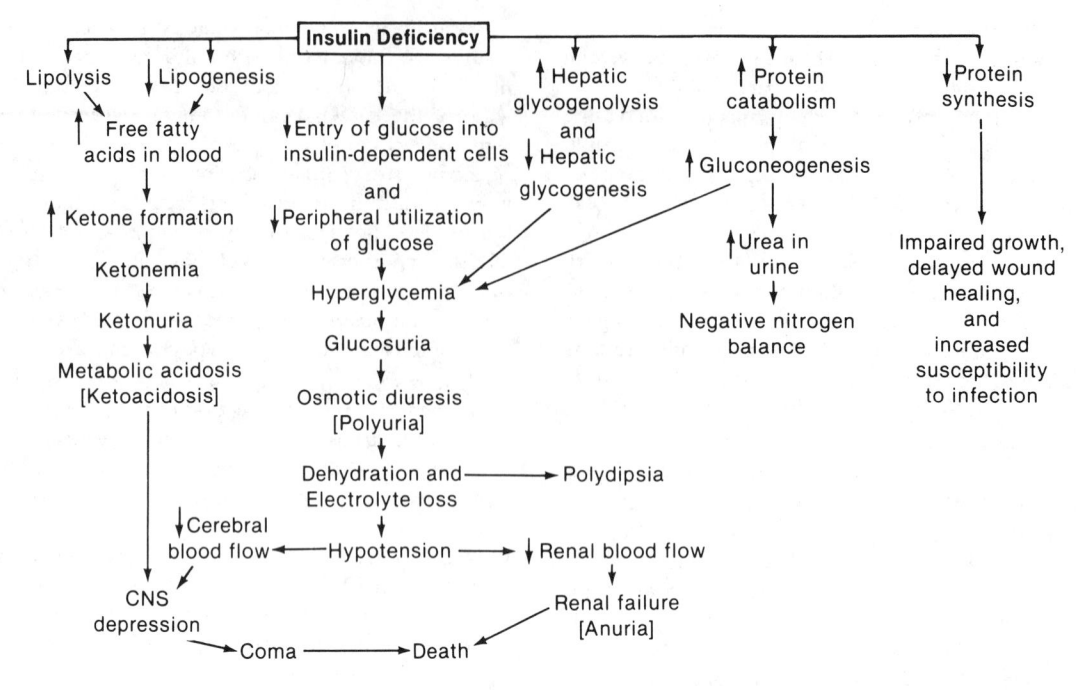

Figure 38-4 Metabolic consequences of severe insulin deficiency.

Immunopathologic mechanisms have been strongly implicated in this type of diabetes. Specific histocompatibility (HLA) antigens have been linked to this disorder, and circulating antibodies to islet cells have been detected in some patients early in the course of the disease.

Viruses such as mumps, coxsackie B4 virus, and rubella have been associated epidemiologically with the onset of type I diabetes. It is possible that an underlying genetic defect of the immune system may predispose an individual to beta cell destruction following these viral infections.

Noninsulin-Dependent (Type II) Diabetes

This type of diabetes mellitus usually has its onset after the age of 40, although it may occur at any age. Obesity is a major risk factor to the development of this disease, beta cell mass may be only moderately reduced, and autoimmunity is not demonstrable. There is no correlation with HLA antigens; however, there is a strong genetic component. Ketosis rarely occurs.

In at least some cases of noninsulin-dependent diabetes, a defect in insulin binding to cellular receptors is likely. Insulin apparently exerts a negative feedback control over its own receptors. In the presence of obesity, certain tissues (such as muscle and adipose tissue) display insensitivity to insulin. Perhaps the hyperinsulinism that results from chronic excessive caloric intake and sustained beta cell stimulation actually reduces the number of available insulin receptors and leads to glucose intolerance.

In addition to obesity and excessive carbohydrate intake, diabetes mellitus may be precipitated by pancreatitis, pregnancy, and endocrine disorders associated with overproduction of GH, glucocorticoids, or catecholamines.

Almost all forms of clinical and experimental diabetes mellitus are associated with increased secretion of glucagon, a potent hyperglycemic hormone whose glycogenolytic, gluconeogenic, lipolytic, and ketogenic actions are intensified by insulin deficiency.

ADRENAL GLANDS

The *adrenal* (suprarenal) glands are paired yellowish masses of tissue situated at the superior pole of each kidney. Each gland consists of two distinct entities—an outer *adrenal cortex* and an inner *adrenal medulla*—that differ in embryologic origin, character, and function.

Adrenal Medulla

The *adrenal medulla* develops from the embryonic ectoderm. It remains functionally associated with the sympathetic nervous system, being essentially a modified sympathetic ganglion whose postganglionic neurons have lost their axons and become secretory.

Histologically, the adrenal medulla contains large, ovoid cells arranged in clumps or irregular cords around numerous blood vessels. The medullary cells, often termed *chromaffin* cells because their granules possess affinity for chromium salts, secrete the catecholamine hormones epinephrine (adrenaline) and norepinephrine (noradrenaline). The principal secretory product is epinephrine, with norepinephrine normally accounting for only 20% of the total secretion.

Adrenal medullary secretion of the catecholamines is physiologically controlled by the posterior hypothalamus. The hormones are stored in cellular granules, bound to adenosine triphosphate (ATP) and protein, and are released in response to the following stimuli: sympathetic nervous system activation, hypoglycemia, pain, hypoxia, hypotension, cold, emotional stress, acetylcholine, histamine, and nicotine.

Epinephrine and norepinephrine are rapidly metabolized to inactive products, principally by the liver and kidneys. Major products of biodegradation include metanephrine, normetanephrine, and vanillylmandelic acid (VMA). These appear in the urine and may be assayed during clinical diagnosis.

ACTIONS OF ADRENAL MEDULLARY HORMONES

Epinephrine and norepinephrine mimic the effects of sympathetic nerve discharge, producing the following effects:

- Direct increase in cardiac rate and myocardial force of contraction
- Elevation of blood pressure
- Dilation of coronary and skeletal muscle blood vessels
- Constriction of the cutaneous and visceral vasculature
- Relaxation of respiratory smooth muscle
- Inhibition of GI motility
- Pupillary dilation (mydriasis)
- Glycogenolysis in liver and muscle
- Lipolysis

The cardiac excitatory effects and the metabolic actions of lipolysis and glycogenolysis are mediated by cyclic AMP, the latter involving the activation of phosphorylase enzyme by protein kinase.

The catecholamines also evaluate the metabolic rate (calorigenic action), stimulate the central nervous system, increase alertness, and stimulate respiration.

CLINICAL DISORDERS

Adrenal medullary function is not essential to life; therefore, hyposecretion of adrenal medullary hormones does not constitute a recognized clinical entity.

Pheochromocytoma

Pheochromocytoma is a chromaffin-cell tumor of the sympathoadrenal system, most commonly involving one of the adrenal glands or both. It is characterized by hypersecretion of the catecholamines epinephrine and norepinephrine, the latter usually dominating. Clinical manifestations of pheochromocytoma include paroxysmal or persistent hypertension, severe headaches, tachycardia, profuse sweating, epigastric pain, nausea, irritability, and dyspnea. Metabolic signs of this disorder include hyperglycemia, increased basal metabolic rate, weight loss, and elevated levels of urinary catecholamines or their metabolites.

Adrenal Cortex

The adrenal cortex develops from the mesoderm during embryonic life. The cells of the adrenal cortex, which are arranged in continuous cords separated by capillaries, are characterized by an abundance of mitochondria, endoplasmic reticulum, and accumulation of lipid.

Adrenal cortical tissue is structurally arranged into three concentric regions or zones: a thin outer zona glomerulosa, a thick middle zona fasciculata, and an inner zona reticularis bordering on the adrenal medulla.

Chemically, the steroid hormones of the adrenal cortex, the *adrenocorticoids*, are all derivatives of cholesterol. The adrenocorticoid hormones are usually divided into three functional groups: the *mineralocorticoids*, such as aldosterone, which regulate electrolyte and water balance; the *glucocorticoids*, such as cortisol, which affect carbohydrate, protein, and fat metabolism; and the *adrenogenital steroids* or *sex hormones*.

The adrenogenital steroids are of three types: *androgens* (such as dehydroepiandrosterone), *estrogens* (such as estradiol), and *progestins* (such as progesterone).

Under normal physiologic conditions the adrenogenital steroids are secreted (under ACTH control) in minute amounts, and therefore they exert minimal effects on reproductive functions. Excessive secretion of adrenal androgens results in precocious pseudopuberty in boys, and causes masculinization of females (*adrenogenital syndrome*).

MINERALOCORTICOIDS

Control of Secretion and Actions

Aldosterone is the principal physiological mineralocorticoid secreted by the zona glomerulosa. Its secretion is regulated primarily by the renin–angiotensin mechanism described in Chapter 28. The plasma concentrations of sodium and potassium are central factors in the control of aldosterone secretion, for low sodium or elevated potassium levels stimulate the zona glomerulosa both directly and indirectly (by way of the renin–angiotensin system). Other factors contributing to the control of aldosterone secretion include blood volume and ACTH, the latter exerting a limited, nonselective stimulatory effect.

Aldosterone plays a major physiological role in the maintenance of electrolyte and fluid balance by promoting the renal tubular reabsorption of sodium and the secretion of potassium and hydrogen. Aldosterone binds to nuclear receptors and stimulates DNA-directed RNA synthesis leading to increased formation of specific proteins involved in sodium transport.

A similar sodium-retaining, potassium-excreting action is exerted on other target tissues, including salivary glands and sweat glands.

GLUCOCORTICOIDS

Control of Secretion and Actions

Glucocorticoid secretion, which occurs primarily in the zona fasciculata, is controlled by ACTH. A variety of stressful stimuli including anxiety, fear, hypoglycemia, hypotension, and hemorrhage increase secretion of adrenocorticotropic hormone–releasing hormone (CRH) from the hypothalamus. CRH promotes ACTH secretion by the adenohypophysis, and ACTH stimulates adrenal cortical secretory activity, thereby elevating blood levels of cortisol (the principal physiological glucocorticoid). Elevated blood levels of free cortisol normally exert a negative feedback control over further secretion of CRH and ACTH. Prolonged ACTH secretion results in hypertrophy and hyperplasia of the adrenal cortex and excessive secretion of all adrenocorticoid hormones. The metabolic and physiological actions of the glucocorticoids are summarized below. The pharmacologic actions and clinical uses of these hormones are discussed in Chapter 43.

- *Carbohydrate metabolism:* Glucocorticoids stimulate hepatic gluconeogenesis and inhibit peripheral uptake and utilization of glucose, thereby promoting hyperglycemia. Hepatic glycogenesis is also enhanced.
- *Protein metabolism:* Glucocorticoids exert protein catabolic and antianabolic actions, promoting the breakdown of existing proteins while inhibiting the incorporation of amino acids into new proteins, except in the liver, where protein synthesis is stimulated.
- *Lipid metabolism:* Glucocorticoids inhibit lipogenesis and favor mobilization of fats from adipose tissues. When present in large amounts, these hormones favor redistribution of adipose stores by promoting loss of fat from the extremities, and accumulation of fat depots in central body regions (e.g., "moon face" and "buffalo hump" formation).
- *Blood and immunologic effects:* Glucocorticoids inhibit the immune response, cause involution of lymphoid tissue, and reduce blood levels of lymphocytes, eosinophils, and basophils. These hormones also stimulate erythropoiesis and elevate circulating levels of platelets and neutrophils.

- *GI tract effects:* Glucocorticoid hormones stimulate gastric acid and pepsin secretion and inhibit the production of protective mucus, thereby favoring development of gastric ulcers.

DISORDERS OF THE ADRENAL CORTEX

Addison's Disease

Addison's disease (chronic adrenocortical insufficiency) may result from idiopathic adrenocortical atrophy, adrenocortical destruction by disease (e.g., tuberculosis or cancer), or deficiency of ACTH or CRH secretion.

Weakness and fatigability are early signs of the disease, and weight loss, dehydration, and hypotension are characteristic. Emotional changes and GI disturbances (such as anorexia, nausea, vomiting, diarrhea) frequently occur. Hyperpigmentation is a major characteristic of primary adrenocortical insufficiency, with increased pigmentation being prominent on skin folds, pressure points (bony prominences), extensor surfaces, nipples, perineum, tongue, and buccal mucosa.

In Addison's disease, aldosterone (mineralocorticoid) deficiency results in increased excretion of sodium and retention of potassium. The salt and water depletion causes severe dehydration, reduced circulatory volume, hypotension, and eventual circulatory collapse.

Glucocorticoid (cortisol) deficiency leads to reduced gluconeogenesis, hypoglycemia, diminished hepatic glycogen, and extreme insulin sensitivity. The inability to withstand stress (such as infection, trauma, surgery) may result in acute adrenal insufficiency (adrenal crisis).

Cushing's Syndrome

Cushing's syndrome is a clinical state characterized by glucocorticoid excess resulting from adrenocortical tumors, hypersecretion of ACTH, or from the administration of large amounts of exogenous corticosteroids or ACTH.

Clinical manifestations of this syndrome include truncal obesity, moon face, and buffalo hump, resulting from the characteristic redistribution of fat from the extremities to central body regions (abdomen, face, and upper back). The increased central subcutaneous fat depots stretch the skin, rupturing the subdermal tissue and causing formation of purple striae.

Excessive protein catabolism results in protein depletion and causes thin skin, muscular wasting, easy bruising, and poor wound healing. Osteoporosis develops, predisposing the patient to fractures and skeletal deformities.

Increased gluconeogenesis and decreased peripheral utilization of glucose result in hyperglycemia and glucose intolerance, and frank diabetes mellitus may develop in genetically predisposed individuals.

Hypertension and renal calculi frequently occur, and psychiatric disturbances are common.

Primary Hyperaldosteronism (Conn's Syndrome)

Conn's syndrome, a clinical state resulting from excessive production of the mineralocorticoid aldosterone, is generally characterized by potassium depletion, sodium retention, hypertension, polyuria, fatigue, and muscular weakness. Hypokalemic alkalosis and tetany may also be observed.

Gonadal Hormones

The physiological and metabolic actions of the gonadal hormones, together with their clinical uses, are reviewed in Chapter 44 (Estrogens and Progestins) and Chapter 46 (Androgens and Anabolic Steroids). The menstrual (endometrial) cycle is presented schematically in Chapter 45, Figure 45-1.

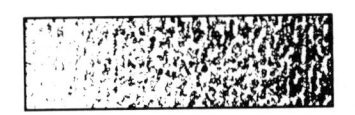

39 HYPOPHYSIAL HORMONES

The *hypophysis*, or pituitary gland, is composed of two major divisions, the *adenohypophysis* (anterior lobe), which contains at least six hormones, and the *neurohypophysis* (posterior lobe), which contains two hormones. Virtually no bodily function is exempt from the influence of at least one of these eight hypophysial hormones, which collectively serve to regulate and integrate the physiological processes necessary for the maintenance of homeostasis. The synthesis, storage, release, and function of these hormones are reviewed in Chapter 38.

HORMONES OF THE ADENOHYPOPHYSIS

Of the six principal hormones of the adenohypophysis, growth hormone (GH), adrenocorticotropic hormone (ACTH), and thyroid stimulating hormone (TSH) are available clinically as purified preparations. Growth hormone is a purified polypeptide of recombinant DNA origin containing the identical sequence of the 191 amino acids constituting endogenous growth hormone. Adrenocorticotropic hormone is a 39 amino acid polypeptide extracted from pituitary glands of animals. Thyroid stimulating hormone is a purified extract of the hormone from bovine pituitary glands. Since these three hormones are peptides, they must be given parenterally, because they would be quickly destroyed in gastric juice if taken by mouth. Further, since ACTH and TSH are naturally derived products, their use is associated with the possibility of allergic reactions. GH is now prepared synthetically and is virtually devoid of hypersensitivity problems.

The two adenohypophysial gonadotropins, *follicle stimulating hormone* (FSH) and *luteinizing hormone* (LH), are extracted from the urine of pregnant and postmenopausal women. The commercial preparation, human menopausal gonadotropin (HMG), is used in the treatment of infertility and cryptorchidism (undescended testes) and is discussed in Chapter 45. The remaining adenohypophysial hormone, *prolactin* (luteotropic hormone, LTH), is unavailable for therapeutic use.

All adenohypophysial hormones except GH exert their effects on *selective* target organs, such as the adrenal cortex, thyroid gland, or gonads. For many of the reasons mentioned above, replacement therapy in cases of hormonal deficiency states is usually best accomplished by supplying the individual target gland hormones (thyroxine, hydrocortisone, estrogen, progesterone) instead of the pituitary hormones. In the case of the gonadal hormones, moreover, the individual purified hypophysial hormones are not clinically available.

Adrenocorticotropic Hormone (ACTH)

Corticotropin Injection
ACTH, Acthar

Repository Corticotropin Injection
ACTH Gel, Cortigel, Cortrophin Gel, Cotropic Gel, H.P. Acthar Gel

Corticotropin Zinc Injection
Cortrophin-Zinc

A polypeptide containing 39 amino acids, extracted from the pituitary glands of several animals, ACTH is commercially available either as a stable aqueous solution for injection, and aqueous solution containing gelatin to delay absorption and prolong the action, or a zinc hydroxide complex to prevent tissue destruction, which also prolongs the effect. A synthetic subunit (i.e., 24 amino acids) of ACTH, available as cosyntropin, is used to test for adrenocortical insufficiency. Cosyntropin is reviewed in Chapter 76. A second diagnostic agent, metyrapone, can also be employed to ascertain whether pituitary secretion of ACTH is adequate and is likewise considered in Chapter 76.

MECHANISM
Stimulates the adrenal cortex to produce and secrete all of its hormones; activates adrenyl cyclase in adrenal cortical tissue, thus increasing cyclic adenosine monophosphate (AMP) levels, which enhances the synthesis of adrenal steroids, principally cortisone and hydrocortisone

USES
Management of severe myasthenia gravis and acute exacerbations of multiple sclerosis

Treatment of nonsuppurative thyroiditis, tuberculous meningitis (with appropriate antibacterial therapy), trichinosis with neurologic or myocardial involvement, and hypercalcemia associated with cancer

Diagnostic testing of adrenocortical function (cosyntropin is the preferred agent—see Chap. 76)

Treatment of rheumatic, collagen, dermatologic, allergic, hematologic, respiratory, edematous, and neoplastic disorders, *only as an alternative* to more specific glucocorticoid therapy—see Chap. 43)

DOSAGE
Adrenal responsiveness must first be verified.

Diagnosis: 10 U to 25 U/500 mL 5% dextrose by IV infusion over 8 hours

Treatment of deficiency states: regular injection: 20 U four times a day IM or SC

Repository injection: 40 U to 80 U every 1 to 3 days IM or SC

Myasthenia: 100 U/day to a total of 2000 U

Multiple sclerosis: 80 U to 120 U/day for 2 to 3 weeks IM

FATE
Readily absorbed from injection sites; effects are rapid following IM or IV injection and persist for 2 to 4 hours. Duration with repository injection is 24 to 48 hours. Half-life following IV injection is 20 to 30 minutes; binds to plasma proteins; excreted largely by the kidney

SIGNIFICANT ADVERSE REACTIONS
(Usually observed with prolonged use)

GI: ulceration and hemorrhage (cause and effect relationship not established), pancreatitis, abdominal distention

Musculoskeletal: weakness, osteoporosis, steroid myopathy, loss of muscle mass, vertebral compression fractures

Dermatologic: erythema, petechiae, ecchymoses, delayed wound healing, sweating, hyperpigmentation, acneiform reactions, thinning skin

CNS: convulsions, vertigo, headache, insomnia, depression, mood swings, euphoria, personality alterations

Endocrine: menstrual irregularities, hirsutism, diabetes, decreased carbohydrate tolerance, growth suppression

Electrolyte: hypernatremia, hypokalemia, hypocalcemia, fluid retention

Cardiovascular: hypertension, necrotizing angiitis

Other: subcapsular cataracts, increased intraocular pressure, exophthalmos, negative nitrogen balance, allergic reactions

CONTRAINDICATIONS

Osteoporosis, scleroderma, systemic fungal infections, peptic ulcer, ocular herpes simplex, recent surgery, congestive heart failure, hypertension, IV use (except diagnostic testing), alone in active tuberculosis, and sensitivity to proteins of porcine origin. *Cautious use* in patients with diabetes, hypothyroidism, cirrhosis, infections, diverticulitis, renal insufficiency, myasthenia gravis, in pregnant and lactating women, and in emotionally unstable individuals

> **NOTE**
> Undertake immunization procedures with extreme caution during ACTH therapy because lack of antibody response and neurologic complications have been reported. Do not vaccinate against smallpox during treatment with ACTH.

INTERACTIONS

Increased requirements for hypoglycemic agents may occur with use of ACTH, owing to the hyperglycemic action of corticosteroids

ACTH may enhance the hypoprothrombinemic action of aspirin

Marked hypokalemia may result if ACTH is given with diuretics that cause potassium loss

ACTH may antagonize oral antagonize oral anticoagulants

The adverse effects of vaccines may be enhanced by ACTH (see *Note:* above)

NURSING CONSIDERATIONS

Nursing Alerts
- Question administration of full therapeutic doses if renal responsiveness has not been verified by a rise in plasma or urinary corticosteroid values following an IM or SC test injection.
- Be prepared to assist with skin sensitivity test, which should be performed in any patient with suspected sensitivity to proteins of porcine origin. Observe patient closely for sensitivity reaction during IV infusion or immediately following IM or SC injection.
- Ensure that ACTH therapy is not abruptly discontinued. The dosage should be reduced gradually to minimize the relative adrenal cortical insufficiency that can result from prolonged ACTH therapy. Full dosage should be reinstituted if periods of stress occur during withdrawal.
- Assess patient frequently for signs of electrolyte imbalances (e.g., thirst, weakness, muscle cramping), sodium or water retention, or psychic changes (e.g., mood swings, insomnia, depression, euphoria).

- Monitor blood pressure regularly during therapy.
- In evaluating patient's response, keep in mind that it may take several days for maximal therapeutic effects to develop. If an immediate effect is desired, more rapidly acting steroids should be used.

1. Inject repository forms deeply IM. They should not be administered IV. The zinc repository form should not be given SC.
2. Reconstitute prepared powder with sterile water for injection or sterile saline solution. Refrigerate. Discard unused portion after 24 hours.

PATIENT EDUCATION

1. Emphasize the importance of notifying physician if illness or infection develops because ACTH can induce immunosuppression. Proper anti-infective therapy should be administered in the presence of an infection.
2. Instruct patient to report any weight gain or signs of edema.

Synthetic Growth Hormone (GH)

Somatrem

Humatrope, Protropin

Somatrem is a synthetic polypeptide hormone obtained by a recombinant DNA technique containing the identical sequence of 191 amino acids comprising endogenous growth hormone plus an additional amino acid, methionine. It is useful in treating growth retardation in children lacking endogenous growth hormone.

MECHANISM

Increases linear bone growth in a manner therapeutically equivalent to that of endogenous human growth hormone; skeletal growth is enhanced and the length of long bones is increased at the epiphyses; increases number and size of skeletal muscle cells and red cell mass; enhances cellular protein synthesis and nitrogen retention and decreases blood urea nitrogen; increases synthesis of chondroitin sulfate and collagen, and elevates serum levels of phosphate; facilitates urinary calcium excretion and enhances GI absorption of calcium, thus serum calcium levels are relatively unchanged. Potassium and sodium retention can also occur; large doses may raise blood glucose levels, lower glucose tolerance, and lower sensitivity to exogenous insulin, leading to a diabetogenic state; anabolic effects of growth hormone are apparently mediated by a group of substances termed *somatomedins,* peptides whose hepatic synthesis is stimulated by growth hormone; somatomedins promote uptake of sulfate into cartilage and appear to be the mediators of cellular processes involved with bone growth

USES

Treatment of growth failure due to a deficiency of pituitary growth hormone (hypopituitary dwarfism)

DOSAGE

Up to 0.1 mg/kg (0.2 U/kg) IM three times a week for 6 to 36 months

NOTE:
Before initiating treatment, document growth hormone deficiency by failure of serum growth hormone concentration to rise above 5 mg to 7 mg/mL in response to at least two standard stimuli (e.g., insulin-induced hypoglycemia, IV arginine (see Chap. 76), oral levodopa, or IM glucogon)

SIGNIFICANT ADVERSE REACTIONS
Myalgia, pain and swelling at injection site, hyperglycemia, ketosis, hypothyroidism

CONTRAINDICATIONS
Patients with closed epiphyses, progressive intracranial lesions or tumors. *Cautious use* in patients with diabetes

INTERACTIONS
Accelerated epiphyseal closure (fusion of ends of long bones) can occur if somatrem is combined with androgens or thyroid hormones
Hydrocortisone and other antiinflammatory steroids may inhibit the response to somatrem
Somatrem may decrease responsiveness to insulin or to oral hypoglycemic agents by increasing blood glucose levels

NURSING CONSIDERATIONS

Nursing Alerts
- Check results of bone age assessments, which should be performed annually, especially in patients receiving concurrent thyroid or androgen therapy, because premature epiphyseal closure can occur.
- Monitor patient for possible development of hypotension, tachycardia, or atrial arrhythmias.
- Be alert for indications of hypercalciuria (e.g., flank pain, renal colic, chills, fever, urinary frequency, hematuria), especially during first 2 to 3 months of therapy.
- Monitor results of thyroid function tests, which should be performed periodically.

1. Administer IM, not SC, because lipoatrophy or lipodystrophy can occur with SC injection, and the likelihood of developing neutralizing antibodies is increased.
2. Reconstitute each vial with 5 mL of bacteriostatic water for injection. Do *not* shake vial vigorously. Store in refrigerator. Discard after 1 month.

Thyroid Stimulating Hormone (TSH)

Thyrotropin
Thytropar

A purified extract of TSH isolated from bovine pituitary glands, this preparation contains no significant amounts of other pituitary hormones.

MECHANISM
Increases uptake of iodide by the thyroid gland, enhances formation of thyroid hormones, and increases release of thyroid hormones from the thyroid gland; in large doses, produces hyperplasia of thyroid glandular tissue, which is readily reversible upon termination of the drug

USES
Differentiation between primary and secondary hypothyroidism
Differentiation of primary hypothyroidism from euthyroidism (normal thyroid function) following thyroid suppression by thyroid replacement therapy
Diagnosis of decreased thyroid reserve

DOSAGE
10 U (contents of 1 vial) IM or SC daily for 1 to 3 days depending on condition. A radioiodine study is performed 24 hours after the last injection; no response is noted in thyroid failure but a substantial response occurs in pituitary failure

FATE
Effect on the thyroid is evident within 8 hours in normal individuals and reaches a maximum within 24 to 48 hours

COMMON SIDE EFFECTS
Nausea, vomiting, headache, urticaria

SIGNIFICANT ADVERSE REACTIONS
Transitory hypotension, tachycardia, thyroid gland swelling, anaphylactic reaction

CONTRAINDICATIONS
Coronary thrombosis, untreated Addison's disease. *Cautious use* in patients with angina pectoris, cardiac failure, hypopituitarism, adrenal cortical insufficiency

NURSING CONSIDERATION
1. Prepare solution by adding 2 mL sterile physiologic saline solution to vial containing 10 U thyrotropic activity. Solution may be kept for up to 2 weeks if refrigerated.

HORMONES OF THE NEUROHYPOPHYSIS

The *neurohypophysis* or posterior lobe of the pituitary contains two hormones, oxytocin and vasopressin, both of which are available for clinical use. In addition, posterior pituitary injection, a preparation possessing the activity of *both* oxytocin and vasopressin is also available.

Oxytocin exerts two principal actions in the body: contraction of uterine smooth muscle (oxytocic effect) and contraction of the myoepithelial cells surrounding the ducts of the mammary gland, resulting in ejection of milk (galactokinetic effect). The sensitivity of the uterus to the effects of oxytocin is dependent on both the stage of gestation (maximal at term and immediately postpartum) and the existing balance of female sex hormones (increased in the presence of estrogen and reduced in the presence of progesterone). Natural oxytocin is no longer available for clinical use and has been replaced by a synthetic derivative. It is most frequently employed to enhance uterine contractions during labor. Although not derived from pituitary sources, two other drugs used for their oxytocic effects, ergonovine and methylergonovine, are also considered in this chapter.

Vasopressin is sometimes referred to as the antidiuretic hormone (ADH) because it promotes reabsorption of water from the distal tubules and collecting ducts of the kidney. Its other pharmacologic effects include contraction of vascular smooth muscle, especially of the portal and splanchnic (visceral) vessels, and a direct spasmogenic effect on gastrointestinal smooth muscle. Available preparations of vasopressin include a synthetic derivative of the naturally occurring hormone possessing marked pressor and antidiuretic activity and two structural analogs, desmopressin and lypressin, which exhibit relatively selective antidiuretic activity with minimal pressor effects. These drugs are reviewed individually in this chapter.

Posterior Pituitary Injection

Pituitrin-S

Posterior pituitary injection is a sterile aqueous extract of pituitary glands of domesticated animals containing the equivalent of 20 United States Pharmacopeial (USP) units per mL.

MECHANISM
Possesses oxytocic, vasopressor, smooth muscle spasmogenic, and antidiuretic activity

USES
Control of postoperative ileus and to facilitate expulsion of gas before pyelography
As aid to achieving hemostasis in surgical procedures or esophageal varices
Treatment of enuresis of diabetes insipidus

DOSAGE
SC, IM, 5 U to 20 U (average 10 U)

COMMON SIDE EFFECTS
Facial pallor, uterine cramping, GI spasms

SIGNIFICANT ADVERSE REACTIONS
Tinnitus, mydriasis, anxiety, diarrhea, urticaria, albuminuria, angioedema, eclamptic episodes, loss of consciousness, and anaphylaxis

CONTRAINDICATIONS
Toxemia of pregnancy, cardiac disease, hypertension, epilepsy, and advanced arteriosclerosis.

Do not use for treatment of surgical shock because the vasoconstriction and increased peripheral resistance are accompanied by decreased coronary blood flow and cardiac output, further aggravating the conditions that may have been responsible for shock. *Cautious use* in patients with arrhythmias or coronary insufficiency and in persons using barbiturates (see Interactions)

INTERACTIONS
Increased incidence of cardiac arrhythmias and coronary insufficiency can occur if Pituitrin is combined with barbiturates or general anesthetics
Antidiuretic effects can be potentiated by chlorpropamide, clofibrate, and carbamazepine

NURSING CONSIDERATION

Nursing Alert
- Question use of drug to assist labor. Such use is not recommended because the drug action is rather short-lived, and there is a high risk of fetal distress or asphyxia and uterine rupture.

Vasopressin
Pitressin Synthetic

Vasopressin Tannate
Pitressin Tannate In Oil

A synthetic compound structurally identical to naturally occurring vasopressin possessing vasopressor and antidiuretic activity, vasopressin injection is available as an aqueous solution containing 20 pressor units (U) per milliliter. Vasopressin tannate injection is a water-insoluble tannate salt of vasopressin suspended in peanut oil, containing 5 pressor units per milliliter and having a prolonged (36–72 h) duration of action.

The principal indication for these agents is the treatment of diabetes insipidus, a condition characterized by excretion of excessive quantities of dilute urine (polyuria) and extreme thirst (polydipsia). Insufficient ADH secretion from the neurohypophysis is often the cause of this condition, and vasopressin provides replacement therapy to correct the symptoms. Occasionally, however, the problem is unresponsiveness of the renal tubules to the action of vasopressin and, in these cases, vasopressin is ineffective in treating the condition. Successful therapy of this latter type of diabetes insipidus is difficult, but clinical benefit has been reported with use of thiazide diuretics and chlorpropamide. Vasopressin is also used to reduce excessive bleeding especially that associated with esophageal varices, because of its ability to strongly contract vascular smooth muscle.

MECHANISM
Increases distal tubular reabsorption of water by increasing the permeability of the tubular epithelium via activation of cyclic AMP in cells of the renal collecting ducts; enhances contraction of vascular and nonvascular smooth muscle, thereby decreasing peripheral blood flow and increasing GI, urinary, and uterine smooth muscle spasm; constriction of coronary arteries may precipitate or worsen existing angina

USES
Treatment of diabetes insipidus of central (hypophysial) origin
Prevention and treatment of postoperative abdominal distention
Dispersion of gas shadows to aid abdominal roentgenography
Control of bleeding esophageal varices and hemorrhage due to abdominal surgery

DOSAGE
Vasopressin Injection

Diabetes insipidus: 5 U to 10 U 2 to 3 times a day IM, SC, or intranasally on cotton pledgets
Abdominal distention: 5 U IM initially; increase to 10 U every 3 to 4 hours as necessary
Abdominal roentgenography: 10 U IM 2 hours and ½ hour before films are exposed
Bleeding episodes: 20 U by IV infusion (or occasionally intra-arterially) over 5 to 10 minutes

Vasopressin Tannate in Oil
0.3 mL to 1 mL (1.5 U–5 U) IM; repeat as needed every 24 to 96 hours

FATE
Duration of action with aqueous injection is 2 hours to 8 hours; effects of tannate injection persist 36 hours to 96 hours, primarily because of slow, cumulative absorption from IM injection

site; rapidly removed from the plasma (half-life 15 min); inactivated by the liver and kidneys and excreted in the urine as metabolites and unchanged drug

COMMON SIDE EFFECTS

Facial pallor, nausea, GI disturbances, and abdominal or uterine cramping

SIGNIFICANT ADVERSE REACTIONS

Vertigo, sweating, headache, vomiting, urticaria, bronchoconstriction, hypersensitivity reactions, anaphylactic reaction, and anginal pain

Following nasal insufflation: congestion, irritation, rhinorrhea, headache, conjunctivitis, and mucosal ulceration

CONTRAINDICATIONS

Chronic nephritis, advanced arteriosclerosis, and severe coronary artery disease. *Cautious use* in patients with epilepsy, asthma, migraine, heart failure, angina, renal disease, goiter, and in elderly, very young, or pregnant patients

INTERACTIONS

Action of vasopressin may be potentiated by hypoglycemics, acetaminophen, fludrocortisone, ganglionic blocking agents, neostigmine, and general anesthetics

Antidiuretic activity can be increased by chlorpropamide, clofibrate, or carbamazepine

Antidiuretic action of vasopressin may be reduced by alcohol, epinephrine, cyclophosphamide, heparin, and lithium

NURSING CONSIDERATIONS

Nursing Alerts

- Have appropriate treatment available (e.g., nitroglycerin, oxygen, antiarrhythmics) if used for patient with coronary artery disease because anginal attacks and myocardial infarction can occur.
- Inject vasopressin tannate IM only, never IV.
- Be alert for early symptoms of water intoxication (nausea, vomiting, drowsiness, listlessness, headache, confusion) because convulsions and coma can occur. If symptoms appear, drug should be withdrawn, and fluid intake should be restricted until specific gravity of urine is at least 1.015 and polyuria occurs. Diuretics may be used with caution.

1. Before therapy is initiated, obtain baseline values for blood pressure, weight, and intake/output ratio. Monitor values regularly (daily, if possible) during therapy, and report any sudden changes.
2. Warm injection to body temperature before administering. Shake tannate suspension vigorously to ensure uniform dispersion. Inform patient that tannate injection may be painful. Observe for development of allergic reactions to both the vasopressin and the vehicle.
3. Administer 1 or 2 glasses of water with a large dose of vasopressin to reduce side effects such as cramping, skin blanching, and nausea.
4. Do not administer tannate salt more frequently than every 36 to 48 hours because the polyuria and thirst of diabetes insipidus are controlled for 36 to 72 hours following a single dose. Note that the tannate injection is indicated *only* for treatment of diabetes insipidus.
5. When drug is used to relieve abdominal distention, assess patient for appearance of peristaltic sounds, passage of flatus, and return of normal pattern of bowel movements. Abdominal measurements should be obtained prior to and during treatment.

Desmopressin Acetate

DDAVP, Stimate

A synthetic analog of vasopressin, desmopressin acetate is used as an intranasal spray or by injection; it possesses prolonged, potent antidiuretic activity with little vasopressor or oxytocic action at normal doses.

MECHANISM

Provides replacement therapy for antidiuretic hormone in treating polyuria and polydipsia; elicits a dose-related increase in Factor VIII levels

USES

Treatment of diabetes insipidus of central (hypophysial) origin

Treatment of polyuria and polydipsia associated with trauma or surgery of the pituitary gland

Treatment of hemophilia A and certain forms of von Willebrand disease where Factor VIII levels are at least 5% or greater (parenteral administration)

DOSAGE

Inhalation

Drug is supplied with a flexible calibrated plastic tube (rhinyle); desired quantity of solution is drawn into tube, one end is inserted into nostril, and patient blows on other end to deposit drug deep into nasal cavity; infants and young children may require assistance (e.g., air-filled syringe attached to tube).

Adults: 0.1 mL to 0.4 mL/day, either as a single dose or in 2 or 3 divided doses

Children (under 12): 0.05 mL to 0.3 mL/day in a single or 2 divided doses

IV, SC

Diabetes insipidus: 0.5 mL to 1.0 mL daily in 2 divided doses

Hemophilia A/von Willebrand disease: 0.3 µg/kg by slow IV infusion over 15 to 30 minutes. In adults, use 50 mL of sterile saline diluent; in children less than 10 kg, use 10 mL diluent.

FATE

Antidiuretic effect persists for 8 to 20 hours; increases in Factor VIII levels are evident within 30 minutes, and levels are maximal within 90 to 120 minutes; drug is metabolized by the liver and kidney and excreted in the urine

COMMON SIDE EFFECTS

Nasal irritation and congestion with inhalation

SIGNIFICANT ADVERSE REACTIONS

(Usually with high doses only) Headache, nausea, flushing, rhinitis, abdominal cramping, vulval pain, and hypertension; erythema, swelling, and burning have occurred at the site of injection

CONTRAINDICATIONS

Hemophilia B, type IIB von Willebrand disease (platelet aggregation may be increased). *Cautious use* in persons with coronary artery disease or hypertension, and in pregnant or nursing women and the elderly

NURSING CONSIDERATION
1. Assist patient in planning a schedule for fluid intake if oral fluids must be reduced to decrease the possibility of water intoxication and hyponatremia. A diuretic may be administered if excessive fluid retention occurs.

PATIENT EDUCATION
1. Provide complete instructions for administering medication (see Dosage), and ensure that patient understands how to use the calibrated plastic tube (rhinyle).

Lypressin
Diapid

A synthetic vasopressin, lypressin possesses little or no vasopressor or oxytocic activity. It is stable in aqueous solution and administered in the form of a nasal spray containing 50 USP posterior pituitary pressor U/mL. It provides replacement therapy for antidiuretic hormone, and is used to treat symptoms of diabetes insipidus in patients who are unresponsive to or intolerant of other forms of replacement therapy, or who experience allergic reactions or other adverse reactions with systemically administered vasopressin.

One or two sprays are administered in each nostril 4 times a day, with an additional dose at bedtime to eliminate nocturia if needed (one spray provides approximately 2 USP posterior pituitary pressor U). Administering more than 2 or 3 sprays in each nostril usually results in wastage, the unabsorbed excess draining into the digestive tract to be inactivated. If a higher dosage is indicated, increase frequency of usage rather than number of sprays with each use. Instruct patient to clear nasal passages before administering, hold bottle upright when spraying, and keep head in an upright position.

The maximal antidiuretic effect occurs within 30 minutes to 60 minutes and effects usually persist for 4 hours to 6 hours. Side effects are mild and infrequent; nasal irritation, congestion, pruritus, and rhinorrhea have been reported. Systemic adverse effects are minimal; however, large or frequent doses may eventually cause headache, heartburn, abdominal cramping, drowsiness, and dyspnea. Cautious use is necessary in patients with coronary artery disease. The effectiveness of intranasal lypressin may be impaired in the presence of nasal congestion, allergic rhinitis, or upper respiratory infections, since absorption may be reduced; larger doses may be required.

Oxytocin, parenteral
Pitocin, Syntocinon

Oxytocin, nasal
Syntocinon

Oxytocin is a synthetic peptide possessing the pharmacologic effects of the endogenous hormone. It is available as an injection for IM or IV use containing 10 U/mL, and as a nasal spray containing 40 U/mL.

MECHANISM
Direct spasmogenic effect on uterine smooth muscle; increases permeability of the cell membranes of myofibrils to sodium ions, thereby augmenting contractile activity; also contracts myoepithelial cells surrounding the ducts and alveoli of the mammary gland, facilitating ejection of milk from the properly primed gland; large doses may exhibit antidiuretic activity

USES
Initiation or augmentation of uterine contractions to assist in delivery of the fetus for *valid fetal or maternal reasons only,* such as the following:
  Maternal diabetes
  Rh problems
  Uterine inertia
  Premature rupture of membranes
  Preeclampsia or eclampsia
Facilitation of uterine contractions during third stage of labor
Control of postpartum hemorrhage
Management of inevitable, incomplete, or missed abortion
Aid in milk let-down during breast-feeding or relief or postpartum breast engorgement (*only* indication for the nasal spray)

DOSAGE
Injection

Induction or enhancement of labor: 0.001 U to 0.002 U/min (0.1 mL–0.2 mL/min of a 1:1000 dilution; see below) by IV infusion; increase gradually in 0.001-U to 0.002-U/min increments at 15-minute to 30-minute intervals until a desirable contraction pattern has been established; adjust rate according to uterine response. *Dilution*—1-mL ampule (10U) added to 1000 mL of 0.9% aqueous sodium chloride or other suitable IV fluid; use constant infusion pump to accurately control dose

Postpartum uterine bleeding: IV—10 U to 40 U/1000-mL diluent infused at a rate to control bleeding; IM—10 U after delivery of the placenta

Incomplete abortion: 10 U/500 mL diluent infused IV at a rate of 0.020 U to 0.040 U/minute

Nasal Spray
One spray into one nostril or both nostrils 2 to 3 minutes before nursing or pumping of breasts

FATE
Onset of effect is within 1 minute with IV infusion, 3 to 7 minutes with IM injection, and 5 to 10 minutes with nasal spray; nasal absorption is erratic; short plasma half-life (several minutes); rapidly cleared from the plasma by the liver, kidney, and mammary gland; primarily excreted as metabolites by the kidney, with small amounts as active drug

SIGNIFICANT ADVERSE REACTIONS
Fetus
Bradycardia, arrhythmias, neonatal jaundice, hypoxia, and trauma from too rapid expulsion

Mother
Arrhythmias, nausea, vomiting, pelvic hematoma, afibrinogenemia, uterine hypertonicity or spasm, uterine rupture, anaphylactic reaction, subarachnoid hemorrhage, hypertension, water intoxication, convulsions, and postpartum hemorrhage

CONTRAINDICATIONS
Unfavorable fetal position, significant cephalopelvic disproportion, fetal distress where delivery is not imminent, hypertonic uterine patterns, undilated cervix, prolonged use in uterine inertia or severe toxemia, conditions in which vaginal delivery is contraindicated (e.g., prolapsed cord, total placenta praevia, vasa praevia), previous cervical or uterine surgery, invasive cervical carcinoma, dead fetus, and abruptio placentae. *Cau-*

tious use: except in unusual circumstances, do not use in prematurity, partial placenta praevia, previous surgery on the cervix or uterus, overdistention of the uterus, grand multiparity, or history of uterine sepsis

INTERACTONS
Severe persistent hypertension can occur if oxytocin is given in the presence of other vasopressor drugs (e.g., epinephrine, ephedrine, methoxamine, or metaraminol)

Estrogens may augment and progestins may decrease the uterine spasmogenic action of oxytocin

Oxytocin can be potentiated by cyclophosphamide

NURSING CONSIDERATIONS

Nursing Alerts
- Ensure that oxytocin used for induction of labor is given only by IV infusion and administered by trained personnel. A physician should be readily available at all times to manage complications.
- Monitor uterine contractions, fetal heart rate, and maternal blood pressure and pulse regularly during infusion.
- Carefully regulate infusion flow rate to obtain optimal contractions. If contractions are frequent (less than 2-min intervals), prolonged, or excessive (greater than 50 mm Hg), the infusion should be stopped to prevent fetal anoxia, the patient should be placed on her side, and oxygen should be ready for administration. Effects diminish rapidly because oxytocin is short-acting.
- During prolonged infusion, assess patient for early signs of water intoxication (confusion, headache, and drowsiness) due to ADH effect of oxytocin. Intake/output ratio should be checked during labor, and edema and anuria should be promptly noted.
- If local anesthetics containing epinephrine are used during labor in patient receiving oxytocin, be alert for development of severe hypertension. Symptoms may include throbbing headache, palpitations, sweating, fever, vomiting, stiff neck, photophobia, and chest pain.
- Do not administer *undiluted* solution IV, nor give oxytocin by more than one route of administration at any one time.

1. Begin IV infusion with non-oxytocin-containing solution (e.g., physiologic electrolyte solution). Oxytocin solution is then added to the system. A constant infusion pump is used to accurately regulate infusion rate. Flow rate should not exceed 2 mL/min.
2. When drug is given IM (deep deltoid injection), have magnesium sulfate available to relax myometrium if necessary.

PATIENT EDUCATION
1. Instruct patient using nasal spray to clear nasal passages before spraying, to hold bottle upright, and to maintain a sitting or standing position.

Nonhypophyseal Oxytocics

In addition to oxytocin, other compounds also possess a uterine spasmogenic action and are used for some of the same indications as oxytocin, particularly to control postpartum atony and hemorrhage. Ergonovine, an alkaloid obtained from ergot, a fungus that grows on the rye plant, and methylergonovine, a semisynthetic derivative of ergonovine, exert a somewhat more prolonged oxytocic action than oxytocin itself and appear to be more selective spasmogens for uterine smooth muscle.

Ergonovine
Ergotrate

MECHANISM
Direct stimulating effect on smooth muscle of the uterus; small doses increase force and frequency of uterine contractions, but normal relaxant phase follows; larger doses produce sustained, forceful contractions, with markedly elevated resting tone; cerebral vasoconstriction is moderate, although less than that observed with ergotamine, a related alkaloid used in migraine (see Chap. 14)

USES
Management of postpartum or postabortion hemorrhage or uterine atony

Investigational uses include alternate therapy of migraine (especially when use of ergotamine causes paresthesias) and diagnosis of Prinzmetal's variant angina during coronary arteriography (provokes reversible coronary artery spasms)

DOSAGE
Oral: 0.2 mg to 0.4 mg 2 to 4 times a day until danger of atony has passed (usually 48 hr)

IM: 0.2 mg following placental delivery; may repeat in 2 to 4 hours as needed

IV: 0.2 mg for excessive uterine bleeding

Diagnosis of Prinzmetal's angina: 0.05 mg to 0.2 mg IV during coronary arteriography

FATE
Well absorbed orally, sublingually, and parenterally; onset of action is 30 to 60 seconds IV, 3 to 7 minutes IM, and 8 to 10 minutes orally; uterine contractions may continue for up to 3 to 4 hours

SIGNIFICANT ADVERSE REACTIONS
(Most frequent with IV administration) Nausea, vomiting, weak and rapid pulse, paresthesias, allergic reactions (including shock), hypertension, tinnitus, headache, dyspnea, cramping, dizziness, confusion, decreased lactation, and muscle weakness

CONTRAINDICATIONS
For induction of labor, threatened spontaneous abortion, severe hypertension, toxemia of pregnancy. *Cautious use* in patients with heart disease, hypertension, mitral valve stenosis, renal or hepatic impairment, obliterative vascular disease, or sepsis

INTERACTIONS
Blood pressure may be further elevated if ergonovine is combined with vasopressors or other oxytocics

Oxytocic action may be attenuated by hypocalcemia

NURSING CONSIDERATIONS

Nursing Alerts
- Expect to administer IV only in extreme emergencies because danger of hypertension and severe nausea and vomiting is increased with IV use.

- Monitor blood pressure, pulse, vaginal blood flow, and uterine response following injection until condition has stabilized. Report marked changes in pulse or blood pressure.
- Monitor patient for early symptoms of ergot poisoning (ergotism) such as vomiting, cramping, headache, or confusion. To avoid development of ergotism, the drug should not be used for prolonged periods.
- Evaluate degree of cramping experienced. Although cramping is usually an indication of drug effectiveness, persistent or severe cramping may indicate a need for dosage reduction.
- Use with extreme caution before delivery of the placenta, and only in the presence of a staff member well versed in the use of ergonovine, because very high uterine tone may be produced.

1. Store injection in cool place, and do not use solution over 60 days old.

Methylergonovine

Methergine

(CAN) Methylergobasine

MECHANISM
Direct spasmogenic action on uterine smooth muscle; weak cerebral vasoconstrictive action

USES
Management of postpartum atony, hemorrhage, or subinvolution of the uterus following delivery of the placenta
Facilitation of labor (given in the second stage following delivery of the anterior shoulder)

DOSAGE
Oral: 0.2 mg 3 or 4 times a day for a maximum of 1 week
IM, IV: 0.2 mg after delivery of the anterior shoulder, after delivery of placenta, or during the puerperium; may repeat as required at 2- to 4-hour intervals

FATE
Well absorbed orally or parenterally; onset of action is 5 to 10 minutes orally and IM and almost immediate with IV injection

SIGNIFICANT ADVERSE REACTIONS
Nausea, vomiting, hypertension, dizziness, tinnitus, sweating, palpitation, chest pain, and dyspnea

CONTRAINDICATIONS
See ergonovine

INTERACTIONS
See ergonovine

NURSING CONSIDERATIONS

Nursing Alert
- When drug is used IV, administer slowly and monitor blood pressure closely. Drug should not be administered IV routinely because risk of hypertension and cerebral vascular accident is increased.

1. Discard solution if discolored. Store in cool place, and protect from light.

Selected Bibliography

Altura BM, Altura BT: Actions of vasopressin, oxytocin and synthetic analogs on vascular smooth muscle. Fed Proc 43:80, 1984

Brownstein MJ: Biosynthesis of vasopressin and oxytocin. Annu Rev Physiol 45:129, 1983

Chrousos GP, et al: Clinical applications of corticotropin releasing factor. Ann Intern Med 102:344, 1985

Gash DM, Thomas GJ: What is the importance of vasopressin in memory processes. Trends Neurosci 6:197, 1983

Hays RM: Alteration of luminal membrane structure by antidiuretic hormone. Am J Physiol 245:1289, 1983

Hintz RL: The somatomedins. Adv Pediatr 28:293, 1981

Hintz RL, Rosenfeld RG: Clinical uses of synthetic growth hormone. Hosp Pract 18:115, 1983

McCann SM: Control of anterior pituitary hormone release by brain peptides. Neuroendocrinology 31:355, 1980

Meisenberg G, Simmons WH: Centrally-mediated effects of neurohypophyseal hormones. Neurosci Biobehav Rev 7:263, 1983

Reichlin S: Somatostatin. N Engl J Med 309:1495, 1556, 1983

Share L, Crofton JT: The role of vasopressin in hypertension. Fed Proc 43:103, 1984

Sklar AH, Schrier RW: Central nervous system mediators of vasopressin release. Physiol Rev 63:1243, 1983

VanVliet G, Styne DM, Kaplan SL, Grumbach MM: Growth hormone treatment for short stature. N Engl J Med 309:1016, 1983

Zimmerman EA, Nilaver G, Hou-Yu A, Silverman AJ: Vasopressinergic and oxytocinergic pathways in the central nervous system. Fed Proc 43:91, 1984

SUMMARY. HYPOPHYSIAL HORMONES

Drug	Preparations	Usual Dosage Range
Adenohypophysis		
Corticotropin injection ACTH, Acthar	Powder for injection: 25 U/mL, 40 U/mL	20 U 4 times/day SC or IM 10 U 25 U/500 mL 5% dextrose infused IV over 8 h for diagnostic purposes
Corticotropin repository ACTH Gel, Cortigel, Cortrophin Gel, Cortropic Gel, H.P. Acthar Gel	Injection: 40 U/mL, 80 U/mL	40 U to 80 U IM or SC every 1 to 3 days
Corticotropin zinc Cortrophin-Zinc	Injection: 40 U/mL with 2 mg zinc/mL	40 U to 80 U IM (only) every 1 to 3 days
Somatrem Humatrope, Protropin	Powder for injection: 5 mg (10 U) per vial	Up to 0.1 mg/kg IM 3 times a week for 6 to 36 months
Thyrotropin Thytropar	Powder for injection: 10 U/vial with diluent	10 U IM or SC daily for 1 to 3 days depending on condition
Neurohypophysis		
Posterior pituitary injection Pituitrin-S	Injection: 20 U/mL	5 U to 20 U (average 10 U) IM or SC
Vasopressin Pitressin synthetic	Injection: 20 U/mL	*Diabetes insipidus:* 5 U to 10 U 2 to 3 times/day IM, SC, or intranasally on cotton pledgets *Abdominal distention:* 5 U IM, increased to 10 U every 3 to 4 h as needed *Roentgenography:* 10 U IM 2 h and ½ h before film
Vasopressin tannate Pitressin tannate in oil	Injection: 5 U/mL	*Diabetes insipidus:* 0.3 mL to 1 mL (1.5 U–5 U) IM only every 24 to 96 h as needed
Desmopressin acetate DDAVP, Stimate	Nasal solution: 0.1 mg/mL Injection: 4 µg/mL	*Inhalation:* Adults: 0.1 mL to 0.4 mL/day either a single dose or in 2 to 3 divided doses; children (under 12): 0.05 mL to 0.3 mL/day in 2 divided doses IV, SC Diabetes insipidus: 0.5 mL to 1.0 mL daily in 2 divided doses Hemophilia A/von Willebrand disease: 0.3 µg/kg by slow infusion (15–30 min) in sterile saline diluent (adults—50 mL; children—10 mL)
Lypressin Diapid	Nasal spray: 0.185 mg/mL	1 to 2 sprays in each nostril 4 times/day with an additional dose at bedtime if needed to control nocturia
Oxytocin Pitocin, Syntocinon	Injection: 10 U/mL	*Induction of labor:* 0.001 U to 0.002 U/min by slow IV infusion; increase gradually until optimal effect is noted *Postpartum uterine bleeding:* 10 U to 40 U/1000 mL by constant IV infusion or 10 U IM after delivery of placenta *Incomplete abortion:* 10 U/500 mL infused IV at a rate of 0.020 U to 0.040 U/min
Oxytocin, synthetic, nasal Syntocinon	Nasal spray: 40 U/mL	1 spray into one or both nostrils 2 to 3 min before nursing or pumping of breast
Nonhypophysial Oxytocics		
Ergonovine Ergotrate	Tablets: 0.2 mg Injection: 0.2 mg/mL	0.2 mg to 0.4 mg orally 2 to 4 times/day until danger of atony has passed 0.2 mg IM or IV
Methylergonovine Methergine	Tablets: 0.2 mg Injection: 0.2 mg/mL	0.2 mg orally 3 to 4 times/day 0.2 mg IM or IV, repeat every 2 to 4 hours as required

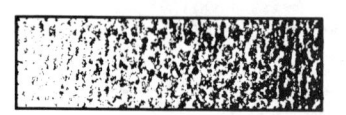

40 THYROID HORMONES AND ANTITHYROID DRUGS

The endogenous thyroid hormones thyroxine (T₄) and triiodothyronine (T₃) are important in normal physical and mental growth and development and in regulating the metabolic activity of essentially every cell of the body. They affect a wide range of physiological activities including central nervous system, cardiovascular, and gastrointestinal function; carbohydrate, lipid, and protein metabolism; temperature regulation; muscle activity; water and electrolyte balance; and reproduction. Unlike many other hormones, however, they do not act upon discrete target organs but exert a diffuse effect throughout the body. Their onset of action is slow and their activity prolonged; thus, they generally provide long-term regulation of bodily functions rather than moment-to-moment control.

The synthesis, storage, and release of the thyroid hormones by the thyroid gland are regulated in large part by the thyroid stimulating hormone (TSH) of the adenohypophysis; this schema is discussed in the review of endocrine function in Chapter 38. The principal clinical application of the thyroid hormones is in the treatment of *hypo*thyroidism. This disease, characterized by reduced or absent secretion of endogenous thyroid hormones, can be clinically subdivided into cretinism (fetal or neonatal hypothyroidism) and myxedema (adult hypothyroidism), and each of these conditions is reviewed in Chapter 38. It should be noted that use of thyroid hormones in hypothyroidism merely constitutes replacement therapy and does not effect a cure. Because normal thyroid function is usually not reestablished, clinical benefit is attained only so long as thyroid hormones are supplied.

Several types of thyroid hormone preparations are available, both natural extracts of animal thyroid glands and synthetic derivatives. The natural animal extracts exhibit more variation in potency than the synthetic derivatives and are much less frequently used today.

The available thyroid preparations are:

- *Desiccated thyroid:* powdered, dried thyroid glands of domesticated animals, standardized on the basis of iodine content
- *Thyroglobulin:* purified extract of porcine thyroid gland, standardized by iodine content and bioassayed for metabolic activity
- *Levothyroxine sodium:* sodium salt of the synthetic *l*-isomer of thyroxine (T₄)
- *Liothyronine sodium:* sodium salt of the synthetic *l*-isomer of triiodothyronine (T₃)
- *Liotrix:* combination of levothyroxine sodium and liothyronine sodium in a 4:1 ratio, on a weight basis

The pharmacology of the thyroid hormones is discussed as a group, because their overall effects are similar. Individual drugs are then listed in Table 40-1.

Secretion of excessive amounts of thyroid hormones reflects a *hyper*thyroid state, the most common cause of which is overstimulation of the gland by circulating immunoglobulins synthesized by B lymphocytes. One such antibody is thyroid stimulating immunoglobulin (TSI), also known as long-acting thyroid stimulator (LATS), which interacts with receptor sites in the thyroid cell to stimulate hormonal output.

Therapy of hyperthyroidism includes surgical removal of a part of the gland (subtotal thyroidectomy), use of radioactive iodide (^{131}I) to destroy thyroid tissue, or administration of antithyroid drugs that interfere with synthesis and release of thyroid hormones. The antithyroid drugs methimazole and propylthiouracil are reviewed in this chapter and listed in Table 40-2, and a discussion of ^{131}I is also presented.

Certain types of thyroid disorders can also be effectively treated with elemental iodine preparations, and these products are considered at the end of the chapter.

Two other thyroid-related drugs are protirelin, a synthetic thyrotropin-releasing hormone, and thyrotropin, a highly purified form of thyroid stimulating hormone of bovine origin. These two agents are used for diagnosis of thyroid dysfunction and are reviewed in Chapter 76 along with other diagnostic drugs.

Effective treatment of thyroid disorders depends on accurate assessment of the thyroid state. Several laboratory parameters used to ascertain thyroid functioning are listed below, with average (normal) values given beside each test.

Commonly Used
- *Free thyroxine index:* 1.4 ng/dL to 4.2 ng/dL
- *Resin uptake of radioactive T₃ in vitro (RT₃U):* 27% to 37% uptake of T₃
- *TSH levels:* up to 5 µU/mL
- *Radioimmunoassays for T₃ and T₄:*
    T₃—80 ng/dL to 100 ng/dL (adults)
    T₄—5 µg/dL to 12 µg/dL (adults)

Infrequently Used
- *Basal metabolic rate (BMR):* ±10%
- *Protein-bound iodine (PBI):* 4 µg/dL to 8 µg/dL serum
- *Radioactive iodine uptake:* 5% to 10% at 2 hours; 10% to 20% at 6 hours; 20% to 40% at 24 hours
- *Thyroxine-binding globulin levels:* 10 µg/dL to 26 µg/dL
- *Free T₃ index (FT₃I):* 20 ng/dL to 60 ng/dL

Because of the possibility of false increases or decreases in the readings of any one of these tests related to other medications taken by the patient (see Interactions for Thyroid Hormones), or the presence of certain disease states (e.g., hepatitis, nephrosis), *several* tests should be performed before a diagnosis is made, and the results should be used only in combination with a thorough clinical assessment of the patient.

Thyroid Hormones

Levothyroxine
Liothyronine
Liotrix
Thyroglobulin
Thyroid, dessicated

MECHANISM
Incompletely understood, but multiple sites and mechanisms are probably involved; probably bind to receptors on cellular surfaces, increasing uptake of glucose and amino acids; may also diffuse into cells and interact with receptors on mitochondria and chromatin material; increased mRNA synthesis can occur,

leading to accelerated protein synthesis; appear to stimulate sodium-potassium-ATPase directly, thus facilitating membrane transport of sodium and potassium and increasing cellular utilization of oxygen; effects of these hormones include increases in body temperature, respiratory rate, heart rate, cardiac output, blood volume, carbohydrate, fat and protein metabolism, and enzymatic activity; conversely, serum cholesterol levels may be reduced

USES

Replacement or substitution therapy of primary hypothyroidism (e.g., cretinism; myxedema; nontoxic goiter; hypothroid state of childhood, pregnancy, or old age) or of secondary hypothyroidism (e.g., surgery, radiation, drug-induced)

Adjuncts to thyroid-inhibiting agents when they are used to reduce release of thyrotropic hormones in treatment of thyrotoxicosis (Thyroid drugs prevent development of goiter and hypothyroidism.)

Differentiation of hyperthyroidism from euthyroidism (T_3 only—T_3 suppression test)

Prevention or treatment of euthyroid goiters such as thyroid nodules, multinodular goiter, or chronic, lymphocytic thyroiditis

Adjunctive therapy of follicular and papillary carcinoma of the thyroid, in conjunction with radioactive iodine

DOSAGE

See Table 40-1

FATE

Oral absorption is variable, T_3 being absorbed to a greater extent (95% within 4 h) than T_4 (50%–75%). Onset of action is within 6 hours to 8 hours for T_3 but much slower with T_4 (2 to 3 days). Peak effects may require up to 8 to 10 days to develop, however. Plasma half-lives are 1 to 2 days for T_3 and 6 to 7 days for T_4. Both hormones are highly bound (99%–100%) to plasma proteins (thyroxine-binding globulin, thyroxine-binding prealbumin, and albumin). Approximately 35% of T_4 is deiodinated in the periphery to T_3. Drugs are metabolized by the liver and in other tissues and excreted in the urine (70%–80%) or bile (20%–30%) both as free drug and conjugated metabolites

COMMON SIDE EFFECTS

(If dosage is excessive) Palpitations, nervousness, sweating, and tachycardia

SIGNIFICANT ADVERSE REACTIONS

(Usually result of overdosage or too-rapid increase in dosage) Headache, diarrhea, fever, arrhythmias, anginal pain, tremors, insomnia, menstrual irregularities, heat intolerance, allergic skin reactions, congestive heart failure, and shock

CONTRAINDICATIONS

Thyrotoxicosis, nephrosis, hypogonadism, hyperthyroidism, hypoadrenalism, cardiovascular diseases uncomplicated by hypothyroidism, and for treating obesity, infertility, or depression, as there is no conclusive evidence of benefit in these conditions. *Cautious use* in the presence of angina, arrhythmias, diabetes mellitus, or adrenocortical insufficiency

INTERACTIONS

Thyroid hormones can enhance the cardiovascular effects of catecholamines, possibly resulting in angina or arrhythmias

Highly protein-bound drugs may compete with thyroid hormones for plasma protein binding sites, resulting in increased plasma levels of thyroid hormones

Thyroid hormones can potentiate the effects of oral anticoagulants by increasing catabolism of vitamin K-dependent clotting factors

Thyroid hormones may increase blood sugar levels, thus increasing requirements for insulin and oral hypoglycemic drugs

Estrogens may decrease plasma levels of free T_4 by increasing levels of thyroid-binding globulin

Thyroid hormone therapy may decrease the effectiveness and increase the likelihood of toxicity of the digitalis glycosides

The activity of tricyclic antidepressants can be enhanced by thyroid hormones, possibly resulting in cardiac arrhythmias

Tachycardia and hypertension may occur with ketamine in patients receiving thyroid hormones

NURSING CONSIDERATIONS

Nursing Alerts

- In patient with cardiovascular disease, including hypertension, assess cardiovascular status frequently for indications of possible complications (e.g., chest pain, dyspnea). Therapy should be initiated with small doses.
- Expect therapy to be initiated with small doses because hypothyroid patient is extremely sensitive to thyroid hormone. Dosage changes should be made gradually. Earliest clinical responses in adult are usually diuresis, increased appetite, and increased pulse.
- Monitor patient for development of signs of overdosage, such as irritability, nervousness, sweating, tachycardia, increased bowel motility, or menstrual irregularities. If these occur, the drug should be stopped for several days, then reinstituted at a lower dosage.
- Monitor sleeping pulse and basal morning temperature, as indicated, because they are important guides to treatment, and the maintenance dosage may be higher in an actively growing child than in an adult.
- Monitor pulse rate and rhythm during periods of dosage adjustment. Notify physician if rate exceeds 100 or if there is a marked change in rate or rhythm because drug may need to be withheld.

1. Test urine of diabetic patient regularly during therapy because dosage of antidiabetic drugs may need to be increased.
2. Evaluate effects of concomitantly administered oral anticoagulants. Their action may be enhanced by thyroid hormone, necessitating a dosage reduction.

PATIENT EDUCATION

1. Suggest taking drug, which is used once a day, in the morning, if possible, to minimize the possibility of sleep disturbances.
2. Stress the importance of taking drug regularly even when feeling well. Replacement therapy is usually a lifelong requirement.
3. Warn juvenile hypothyroid patient and parents that initial response to therapy may be dramatic (excessive hair loss, rapid growth, assertiveness). These reactions tend to abate with continued therapy.
4. Instruct parents of juvenile taking thyroid hormone to monitor growth regularly. Too-rapid increases in height

can result in premature closure of epiphyses and resultant skeletal deformities.
5. Explain, as appropriate, that both pharmacologic and toxicologic effects may persist for 10 to 14 days after withdrawal of T_3 and for 4 to 6 weeks after withdrawal of T_4.

ANTITHYROID DRUGS (THIOAMIDES)

Methimazole
Propylthiouracil

The antithyroid drugs impair the synthesis of the thyroid hormones T_3 and T_4 in the thyroid gland and are used in the treatment of hyperthyroid states. Unlike other means of hyperthyroid therapy, such as subtotal thyroidectomy or treatment with ^{131}I, antithyroid drugs do not tend to damage thyroid tissue beyond repair and thus are usually the initial treatment of choice. Long-term therapy may produce remission of the disease in some cases, but relapse is not uncommon. Patients who fail to respond fully to drug therapy or who show evidence of relapse should be considered as candidates for either surgery or radioisotope therapy.

Because the antithyroid drugs do not interfere with the release or activity of previously formed thyroid hormones, their clinical effects are delayed for several weeks, until body stores of preformed T_4 and T_3 are exhausted. Likewise, the action of exogenously administered thyroid hormones is unimpaired by antithyroid drugs.

Several kinds of compounds are capable of exerting an antithyroid effect. Large amounts of the iodide ion (6 mg–10 mg/day) can suppress release of thyroid hormones from the gland and are thus occasionally used for treating some forms of hyperthyroidism and for reducing the size and vascularity of the gland before thyroidectomy. Certain monovalent inorganic anions (e.g., perchlorate, thiocyanate, periodate) block uptake of iodide by the gland and can exert an antithyroid action. They are rarely used clinically, however, because more effective and less toxic drugs are available. The principal antithyroid agents are the thioamide derivatives methimazole and propylthiouracil and they are discussed below, then summarized in Table 40-2.

MECHANISM

Inhibit the biosynthesis of thyroid hormones by inhibiting the peroxidase enzyme system that catalyzes the conversion of iodide to iodine thus reducing the concentration of free iodine available for reaction with tyrosine; may also block oxidative coupling of mono- and diiodotyrosine to form T_3 and T_4 (see Chap. 38) and can partially inhibit conversion of T_4 to T_3 in the periphery; do *not* inactivate existing T_3 and T_4 nor interfere with the action of exogenous thyroid hormones.

Drug-induced depression of circulating hormone levels results in compensatory increase in TSH release from the adenohypophysis. Excess TSH increases size and vascularity of thyroid gland (goitrogenic action).

Table 40-1
Thyroid Hormones

Drug	Preparations	Usual Dosage Range	Nursing Implications
Thyroid, desiccated Armour Thyroid, S-P-T, Thyrar	Tablets: 16 mg, 32 mg, 65 mg, 98 mg, 130 mg, 195 mg, 260 mg, 325 mg Coated tablets: 32 mg, 65 mg, 130 mg, 195 mg Capsules (timed-release): 65 mg, 130 mg, 195 mg, 325 mg	*Adults* Myxedema: 16 mg/day for 2 wk; 32 mg/day for 2 wk; then 65 mg/day; increase daily dosage at monthly or greater intervals on basis of laboratory tests; usual range 65 mg–195 mg/day Hypothyroidism without myxedema: 65 mg/day increased by 65 mg every 30 days until desired response *Children* Dosage regimen same as adults, with increments made at 2-wk intervals; maintenance doses may be higher in growing child than in adult	Dessicated animal thyroid glands containing active thyroid hormones (T_3 and T_4) in their natural state and ratio; potency can vary significantly from lot to lot; clinical effects develop slowly and are very prolonged; caution in transferring patient from thyroid to T_3 alone—discontinue thyroid, begin T_3 at very low doses and gradually increase dosage levels; drug should be stored in dark, moisture-free bottles
Thyroglobulin Proloid	Tablets: 32 mg, 65 mg, 100 mg, 130 mg, 200 mg	Initially 32 mg/day; increase at 2–3-wk intervals until optimal response is attained; usual maintenance dosage range 65 mg/day–200 mg/day	Purified extract of hog thyroid containing T_4 and T_3 in an approximate 2.5:1.0 ratio; biologically assayed and standardized in animals; action is similar to that of desiccated thyroid with comparable onset and duration

Continued

Table 40-1
Thyroid Hormones (continued)

Drug	Preparations	Usual Dosage Range	Nursing Implications
Levothyroxine sodium—T₄ Levothroid, Levoxine Synthroid, Synthrox, Syroxine (CAN) Eltroxin	Tablets: 0.025 mg, 0.05 mg, 0.075 mg, 0.1 mg, 0.125 mg, 0.15 mg, 0.175 mg, 0.2 mg, 0.3 mg Injection: 200 μg/vial, 500 μg/vial	*Oral* Adults: 0.1 mg/day initially; increased by 0.05-mg–0.1-mg increments every 1–3 wk until desired response is obtained; in elderly, myxedematous, or cardiovascular patients, initial dose 0.025 mg with 0.025-mg–0.05-mg increments as needed; usual range 0.1 mg–0.2 mg/day Children: 0.025 mg–0.05 mg initially, with increments of 0.05 mg–0.1 mg/day at 1–3-wk intervals until desired response is obtained; usual range 0.2 mg–0.4 mg/day *Parenteral* Myxedematous coma: 0.2 mg–0.5 mg IV first day; 0.1 mg–0.3 mg second day if necessary; daily injections maintained until patient can accept a daily oral dose	Synthetic monosodium salt of the naturally occurring L-isomer of thyroxine; 0.1 mg is equivalent to 65 mg of desiccated thyroid; used orally for hypothyroid replacement therapy and IV for treatment of myxedema coma or stupor demanding immediate replacement; may be given IM when oral route is not feasible; slower onset and longer duration than synthetic T₃; discontinue T₄ before switching to T₃; conversely, begin T₄ several days before stopping T₃; parenteral solution is prepared with sodium chloride injection and shaken until clear, use immediately; administer IV cautiously to patients with heart disease; inject slowly in small doses and carefully observe patient
Liothyronine sodium—T₃ Cytomel, Cyronine	Tablets: 5 μg, 25 μg, 50 μg	*Adults and children over 3 yr* Mild hypothyroidism: 25 μg/day initially; increase by 12.5 μg/day–25 μg/day every 1–2 wks; usual maintenance is 25 μg–75 μg/day in divided doses Myxedema: 5 μg/day initially; increased by 5 μg–10 μg/day every 1–2 wk; usual maintenance is 50 μg–100 μg/day Simple nontoxic goiter: *see* Myxedema T₃ suppression test: 75 μg–100 μg/day for 7 days; then repeat ¹³¹I uptake test; in hyperthyroid patient, uptake is not affected; in normal patient, uptake will fall to less than 20% *Children under 3 yr* Cretinism: initially 5 μg/day; increase by 5 μg every 3–4 days until desired response is achieved; infants a few months old require about 20 μg/day; at 1 yr, 50 μg/day is required	Synthetic form of the naturally occurring L-triiodothyronine (T₃); 25 μg is equivalent to 65 mg of desiccated thyroid; possesses similar actions and uses of other thyroid hormones but has a more rapid onset of maximal effect and shorter duration (half-life 1–2 days), allowing quicker dosage adjustments; serum TSH levels are most reliable laboratory index for monitoring T₃ replacement; also used in T₃ suppression test to differentiate borderline hyperthyroid from euthyroid (normal); useful in patients allergic to naturally extracted derivatives; be alert for possible additive effects due to residual action of longer-acting thyroid drugs when T₃ is substituted for them; drug may be cardiotoxic—use with caution in patients with cardiac disease
Liotrix Euthroid, Thyrolar	Tablets containing T₄ and T₃ in a fixed 4:1 ratio | T₄ (μg) | T₃ (μg) | Thyroid equivalent (mg) | |---|---|---| | 12.5 | 3.1 | 15 | | 25 | 6.25 | 30 | | 30 | 7.5 | 30 | | 50 | 12.5 | 60 | | 60 | 15 | 60 | | 100 | 25 | 120 | | 120 | 30 | 120 | | 150 | 37.5 | 180 | | 180 | 45 | 180 |	Dosage given in thyroid equivalents Initially 15 mg–30 mg/day; increased gradually every 1–2 wks until desired response is obtained Replacement therapy for other thyroid products is based on the equivalency: 60 mg liotrix = 65 mg desiccated thyroid or thyroglobulin = 0.1 mg T₄ = 25 μg T₃	A constant mixture of synthetic T₄ and T₃ in a fixed 4:1 ratio by weight; although the product is claimed to more closely approximate the endogenous ratio of T₄:T₃, when differences in potency, absorption, binding, peripheral conversion of T₄ to T₃, and metabolism are considered, the fixed ratio offers *no* apparent advantage over other thyroid hormones used at optimal doses (except in those few intolerant persons); tablets have a shelf life of 2 yr

USES

Treatment of hyperthyroidism (most effective in milder cases in which thyroid gland is not excessively enlarged)

Preparation for subtotal thyroidectomy or radioactive iodide therapy (to reduce hyperthyroidism and to lessen surgical risks)

DOSAGE

See Table 40-2

FATE

Well absorbed orally and oral bioavailability is high; concentrated in the thyroid gland; peak serum levels occur within 1 hour; plasma half-lives are relatively short (2–3 h) but do *not* reflect duration of antithyroid effect, which is due to action within the thyroid gland; dosing frequency is every 6 hours to 8 hours; propylthiouracil is excreted by the kidneys more quickly than methimazole

COMMON SIDE EFFECTS

Skin rash, itching, nausea, epigastric distress

SIGNIFICANT ADVERSE REACTIONS

Paresthesias, arthralgia, myalgia, loss of taste, loss of hair, dizziness, drowsiness, neuritis, edema, skin pigmentation, lymphadenopathy, sialadenopathy, and jaundice

Less commonly: agranulocytosis (0.5%), granulocytopenia, thrombocytopenia, drug fever, lupuslike reaction, hepatitis, periarteritis, hypoprothrombinemia, and bleeding

Goitrogenic action is indicated by enlarged thyroid, periorbital edema, fatigue, paresthesias, muscle cramps, cool skin, sensitivity to cold, and bradycardia.

CONTRAINDICATIONS

Nursing mothers. *Cautious use* in patients with liver dysfunction or bleeding tendencies and in pregnant women

INTERACTIONS

Antithyroid drugs can magnify the effects of oral anticoagulants by causing hypoprothrombinemia

Use cautiously in the presence of other drugs known to cause agranulocytosis, e.g., antidepressants, carbamazepine, clofibrate, indomethacin, methyldopa, meprobamate, phenothiazines, phenylbutazone, procainamide, quinidine, tetracyclines, and tolbutamide

NURSING CONSIDERATIONS

Nursing Alerts

- Monitor results of prothrombin times, which should be performed regularly during therapy, for hypoprothrombinemia.
- Expect to use smallest effective dose during pregnancy because drugs readily cross placental barrier and may produce goiter and cretinism in developing fetus. The drug should be discontinued, if possible, 2 to 3 weeks before delivery. Thyroid hormones and antithyroid drugs are often given concurrently during pregnancy to prevent hypothyroidism in mother and fetus.

1. In patient receiving antithyroid drug, expect to administer iodine (e.g., Lugol's solution, potassium iodide solution) for 7 to 10 days before thyroidectomy to reduce size and vascularity of the thyroid gland.

PATIENT EDUCATION

1. Stress the importance of adhering to prescribed dosage regimen.
2. Warn patient that use of OTC preparations containing iodide (e.g., cough syrups, asthma preparations) may interfere with effectiveness of antithyroid drug.
3. Teach patient how to monitor pulse and weight. Increased pulse, weight loss, anxiety, or tremor, possible indications of inadequate response, should be reported to drug prescriber.
4. Instruct patient to report development of sore throat, rash, fever, headache, or malaise immediately because these may be early indications of developing blood dyscrasia. If they occur, drug should be discontinued, and hematologic studies should be performed.
5. Instruct patient to report appearance of petechiae, ecchymoses, or any other unexplained bleeding because drugs can cause hypoprothrombinemia.
6. Instruct patient and family to be alert for indications of overdosage (e.g., depression, nonpitting edema, cold intolerance) and to notify health care provider if any occur.
7. Instruct mother taking antithyroid drug not to nurse infant.
8. Inform patient that thyroid hormone may be added to the regimen to prevent goiter when euthyroid state is attained.
9. Explain that therapy usually lasts 1 to 2 years, whereupon about 50% of patients have attained remission.
10. Instruct patient in remission to continue monitoring pulse and weight and to report any significant changes.

RADIOACTIVE IODIDE

Radioactive Sodium Iodide—^{131}I

Iodotope

Of the several radioactive isotopes of iodine, ^{131}I is the most widely used clinically. Although its major indication is the treatment of certain types of hyperthyroidism, it has also been successfully employed for therapy of thyroid carcinoma.

MECHANISM

Rapidly and efficiently taken up by the thyroid gland, incorporated into T_3 and T_4 and stored in the follicle of the gland; emits both beta radiation, which penetrates only a few mm of tissue and thus remains localized in the thyroid gland, and small amounts of longer wave length gamma radiation, which can be detected and measured externally; beta radiation destroys thyroid tissue, leading to a gradual reduction in thyroid hormone secretion; some degree of *hypo*thyroidism almost always occurs

USES

Treatment of hyperthyroidism, especially in patients over 30 years of age whose condition does not respond to other antithyroid medications

Treatment of thyroid carcinoma and metastases (effectiveness is questionable in all cases because some thyroid neoplasms, e.g., giant cell, spindle cell, and amyloid solid carcinomas, do *not* concentrate sufficient iodide ion)

Table 40-2
Antithyroid Drugs

Drug	Preparations	Usual Dosage Range	Nursing Implications
Methimazole Tapazole	Tablets: 5 mg, 10 mg	Adults: 15 mg–60 mg initially depending on degree of hyperthyroidism in 3 daily doses at 8-h intervals; maintenance is 5 mg–15 mg/day Children: 0.4 mg/kg initially in 3 divided doses at 8-h intervals; maintenance is ½ initial dose	More potent than propylthiouracil, longer duration of action, and somewhat more toxic; skin rash is an indication for discontinuing drug
Propylthiouracil (CAN) Propyl-Thyracil	Tablets: 50 mg	Adults: 100 mg initially 3 times/day every 8 h; maintenance is 100 mg–150 mg/day Children (over 10 yr): 50 mg–100 mg 3 times/day every 8 h Children (6–10 yr): 50 mg–150 mg/day in divided doses	Least toxic antithyroid drug; administer with meals to reduce GI distress; monitor prothrombin time regularly during therapy, because drug can cause hypoprothrombinemia

DOSAGE
Dose is measured in millicuries (mCi) and varies depending on indication, size of the thyroid, uptake of a small initial tracer dose, and rate of release of radioactive iodine from the gland. Average doses are:

Hyperthyroidism: 4 mCi to 10 mCi as a single dose; a second dose may be given 6 to 12 months later depending on thyroid status

Thyroid carcinoma: 50 mCi to 150 mCi

Usually administered orally as a solution (colorless and tasteless) or as capsules

FATE
Rapidly absorbed when taken orally, and quickly and efficiently concentrated by the thyroid gland as well as by the stomach and salivary glands; radioactivity can be detected in the thyroid within minutes. Half-life of ^{131}I isotope is 8 days. Thyroid function begins to decrease within 2 weeks; maximum effects are observed in 8 to 12 weeks; excreted mainly by the kidneys

COMMON SIDE EFFECTS
Hypothyroidism (see Nursing Alerts), tenderness and soreness over the thyroid area, nausea, dysphagia, cough

SIGNIFICANT ADVERSE REACTIONS
Vomiting, sialoadenitis, thinning of the hair, acute thyroid crisis, chromosomal abnormalities, bone marrow depression, leukemia, anemia, leukopenia, and thrombocytopenia. Destruction of excessive thyroid tissue can lead to symptoms of hypothyroidism such as weakness, fatigue, cold intolerance, peripheral edema, bradycardia, dyspnea, puffiness of the skin, and anginalike pain

CONTRAINDICATIONS
Pregnant and nursing mothers, very young children, preexisting vomiting and diarrhea, and persons with recent myocardial infarction. *Cautious use* in women of childbearing age

INTERACTIONS
Uptake of ^{131}I by thyroid gland can be impaired by recent intake of iodine in any form (e.g., x-ray contrast media; see Chap. 76) or by use of thyroid or antithyroid drugs

NURSING CONSIDERATIONS

Nursing Alerts
- Observe proper procedures for handling and administering radioactive materials.
- Monitor results of thyroid function studies, which should be performed periodically to detect possible development of hypothyroidism.

1. Expect antithyroid drug therapy to be discontinued for 3 to 4 days before administration of radioiodide.
2. Note that solution may darken upon standing, but this does not affect potency.

PATIENT EDUCATION
1. Explain that several treatments with ^{131}I may be required to adequately control hyperthyroidism. If therapy is inadequate, it is usually apparent within 2 to 3 months (patient remains hyperthyroid).
2. Reassure patient that, with usual doses, no special radiation precautions are necessary because radioactivity is minimal.
3. Explain that thyroid hormone replacement therapy may be needed after treatment with ^{131}I to minimize the incidence and severity of hypothyroidism. Hypothyroidism often develops insidiously, but it probably occurs in *almost everyone* receiving ^{131}I. It may not, however, become manifest for years. Stress the importance of continuing thyroid replacement therapy for as long as necessary if hypothyroidism develops.

IODINE/IODIDE COMPOUNDS

Potassium Iodide
Sodium Iodide
Strong Iodine Solution

At one time, iodine and iodide were commonly used for treatment for hyperthyroidism. Despite the rapid beneficial action, effects were short-lived, and within a few weeks symptoms usually returned and in many instances were intensified. Largely for this reason, these drugs have only a limited therapeutic application today; they are primarily used adjunctively to reduce the size and vascularity of the thyroid gland *before thyroidectomy*. In addition, potassium iodide is used in radiation emergencies to block uptake of radioactive iodide by the thyroid gland. Available compounds include strong iodine solution (5% iodine and 10% potassium iodide), sodium iodine injection, saturated solution of potassium iodide (SSKI), and tablets or solution containing potassium iodide in different amounts. The pharmacology of these agents is discussed in general terms and individual drugs are then listed in Table 40-3. In addition, certain iodide-containing products useful as expectorants are detailed in Chapter 54.

MECHANISM
Not completely established; may suppress release of thyroid hormones from thyroglobulin and interfere with synthesis of thyroid hormones; improvement in symptoms is rapid, hence these drugs are of value in treating thyroid storm; reduce size and vascularity of the thyroid gland and increase quantity of bound iodine within the gland

USES
Preparation for thyroidectomy in hyperthyroid patients, in conjunction with an antithyroid drug (reduce size and vascularity of gland)
Acute treatment of thyrotoxic crisis (thyroid storm) or neonatal thyrotoxicosis
Provide a thyroid-blocking action in a radiation emergency
Symptomatic treatment of pulmonary diseases characterized by accumulation of excessive mucus (see Chap. 54)

DOSAGE
See Table 40-3

FATE
Well absorbed when taken orally; effects usually noted within 24 hours to 48 hours and maximal effect occurs within 10 days to 14 days; cleared from plasma primarily by thyroid uptake; eliminated in either urine or feces by way of the bile

COMMON SIDE EFFECTS
Unpleasant metallic taste, GI distress

Table 40-3
Iodine/Iodide Compounds

Drug	Preparations	Usual Dosage Range	Nursing Implications
Potassium iodide Iosat,[a] PIMA, Thyro-Block[a]	Liquid: 500 mg/15 mL Syrup: 325 mg/5 mL Enteric-coated tablets: 300 mg Solution: 21 mg/drop[a] Tablets: 130 mg[a]	Expectorant: 300 mg–1000 mg 2–3 times/day Radiation emergency: Adults— 130 mg daily Children (under age 1)—65 mg daily	Useful for hyperthyroidism, thyrotoxic crisis (with antithyroid drugs), preoperatively for thyroidectomy, and to facilitate bronchial drainage and cough in chronic pulmonary diseases; also used in radiation emergencies to block uptake of radioactive iodine by the thyroid gland; discontinue if skin rash appears; *see also* Chap. 54
Saturated solution potassium iodide SSKI	Solution: 1 g/mL	0.3 mL–0.6 mL 4–12 times/day diluted in water, juice, or milk	Used presurgically for reducing size and fragility of thyroid gland; do not allow to stand uncovered for prolonged periods because solution may evaporate; slight discoloration of solution does not affect potency
Sodium iodide Several manufacturers	Injection: 10%	Thyroid crisis: 2 g/day by IV infusion	Primarily used for acute treatment of thyroid crisis; be alert for development of acute iodism (e.g., metallic taste, stomatitis, sneezing, vomiting, swollen salivary glands), and pulmonary edema
Strong iodine solution Lugol's solution	Solution: 5% iodine and 10% potassium iodide	0.1 mL–0.3 mL (approximately 2–6 drops) 3 times/day (usually for 10–14 days before thyroidectomy)	Principally used to prepare thyroid gland for surgery; also used with an antithyroid drug for treating thyrotoxic crisis; discontinue if signs of iodism appear (see above); administer solution diluted in juice, milk, or water, preferably after meals

[a] Available only to state and federal agencies for radiation emergencies

SIGNIFICANT ADVERSE REACTIONS

Gum soreness, mucosal ulceration, salivary gland enlargement, excessive salivation, rhinitis, fever, joint pain, dyspnea, edema, skin rash, vomiting, headache, and goiter

IV administration can result in acute iodide poisoning, characterized by edema (bronchial, laryngeal); mucosal hemorrhaging; serum sickness; acneiform, maculopapular, vesicular or bullous eruptions; and generalized inflammation.

CONTRAINDICATIONS

Potassium iodide is contraindicated in hyperkalemia; sodium iodide is contraindicated in pulmonary tuberculosis. *Cautious use* in pregnant women

INTERACTIONS

Lithium may enhance the hypothyroid action of potassium iodide

Estrogens and progestins can increase protein-bound iodine

NURSING CONSIDERATIONS

Nursing Alert

- Be alert for development or exacerbation of hyperthyroidism if ^{131}I is given following iodine solution because large amounts of stored hormone may be released if gland is destroyed by radiation.

1. Observe patient for development of goiter. Withdrawal of iodide or administration of thyroid hormone will correct the condition, although the mechanism is incompletely understood.
2. Question administration of ^{131}I to patient recently treated with iodine/iodides because the thyroid gland will be saturated and unable to take up the radioiodide.

PATIENT EDUCATION

1. Warn patient not to indiscriminately use OTC drugs containing iodides (e.g., cough or asthma preparations, salt substitutes) because they may increase response to iodide therapy.
2. Stress the importance of adhering to prescribed dosage regimen when drug is used before thyroidectomy to avoid possible loss of iodide effectiveness and gland enlargement.
3. Advise patient to consult physician concerning need for restriction of iodine-rich foods (e.g., seafoods, vegetables) or iodized salt.

Selected Bibliography

Cooper DS: Antithyroid drugs. N Engl J Med 311:1353, 1984

Dunn JT: Choice of therapy in young adults with hyperthyroidism of Graves' disease: A brief case-directed poll of 54 thyroidologists. Ann Intern Med 100:891, 1984

Evangelisti J, Thorpe C: Thyroid storm—A nursing crisis. Heart Lung 12:184, 1983

Horita A, Carino MA, Lai H: Pharmacology of thyrotropin releasing hormone. Annu Rev Pharmacol Toxicol 26:311, 1986

Larsen PR: Thyroid pituitary interaction: Feedback regulation of thyrotropin secretion by thyroid hormones. N Engl J Med 306:23, 1982

Morkin E, Flink IL, Goldman S: Biochemical and physiological effects of thyroid hormones on cardiac performance. Prog Cardiovasc Dis 25:435, 1983

Murphy D: Iodide—An Rx for radiation accident. Am J Nurs 82:96, 1982

Nunez J, Pommier J: Formation of thyroid hormones. Vitam Horm 39:175, 1982

Oppenheimer JH: Thyroid hormone action at the nuclear level. Ann Intern Med 102:374, 1985

Slingerland DW, Burrows BA: Long-term antithyroid treatment in hyperthyroidism. JAMA 242:2408, 1979

Sterling K: Thyroid hormone action at the cell level. N Engl J Med 300:117, 1979

Wake MM, Brensinger JF: The nurse's role in hypothyroidism. Nurs Clin North Am 15:453, 1980

SUMMARY. THYROID HORMONES AND ANTITHYROID DRUGS

Drug	Preparations	Usual Dosage Range
Thyroid hormones	See Table 40-1	
Antithyroid drugs	See Table 40-2	
Radioactive iodide— ^{131}I Iodotope	Solution or capsules containing a known amount of ^{131}I in mCi suitable for oral or IV administration	Highly variable *Average doses* Hyperthyroidism: 4 mCi to 10 mCi Carcinoma: 50 mCi to 150 mCi
Iodine/iodide products	See Table 40-3	

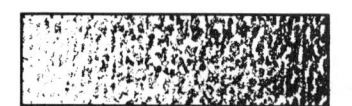

41 PARATHYROID DRUGS, CALCITONIN, AND CALCIUM

Calcium, the most abundant cation in the body, plays an important role in many vital physiological processes, including bone formation, blood coagulation, muscle contraction, nerve conduction, hormone secretion, and enzyme activity. The level of free calcium and phosphate in the blood is dependent on a complex series of interactions among several substances, most important of which are parathyroid hormone (PTH) and vitamin D. PTH is a polypeptide synthesized by the parathyroid glands and is secreted in response to reductions in serum calcium. PTH elevates plasma calcium levels by increasing resorption of calcium ions from bone, by promoting renal tubular reabsorption of calcium, and by enhancing calcium absorption from the GI tract (see Chap. 38). *Vitamin D* is the term commonly applied to two biologically similar substances, ergocalciferol (D_2) and cholecalciferol (D_3). Its major actions on calcium metabolism are essentially identical to those of PTH, namely, increased resorption from bone and enhanced GI absorption. A third endogenous substance, *calcitonin,* can also influence calcium and phosphate metabolism. Calcitonin is a polypeptide secreted by the parafollicular (C) cells of the thyroid gland in response to a rise in serum calcium levels. It lowers serum calcium by inhibiting bone resorption and promotes renal excretion of calcium, probably by interfering with renal tubular reabsorption of the ion.

Serum levels of calcium are normally maintained within a narrow range (10 ± 1 mg/dl) and deviation from this level results in the appearance of symptoms of either hypercalcemia or hypocalcemia. *Hyper*calcemia may be related to hyperparathyroidism, excessive vitamin D intake, malignant tumors, or hyperthyroidism. It is characterized by vomiting, constipation, muscle weakness, electrocardiographic abnormalities, and deposition of calcium in soft tissues such as the kidney. Significant elevations in serum calcium can lead to progressive loss of sensation and eventually coma. Principal causes of *hypo*calcemia are hypoparathyroidism, inadequate vitamin D levels, and dietary calcium deficiency. Symptoms include muscle twitching, tetanic spasms, and convulsions.

Drugs discussed in this chapter are used to regulate body calcium stores, provide replacement for inadequate calcium, and to treat Paget's disease, a decalcification of bone leading to skeletal deformities, joint impairment, and development of vascular fibrous tissue in marrow spaces. Although once used clinically, bovine extracts of parathyroid hormone are no longer available, because tolerance usually developed quickly, and allergic reactions were noted in a number of patients. Synthetic calcitonin and a nonhormonal substance, etidronate, two drugs used in moderate to severe forms of Paget's disease, are reviewed individually below. Mention is also made of plicamycin, an antibiotic used to treat hypercalcemia and hypercalciuria in patients whose condition is not responsive to conventional treatment. Plicamycin is also used to treat testicular tumors, and that aspect of its pharmacology is reviewed in Chapter 72. Oral calcium salts, employed as dietary supplements for calcium deficiency states, are also considered in this chapter. Preparations with vitamin D–like activity (calcifediol, calcitriol, dihydrotachysterol) can be used to control hypocalcemic states related to a number of conditions, and these agents are discussed with the other fat-soluble vitamins in Chapter 74.

Calcitonin, salmon
Calcimar, Miacalcin
Calcitonin, human
Cibacalcin

The calcitonin products available for clinical use are synthetic compounds that resemble the polypeptide hormones of salmon calcitonin and human calcitonin.

Salmon calcitonin is considerably more potent in humans than is human calcitonin, and it is also longer acting, perhaps because it is cleared from the circulatory system more slowly. However, circulating antibodies to salmon calcitonin can form, and its efficacy may decline with continued use. The risk of reduced effectiveness due to antibody formation appears to be less with synthetic human calcitonin, and this product may be effective in patients who have developed resistance to nonhuman calcitonin.

MECHANISM

Decreases serum calcium levels by directly inhibiting osteoclastic bone resorption (effects become less intense with prolonged administration—possibly owing to development of neutralizing antibodies); bone turnover rate is slowed and serum alkaline phosphatase levels fall; increases renal excretion of calcium and phosphorus by blocking their tubular reabsorption; transiently but markedly reduces output of gastric and pancreatic secretions such as hydrochloric acid, gastrin, trypsin, and amylase

USES

Treatment of moderate to severe Paget's disease (osteitis deformans), characterized by polyostotic involvement and elevated serum alkaline phosphatase and urinary hydroxyproline excretion

Treatment of hypercalcemia, especially hypercalcemic emergencies (salmon calcitonin)

Adjunctive treatment of postmenopausal osteoporosis, in conjunction with adequate calcium and vitamin D intake (salmon calcitonin)

DOSAGE
Salmon Calcitonin

Paget's disease: initially 100 U/day SC (preferred) or IM; maintenance 50 U to 100 U daily or on alternate days

Hypercalcemia: initally 4 U/kg/12 hours SC or IM; may increase to 8 U/kg/12 hours after 1 day to 2 days, then to a maximum of 8 U/kg/6 hours if response is still unsatisfactory

Postmenopausal osteoporosis: 100 U/day SC or IM in conjunction with supplemental calcium and an adequate vitamin D intake

Skin testing for allergy: 0.1 mL of a 10-U/mL-dilution intracutaneously of the forearm; appearance of more than mild erythema or wheal indicates a positive allergic response.

Human Calcitonin

Paget's disease: initially 0.5 mg/day SC; usual dosage range is 0.25 mg/day to 0.5 mg 2 to 3 times a week: more severe cases may require 0.5 mg twice a day; treatment may be continued for 6 months

FATE
Calcium-lowering effect occurs within 2 hours after injection and persists for 6 to 8 hours; when given every 12 hours, the calcium-lowering effect lasts for up to 8 days. Calcitonin is rapidly converted to smaller fragments in the kidneys, blood, and other organs, and these fragments are excreted in the urine

COMMON SIDE EFFECTS
Nausea, vomiting, local inflammatory reaction at injection site, facial flushing, paresthesias, urinary frequency

SIGNIFICANT ADVERSE REACTIONS
Diuresis, urticaria, skin rash, diarrhea, abdominal pain, salty taste, chills, dyspnea, dizziness, hypocalcemic tetany. Since calcitonin is a protein, systemic allergic reactions can occur and are more common with salmon calcitonin. In addition, antibodies to calcitonin may form with repeated use, reducing its efficacy. This latter effect is seen more frequently with salmon calcitonin as well.

CONTRAINDICATIONS
In young children, pregnancy, and nursing mothers. *Cautious use* in osteoporosis *without adequate calcium and vitamin D supplementation,* and in persons with renal dysfunction or pernicious anemia

INTERACTIONS
Calcitonin may antagonize the hypercalcemic action of PTH, dihydrotachysterol, and vitamin D
The effects of calcitonin can be augmented by androgens

NURSING CONSIDERATIONS

Nursing Alert
- Ensure that proper materials (e.g., epinephrine, antihistamines, oxygen) are available to treat allergic reactions. Have parenteral calcium available to treat hypocalcemic tetany that may develop, especially during initial stages of therapy.

1. Help evaluate drug effect by monitoring results of serum alkaline phosphatase and 24-hour urinary hydroxyproline levels, which should be measured periodically, and assessing patient for symptoms. Biochemical abnormalities and bone pain should decrease during the first few months of therapy. Dosages beyond 100 U/day do not, however, result in improved clinical response.

PATIENT EDUCATION
1. Teach patient proper technique for handling and injecting drug at home.
2. Reassure patient that the nausea and vomiting that may occur during initial stages of therapy disappear as treatment continues.
3. Stress the importance of continuing therapy even when clinical symptoms have abated.

Etidronate
Didronel
A nonhormonal substance, etidronate acts primarily to reduce the rate of bone turnover. It is principally used orally for symptomatic treatment of Paget's disease

MECHANISM
Absorbs onto calcium hydroxyapatite crystals, disrupting both crystal growth and resorption, depending on concentration of drug; decreases urinary hydroxyproline excretion and serum alkaline phosphatase; also reported to reduce vascularity of Pagetic bone and to decrease elevated cardiac output associated with active Paget's disease

USES
Treatment of moderate to severe Paget's disease (osteitis deformans); symptomatic improvement occurs in approximately three out of five patients
Reduction of heterotopic bone ossification due to spinal cord injury or that complicating total hip replacement
Treatment of hypercalcemia of malignancy (given IV following rehydration and use of loop diuretics to restore urine output)

DOSAGE
Oral
Paget's disease: Initially 5 mg to 10 mg/kg/day for up to 6 months or 11 mg to 20 mg/kg/day for up to 3 months (maximum dose 20 mg/kg/day); retreatment at the same doses may be initiated after at least a 3-month drug-free period if reactivation of the disease has occurred
Heterotopic ossification due to spinal cord injury: 20 mg/day for 2 weeks, followed by 10 mg/kg/day for 10 weeks, instituted as soon as possible following the injury
Heterotopic ossification complicating total hip replacement: 20 mg/kg/day for 1 month preoperatively; then 20 mg/kg/day for 3 months postoperatively
IV Infusion
Hypercalcemia of malignancy: 7.5 mg/kg/day for 3 successive days, given over at least 2 hours. Daily dosage is diluted in at least 250 mL sterile saline; may repeat after 7 days. Oral tablets may be started the day following the last infusion at a dose of 20 mg/kg/day for up to 30 days

FATE
Very poorly absorbed if taken orally (1% at 5 mg/kg); cleared from the blood within 6 hours; one half absorbed dose is excreted in the urine within 24 hours, the remainder being adsorbed onto bone and very slowly eliminated; half-life on bone is 3 to 6 months; unabsorbed drug is eliminated in the feces; most of an infused dose is excreted in the urine

COMMON SIDE EFFECTS
Loose stools, nausea

SIGNIFICANT ADVERSE REACTIONS
Increased bone pain at previously asymptomatic sites, demineralization of bone leading to fractures

CONTRAINDICATIONS
No absolute contraindications. *Cautious use* in patients with renal impairment, enterocolitis, long-bone fractures (may retard fracture healing), in children and in pregnant or nursing women

NURSING CONSIDERATIONS

Nursing Alerts
- Seek clarification if recommended dosage regimen is exceeded because the incidence of untoward reactions

(e.g., GI distress, bone pain, fractures) rises dramatically at elevated doses.
- If fracture occurs, expect drug to be discontinued and resumed only after fracture heals completely.

1. Monitor results of urinary hydroxyproline and serum alkaline phosphatase tests, which should be performed periodically during therapy. Usually, the first evidence of clinical benefit is reduced urinary hydroxyproline excretion. Serum alkaline phosphatase is also lowered by 30% in most patients.
2. Question prophylactic use in asymptomatic patient because there is no evidence to support this. Most patients with mild symptoms can be effectively treated with analgesics.

PATIENT EDUCATION

1. Instruct patient to take drug on an empty stomach, 2 hours before meals, unless GI distress is extreme, because food impairs absorption.
2. Inform patient that response to therapy is gradual and continues for months after drug is stopped. Consequently, dosage is usually increased cautiously, treatment is usually not resumed until evidence of disease recurrence is clear, and therapy should not be reinstituted before at least 3 drug-free months have passed.
3. Stress the need to maintain an adequate intake of calcium and vitamin D through dietary sources, calcium supplementation, or both.

Plicamycin

Mithracin

Plicamycin (also known as mithramycin) is an antibiotic produced by *Streptomyces plicatus*. It is employed by IV infusion to treat hypercalcemia and hypercalciuria in patients whose condition is not responsive to conventional therapy, such as those with advanced neoplasms. Because of its potential to elicit serious toxicity (thrombocytopenia, hemorrhage, liver or kidney dysfunction), however, the drug's potential benefit must be carefully weighed against the risk. Plicamycin is contraindicated in patients with thrombocytopenia, coagulation disorders, increased susceptibility to bleeding, and bone marrow depression. Platelet counts, prothrombin time, and bleeding time must be determined frequently during therapy and for several days following the last dose. Epistaxis or hematemesis may be early indications of a developing hemorrhagic syndrome and should be reported immediately. GI symptoms (nausea, diarrhea, anorexia, stomatitis) represent the most frequent side effects. The recommended dose is 25 µg/kg/day by IV infusion over 4 to 6 hours for 3 or 4 days. If the desired degree of reversal of hypercalcemia is not attained, the dosage may be repeated at intervals of one week or more. Normal calcium balance can often be maintained with single weekly doses or 2 to 3 doses/week. Rapid IV injections should be avoided, because the incidence of GI disturbances is much greater with this method. Extravasation of the solution should be avoided, because local irritation, cellulitis, and possibly thrombophlebitis can occur. Moderate heat applied to the site of extravasation may help disperse the compound and minimize discomfort.

Plicamycin is also employed in the treatment of testicular neoplasms, and that application is considered in detail in Chapter 72.

NURSING CONSIDERATIONS
See Antineoplastic Agents and Natural Products in Chapter 72.

PATIENT EDUCATION
See Antineoplastic Agents and Natural Products in Chapter 72.

ORAL CALCIUM SALTS

Calcium Carbonate
Calcium Glubionate
Calcium Gluconate
Calcium Lactate
Dibasic Calcium Phosphate
Tricalcium Phosphate

Adequate intake of calcium is essential for normal homeostasis and is particularly critical during periods of active bone growth—for example, during childhood, adolescence, pregnancy, or lactation. In addition, sufficient calcium intake is necessary for the prevention and treatment of disease-induced calcium deficiency states such as hypoparathyroidism, postmenopausal osteoporosis, and tetany of the newborn. The use of oral calcium supplements, particularly as they apply to the adjunctive treatment of calcium deficiency states resulting from hypoparathyroidism, is discussed here. In contrast, parenteral therapy with calcium is indicated for treatment of hypocalcemic states requiring a *prompt* elevation in plasma calcium, for example, neonatal tetany, severe vitamin D deficiency, and systemic alkalosis. Parenteral calcium therapy is reviewed along with other parenteral electrolytes in Chapter 75. The pharmacology of the oral calcium preparations is described for the group, then individual drugs are listed in Table 41-1.

MECHANISM
Replace deficient calcium stores in the body; presence of sufficient calcium is essential for bone development, blood coagulation, muscle contraction, cardiac functioning, and many other physiological processes

USES
Prevention or treatment of calcium deficiency states, such as those associated with hypoparathyroidism, osteoporosis, rickets, and osteomalacia

Supplementation of dietary calcium insufficiency such as may occur during childhood, pregnancy, lactation, and in the postmenopausal woman

DOSAGE
See Table 41-1

FATE
Absorption is good when taken orally provided adequate levels of vitamin D and PTH are present; solubility (and thus absorption rate) is increased in acidic pH; excretion occurs largely in urine

COMMON SIDE EFFECTS
Occasional GI distress

Table 41-1
Oral Calcium Salts

Drug	Preparations	Usual Dosage Range	Nursing Implications
Calcium carbonate Several manufacturers	Tablets: 650 mg, 667 mg, 750 mg, 1.25 g, 1.5 g Chewable tablets: 625 mg, 750 mg, 1.25 g, 1.5 g Capsules: 1.5 g Oral suspension: 1.25 g/5mL	1 g–1.5 g 3 times/day (maximum 8 g/day)	Contains 40% calcium; very potent antacid (*see* Chap. 48); high incidence of constipation; tablet may be chewed before swallowing or dissolved in mouth and followed by water
Calcium glubionate Neo-Calglucon	Syrup: 1.8 g/5 mL	Adults: 15 mL, 3 times/day Pregnant women: 15 mL 4 times/day Children: 10 mL 3 times/day Infants: 5 mL 5 times/day	Contains 6.5% calcium; GI disturbances are rare; administer before meals to enhance absorption
Calcium gluconate	Tablets: 500 mg, 650 mg, 975 mg, 1 g	Adults: 1 g–2 g orally 3–4 times/day	Contains 9% calcium; GI irritation is minimal, but drug may be constipating
Calcium lactate	Tablets: 325 mg, 650 mg	325 mg–1.3 g 3 times/day	Contains 13% calcium; tablets may be dissolved in hot water, then cool water added to taste; absorption may be enhanced by lactose; administer with meals
Dibasic calcium phosphate dihydrate (dicalcium phosphate)	Tablets: 486 mg	1–3 tablets 2–3 times/day	Contains 23% calcium; administer with meals
Tricalcium phosphate Posture	Tablets: 300 mg, 600 mg	1–2 tablets 2–4 times/day	Contains 39% calcium

SIGNIFICANT ADVERSE REACTIONS

Hypercalcemia (nausea, vomiting, abdominal pain, constipation, polyuria, fatigue, muscle weakness, bradycardia, arrhythmias, confusion), and hypercalciuria

CONTRAINDICATIONS

Renal calculi, hypercalcemia. *Cautious use* in persons with a history of renal stones, cardiac arrhythmias, or renal insufficiency and to persons receiving digitalis glycosides (see Interactions)

INTERACTIONS

GI absorption of calcium can be enhanced by vitamin D and impaired by corticosteroids, phosphorus (e.g., milk, dairy products), oxalic acid (e.g., spinach, rhubarb), and phytic acid (e.g., bran cereals)

Calcium may reduce the muscle-relaxing effects of neuromuscular blocking agents

Elevated serum calcium levels may increase digitalis toxicity

Oral calcium products can retard the oral absorption of tetracyclines, phenytoin, and iron salts

Calcium may antagonize the action of calcium channel blocking drugs (see Chap. 32)

PATIENT EDUCATION

1. Advise patient to take oral calcium half hour before meals or 1 to 1.5 hours after meals to increase utilization.
2. Explain that frequent blood and urine tests may be required during prolonged therapy to avoid hypercalcemia and hypercalciuria.

Selected Bibliography

Anghileri LJ, Tuffer-Anghileri AM (eds): The Role of Calcium in Biological Systems. Boca Raton, Fla, CRC Press, 1982

Austin LA, Heath H: Calcitonin: Physiology and pathophysiology. N Engl J Med 304:269, 1981

Broadus AE, Rasmussen H: Clinical evaluation of parathyroid function. Am J Med 70:475, 1981

Deftos LJ, First BP: Calcitonin as a drug. Ann Intern Med 95:192, 1981

Elliott GI, KcKenzie MW: Treatment of hypercalcemia. Drug Intell Clin Pharm 17(1):12, 1981

Krane SM: Etidronate disodium in the treatment of Paget's disease of bone. Ann Intern Med 96(5):619, 1982

Neimark J: Beyond calcium: Why milk is just a start. Am Health 5(8):53, 1986

Rosen JF, Chesney RW: Circulating calcitrol concentrations in health and disease. J Pediatr 103:1, 1983

Stewart AF: Therapy of malignancy-associated hypercalcemia. Am J Med 74:475, 1983

Synthetic calcitonin for postmenopausal osteoporosis. Med Lett Drugs Ther 27:53, June, 1985

VanDop C, Bourne HR: Pseudohypoparathyroidism. Annu Rev Med 34:259, 1983

SUMMARY. PARATHYROID DRUGS, CALCITONIN AND CALCIUM

Drug	Preparations	Usual Dosage Range
Calcitonin, salmon Calcimar, Miacalcin	Injection: 100 U/mL, 200 U/mL	100 U/day, SC or IM; maintenance, 50 U–100 U/day or on alternate days Hypercalcemia: 4 U–8 U/kg every 6–12 h SC or IM
Calcitonin, human Cibacalcin	Injection: 0.5 mg/vial	0.5 mg/day SC; range is 0.25 mg/day–0.5 mg twice a day
Etidronate Didronel	Tablets: 200 mg, 400 mg Injection: 300 mg/6 mL	*Oral* Paget's disease: initially 5–10 mg/kg/day for up to 6 mo; retreatment after a 3-mo drug-free period if symptoms return Heterotopic ossification (spinal injury): 20 mg/kg/day for 2 wk then 10 mg/kg/day for 10 wk Heterotopic ossification (hip replacement): 20 mg/kg/day for 1 mo before and 3 mo following surgery *IV* 7.5 mg/kg/day for 3 successive days, given over 2 h; may repeat in 7 days
Plicamycin Mithracin	Injection: 2.5 mg/vial	Hypercalcemia: 0.025 mg/kg/day for 3–4 days; repeat at 1-wk intervals as necessary Testicular carcinoma: 0.025 mg–0.03 mg/kg/day for 8–10 days *or* 0.025 mg to 0.05 mg/kg/day on alternate days for 3 to 8 doses
Oral calcium salts	*See* Table 41-1	

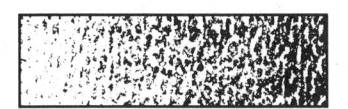

42 ANTIDIABETIC AND HYPERGLYCEMIC AGENTS

Alterations in blood glucose levels can occur in a variety of disease states as well as with the use of many drugs; in most cases these changes represent undesired side effects of the compounds. A few drugs, however, are employed specifically for their ability to lower or raise blood glucose levels and thus are termed *hypoglycemic* and *hyperglycemic agents,* respectively.

Hypoglycemic drugs produce a decline in blood and urinary levels of glucose and are used principally in the treatment of diabetes mellitus, a chronic metabolic disorder characterized by a deficiency of *functional* insulin and elevated levels of glucose in the blood (hyperglycemia) and urine (glycosuria). The etiology and types of diabetes mellitus and the associated metabolic disturbances are reviewed in Chapter 38. Drug therapy of diabetes mellitus may be undertaken by either providing replacement insulin or by oral administration of synthetic sulfonamide-related hypoglycemic drugs (sulfonylureas), which increase release of endogenous insulin and increase the number and affinity of insulin receptors on body cells.

The antidiabetic drugs considered in this chapter include the several kinds of insulin preparations, which are indicated in absolute insulin-deficient forms of diabetes (type I, insulin-dependent diabetes or juvenile-onset diabetes; see Chap. 38) and the oral hypoglycemic drugs, which are used mainly in milder diabetes, frequently associated with obesity, in which insulin levels are near normal but the hormone is relatively ineffective (type II, non-insulin-dependent diabetes or maturity-onset diabetes; see Chap. 38).

Successful treatment of diabetes mellitus, however, requires more than mere drug therapy. Among the many adjunctive measures that should be considered in properly managing the diabetic state are:

- Weight reduction
- Regulation of the diet
- Proper amounts of exercise
- Maintenance of good hygiene
- Education of the patient about proper monitoring procedures to avoid untoward effects.

In fact, milder forms of type II diabetes can be adequately controlled in many instances without resorting to drugs, simply by weight loss and careful regulation of the diet. Drug treatment of diabetes mellitus, when necessary, is a highly individual matter and requires accurate diagnosis, continual monitoring of the patient, and proper drug dosage modifications as necessitated by changes in patient status.

On the other hand, drugs that elevate blood glucose levels can be employed to reverse hypoglycemia resulting from diseases (such as pancreatic carcinoma, hormonal imbalances, liver and kidney dysfunction) or antidiabetic drug overdosage. Parenteral glucose is the most effective agent for elevating blood glucose levels and should be employed in acute situations whenever feasible. Glucagon, a purified peptide extracted from pancreatic alpha (A) cells; diazoxide, a thiazide derivative that blocks insulin release; and oral administration of glucose as a gel or chewable tablet may also be employed. These compounds are also reviewed in this chapter.

INSULINS

Insulin injection
Insulin Zinc suspension
Insulin Zinc suspension, extended
Insulin Zinc suspension, prompt
Isophane Insulin suspension
Protamine Zinc Insulin suspension

Endogenous insulin is a 51 amino acid polypeptide hormone secreted by the beta (B) cells of the islets of Langerhans of the pancreas. The clinically available insulin preparations include purified extracts from beef or pork pancreas that possess biological effects qualitatively identical to those of human insulin, differing from human insulin by only three (beef) or one (pork) amino acid in the sequence. In addition, *"human"* insulin (i.e., having the *exact* amino acid sequence of endogenous insulin) is now available; it is derived by either recombinant DNA techniques utilizing strains of *Escherichia coli* or chemical modification of animal-extracted pork insulin to replace the lone amino acid that is different from that of human insulin.

All commercially available insulins extracted from animal sources contain certain quantities of the prohormone proinsulin and possibly other proteins or substances resulting from incomplete conversion of the prohormone. These "contaminants" may contribute to the immunogenic reactions that some insulin users experience, such as lipodystrophy and other local and systemic allergic reactions. Generally, beef-derived insulins are somewhat more immunologic than pork-derived products. All commercially available insulins in the United States contain less than 25 parts per million (ppm) of proinsulin and are termed *single-peak* insulins because their purification by gel chromatography yields a single spectrographic peak

Purification techniques used to remove the allergenic contaminants have been refined to the point that a new class of further purified single-peak insulins is available. These products, indicated by the term *purified insulin* on the label, contain less than 10 ppm of proinsulin and may elicit even fewer allergic reactions in hypersensitive patients than conventional single-peak insulins. The newer "human" insulins, as indicated above, are prepared synthetically and are virtually free of contaminants. They appear to be as effective as the conventional insulins and may be less immunogenic than the beef or pork insulins in certain patients because of their lack of contaminants.

Most diabetic patients do equally well on conventional single-peak insulin or purified insulin. Generally, candidates for the purified insulins are those patients who exhibit local or systemic allergic reactions or severe lipodystrophy with conventional insulin preparations. A few patients may require dosage adjustments when switched from conventional to highly purified insulins, because the highly purified preparations are less bound by insulin antibodies. All stabilized diabetic patients being switched to a purified insulin preparation should be monitored closely to determine if a dosage modification is required. The possible advantages of human insulin over purified porcine insulin remain to be definitely established, and the number of patients who absolutely require human insulin remains quite small. Should the methods for synthesizing human insulins become more cost-effective than animal-extraction procedures over time, however, the use of human insulin products will greatly increase.

Several types of insulin preparations are available in addition to regular insulin. These modified forms of insulin have been formulated to display differences in onset, peak, and duration of action, thereby allowing the physician to carefully control the response in each patient. The time course of action of the different insulins is largely dependent on the physical properties of the different preparations, such as the presence of conjugating metals or proteins (e.g., zinc, protamine), the types of buffers used, and the pH of the medium. Thus, insulin preparations can conveniently be divided into three groups according to their onset and duration of action. This classification is outlined in Table 42-1, where several characteristics of the different insulins are listed. All available insulin preparations are presented in Table 42-2, where specific indications and other pertinent information are given for each individual drug.

Insulin preparations are standardized on the basis of their hypoglycemic action in fasted rabbits, and doses are measured in units (U). One insulin unit (U) possesses the activity of 1/24 mg of Zinc Insulin Crystals Reference Standard. Insulin is marketed in 10-mL vials containing 40 U/mL or 100 U/mL as well as a 20-mL concentrated solution containing 500 U/mL. The U100 insulins have virtually replaced the older U40 insulins today, because they allow for greater ease in measuring the correct dosage. Most insulin preparations available today are stable at room temperature, unlike the older preparations which had to be refrigerated; however, it is probably still advisable to store the bottle in the refrigerator. In addition, the mixing of certain types of insulins in the same syringe can now be accomplished without incompatibility problems (see Dosage).

MECHANISM
Facilitates uptake of glucose by cells of striated muscle and adipose tissue, probably by activating a carrier system for transport of glucose across the cell membrane; stimulates glycogen synthesis in muscle and liver by increasing enzyme activity, and suppresses gluconeogenesis; enhances formation of triglycerides and retards release of free fatty acids from adipose tissue; facilitates incorporation of amino acids into muscle protein and may thus promote protein synthesis; restoration of efficient glucose utilization decreases hyperglycemia, reduces glucosuria, and prevents diabetic acidosis and coma

USES
Treatment of diabetes mellitus, especially the insulin-dependent (type I) type and complicated forms of non-insulin dependent (i.e., maturity-onset; type II) diabetes not adequately controlled by diet and weight loss

Emergency treatment of severe ketoacidosis or diabetic coma (regular insulin, IM or IV)

Induction of hypoglycemic shock for therapy of certain psychiatric states (essentially obsolete)

DOSAGE
Must be individually titrated on the basis of blood glucose, urinary glucose, and ketone determinations. The various insulin preparations are listed in Table 42-2 along with their source and nursing implications. The drug is given SC, and sites of administration are rotated to minimize the occurrence of lipodystrophy (localized hollowing of the skin at injection sites, presumably because of alterations in lipid metabolism).

Preparations available as suspensions should be rolled gently between the hands before administration to facilitate uniform dispersion; vigorous shaking should be avoided, because frothing may lead to withdrawal of improper amounts of drug for injection.

Compatability of Admixtures
Certain types of insulin may be mixed in the same syringe. If regular insulin is used, it should always be drawn into the syringe first. Regular insulin may be mixed with protamine zinc insulin in any proportion. Mixtures of regular insulin with NPH or lente insulins should be injected immediately

Table 42-1
Characteristics of Insulin Preparations

Drug	Synonym	Onset	Peak Action	Duration
Rapid Acting				
Insulin injection	Regular insulin	½ hour to 1 hour	2 hours to 4 hours	6 hours to 8 hours
Insulin zinc suspension, prompt	Semilente insulin	½ hour to 1 hour	4 hours to 8 hours	12 hours to 16 hours
Intermediate Acting				
Insulin zinc suspension	Lente insulin	1 hour to 2 hours	8 hours to 14 hours	18 hours to 24 hours
Isophane insulin suspension	NPH insulin	1 hour to 1½ hours	6 hours to 12 hours	18 hours to 24 hours
Long Acting				
Insulin zinc suspension, extended	Ultralente insulin	4 hours to 8 hours	12 hours to 24 hours	30 hours to 36 hours
Protamine zinc insulin suspension	Protamine zinc insulin (PZI)	4 hours to 8 hours	14 hours to 20 hours	30 hours to 36 hours

Note: A 70/30 mixture of isophane insulin suspension and regular insulin injection is also available; onset is ½ hour, peak effect is within 4 hours to 8 hours and duration is 18 hours to 24 hours. In addition, a 50/50 mixture of regular insulin injection and isophane insulin suspension is available in Canada, providing faster peak blood levels and a shorter duration of action than the 70/30 mixture.

after mixing, as some regular insulin is bound to either protamine or zinc within the first 15 minutes, possibly altering the onset and duration of action. Semilente, lente, and ultralente insulins may be combined in any proportion, since they are chemically identical.

Insulin can adsorb onto plastic IV infusion sets; the extent of adsorption is approximately 20% to 30% and is inversely proportional to the concentration of insulin. If insulin is administered in this manner, the patient's response should be closely monitored.

FATE
Inactivated when taken orally; absorbed at varying rates from SC injection sites (see Table 42-1 for onset, peak action, and duration of effect); plasma half-life is less than 10 minutes; metabolized by both the liver and the kidneys and excreted in the feces and to a small extent in the urine

COMMON SIDE EFFECTS
Mild hypoglycemia (fatigue, headache, drowsiness, nausea, mild tremor), local allergic reactions at injection site (itching, swelling, erythema)

SIGNIFICANT ADVERSE REACTIONS
Marked hypoglycemia (sweating, tremor, hypothermia, weakness, hunger, palpitations, nervousness, paresthesias, irritability, blurred vision, numbness in mouth, confusion, delirium, convulsions, and loss of consciousness)

Systemic allergic reactions (urticaria, angioedema, anaphylactic episodes), lipodystrophy at injection sites, insulin resistance, and visual disturbances

CONTRAINDICATIONS
Hypersensitivity to specific animal proteins (e.g., bovine, porcine)

INTERACTIONS
Hypoglycemia may be augmented by alcohol, anabolic steroids, anticoagulants, oral hypoglycemics, antineoplastics, monoamine oxidase (MAO) inhibitors, fenfluramine, guanethidine, phenylbutazone, sulfinpyrazone, tetracycline, beta blockers, and salicylates

The hypoglycemic effects of insulin can be antagonized by corticosteroids, thiazide diuretics, dextrothyroxine, dobutamine, diazoxide, epinephrine, estrogens, glucagon, oral contraceptives, phenytoin, and thyroid preparations

Insulin may lower serum potassium levels and can increase the toxicity of digitalis glycosides

NURSING CONSIDERATIONS
See **Plan of Nursing Care** 10 in this chapter. In addition:

Nursing Alert
- Closely monitor patient receiving insulin through a plastic IV infusion set to ensure adequate response because the plastic surface can adsorb 25% to 50% of the dose.

1. Store insulin vials in a cool place. Avoid freezing or high temperatures and protect from strong light.
2. Avoid injecting cold insulin because lipodystrophy and reduced absorption can result.
3. To ensure proper dispersion of particles in suspension preparations, rotate vial and invert end to end several times just before withdrawing each dose. Do *not* shake vigorously because frothing may occur, which could result in withdrawal of an inadequate dose. Regular insulin, which is a solution, does not contain particles.
4. When mixing regular insulin with another insulin in one syringe, withdraw appropriate volume of regular insulin first to avoid contaminating vial of regular insulin, which does not contain protein (i.e., protamine), with insulin that does contain protein (see Table 42-2 for protein content and mixture compatability of different insulins).
5. If regular insulin is mixed with NPH or lente insulin, use immediately because mixture may not be stable beyond 10 to 15 minutes.
6. Administer insulin 15 to 90 minutes before a meal, depending on type (see Table 42-2). If a dose is withheld for any reason, decrease food intake and increase fluid intake.
7. Inject SC into areas with substantial fatty layers.
8. Systematically rotate injection sites to minimize trauma and lipodystrophy at particular sites.
9. Observe injection site for local allergic reaction. Although symptoms usually disappear with continued use, an antihistamine may be used to alleviate local discomfort. Allergic reactions can also be minimized by using pork insulin instead of either beef or mixtures of beef and pork (or vice versa). Switching to the corresponding purified or human insulin are additional alternatives.
10. Discard discolored or clumped solutions or partially used vials that have been open for several weeks.

PATIENT EDUCATION
1. Teach patient techniques involved in insulin administration.
2. Ensure that patient always administers insulin with syringe that corresponds with the strength of the insulin to avoid incorrect dosage. Vial labels and syringe calibrations are color-coded red (U40) and black (U100).
3. Advise patient to carry a sufficient supply of syringes and needles when traveling and to store insulin vial in a cool place.
4. Inform patient that visual disturbances may occur during initial therapy. Eyeglass prescriptions should not be changed for at least several weeks after therapy has been initiated.
5. Warn patient not to use any other medications without consulting the primary health care provider.

ORAL ANTIDIABETIC DRUGS

Acetohexamide
Chlorpropamide
Glipizide
Glyburide
Tolazamide
Tolbutamide

The orally effective antidiabetic agents are sulfonamide derivatives classified as sulfonylureas. The clinically useful oral antidiabetics have similar mechanisms of action, that is, release of endogenous insulin from functional beta cells in the pancreas and enhanced sensitivity of insulin receptor sites on cellular

(Text continued on page 436)

PLAN OF NURSING CARE 10
PATIENTS TREATED WITH ANTIDIABETIC AGENTS

Nursing Diagnosis: Potential Complication: Hypoglycemia secondary to antidiabetic drug therapy
Goal: Hypoglycemia in patient taking antidiabetic agent will be controlled.

Intervention	Rationale	Expected Outcome
Monitor results of serum glucose determinations.	Symptoms of hypoglycemia appear with serum glucose levels below 50 mg/mL.	Low serum glucose will be noted.
Monitor patient for signs and symptoms of hypoglycemia, which include sympathetic and CNS responses: nausea, hunger, dizziness, a vague sense of apprehension, palpitations, tremor, headache, pallor, cool skin, sweating, irritability, agitation, confusion, apathy, double or blurred vision, weakness, and ataxia. Late developments include lethargy, stupor, seizures, coma, and death.	Hypoglycemia triggers epinephrine secretion, which activates the sympathetic nervous system. Because the brain is so dependent on glucose to satisfy its energy requirements, it is particularly vulnerable to glucose deprivation.	Hypoglycemia will be detected promptly.
If mild hypoglycemia develops, have patient ingest food or fluid that contains approximately 10 g of soluble glucose (see below).	Hypoglycemic symptoms are quickly relieved by oral administration of soluble carbohydrates.	Patient's symptoms of hypoglycemia will resolve.
If hypoglycemia is severe: 1. Immediately report patient's condition to appropriate health care provider. 2. Be prepared to administer 10% to 50% glucose IV after blood sample has been drawn to determine glucose level. 3. Be prepared to provide oral carbohydrate supplements as soon as patient is able to ingest them.	If patient is unable to ingest oral carbohydrates, glucose is administered IV. To prevent secondary hypoglycemia, oral carbohydrates are given as soon as possible.	Patient will receive treatment to correct severe hypoglycemia.
Explain to patient why excessive consumption of alcohol should be avoided.	Alcohol may intensify and prolong the effect of hypoglycemic drugs.	Patient will explain the effect of alcohol on blood sugar.
Provide patient with a list of drugs that may add to the hypoglycemic effect of the prescribed drug.	Some drugs, if taken in conjunction with drugs prescribed for diabetes, may intensify their hypoglycemic effect.	Patient will possess list of drugs that lower blood sugar.
Teach patient to recognize symptoms of hypoglycemia (see above).	Symptoms of hypoglycemia progress rapidly. The patient must be able to recognize them quickly in order to institute treatment promptly.	Patient will describe symptoms of hypoglycemia.
Teach patient the timing of the peak effect of prescribed antidiabetic agent; instruct patient to be particularly alert for symptoms of hypoglycemia around this time.	Hypoglycemia is more likely to occur during the drug's peak effect.	Patient will state timing of peak effect and will explain how this relates to hypoglycemia.
Advise patient to carry, or have access to at all times, a source of about 10 g of glucose, such as 2 sugar lumps, 2 or 3 pieces of hard candy, 5 or 6 Lifesaver candies, 4 oz fruit juice or ginger ale, or 1 to 2 tsp of sugar, syrup, honey, or jelly. Products containing 40% glucose as a tablet or a gel (e.g., Glutose, Insta-Glucose, Monojel, B-D Glucose) are also available.	Hypoglycemic reactions should be treated when symptoms are first noted.	Patient will express understanding of need for immediate access to source of soluble glucose and will name at least four sources and corresponding amounts of carbohydrate that meet this need.
Instruct patient to immediately ingest source of glucose if symptoms of hypoglycemia develop, to repeat this in 10 to 15 minutes, if necessary, and to eat slowly absorbed carbohydrate and protein foods such as milk, cheese, and bread after symptoms dissipate.	Treatment of hypoglycemia requires administration of fast-acting carbohydrates followed by slower-acting carbohydrates to replace glycogen stores in the liver and to prevent secondary hypoglycemia from rapid depletion of carbohydrates ingested earlier.	Patient will describe what to do if symptoms of hypoglycemia develop.

Continued

PLAN OF NURSING CARE 10
PATIENTS TREATED WITH ANTIDIABETIC AGENTS (continued)
Nursing Diagnosis: Potential Complication: Hypoglycemia secondary to antidiabetic drug therapy
Goal: Hypoglycemia in patient taking antidiabetic agent will be controlled.

Intervention	Rationale	Expected Outcome
Instruct patient to contact appropriate health care provider if hypoglycemic symptoms fail to subside within 30 minutes after ingestion of carbohydrates.	Prolonged hypoglycemia is associated with diminished oxygen consumption and irreparable nervous system damage.	Patient will explain what to do if hypoglycemic symptoms fail to subside.
Instruct patient to notify appropriate health care provider if hypoglycemic episodes occur frequently.	Dosage adjustment or interventions to correct noncompliance or knowledge deficits may be needed.	Patient will state what to do if hypoglycemic episodes recur.

Nursing Diagnosis: Potential Complication: Ketoacidosis secondary to inadequate antidiabetic drug control
Goal: Ketoacidosis in patient taking antidiabetic agent will be controlled.

Intervention	Rationale	Expected Outcome
Monitor intake and output, urinary glucose and ketone levels, and results of blood sugar determinations. Report signs of hyperglycemia to appropriate health care provider.	With careful monitoring, antidiabetic therapy can be adjusted as needs change. In hyperglycemia, the frequency and quantity of fluid intake and output increase, urine may contain glucose and ketones, and blood sugar is elevated.	Signs of hyperglycemia will be noted.
Monitor patient for indications of ketoacidosis: polyuria, polydipsia, polyphagia, headache, fatigue, drowsiness, weight loss, fruity odor on breath (acetone), nausea, vomiting, abdominal pain, diarrhea, blurred vision, irritability, numbness of fingers and toes, flushing, skin warm and dry, Kussmaul respirations, tachycardia, hypotension, temperature elevation, coma.	Insulin deficiency causes hyperglycemia and deprives cells of glucose. When this happens, metabolism of lipids in adipose tissue and proteins in muscle cells is accelerated to meet energy requirements. Ketones, a product of this metabolism, lead to acidosis and acetone formation. Acidosis and, to a lesser extent, cellular dehydration and electrolyte depletion ultimately result in coma.	Symptoms of ketoacidosis will be detected promptly.
If indications of ketoacidosis occur:		
1. Immediately report patient's condition to appropriate health care provider.		Patient's ketoacidosis will be treated.
2. Prepare to administer regular insulin injection IV (if necessary, 1 g of dextrose may be added for each unit of insulin administered).	In an acute situation, such as acidosis or severe hyperglycemia, prompt insulin action is required. Regular insulin, which is fast-acting and can be given IV, is the drug of choice. Longer-acting preparations should not be used.	
3. Check vital signs frequently until stable.		
4. Monitor results of serum potassium determinations.	Serum potassium levels increase in ketoacidosis as hydrogen ions are exchanged for intracellular potassium. Hydrogen ions enter cells, potassium ions leave.	Serum potassium abnormalities will be noted.
5. Be prepared to administer supplemental potassium as blood glucose falls.	As acidemia is corrected, hypokalemia may develop because potassium shifts from intravascular back to intracellular compartments.	Patient's hypokalemia will be treated.
Teach patient and significant others to recognize symptoms of hyperglycemia, and stress the importance of immediately reporting these to appropriate health care provider.	Although acidosis develops slowly over a period of days, hyperglycemia, which reflects inadequate control of diabetes with the current drug regimen, should be treated as quickly as possible.	Patient and significant others will state symptoms of hyperglycemia and explain what to do if they occur.

Continued

PLAN OF NURSING CARE 10
PATIENTS TREATED WITH ANTIDIABETIC AGENTS (continued)

Nursing Diagnosis: Potential Complication: Ketoacidosis secondary to inadequate antidiabetic drug control
Goal: Ketoacidosis in patient taking antidiabetic agent will be controlled.

Intervention	Rationale	Expected Outcome
Instruct patient to be particularly alert for evidence of hyperglycemia and to notify appropriate health care provider if major changes in living patterns (physical, emotional, situational, or maturational stressors) occur.	Numerous internal and external influences affect blood glucose levels. Because several hormones elevate blood glucose, including cortisol, epinephrine, growth hormone, estrogen, and progesterone, events such as rapid growth, emotional upset, pregnancy, injury, infection, illness, and surgery can precipitate ketoacidosis, especially in juveniles. Additional or supplemental insulin may be required at such times for patients taking insulin or an oral antidiabetic agent.	Patient will explain what to do if life stressors change greatly.
Provide patient with list of drugs that may increase amount of antidiabetic drug required to control blood glucose.	Drugs that increase the amount of antidiabetic drug required to control blood sugar may induce hyperglycemia.	Patient will possess list of drugs that elevate blood sugar.

Nursing Diagnosis: Potential Knowledge Deficit related to antidiabetic drug therapy
Goal: Patient will possess knowledge and skills needed to implement antidiabetic drug therapy and related actions.

Intervention	Rationale	Expected Outcome
See also **Plan of Nursing Care 1 (Knowledge Deficit)** and **2 (Noncompliance).**		
Assist patient to develop plans to stabilize the following: 1. Amount of antidiabetic drug taken and dosage schedule 2. Amount and type of food intake 3. Intervals between food intake 4. Level of exercise 5. Emotional state	Stabilization of these factors helps avert uneven results from dosage of antidiabetic agent by minimizing significant fluctuations in blood glucose. Excessive insulin, reduced food intake, or increased exercise reduce blood glucose. Converse changes may increase blood glucose.	Patient will discuss plans to stabilize factors that affect serum glucose level.
Teach patient how to take insulin, even if oral antidiabetic drug is prescribed.	The patient taking an oral antidiabetic drug may need to administer insulin in an emergency.	Patient will demonstrate correct techniques for insulin self-administration.
Teach patient how to monitor blood glucose and urine glucose and ketones.	Blood glucose and urine glucose and ketone determinations enable the patient to gauge the adequacy of drug control and, for the patient on insulin, to adjust dosage accordingly.	Patient will demonstrate proper procedures for urine and blood glucose monitoring.
Provide patient with a list of drugs that may cause false positive readings for the type of urine or serum glucose test patient is using.	A variety of drugs may cause false readings for certain types of urine or serum glucose tests.	Patient will possess list of drugs that affect urine or serum glucose test results.
Instruct patient to take only drugs prescribed by health care provider who is aware that patient is diabetic.	Antidiabetic agents interact with many other drugs including many OTC preparations, that can either enhance or reduce their effect.	Patient will state action to be taken before using any new drug.
Warn patient taking oral antidiabetic drug to eliminate alcohol consumption.	A disulfiram-like reaction, resulting in vomiting, tachycardia, headache, hypertension, and sweating, may occur if alcohol is ingested by a person taking an oral antidiabetic drug.	Patient will state that alcohol should not be consumed.
Stress the importance of weight control and careful adherence to prescribed diet to successful control of blood sugar.	Normal weight and controlled caloric intake decrease the need for medication and allow the body to use insulin more efficiently.	Patient will verbalize importance of weight control and diet in management of diabetes.

Continued

PLAN OF NURSING CARE 10
PATIENTS TREATED WITH ANTIDIABETIC AGENTS (continued)
Nursing Diagnosis: Potential Knowledge Deficit related to antidiabetic drug therapy
Goal: Patient will possess knowledge and skills needed to implement antidiabetic drug therapy and related actions.

Intervention	Rationale	Expected Outcome
Refer patient to dietitian for instruction regarding prescribed diet.		Patient will receive dietary instruction.
Advise patient to remain under continuous health care supervision.	Drug requirements can change frequently.	Patient will verbalize importance of continuous medical supervision.
Suggest that patient carry some form of medical identification at all times stating condition, drugs taken, dosages, and name and location of primary health care provider.	In an emergency, appropriate treatment can be provided if patient carries medical identification.	Patient will verbalize value of carrying medical identification.

Table 42-2
Insulin Preparations

Drug	Preparations and Sources	Nursing Implications
Rapid Acting		
Insulin injection Regular Insulin, Regular Iletin I **Purified** Regular Purified Pork, Regular Iletin II, Velosulin **Human** Novolin R, Humulin R, Velosulin Human	Injection: 40 U/mL, 100 U/mL (pork, beef and pork) Purified injection: 100 U/mL (beef, pork) Human: 100 U/mL	Short acting; solution is clear; may be administered SC 15–30 min before meals for control of diabetes or IV (only insulin suitable for IV use) for severe ketoacidosis or diabetic coma; give 1 g dextrose/U insulin when administered IV, and monitor blood sugar, blood pressure, and intake/output ratio every hour until stable; be alert for development of rapid hypoglycemia and insulin shock
Insulin injection, concentrated Regular Concentrated Iletin II	Purified injection: 500 U/mL (pork)	Indicated for control of diabetes in patients with marked insulin resistance; may be administered SC or IM; concentrated from pork pancreas, solution is clear and colorless; accuracy in dosage is essential because of potency; marked hypoglycemia can occur
Insulin zinc suspension, prompt Semilente Iletin I, Semilente Insulin **Purified** Semilente Purified Pork	Injection: 40 U/mL, 100 U/mL (beef, beef and pork) Purified injection—100 U/mL (pork)	Suspension of small particles of insulin and zinc chloride; solution is cloudy; administered SC 30 min before meals, usually breakfast; may be mixed only with other lente insulins; mix thoroughly by rolling vial and inverting end to end; do not shake; if suspension is granular or clumped, discard vial
Intermediate Acting		
Insulin zinc suspension Lente Iletin I, Lente Insulin **Purified** Lente Iletin II, Lente Purified Pork **Human** Humulin L, Novolin L	Injection: 40 U/mL, 100 U/mL (beef, beef and pork) Purified injection: 100 U/mL (beef, pork) Human: 100 U/mL	Cloudy suspension containing a mixture of 30% prompt zinc suspension and 70% extended zinc suspension; contains no proteins, thus allergic reactions are rare; administered SC 30–60 min before breakfast; action closely approximates that of NPH insulin, although duration of action may be slightly longer; *see* insulin zinc suspension, prompt for mixing instructions and compatabilities

Continued

Table 42-2
Insulin Preparations (continued)

Drug	Preparations and Sources	Nursing Implications
Isophane insulin suspension NPH insulin, NPH Iletin I **Purified** Insulatard NPH, NPH Iletin II, NPH Purified Pork **Human** Humulin N, Novolin N	Injection: 40 U/mL, 100 U/mL (beef, beef and pork) Purified injection: 100 U/mL (beef, pork) Human: 100 U/mL	Suspension of protamine zinc insulin crystals; administered SC 30 min before breakfast; a second injection in the evening may be required; *see* insulin zinc suspension, prompt for mixing instructions; may be mixed with regular insulin injection, but not lente forms; available in fixed combination with regular insulin injection (70%/30%) as Mixtard, Novolin (70/30), Humulin 70/30 and Mixtard Human 70/30.
Long Acting		
Insulin zinc suspension, extended Ultralente Iletin I, Ultralente Insulin **Purified** Ultralente Purified Beef **Human** Humulin U	Injection: 40 U/mL, 100 U/mL (beef, beef and pork) Purified injection: 100 U/mL (beef) Human: 100 U/mL	Cloudy suspension of large particles of zinc insulin, which delay absorption and prolong effects; no protein and low incidence of allergic reactions; administered SC 30–90 min before breakfast; may be mixed with other lente preparations
Protamine zinc insulin suspension Protamine, Zinc and Iletin I **Purified** Protamine, Zinc and Iletin II	Injection: 40 U/mL, 100 U/mL (beef and pork) Purified injection: 100 U/mL (beef, pork)	Cloudy suspension of fine particles of protamine zinc insulin; administered 30–60 min before breakfast; duration of action may exceed 36 h; balanced diet and regular meals are essential; may be mixed with regular insulin only; clinical effects may be delayed several days, supplemental doses of regular insulin may be needed during that time; hypoglycemia may be gradual in onset and often unnoticed

membranes. However, they display significant differences in the duration of their hypoglycemic action. These differences are detailed in Table 42-3, which lists the available drugs, dosages, and other pertinent characteristics.

The principal indication for the oral antidiabetic agents is management of mild, stable, non-insulin-dependent, maturity-onset (type II) diabetes that cannot be adequately controlled by diet alone. They are of no value in type I, insulin-dependent diabetes, nor in those forms of diabetes complicated by ketoacidosis.

This cautious approach to oral antidiabetic drug therapy has evolved from earlier reports of increased cardiovascular mortality in patients receiving oral antidiabetic drugs compared to patients being controlled with diet or diet plus insulin. Although the conclusions of this study conducted in a number of American clinics some years ago have been challenged, largely the basis of faulty experimental design, the status of oral antidiabetic drugs is still somewhat uncertain. General guidelines for use of oral antidiabetic drugs in type II diabetes are onset of diabetes at age 40 or greater and duration of diabetes of less than 5 years, absence of ketoacidosis and renal or hepatic dysfunction, fasting serum glucose of less than 200 mg/dL, and insulin requirements of less than 40 U/day.

Although the pharmacology of all the oral sulfonylurea drugs is rather similar, certain distinctions can be made among some of the drugs. Therefore, they have been categorized as first generation (acetohexamide, chlorpropamide, tolazamide, tolbutamide) and second generation (glipizide, glyburide) drugs.

Second generation drugs are more lipophilic and and possess a higher intrinsic potency (i.e., are used in lower doses), and they appear to be less easily displaced from protein binding sites than the first generation drugs. The following discussion pertains to all of the sulfonylurea agents; individual drugs are then listed in Table 42-3.

MECHANISM
Stimulate release of preformed endogenous insulin from functional beta cells in the pancreas; also appear to increase the number and sensitivity of insulin receptor sites on tissues, thus increasing the utilization of available insulin; may inhibit hepatic glucose production and reduce serum glucagon concentrations

USES
Treatment of stable, nonketotic, or nonacidotic type II (non-insulin-dependent) diabetes mellitus not adequately controlled by diet and weight reduction
Adjunct to insulin in certain types of *insulin-dependent* diabetes (allows reduced insulin dosage)
Diagnosis of pancreatic insulinoma (tolbutamide)
Adjunctive treatment of diabetes insipidus (chlorpropamide *only*)

DOSAGE
See Table 42-3

FATE

Drugs are well absorbed orally, tolazamide being the most slowly absorbed and having the slowest onset of action (4–6 h) compared to the other drugs (1–2 h); all are highly bound to plasma proteins, the first generation agents being less strongly bound than the second generation drugs; metabolized in the liver to both active and inactive metabolites which are excreted primarily in the urine, except for glyburide, whose metabolites are eliminated in both the bile and urine. *Tolbutamide* is the shortest acting oral hypoglycemic drug (6–12 h) and is given 2 to 3 times a day. The duration of action of *chlorpropamide* is up to 60 hours, whereas the remaining drugs exhibit durations of action ranging from 12 to 24 hours

COMMON SIDE EFFECTS

Mild hypoglycemia (fatigue, drowsiness, headache, weakness, hunger, nervousness), GI distress (anorexia, nausea, abdominal cramps, heartburn)

SIGNIFICANT ADVERSE REACTIONS

Severe hypoglycemia (tachycardia, vomiting, diarrhea, sweating, blurred vision, irritability, delirium, convulsions), dizziness, edema, and hyponatremia

Dermatologic: urticaria, pruritus, photosensitivity, morbilliform or maculopapular rash, erythema multiforme, exfoliative dermatitis

Hepatic: cholestatic jaundice, altered liver function tests, hepatic porphyria

Hematologic (rare): thrombocytopenia, leukopenia, mild anemia, eosinophilia, agranulocytosis

CONTRAINDICATIONS

Insulin-dependent diabetes; severe hepatic or renal dysfunction; uremia; ketosis; acidosis; coma; pregnancy; *severe* cases of stress, fever, infection, or trauma; and before surgery. *Cautious use* in patients with cardiac impairment or adrenal or thyroid dysfunction, in women of childbearing age, in elderly or debilitated patients, and in alcoholics

INTERACTIONS

Effects of oral antidiabetic drugs may be prolonged or enhanced by oral anticoagulants, alcohol, allopurinol, antiinflammatory drugs, chloramphenicol, insulin, MAO inhibitors, probenecid, salicylates, sulfonamides, and other highly protein-bound drugs

Effects of oral antidiabetic drugs may be reduced by beta blockers, calcium channel blockers, diazoxide, estrogens, glucocorticoids, phenobarbital, phenothiazines, phenytoin, sympathomimetics, thiazide diuretics, and thyroxine

Alcohol may elicit a disulfiram-like toxic reaction in patients taking oral antidiabetics (see Chap. 78), and may also produce photosensitivity reactions

Chlorpropamide and possibly other sulfonylureas may prolong the effects of barbiturates

Oral hypoglycemics may increase the metabolism of digoxin

NURSING CONSIDERATIONS

See **Plan of Nursing Care 10** in this chapter. In addition:

Nursing Alerts

- Collaborate with patient and health care team to carefully weigh benefit versus risk before oral antidiabetic drugs are prescribed. Although its controversial results have not been replicated, results of one study showed a higher mortality from cardiovascular disease in patients receiving oral antidiabetic agents than in those treated with diet alone or diet plus insulin.
- When therapy is begun in elderly patient, carefully monitor results of blood and urine glucose tests, which should be obtained daily. Dosage should be adjusted accordingly. Low dosages should be used initially because hyper-responsiveness has been reported.
- Observe patient closely if patient is being transferred from insulin to oral antidiabetic drug. Dosages should be adjusted gradually to avoid precipitating ketosis, acidosis, or coma unless insulin dosage has been 20 U/day or less, in which case it may be discontinued abruptly. Urine should be tested frequently during transition. No transitional period is required when switching between different oral antidiabetic agents. Oral antidiabetic agents are *not*, however, insulin substitutes and should never be employed alone in insulin-dependent diabetes.

1. Administer in the morning whenever possible to minimize nocturnal hypoglycemia. Give with food to decrease GI upset.

PATIENT EDUCATION

See **Plan of Nursing Care 10** in this chapter. In addition:
1. Instruct patient to report immediately any indications of hypersensitivity or hepatic dysfunction (e.g., itching, rash, fever, sore throat, dark urine, light-colored stools, diarrhea, vomiting).
2. Advise patient beginning therapy to avoid excessive sunlight because photosensitivity reactions can occur. Exposure to sun should be gradual until effects of drug are known.

HYPERGLYCEMIC AGENTS

Although the most effective means of elevating the blood sugar level in cases of severe hypoglycemia is direct IV injection of glucose, this method is not always available or feasible. Alternatives include the oral administration of glucose, as a gel or chewable tablet, or *diazoxide,* a thiazide-like drug that inhibits release of insulin from the pancreas and is used in the management of hypoglycemia due to hyperinsulinism. Also, the parenteral use of *glucagon*, a polypeptide produced by pancreatic alpha cells, can increase conversion of glycogen to glucose and stimulate hepatic gluconeogenesis, thereby elevating blood glucose levels.

Most drug-induced hypoglycemic episodes are mild and generally can be reversed by oral ingestion of some form of glucose (such as candy, soda, sweetened orange juice). Only in those instances in which the hypoglycemic response is severe (insulin shock) or prolonged (when symptoms persist longer than 30 min after oral consumption of glucose) is the use of IV glucose or glucagon indicated.

Glucose, oral

B-D Glucose, Glutose, Insta-Glucose, Monoject
(CAN) Glucosal

Although glucose may be administered by IV infusion (see Chap. 75) to provide an immediate source in acute hypoglycemic episodes, symptoms of mild hypoglycemic reactions

Table 42-3
Oral Antidiabetic Drugs

Drug	Preparations	Usual Dosage Range	Nursing Implications
First Generation			
Acetohexamide Dymelor	Tablets: 250 mg, 500 mg	250 mg–1500 mg/day in a single dose or 2 divided doses if over 1000 mg/day	Intermediate acting drug (duration 12–24 h); possesses significant uricosuric activity at therapeutic doses; metabolized to active intermediate by the liver (2.5 times as potent as parent compound); use with caution in renal insufficiency
Chlorpropamide Diabinese (CAN) Apo-Chlorpropamide, Novopropamide	Tablets: 100 mg, 250 mg	Initially 250 mg/day (100 mg–125 mg/day in older patients); maintenance 100 mg–500 mg/day (usual 250 mg/day) depending on condition	Longest acting oral antidiabetic drug (duration up to 60 h); more potent and generally more toxic than other oral drugs; also indicated for treatment of polyuria of diabetes *insipidus*; may enhance effects of ADH; give as a single morning dose, with food, to minimize GI upset; if hypoglycemia occurs, give frequent feedings or glucose for at least 3–5 days, as drug is very long acting, and observe patient closely during this time
Tolazamide Ronase, Tolamide, Tolinase	Tablets: 100 mg, 250 mg, 500 mg	Initially 100 mg–250 mg/day in a single dose depending on fasting blood sugar; maintenance 100 mg–500 mg/day	Intermediate-acting drug (duration 10–14 h); may be effective in patients who do not respond to other sulfonylureas or in some patients with a history of ketoacidosis or coma; close observation of these patients is required; converted to several weakly active metabolites by the liver

Continued

---

can often be controlled by the oral use of glucose as either chewable tablets or a 40% liquid gel-like solution. Glucose is rapidly absorbed from the GI tract, and a rapid increase (i.e., 5–10 min) in blood glucose concentration occurs following oral administration. The recommended dose is 10 g to 20 g, which may be repeated in 10 minutes if required. Glucose is *not* absorbed from the buccal cavity and must therefore be swallowed to be effective. Thus, whenever possible, other drugs should be employed to treat hypoglycemia in the *unconscious* patient, because the swallowing reflex does not always occur, and the absence of the normal gag reflex can lead to aspiration. Occasional reports of nausea have appeared, but the drug is virtually nontoxic when taken as directed. It is not recommended in children under 2 years of age.

Glucagon

MECHANISM
Accelerates synthesis of cyclic AMP, thereby increasing phosphorylase activity with consequent glycogenolysis and increased blood glucose levels; inhibits glycogen synthetase, promotes uptake of amino acids into liver, and stimulates hepatic gluconeogenesis; exerts effects on heart similar to catecholamines, that is, increased rate and force of contraction

USES
- Treatment of severe drug-induced hypoglycemic reactions in diabetic patients or persons undergoing insulin shock therapy (minimal effectiveness in states of starvation, adrenal insufficiency, or chronic hypoglycemia)
- Production of GI hypotonia as a diagnostic aid for radiologic examination of stomach, duodenum, small intestine, and colon

DOSAGE
Hypoglycemia: 0.5 mg to 1 mg SC, IM, or IV; repeat once or twice at 10- to 20-minute intervals if no response has occurred; IV glucose may also be needed to prevent cerebral hypoglycemia

Insulin shock therapy: 0.5 mg to 1 mg SC, IM, or IV after 1 hour of coma; if no response within 15 to 25 minutes, repeat

Diagnostic aid: 0.25 mg to 2 mg IV or IM depending on speed of onset and duration of action desired

Table 42-3
Oral Antidiabetic Drugs (continued)

Drug	Preparations	Usual Dosage Range	Nursing Implications
Tolbutamide Oramide, Orinase (CAN) Apo-Tolbutamide, Mobenol, Novobutamide	Tablets: 250 mg, 500 mg Vials (sodium salt): 1 g with diluent	Initially 1 g–2 g/day orally; maintenance 0.25 g–2 g/day, usually in divided doses IV: 1 g given over 2–3 min	Short-acting drug (duration 6–12 h); mildly goitrogenic at high doses and may reduce radioactive iodide uptake after prolonged administration without producing clinical hypothyroidism; rapidly metabolized to inactive metabolites; useful in patients with kidney disease; Orinase IV is used to diagnose islet cell adenoma (see Chap. 76); in presence of tumor, there is a rapid, marked drop in blood glucose that persists for up to 3 h; IV injection may produce local irritation or thrombophlebitis
Second Generation			
Glipizide Glucotrol	Tablets: 5 mg, 10 mg	Initially 5 mg before breakfast; increase in 2.5 mg–5 mg increments every 7 days until optimal response; maximum daily dose is 40 mg	Peak plasma concentrations occur in 1–3 h. Elimination half-life is 2–4 h, but blood sugar control persists for up to 24 h. Liver metabolism is rapid and extensive. Daily doses greater than 15 mg should be divided and given before meals. Reduce dosage in elderly, debilitated, or malnourished persons, and in the presence of impaired renal or hepatic function
Glyburide Diabeta, Micronase (CAN) Euglucon	Tablets: 1.25 mg, 2.5 mg, 5 mg	Initially, 2.5 mg–5 mg before breakfast; usual maintenance dose is 5 mg–20 mg daily in a single dose or two divided doses; maximum daily dose is 20 mg	Peak plasma levels are attained within 4 h, and effects persist for at least 24 h. Elimination half-life is approximately 10 h. Excreted in the bile and urine, 50% by each route, thus, can be used in patients with renal impairment with greater safety than other oral antidiabetics

FATE
Blood glucose begins to increase and consciousness is restored within 5 to 20 minutes; duration of action is approximately 1 to 2 hours; metabolized in the liver, kidneys, and plasma

SIGNIFICANT ADVERSE REACTIONS
(Rare) Nausea, vomiting, and hypersensitivity reactions; hypokalemia in large doses

CONTRAINDICATIONS
No absolute contraindications. *Cautious use* in patients with a history of insulinoma (increased *hypo*glycemia can occur) and pheochromocytoma (increased blood pressure can occur)

INTERACTION
Glucagon may potentiate the action of oral anticoagulants

NURSING CONSIDERATIONS

Nursing Alerts
- Be prepared to administer supplemental carbohydrates, as needed, to an insulin-dependent (type I) diabetic, who usually does not respond to glucagon with as large an increase in blood glucose as a non-insulin-dependent (type II) diabetic. Also, glucagon is of little benefit in states of starvation, adrenal insufficiency, chronic hypoglycemia, or other conditions in which liver glycogen is unavailable. IV glucose should be available and must be used if patient is in a deep coma or fails to respond to glucagon.
- Expect to begin oral carbohydrates as soon as possible after consciousness is regained in order to restore liver glycogen and prevent secondary hypoglycemia.

1. Be alert for indications of possible hypersensitivity reactions because drug is a protein.
2. Do not mix glucagon solution with solutions containing sodium, potassium, or calcium chlorides because precipitation will occur. Glucagon does not precipitate in dextrose solution.

Diazoxide, oral
Proglycem

Diazoxide is used orally for the management of persistent hypoglycemia due to hyperinsulinism. It is also available for IV injection as Hyperstat for treating hypertensive emergencies (see Chap. 31).

MECHANISM
Inhibits secretion of insulin from the pancreas and may increase glycogen synthesis; effect on insulin release is antagonized by alpha-adrenergic blocking agents; other pharmacologic actions include hyperuricemia, decreased sodium and water excretion, tachycardia, and increased serum free fatty acid levels; as an antihypertensive agent, drug directly relaxes vascular smooth muscle; effects on blood pressure are minimal when it is used orally in therapeutic doses

USES
Management of hypoglycemia due to hyperinsulinism (e.g., islet cell proliferation, hyperplasia, or carcinoma; extrapancreatic malignancy; leucine sensitivity) where other medical or surgical treatment is ineffective or inappropriate

DOSAGE
Initially 3 mg/kg/day in 3 divided doses every 8 hours
Maintenance 3 mg/kg to 8 mg/kg/day in divided doses; infants— 8 mg/kg to 15 mg/kg/day in 2 or 3 equal doses every 8 to 12 hours

FATE
Onset of hyperglycemia is 1 hour; duration is 6 to 8 hours; highly bound to plasma albumin; plasma half-life is 24 to 36 hours in children and adults; excreted in the urine

COMMON SIDE EFFECTS
Sodium and fluid retention, hirsutism, GI distress (nausea, diarrhea, abdominal pain), loss of taste, palpitations, tachycardia, hyperuricemia, skin rash, headache, and weakness

SIGNIFICANT ADVERSE REACTIONS
Cardiovascular: hypotension, chest pain
CNS: anxiety, dizziness, insomnia, extrapyramidal symptoms
Hematologic: thrombocytopenia, neutropenia, eosinophilia, excessive bleeding, decreased hemoglobin
Ocular: transient cataracts, subconjunctival bleeding, blurred vision, scotoma, lacrimation
Hepatic/renal: azotemia, hematuria, proteinuria, decreased urinary output, nephrotic syndrome, increased alkaline phosphatase and SGOT
Other: fever, lymphadenopathy, pancreatitis, galactorrhea, gout, dermatitis, pruritus, loss of scalp hair, paresthesias, hyperglycemia, glycosuria, ketoacidosis

CONTRAINDICATIONS
Functional hypoglycemia, hypersensitivity to sulfonamides or thiazides. *Cautious use* in patients with diabetes, renal dysfunction, impaired cerebral or cardiac circulation, or history of gout, in children and pregnant women, and in persons taking corticosteroids

INTERACTIONS
Hypotensive effects of diazoxide may be intensified by antihypertensives and diuretics

Thiazides may potentiate the hyperglycemic and hyperuricemic action of diazoxide

Effects of diazoxide may be enhanced by other protein-bound drugs (e.g., antiinflammatory agents, anticoagulants, barbiturates, phenytoin, sulfonamides)

Chlorpromazine can strongly potentiate the hyperglycemic effect of diazoxide

The inhibition of insulin release by diazoxide is antagonized by alpha-adrenergic blocking agents

Concurrent use of diazoxide and sulfonylurea antidiabetic drugs may reduce effects of both drugs

Diazoxide may decrease the effects of phenytoin by increasing its hepatic metabolism

NURSING CONSIDERATIONS

Nursing Alerts
- Closely monitor intake/output ratio and check frequently for appearance of edema. Drug can cause significant fluid retention, which may be hazardous in cardiac patient. Conventional diuretic therapy usually controls fluid retention.
- In cases of overdosage, be alert for development of ketoacidosis, which may lead to coma. Overdosage responds promptly to insulin and restoration of fluid and electrolyte balance. Observe patient closely for at least 7 days following suspected overdosage because diazoxide is long-acting.

1. In patient with impaired renal function, in whom dosage should be reduced, monitor results of serum electrolyte determinations, which should be performed often.
2. Collaborate in evaluation of drug effects. Clinical response and blood glucose levels should be monitored frequently until condition is stable. The drug formulation should be changed cautiously because blood levels may be higher with the liquid than with the capsule formulation. Diazoxide should be discontinued if response is not satisfactory within 2 to 3 weeks.

PATIENT EDUCATION
1. Teach patient to monitor urine for sugar and ketones. Abnormalities should immediately be reported to physician.
2. Instruct patient to report any changes in vision because transient cataracts have occurred.
3. Reassure patient that the hirsutism that may occur (mainly on forehead, back, and limbs, especially in children and women) is reversible upon withdrawal of the drug.

Selected Bibliography
Baker DE, Campbell RK: The second generation sulfonylureas: Glipizide and glyburide. Diabetes Educ 11(3):29, 1985
Dillon R: Improved serum profiles in diabetic individuals who massage their insulin injection sites. Diabetes Care 6:399, 1983

Donohue-Porter P: Insulin dependent diabetes mellitus. Nurs Clin North Am 20:191, 1985

Dupre J: Insulin therapy: Progress and prospects. Hosp Pract 18:171, 1983

Eisenbarth GS: Type I diabetes mellitus: A chronic autoimmune disease. N Engl J Med 314:1360, 1986

Essig M: Oral antidiabetic drugs. Nursing 83/13:59, 1983

Flavin K, Haire-Joshu D: Drugs for diabetes: The pharmacologic repertoire. Am J Nurs 86:1244, 1986

Guthrie D, Guthrie R: Nursing Management of Diabetes Mellitus, 2nd ed. St. Louis, CV Mosby, 1982

Hairc-Joshu D, Flavin K, Santiago JV: Intensive conventional insulin therapy. Am J Nurs 86:1251, 1986

Jacobs S, Cuatrecasas P: Insulin receptors. Am Rev Pharmacol Toxicol 23:461, 1983

McCall AL: How drugs work: The new human insulins. Mod Med 53(9):112, 1985

Peden N, Newton RW, Feely J: Oral hypoglycemic agents. Br Med J 286:1564, 1983

Price MJ: Insulin and oral hypoglycemic agents. Nurs Clin North Am 18:687, 1983

Salans LB: Diabetes mellitus: A disease that is coming into focus. JAMA 247:590, 1982

Seltzer HS: Efficacy and safety of oral hypoglycemic agents. Am Rev Med 31:261, 1980

SUMMARY. ANTIDIABETIC AND HYPERGLYCEMIC DRUGS

Drug	Preparations	Usual Dosage Range
Insulins	See Table 42-2	
Oral Antidiabetics	See Table 42-3	
Glucose B-D Glucose, Glutose, Insta-Glucose, Monoject	Gel: 40% Chewable tablets: 5 g	10 g–20 g: repeat in 10 min if necessary
Glucagon Glucagon	Powder for injection: 1 mg, 10 mg (1 mg = 1 U)	0.5 mg–1 mg SC, IM, or IV; may repeat in 10–20 min if no response is noted
Diazoxide, oral Proglycem	Capsules: 50 mg Suspension: 50 mg/mL	Adults: 3 mg/kg–8 mg/kg/day in 2–3 divided doses every 8–12 hours Infants: 8 mg/kg to 15 mg/kg/day in 2–3 divided doses

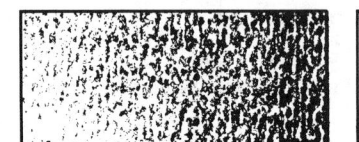

43 ADRENAL CORTICAL STEROIDS

The adrenal cortex secretes a large number of steroidal compounds possessing a variety of physiological actions. These substances are termed *adrenocorticoids,* or simply *corticoids.* According to their predominant action in the body, they may be divided into one of the three following categories:

- Mineralocorticoids (e.g., aldosterone)
- Glucocorticoids (e.g., hydrocortisone)
- Adrenogenital corticoids (e.g., dehydroepiandrosterone)

The *mineralocorticoids,* of which aldosterone is the major endogenous representative, exert their principal action on electrolyte and water metabolism, especially in the kidney; there they facilitate the reabsorption of sodium and water from the urine by the ionic exchange mechanisms in the distal segments of the renal tubules. Aldosterone itself is not available for therapeutic use, and the clinically available mineralocorticoid is fludrocortisone.

The *glucocorticoids* are those compounds that primarily influence carbohydrate, fat, and protein metabolism and thus can elicit varied effects in the body and alter the body's immune response to diverse stimuli. Hydrocortisone and cortisone are the major endogenous glucocorticoids. Metabolic actions of the glucocorticoids include gluconeogenesis, hyperglycemia, increased protein catabolism, decreased utilization of amino acids, impaired lipogenesis, and increased lipolysis. In addition, they can suppress the inflammatory process, and this action is the reason for their major clinical application, the control of symptoms of inflammation. Naturally occurring glucocorticoids (such as cortisone, hydrocortisone) as well as synthetic glucocorticoids (e.g., betamethasone, prednisone) are available for therapeutic use, and they differ primarily in potency and degree of side effects.

The *adrenogenital corticoids* are male and female sex hormones (such as estrogen, progesterone, testosterone) found in very small amounts in the adrenal cortex. Other than dehydroepiandrosterone, a precursor of both testosterone and the estrogens, the adrenogenital corticoids are present in the adrenal cortex in amounts too small to be of clinical significance. The sex hormones are discussed in Chapters 44 to 46.

Although the classification of the major adrenal corticoids into mineralocorticoids and glucocorticoids is convenient for discussion purposes, it represents an oversimplification from a functional standpoint. With the exception of a few potent synthetic glucocorticoids, *complete* separation of mineralocorticoid from glucocorticoid activity has not been achieved and considerable overlapping of activity exists with most compounds, especially when employed in large doses. This overlapping is responsible for many of the side effects associated with adrenal corticosteroid therapy, although in some cases it may represent a desirable extension of the clinical activity of a particular drug. For example, in the treatment of primary adrenal cortical hypofunction (Addison's disease), the mineralocorticoid action (salt and water retention) of glucocorticoid compounds such as hydrocortisone is desirable from a therapeutic point of view. In fact, mineralocorticoid supplementation is often provided with glucocorticoid therapy in the treatment of Addison's disease. On the other hand, a mineralocorticoid action might prove undesirable in the cardiac patient, because salt and water retention may aggravate the already compromised cardiac function.

Regulation of adrenal corticosteroid secretion is reviewed in Chapter 38. Synthesis of adrenal corticoids is controlled primarily by ACTH (corticotropin) released from the adenohypophysis. ACTH itself is used in certain clinical situations and is discussed in Chapter 39; the remaining adrenal cortical drugs are reviewed in this chapter. In addition, aminoglutethimide and trilostane, drugs used in the treatment of adrenal cortical *hyper*function (Cushing's syndrome) are considered at the end of the chapter.

MINERALO-CORTICOIDS

Clinically useful mineralocorticoids possess actions qualitatively similar to those of the major endogenous agent aldosterone; that is, they facilitate the reabsorption of sodium and water from the distal segment of the nephron. They are indicated as partial replacement therapy for adrenocortical insufficiency and for treatment of salt-losing adrenogenital syndrome. The only clinically available drug is fludrocortisone, an orally effective, potent synthetic mineralocorticoid.

Fludrocortisone Acetate
Florinef

MECHANISM
Promotes sodium and water reabsorption in the distal tubule of the nephron, which occurs in conjunction with hydrogen and potassium excretion; may also enhance sodium retention in sweat and salivary glands; small doses can cause marked sodium retention and elevated blood pressure; large doses may promote hepatic deposition of glycogen and may induce a negative nitrogen balance unless protein intake is adequate; also exhibits effects on carbohydrate, fat, and protein metabolism (see Mechanism under Glucocorticoids)

USES
Partial replacement therapy for primary and secondary adrenocortical insufficiency in Addison's disease
Treatment of salt-losing adrenogenital syndrome
Management of severe orthostatic hypotension (e.g., Shy-Drager syndrome)

DOSAGE
Addison's disease: 0.1 mg 3 times/week orally to 0.2 mg/day (usually 0.1 mg/day)
Dose should be reduced to 0.05 mg/day if hypertension develops
Salt-losing adrenogenital syndrome: 0.1 mg/day to 0.2 mg/day
Orthostatic hypotension: 0.1 mg to 0.5 mg/day; dosage is titrated by clinical response or development of ankle edema

FATE
Adequately absorbed orally; metabolized in the liver and excreted mainly in the urine

COMMON SIDE EFFECTS

Hypokalemia (muscle weakness, paresthesias, fatigue), and edema

SIGNIFICANT ADVERSE REACTIONS

(See also under glucocorticoids) Hypertension, pulmonary congestion, cardiac arrhythmias, headaches, arthralgia, muscle paralysis, hypersensitivity reactions

CONTRAINDICATIONS

Treatment of conditions other than those specifically indicated (see Uses), hypertension, cardiac disease, and systemic fungal infections. *Cautious use* in the presence of stress, trauma, or severe illness and in pregnant or nursing women

INTERACTIONS

See glucocorticoids

NURSING CONSIDERATIONS

See glucocorticoids (oral use). In addition:

Nursing Alerts

- Ensure that weight, blood pressure, and electrolyte levels are obtained prior to initiation of therapy and periodically during extended therapy. The physician should be advised of any significant changes.
- Assess patient for indications of excessive hypokalemia (e.g., muscle cramping or weakness, paresthesias, palpitations, fatigue, nausea, polyuria) or drug overdosage (weight gain, edema, hypertension, pulmonary congestion, insomnia). Supplemental potassium therapy may be indicated.

PATIENT EDUCATION

See glucocorticoids (oral use). In addition:
1. Stress the importance of controlling salt intake for optimal drug effects. Excess salt intake increases sodium retention and potassium excretion, reducing drug efficacy and necessitating potassium supplementation.
2. Stress the need to maintain a diet adequate in protein.

GLUCOCORTICOIDS

Alclometasone	Fluocinonide
Amcinonide	Fluorometholone
Beclomethasone	Flurandrenolide
Betamethasone	Halcinonide
Clobetasol	Hydrocortisone
Clocortolone	Medrysone
Cortisone	Methylprednisolone
Desonide	Mometasone
Desoximetasone	Paramethasone
Dexamethasone	Prednisolone
Diflorasone	Prednisone
Flunisolide	Triamcinolone
Fluocinolone	

The glucocorticoids encompass a large number of naturally occurring and synthetic steroids possessing similar pharmacologic actions but differing widely in potency and the type and severity of side effects. The principal naturally occurring adrenal cortical steroids are cortisone and hydrocortisone, and they exhibit both mineralocorticoid (salt-retaining) as well as glucocorticoid (antiinflammatory) effects. As such, they are primarily used as replacement therapy for adrenocortical deficiency states.

Synthetic glucocorticoids are characterized by their greater glucocorticoid potency compared to natural adrenal cortical steroids and by their reduced (and in some cases complete absence of) mineralocorticoid action. The synthetic drugs are used principally for their potent antiinflammatory action and are available in many different dosage forms. The relative potencies of the various systemically employed glucocorticoids are listed in Table 43-1, which compares their oral effectiveness, antiinflammatory activity, and mineralocorticoid potency.

It is important to recognize that the majority of adverse reactions associated with glucocorticoid use occur following the systemic use of these compounds. When a local effect is desired, the drug may be applied topically in several dosage forms (e.g., ointment, cream, lotion, aerosol, nasal spray, ophthalmic drops) or administered by an intralesional or intraarticular injection. A number of different corticosteroids are used topically, and the relative potency of topical steroids is dependent on several factors, including the concentration of drug applied, the basic characteristics of the drug molecule, and the type of vehicle used. For example, fluorinated derivatives (e.g., betamethasone, fluocinonide, halcinonide) are more potent than nonfluorinated agents (e.g., hydrocortisone, desonide) but may have a higher incidence of local adverse effects. A relative potency ranking of the various topical steroid preparations is presented in Table 43-2.

The discussion of glucocorticoids below focuses mainly on their systemic pharmacology. Following this general review of glucocorticoids, individual drugs, both systemic and local, are listed in Table 43-3; the available dosage forms are given along with recommended dose levels for each dosage form, and nursing implications pertaining to each drug are presented.

MECHANISM

Mechanism of antiinflammatory action is not completely established, but may include one or more of the following actions:

- Stabilization of lysosomal membranes, reducing release of tissue-destructive enzymes
- Inhibition of capillary dilation and permeability
- Interference with the biosynthesis, storage, or release of allergic substances (e.g., bradykinin, histamine)
- Suppression of leukocyte migration and phagocytosis
- Inhibition of fibroblast formation and collagen deposition
- Reduction of antibody formation by lymphocytes and plasma cells.

Drugs may also enhance the responsiveness of the cardiovascular system to circulating catecholamines, thereby increasing cardiac output as well as local perfusion pressure. Derivatives possessing mineralocorticoid activity exert effects on fluid and electrolyte balance as well (see Mechanism for fludrocortisone earlier in the chapter)

USES

Replacement therapy in primary or secondary adrenal cortical insufficiency (hydrocortisone is drug of choice)

Treatment of congenital adrenal hyperplasia

Table 43-1
Comparative Activities of Systemic Glucocorticoids

Drug	Equivalent Oral Doses (mg)	Relative Antiinflammatory Activity	Relative Mineralocorticoid Potency
Short Acting			
Cortisone	25	0.8	+ +
Hydrocortisone	20	1	+ +
Intermediate Acting			
Prednisone	5	3–4	+
Prednisolone	5	3	+
Methylprednisolone	4	5	0
Triamcinolone	4	5	0
Long Acting			
Paramethasone	2	10	0
Dexamethasone	0.75	25–30	0
Betamethasone	0.6	25–30	0

Table 43-2
Relative Potencies of Topically Applied Corticosteroids[a]

Generic Name	Trade Name	Dosage Form	Strength (%)
Group I			
Amcinonide	Cyclocort	Ointment	0.1
		Cream	0.1
		Lotion	0.1
Betamethasone Dipropionate	Alphatrex, Diprolene, Diprosone, Maxivate	Ointment	0.05
		Cream	0.05
		Lotion	0.05
Clobetasol Propionate	Temovate	Cream	0.05
		Ointment	0.05
Desoximetasone	Topicort	Cream	0.25
		Ointment	0.25
Diflorasone Diacetate	Florone, Maxiflor, Psorcon	Ointment	0.05
		Cream	0.05
Fluocinolone Acetonide	Synalar HP	Cream	0.2
Fluocinonide	Lidex, Lidex-E	Cream	0.05
		Ointment	0.05
		Solution	0.05
		Gel	0.05
Halcinonide	Halog, Halog-E	Cream	0.1
		Ointment	0.1
		Solution	0.1
Mometasone	Elocon	Cream	0.1
		Ointment	0.1
Group II			
Betamethasone Benzoate	Benisone, Uticort	Cream	0.025
		Ointment	0.025
		Lotion	0.025
Betamethasone Valerate	Betatrex, Beta-Val, Valisone	Ointment	0.1
		Cream	0.1
		Lotion	0.1

Continued

Table 43-2
Relative Potencies of Topically Applied Corticosteroids[a] (continued)

Generic Name	Trade Name	Dosage Form	Strength (%)
Group II			
Desoximetasone	Topicort	Cream	0.05
		Gel	0.05
Triamcinolone Acetonide	Aristocort, Kenalog	Cream	0.5
		Ointment	0.5
Group III			
Fluocinolone Acetonide	Synalar, Synemol	Ointment	0.025
		Cream	0.025
Flurandrenolide	Cordran	Ointment	0.05
		Cream	0.05
		Lotion	0.05
Halcinonide	Halog	Cream	0.025
Triamcinolone Acetonide	Aristocort, Kenalog	Ointment	0.1
		Cream	0.1
		Lotion	0.1
Group IV			
Betamethasone Valerate	Betatrex, Valisone	Cream	0.01
Clocortolone Pivalate	Cloderm	Cream	0.1
Fluocinolone Acetonide	Synalar, Synemol	Cream	0.01
		Solution	0.01
Flurandrenolide	Cordran	Cream	0.025
		Ointment	0.025
Hydrocortisone Valerate	Westcort	Ointment	0.2
		Cream	0.2
Triamcinolone Acetonide	Aristocort, Kenalog	Cream	0.025
		Lotion	0.025
		Ointment	0.025
Group V			
Alclometasone, Dipropionate	Aclovate	Cream	0.05
		Ointment	0.05
Desonide	DesOwen, Tridesilon	Cream	0.05
Dexamethasone	Hexadrol	Cream	0.05
Hydrocortisone	Alphaderm, Hytone, Cortril, Cort-Dome	Cream	1.0
		Ointment	1.0
		Lotion	1.0
Methylprednisolone, Acetate	Medrol	Ointment	1.0

[a]Group I drugs are the most potent; group V drugs are the least potent. Drugs in each group are listed alphabetically; there is no significant difference among agents in each group.

Symptomatic treatment of various inflammatory, allergic, or immunoreactive disorders including the following:
  Rheumatic: rheumatoid arthritis, bursitis, osteoarthritis, acute gouty arthritis, tenosynovitis, synovitis, ankylosing spondylitis
  Collagen: acute rheumatic carditis, systemic lupus erythematosus
  Allergic: allergic rhinitis, bronchial asthma, status asthmaticus, dermatitis, serum sickness, drug hypersensitivity
  Dermatologic: erythema multiforme (Stevens–Johnson syndrome) exfoliative dermatitis, severe psoriasis, angioedema, urticaria, chronic eczema
  Ophthalmic: conjunctivitis, keratitis, iritis, uveitis, acute optic neuritis, chorioretinitis, allergic corneal marginal ulcers
  Gastrointestinal: ulcerative colitis, regional enteritis
  Hematologic/neoplastic: thrombocytopenic purpura, hemolytic anemia (autoimmune), erythroblastopenia, leukemias, Hodgkin's disease, multiple myeloma
  Other: nephrotic syndrome, gout, hypercalcemia, multiple sclerosis, acute myasthenic episodes, anaphylactic shock, tuberculous meningitis, nonsuppurative thyroiditis
Testing of adrenal cortical hyperfunction and treatment of cerebral edema associated with brain tumors, craniotomy, or trauma (dexamethasone only)

Treatment of pulmonary emphysema with bronchospasm and edema, treatment of diffuse interstitial pulmonary fibrosis, control of postoperative dental inflammatory reactions, and in conjunction with diuretics in refractory congestive heart failure (triamcinolone *only*)

Investigational uses include prevention of cisplatin-induced vomiting (dexamethasone), prevention of respiratory distress syndrome in premature neonates (betamethasone), treatment of septic shock (methylprednisolone IV), prevention or treatment of acute mountain sickness (dexamethasone), and diagnosis of depression (dexamethasone)

DOSAGE
See Table 43-3

FATE
Most drugs are well absorbed from the GI tract and circulate in the blood partially bound to plasma proteins; duration of action varies among derivatives; metabolized in the liver and excreted largely by the kidneys in conjugated form; induction of hepatic enzymes will increase the metabolic clearance of glucocorticoids; renal clearance is accelerated when plasma levels are increased. (See Table 43-3 for specific data for individual drugs)

COMMON SIDE EFFECTS
Salt and water retention, sweating, increased appetite

SIGNIFICANT ADVERSE REACTIONS
GI: vomiting, peptic ulcer, pancreatitis, abdominal distention, ulcerative esophagitis
Cardiovascular: hypertension, arrhythmias, congestive heart failure, shock, thrombophlebitis, fat embolism
Dermatologic: petechiae, ecchymoses, purpura, hirsutism, acne, thinning of skin, striae, fatty redistribution in subcutaneous layers, impaired wound healing, abnormal pigmentation
Musculoskeletal: osteoporosis, muscle weakness, tendon rupture, vertebral compression fractures, spontaneous fractures, steroid myopathy
Neurologic: vertigo, headache, syncope, personality changes, irritability, insomnia, convulsions, catatonia
Fluid/electrolyte: hypokalemia, hypocalcemia, alkalosis
Endocrine: menstrual irregularities, growth retardation, decreased carbohydrate tolerance, steroid diabetes
Ophthalmic: posterior subcapsular cataracts, glaucoma, exophthalmos
Other: increased susceptibility to or masking of infections, fatty embolism, negative nitrogen balance, hypersensitivity and anaphylactic reactions, renal stones, leukocytosis

CONTRAINDICATIONS
Systemic glucocorticoids are contraindicated in the presence of active peptic ulcer, systemic fungal infection, active tuberculosis, and in combination with any live virus vaccine; *IM* administration is contraindicated in thrombocytopenic purpura; *ocular and topical* administration are contraindicated in the presence of herpes simplex, tubercular, or other viral infections of the eye or skin. *Cautious use* in patients with hypothyroidism, ulcerative colitis, fresh intestinal anastomoses, diverticulitis, cirrhosis, active or latent peptic ulcer, diabetes mellitus, chronic nephritis, hypertension, congestive heart failure, osteoporosis, renal insufficiency, thrombophlebitis, glaucoma, myasthenia gravis, convulsive disorders, metastatic carcinoma, pyogenic infections, Cushing's syndrome, vaccinia or varicella infections, and in pregnant or nursing women

> **WARNING**
> *Note:* Steroids should not be injected into a joint suspected of being infected or unstable, since frequent intra-articular injections can damage joint

INTERACTIONS
The pharmacologic effects of corticosteroids may be reduced by barbiturates, phenytoin, ephedrine, and rifampin, drugs that enhance the metabolic clearance of steroids

Corticosteroids may increase the dosage requirements for insulin and oral antidiabetic agents, isoniazid, salicylates, and oral anticoagulants

Increased intraocular pressure can result from combinations of corticosteroids and anticholinergics, tricyclic antidepressants, or adrenergics

Excessive hypokalemia has resulted from concomitant use of corticosteroids and potassium-depleting diuretics or amphotericin

Corticosteroids can increase digitalis toxicity as a result of potassium loss

The antiinflammatory action of corticosteroids may be enhanced by estrogens because of reduced hepatic clearance

GI absorption of corticosteroids can be impaired by cholestyramine and colestipol

Corticosteroids may increase the pharmacologic effects of theophylline

Concurrent use of corticosteroids and salicylates may result in reduced salicylate levels and increased likelihood of gastric ulceration

NURSING CONSIDERATIONS

Nursing Alerts
- Be alert for possibility of hypersensitivity reactions with parenteral use. Severe anaphylactic reactions have been reported.
- Assess patient's mental status carefully for signs of change (e.g., euphoria, insomnia, depression, mood swings) because emotional aberrations may occur. Glucocorticoids should be used cautiously in persons with a history of emotional instability.

1. Ensure that baseline values for blood pressure, weight, intake/output ratio, blood glucose, and serum potassium are obtained before therapy is initiated. These values should also be determined at regular intervals thereafter.
2. Collaborate with health care team in evaluating drug effects. Dosage should be individually adjusted for each patient on the basis of the disease state being treated and the clinical response. Initial dosage should be adjusted and then maintained until a satisfactory response is evident. Dosage may then be gradually reduced to lowest effective level. Alternate-day therapy is generally preferred, where feasible, to minimize adrenal suppression.
3. Monitor diabetic patients closely because hyperglycemia can occur.
4. Monitor weight and height of pediatric patient because drugs can suppress normal growth pattern.
5. If signs and symptoms of toxicity occur without obvious cause, determine if patient has a history of excessive use of OTC topical corticosteroid preparations.

PATIENT EDUCATION

1. Instruct patient to take drug with food or milk in a single daily morning dose, preferably before 9:00 A.M. Corticosteroids suppress adrenal function least when given at the time of maximal adrenocortical activity, which is early morning.
2. To effect a changeover from daily to alternate-day dosing, provide patient with schedule of doses to be taken each day. Alternate-day therapy is usually accomplished by administering twice the daily maintenance dose every other morning. Long-acting drugs should *not* be employed in alternate-day therapy.
3. Reassure patient that sudden worsening of condition during periods of dosage adjustment is temporary.
4. Inform patient that drug requirements may be increased during periods of stress. Supplementary doses of a rapid-acting agent should be administered during these periods.
5. Emphasize the importance of trying to avoid infections and of notifying physician immediately if one is suspected (e.g., slow wound healing, prolonged inflammation, persistent fever, sore throat). Glucocorticoids may mask some signs of infection, encourage their spread, and decrease patient's resistance. Appropriate antibiotic therapy is essential.
6. Instruct patient receiving long-term therapy to obtain periodic ophthalmic examinations and to report any visual disturbances immediately because cataracts, glaucoma, or optic nerve damage may occur.
7. Urge patient to advise physician if gastric distress is severe or persistent because gastric ulceration may occur. Supplemental antacids may alleviate GI distress.
8. Encourage patient to use a firm mattress and bedboard and to report persistent backache or chest pain, which may indicate the presence of spontaneous vertebral or rib fractures.
9. Instruct patient to notify physician if excessive weight gain, edema, hypertension, muscle weakness, or bone pain occurs.
10. Ensure that patient undergoing high-dose therapy understands that immunizations are contraindicated (antibody response is impaired, and neurologic complications could occur).
11. Inform female patients that menstrual irregularities may develop.
12. Stress the importance of adhering to prescribed dosage regimen and the danger of sudden termination of usage. Following extended therapy, corticosteroids should be withdrawn gradually to minimize the risk of adrenal suppression.
13. Teach patient symptoms of adrenal insufficiency (e.g., nausea, dyspnea, fever, hypotension, myalgia, hypoglycemia) and instruct patient to notify physician if they occur. Supplementary steroids may be needed to reverse the symptoms.
14. Suggest that patient carry information describing condition treated and drug and dosage taken.
15. Warn patient not to overuse an injected joint following cessation of pain because the inflammatory focus may still be present, and further deterioration may occur with overactivity.
16. Instruct patient to moderate salt intake.
17. Encourage patient to regularly include potassium-rich foods in diet (see hypokalemia in **Plan of Nursing Care 9 in Chap. 37**), especially if taking a glucocorticoid with significant mineralocorticoid activity (see Table 43-1).
18. Warn patient to avoid licorice because it may intensify hypokalemia.

ADRENAL STEROID INHIBITORS

Two drugs that inhibit the synthesis of adrenal steroids, aminoglutethimide and trilostane, are available for treating selected cases of Cushing's syndrome (adrenocortical hyperfunction). They are reviewed below.

Aminoglutethimide
Cytadren

MECHANISM

Inhibits the conversion of cholesterol to delta-5-pregnenolone, thus impairing normal synthesis of adrenal steroids; probably acts by binding to cytochrome P-450

USES

Suppression of adrenal function in selected patients with adrenocortical hyperfunction (Cushing's syndrome). Usually given only until more definitive therapy (i.e., surgery) can be undertaken

Investigational uses include treatment of advanced mammary carcinoma in postmenopausal women and metastatic prostatic carcinoma

DOSAGE

Initially 250 mg 4 times a day; may increase in increments of 250 mg/day at intervals of 1 to 2 weeks to a total daily dose of 2 g; may be necessary to provide mineralocorticoid replacement therapy (e.g., fludrocortisone)

FATE

Well absorbed orally; plasma half-life is initially 12 to 16 hours but decreases to 6 to 8 hours with continued therapy; eliminated as both unchanged drug and metabolites in the urine

COMMON SIDE EFFECTS

Drowsiness, skin rash, nausea, anorexia, headache, dizziness

SIGNIFICANT ADVERSE REACTIONS

Hematologic: neutropenia, transient leukopenia, pancytopenia, thrombocytopenia
Cardiovascular: orthostatic hypotension, tachycardia
GI: vomiting
Dermatologic: pruritus, urticaria
Other: adrenal insufficiency, hypothyroidism, hirsutism, fever, myalgia, altered liver function tests, cholestatic jaundice

CONTRAINDICATIONS

Sensitivity to glutethimide (Doriden). *Cautious use* in patients with hypothyroidism, liver disease, or acute illness and in pregnant or nursing women

INTERACTIONS

Aminoglutethimide can accelerate the metabolism of dexamethasone

(Text continued on page 452)

Table 43-3
Glucocorticoids

Drug	Preparations	Usual Dosage Range	Nursing Implications
Alclometasone Aclovate	Ointment: 0.05% Cream: 0.05%	Apply to affected area 2–3 times/day	Synthetic corticosteroid used for treatment of inflammatory and pruritic manifestations of steroid-responsive dermatoses; side effects inlcude localized itching, burning, erythema, dryness, irritation, and rash
Amcinonide Cyclocort	Cream: 0.1% Ointment: 0.1% Lotion: 0.1%	Apply 2–3 times/day	Effective against steroid-responsive dermatoses; drug is formulated in nonsensitizing hydrophilic base
Beclomethasone Beclovent, Beconase, Vancenase, Vanceril (CAN) Propaderm	Aerosol for oral inhalation: 42 µg/dose Aerosol for intranasal inhalation: 42 µg/dose	*Oral inhalation* Adults: 2 inhalations 3–4 times day (maximum 20/day) Children: 1–2 inhalations 3–4 times a day (maximum 10/day) Nasal inhalation: 1 inhalation 2–4 times a day	Synthetic corticosteroid related to prednisolone; used by oral inhalation for long-term management of bronchial asthma not controlled by bronchodilators and other nonsteroidal drugs (see Chap. 55) dry mouth, hoarseness, and localized fungal infections of mouth and pharynx can occur; danger of adrenal insufficiency if patients are transferred from oral to inhaled steroids too quickly or during periods of stress; oral steroids should be available at all times; *not* indicated for relief of acute asthmatic attack; intranasal solution is used for relief of symptoms of seasonal or perennial rhinitis, minimal systemic effects; do not use in children under 12; nasal irritation and dryness are most common side effects; effects are evident only with several days use; patients with blocked nasal passages should use a decongestant (see Chap. 12) prior to administration; do *not* use longer than 3 wk if no effect
Betamethasone Celestone (CAN) Betnelan **Betamethasone Phosphate** Betameth, Celestone Phosphate, Cel-U-Jec, Selestoject (CAN) Betnesol **Betamethasone Benzoate** Benisone, Uticort (CAN) Beben **Betamethasone Dipropionate** Alphatrex, Diprolene, Diprosone, Maxivate **Betamethasone Valerate** Betatrex, Beta-Val, Valisone, Valnac (CAN) Betacort, Betaderm, Betnovate, Celestoderm, Ectosone, Metaderm	Tablets: 0.6 mg Syrup: 0.6 mg/5 mL Injection: 4 mg/mL Respository injection: 3 mg acetate and 3 mg phosphate/mL Cream: 0.01%, 0.025%, 0.05%, 0.1% Ointment: 0.025% Cream: 0.025% Lotion: 0.025% Gel: 0.025% Ointment: 0.05% Cream: 0.05% Lotion: 0.05% Aerosol: 0.01% Ointment: 0.1% Cream: 0.1% Lotion: 0.1%	Oral: 0.6 mg–7.2 mg/day IM, IV (phosphate only): up to 9 mg/day IM (respository): 0.5 mg–9.0 mg/day Intraarticular: 2 mg–8 mg (0.25 mL–2 mL) depending on joint size and disease Topical: 1–3 times/day	Long-acting agent with no mineralocorticoid activity; phosphate salt has a prompt onset of action and is given IV or IM; may be combined with acetate salt (prolonged action) for respository IM injections, given every 3–10 days into joints, lesions, or bursae; up to 2 mL may be injected into very large joints; *not used* in Addison's disease where salt- and water-retaining action is desirable; used topically for dermatoses, pruritis, and psoriatic lesions; use aerosol *cautiously* because systemic absorption may be substantial, resulting in increased adverse effects. Dipropionate is available in a specially formulated waxy vehicle that enhances drug absorption (Diprolene)

Continued

Table 43-3
Glucocorticoids (continued)

Drug	Preparations	Usual Dosage Range	Nursing Implications
Clobetasol Temovate (CAN) Dermovate	Cream: 0.05% Ointment: 0.05%	Apply twice a day	Very potent topical corticosteroid; limit treatment to 14 days; adrenal suppression has occurred with doses as low as 2 g/day; use very sparingly and *do not* cover with occlusive dressings
Clocortolone Cloderm	Cream: 0.1%	Apply 1–3 times/day	Indicated for relief of inflammatory manifestations of corticosteroid responsive dermatoses
Cortisone Cortone	Tablets: 5 mg, 10 mg, 25 mg Injection: 25 mg/mL, 50 mg/mL	Oral, IM: 20 mg–300 mg/day; reduce to lowest effective dosage	Short-acting glucocorticoid with prominent mineralocorticoid activity; it is largely converted to hydrocortisone, which is responsible for most of its pharmacologic action
Desonide Des Owen, Tridesilon	Cream: 0.05% Ointment: 0.05%	Apply 2–3 times/day	Possesses antiinflammatory, antipruritic, and vasoconstrictive activity; discontinue if irritation develops; less potent than most other topical steroids
Desoximetasone Topicort	Cream: 0.05%, 0.25% Gel: 0.05%	Apply 1–2 times/day	Higher strength (0.25%) cream is very potent; weaker strength cream (Topicort LP) and gel are of moderate potency
Dexamethasone Decadron, Hexadrol and other manufacturers (CAN) Deronil, Dexasone	Tablets: 0.25 mg, 0.5 mg, 0.75 mg, 1.0 mg, 1.5 mg, 2 mg, 4 mg, 6 mg Oral solution: 0.5 mg/5 mL Elixir: 0.5 mg/5 mL Drops: 0.5 mg/0.5 mL Injection: 4 mg/mL, 10 mg/mL, 20 mg/mL, 24 mg/mL Repository injection: (acetate salt): 8 mg/mL, 16 mg/mL Ophthalmic solution: 0.1% Ophthalmic suspension: 0.1% Ophthalmic ointment: 0.05%, 0.1% Cream: 0.1% Gel: 0.1% Aerosol: 0.01%, 0.04% Aerosol (Respihaler): 12.6 g (84 μg/dose) Aerosol (Turbinaire): 12.6 g (84 μg/dose)	Oral: 0.75 mg–9 mg/day Children: 0.2 mg/kg/day Parenteral: 1/3–1/2 oral dose/12 h (usual range 0.5–5 mg/day) Repository injection: 8 mg–16 mg IM every 1–3 wk Intraarticular, intralesion, or soft-tissue injection: 0.4 mg–6 mg depending on area Ophthalmic: 1–2 drops *or* thin film of ointment 3–4 times/day Topical: 2–4 times/day as needed Respihaler: 2–3 inhalations 3–4 times/day Turbinaire: 2 sprays in nostril 2–3 times/day	Widely used, potent corticosteroid; long-acting, and *not* recommended for alternate-day dosing; phosphate salt is freely soluble and is given IM or IV; prompt onset of action; acetate salt is highly insoluble and has a prolonged effect when given IM; aerosol therapy may result in nasal or bronchial irritation, drying of mucosa, rebound congestion, asthmatic-like reaction, and other systemic effects; Turbinaire aerosol is used for nasal inflammation, whereas Respihaler aerosol is indicated for bronchial asthma; available with lidocaine for soft-tissue injection (e.g., bursitis, tenosynovitis); systemic adverse effects may follow long-term or high-dose topical intralesional, or inhalation therapy; *protect eyes* from topical spray in the face area; discontinue ophthalmic use if eye irritation develops
Diflorasone Florone, Maxiflor, Psorcon (CAN) Flutone	Ointment: 0.05% Cream: 0.05%	Apply 2–3 times/day	Used in steroid-responsive dermatoses; cream is in an emulsified hydrophilic base
Flunisolide AeroBid, Nasalide (CAN) Bronalide, Rhinalar	Aerosol: 7 g (250 μg/dose) Nasal spray: 25 μg/dose	*Oral inhalation* Adults: 2 inhalations twice/day (maximum 2 mg/day) Children (age 6–15): 1–2 inhalations twice/day (maximum 1 mg/day) *Nasal inhalation* Adults: 2 sprays each nostril 2–3 times/day	Oral inhalation used to control steroid-dependent bronchial asthma—see Chap. 55 (*not* for relief of acute attacks); transfer from oral steroids should be done *gradually*; during periods of stress or severe asthma attacks, oral steroids should be reinstituted;

Continued

Table 43-3
Glucocorticoids (continued)

Drug	Preparations	Usual Dosage Range	Nursing Implications
		Children (age 6–14): 1 spray 3 times/day or 2 sprays twice/day	side effects include cough, dry mouth, hoarseness, and local fungal infections; nasal spray is used to relieve symptoms of rhinitis; *not* recommended in children under age 6; discontinue after 3 wk if no improvement is noted; after clinical effect is observed reduce to lowest effective maintenance dosage
Fluocinolone Fluocet, Fluonid, Flurosyn, Synalar, Synemol (CAN) Dermalar, Fluoderm, Fluolar	Ointment: 0.025% Cream: 0.01%, 0.025%, 0.2% Solution: 0.01%	Apply 2–4 times/day in a thin layer	Possesses moderate antiinflammatory and antipruritic activity; high potency cream (0.2%) should be used for short periods only; also available with neomycin (Neo-Synalar)
Fluocinonide Lidex, Lidex-E (CAN) Lidemol, Lyderm, Topsyn	Ointment: 0.05% Cream: 0.05% Gel: 0.05% Solution: 0.05%	Apply 3–4 times/day	Used for antiinflammatory action in steroid responsive dermatoses; one of the more potent topical corticosteroids; available in several different vehicles
Fluorometholone Fluor-Op, FML Liquifilm	Ophthalmic suspension: 0.1% Ophthalmic ointment: 0.1%	Ophthalmic: 1–2 drops or small ribbon of ointment 3–4 times/day	Be alert for ocular irritation and discontinue drug; transient burning may occur when first applied
Flurandrenolide Cordran (CAN) Drenison	Ointment: 0.025%, 0.05% Cream: 0.025%, 0.05% Lotion: 0.05% Tape: 4 µg/cm^2	Apply 2–3 times/day Tape: Cut tape to size of area; apply to clean dry skin and replace every 12 h	Good antiinflammatory, antipruritic, and vasoconstrictive activity; ointment is slightly more effective than cream; both preparations are available with neomycin (Cordran-N); for use in dermatoses complicated by bacterial infections; tape is usually removed every 12 h but may be left in place for 24 h if well tolerated; if irritation or infection develops, remove tape and inform physician
Halcinonide Halog, Halog E	Ointment: 0.1% Cream: 0.025%, 0.1% Solution: 0.1%	Apply 2–3 times/day in a thin film	Similar to most other topical corticosteroids; ointment is formulated in a polyethylene and mineral oil gel base; cream (0.1%) is available in a vanishing base (Halog E)
Hydrocortisone Cort-Dome, Cortef, and several other manufacturers (CAN) Cortamed, Cortiment	Tablets: 5 mg, 10 mg, 20 mg Oral suspension: 10 mg/5 mL Injection: 25 mg/mL 50 mg/mL; 100 mg/vial, 250 mg/vial, 500 mg/vial, 1000 mg/vial Respository injection (acetate): 25 mg/mL, 50 mg/mL Enema: 100 mg/60 mL Rectal foam aerosol: 90 mg/application Ointment: 0.1%, 0.2%, 0.5%, 1%, 2.5% Cream: 0.1%, 0.2%, 0.25%, 0.5%, 1%, 2.5% Lotion: 0.25%, 0.5%, 1%, 2%, 2.5% Gel: 1% Aerosol spray: 0.5%	Oral: 20 mg–240 mg/day in divided doses Parenteral: 1/3–1/2 oral dose every 12 h *Acute adrenal insufficiency* Adults: 100 mg IV followed by 100 mg/8 h in IV fluids Children: 1 mg–2 mg/kg IV bolus, then 150 mg–250 mg/day IV in divided doses Enema: 100 mg/night for 21 days Intralesional, intraarticular, or soft-tissue injection: 10 mg–50 mg depending on area Ophthalmic: A thin film of ointment 3–4 times/day Topical: A thin film or spray onto area 2–4 times/day	Short-acting corticosteroid possessing mineralocorticoid activity; similar in action but less potent than many other synthetic derivatives; local injection as acetate provides long-lasting effect owing to low solubility; phosphate and succinate salts are water soluble and may be given IV; topical hydrocortisone preparations of 0.5% or weaker are available over-the-counter; available with neomycin in cream and ointment (Neo-Cort-Dome, Neo-Cortef)

Continued

Table 43-3
Glucocorticoids (continued)

Drug	Preparations	Usual Dosage Range	Nursing Implications
Medrysone HMS Liquifilm	Ophthalmic suspension: 1%	1–2 drops 2–4 times/day as needed	Used for steroid-responsive inflammatory conditions of the eye; discontinue drug if irritation develops; prolonged use has resulted in cataract formation; shake suspension well before using
Methylprednisolone Medrol and other manufacturers	Tablets: 2 mg, 4 mg, 8 mg, 16 mg, 24 mg, 32 mg Injection: 40 mg/mL, 125 mg/2 mL, 500 mg/8 mL, 1000 mg/16 mL Repository injection (acetate): 20 mg/mL, 40 mg/mL, 80 mg/mL Powder for injection: 2000 mg/vial Enema: 40 mg Ointment: 0.25%, 1%	*Adults* Oral: 4 mg–48 mg/day in divided doses Repository injection: 40 mg–120 mg IM every 1–4 wk depending on condition Intraarticular: 4 mg–80 mg depending on joint size Injection: 10 mg–40 mg IV over several minutes; subsequent doses may be given IM or IV *Children* No less than 0.5 mg/kg/day Topical: 2–3 times/day	Available as base (tablets), sodium succinate (rapid acting injection) or acetate (repository injection, topical ointment); use alternate-day regimen when administered over extended periods; do *not* inject acetate salt IV
Mometasone Elocon	Cream: 0.1% Ointment: 0.1%	Apply thin film once a day	Potent topical steroid used for steroid-responsive dermatoses; do *not* use occlusive dressings
Paramethasone Haldrone	Tablets: 1 mg, 2 mg	2 mg–24 mg/day in divided doses depending on severity of condition	Approximately 10 times more potent than hydrocortisone, with minimal mineralocorticoid activity; hypocalcemia is common with prolonged high dosage
Prednisolone Several manufacturers	*Oral* Tablets: 5 mg Oral liquid: 5 mg/5 mL *Injection* Sodium phosphate: 20 mg/mL Acetate: 25 mg/mL, 50 mg/mL, 100 mg/mL Tebutate—20 mg/mL *Ophthalmic drops:* 0.12%, 0.125%, 0.5%, 1%	Oral: 5 mg–60 mg/day up to 200 mg/day for acute exacerbation of multiple sclerosis Systemic injection: IM (acetate, sodium phosphate) or IV (sodium phosphate *only*)—4 mg–60 mg/day Intralesional, intraarticular, or soft-tissue injection: 4 mg–30 mg (tebutate) *or* 5 mg–100 mg (acetate) Ophthalmic: 1–2 drops into conjunctival sac every 4 h	Synthetic derivative of hydrocortisone, approximately 5 times more potent; administer orally with meals to minimize GI irritation; sodium and water retention is minimal with normal doses; alternate-day therapy is advisable with prolonged use to reduce incidence of adverse effects; ophthalmic use may increase intraocular pressure; *frequent ocular examinations* are advisable during extended therapy; injections are available as phosphate (rapid onset; short duration), acetate (prolonged action), tebutate (prolonged action), and a combination of acetate and phosphate (prompt onset and prolonged effect)
Prednisone Several manufacturers	Tablets: 1 mg, 2.5 mg, 5 mg, 10 mg, 20 mg, 25 mg, 50 mg Syrup: 5 mg/5 mL Oral concentrate: 5 mg/mL	Adults: 5 mg–60 mg/day in divided doses Children: 0.1–0.15 mg/kg/day divided every 12 h	Synthetic derivative of hydrocortisone; therapeutic action is due to metabolism to prednisolone; use with *caution* in patients with liver disease; may induce sodium and water retention and potassium loss, especially at high doses; administer on alternate days during prolonged therapy; frequently combined with antineoplastic drugs in certain forms of carcinoma (see Chap. 72)

Continued

Table 43-3
Glucocorticoids (continued)

Drug	Preparations	Usual Dosage Range	Nursing Implications

Triamcinolone
Aristocort, Azmacort, Kenalog, and other manufacturers
(CAN) Triaderm, Triamcort
	Tablets: 1 mg, 2 mg, 4 mg, 8 mg
	Syrup: 2 mg/5 mL, 4 mg/5 mL
	Suspension: 3 mg/mL
	Injection: 25 mg/mL, 40 mg/mL
	Repository injection: 5 mg/mL, 10 mg/mL, 20 mg/mL, 40 mg/mL
	Ointment: 0.025%, 0.1%, 0.5%
	Cream: 0.025%, 0.1%, 0.5%
	Dental paste: 0.1%
	Lotion: 0.025%, 0.1%
	Topical spray: approximately 0.2 mg per spray
	Oral inhaler: approximately 100 µg are delivered with each activation
		Oral: 4 mg–60 mg/day depending on condition
		Repository injection (IM): 40 mg once a week
		Intralesional, intraarticular injection:
		  Diacetate: 5 mg–40 mg
		  Acetonide: 2.5 mg–15 mg
		  Hexacetonide: 2 mg–20 mg
		Topical: 2–4 times/day as needed
		Inhalation: 2 inhalations 3–4 times/day
			Synthetic corticosteroid approximately 5 times more potent than hydrocortisone; no significant mineralocorticoid activity at normal doses; diacetate has an intermediate onset and moderate duration of action; acetonide and hexacetonide derivatives possess a slow onset and prolonged duration of action; do *not* use in children; injections should be made IM—do *not* administer IV; oral inhalation (Azmacort) is used in steroid-responsive bronchial asthma (see Chap. 55)

NURSING CONSIDERATIONS

Nursing Alerts
- Monitor results of serum cortisol levels. Either drug overdosage or increased levels of stress may induce adrenal insufficiency.
- Assess patient carefully for indications of adrenocortical hypofunction (e.g., fatigue, nausea, vomiting, anorexia, diarrhea), especially under conditions of stress, trauma, surgery, or acute illness. It may be necessary to administer a mineralocorticoid (see Dosage).
- Monitor results of thyroid function tests, which should be performed at regular intervals, and observe for clinical signs of hypothyroidism (fatigue, hypotension, weakness). Supplementary thyroid drugs may be required.
- Monitor blood pressure because orthostatic hypotension may occur.

1. Ensure that baseline hematologic studies are performed. They should also be repeated at regular intervals during therapy.
2. Monitor results of liver function tests and serum electrolyte determinations, which should be obtained periodically during therapy.

PATIENT EDUCATION
1. Instruct patient to perform hazardous tasks cautiously because dizziness, faintness, ataxia, or weakness may occur.
2. Teach patient appropriate interventions to minimize symptoms of orthostatic hypotension (see **Plan of Nursing Care 8 in Chap. 31**).
3. Inform patient that nausea and loss of appetite can occur during early therapy. If these effects are pronounced or prolonged, the physician should be consulted.
4. Instruct patient to notify physician if side effects (e.g., skin rash, drowsiness) become severe because a dosage reduction or temporary discontinuation of drug may be warranted.

Trilostane
Modastrane

MECHANISM
Lowers circulating glucocorticoid levels by inhibiting enzyme systems essential for their production; exhibits *no* intrinsic hormonal activity

USE
Temporary treatment of adrenocortical hyperfunction (Cushing's syndrome) until more definitive measures (e.g., surgery) can be undertaken

DOSAGE
Initially, 30 mg 4 times/day; increase gradually at 3-day to 4-day intervals; doses generally do not exceed 360 mg/day; discontinue therapy if no response occurs within 2 weeks

COMMON SIDE EFFECTS
Abdominal discomfort, cramping, diarrhea, headache, flushing, burning sensation of the oral or nasal mucosa

SIGNIFICANT ADVERSE REACTIONS
Nasal stuffiness, bloating, belching, lacrimation, muscle and joint pain, skin rash, erythema, fever, paresthesias, fatigue

CONTRAINDICATIONS
Adrenal insufficiency, severe renal or hepatic disease, pregnancy. *Cautious use* in patients with acute illness, in nursing mothers and in persons receiving other drugs that may suppress adrenal function

INTERACTIONS
Concurrent use of trilostane and aminoglutethimide or mitotane can cause severe adrenocortical hypofunction

NURSING CONSIDERATIONS
See aminoglutethimide

PATIENT EDUCATION
See aminoglutethimide

Selected Bibliography

Adams CE: Pulling your patient through an adrenal crisis. RN 46(10):36, 1983

Baxter JD, Rosseau GG (eds): Glucocorticoid Hormone Action. New York, Springer-Verlag, 1979

Baylink DJ: Glucocorticoid-induced osteoporosis. N Engl J Med 309:306, 1983

Cornell RC, Stoughton RB: The use of topical steroids in psoriasis. Dermatol Clin 2:397, 1984

Corticotropin-releasing factor (symposium). Fed Proc 44:145, 1985

Cupps TR, Fauci AS: Corticosteroid-mediated immunoregulation in man. Immunol Rev 65:133, 1982

Donham J: The weakness of steroids. Am J Nurs 86:917, 1986

Gotch PM: Teaching patients about adrenal corticosteroids. Am J Nurs 81:78, 1981

Larson CA: The critical path of adrenocortical insufficiency. Nursing '84 14:66, 1984

Messer J, Reitman D, Sacks HS et al: Association of adrenocorticosteroid therapy and peptic ulcer disease. N Engl J Med 309:21, 1983

Miller JA, Munro DD: Topical corticosteroids: Clinical pharmacology and therapeutic use. Drugs 19:119, 1980

Schleimer RP: The mechanisms of anti-inflammatory steroid action in allergic diseases. Annu Rev Pharmacol Toxicol 25:381, 1985

Young C: Drugs: Actions and reactions—topical corticosteroids. J Enterost Therapy 11:245, Nov—Dec, 1984

SUMMARY. ADRENAL CORTICAL STEROIDS

Drug	Preparations	Usual Dosage Range
Fludrocortisone Florinef	Tablets: 0.1 mg	Initially, 0.1 mg/day (Range 0.1 mg 3 times/wk to 0.2 mg/day up to 0.5 mg/day for orthostatic hypotension)
Glucocorticoids	See Table 43-3	
Aminoglutethimide Cytadren	Tablets: 250 mg	Initially 250 mg 4 times/day; increase in increments of 250 mg/day at 1–2 wk intervals; maximum 2 g/day
Trilostane Modastrane	Capsules: 30 mg, 60 mg	Initially, 30 mg 4 times/day; increase gradually to a maximum of 360 mg/day

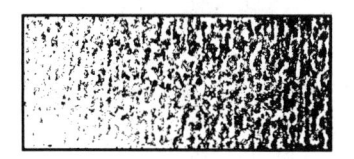

44 ESTROGENS AND PROGESTINS

The female hormones may be categorized into two types—estrogens and progestins. Both groups consist of steroidal compounds secreted by the ovaries, beginning around the time of puberty, as well as by the placenta during pregnancy, and in much lesser amounts by the adrenal cortex. The female sex hormones play a major role in the development and maintenance of the reproductive system and also affect the functioning of many other physiological systems.

ESTROGENS

Chlorotrianisene
Conjugated estrogens
Dienestrol
Diethylstilbestrol
Esterified estrogens
Estradiol
Estrone
Estropipate
Ethinyl estradiol
Polyestradiol phosphate
Quinestrol

The *estrogens* are a group of both naturally occurring and synthetic derivatives that exhibit similar pharmacologic and toxicologic effects, differing primarily in suitability for a particular route of administration, potency, and therapeutic indications. One useful classification for the estrogens divides them into the following categories:

- *Natural (endogenous) estrogens* (e.g., estradiol, estriol, estrone)
- *Esters and conjugates of natural estrogens* (e.g., estradiol valerate, estropipate, polyestradiol phosphate, conjugated estrogens)
- *Semisynthetic and synthetic estrogens* (e.g., ethinyl estradiol, chlorotrianisene, dienestrol, diethylstilbestrol)

The *naturally occurring estrogens* are synthesized principally in the ovary and are secreted during the early phase of the menstrual cycle through the synergistic action of follicle-stimulating hormone (FSH) and luteinizing hormone (LH) on the maturing ovarian follicle. The *endogenous* estrogens are composed of several related substances, the principal one being estradiol, which is the most potent. Estradiol is rapidly converted to estrone, which is approximately one half as potent. Estrone in turn is metabolized to estriol, the weakest in action of the three. These endogenous estrogens promote the growth and development of the endometrium and exert a wide range of effects on other body structures (see Mechanism).

Naturally occurring estrogens are poorly absorbed when administered orally, are rapidly inactivated, and are quickly eliminated, and thus are largely unsuited for oral therapy. Estradiol is available for injection as either the cypionate or valerate salt in an oily vehicle (long-acting), whereas estrone is available in either an aqueous suspension (short-acting) or oily vehicle (long-acting). Crystalline estrone sulfate stabilized with piperazine (estropipate) can be used as a vaginal cream, as can dienestrol, a synthetic estrogen. Orally effective estrogens include micronized estradiol, estropipate, conjugated and esterified estrogenic substances, and a number of semisynthetic and synthetic derivatives. Estradiol is also available in the form of a transdermal patch. Two very potent orally effective semisynthetic estrogens, ethinyl estradiol and mestranol, are the only estrogens found in the combination oral contraceptive formulations, and these products are reviewed in Chapter 45.

Principal indications for use of estrogens include relief of the symptoms of menopause, symptomatic management of atrophic vaginitis, treatment of primary female hypogonadism and ovarian failure, palliation of certain types of carcinoma, suppression of lactation, relief of postpartum breast engorgement, and control of abnormal uterine bleeding due to hormonal imbalance. In addition, certain estrogens are used in combination with progestins for contraception. Of these uses, the treatment of menopause has been a somewhat controversial application for estrogens, and a division of opinion still exists on the safety and efficacy of oral estrogen replacement therapy for menopausal symptoms. There is fairly general agreement that *low-dose* oral estrogen therapy can reduce the incidence and severity of vasomotor symptoms associated with the menopause (such as sweating, flushing, "hot flashes") and that topical application is effective in retarding the atrophic changes in the vaginal epithelium (as in senile vaginitis). Conversely, little evidence supports the use of estrogenic substances for the control of the mental and emotional changes that often accompany the onset of menopause.

The use of estrogens to retard the progression of osteoporosis in postmenopausal women has been the subject of some debate; however, the current consensus seems to favor use of low doses of estrogen together with supplemental calcium as a safe and effective means of retarding bone loss and reducing the incidence of spontaneous fractures. The estrogen is usually given for 25 days each month and a progestin is added for the last 10 days for reasons outlined below. Most clinicians prescribe supplemental calcium as well, and it appears that the dosage necessary to maintain a positive calcium balance in perimenopausal and postmenopausal women is 1.0 g to 1.5 g of calcium per day. Concurrent use of vitamin D is also recognized as safe and effective, but dosage should be restricted to 400 U/day or less. Large doses of vitamin D have actually been demonstrated to *increase* bone resorption. Use of other therapeutic agents, such as calcitonin or sodium fluoride, is much less generally accepted.

Evidence indicates that estrogen therapy is most effective if begun as soon as possible after the onset of menopause. Further, estrogen supplementation, once begun, is probably a lifelong program, as bone resorption resumes shortly after the estrogen is stopped and some reports indicate that bone loss may be *accelerated* if estrogen is employed and then withdrawn.

The principal hazards associated with estrogen replacement therapy are thromboembolic complications, gallbladder disease, hypertension and, most critically, endometrial carcinoma. Estimates of the risk of endometrial carcinoma range from 5 times to 14 times greater than in nonusers according to the dosage being used and the duration of therapy. Current recommendations call for use of small doses of estrogens (i.e., 0.3 to 0.625 mg of conjugated estrogens) in conjunction with calcium and addition of a progestin from days 15 to 25 of the dosage cycle. Progestin treatment has been shown to reduce (and perhaps even eliminate) the risk of endometrial carcinoma but can increase the frequency of cyclic withdrawal bleeding.

The use of estrogens in postmenopausal women must be undertaken cautiously, minimal effective doses must be used, and cyclic administration should be employed. Therapy should be reevaluated at 6-month intervals and dosage adjustments made if necessary. Appropriate laboratory tests and a physical examination should be performed before initiating therapy and at regular intervals thereafter.

The discussion of the estrogens considers the agents as a group. Individual drugs and dosages are listed in Table 44-1 along with nursing implications pertaining to each individual drug.

MECHANISM

Produce thickening and increase development of blood vessels and glands of the endometrium; increase volume and acidity of cervical and vaginal secretions; promote growth and cornification of vaginal epithelium and enhance glycogen deposition; accelerate uterine motility; assist growth and development of the duct system of the mammary glands; increase sensitivity of uterus to oxytocin; metabolic actions include a protein anabolic action, accelerated closure of the epiphyses, decreased bone resorption rate, increased serum triglycerides, decreased serum cholesterol and low-density lipoproteins, and enhanced sodium and water retention; reduce platelet adhesiveness and increase levels of vitamin K–dependent clotting factors; *large doses* reduce release of FSH and prolactin from the anterior pituitary by negative feedback, thus inhibiting follicular maturation and lactation; appear to increase release of LH, assisting ovulation; biochemical actions of estrogens are apparently due to their interaction with receptor proteins on estrogen-responsive tissues (e.g., breasts, genitalia); as a result, there is increased synthesis of DNA, RNA, and several proteins that alter the function of these tissues; receptor effects are blocked by inhibitors of RNA or protein synthesis

USES

(See Table 44-1 for specific indications for each drug)

Relief of vasomotor and atrophic symptoms of the menopause and prevention of osteoporotic changes

Treatment of atrophic vaginitis and kraurosis vulvae (dryness and pruritus of female genitalia)

Replacement therapy in female hypogonadism, female castration, and primary ovarian failure

Palliative treatment of advanced prostatic carcinoma, and mammary carcinoma in women who are at least 5 years postmenopausal (see Chap. 72)

Relief of postpartum breast engorgement (benefit versus risk must be critically weighed; largely obsolete use)

Control of abnormal uterine bleeding due to lack of estrogen secretion

Relief of severe acne resistant to more conventional therapy (investigational use in female patients only)

Postcoital contraception (*emergency* use only; see diethylstilbestrol, Table 44-1)

DOSAGE

See Table 44-1

FATE

Estradiol is metabolized to estrone and further to estriol in vivo, then is conjugated and excreted in the urine. Natural estrogens are rapidly inactivated in the GI tract. Esterification of natural estrogens delays metabolism and prolongs action. Aqueous solution of estrogens provides rapid onset and relatively short duration of action. Suspensions or solutions in oil allow slower absorption from IM injection sites, delayed onset, and prolonged duration of action. Oral absorption of synthetic estrogens is good, and they are less rapidly inactivated than natural derivatives. They circulate in both free and conjugated forms, which are 50% to 75% protein bound. Metabolism of estrogens occurs primarily in the liver; less active conjugated products are produced. Estrogens are excreted largely in the urine, although some excretion occurs by way of the bile

COMMON SIDE EFFECTS

Nausea, fluid retention, "breakthrough" (midcycle) menstrual bleeding, change in menstrual flow, and breast fullness or tenderness

SIGNIFICANT ADVERSE REACTIONS

> **WARNING**
>
> Use of estrogens is associated with an increased risk of endometrial carcinoma. The risk is dose and duration dependent, and is estimated to be between 5 times and 14 times that of nonusers. There appears to be no difference in risk between "natural" and synthetic estrogens. Cyclical progestin therapy (i.e., days 15 to 25) appears to significantly reduce this risk.
>
> Use of estrogens during early pregnancy may damage the fetus. Female offspring exposed in utero to diethylstilbestrol display an increased incidence of cervical or vaginal adenocarcinoma. Congenital anomalies have also been reported in male offspring whose mothers ingested the drug. Patients using estrogens must be apprised of the risks of becoming pregnant while taking the drugs

GI: vomiting, abdominal cramps, bloating, diarrhea, anorexia, cholestatic jaundice, colitis

Dermatologic: skin rash, pruritus, hirsutism, chloasma, melasma, erythema multiforme, erythema nodosum, alopecia, acne

CNS: irritability, depression, headache, migraine attacks, dizziness, insomnia, paresthesias

Genitourinary: in females, dysmenorrhea, amenorrhea, vaginal candidiasis, increased cervical secretions, cystitis-like reaction, endometrial hyperplasia, increase in size of uterine fibromyomata; in males, feminization of genitalia, testicular atrophy, impotence

Other: gallbladder disease, thromboembolic complications, hepatic adenoma, hypertension, hypercalcemia, decreased carbohydrate tolerance, aggravation of porphyria, changes in libido, pain at injection site, sterile abscess,

(See also under Oral Contraceptives, Chapter 45)

CONTRAINDICATIONS

Pregnancy, known or suspected breast cancer in premenopausal women, estrogen-dependent neoplasia, undiagnosed genital bleeding, a history of or active thromboembolic disease, incomplete bone growth, or epiphyseal closure. *Cautious use* in persons with cerebrovascular or coronary artery disease, severe hypertension, epilepsy, migraine, renal or hepatic dysfunction, diabetes mellitus, depression or other emotional disturbances, gallbladder disease, metabolic bone disease associated with hypercalcemia, thyroid dysfunction, endometriosis, and in patients with a history of jaundice or a family history of breast or genital cancer

INTERACTIONS

See also Interactions under oral contraceptives in Chapter 45

Estrogens may reduce the effectiveness of oral anticoagulants, chenodiol, and insulin, thereby increasing dosage requirements

The incidence of adverse effects with tricyclic antidepressants may be increased by estrogens

The effects of estrogens may be attenuated by phenobarbital, phenytoin, carbamazepine, primidone, rifampin, and other drugs that can induce hepatic microsomal enzymes, thus accelerating the metabolism of estrogens

Estrogens increase the effects of oxytocin on the uterus

Estrogens can alter many laboratory values; for example, they may increase prothrombin, thyroid-binding globulin, serum triglycerides, phospholipids, sulfobromophthalein retention, and norepinephrine-induced platelet aggregability, and they may decrease serum folate levels, glucose tolerance, pregnanediol excretion, antithrombin III levels, and triiodothyronine (T_3) uptake; in addition, estrogens may cause an impaired response to the metyrapone test

NURSING CONSIDERATIONS

Nursing Alert

- Ensure that a comprehensive patient history and physical examination are completed before therapy is initiated. If therapy is prolonged, physical examination should be repeated at regular intervals. Estrogen should be administered very cautiously to patients with a family history of breast cancer or thromboembolic or other cardiovascular disorders.

1. Provide emotional support as needed for menopausal patient, and be prepared to discuss fears concerning use of estrogen and its possible adverse effects, including cancer and thromboembolic complications.
2. Interpret results of laboratory studies cautiously because estrogen use can alter many of them (see Interactions).

PATIENT EDUCATION

1. Strongly encourage patient to curtail smoking during therapy because the risk of cardiovascular complications increases with amount of smoking (and age).
2. Explain to menopausal patient that the lowest effective dose is used to control symptoms and that estrogen is administered on a cyclic schedule whenever possible to minimize untoward reactions. If therapy is extended, patient should obtain Pap smear periodically and report abnormal vaginal bleeding immediately.
3. Explain to postmenopausal woman taking estrogen *cyclically* that withdrawal bleeding is normal and does not indicate return of fertility.
4. Reassure patient that the nausea that often occurs early in therapy will disappear within 1 to 2 weeks.
5. Teach patient signs of embolic disorders (e.g., severe headache, chest pains, dyspnea, calf pain, leg swelling, visual disturbances). If these occur, drug should be discontinued and physician should be notified immediately.
6. Stress the importance of health care supervision during treatment because the potential for adverse reactions is considerable, and early detection is important.
7. Instruct female patients to inform physician immediately if pregnancy is suspected. Estrogen use should be avoided during pregnancy because fetal abnormalities have occurred.
8. Alert patient and significant others to note behavioral changes or signs of depression. If any occur, unless the drug is absolutely necessary, it should be discontinued to avoid further psychological deterioration.
9. Instruct patient to be alert for signs of developing jaundice (yellow skin or sclera, itching, darkened urine, light-colored stools) and to discontinue drug if they occur.
10. Advise patient to report symptoms of abdominal distress because gallbladder disease and benign hepatic adenomas can occur.
11. Instruct patient to inform physician if fluid retention or weight gain occur because dose may have to be adjusted.
12. Warn diabetic patient that estrogen may increase hypoglycemic drug requirements by decreasing glucose tolerance.
13. Inform female patients that vaginal candidiasis may occur and should be treated with an appropriate antifungal agent. Symptoms include thick, whitish vaginal secretion and local inflammation.
14. Reassure male that signs of feminization and impotence that may occur during therapy are reversible upon cessation of drug.

PROGESTINS

Hydroxyprogesterone   Norethindrone
Medroxyprogesterone   Norgestrel
Megestrol   Progesterone

The term *progestins* refers to a group of naturally occurring and synthetic steroids having the physiological effects of progesterone, the principal endogenous progestational hormone. Progesterone is normally secreted by the corpus luteum and also by the placenta during pregnancy, and it elicits a variety of actions in the body, which are reviewed under Mechanism. Because it is rapidly inactivated following oral ingestion, progesterone is administered intramuscularly only, in either an aqueous or an oily vehicle. A number of synthetic progestational steroids are also available. These drugs exhibit effects qualitatively similar to progesterone itself but differ from the endogenous progestin in that they possess greater potency, longer duration of action, and in some cases, oral or sublingual effectiveness.

Primary indications for the various progestins are amenorrhea, abnormal uterine bleeding, endometriosis, and endometrial carcinoma. In addition, several of the orally effective synthetic derivatives are used either alone or in fixed combinations with estrogen for the prevention of conception. A discussion of the oral contraceptive agents is presented in Chapter 45.

An earlier use for progestational drugs is no longer considered a valid indication for these compounds: Progestins were formerly employed during the first trimester of pregnancy in an

Table 44-1
Estrogens

Drug	Preparations	Usual Dosage Range	Nursing Implications
Chlorotrianisene Tace	Capsules: 12 mg, 25 mg, 72 mg	*Menopause:* 12 mg–25 mg/day cyclically for 30 days *Hypogonadism:* 12 mg–25 mg/day cyclically for 21 days, followed by 100 mg progesterone IM *Prostatic carcinoma:* 12 mg–25 mg/day *Breast engorgement:* 12 mg 4 times/day for 7 days *or* 50 mg every 6 h for 6 doses *or* 72 mg twice a day for 2 days	Synthetic estrogen with delayed onset and prolonged duration of action; stored in adipose tissue; 72-mg capsule is used only for postpartum breast engorgement in non-nursing mothers; first dose should be given within 8 h of delivery; drug is not recommended for mammary carcinoma, because it induces uterine bleeding and endometrial hyperplasia (see Chap. 72)
Conjugated Estrogens Estrocon, Premarin, Progens (CAN) C.E.S.	Tablets: 0.3 mg, 0.625 mg, 0.9 mg, 1.25 mg, 2.5 mg Injection: 25 mg/vial with 5 mL diluent Vaginal cream: 0.625 mg/g	*Menopause:* 0.3 mg–0.625 mg/day cyclically with progestins on days 15–25 *Hypogonadism, ovarian failure:* 2.5 mg–7.5 mg/day in divided doses for 20 days; oral progestin during last 5 days *Prostatic carcinoma:* 1.25 mg–2.5 mg 3 times/day for several weeks (maintenance ½ initial dose) *Breast cancer:* 10 mg 3 times/day for 2–5 mo as needed to obtain desired response *Vaginitis, kraurosis vulvae:* Insert vaginal cream 1–2 times/day *Abnormal uterine bleeding:* 25 mg IV or IM; repeat in 6 h if necessary	Water-soluble mixture of conjugated estrogens (sodium estrone sulfate, 50%–65%, and sodium equilin sulfate, 20%–35%) obtained from the urine of pregnant mares; most commonly used orally for menopausal symptoms although vaginal cream is employed for atrophic vaginitis and pruritus vulvae and injection can be used to control abnormal uterine bleeding due to hormonal imbalance; perform IV injection slowly to minimize flushing; do *not* use if solution is darkened or a precipitate is noted; solution is incompatible with other solutions having an acid *p*H; it is also available in combination with meprobamate (Milprem and PMB; see Chap. 72)
Dienestrol DV, Estraguard, Ortho Dienestrol	Vaginal cream: 0.01%	*Atrophic vaginitis, kraurosis vulvae:* 1–2 applicators of cream daily for 1–2 wk, then 1 applicator every other day	Synthetic estrogen employed vaginally; systemic absorption may be significant during prolonged use
Diethylstilbestrol (DES)	Tablets: 1 mg, 5 mg Enteric-coated tablets: 0.1 mg, 0.25 mg, 0.5 mg, 1 mg, 5 mg	*Menopause:* 0.2 mg–0.5 mg/day cyclically *Hypogonadism:* 0.2 mg–0.5 mg/day cyclically *Prostatic carcinoma:* 1 mg–3 mg/day *Breast cancer:* 15 mg/day *Postcoital contraception:* 25 mg twice a day for 5 days (emergency use *only*)	Potent synthetic estrogen given orally; frequently produces nausea, vomiting, and headache; should be administered cyclically when given for prolonged periods; contraindicated during pregnancy, because drug has been implicated in causing vaginal and cervical cancer in offspring of women receiving the drug during first trimester; as a postcoital contraceptive, must be given within 24–72 h of intercourse.
Diethylstilbestrol Diphosphate Stilphostrol (CAN) Honvol	Tablets: 50 mg Injection: 0.25 g/5 mL	*Advanced prostatic carcinoma:* 50 mg–200 mg orally 3 times/day *or* 0.5 g by IV infusion first day, then 1 g/day on subsequent 5 days; maintenance 0.25 g–0.5 g 1–2 times/week	High-dose diethylstilbestrol used for treatment of prostatic carcinoma unresponsive to other estrogens; be alert for early signs of thrombotic complications; for IV administration, dissolve 0.5 g–1 g of drug in 300 mL saline or dextrose and infuse *slowly* (20–30 drops a min) during first 10–15 min; adjust rate thereafter so that entire amount is given over 1 h (see Chap. 72)

Continued

Table 44-1
Estrogens (continued)

Drug	Preparations	Usual Dosage Range	Nursing Implications
Esterified Estrogens Estratab, Menest	Tablets: 0.3 mg, 0.625 mg, 1.25 mg, 2.5 mg	*Menopause:* 0.3 mg–0.625 mg/day *Hypogonadism, ovarian failure:* 2.5 mg–7.5 mg/day in divided doses for 20 days, then stop for 10 days *Prostatic carcinoma:* 1.25 mg–2.5 mg 3 times/day; maintenance—reduce by half after several weeks *Breast cancer:* 10 mg 3 times/day for 3 mo	Mixture of sodium estrone sulfate (75%–85%) and sodium equilin sulfate (6%–15%); action is similar to conjugated estrogens; also available with chlordiazepoxide as Menrium
Estradiol, Oral Estrace	Tablets: 1 mg, 2 mg	*Menopause:* 1 mg–2 mg/day orally for 3 wk; then 1 wk off *Breast cancer:* 10 mg 3 times/day for 3 mo *Prostatic carcinoma:* 1 mg–2 mg 3 times/day	Estrogenic hormone derived from estrone but more potent; readily absorbed orally; available in salt form for injection (see below) providing slow onset and more prolonged duration of action
Estradiol Cypionate Depo-Estradiol, and other manufacturers	Injection: 1 mg/mL, 5 mg/mL	*Menopause:* 1 mg–5 mg IM every 3–4 wk *Hypogonadism:* 1.5 mg–2 mg once a month	Salt of estradiol in cottonseed oil providing a depot effect; duration of action 3–6 wk; administered IM only (see Chap. 72)
Estradiol Valerate Delestrogen, and other manufacturers (CAN) Femogex	Injection: 10 mg/mL, 20 mg/mL, 40 mg/mL	*Menopause:* 10 mg–20 mg IM every 4 wk *Hypogonadism, ovarian failure:* 10 mg–20 mg IM every 4 wk *Prostatic carcinoma:* 30 mg every 1–2 wk	Salt of estradiol in sesame or castor oil provides 2–3 wk of estrogenic activity following a single IM dose (see Chap. 72)
Estradiol Transdermal System Estraderm	Transdermal patch releasing either 0.05 mg/24 h *or* 0.1 mg/24 h	Apply patch to skin twice weekly; usually given on a cyclic schedule (i.e., 3 wk on, 1 wk off)	Transdermal patch used to control vasomotor symptoms of the menopause, atrophic vaginitis, kraurosis vulvae, and symptoms of primary ovarian failure and female hypogonadism; system is placed on a clean, dry area of skin, preferably the abdomen; do not apply to breasts; rotate application sites; apply patch immediately after opening pouch and ensure good contact between patch and skin
Estrone Theelin Aqueous, and other manufacturers (CAN) Femogen	Injection: 2 mg/mL, 5 mg/mL	*Menopause:* 0.1 mg–0.5 mg IM 2–3 times/wk *Hypogonadism, ovarian failure:* 0.1 mg–2 mg/week IM in single or divided doses *Prostatic carcinoma:* 2 mg–4 mg IM 2–3 times/wk	Estrogenic hormone derived from both natural and synthetic sources; response to therapy for prostatic carcinoma should become apparent within 3 mo; if response occurs, continue drug until disease again becomes progressive (see Chap. 72)
Estropipate Ogen	Tablets: 0.625 mg, 1.25 mg, 2.5 mg, 5 mg (equivalent to 0.75 mg, 1.5 mg, 3 mg and 6 mg estropipate, respectively) Vaginal cream: 1.5 mg/g	*Menopause:* 0.625 mg–5 mg/day cyclically each month *Hypogonadism, ovarian failure:* 1.25 mg–7.5 mg/day for 3 wk, followed by 8–10-day rest period; repeated as needed *Atrophic vaginitis:* 1 g–2 g vaginal cream daily	Crystalline form of estrone solubilized as sulfate and stabilized with piperazine, making preparation orally effective; tablets contain 83% sodium estrone sulfate equivalent; formerly known as piperazine estrone sulfate

Continued

Table 44-1
Estrogens (continued)

Drug	Preparations	Usual Dosage Range	Nursing Implications
Ethinyl Estradiol Estinyl, Feminone	Tablets: 0.02 mg, 0.05 mg, 0.5 mg	*Menopause:* 0.02 mg–0.05 mg/day for 21 days cyclically each month *Hypogonadism:* 0.05 mg 1–3 times/day for 2 wk, followed by an oral progestin for 2 wk *Breast cancer:* 1 mg 3 times/day *Prostatic carcinoma:* 0.15 mg–2 mg/day	Potent, orally effective synthetic estrogen is found in many oral contraceptives (see Chap. 45); also used for menopausal symptoms, female hypogonadism, and certain carcinomas (see Chap. 72)
Polyestradiol Phosphate Estradurin	Injection: 40 mg/vial with 2 mL diluent	*Advanced prostatic carcinoma:* 40 mg IM every 2–4 wk up to 80 mg	Provides a stable level of active estrogen over a prolonged period; quickly cleared from blood (24 h) and passively stored in reticuloendothelial system; estradiol levels are maintained constant by continuous replacement from storage sites; increasing the dose prolongs the duration of action but does not significantly enhance the response; may produce temporary burning at IM injection site; clinical response should be evident within 3 mo; continue drug until disease becomes progressive (see Chap. 72)
Quinestrol Estrovis	Tablets: 100 μg	*Menopause, hypogonadism, ovarian failure, kraurosis vulvae, atrophic vaginitis:* 100 μg once daily for 7 days, then 100 μg to 200 μg once a week thereafter	A derivative of ethinyl estradiol that is stored in body fat and slowly released, thus providing a prolonged duration of action; once-weekly administration is as effective as cyclic therapy with shorter-acting estrogens, and may improve patient compliance

attempt to prevent habitual abortion or to treat threatened abortion. There is no conclusive evidence that such treatment is effective, however, and several reports have suggested that fetal damage (i.e., congenital heart or limb-reduction defects) and delayed spontaneous abortion of defective ova can result from use of progestational agents during early pregnancy. If inadvertantly exposed to progestins during the initial stages of pregnancy, patients should be apprised of the potential risks to the fetus.

The discussion of the progestational drugs treats them as a group, inasmuch as their pharmacology is similar. Individual drugs are listed in Table 44-2.

MECHANISM
Induce biochemical changes in the endometrium in preparation for implantation of the fertilized egg; inhibit secretion of pituitary gonadotropins (primarily LH), preventing maturation of the follicle and ovulation; stimulate cervical mucus secretion; decrease sensitivity of uterus to oxytocin and facilitate development of secretory apparatus in mammary gland; metabolic actions include increased body temperature, decreased plasma level of amino acids, and elevated basal insulin levels

USES
(*See* Table 44-2 for specific indications for each drug)
Treatment of primary and secondary amenorrhea and dysmenorrhea
Control of abnormal uterine bleeding due to hormonal imbalance, in the absence of organic pathology
Treatment of endometriosis
Palliative and adjunctive treatment of advanced, inoperable, or metastatic breast or endometrial carcinoma (see Chap. 72)
Prevention of conception (alone or combined with estrogens; see Chap. 45)
Investigational uses include use of medroxyprogesterone acetate for relief of menopausal symptoms and to stimulate respiration in obstructive sleep apnea, and use of progesterone suppositories or oral progestins for treatment of premenstrual syndrome (PMS)

DOSAGE
See Table 44-2

FATE
Progesterone is quickly inactivated when given orally. Other derivatives are rapidly absorbed following oral administration

Table 44-2
Progestins

Drug	Preparations	Usual Dosage Range	Nursing Implications
Hydroxyprogesterone Caproate Duralutin and other manufacturers	Injection: 125 mg/mL, 250 mg/mL	*Amenorrhea, uterine bleeding:* 375 mg IM; if no bleeding after 21 days, begin cyclic therapy with estradiol and repeat every 4 wk for 4 cycles *Uterine adenocarcinoma:* 1 g or more IM initially; repeat 1 or more times each week (maximum 7/g/wk; stop when relapse occurs or after 12 wk with no response *Test for endogenous estrogen production:* 250 mg IM; repeat in 4 wk; bleeding 7–14 days after injection indicates presence of endogenous estrogen	Long-acting synthetic progestin, available in either sesame oil or castor oil; duraton of acton is approximately 10–17 days; devoid of estrogenic activity and does not prevent conception; may produce dyspnea, coughing, constriction of the chest, and allergic-like reactions, especially at high doses; solution should be protected from light and stored at room temperature (*see also* Chap. 72)
Medroxyprogesterone Acetate Amen, Curretab, Cycrin, Depo-Provera, Provera	Tablets: 2.5 mg, 5 mg, 10 mg Injection (Depo-Provera): 100 mg/mL, 400 mg/mL	*Amenorrhea:* 5 mg–10 mg/day orally for 5–10 days *Uterine bleeding:* 5 mg–10 mg/day for 5–10 days beginning on 16th or 21st day of cycle *Endometrial or renal carcinoma:* 400 mg–1000 mg/wk IM; maintenance therapy following improvement 400 mg a mo	Synthetic progestin used orally for inducing secretory changes in the estrogen-primed endometrium and IM in a depot-injectable form for adjunctive therapy of inoperable, recurrent, or metastatic endometrial or renal carcinoma; also has been used orally to stimulate respiration in the obesity–hypoventilation syndrome; has produced malignant mammary nodules in dogs; the human significance of this finding is not established (*see* Chap. 72)
Megestrol Acetate Megace, Palace	Tablets: 20 mg, 40 mg	*Breast or endometrial carcinoma:* 40 mg–80 mg 4 times/day for at least 2 mo	Orally effective synthetic progestin indicated for palliative treatment or advanced breast or endometrial carcinoma; malignant breast tumors have occurred in megestrol-treated dogs; no serious side effects have been reported in humans in doses as high as 800 mg a day (*see* Chap. 72)
Norethindrone Micronor, Norlutin, Nor-Q.D.	Tablets: 0.35 mg, 5 mg	*Amenorrhea, uterine bleeding:* 5 mg–20 mg/day from day 5–25 of cycle *Endometriosis:* 10 mg/day for 2 wk, then increase by 5 mg/day every 2 wk to 30 mg/day *Contraception:* 0.35 mg daily	Synthetic progestin possessing androgenic, anabolic, and antiestrogenic properties, especially in high doses; component of several oral contraceptive products and used alone (0.35 mg) as well as a progestin-only contraceptive (*see* Chap. 45)
Norethindrone Acetate Aygestin, Norlutate	Tablets: 5 mg	*Amenorrhea, uterine bleeding:* 2.5 mg–10 mg/day from day 5–25 of cycle *Endometriosis:* 5 mg/day for 2 wk; then increase by 2.5 mg/day every 2 wk to 15 mg/day	Potent synthetic progestin possessing androgenic, anabolic, and *anti*estrogenic activity; component of several oral contraceptive drugs (*see* Chap. 45)
Norgestrel Ovrette	Tablets: 0.075 mg	*Contraception:* 0.075 mg a day	Potent progestational hormone used as a progestin-only oral contraceptive ("mini-pill") (*see* Chap. 45)

Continued

Table 44-2
Progestins (continued)

Drug	Preparations	Usual Dosage Range	Nursing Implications
Progesterone Bay Progest, Femotrone Gesterol-50, Progestaject	*Injection:* Aqueous: 25 mg/mL, 50 mg/mL Oil: 25 mg/mL, 50 mg/mL, 100 mg/mL	*Amenorrhea:* 5 mg–10 mg IM for 6–8 consecutive days *Uterine bleeding:* 5 mg–10 mg/day IM for 6 days	Endogenous progestin possessing *anti*estrogenic activity; large doses may have a catabolic action and produce loss of sodium and chloride; warm solution before injecting to assure dissolution of all particles; should not be used for diagnosis of pregnancy; suppositories have been used for treatment of premenstrual syndrome (PMS) but are not approved for this indication

or aqueous IM injection; metabolized by the liver and excreted both in the urine and feces

COMMON SIDE EFFECTS
(Usually seen with large doses) Fluid retention, break-through bleeding

SIGNIFICANT ADVERSE REACTIONS
(Usually seen with prolonged use or high doses) Menstrual flow irregularities, amenorrhea, cervical erosion, changes in cervical secretion, altered libido, masculinization of the female fetus, edema, weight gain, breast tenderness, hirsutism, alopecia, rash, melasma, decreased glucose tolerance, photosensitivity, cholestatic jaundice, pruritus, diarrhea, depression, nervousness, migraine, coughing, dyspnea, allergic reactions, and retinal vascular lesions. In addition, thromboembolic episodes with medroxyprogesterone.
See also Oral Contraceptives (Chap. 45)

CONTRAINDICATIONS
Thromboembolic disorders, markedly impaired liver function, known or suspected genital or breast malignancy, undiagnosed vaginal bleeding, missed abortion, and cerebral apoplexy. *Cautious use* in patients with diabetes, migraine, epilepsy, cardiac or renal disease, asthma, and psychoses

INTERACTIONS
Progestins can impair the action of sympathomimetic drugs by enhancing their metabolism and can reduce the effectiveness of hypoglycemic agents by decreasing glucose tolerance
The effects of progestins may be reduced by barbiturates, phenylbutazone, and phenytoin

NURSING CONSIDERATION
1. Interpret results of laboratory tests for hepatic or endocrine function cautiously because progestins may alter the values.

PATIENT EDUCATION
1. Discuss the need for pretreatment and periodic follow-up examinations of the breast and pelvic region, including a Pap smear. Teach breast self-examination.
2. Suggest that oral progestin be taken with food to minimize GI distress.
3. Alert patient receiving IM injection that pain or local allergic reaction can occur, but that these side effects are generally transient.
4. Explain the difference between normal withdrawal bleeding (3–4 days following discontinuation of drug) and breakthrough bleeding or spotting (during course of drug therapy). The latter type of bleeding should be reported because dosage may need to be adjusted.
5. Teach patient how to recognize, and stress the importance of immediately reporting, early manifestations of thromboembolic complications (e.g., chest or calf pain, dyspnea, numbness in arm or leg, edema, dizziness, visual disturbances). Drug should be discontinued if these occur.
6. Apprise patient of danger to fetus if a progestin is taken during initial months of pregnancy. Health care provider should be informed immediately if pregnancy is suspected in a woman taking progestin.
7. Instruct patient to note, and report to physician, occurrence of any visual changes, diplopia, ptosis, or headache. If ophthalmic examination reveals retinal vascular lesions or papilledema, drug should be discontinued.
8. Instruct patient to observe for symptoms of jaundice (dark urine, pruritus, yellowish skin or sclera) and to report them immediately.
9. Teach patient to monitor weight regularly and to observe for signs of edema. Significant weight variations should be reported.
10. Explain that vaginal itching or burning may indicate local candidal infection, which should be treated with appropriate antifungal medication (see Chap. 72).
11. Instruct diabetic patient to monitor urine or blood sugar carefully and to report any changes because progestins may reduce glucose tolerance.
12. Advise significant others to closely observe patient with a history of depression for mood changes or signs of recurring depression.

Selected Bibliography
Aloia JF et al: Risk factors for postmenopausal osteoporosis. Am J Med 78:95, 1985
Ettinger B, Genant HK, Cann CE: Postmenopausal bone loss is prevented by treatment with low dose estrogen with calcium. Ann Intern Med 106:40, 1987

Frank EP: What are nurses doing to help PMS patients? Am J Nurs 86:137, 1986

Gambrell RD: Menopause: Benefits and risks of estrogen–progestogen replacement therapy. Fertil Steril 37:457, 1982

Gambrell RD, Maier RC, Sanders BI: Decreased incidence of breast cancer in postmenopausal estrogen–progestogen users. Obstet Gynecol 62:435, 1983

Hammond MG: Managing menopausal signs and symptoms. Drug Ther 14(12):35, 1984

Horsman A, Jones M, Francis R, Nordin C: The effect of estrogen dose on postmenopausal bone loss. N Engl J Med 309:1405, 1983

Judd HL, Meldrum DR, Deftos LJ, Henderson BE: Estrogen replacement therapy: Indications and complications. Ann Intern Med 98:195, 1983

Kalkhoff RK: Metabolic effects of progesterone. Am J Obstet Gynecol 142:735, 1982

Kase NG: Progestin therapy for perimenopausal women. J Reprod Med 27:522, 1982

Ladewig PA: Protocol for estrogen replacement therapy in menopausal women. Nurse Pract 10(10):44, 1985

Licata AA: New ideas in diagnosis and treatment of osteoporosis. Mod Med 55:95, 1987

Mann JI: Progestogens in cardiovascular disease: An introduction to the epidemiologic data. Am J Obstet Gynecol 142:752, 1982

Meade TW: Effects of progestogens on the cardiovascular system. Am J Obstet Gynecol 142:776, 1982

O'Brien PM: The premenstrual syndrome: A review of the present status of therapy. Drugs 24:140, 1982

Quigley MM: Postmenopausal hormone R_x: Time for a fresh clinical look. Mod Med 54(8):34, 1986

Raisz LG, Smith JA: Prevention and therapy of osteoporosis. Ration Drug Ther 19(8):1, 1985

Raunikar V: Osteoporosis: A Strategy for management. Mod Med 56:62, 1988

Riis B, Thomsen K, Christiansen C: Does calcium supplementation prevent postmenopausal bone loss? A double-blinded, controlled clinical study. N Engl J Med 316(4):173, 1987

Ryan KJ: Postmenopausal estrogen use. Annu Rev Med 33:171, 1982

Stampfer MJ et al: A prospective study of postmenopausal estrogen therapy and coronary heart disease. N Engl J Med 313:1044, 1985

45 DRUGS USED IN FERTILITY CONTROL

Several different kinds of pharmacologic agents are employed to control female fertility. They may be grouped according to their action as the following:

- *Steroid contraceptives* (e.g., estrogen–progestin combinations)
- *Ovulation stimulants* (e.g., clomiphene, menotropins)
- *Abortifacients* (e.g., prostaglandins, sodium chloride 20%)

Steroid contraceptives are the most effective drug-based means of preventing conception and are widely used. They are discussed in detail below. Ovulation stimulants are drugs capable of inducing ovulation in infertile women, provided ovarian responsiveness is adequate. These agents are likewise considered in detail in this chapter. Drugs used to abort a fetus include several prostaglandin derivatives as well as hypertonic sodium chloride solution. These agents are also reviewed in this chapter.

STEROID CONTRACEPTIVES

The widest application for estrogens and progestins is in the prevention of pregnancy. Combinations of estrogens and progestins, commonly referred to as oral contraceptives or "the pill," are the most frequently employed and most effective means for preventing pregnancy in fertile women. The many fixed-combination products differ both in the amount and potency of the two components and in the relative estrogen-progestin activity ratio.

Three basic types of combination oral contraceptives are currently available:

- *Monophasic:* a fixed dose of estrogen and progestin in every tablet; the majority of oral contraceptives are of this type
- *Biphasic* (e.g., Ortho-Novum 10/11, Nelova 10/11): a fixed amount of estrogen in every tablet; the amount of progestin in the first 10 tablets is half the amount in the remaining 11 tablets
- *Triphasic* (e.g., Ortho-Novum 7/7/7, Tri-Norinyl, Triphasil): amounts of estrogen *and* progestin vary throughout the tablets

The latter two types, biphasic and triphasic, are formulated to deliver the hormones in a manner that more closely resembles their physiologic secretion than is possible with the monophasic preparations. However, contraceptive efficacy is *equivalent* for all three types of products, and the potential advantages of phasic delivery of the hormones remains to be definitively established.

The two estrogens that are found in all of the oral contraceptives, either ethinyl estradiol or mestranol, are essentially equivalent in their activity. They are present in varying amounts in the different products, as indicated in Table 45-1. The most popular products are those that contain relatively low amounts of estrogens (i.e., 35 μg of ethinyl estradiol or 50 μg of mestranol), because they are associated with a lower incidence of estrogen-related side effects than combinations containing 50 μg to 100 μg of estrogen and are equally effective.

The progestin component of these preparations, however, may comprise one of five different compounds, which vary not only in potency but also in degree of estrogenic, antiestrogenic, and androgenic activity. Although contraceptive efficacy varies little among the currently available oral contraceptive combinations, frequency and severity of side effects are often related to the relative strength of the estrogen or progestin component. Achieving the proper hormonal balance of estrogen–progestin activity in each individual can often significantly reduce the degree of untoward effects and thus maximize patient compliance. Table 45-2 presents the important side effects resulting from either estrogen or progestin excess and provides a listing of currently available oral contraceptives grouped according to their relative estrogen: progestin ratio.

Although the fixed estrogen–progestin combination products are generally recognized as being the most effective nonsurgical means of contraception, other types of steroidal and nonsteroidal products are used to prevent conception. Progestin-only oral contraceptives (the "mini-pill") are claimed to elicit fewer adverse effects than the combination products, but are also somewhat less effective, having approximately a threefold higher incidence of pregnancy than the estrogen–progestin combinations.

Another steroidal preparation is the intrauterine progesterone contraceptive system, a T-shaped device containing a reservoir of progesterone that is continuously released in small amounts into the uterine cavity following implantation. The unit is effective for up to 1 year. Contraceptive efficacy is equivalent to that of progestin-only drugs.

Diethylstilbestrol (DES), a synthetic estrogen (see Chap 44), has been effective as a postcoital contraceptive in large doses (25 mg twice a day for 5 days), provided the drug is given within 72 hours after intercourse. At these dosages, DES apparently blocks implantation of the fertilized ovum. Because of the hazards of such large doses of DES, this method of contraception is not recommended for routine use but should be restricted to emergency situations, such as rape or incest.

Many other chemical (spermicidal foams, gels, and creams) and mechanical (diaphragm, intrauterine device, condom) methods of contraception are available. Although usually somewhat less reliable than steroidal drugs, these methods do not present so great a risk of serious untoward reactions as does the use of steroid drugs. Choice of a contraceptive method is a highly personal one, and the advantages and disadvantages of the available methods should be clearly understood by both prescriber and user before a decision is reached.

Fertility control is widely practiced and is highly successful in most instances. However, serious and occasionally fatal adverse effects have occurred in some women taking these drugs. Proper dosing of fertility control drugs is essential for their safe and effective use, and these drugs should always be prescribed and monitored by persons aware of their pharmacologic actions and toxicologic potential as well as the pituitary hormone–ovarian relationship. A graphic representation of the menstrual (endometrial) cycle and the hormonal influences upon ovarian function and endometrial growth and development is presented in Figure 45-1. In addition, patient education is a vital component of a safe and successful contraceptive regimen (see Nursing Considerations), and all persons receiving contraceptives for the first time should be given the literature included in the package, and encouraged to read it.

(Text continued on page 466)

Table 45-1
Oral Contraceptives

Drug	Estrogen	Progestin
Estrogen Dominant		
Enovid-E	mestranol 100 μg	norethynodrel 2.5 mg
Norinyl 2 mg	mestranol 100 μg	norethindrone 2 mg
Ovulen	mestranol 100 μg	ethynodiol diacetate 1 mg
Intermediate Estrogen–Low Progestin		
Norinyl 1 + 80	mestranol 80 μg	norethindrone 1 mg
Norlestrin 1/50	ethinyl estradiol 50 μg	norethindrone 1 mg
Ovcon-50	ethinyl estradiol 50 μg	norethindrone 1 mg
Intermediate Estrogen–Intermediate Progestin		
Demulen 1/50	ethinyl estradiol 50 μg	ethynodiol diacetate 1 mg
Enovid 5 mg	mestranol 75 μg	norethynodrel 5 mg
Norlestrin 2.5/50	ethinyl estradiol 50 μg	norethindrone 2.5 mg
Ovral	ethinyl estradiol 50 μg	norethindrone 0.5 mg
Low Estrogen–Low Progestin		
Brevicon	ethinyl estradiol 35 μg	norethindrone 0.5 mg
Genora 1/35	ethinyl estradiol 35 μg	norethindrone 1 mg
Genora 1/50	mestranol 50 μg	norethindrone 1 mg
Gynex 0.5/35E	ethinyl estradiol 35 μg	norethindrone 0.5 mg
Gynex 1/35E	ethinyl estradiol 35 μg	norethindrone 1 mg
Loestrin 1/20	ethinyl estradiol 20 μg	norethindrone 1 mg
Modicon	ethinyl estradiol 35 μg	norethindrone 0.5 mg
N.E.E.	ethinyl estradiol 35 μg	norethindrone 1 mg
Nelova 0.5/35E	ethinyl estradiol 35 μg	norethindrone 0.5 mg
Nelova 1/35E	ethinyl estradiol 35 μg	norethindrone 1 mg
Nelova 10/11	ethinyl estradiol 35 μg	norethindrone (10 tablets 0.5 mg; 11 tablets 1 mg)
Norcept-E 1/35	ethinyl estradiol 35 μg	norethindrone 1 mg
Norethin 1/35E	ethinyl estradiol 35 μg	norethindrone 1 mg
Norethin 1/50M	mestranol 50 μg	norethindrone 1 mg
Norinyl 1 + 50	mestranol 50 μg	norethindrone 1 mg
Norinyl 1 + 35	ethinyl estradiol 35 μg	norethindrone 1 mg
Ortho-Novum 1/50	mestranol 50 μg	norethindrone 1 mg
Ortho-Novum 1/35	ethinyl estradiol 35 μg	norethindrone 1 mg
Ortho-Novum 10/11	ethinyl estradiol 35 μg	norethindrone (10 tablets 0.5 mg; 11 tablets 1 mg)
Ortho-Novum 7/7/7	ethinyl estradiol 35 μg	norethindrone (7 tablets 0.5 mg; 7 tablets 0.75 mg; 7 tablets 1.0 mg)
Ovcon-35	ethinyl estradiol 35 μg	norethindrone 0.4 mg
Tri-Levlen, Triphasil	ethinyl estradiol (6 tablets 30 μg; 5 tablets 40 μg; 10 tablets 30 μg)	levonorgestrel (6 tablets 0.05 mg; 5 tablets 0.075 mg; 10 tablets 0.125 mg)
Tri-Norinyl	ethinyl estradiol 35 μg	norethindrone (7 tablets 0.5 mg; 9 tablets 1 mg; 5 tablets 0.5 mg)
Low Estrogen–Intermediate Progestin		
Levlen	ethinyl estradiol 30 μg	levonorgestrel 0.15 mg
Lo/Ovral	ethinyl estradiol 30 μg	norgestrel 0.3 mg
Nordette	ethinyl estradiol 30 μg	levonorgestrel 0.15 mg
Progestin Dominant		
Demulen 1/35	ethinyl estradiol 35 μg	ethynodiol deacetate 1 mg
Loestrin 1.5/30	ethinyl estradiol 30 μg	norethindrone 1.5 mg
Progestin Only		
Micronor		norethindrone 0.35 mg
Nor-Q.D.		norethindrone 0.35 mg
Ovrette		norgestrel 0.075 mg

Table 45-2
Hormonal Balance of Oral Contraceptive Products and Relation to Adverse Effects

Hormone Balance

Estrogen dominant: Enovid-E, Norinyl 2 mg, Ovulen

Intermediate estrogen–low progestin: Norinyl 1 + 80, Norlestrin 1/50, Ovcon-50

Intermediate estrogen–intermediate progestin: Demulen 1/50, Enovid 5 mg, Norlestrin 2.5/50, Ovral

Low estrogen-low progestin: Brevicon, Genora 1/35, 1/50, Gynex 0.5/35E, 1/35E, Loestrin 1/20, Modicon, N.E.E., Nelova 0.5/35E, 1/35E, Norcept-E 1/35, 10/11, Norethin 1/35E, 1/50M, Norinyl 1 + 35 and 1 + 50, Ortho-Novum 1/35, 1/50, 10/11 and 7/7/7, Ovcon-35, Tri-levlen, Triphasil, Tri-Norinyl

Low estrogen–intermediate progestin: Levlen, Lo/Ovral, Nordette

Progestin dominant: Demulen 1/35, Loestrin 1.5/30

Adverse Effects

Estrogen excess: Cervical mucorrhea, edema, nausea, bloating, breast tenderness, migraine, hypertension, chloasma

Estrogen deficiency: Early or midcycle breakthrough bleeding, spotting, nervousness, hypomenorrhea

Progestin excess: Acne, depression, hirsutism, fatigue, increased appetite, weight gain, monilial vaginitis, oily skin, pruritis, hypomenorrhea

Progestin deficiency: Late-cycle bleeding, dysmenorrhea, delayed withdrawal bleeding

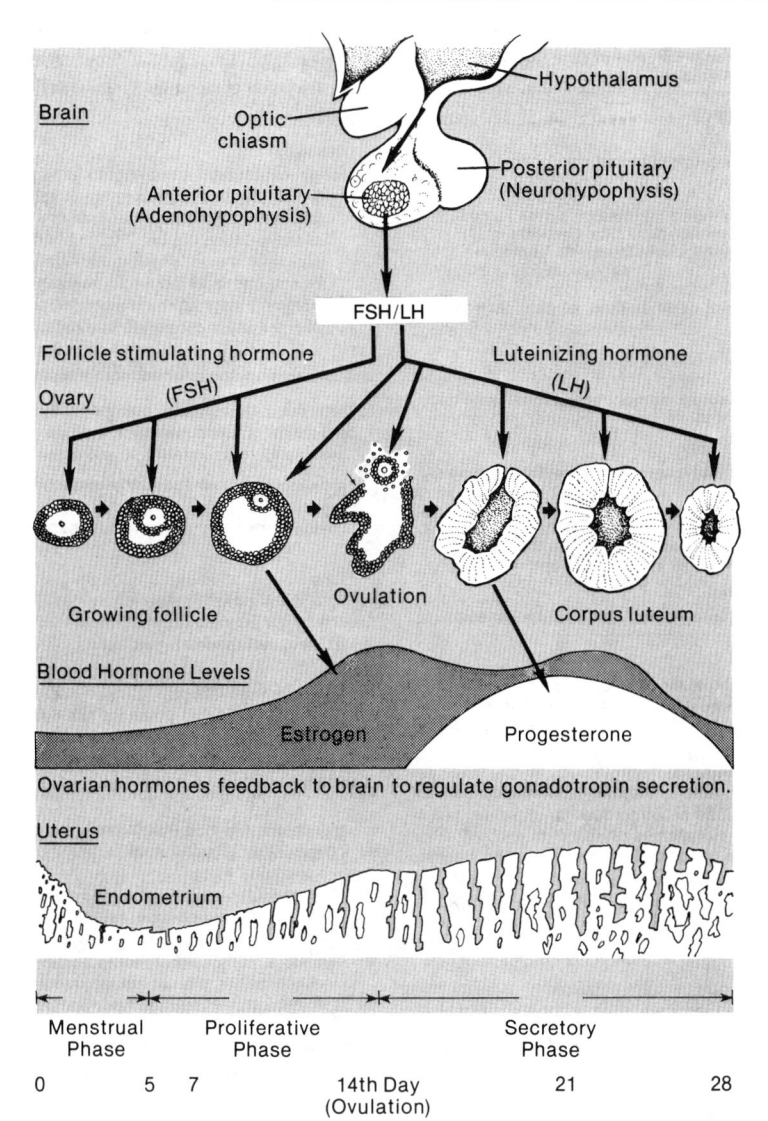

Figure 45–1 The menstrual (endometrial) cycle.

The oral contraceptives are discussed as a group, inasmuch as they are essentially alike in their pharmacologic action. A complete list of available products is given in Table 45-1, along with their respective estrogen and progestin content. A review of the intrauterine progestin system is also presented.

Oral Contraceptives

MECHANISM

Interfere with follicular maturation (estrogen decreases release of FSH) and inhibit ovulation (progestin suppresses release of LH)—(see Fig. 45-1); induce structural and biochemical changes in the endometrium making it unfavorable for implantation of the fertilized ovum; progestins reduce the amount and increase the viscosity of cervical mucus, thus interfering with motility of sperm cells; many also impair the ciliary and peristaltic activity of the fallopian tubes, impeding movement of the ova

USES

Prevention of pregnancy
Treatment of menstrual irregularities (see Progestins, Chap. 44)

DOSAGE

> NOTE
>
> Because of the association between the dose of estrogen and the risk of thromboembolism and possibly hypertension, patients should be given a preparation containing *50 μg or less* of estrogen

Estrogen–progestin combinations: 1 tablet daily for 21 days beginning on cycle day 5 (day 1 is first day of bleeding); some products are supplied as 28-tablet packs, the last 7 tablets being inert or containing only iron, allowing continuous daily dosage for the entire 28-day cycle; resume next course of therapy 7 days after cessation of previous course, whether or not menstrual flow has occurred
Progestin-only products: 1 tablet daily without interruption

Although the likelihood of ovulation is minimal if one tablet is missed, it increases with each succeeding day that a dose is missed. If *one* tablet is missed, it may be taken later that day or 2 tablets may be taken the following day. If tablets are missed for 2 consecutive days, 2 tablets should be taken daily for the next 2 days before resuming the regular schedule. If 3 consecutive days of therapy are missed, a new package of tablets should be started 7 days after the last tablet was taken and alternative means of birth control should be used until resumption of therapy.

FATE

Ethinyl estradiol is rapidly absorbed and undergoes significant first-pass hepatic metabolism; *mestranol* is converted to ethinyl estradiol, which is highly bound to plasma proteins (97%–98%); plasma half-life ranges from 6 to 18 hours; The drugs are excreted in both the bile and the urine.
Progestins are well absorbed orally. Norethynodrel and ethynodiol diacetate are converted to norethindrone. Peak plasma levels occur in 0.5 to 3 hours. Progestins are bound to plasma proteins and are primarily metabolized in the liver

COMMON SIDE EFFECTS

(Depends to a large extent on the estrogen–progestin ratio—see Table 45-2) Nausea, vomiting, headache, fluid retention, weight gain, dizziness, breast tenderness, breakthrough bleeding, leg cramps

SIGNIFICANT ADVERSE REACTIONS

> WARNING
>
> Use of oral contraceptives has been associated with increased risk of thromboembolic episodes, hemorrhagic stroke, hypertension, myocardial infarction, hepatic tumors, visual disturbances, gallbladder disease, and fetal abnormalities. In addition, cigarette smoking *significantly* increase the risk of cardiovascular side effects

GI/hepatic: abdominal cramping, diarrhea, benign adenomas and other hepatic lesions, cholelithiasis, and cholestatic jaundice
Genitourinary: dysmenorrhea, amenorrhea, infertility after discontinuation, change in cervical secretions, increased urinary tract and vaginal infections
Ophthalmic: neuroocular lesions (e.g., retinal thrombosis, optic neuritis), papilledema, change in corneal curvature, intolerance to contact lenses
CNS: migraine, depression, menstrual tension, fatigue
Other: rash, chloasma, reduced lactation, impaired carbohydrate tolerance, altered laboratory values (e.g., liver function, thyroid function, serum triglycerides, blood glucose)

CONTRAINDICATIONS

Thromboembolic disorders, coronary artery or cerebrovascular disease, myocardial infarction or history of these disorders, known or suspected breast or other estrogen-dependent carcinoma, undiagnosed vaginal bleeding, known or suspected pregnancy, severe liver disease, or liver tumors. *Cautious use* in women with diabetes, hypertension, obesity, migraine, depression, anemia, amenorrhea and porphyria

> WARNING
>
> Pregnancy must be ruled out before beginning an oral contraceptive regimen, because fetal damage can occur if these agents are used during early pregnancy

INTERACTIONS

See Estrogens and Progestins, Chapter 44. In addition:

Increased incidence of breakthrough bleeding and possibly reduced contraceptive efficacy may occur with barbiturates, penicillin, ampicillin, chloramphenicol, sulfonamides, tetracycline primidone, phenytoin, carbamazepine, rifampin, isoniazid, meprobamate, griseofulvin, phenylbutazone, or nitrofurantoin
Oral contraceptives may impair the effectiveness of anticonvulsants, anticoagulants, antihypertensives, tricyclic antidepressants, hypoglycemics, and certain vitamins (folic acid, B_6)
Oral contraceptives may impair the metabolism of caffeine, chlordiazepoxide, corticosteroids, diazepam, metoprolol, imipramine, phenytoin, and phenylbutazone
The metabolism of acetaminophen, lorazepam, and oxazepam may be accelerated by oral contraceptives
Use of aminocaproic acid with oral contraceptives may increase clotting factors, leading to a hypercoagulable state
Concurrent use of troleandomycin and oral contraceptives may result in jaundice

NURSING CONSIDERATIONS

See estrogens and progestins, Chapter 44. In addition:
1. Assess patient for indications of hormonal imbalance. If a certain pattern of side effects persists (see Table 45-2), the oral contraceptive formulation may need to be changed.

PATIENT EDUCATION

See estrogens and progestins, Chapter 44. In addition:
1. Discuss the need to rule out pregnancy before therapy is initiated or before therapy is continued if pregnancy is suspected.
2. Inform patient that the combination with the lowest effective and tolerable estrogen content is usually prescribed because a positive correlation exists between dosage of estrogen and risk of both thromboembolism and endometrial carcinoma.
3. Explain that pregnancy should always be suspected if withdrawal bleeding does not occur following each course of therapy.
4. Provide user with patient information contained in each package. Carefully review material with patient to ensure that she understands it.
5. Suggest that patient use an additional method of contraception during first week of administration in initial cycle of therapy.
6. Suggest that medication be taken at the same time every day to minimize possibility of missing a dose.
7. Explain actions to be taken if doses of medication are missed (see information at end of Dosage section, above).
8. Explain to patient taking progestin-only product that breakthrough bleeding and altered menstrual pattern are more likely to occur than with a combination product.
9. Instruct patient to report any abnormal vaginal bleeding immediately. If bleeding is sparse (e.g., spotting), medication may be continued uninterrupted, but physician should be notified if spotting continues past the second month. If flow is heavy (e.g., menstrual-like), patient should discontinue medication and begin a new package of tablets on the fifth day after the start of new bleeding.
10. Alert patient that menstrual flow may be greatly reduced after several months of therapy.
11. When pregnancy is desired, instruct patient to terminate oral contraceptives and use alternative means of birth control for an additional 3 months to minimize risk of congenital abnormalities from residual effects of steroidal hormones.

Intrauterine Progesterone Contraceptive System

Progestasert

The intrauterine progesterone contraceptive system is a T-shaped intrauterine device (IUD) containing 38 mg progesterone dispersed in silicone oil. Following insertion of the unit into the uterine cavity, progesterone is continuously released at an average rate of 65 µg/day. The contraceptive effectiveness approximates that of progestin-only tablets and is retained for a period of 1 year, after which the system must be replaced. The system acts to suppress proliferation of endometrial tissue, creating an environment unfavorable for implantation; it may also decrease sperm survival time, possibly by altering cervical mucus; it does not appear to prevent ovulation.

The intrauterine progesterone system is contraindicated in the presence of pregnancy or suspicion of pregnancy, previous ectopic pregnancy, pelvic inflammatory disease, sexually transmitted disease, previous pelvic surgery, uterine abnormalities, uterine or cervical malignancy, vaginal bleeding of undetermined origin, and acute cervicitis.

Adverse reactions associated with the system include dysmenorrhea, amenorrhea, cervical erosion, pelvic infection, vaginitis, endometritis, spotting, prolonged menstrual flow, delayed menses, dyspareunia, septicemia, septic abortion, cervical or uterine perforation, ectopic pregnancy, and pain, bleeding, bradycardia, or syncope upon insertion.

The device should be inserted during or immediately following menstruation to ensure that pregnancy has not occurred. An increased risk of pelvic inflammatory disease (PID) is associated with the use of intrauterine devices. Users should be apprised of the usual symptoms of PID (fever, nausea, vomiting, abdominal pain, malaise, purulent vaginal discharge) and if these are present, should report to their physician.

NURSING CONSIDERATIONS

Nursing Alerts
- If pregnancy occurs with the system in place, provide emotional support as needed, and explain that the device will be removed by its threads if possible. Termination of the pregnancy should be considered if the system cannot be removed because risk of spontaneous abortion and sepsis is considerable.
- Be alert for delayed menses, unilateral pelvic pain, and falling hematocrit, possible indications of an ectopic fetus, because incidence of ectopic pregnancy is higher in patient with an IUD in place.

PATIENT EDUCATION
1. Instruct patient not to pull on threads or to attempt to remove unit once it is inserted.
2. Explain that reexamination is required within 3 months after insertion to ensure that unit is in place.

OVULATION STIMULANTS

Although an infrequent cause of infertility, anovulation, when it occurs, has responded to the use of ovulation-stimulating drugs, and conception has been made possible in previously anovulatory women. Because therapy with these agents is expensive, often tedious, and potentially hazardous, selection of patients with a reasonable expectation for success is important. Thus, women with primary ovarian failure, uterine abnormalities, fallopian tube obstruction, or endometrial carcinoma should be excluded as potential candidates. Likewise, impaired or absent sperm production in the partner should be ruled out. When careful patient selection is observed, 25% to 50% of women completing a course of therapy can be expected to conceive. However, treatment with ovulation-inducing drugs is not without its hazards, such as ovarian enlargement, often accompanied by pain and ascites. The incidence of early abortion is increased with use of these drugs, and the occurrence of multiple pregnancies with recommended dosage schedules has been estimated as high as 20%.

Ovulation-inducing agents include clomiphene, a drug capable of increasing release of FSH and LH from the adenohypophysis, and human menopausal gonadotropins (HMG, menotropins) and urofollitropin, two preparations that are purified extracts of FSH and LH. Clomiphene is used alone, whereas HMG therapy and urofollitropin therapy are followed by an injection of human chorionic gonadotropin (HCG) to induce ovulation. These drugs are reviewed individually below.

Clomiphene

Clomid, Milophene, Serophene

A nonsteroidal synthetic estrogen possessing weak estrogenic as well as antiestrogenic activity, clomiphene stimulates release of FSH and LH from the adenohypophysis and thus requires both a functioning pituitary and a responsive ovary for its therapeutic effect. A single ovulation is induced by each 5-day course of treatment, and the majority of patients who are going to respond will do so with the first course of therapy. A second and third course may be tried if conception has not occurred, but treatment beyond three courses in patients exhibiting no evidence of ovulation or who do not conceive is not recommended. Approximately 30% to 40% of women with ovulatory dysfunction conceive with a course of clomiphene therapy.

MECHANISM

Binds to estrogenic receptors in the cytoplasm, thus decreasing the number of available estrogenic receptor sites (antiestrogenic action); action is interpreted by the hypothalamus and pituitary as a sign that estrogen levels are low, and the secretion of FSH and LH is increased in response to the removal of the negative feedback; increased release of FSH and LH stimulates maturation of the follicle, ovulation, and development of the corpus luteum

USES

Treatment of ovulatory failure in properly selected patients desiring pregnancy, whose partners are fertile

Treatment of male infertility (investigational use)

DOSAGE

Female infertility: beginning on the fifth day of the cycle, 50 mg/day for 5 days (therapy may be started anytime in amenorrheic women); if ovulation does not occur, a second and third course of therapy (at 100 mg/day for 5 days) may be tried, with a minimum 30-day interval between treatment courses. Treatment beyond three courses of therapy is *not* recommended

Male infertility: 25 mg/day for 25 days or 100 mg 3 times a week (e.g., Mon, Wed, and Fri)

FATE

Well absorbed when taken orally; metabolized in the liver and excreted largely in the feces, both as metabolites and unchanged drug

COMMON SIDE EFFECTS

Ovarian enlargement, abdominal discomfort, bloating, vasomotor symptoms (e.g., hot flashes, flushing), breast tenderness

SIGNIFICANT ADVERSE REACTIONS

Nausea, vomiting, diarrhea, visual disturbances (e.g., blurring, photophobia, diplopia, scotomata), headache, nervousness, lightheadedness, vertigo, insomnia, depression, abnormal uterine bleeding, ovarian hemorrhage, urinary frequency, rash, dermatitis, fluid retention, weight gain; increased incidence of early abortion and multiple births (approximately 7%)

CONTRAINDICATIONS

Pregnancy, liver dysfunction or history of liver disease, ovarian cysts, thrombophlebitis, and abnormal uterine or vaginal bleeding. *Cautious use* in thyroid disorders (see Interactions)

INTERACTIONS

Clomiphene can elevate levels of serum thyroxine and thyroxine-binding globulin

NURSING CONSIDERATIONS

1. Ensure that recommended procedures (e.g., complete pelvic examination, endometrial biopsy, liver function tests) have been completed and the cause of any abnormal bleeding has been determined before initiating administration.
2. Question dosage that exceeds 100 mg/day for 5 days because effectiveness is not enhanced with higher doses, but the incidence of untoward reactions and the danger of multiple births is increased.

PATIENT EDUCATION

1. Teach patient how to use a basal thermometer to ascertain time of ovulation.
2. Explain the importance of properly timed sexual intercourse for conception.
3. Instruct patient to report development of any visual disturbances. If they occur, treatment should be discontinued, and a complete ophthalmologic examination should be performed.
4. Caution patient against engaging in hazardous activities because blurred vision, dizziness, and lightheadedness may occur.
5. Instruct patent to report development of pelvic or abdominal pain. Patient should be examined for ovarian enlargement if this occurs.

Menotropins (human menopausal gonadotropins—HMG)

Pergonal

A purified preparation of gonadotropins extracted from the urine of postmenopausal women, menotropins is biologically standardized for FSH and LH activity. It is frequently referred to as human menopausal gonadotropins or HMG and provides an exogenous source of pituitary gonadotropins and thus, unlike clomiphene, does not require the presence of functional hypophysial gonadotropins for its activity. Treatment with menotropins usually results only in follicular growth and maturation; subsequent ovulation is effected by sequential administration of HCG (see Chorionic Gonadotropin, below) when sufficient follicular maturation has occurred.

MECHANISM

Provides a source of FSH and LH, thus promoting growth of ovarian follicles in women who do not have primary ovarian failure (see Fig. 45-1); does not usually elicit ovulation, which must be induced by injection of HCG, a polypeptide-possessing significant LH activity (see below)

USES

Treatment of infertility in women with primary or secondary amenorrhea (with or without galactorrhea), polycystic ovary syndrome, anovulatory cycles, or irregular menses (*not* effective in primary ovarian failure)

Stimulation of spermatogenesis in men who have primary or secondary hypogonadotropic hypogonadism

DOSAGE

Women (must be individually adjusted): usually, 1 ampule/day (75 U each of FSH and LH) IM for 9 to 12 days, followed by HCG, 10,000 U IM 1 day after the last dose of HMG; if ovulation occurs without pregnancy, may repeat course of therapy twice with same dosage levels at monthly intervals. If ovulation does not occur, repeat treatment with 2 ampules/day (150 U each of FSH and LH) for 3 to 12 days, followed by 10,000 U HCG IM. Do *not* exceed 2 ampules/day

Men (to increase spermatogenesis): HCG alone (5000 IU 3 times/wk for 4–6 mo); then, 1 ampule menotropins IM 3 times/wk and HCG, 2000 IU, twice a week for 4 months

COMMON SIDE EFFECTS
Mild uncomplicated ovarian enlargement, with or without abdominal pain (20% incidence)

SIGNIFICANT ADVERSE REACTIONS
(Usually with larger doses) Ovarian hyperstimulation syndrome (e.g., abdominal pain, ascites, pleural effusion, sudden ovarian enlargement), fever, nausea, vomiting, diarrhea, hemoperitoneum, arterial thromboembolism (rare), and ovarian cysts

Multiple births have occurred with HMG–HCG treatment; occasional gynecomastia in men

CONTRAINDICATIONS
Primary ovarian failure, pregnancy, ovarian cysts or enlargement *not* due to polycystic ovary syndrome, thyroid or adrenal dysfunction, intracranial lesion, abnormal bleeding of unknown origin, and infertility due to factors other than anovulation

In men, primary testicular failure and infertility *not* due to hypogonadotropic hypogonadism

PATIENT EDUCATION
1. Advise patient that administration of HMG–HCG or urofollitropin–HCG (see below) should be undertaken only by persons trained in their use, knowledgeable about the necessary estrogen and progesterone assays required to monitor hormonal status, and thoroughly familiar with treatment of female infertility.
2. Explain that a thorough gynecologic examination and endocrinologic evaluation are performed before therapy is initiated. Pregnancy and primary ovarian failure must be ruled out and the cause of any abnormal vaginal bleeding determined. Evaluation of the male partner is likewise essential.
3. Teach patient signs of ovarian hyperstimulation (see Significant Adverse Reactions). Advise patient to notify physician if signs occur and refrain from sexual intercourse. Mild ovarian enlargement generally regresses within 2 to 3 weeks.
4. Inform patient that she will probably be examined every other day during treatment and for at least 2 weeks posttreatment for signs of excessive ovarian stimulation. Most ovarian hyperstimulation is noted 7 to 10 days after ovulation.
5. Explain that HCG should not be administered if ovaries are abnormally enlarged or if estrogen excretion is greater than 100 μg/24 h on the last day of HMG (or urofollitropin) therapy because risk of excessive ovarian stimulation is greatly increased.
6. Encourage patient to have sexual intercourse daily beginning the day HCG is administered until ovulation has occurred, as indicated by indices of increased progesterone production.

Urofollitropin
Metrodin

Urofollitropin is a purified preparation of gonadotropin extracted from the urine of postmenopausal women.

MECHANISM
Stimulates ovarian follicular growth in women who do not have primary ovarian failure; treatment results in follicular growth and maturation only; ovulation is effected by subsequent administration of HCG (see below) where laboratory assessment indicates that sufficient follicular maturation has occurred

USE
Induction of ovulation in patients with polycystic ovarian disease who display elevated LH : FSH ratio and whose condition has not responded to clomiphene therapy; treatment with urofollitropin must be followed by administration of HCG to induce ovulation from the mature follicle

DOSAGE
75 U/day IM for 7 to 12 days followed by 5,000 U to 10,000 U of HCG 1 day after the last urofollitropin dose

If there is evidence of ovulation but no pregnancy, the above course of therapy may be repeated at least twice at monthly intervals before increasing the dose of urofollitropin to 150 U/day for 3 additional monthly treatments. Do *not* increase the dose further.

COMMON SIDE EFFECTS
Abdominal pain and distention; ovarian enlargement; rash, pain, swelling, or irritation at injection site

SIGNIFICANT ADVERSE REACTIONS
Nausea, vomiting, diarrhea, abdominal cramping, bloating, headache, breast tenderness, fever, muscle aching, chills, malaise, fatigue, dry skin, hair loss, and ectopic pregnancy. Thromboembolic episodes have occurred with the similar-acting drug menotropins and must be considered a possibility with urofollitropin as well.

Multiple births have occurred with a frequency estimated to be in the range of 15% to 20%.

Sudden ovarian enlargement, occasionally accompanied by ascites and pleural effusion, has been reported in approximately 5% of treated patients

CONTRAINDICATIONS
Presence of high levels of FSH or LH, indicating primary ovarian failure; thyroid or adrenal dysfunction; intracranial lesions; abnormal bleeding of undetermined origin; ovarian cysts; pregnancy. *Cautious use* in persons with thromboembolic disorders and in nursing mothers

PATIENT EDUCATION
See menotropins.

Human Chorionic Gonadotropin
A.P.L., Chorex, Corgonject-5, Chorigon, Choron-10, Follutein, Glukor, Gonic, Pregnyl, Profasi HP
(CAN) Autuitrin

A purified polypeptide hormone, HCG is produced by the human placenta and extracted from the urine of women during the first trimester of pregnancy. The effect of HCG is due primarily to its LH-like activity, although it exhibits a slight degree of FSH-like activity as well.

MECHANISM

Stimulates the corpus luteum of the ovaries to produce progesterone, and triggers ovulation from FSH-primed follicles (see Fig. 45-1). In males, stimulates the interstitial cells of the testes to produce androgens, thus promoting development of secondary sex characteristics and descent of the testicles

USES

Induction of ovulation in the anovulatory female who has been properly pretreated with HMG or urofollitropin

Treatment of cryptorchidism (undescended testes) in instances *not* due to anatomical obstruction; therapy is usually instituted between ages 4 and 9 years

Treatment of male hypogonadism secondary to a pituitary deficiency

DOSAGE

(Highly individualized; IM only; dosage measured in USP units)

Induction of Ovulation

5000 U to 10,000 U 1 day following last dose of HMG or urofollitropin

Cryptorchidism

4000 U three times a week for 3 weeks *or*

5000 U every other day for four injections *or*

15 injections of 500 U to 1000 U over 6 weeks *or*

500 U three times a week for 4 to 6 weeks; if unsuccessful, repeat after 1 month with 100 U per injection

Hypogonadism

500 U to 1000 U three times a week for 3 weeks, then twice a week for 3 weeks *or*

1000 U to 2000 U three times a week *or*

4000 U three times a week for 6 months to 9 months, then 2000 U three times a week for 3 months

COMMON SIDE EFFECTS

Headache, restlessness

SIGNIFICANT ADVERSE REACTIONS

Depression, fatigue, ovarian hyperstimulation, thromboembolism, fluid retention, gynecomastia, pain at injection site, and sexual precocity in prepubertal patients

CONTRAINDICATIONS

Androgen-dependent neoplasms (e.g., prostatic cancer), precocious puberty. *Cautious use* in patients with cardiac or renal disease, asthma, migraine, or epilepsy

NURSING CONSIDERATIONS

Nursing Alert

- Assess patient being treated for cryptorchidism for signs of precocious puberty. Drug should be discontinued if signs appear.

1. Question prescription of HCG for treatment of obesity. Although drug is sometimes used to treat obesity, there is no substantial evidence that HCG alters fat mobilization or distribution, retards appetite, or reduces hunger associated with low-calorie diets.

PATIENT EDUCATION

1. Explain to child and parents that cryptorchidism that does not respond to HCG within a reasonable period of time (6–12 wk) usually requires surgical intervention because excessive treatment with HCG may damage a mechanically obstructed undescended testis.
2. Instruct patient to notify physician if edema becomes problematic. Dosage reduction usually eliminates fluid retention.

ABORTIFACIENTS

Termination of pregnancy can be accomplished by both mechanical and pharmacologic methods. During the early weeks of pregnancy, there is no safe and reliable method for pharmacologically inducing fetal expulsion, and suction curettage is the commonly performed procedure. Beginning at about the start of the second trimester, however, pharmacologic methods are usually employed; these consist of injections of hypertonic saline solution into the amniotic sac, IM administration of a prostaglandin salt, or use of a prostaglandin (E_2) vaginal suppository. Certain prostaglandins (PGE_2, $PGF_{2\alpha}$) have been detected in amniotic fluid during labor or spontaneous abortion and appear to play a role in fetal expulsion by facilitating myometrial contractions. These observations have led to the development of prostaglandin preparations for the induction of second trimester elective abortion. Currently available drugs can be used by IM injection or by insertion of a vaginal suppository. These agents are preferable to intraamniotic injection of hypertonic sodium chloride (see below) because they have a more rapid onset of action and a lower incidence of side effects. The prostaglandins used as abortifacients are reviewed as a group, followed by a listing of individual drugs and dosages in Table 45-3.

Prostaglandin Abortifacients

Carboprost Tromethamine

Hemabate

Dinoprostone

Prostin E_2

MECHANISM

Elicit contractions of the gravid uterus, probably by a direct stimulation of the myometrium; may produce a regression of corpus luteum function; also increase contractile activity of the GI tract and other smooth muscle, especially following systemic injection

USES

Termination of pregnancy from the 12th through the 20th gestational week

Production of uterine evacuation in cases of missed abortion or fetal death up to 28 weeks gestational age (dinoprostone only)

Management of nonmetastatic gestational trophoblastic disease (benign hydatidiform mole)—dinoprostone only

Induction of labor and initiation of cervical ripening prior to induction of labor (dinoprostone vaginal suppositories—investigational use only)

DOSAGE

See Table 45-3

FATE
Drugs are widely distributed in both fetal and maternal bodies; half-life in amniotic fluid is several hours, but much shorter in plasma; metabolized by maternal liver and excreted largely in the urine

COMMON SIDE EFFECTS
Vomiting, diarrhea, nausea, headache, shivering, chills, hyperthermia, flushing, abdominal cramps

SIGNIFICANT ADVERSE REACTIONS
(Not all are clearly drug related)

GI: hiccups, dry throat, choking sensation, pharyngitis, laryngitis, taste alterations
CNS: paresthesia, weakness, drowsiness, tremor, dizziness, lethargy, anxiety, blurred vision, tinnitus, vertigo, sleep disorders
Cardiovascular: hypertension (*hypo*tension with dinoprostone), chest pain, arrhythmias, bradycardia, palpitations, congestive heart failure, cardiac arrest
Respiratory: coughing, wheezing, dyspnea, hyperventilation, asthma-like reactions, pulmonary embolism
Genitourinary: endometritis, urinary tract infection, perforated cervix or uterus, uterine or vaginal pain, urinary incontinence, hematuria
Other: sweating, hot flashes, muscle pain, leg cramps, joint pain, stiff neck, diplopia, polydipsia, rash, aggravation of diabetes, uterine infections

CONTRAINDICATIONS
Acute pelvic inflammatory disease; active cardiac, pulmonary, hepatic, or renal disease. *Cautious use* in patients with asthma, hypertension, heart disease, diabetes, glaucoma, epilepsy, renal or hepatic impairment, anemia, jaundice, vaginitis, and cervicitis

NOTE
Prostaglandin-induced abortion is not always complete. If incomplete, other measures should be taken to ensure complete expulsion (e.g., hypertonic sodium chloride; see below)

INTERACTIONS
Aspirin and other antiinflammatory drugs may prolong the time required for fetal expulsion with prostaglandins

The activity of oxytocin may be enhanced by prostaglandin abortifacients

NURSING CONSIDERATIONS

Nursing Alerts
- Administer drugs only in a hospital or other health care facility where trained personnel, intensive care, and acute surgical facilities are available.
- Anticipate the possibility of a liveborn fetus, especially if drugs are given near the end of the second trimester because prostaglandins, unlike hypertonic saline, are not usually lethal to the fetus.
- Expect pregnancy to be terminated by other means, such as hypertonic sodium chloride (see below), if these drugs fail because prostaglandins can damage the fetus.

1. Be prepared for the possibility of transient pyrexia with IM injection of carboprost. Temperature elevations greater than 2°F have been noted in approximately one-eighth of patients receiving the drug. Supplemental fluids are recommended, but other modes of treatment are usually unnecessary because temperature reverts to normal shortly after therapy is discontinued.
2. As appropriate, advocate pretreatment of patient with antiemetic and antidiarrheal medication to minimize incidence of nausea, vomiting, and diarrhea.

Table 45-3
Prostaglandin Abortifacients

Drug	Preparations	Usual Dosage Range	Nursing Implications
Carboprost Tromethamine Hemabate	Injection: 250 μg/mL	Initially 250 μg IM; repeat at 1.5–3.5 h intervals; may increase to 500 μg per dose if necessary; maximum dose 12 mg *Refractory postpartum bleeding:* Initially, 250 μg IM; if necessary, additional doses, may be given at 15–90 min intervals to a maximum of 2 mg	Administer deeply IM; abortion is incomplete in about 20% of cases; may produce transient elevation in body temperature (1°–3°F), which persists only as long as drug is being given; forced fluids are recommended during hyperpyrexia; an optional test dose of 100 μg (0.4 ml) may be give initially to ascertain hypersensitivity to drug
Dinoprostone Prostin E2	Vaginal suppository: 20 mg	Insert 1 suppository high into vagina; repeat at 3–5-h intervals until abortion occurs	Keep patient supine for at least 10 min following insertion; vomiting occurs in about two thirds of all patients, and diarrhea in approximately half, provide assistance as needed; nausea, headache, chills, and hypotension (20 mm Hg–30 mm Hg) have also been noted frequently

3. Following drug administration, monitor uterine activity, and monitor cardiovascular status for signs of vasomotor disturbance (e.g., bradycardia, pallor, rapid fall in blood pressure).

Sodium Chloride

20% sodium chloride solution

Intraamniotic injection of hypertonic sodium chloride can be used for second trimester abortion but has been largely replaced by the prostaglandins, which are both safer and more effective. The principal indication for sodium chloride injection is in the patient desiring abortion who has not responded successfully or completely to one of the prostaglandins. When prostaglandin-induced abortion is incomplete, however, injection of hypertonic saline should be delayed until the uterus is no longer contracting. The volume of solution instilled should not exceed the volume of amniotic fluid removed. Injection should be performed at a relatively slow rate and fluid samples taken at regular intervals to ensure that the injection catheter remains in the amniotic cavity. The maximum dose is considered to be 250 mL. Inadvertent intravascular injection should be avoided, because sudden, severe hypernatremia may result, possibly leading to cardiovascular shock, extensive hemolysis, and renal necrosis. The drug should be administered only in a medical unit with intensive care facilities readily available. If labor has not begun within 48 hours after instillation, a reevaluation of the patient's status is indicated.

Selected Bibliography

Alexander NB, Cotanct PH: The endocrine basis of infertility in women. Nurs Clin North Am 15:511, 1980

Bronson RA: Oral contraception: Mechanism of action. Clin Obstet Gynecol 24:869, 1981

Cancer and Steroid Hormone Study Group: Oral contraceptive use and the risk of breast cancer. N Engl J Med 315(7):405, 1986

Dickerson J: The pill, a closer look. Am J Nurs 83(10):1392, 1983

Friedman BM: Infertility work up. Am J Nurs 81:2041, 1981

Goldzieher JW (ed): Advances in oral contraception: An international review of levonorgestrel and ethinyl estradiol. J Reprod Med 28:53, 1983

Jordan VC: Biochemical pharmacology of antiestrogen action. Pharmacol Rev 36:245, 1984

Kanell RG: Oral contraceptives: the risks in perspective. Nurse Pract 9(9):25, 1984

Meade TW: Oral contraceptives, clotting factors and thrombosis. Am J Obstet Gynecol 142:758, 1982

Oral contraceptives and the risk of cardiovascular disease. Med Lett Drugs Ther 25:69, 1983

Price MC, Henderson BE, Krailo MD, et al: Breast cancer in young women and use of oral contraceptives: possible modifying effect of formulation and age at use. Lancet 2:920, 1983

Rahwan RG: Antiabortifacient and fertility-inducing drugs. Am J Pharm Ed 49:86, 1985

Sands CD, Robinson JD, Orlando JB: The oral contraceptive PPI: Its effect on patient knowledge, feelings, and behavior. Drug Intell Clin Pharm 18:730, 1984

Speroff L: Formulation of oral contraceptives: Does the amount of estrogen make any clinical difference. Johns Hopkins Med J 150:170, 1982

Stedel BV: Oral contraceptives and cardiovascular disease. N Engl J Med 305:612,672, 1981

Weiss NS, Sayvetz TA: Incidence of endometrial cancer in relation to the use of oral contraceptives. N Engl J Med 302:551, 1980

Wynn V: Cardiovascular effects and progestins in oral contraceptives. Am J Obstet Gynecol 142:718, 1982

SUMMARY. DRUGS USED IN FERTILITY CONTROL

Drug	Preparations	Usual Dosage Range
Oral Contraceptives	See Table 45-1	
Intrauterine Progesterone Contraceptive System Progestasert	T-shaped IUD containing 38 mg progesterone; releases 65 μg/day	Insert system into uterine cavity; replace after 1 yr
Clomiphene Clomid, Milophene, Serophene	Tablets: 50 mg	50 mg/day for 5 days; if no response, 100 mg/day for 5 days the second and third months
Menotropins (Human Menopausal Gonadotropins—HMG) Pergonal	Injection: containing 75 U FSH activity and 75 U LH activity per ampule	2 mL/day IM for 9–12 days, followed by 10,000 U HCG 1 day after last dose of HMG; may repeat twice at monthly intervals if ovulation has occurred
Urofollitropin Metrodin	Powder for injection: 0.83 mg (75 U FSH) per ampule	75 U/day for 7–12 days, followed by 5,000–10,000 U of HCG 1 day after last dose of urofollitropin
Human Chorionic Gonadotropin (HCG) Several manufacturers	Powder for injection: 200 U/mL 500 U/mL, 1000 U/mL, 2000 U/mL	*Induction of ovulation:* 5,000 U–10,000 U IM 1 day following last dose of HMG *or* urofollitropin *Cryptorchidism:* highly individualized; see text

Continued

SUMMARY. DRUGS USED IN FERTILITY CONTROL (continued)

Drug	Preparations	Usual Dosage Range
		Hypogonadism: 500 U–1000 U 3 times/wk for 6 wk *or* 1000 U–2000 U 3 times/wk *or* 4000 U 3 times/wk for 6–9 mo, then 2000 U 3 times/wk for 3 mo (also highly individualized)
Prostaglandin Abortifacients	*See* Table 45-3	
Sodium Chloride	Injection: 20%	Instill at a slow rate into the amniotic cavity, replacing amniotic fluid in equal amounts; maximum dose 250 mL
20% sodium chloride solution		

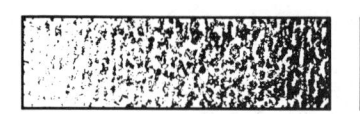

46 ANDROGENS AND ANABOLIC STEROIDS

The term *androgen* refers to a number of naturally occurring or synthetic steroidal compounds exhibiting the masculinizing and tissue-building (anabolic) actions of testosterone, the principal endogenous physiological androgenic hormone. Testosterone is produced in and secreted by the interstitial (Leydig) cells of the testes under the stimulus of interstitial cell–stimulating hormone (ICSH), which is identical to the luteinizing hormone (LH) of the female.

Testosterone is responsible for the development and support of the male sex organs and the appearance of the male secondary sex characteristics (e.g., deep voice, body hair), at the time of puberty. In addition, testosterone exerts a protein anabolic action, thus stimulating growth of skeletal muscle tissue; reduces excretion of sodium, potassium, chloride, nitrogen, and phosphorus; and enhances growth of long bones in prepubertal males. However, it also accelerates the ossification (hardening) process at the ends of long bones, eventually resulting in a conversion of cartilage into bone in the active growth areas (epiphyses) and cessation of further bone growth. For this reason, use of large amounts of androgens in young boys may actually cause a *reduction* of full potential growth by inducing a premature closing of the epiphyses after an initial growth spurt. Likewise, androgenic therapy in young males can result in precocious puberty, that is, premature development of the male sex organs and secondary sex characteristics, with possible attendant psychological trauma.

Other physiologic actions of testosterone include increased sebaceous gland activity, thickening of the vocal cords, darkening of the skin, loss of subcutaneous fat, and increased skin vascularization. In addition, psychologic and behavioral changes occur as production of testosterone is increased.

Testosterone itself, although adequately absorbed from the GI tract, is not administered orally because it is rapidly inactivated by the liver. Thus, very large oral doses (e.g., 400 mg/day) are needed to provide clinically effective blood levels. Testosterone may be given by IM injection (aqueous suspension); however, it is relatively short acting when administered by this route, again owing to rapid metabolism. Several esters of testosterone (propionate, cypionate, enanthate) exhibit greater stability and slower metabolism and, when injected IM in an oily vehicle, display a prolonged duration of action. Other structural modifications of testosterone (e.g., methyltestosterone, fluoxymesterone) can increase potency and confer resistance to hepatic metabolism, thus permitting use by the oral or buccal route.

A group of synthetic steroids structurally related to testosterone have been developed that display some separation of anabolic from androgenic activity, although the degree of separation is incomplete and variable. These compounds are termed *anabolic steroids* and have been used for a variety of conditions in which an anabolic activity is desired, such as retarded growth and development in children; senile, postmenopausal, or corticosteroid-induced osteoporosis; debilitation resulting from trauma, surgery, or illness; and certain types of anemia (e.g., aplastic).

Much attention has been focused in recent years on the use of anabolic steroids by athletes for the purpose of enhancing their performance. In conjunction with sufficient caloric and protein intake, anabolic steroids can increase muscle mass and appear to provide a competitive edge in those athletic activities that depend on strength, such as weight lifting or football. However, the serious health hazards associated with steroid use, such as hepatotoxicity, fluid retention, endocrine disorders, and blood lipid changes argue strongly against the use of these agents strictly for athletic purposes. Any gain in performance with utilization of anabolic steroids is achieved at the expense of incurring serious and potentially life-threatening physiological damage and there can be no justification for the use of steroids in otherwise healthy athletes.

Although these compounds exhibit a higher anabolic: androgenic ratio than testosterone or methyltestosterone, excessive dosage or prolonged administration is associated with most of the same untoward effects as seen with testosterone itself. Thus, use of anabolic steroids, especially in women and children, should be closely supervised and restricted to those valid medications listed below.

Other steroids that bear structural resemblance to testosterone but exhibit reduced androgenic activity are used in the treatment of advanced or metastatic breast cancer in postmenopausal women. These drugs, dromostanolone and testolactone, are reviewed in Chapter 72. The rest of the androgenic and anabolic steroids are discussed here as a group and then are listed in Table 46-1 with their specific indications and recommended dosages. Finally, danazol, a synthetic androgen possessing antigonadotropic and androgenic activity that is used in the treatment of endometriosis, is reviewed at the end of this chapter.

ANDROGENS AND ANABOLIC STEROIDS

Ethylestrenol
Fluoxymesterone
Methandrostenolone
Methyltestosterone
Nandrolone
Oxandrolone
Oxymetholone
Stanozolol
Testosterone

MECHANISM

Increase synthesis of RNA and cellular protein; testosterone itself is converted to its active metabolite dihydrotestosterone, in some tissues while at other sites it is active itself; other derivatives also enhance RNA and protein synthesis directly; stimulate growth of muscle, bone, skin, and hair and accelerate closure of epiphyses at ends of long bones; increase production of red blood cells; decrease excretion of nitrogen, phosphorus, sodium, and probably also calcium and potassium; temporarily arrest progression of estrogen-dependent carcinomas; *large doses* can suppress pituitary gonadotropin secretion, and decrease spermatogenesis through feedback inhibition of FSH

USES
(See Table 46-1 for specific indications)

Replacement therapy in androgen deficiency states, such as testicular hypofunction, pituitary dysfunction, eunuchism (complete testicular failure), eunuchoidism (partial testicular failure), cryptorchidism, castration, or male climacteric

Treatment of low sperm count or impotence due to androgen deficiency (low doses only)

Palliative therapy of androgen-responsive inoperable breast cancer in 1- to 5-year postmenopausal women

Induction of a positive nitrogen balance in those conditions in which an anabolic action is desired, for example, retarded growth and physical development in children, osteoporosis, anemia, corticosteroid-induced catabolism, and debilitation resulting from injury, trauma, illness, and other causes

NOTE
Anabolic steroids are dangerous drugs that can cause serious adverse effects, and their use has resulted in death. Although muscle mass and muscle strength may increase, data suggesting that there is a corresponding significant improvement in athletic prowess are inconclusive. Much of the increased body weight noted with use of these drugs is probably the result of increased sodium and fluid retention. In addition, increases in muscle mass are *not* accompanied by increases in tendon strength, and ruptured tendons are common if the muscle mass becomes too great for the tendon to support under higher physical demand.

Nitrogen retention and increased body mass can occur with *females* taking anabolic steroids, but the inevitable virilizing side effects must be recognized and seem a high price to pay for possible improvement in athletic performance. Moreover, use of other drugs with anabolic steroids, such as diuretics to reduce fluid retention, can further increase the likelihood of toxicity, and resultant electrolyte imbalances may have serious adverse consequences. Use of anabolic steroids for improving athletic prowess should be *strongly* discouraged

DOSAGE
See Table 46-1

FATE
Testosterone is adequately absorbed when given orally, but as much as 50% of a dose undergoes first-pass hepatic metabolism and very high doses are necessary to achieve effective plasma levels. Synthetic androgens are less extensively metabolized and exhibit longer half-lives. Esterification of testosterone increases its stability, and when administered in an oily vehicle it possesses a long duration of action (2–4 wk). Testosterone is highly (98%) bound to plasma proteins, especially testosterone estradiol–binding globulin. Androgens are metabolized in the liver, and conjugated metabolites are excreted largely in the urine

COMMON SIDE EFFECTS
Female virilization (e.g., hirsutism, voice changes, clitoral enlargement), amenorrhea, changes in libido, flushing, nausea with oral preparations; gynecomastia in males

SIGNIFICANT ADVERSE REACTIONS

WARNING
Use of androgens or anabolic steroids can result in development of peliosis hepatis, a condition in which the liver and spleen may become engorged with blood-filled cysts. Liver failure has resulted, and intraabdominal hemorrhage has also occurred. Liver cell tumors have been reported, and although these are usually benign, fatal malignant tumors can occur. Adverse serum lipid changes, such as decreased high-density lipoproteins and elevated low-density lipoproteins, have also been noted with androgen therapy. Cholestatic hepatitis and jaundice can occur with fluoxymesterone and methyltestosterone at relatively low doses; the drug-induced jaundice is reversible when the medication is discontinued

Males
Prepubertal: phallic enlargement, increased erections, premature closing of epiphyses
Postpubertal: impotence, testicular atrophy, bladder irritability, decreased sperm count, epididymitis, chronic priapism, gynecomastia

Females
Male pattern baldness, menstrual irregularities, suppression of ovulation or lactation

Both sexes
Acne; oily skin; excitation; insomnia; anxiety; depression; headache; paresthesia; chills; leukopenia; polycythemia; hypercalcemia; pain; swelling, urticaria, and irritation at injection sites; jaundice; hepatic necrosis; sodium and water retention; increased serum cholesterol; in addition, *oral* preparations may cause vomiting and ulcer symptoms; alterations can occur in many clinical laboratory tests

CONTRAINDICATIONS
Pregnancy, lactation, known or suspected prostatic or breast cancer in males; in addition, *anabolic hormones* are also contraindicated in prostatic hypertrophy, pituitary insufficiency, history of myocardial infarction, hepatic dysfunction, nephrosis, hypercalcemia, and in elderly asthenic males who may react adversely to overstimulation. *Cautious use* in persons with hypertension, coronary artery disease, gynecomastia, renal dysfunction, hypercholesterolemia, and in prepubertal males

INTERACTIONS
Androgens may decrease oral anticoagulant dosage requirements

Barbiturates and other hypnotics, phenytoin, and phenylbutazone may decrease the action of androgens by accelerating their metabolic breakdown

Androgens can antagonize the action of calcitonin and parathyroid hormone

Corticosteroids may increase the severity of androgen-induced edema

Anabolic steroids may decrease blood glucose in diabetics, reducing insulin or oral hypoglycemic drug requirements

NURSING CONSIDERATIONS

Nursing Alerts

- If symptomatic hypercalcemia occurs (e.g., vomiting, constipation, loss of muscle tone, polyuria, lethargy), provide copious fluids to prevent formation of renal calculi. The drug should be discontinued, and symptoms should be treated with appropriate medications. All patients should be tested regularly for development of hypercalcemia, which occurs mainly in patients who are bedridden or immobilized or those who have metastatic breast cancer. In the latter, elevated calcium levels usually indicate bone metastases.
- Notify physician if liver tests are abnormal, signs of excessive sexual stimulation occur (e.g., priapism), or vaginal bleeding develops because the drug should be discontinued. Observe for signs of jaundice (yellow skin or sclerae, itching) or excessive stimulation in the elderly patient.

1. Monitor results of liver function tests, serum cholesterol determinations, and tests for serum calcium levels, which should be performed periodically during therapy.
2. Assist with evaluation of drug effects. Anabolic steroids should not be administered for longer than 90 days without careful patient reassessment.
3. Cautiously interpret results of the following laboratory tests because androgens may alter their values: liver function, thyroid function, glucose tolerance, blood coagulation, creatinine excretion, serum cholesterol, and the metyrapone test.

PATIENT EDUCATION

1. Suggest that oral tablets be taken with food to minimize GI distress. Buccal tablets should be allowed to dissolve between gum and cheek or under the tongue, but should not be swallowed. Instruct patient not to eat, drink, or smoke while tablet is in place.
2. Instruct female patient to report signs of virilization (see Common Side Effects) to physician because they may necessitate termination of therapy. Some changes (e.g., voice deepening, hirsutism) may be irreversible even when drug is discontinued.
3. Advise male patient to notify physician if priapism, reduced ejaculatory volume, impotence, or gynecomastia occurs. These symptoms may be controlled by dosage reduction or temporary cessation of therapy.
4. When an anabolic steroid is given to a prepubertal male, instruct parents to carefully observe for signs of premature sexual development. Rate of bone growth and maturation should be periodically checked radiologically to minimize danger of premature fusion of epiphyses.
5. Instruct patient on prolonged therapy to note signs of development of excessive fluid retention (e.g., edema, weight gain). If these occur, the drug should be temporarily withdrawn or a diuretic administered.
6. Instruct diabetic patient to be alert for signs of hypoglycemia (sweating, tremor, anxiety, vertigo) and to adjust antidiabetic drug dosage accordingly.
7. Instruct patient taking anticoagulants to report signs of bleeding (e.g., petechiae, ecchymoses) because dosage of anticoagulant drug may have to be reduced.
8. Encourage bedridden patient to perform exercises regularly to minimize development of hypercalcemia.
9. When appropriate, explain that anabolic steroids do not significantly enhance athletic ability and should not be used to improve performance or stamina because the risk far outweighs the potential benefit.

Danazol

Danocrine

(CAN) Cyclomen

A synthetic derivative of 17-alpha-ethinyl testosterone, danazol inhibits the release of gonadotropins from the pituitary gland and exhibits a weak androgenic effect. No estrogenic or progestational activity has been demonstrated. Danazol provides alternative therapy for endometriosis in those women who cannot tolerate or who fail to respond to other forms of treatment, and it may also be employed in severe fibrocystic breast disease and hereditary angioedema.

MECHANISM

Suppresses release of FSH and LH from the adenohypophysis; inhibits enzymes necessary for biosynthesis of gonadal hormones; may also compete with sex steroids for binding sites on body tissues; lack of ovulation and associated amenorrhea results in atrophy of endometrium and resolution of endometrial lesions

USES

Treatment of endometriosis in those patients who cannot tolerate or who fail to respond to other means of therapy (*not* indicated in cases in which surgery is the treatment of choice)

Symptomatic treatment of severe fibrocystic breast disease

Prevention of attacks of all types (e.g., cutaneous, laryngeal, abdominal) of hereditary angioedema

Treatment of gynecomastia, infertility, and menorrhagia (investigational use only)

DOSAGE

NOTE

Begin therapy during menstruation, if possible, to ensure that patient is not pregnant. Otherwise, perform pregnancy test before initiating therapy if possibility of pregnancy exists. Also, rule out carcinoma of the breast before initiating therapy for fibrocystic breast disease. If any nodule persists or enlarges during therapy, discontinue drug and perform appropriate tests

Endometriosis

200 mg to 400 mg twice a day for 3 to 9 months; may reinstitute therapy if symptoms recur

Fibrocystic Breast Disease

100 mg to 400 mg/day in two divided doses for 3 to 6 months

Hereditary Angioedema

Initially, 200 mg two to three times/day; reduce dosage at 1- to 3-month intervals if clinical response is favorable.

COMMON SIDE EFFECTS

Flushing, sweating, vaginitis

SIGNIFICANT ADVERSE REACTIONS

Virilization (acne, oily skin, hirsutism, deepening of the voice, decrease in breast size, clitoral hypertrophy), vaginal bleeding, edema, weight gain, nervousness; other effects for which a direct causal relationship has not been established are loss of hair, changes in libido, pelvic pain, muscle cramps, back, neck,

Table 46-1
Androgens and Anabolic Steroids

Drug	Preparations	Usual Dosage Range	Nursing Implications
Androgens			
Fluoxymesterone Android-F, Halotestin, Ora-Testryl	Tablets: 2 mg, 5 mg, 10 mg	*Hypogonadism, impotence:* 5 mg–20 mg/day *Delayed puberty:* 2 mg/day initially; increase gradually as necessary, up to 20 mg/day *Breast cancer:* 10 mg–40 mg/day in divided doses *Postpartum breast engorgement:* 2.5 mg shortly after delivery; thereafter, 5 mg–10 mg/day in divided doses for 4–5 days	Potent, orally effective, short-acting derivative of testosterone, approximately five times more active than testosterone itself; minimal sodium and water retention but frequent GI distress (administer drug with food); be alert for symptoms suggestive of peptic ulcer; confirmatory tests should be performed (see also Chap. 72)
Methyltestosterone Android, Metandren, Oreton, Testred, Virilon	Tablets *Oral:* 10 mg, 25 mg *Buccal:* 5 mg, 10 mg Capsules: 10 mg	*Male hypogonadism impotence, male climacteric:* 10 mg–40 mg/day (oral) *or* 5 mg–20 mg/day (buccal) *Cryptorchism:* 30 mg/day (oral) *or* 15 mg/day (buccal) *Postpartum breast pain and engorgement:* 80 mg/day (oral) *or* 40 mg/day (buccal) for 3–5 days *Breast cancer:* 200 mg/day (oral) *or* 100 mg/day (buccal)	Orally effective, short-acting androgen somewhat less effective than testosterone esters; does not produce full sexual maturation in prepubertal testicular failure unless patient has been pretreated with testosterone; creatinuria is a common finding, although its significance is not known; buccal tablets should be placed between cheek and gum and allowed to dissolve, *not* chewed or swallowed, patient should avoid eating, drinking, or smoking for at least 1 h after ingestion; instruct patient to report any inflammation or pain in oral cavity following drug usage; good oral hygiene should be stressed to reduce infection or irritation (see also Chap 72)
Testosterone, Aqueous Andronaq-50, Andro 100, Histerone, Testamone 100, Testaqua, Testoject (CAN) Malogen	Injection (aqueous): 25 mg, 50 mg, 100 mg/mL	*Male hypogonadism, impotence, male climacteric:* 25 mg–50 mg IM 2–3 times/wk *Postpartum breast engorgement:* 25 mg–50 mg/day for 3–4 days *Breast cancer:* 50 mg–100 mg 3 times/wk	Male sex hormone used as replacement therapy in deficiency states, for relief of breast engorgement and treatment of mammary carcinoma in women; inject IM only deep into gluteal muscle; if crystals are present in the vial, warming and shaking will disperse them; absorption is slow and effects persist for several days; do *not* administer more frequently than recommended; regression of mammary tumors should be apparent within 3 mo; occasionally, acceleration of tumor growth is encountered, in which case discontinue immediately; in some of these cases, estrogens will then cause regression (see also Chap. 72)
Testosterone Propionate Testex (CAN) Malogen in Oil	Injection (in oil): 25 mg, 50 mg, 100 mg/mL	IM: *see* Testosterone, aqueous	Ester of testosterone formulated in an oily vehicle; absorption may be somewhat slower than testosterone aqueous, but duration of action is comparable

Continued

Table 46-1
Androgens and Anabolic Steroids (continued)

Drug	Preparations	Usual Dosage Range	Nursing Implications
Testosterone Cypionate Andro-Cyp, Andronate, Andronaq-LA, depAndro, Depo-Testosterone, Depotest, Duratest, Testa-C, Testadiate-Depo, Testoject-LA, Testred **Testosterone Enanthate** Andro-L.A., Andropository, Andryl, Delatest, Delatestryl, Durathate, Everone, Testone L.A., Testrin-P.A. (CAN) Malogex	Injection (in oil): 50 mg, 100 mg, 200 mg/mL	*Hypogonadism, male climacteric:* 50 mg–400 mg IM every 2–4 wk *Oligospermia:* 100 mg–200 mg every 4–6 wk *Delayed puberty:* 50 mg–200 mg every 2–4 wk *Inoperable mammary cancer:* 200 mg–400 mg every 2–4 wk	Long-acting esters of testosterone providing a therapeutic effect for approximately 4 wk with single injection; *not* recommended for use in treating *metastatic* breast carcinoma; inject *deep* into gluteal muscle; shaking and warming of vial will redissolve any crystals that have formed; use of a wet needle or syringe may cloud solution but potency is unaffected
Anabolic Steroids			
Ethylestrenol Maxibolin	Tablets: 2 mg Elixir: 2 mg/5 mL	*Weight gain, osteoporosis, anemias* Adults: 4 mg–8 mg/day initially if needed Children: 2 mg/day (range 1 mg–3 mg/day	Anabolic steroid given for a 6-wk period, then stopped for 4 wk; if indication for its use is still evident, it may be resumed for additional 6-wk period; in children, x-rays should be taken before reinstating therapy to determine stage of bone maturation
Methandrostenolone Methandrostenolone	Tablets: 2.5 mg, 5 mg	Adults: 5 mg initially; usual maintenance dose 2.5 mg–5 mg/day	Used as adjunctive therapy in senile and postmenopausal osteoporosis; intermittent therapy is recommended for long-term use
Nandrolone Decanoate Anabolin L.A., Androlone-D, Deca-Durabolin, Decolone, Hybolin, Nandrobolic L.A., Neo-Durabolic	Injection (in oil): 50 mg, 100 mg, 200 mg/mL	*Osteoporosis, tissue building, anemia* (investigational) Adults: 50 mg–200 mg IM every 3–4 wk Children: 25 mg–50 mg every 3–4 wk *Metastatic breast cancer:* 100 mg–200 mg/wk	Long-acting ester of nandrolone (duration 3–4 wk); rated *possibly* effective for adjunctive therapy of senile or postmenopausal osteoporosis, for increasing tissue building activity postsurgically, for control of metastatic breast carcinoma, and in certain types of refractory anemia
Nandrolone Phenpropionate Anabolin I.M., Androlone, Durabolin, Hybolin Improved, Nandrobolic	Injection (in oil): 25 mg, 50 mg/mL	*Metastatic breast cancer:* 25 mg–100 mg/wk IM *Osteoporosis, anemia, tissue building:* (investigational) Adults: 50 mg–100 mg/wk Children: 12.5 mg–25 mg every 2–4 wk	Synthetic androgen with high anabolic–androgenic ratio; effects persist 1–3 wk; injection should be made deeply into gluteal muscle in adults; intermittent therapy is recommended, with 4–8-wk rest periods every 4 mo (see Chap. 72)
Oxandrolone Anavar	Tablets: 2.5 mg	*Osteoporosis, tissue building* Adults: 2.5 mg 2–4 times/day (up to 20 mg a day) for 2–4 wk; repeat after a rest period if desired Children: 0.25 mg/kg/day	Synthetic anabolic steroid with low androgenic activity; used frequently to help promote weight gain following trauma, severe illness, major surgery, or prolonged corticosteroid administration; do not administer longer than 3 mo
Oxymetholone Anadrol-50 (CAN) Anapolin 50	Tablets: 50 mg	*Anemias:* (adults and children): 1 mg–2 mg/kg/day to a maximum of 5 mg/kg/day (highly individual)	Synthetic anabolic steroid used primarily for anemias due to deficient red cell production, congenital or acquired aplastic anemia, and anemias resulting from administration of myelotoxic drugs; a minimum of 3–6 mo should be allowed,

Continued

Table 46-1
Androgens and Anabolic Steroids (continued)

Drug	Preparations	Usual Dosage Range	Nursing Implications
			because response is often slow; following remission, some patients may be able to stop drug, while others may require a minimum daily dosage
Stanozolol Winstrol	Tablets: 2 mg	*Hereditary angioedema* (adults): Initially 2 mg 3 times/day; decrease gradually to maintenance dosage of 2 mg/day	Primarily used to decreased frequency and severity of attacks of hereditary angioedema; exhibits minimal androgenic effects at normal doses; administer with meals to decrease GI distress

or leg pain, skin rash, nasal congestion, nausea, vomiting, gastroenteritis, dizziness, headache, tremor, paresthesias, and visual disturbances

CONTRAINDICATIONS
Pregnancy, lactation, undiagnosed vaginal bleeding, and markedly impaired cardiac, hepatic, or renal function. *Cautious use* in patients with migraine, epilepsy, hypertension, cardiac disease, and mild to moderate renal dysfunction

INTERACTIONS
Danazol may prolong prothrombin time in patients stabilized on warfarin
Therapy with danazol may increase insulin requirements and result in abnormal glucose tolerance tests

PATIENT EDUCATION
1. Reassure patient that drug-induced anovulation and amenorrhea are reversible within 60 to 90 days after therapy is terminated.
2. Instruct patient to inform physician if signs of virilization develop. Some of these may be irreversible.

Selected Bibliography
Barbieri RL, Ryan KJ: Danazol: Endocrine pharmacology and therapeutic applications. Am J Obstet Gynecol 141:453, 1981
Danazol and other androgens for hereditary angioedema. Med Lett Drugs Ther 23:83, 1981
Duncan DJ, Shaw EB: Anabolic steroids: Implications for the nurse practitioner. Nurse Pract 10(12):8, 1985
Griffin JE, Leshin M, Wilson JD: Androgen resistance syndromes. Am J Physiol 243:81, 1982
Mandanes AE, Farber M: Danazol. Ann Intern Med 96:625, 1982
Marchant DJ: Evaluation, diagnosis and treatment of the fibrocystic breast. Mod Med 55:42, 1987
Neumann F: Pharmacology and clinical use of antiandrogens. Ir J Med Sci 15:61, 1982
Pardridge WM, Gorski RA, Lippe BM, Green R: Androgens and sexual behavior. Ann Intern Med 96:488, 1982
Perlmutter G, Lowenthal DT: Use of anabolic steroids by athletes. Am Fam Physician 32:203, 1985
Ryan AJ: Anabolic steroids are fool's gold. Fed Proc 40:2682, 1982
Wilson JD, Griffin JE: The use and misuse of androgens. Metabolism 29:1278, 1980

SUMMARY. ANDROGENS AND ANABOLIC STEROIDS

Drug	Preparations	Usual Dosage Range
Androgens and Anabolic Steroids	See Table 46-1	
Danazol Danocrine	Capsules: 50 mg, 100 mg, 200 mg	*Endometriosis:* 200 mg to 400 mg twice a day for 3 months to 9 months *Fibrocystic breast disease:* 100 mg to 400 mg a day in two divided doses for 3 months to 6 months *Angioedema:* 200 mg initially, two to three times/day; reduce dosage at 1-month to 3-month intervals if clinical response is favorable

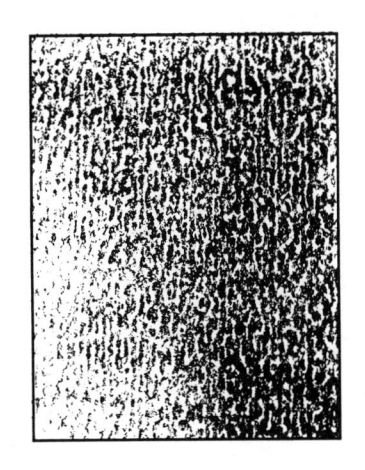

VI Drugs Acting on Gastrointestinal Function

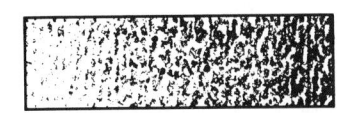

47 GASTROINTESTINAL PHYSIOLOGY: A REVIEW

The digestive system functions to provide body cells with water, electrolytes, vitamins, and nutritive substances. During passage through the GI tract, ingested carbohydrates, fats, and proteins are converted into smaller, absorbable units by the action of digestive enzymes aided by specialized secretions such as bile and hydrochloric acid.

The luminal contents of the digestive tract are transported and effectively mixed with digestive secretions and mucus by specialized muscular movements. GI motility and secretion are affected by a complex interaction of intrinsic and extrinsic neural influences and by several peptide hormones. This chapter briefly reviews the important anatomic features of the GI tract, then explores in detail the principal physiologic functions of the digestive system.

ORGANIZATION OF THE DIGESTIVE SYSTEM

Gastrointestinal Tract

The GI tract (digestive tract or alimentary canal) is a continuous muscular tube lined with mucous membrane, extending from the mouth to the anus, with regional anatomic and functional modifications as outlined in Tables 47-1 and 47-2. The digestive tract includes the mouth, pharynx, esophagus, stomach, and the small and large intestines.

Accessory Organs of Digestion

The salivary glands, pancreas, liver, and gallbladder contribute exocrine secretions essential to the chemical breakdown of food. Digestion is also aided mechanically by the teeth, tongue, and cheeks.

GENERAL HISTOLOGY OF THE GASTROINTESTINAL TRACT

The walls of the organs making up the digestive tract contain four basic layers (tunics) of tissue. From the lumen outward they are as depicted in the following sections.

Tunica Mucosa

The tunica mucosa or mucous membrane consists of a lining *epithelium*, which is in direct contact with the luminal contents. The epithelium may be protective, secretory, or absorptive. Histologically, the epithelium is stratified squamous in the mouth, pharynx (except for the nasopharynx), esophagus, and anal canal. It is simple columnar in the stomach and intestines.

A loose connective tissue, the *lamina propria*, supports the epithelium and binds it to the underlying smooth muscle, the *muscularis mucosa*.

Tunica Submucosa

This loose connective tissue layer contains blood vessels, lymphatic tissue, and the nerve *plexus of Meissner* (submucosal plexus).

Tunica Muscularis (Muscularis Externa)

Characteristically, the tunica muscularis is composed of two layers of smooth muscle, an inner, somewhat thicker circular layer and an outer longitudinal layer. Between these lies the *plexus of Auerbach* (myenteric plexus) which contains autonomic nerve fibers and ganglia.

Tunica Serosa or Adventitia

Generally, the outermost tunic is a serious membrane or *serosa* (visceral peritoneum) composed of loose connective tissue covered by a layer of squamous mesothelial cells. In certain parts of the digestive tract (such as the esophagus and rectum) where the connective tissue is not covered by mesothelial cells, the outer tunic is termed the *adventitia*.

FUNCTIONAL OVERVIEW

The principal activities of the digestive system include (1) motility, (2) secretion, (3) digestion, and (4) absorption.

Motility

Muscular movements propel materials through the digestive tract, aid in the mechanical breakdown of food, promote mixing of luminal contents with mucus and digestive secretions, and facilitate absorption by renewing the absorptive surface.

The motor functions of the alimentary canal are of two basic types: *mixing* and *propulsive*. These movements are subject to intrinsic and extrinsic neural influences as well as to hormonal regulation.

The alimentary canal is extensively innervated by autonomic nerve fibers belonging to both the sympathetic and parasympathetic divisions. Autonomic elements are represented in the intrinsic nerve supply, the submucosal plexus (of Meissner) and more extensively in the myenteric plexus (of Auerbach). The nerves maintain muscle tone and regulate the force and velocity of muscular contractions.

GI motility is generally increased by parasympathetic (vagal and sacral nerve) stimulation and inhibited by sympathetic activation. Only the sphincters respond in an opposite manner, being relaxed by parasympathetic stimulation and contracted by sympathetic stimulation.

The motor functions of individual digestive organs are summarized in Table 47-2.

Secretion

The major secretions of the digestive system are saliva, gastric juice, intestinal juice, pancreatic juice, and bile. These are produced by specialized exocrine glands associated with specific components of the digestive tract. Basically, each secretion consists of water, electrolytes, and one or more active organic constituents. *Mucin*, the active constituent of mucus, is produced by all segments of the digestive tract. Mucus lubricates and protects each region of the alimentary canal from chemical and mechanical irritation.

Table 47-1
Anatomical and Histologic Features of the Major Organs of the Digestive Tract

Organ	Gross Anatomic Features	Histologic Features
Esophagus	Muscular tube continuous with the pharynx	Mucosal epithelium is nonkeratinizing *stratified squamous*. Composition of the tunica muscularis: upper one-third—striated muscle; middle one-third—striated and smooth muscle; and lower one-third—smooth muscle. Outer layer—adventitia
Stomach	*Cardia*—portion surrounding the lower esophageal sphincter *Fundus*—rounded upper portion lying above the entrance of the esophagus *Body*—dilated (major) central region *Pyloric antrum*—tapering distal portion terminating at the pyloric sphincter *Greater curvature*—Large convex curvature on the lateral border *Lesser curvature*—smaller, concave curvature on the medial border The empty (contracted) stomach exhibits longitudinal folds of mucosa termed *rugae*	Mucosal epithelium is *simple columnar*. Tunica muscularis contains three layers of smooth muscle; an inner *oblique*, a middle *circular*, and an outer *longitudinal*. Outer layer is a *serosa* formed by the visceral peritoneum, which reflects from the greater and lesser curvatures as the greater and lesser omenta.
Small Intestine	*Duodenum*—first 25 cm, which receives the common bile duct and the pancreatic duct *Jejunum*—middle segment representing about two fifths of the small intestine *Ileum*—remaining three fifths, rich in lymphatic aggregates (Peyer's patches)	Mucosal epithelium is *simple columnar*. Submucosa contains Brunner's glands. Outer layer is a *serosa* (except in duodenum) Absorptive surface area is increased by the following structural features: • *Plicae circulares* (valves of Kerckring)—circular folds of the mucosa and submucosa projecting into the lumen • *Villi*—fingerlike projections of mucous membrane containing a blood capillary and a lacteal (lymphatic) • *Microvilli*—microscopic projections of the free surfaces of lining epithelial cells
Large Intestine	*Cecum*—blind pouch from which the vermiform appendix is suspended *Colon* (ascending, transverse, descending and sigmoid) Rectum Anal canal	Mucosal epithelium is *simple columnar*. Outer layer is a *serosa* except for the rectum and anal canal, which are covered by adventitia. Prominent morphologic features include: • *Taeniae coli*—three strap-like bands of longitudinal smooth muscle • *Haustra*—sacculations or pouches giving the colon a scalloped appearance • *Epiploic appendages*—fat-filled tabs suspended from the colon

Digestive secretions are produced in response to both mechanical and chemical stimulation. Nervous and humoral (hormonal) mechanisms control the rate and, in some instances, the relative composition of secretions. Generally, parasympathetic activity promotes GI secretion.

The major digestive secretions are characterized in Table 47-2.

CONTROL OF GASTRIC SECRETION

Gastric secretion, which occurs in three phases, cephalic, gastric, and intestinal, is controlled by neural and humoral mechanisms.

The *cephalic phase*, which occurs before food enters the stomach, may be initiated by the thought, sight, smell, or taste of food. This phase, which is mediated by the vagus (10th cranial)

Table 47-2
Major Activities of the Digestive Tract

Organ	Motor Activity	Secretion	Digestion	Absorption
Mouth	Chewing (mastication)—ingested food is subdivided into small particles by the teeth and mixed with saliva to form a bolus. Swallowing (deglutition)—oral phase of swallowing is initiated voluntarily as the tongue forces the bolus toward the oropharynx.	Saliva is secreted by buccal and salivary glands (parotid, submaxillary, and sublingual) in response to the sight, smell, or taste of food. Saliva moistens the mucous membranes, cleanses the mouth and teeth, lubricates the food to facilitate chewing and swallowing, and enhances the taste of food.	Digestion of complex carbohydrates (starches) is initiated by salivary amylase (ptyalin).	Certain drugs (e.g., nitroglycerin) are absorbed sublingually.
Pharynx	Swallowing (pharyngeal phase)—swallowing proceeds reflexly as the bolus enters the oropharynx and continues through the laryngopharynx into the esophagus.			
Esophagus	Swallowing (esophageal phase)—swallowing continues reflexly, coordinated by a swallowing center in the medulla. Bolus passes along the esophagus into the stomach through peristalsis.	Esophageal glands secrete mucus to facilitate passage of bolus and protect the mucosa.		
Stomach	Receptive relaxation—stomach adapts to increased volume without an increase in intragastric pressure Reservoir function—stomach stores contents ingested in a meal and allows partial digestion and gradual emptying into the intestine. Mixing function—mixing waves, aided by peristaltic waves, macerate the bolus, mix it with gastric juice, and reduce it into chyme. Propulsive function—peristaltic waves force the chyme through the pyloric sphincter into the duodenum. Gastric emptying—chyme leaves the stomach at a rate consistent with the most effective rates of digestion and absorption by the small intestine. The rate of gastric emptying is influenced by the physical and chemical composition of chyme (e.g., volume, viscosity, acidity, osmotic pressure). Hormonal and neural factors, including emotional state, can affect the gastric emptying rate.	Gastric juice contains: *Mucus* (secreted by mucous cells)—protects the stomach wall from autodigestion *Hydrochloric acid* (secreted by parietal or oxyntic cells)—converts pepsinogen into active pepsin; provides optimal pH for pepsin activity; inactivates ptyalin; bacteriostatic action *Renin:* the milk-curdling enzyme that acts on the milk protein; of little importance in humans *Pepsinogen:* (secreted by chief or zymogenic cells)—inactive form of the proteolytic enzyme pepsin *Intrinsic factor* (secreted by oxyntic or parietal cells)—forms a complex with vitamin B_{12} to allow intestinal absorption (cyanocobalamin)	Protein digestion—pepsin begins the digestion of proteins by attacking certain amino-acid linkages and reducing proteins into proteoses and peptones. Fat digestion—gastric lipase acts principally on tributyrin and is not considered to contribute significantly to the digestion of fats.	Certain drugs (e.g., alcohol, aspirin), some water, and a few electrolytes are absorbed from the stomach.

Continued

Table 47-2
Major Activities of the Digestive Tract (continued)

Organ	Motor Activity	Secretion	Digestion	Absorption
Small intestine	Segmentation—these fairly regular localized contractions of the circular smooth muscle mix the chyme with pancreatic, intestinal, and hepatobiliary secretions. Peristalsis—peristaltic waves propel the intestinal contents onward at a rate suitable for optimal absorption.	*Succus entericus* (intestinal juice)—intestinal glands secrete a slightly alkaline fluid containing water, mucus, and enzymes that complete the digestion of carbohydrates, fats, and proteins. *Bile* (produced by the liver and concentrated by the gallbladder) and *pancreatic juice* are delivered to the duodenum by the common bile duct and pancreatic ducts, respectively.	*Fats* are emulsified by bile and are digested principally by pancreatic lipase. *Carbohydrates* are digested by pancreatic amylase and by intestinal disaccharidases. Proteolytic enzymes produced by the pancreas and the small intestine digest *proteins* (see Table 47-4). Enterokinase converts pancreatic trypsinogen into active trypsin. Nucleic acids are broken down by pancreatic and intestinal nucleases.	Water, electrolytes, vitamins, and nutrients (products of carbohydrates, fat, and protein digestion) are absorbed readily from the small intestine (particularly the duodenum and jejunum), as are most orally administered drugs. Bile salts and vitamin B_{12} are absorbed from the ileum.
Large intestine	Haustral churning—haustral (segmenting) contractions promote water and electrolyte absorption. Peristalsis—peristaltic waves move the contents along the length of the large intestine. Mass peristalsis—strong propulsive contractions drive the luminal contents into the sigmoid colon and rectum. Defecation—reflex evacuation of the bowel initiated by distention of the rectum; reflex is integrated by the sacral segments of the spinal cord.	*Mucus* is secreted to protect the mucosa from chemical and mechanical trauma, and to lubricate the colonic contents, thereby facilitating passage of feces.		Water is absorbed, thereby reducing the contents from a semifluid to a semisolid mass. Some electrolytes and certain vitamins (B and K) synthesized in the colon are absorbed. Organic products of bacterial action (e.g., indole and skatole) are absorbed and transported to the liver for biotransformation to less toxic substances. Rectally administered drugs are absorbed from the rectum.

nerve (and may therefore be abolished by vagotomy), elicits secretion of gastric juice high in acid and pepsin content.

The *gastric phase* of secretion, which is mediated mainly by the hormone gastrin, takes place while food is present in the stomach. Gastrin is released from the pyloric antrum in response to mechanical distention or chemical stimulation (protein digestion products, alcohol, caffeine, others). Gastrin release is a major stimulus to acid secretion. In the absence of a basal level of histamine, gastrin alone has little effect on acid secretion. The parietal cells contain separate receptors for gastrin, acetylcholine, and histamine, suggesting a synergistic effect. The histamine receptors on the parietal cells are blocked by the histamine-2 (H_2) antagonists (see Chap. 14). Other actions of gastrin are listed in Table 47-3.

Excessive gastric acidity (pH less than 2) inhibits gastrin secretion. The buffering actions of proteins and polypeptides in the stomach help prevent a rapid decline in gastric pH, thereby promoting the secretion of gastrin.

The *intestinal phase* of gastric secretion regulation is largely inhibitory. Both neural and hormonal mechanisms are involved in this control of gastric secretion and gastric emptying. Distention of the duodenum and the arrival of acidic chyme, hypertonic or hypotonic fluid, and protein digestion products triggers the enterogastric reflex, which inhibits gastric secretion

and gastric motility. The above-mentioned stimuli, as well as the presence of fats, also promote the release of intestinal hormones (secretin, cholecystokinin, gastric inhibitory peptide) that reduce gastric secretory activity.

Digestion

Most substances ingested in the diet are structurally complex carbohydrates, fats, or proteins, which cannot be absorbed and utilized by the body in their natural states. During the process of digestion these complex organic constituents are chemically broken down into molecules that can be absorbed readily into body fluids. Specific digestive enzymes from the salivary glands, stomach, small intestine, and pancreas hydrolyze (1) complex carbohydrates into simple sugars; (2) fats into monoglycerides, fatty acids, and glycerol; and (3) proteins into amino acids.

The digestion of carbohydrates is initiated in the mouth by salivary amylase and is completed in the small intestine by pancreatic amylase and intestinal disaccharidases. Proteins are broken down by the combined actions of gastric, pancreatic, and intestinal proteolytic enzymes. Fats are emulsified by bile and are hydrolyzed mainly by pancreatic lipase.

The major digestive enzymes are presented in Table 47-4.

Table 47-3
Major Hormones and Regulatory Peptides of the Digestive Tract

Hormone	Source	Stimulus for Secretion	Major Actions
Gastrin	Gastric mucosa of pyloric antrum	Presence of food (particularly protein) Antral distention Vagal stimulation	Stimulates gastric acid and pepsinogen secretion by the gastric mucosa Promotes antral motility
Secretin	Duodenal and jejunal mucosa	Acidic chyme	Stimulates secretion of a watery, alkaline (bicarbonate-rich) pancreatic juice Inhibits gastric secretion Inhibits gastrin-induced release of gastric acid
Cholecystokinin (CCK)	Duodenal and jejunal mucosa	Products of fat and protein digestion Long-chain fatty acids Amino acids (tryptophan and phenylalanine)	Stimulates gallbladder contraction and relaxes the sphincter of Oddi to promote bile flow into the duodenum Stimulates secretion of pancreatic enzymes
Gastric inhibitory peptide (GIP)	Duodenal and jejunal mucosa	Presence of fats and carbohydrates	Stimulates insulin secretion Inhibits gastric acid secretion

Note: Other gut regulatory peptides and hormones include gastrin-releasing peptide (GRP), vasoactive intestinal peptide (VIP), motilin, pancreatic polypeptide, somatostatin, substance P, and neurotensin.

Absorption

Absorption involves the transport of substances (water, electrolytes, vitamins, and products of digestion) across the wall of the digestive tract into the blood or lymph. Mechanisms of transport include diffusion, osmosis, active transport, and pinocytosis.

The proximal small intestine is the major site of absorption of vitamins, water, electrolytes, and nutrients. With the exception of vitamin B_{12} (cyanocobalamin) and the bile salts, which are absorbed mainly from the terminal ileum, most substrates are absorbed from the duodenum and upper jejunum. Intestinal villi, richly endowed with blood capillaries and lymphatic vessels (lacteals), provide an extensive surface area that greatly facilitates absorption. Epithelial cells lining the small intestine exhibit microvilli that further increase the absorptive surface. Finally, the epithelium of the small intestine contains a variety of specialized transport systems for certain substrates (such as amino acids and glucose).

Absorption through the gastric mucosa is limited. Aspirin and alcohol are, however, rapidly absorbed from the stomach.

ABSORPTION OF CARBOHYDRATES

Carbohydrates are absorbed mainly in the form of monosaccharides (pentoses or hexoses), principally from the duodenum and upper jejunum. Glucose and galactose are absorbed by an active carrier system intimately linked to the sodium transport mechanism. Fructose is transported by facilitated diffusion, whereas the remaining monosaccharides are transported by simple passive diffusion.

ABSORPTION OF FATS (LIPIDS)

The products of fat digestion—fatty acids, glycerol, and monoglycerides—are absorbed mainly in the duodenum. Fatty acids containing fewer than 12 carbons are transported directly into the portal blood. Those containing more than 12 carbons are transported into the lymphatics (lacteals) in the form of chylomicrons.

Glycerol may pass into the liver to be used for glycogen synthesis, it may be oxidized by the intestinal mucosal cells, or it may be utilized for intracellular resynthesis of triglycerides.

Certain essential fat-soluble substances and vitamins A, D, E, and K require bile for their absorption. Water-soluble aggregates containing fatty acids, monoglycerides, and bile salts are called *micelles*.

ABSORPTION OF PROTEINS

Ingested proteins are absorbed mainly as amino acids from the duodenum and jejunum. Three active, carrier-mediated transport systems for amino acids have been characterized. Some dipeptides and tripeptides are also actively transported.

Occasionally, whole proteins may be absorbed from the intestine through pinocytosis. For example, gamma globulins (antibodies) ingested by a suckling infant are absorbed intact in this manner.

ABSORPTION OF WATER

The net absorption of water from the intestines is variable, being greatly affected by the osmotic pressure and electrolyte composition of the intestinal contents. The transport of water occurs mainly through osmosis, with the driving force for water absorption being generated by the active transport of various solutes (such as glucose, amino acids, and electrolytes). Pinocytotic vacuoles have also been proposed as bulk carriers of water together with certain solutes. Water is absorbed principally in the upper small intestine and to a limited extent in the colon.

ABSORPTION OF ELECTROLYTES

The electrolytes absorbed from the intestine include minerals ingested in the diet and electrolyte constituents of various digestive juices.

Table 47-4
Major Digestive Enzymes

Source	Enzyme	Activator	Substrate	Action
Salivary glands	Salivary amylase (ptyalin)		Starch, glycogen	Initiates digestion of carbohydrates, converting starch into dextrins and disaccharides
Gastric glands	Pepsin (pepsinogen[a])	HCl	Proteins, polypeptides	Converts proteins and polypeptides into smaller polypeptides (proteoses and peptones)
Exocrine pancreas	Trypsin (trypsinogen[a])	Enterokinase	Proteins, polypeptides	Converts proteins and polypeptides into smaller peptides and amino acids
	Chymotrypsin (chymotrypsinogen[a])	Trypsin	Proteins, polypeptides	Converts proteins and polypeptides into smaller peptides and amino acids
	Carboxypeptidase (procarboxypeptidase[a])	Trypsin	Polypeptides	Converts polypeptides into smaller peptides and amino acids
	Pancreatic amylase (amylopsin)	Chloride ion	Starch, glycogen, dextrins	Converts complex carbohydrates into disaccharides
	Pancreatic lipase (steapsin)	Emulsifying agents	Triglycerides	Converts fats into fatty acids and glycerol
	Ribonuclease		RNA	Converts RNA into nucleotides
	Deoxyribonuclease		DNA	Converts DNA into nucleotides
Intestinal mucosa	Enterokinase		Trypsinogen	Converts trypsinogen into the active proteolytic enzyme trypsin
	Aminopeptidase		Polypeptides	Converts polypeptides into smaller units
	Dipeptidase		Dipeptides	Complete protein digestion by converting dipeptides into absorbable amino acids
	Disaccharidase		Disaccharides	Convert disaccharides into absorbable monosaccharides
	Sucrase		Sucrose	Converts sucrose into glucose and fructose
	Lactase		Lactose	Converts lactose into glucose and galactose
	Maltase (isomaltase)		Maltose	Converts maltose into glucose
	Intestinal lipase		Monoglycerides	Converts fats into fatty acids and glycerol
	Nuclease (nucleotidase)		Nucleotides	Convert nucleotides into nucleosides and phosphates

[a]Inactive form of the enzyme

Monovalent ions, such as potassium and chloride, are absorbed more readily than divalent ions, such as calcium and magnesium. Sodium, calcium, and iron are absorbed actively; potassium, magnesium, and bicarbonate are transported passively.

Calcium and iron are absorbed by special mechanisms largely in accordance with the body's needs. The rate of calcium absorption from the duodenum is greatly enhanced by vitamin D. Iron can be absorbed only in the reduced, ferrous (Fe^{+2}) state, and its absorption is increased when the body's iron stores are low and erythrocyte production is increased.

ABSORPTION OF VITAMINS

The water-soluble vitamins (B and C) are readily absorbed in the upper portions of the small intestine. Vitamin B_{12} (cyanocobalamin), however, requires a special mechanism for absorption. Vitamin B_{12} forms a complex with *intrinsic factor*, a mucoprotein produced by the gastric parietal cells. The vitamin B_{12}–intrinsic factor complex is taken up by the mucosal cells through pinocytosis, and the vitamin B_{12} is then liberated for uptake into the blood. Failure to elaborate intrinsic factor impairs absorption of vitamin B_{12} and results in pernicious anemia.

The fat-soluble vitamins (A, D, E, and K) require bile for proper absorption. Lack of bile or pancreatic lipase may impair adequate absorption of these fat-soluble vitamins.

VOMITING (EMESIS)

Vomiting is the reflex expulsion of the gastric contents through the mouth. Vomiting involves a complex sequence of visceral and somatic events coordinated by a *vomiting center* in the medulla.

The medullary vomiting center may be stimulated through five pathways:

- The chemoreceptor trigger zone (CTZ)
- Cortical stimulation
- Disturbances of the inner ear
- Visceral stimulation
- Nodose ganglion stimulation

Chemoreceptor Trigger Zone

Located in the floor of the fourth ventricle of the brain near the vomiting center, the CTZ may be stimulated by the following:

- Drugs, chemicals, and toxins (e.g., cardiac glycosides and apomorphine)
- Pathologic states (e.g., uremia and diabetic ketoacidosis)
- Variations in gonadotropin and progesterone levels (e.g., pregnancy)
- Radiation

The CTZ exerts a tonic influence on the vomiting center, maintaining a state of excitability to other incoming vestibular impulses (see below).

Drug-, chemical-, or toxin-induced neuronal excitation of the CTZ is probably mediated by the release of dopamine from surrounding cells (e.g., astrocytes) that form synaptic connections with the neurons of the CTZ.

Cortical Stimulation

Emesis may follow cortical stimulation induced by *psychic factors,* such as unpleasant scenes or disagreeable odors, or *increased intracranial pressure,* for example, hydrocephalus, brain tumors, or inflammation.

Disturbances of the Inner Ear (Labyrinth)

Motion (through mechanical stimulation of receptors in the labyrinths of the ear) and disorders affecting the vestibular apparatus may produce emesis. Impulses are carried by the vestibulocochlear (8th cranial) nerve and are transmitted through the cerebellum and CTZ to the vomiting center. Acetylcholine is thought to be the neurotransmitter involved with impulse transmission along the labyrinthine pathway to the vomiting center.

Visceral Stimulation

Afferent impulses from the abdominal viscera may be generated by *visceral distention* or *visceral irritation,* and these impulses can *directly* stimulate the vomiting center. Destruction of the CTZ abolishes vomiting of labyrinthine origin (suggesting a modulatory role for the CTZ in vestibular activation of the vomiting center) but does not alter the emetic effect of visceral stimulation.

Nodose Ganglion

Certain drugs may produce vomiting by stimulating the nodose ganglion of the vagus (10th cranial) nerve.

Following stimulation of the vomiting center, the esophagus, gastroesophageal sphincter, and the body of the stomach relax, while the pyloric antrum and duodenum contract. Forced inspiration follows, and sudden, powerful contraction of the diaphragm and abdominal muscles generates increased intragastric pressure that propels the gastric contents through the esophagus and pharynx into the mouth. Reflex elevation of the soft palate prevents the vomitus from entering the nasopharynx, and closure of the glottis prevents pulmonary aspiration.

Emesis is often preceded by nausea and profuse salivary secretion. Severe nausea may be accompanied by sweating, pallor of the skin, and dizziness.

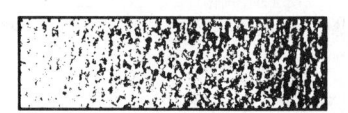

48 ANTACIDS, ANTIULCER DRUGS

The drugs reviewed in this chapter—antacids, other anti-ulcer drugs, and antiflatulents—represent the most widely used group of medications for the treatment of upper GI disorders, ranging from mild indigestion and heartburn to peptic ulcer.

The principal action of antacids is to neutralize acidity, thus raising gastric pH. Increasing the pH results in progressive inhibition of the proteolytic activity of pepsin, thereby reducing its digestive action on the gastric mucosa. Consequently, antacids can reduce pain that results when mucosal nerve endings are activated by excessive gastric acid. They can also promote healing of damaged or ulcerated mucosa by protecting it from the destructive effects of pepsin.

The efficacy of antacids depends on many factors, most importantly their acid-neutralizing capacity, formulation, and dosage schedule. Among the commercially available antacid preparations, there is nearly a 20-fold difference in acid-neutralizing capacity. Sodium bicarbonate and calcium carbonate possess the greatest neutralizing capacity, whereas aluminum phosphate and magnesium trisilicate are considerably weaker.

It is important to recognize, however, that the most potent preparation may not always be the most suitable in terms of potential toxicity (diarrhea, constipation, hypercalcemia, systemic alkalosis), patient acceptance (taste, consistency), sodium content (danger in cardiovascular conditions), or cost. For example, persons with conditions such as edema, hypertension, or congestive heart failure in which low salt intake is required, should be given antacid preparations containing little or no sodium such as Riopan Plus. Magnesium-containing antacids, on the other hand, may cause central nervous system (CNS) toxicity in patients with renal failure and may intensify chronic diarrhea; thus they should be avoided in these conditions. Antacids containing aluminum require cautious use in the presence of constipation or gastric outlet obstruction because they may further reduce gastric emptying. Preparations containing calcium carbonate or sodium bicarbonate are indicated only for short-term therapy, because their side effects (e.g., systemic alkalosis, rebound hyperacidity, milk–alkali syndrome) are significantly enhanced during prolonged treatment.

Aluminum-containing antacids bind phosphate ions in the intestine, causing accelerated elimination with the danger of hypophosphatemia. However, clinical advantage is taken of this property in the use of aluminum carbonate gel for prevention of phosphatic urinary stones or in the management of hyperphosphatemia associated with advanced renal failure.

Product formulation (suspension, tablet, powder) may also be a determining factor in the effectiveness and acceptance of antacids—liquid suspensions generally providing the best neutralizing action. Dosage schedules should be based on the type and severity of the condition being treated; both the frequency and duration of therapy should be sufficient to provide maximum therapeutic benefit with minimal untoward reactions.

Failure of antacid therapy is frequently related to poor selection, inadequate dosage, or improper administration and can be avoided in most cases by judicious choice of an agent appropriate for both the patient and the condition. Selection of an appropriate antacid regimen requires consideration of many factors, and persons should be cautioned against indiscriminate use of these widely available and easily obtainable products.

Antacids are usually administered as one of the many available combination products, inasmuch as these products generally provide good acid-neutralizing activity with a reduced incidence of side effects as compared with the individual components themselves. A popular pairing of antacids is aluminum hydroxide and magnesium hydroxide, a mixture that significantly reduces the occurrence of the constipation and diarrhea frequently observed with aluminum (constipation) and magnesium (diarrhea) alone.

Antacid drugs are discussed as a group, then listed individually in Table 48-1, in which the major uses and characteristics (including acid-neutralizing capacity [ANC], where established) of each drug are presented. Because most antacid preparations are combination products, the composition of the most commonly used combination products, including sodium content and ANC, is given in Table 48-2. Another antiulcer drug discussed in this chapter is sucralfate, a sulfated sucrose–aluminum hydroxide complex that appears to form a protective barrier over the ulcerated area. In addition, reviews of simethicone, an antiflatulent drug used to relieve symptoms associated with excessive production of gas in the digestive tract, and charcoal, an adsorbent, are presented at the end of the chapter.

Several other classes of drugs have been employed in treating peptic ulcer disease and are discussed in previous chapters. Thus, anticholinergics may be found in Chapter 11, the histamine$_2$ receptor blockers are reviewed in Chapter 14, and the tricyclic antidepressants are considered in Chapter 24.

New approaches to the treatment of ulcer disease are currently being evaluated, and two other types of drugs have shown great promise as antiulcer agents. The first of these is omeprazole, which inhibits the parietal cell membrane pump (the so-called proton pump) that represents the final process involved in the secretion of gastric hydrochloric acid. Omeprazole exerts a sustained inhibitory action on acid secretion, in excess of that obtained with the histamine$_2$ antagonists, and promotes prompt healing of ulcerated areas. The second group of potential antiulcer drugs are synthetic derivatives of prostaglandin E that appear to exert both an antisecretory and a cytoprotective effect on the gastric mucosa.

ANTACIDS

Aluminum carbonate
Aluminum hydroxide
Aluminum phosphate
Calcium carbonate
Dihydroxyaluminum sodium carbonate
Magaldrate
Magnesium hydroxide
Magnesium oxide
Sodium bicarbonate

MECHANISM

Neutralize gastric acidity and usually elevate gastric pH above 3 to 4; proteolytic activity of pepsin on gastric mucosa is suppressed above pH 4 and totally abolished above pH 7 to 8; elevated pH also induces the pyloric antrum to release gastrin; acid neutralization may increase lower esophageal sphincter tone; antacids do not appear to "coat" the mucosal barrier but can bind bile acids (especially the aluminum products), although the contribution of this latter action to the therapeutic effects of the drugs is unclear

USES

Symptomatic treatment of GI symptoms associated with hyperacidity (e.g., heartburn, acid indigestion)

Treatment of hyperacidity associated with gastritis, peptic ulcer, hiatal hernia, esophagitis

Prophylaxis of GI bleeding or stress ulcers

Reduction of phosphate absorption in hyperphosphatemia and chronic renal failure (investigational use for aluminum hydroxide and aluminum carbonate)

DOSAGE

See Table 48-1

FATE

Most preparations (except sodium bicarbonate) are not appreciably absorbed from the GI tract and are excreted largely in the feces. Calcium and magnesium products can form chloride salts by reaction with hydrochloric acid, which may be partly absorbed and require elimination by the kidneys. The presence of food can prolong the action of antacids. Thus, antacids taken on an empty stomach have a duration of action of 30 minutes, whereas if they are taken 1 hour after meals, their duration is approximately 3 hours.

COMMON SIDE EFFECTS

Diarrhea (magnesium products), constipation (aluminum and calcium products)

SIGNIFICANT ADVERSE REACTIONS

Aluminum: intestinal impaction, phosphate depletion (anorexia, weakness, impaired reflexes, depression, tremors, bone pain, osteomalacia)

Magnesium: profound diarrhea, dehydration, hypermagnesemia (nausea, vomiting, impaired reflexes, hypotension, respiratory depression—high risk in patients with impaired renal function), bradyarrhythmias, renal stones (magnesium trisilicate)

Calcium carbonate: rebound hyperacidity, milk–alkali syndrome (metabolic alkalosis, hypercalcemia, vomiting, confusion, headache, renal insufficiency), renal calculi, neurologic impairment, GI hemorrhage, fecal impaction

Sodium bicarbonate: systemic alkalosis, sodium overload, milk–alkali syndrome, rebound hypersecretion

CONTRAINDICATIONS

Depend on individual product (see Table 48-1). *Cautious use* of magnesium-containing products in renal insufficiency and of aluminum-containing products in gastric outlet obstruction. Products high in sodium (see Tables 48-1 and 48-2) must be used cautiously in hypertension, congestive heart failure and in persons on sodium-restricted diets

INTERACTIONS

> NOTE
>
> Owing to the adsorptive capacity of most antacids and their ability to alter gastric pH, other drugs should not be administered within 1 to 2 hours of antacid ingestion, if possible

Antacids (esp. magnesium–aluminum combinations) can impair the absorption of tetracyclines, digoxin, phenothiazines, indomethacin, phenylbutazone, isoniazid, benzodiazepines, captopril, chloroquine, cimetidine, valproic acid, corticosteroids, phenytoin, oral iron products, and salicylates

Antacids can increase the effects of pseudoephedrine, levodopa, and meperidine by *facilitating* their intestinal absorption, and can enhance the effects of amphetamines and quinidine by decreasing their urinary excretion

PATIENT EDUCATION

See Table 48-1 for specific information on each drug.

1. Inform patient that the efficacy of liquid antacid is significantly greater than that of tablets or capsules. If drug is taken in tablet form, instruct patient to chew *thoroughly* before swallowing and to drink a small amount of water afterwards.
2. Explain that antacid is optimally effective during long-term therapy if administered 1 and 3 hours after meals and at bedtime. Food acts as a buffer to gastric acid for approximately 60 minutes, and the presence of food can enhance the action of antacids. Thus, the duration of action of antacids taken on an empty stomach is 30 minutes, whereas it is approximately 3 hours if they are taken 1 hour after meals.
2. Urge patient to report GI pain that persists longer than 72 hours or the presence or tarry stools because these symptoms may indicate ulcer perforation, gastric hemorrhage, or other serious complications.
3. Inform patient that diarrhea or constipation may occur, depending on particular antacid used, and should be treated early.
4. Advise patient on restricted or low sodium diet (e.g., for hypertension, congestive heart failure, edema, pregnancy) that a low sodium preparation should be used.
5. Warn patient with significant renal impairment that magnesium- or calcium-containing products are contraindicated because hypermagnesemia and hypercalcemia can occur. See Significant Adverse Reactions for symptoms.
6. Explain that milk has no antacid properties and may increase acid production.
7. Instruct patient to avoid coffee, other caffeine-containing beverages, and alcohol. The value of bland diets, other than during the acute symptomatic period, is unproven. A *reasonable* diet is far more acceptable than a bland diet, and compliance is accordingly better.
8. Suggest small, frequent meals or snacks. They may be tolerated better than larger meals consumed twice a day, and they result in less gastric acid secretion.

Sucralfate

Carafate

(CAN) Sulcrate

Sucralfate is a complex of sulfated sucrose and aluminum hydroxide used orally for the short-term treatment of duodenal ulcers. Because it is not absorbed from the GI tract, it is virtually free of systemic side effects. It requires an acidic environment for optimal activity, so it should not be administered simultaneously with antacids or H_2 antagonists, because its effectiveness may be somewhat reduced.

(Text continued on page 498)

Table 48-1
Antacids

Drug	Preparations	Sodium Content	Acid Neutralizing Capacity (mEq)
Aluminum Carbonate Gel, Basic Basaljel	Suspension (equivalent to 400 mg of aluminum hydroxide per 5 mL)	0.58 mg/mL	14
	Extra-strength suspension (equivalent to 1000 mg of aluminum hydroxide per 5 mL)	4.6 mg/mL	22
	Capsules and swallow tablets (equivalent to 500 mg of aluminum hydroxide)	2.8 mg/capsule 2.8 mg/tablet	12 13
Aluminum Hydroxide Gel ALternaGEL, Alu-Cap, Alu-Tab, Amphojel, Dialume	Suspension: 320 mg/5 mL	0.5 mg/mL	10
	Concentrated suspension: 600 mg/5 mL	0.5 mg/mL	16
	Capsules: 475 mg, 500 mg	1 mg/capsule	10
	Tablets: 300 mg, 600 mg	300 mg–1.8 g 600 mg–2.9 g	8 16
Aluminum Phosphate Gel Phosphaljel	Suspension: 233 mg/5 mL	1.4 mg/mL	
Calcium Carbonate Alka-Mints, Chooz, Dicarbosil, Tums, and various other manufacturers (CAN) Apo-Cal, Calcite	Tablets: 650 mg Chewable tablets—350 mg, 420 mg, 500 mg, 750 mg, 850 mg	Less than 2 mg/tablet	350 mg—7 500 mg—10 750 mg—15
Dihydroxyaluminum Sodium Carbonate Rolaids	Chewable tablets: 334 mg	53 mg/tablet	7–8
Magaldrate Lowsium, Riopan	Suspension: 540 mg/5 mL	Less than 0.1 mg/5 mL	13–14
	Tablets: 480 mg Chewable tablets: 480 mg	Less than 0.1 mg/tablet or chewable tablet	13–14
Magnesium Hydroxide Milk of Magnesia, M.O.M	Tablets: 325 mg Liquid: 390 mg/5 mL	0.1 mg/5 mL	10–14

Usual Dosage Range

Antacid: 2 capsules or tablets, 2 tsp of regular suspension or 1 tsp extra-strength suspension 4–8 times a day

Prevention of phosphate stones: 2 capsules or tablets 1 h after meals and at bedtime *or* 1–2 tbsp suspension in water or juice 1 h after meals and at bedtime

600 mg 3–6 times/day between meals and at bedtime

Hypophosphatemia in children: 50–150 mg/kg/24 h in divided doses every 4–6 h

15 mL–30 mL every 2 h between meals and at bedtime

0.5 g–1.5 g 3–6 times a day as needed

1–2 tablets 3–6 times/day as needed

480 mg–1080 mg 3–6 times a day between meals and at bedtime

Antacid: 5 mL–15 mL *or* 2–4 tablets 4 times/day
Cathartic
   Adults: 15 mL–30 mL
   Children: 5 mL–30 mL

Nursing Implications

Used as an antacid and for preventing development of urinary phosphate stones; exhibits strong phosphate-binding capacity, increasing fecal and decreasing urinary phosphate excretion; periodic determinations of serum electrolytes, especially calcium and phosphate, should be performed; low phosphate diet is recommended; excessive doses can lead to phosphate depletion (weakness, tremors, bone pain, demineralization); be alert for signs of urinary infection (fever, chills, dysuria); high fluid intake should be maintained

Antacid with moderate acid-neutralizing capacity; does not produce acid rebound or alkalosis; possesses phosphate-binding capacity although to a lesser degree than aluminum carbonate; constipation is a frequent side effect; do *not* use for prolonged periods in patients with low serum phosphate or those on a low sodium diet

No longer labeled for use as an antacid; only used to reduce fecal excretion of phosphates

Very effective antacid, possessing high neutralizing capacity, rapid onset, and relatively prolonged duration of action; does not cause systemic alkalosis but is constipating and may elicit acid rebound and gastric hypersecretion; converted to calcium chloride by gastric acid, which may be absorbed in sufficient quantities to produce hypercalcemia with prolonged treatment; long-term use with foods high in vitamin D (e.g., milk) may lead to milk–alkali syndrome (see Significant Adverse Reactions); contains 40% calcium; use with caution in persons receiving thiazide diuretics, which may reduce calcium excretion

Converted to aluminum hydroxide in the presence of gastric acid, releasing carbon dioxide; gives rapid but transient neutralizing effect; because of high sodium content, use with caution in sodium-restricted patients

A *chemical* combination of magnesium and aluminum hydroxides equivalent to 28%–39% magnesium oxide and 17%–25% aluminum oxide; has somewhat lower neutralizing capacity than a physical mixture of the two ingredients; does not elicit acid rebound or systemic acidosis; has a low incidence of diarrhea and constipation, and very low sodium content; available with simethicone as Riopan Plus

Used as an antacid in small doses or as a cathartic in slightly higher doses; elicits prompt and sustained neutralization of gastric acid without marked acid rebound or systemic alkalosis; however, laxative action is commonly observed at higher doses, thus drug is often combined with aluminum or calcium antacids; also available as an emulsion containing mineral oil (Haley's MO); laxative dose should be given at bedtime, followed by a full glass of water (see Chap. 50)

Continued

Table 48-1
Antacids (continued)

Drug	Preparations	Sodium Content	Acid Neutralizing Capacity (mEq)
Magnesium Oxide Mag-Ox 400, Maalox, Par-Mag, Uro-Mag	Tablets: 400 mg, 420 mg Capsules: 140 mg Powder	NA[a]	21
Sodium Bicarbonate Bell/ans, Soda Mint	Tablets: 325 mg, 520 mg, 650 mg	27% sodium	

[a]NA = Sodium content is not available.

Table 48-2
Antacid Combinations

Trade Name	Dosage Form	Aluminum Hydroxide	Calcium Carbonate	Magnesium Oxide or Hydroxide
Algicon	Tablet	360 mg		
Alka-Seltzer	Tablet			
Alkets	Tablet		780 mg	65 mg
Almacone	Tablet	200 mg		200 mg
	Liquid	40 mg/mL		40 mg/mL
Almacone II	Liquid	80 mg/mL		80 mg/mL
Alma-Mag	Liquid	40 mg/mL		40 mg/ml
Aludrox	Tablet	233 mg		83 mg
	Liquid	61.4 mg/mL		20.6 mg/mL
Alumid	Liquid	45 mg/mL		40 mg/mL
Alumid Plus	Liquid	40 mg/mL		40 mg/mL
Bisodol	Tablet Powder		194 mg	178 mg
Bromo Seltzer	Granules			
Camalox	Tablet	225 mg	250 mg	200 mg
	Liquid	45 mg/mL	50 mg/mL	40 mg/mL
Citrocarbonate	Effervescent powder			
Delcid	Liquid	120 mg/mL		133 mg/mL
Di-Gel	Liquid	40 mg/mL		40 mg/mL

Usual Dosage Range	Nursing Implications
280 mg–1.5 g with water or milk 4 times/day	Slow-acting antacid with prolonged effects; high neutralizing capacity, but frequently elicits nausea and diarrhea; in large doses has been used as a cathartic; also used in powder form; available as light and heavy magnesium oxide; *light* is 5 times bulkier than *heavy* but possesses greater neutralizing power owing to larger surface area
0.3 g–2 g as needed 1–4 times a day	Systemic, absorbable antacid, with a short duration of action; its use should be discouraged because it frequently elicits acid rebound, belching (owing to liberated carbon dioxide), and gastric distention and may cause systemic alkalosis; high sodium content precludes its use in patients with hypertension or cardiac or renal disease; large doses may cause phosphaturia

Simethicone	Other	Sodium Content	Acid Neutralizing Capacity (mEq)
	Magnesium carbonate 320 mg	5 mg/tablet	17–18
	Sodium bicarbonate 958 mg; citric acid 832 mg; potassium bicarbonate 312 mg	284 mg/tablet	10–11
	Magnesium carbonate 130 mg		
20 mg			
4 mg/mL		0.15 mg/mL	10
6 mg/mL		0.3 mg/mL	20
5 mg/mL			
		1.4 mg/tablet	10
		0.46 mg/mL	12
		0.28 mg/mL	
4 mg/mL			
	Sodium bicarbonate 129 mg/g; magnesium carbonate 95 mg/g	31 mg/g	15
	Sodium bicarbonate 2.8 g/dose; citric acid 2.2 g/dose; acetaminophen 0.325 g/dose	0.75 g/dose	
		1 mg/tablet	18
		0.24 mg/mL	18
	Sodium citrate 1.82 g and sodium bicarbonate 0.78 g per 3.9-g dose	700 mg/dose	
		3 mg/mL	42
4 mg/mL		1 mg/mL	11

Continued

Table 48-2
Antacid Combinations (continued)

Trade Name	Dosage Form	Aluminum Hydroxide	Calcium Carbonate	Magnesium Oxide or Hydroxide
Di-Gel (Advanced Formula)	Tablet		280 mg	128 mg
ENO	Powder			
Gaviscon	Tablet	80 mg		
Gaviscon-2	Tablet	160 mg		
Gaviscon	Liquid	6.3 mg/mL		
Gaviscon Extra Strength	Tablet	160 mg		
Gelusil	Tablet	200 mg		200 mg
	Liquid	40 mg/mL		40 mg/mL
Gelusil-II	Tablet	400 mg		400 mg
	Liquid	80 mg/mL		80 mg/mL
Gelusil-M	Tablet	300 mg		200 mg
	Liquid	60 mg/mL		40 mg/mL
Glycate	Tablet		300 mg	
Kolantyl	Wafer	180 mg		170 mg
	Liquid	30 mg/mL		30 mg/mL
Lowsium Plus	Tablet			
	Liquid			
Maalox	Liquid	45 mg/mL		40 mg/mL
Maalox Extra Strength	Whip	131 mg/g		120 mg/g
Maalox No. 1	Tablet	200 mg		200 mg
Maalox No. 2	Tablet	400 mg		400 mg
Maalox TC	Tablet	600 mg		300 mg
Maalox Plus	Tablet	200 mg		200 mg
	Liquid	45 mg/mL		40 mg/mL
Maalox Plus Extra Strength	Liquid	100 mg/mL		90 mg/mL
Magnatril	Tablet	260 mg		130 mg
	Liquid	52 mg/mL		26 mg/mL
Marblen	Tablet		520 mg	
	Liquid		104 mg/mL	
Mylanta	Tablet	200 mg		200 mg
	Liquid	40 mg/mL		40 mg/mL
Mylanta II	Tablet	400 mg		400 mg
	Liquid	80 mg/mL		80 mg/mL
Remegel	Chewable squares			
Riopan Plus	Tablet			
	Liquid			
Riopan Extra Strength	Liquid			
Riopan Plus 2	Liquid			
	Tablet			
Rulox No. 1	Tablet	200 mg		200 mg
Rulox No. 2	Tablet	400 mg		400 mg
Rulox	Liquid	45 mg/mL		40 mg/mL
Silain-Gel	Liquid	56.4 mg/mL		57 mg/mL
TC	Liquid	120 mg/mL		60 mg/mL
Tempo	Tablet	133 mg	414 mg	81 mg
Titralac	Tablet		420 mg	
	Liquid		200 mg/mL	
Win-Gel	Tablet	180 mg		160 mg
	Liquid	36 mg/mL		32 mg/mL

Simethicone	Other	Sodium Content	Acid Neutralizing Capacity (mEq)
20 mg			
	Sodium tartrate 324 mg/g and sodium citrate 235 mg/g	104 mg/g	
	Magnesium trisilicate 20 mg plus alginic acid and sodium bicarbonate	19 mg/tablet	0.5
	Magnesium trisilicate 40 mg plus alginic acid and sodium bicarbonate	37 mg/tablet	
	Magnesium carbonate 27.5 mg/mL	2.6 mg/mL	1
	Magnesium carbonate 105 mg		
25 mg		0.8 mg/tablet	11
5 mg/mL		0.14 mg/mL	12
30 mg		2.1 mg/tablet	21
6 mg/mL		0.26 mg/mL	24
25 mg		1.3 mg/tablet	12–13
5 mg/mL		0.24 mg/mL	15
	Glycine 150 mg		
		2 mg/tablet	10–11
		<1 mg/mL	10–11
20 mg	magaldrate 480 mg		
4 mg/ml	magaldrate 96 mg/mL		
		0.27 mg/mL	13–14
		0.7 mg/tablet	9–10
		1.4 mg/tablet	18
		0.5 mg/tablet	28
25 mg		0.8 mg/tablet	11–12
5 mg/mL		0.26 mg/mL	13–14
8 mg/mL		0	
	Magnesium trisilicate 455 mg		
	Magnesium trisilicate 52 mg/mL		
	Magnesium carbonate 400 mg	3.2 mg/tablet	18
	Magnesium carbonate 80 mg/mL	0.6 mg/mL	18
20 mg		0.77 mg/tablet	11–12
4 mg/mL		0.14 mg/mL	12–13
30 mg		1.3 mg/tablet	23
6 mg/mL		0.23 mg/mL	25–26
	Aluminum hydroxide/ magnesium carbonate complex 476 mg	25 mg/square	13–14
20 mg	Magaldrate 480 mg	0.1 mg/tablet	13–14
4 mg/mL	Magaldrate 180 mg/mL	Less than 0.02 mg/mL	15
	Magaldrate 216 mg/mL	0.06 mg/mL	30
6 mg/mL	Magaldrate 216 mg/mL	0.06 mg/mL	30
20 mg	Magaldrate 1080 mg	0.1 mg/tablet	
		0.16 mg/mL	12
5 mg/mL		0.96 mg/mL	15
		0.16 mg/mL	27–28
20 mg		2.5 mg/tablet	14
	Glycine 180 mg	<0.3 mg/tablet	7–8
	Glycine 60 mg/mL	2.2 mg/mL	19
		2.5 mg/tablet	12
		0.5 mg/mL	11–12

MECHANISM
Not completely established; possible actions include formation of an ulcer-adherent complex with exudative material at the ulcer site, thus protecting the ulcerated area from further attack by acid, pepsin, and bile salts; may also inhibit activity of pepsin; does not appear to neutralize gastric acid

USES
Short-term (i.e., up to 8 weeks) treatment of duodenal ulcers
Investigational uses include treatment of gastric ulcers and prophylaxis of duodenal and gastric ulcers

DOSAGE
1 g (1 tablet) four times a day on an empty stomach

FATE
Minimally absorbed from GI tract and eliminated primarily in the feces; absorbed fraction is excreted principally in the urine

COMMON SIDE EFFECT
Constipation

SIGNIFICANT ADVERSE REACTIONS
(Rare) Diarrhea, nausea, GI distress, indigestion, dry mouth, rash, pruritus, dizziness, vertigo, and sleepiness

INTERACTIONS
Sucralfate may reduce GI absorption of tetracyclines, cimetidine, and phenytoin

PATIENT EDUCATION
1. Inform patient that sucralfate tablets should be taken at least 1 hour before meals and at bedtime to obtain maximal benefit.
2. Advise patient that antacids may be used to control pain, but they should not be used within ½ hour of sucralfate.

Antiflatulents

Drugs used to reduce the symptoms resulting from excess production of gas in the GI tract are termed *antiflatulents*. Simethicone is a silicone derivative commonly found in combination with antacids (see Table 48-2), although it is available alone in tablet and liquid form. Charcoal is an adsorbent used as tablets or capsules for a variety of indications, including the relief of indigestion and bloating resulting from accumulation of intestinal gas.

Simethicone
Gas-X, Mylicon, Phazyme, Silain
(CAN) Ovol

MECHANISM
Alters the surface tension of gas bubbles, causing coalescence of the gas, thereby facilitating its elimination by belching or flatus

USES
Adjunctive treatment of conditions associated with retention of excessive gas (e.g., dyspepsia, peptic ulcer, spastic colon, diverticulitis, or postoperative gaseous retention)

DOSAGE
Capsules or tablets: 40 mg to 125 mg four times a day
Drops: 40 mg four times a day

PATIENT EDUCATION
1. Inform patient that drug should be taken after each meal and at bedtime. Tablets should be chewed thoroughly because complete particle dispersion facilitates the antiflatulent action.
2. Advise patient to consult health care provider if symptoms are not relieved within several days because continual passage of gas may indicate a more serious underlying condition.

Charcoal
Charcocaps

MECHANISM
Adsorbs toxins and gas onto surface of particles, thereby relieving cramping, diarrhea, and flatulence

USES
Temporary relief of indigestion, bloating, cramping, and flatulence
Prevention of nonspecific pruritus associated with kidney dialysis treatment

NOTE
Charcoal may be "activated" by exposing it to an oxidizing gas at high temperatures; this activated product is used as a powder or suspension for emergency treatment of poisoning with many drugs and other chemicals

DOSAGE
975 mg to 3.9 g three or four times a day, followed by a small amount of water

PATIENT EDUCATION
1. Warn patient not to take for more than 3 days and to use only when condition is acute. Charcoal can absorb nutrients, digestive enzymes, and other essential substances.
2. Instruct patient to chew or dissolve tablets in the mouth before swallowing.
3. Instruct patients to administer to children under 3 years of age only if directed by a health care provider.

Selected Bibliography
Adams MH, Ostrosky JD, Kirkwood CF: Therapeutic evaluation of omeprazole. Clin Pharm 7:725, 1988

Berardi RR, Savitsky ME, Nostrant TT: Maintenance therapy for the prevention of recurrent peptic ulcers. Drug Intell Clin Pharm 21:493, 1987

Garnett WR: Sucralfate—Alternative therapy for peptic ulcer disease. Clin Pharm 1:307, 1982

Halter F (ed): Antacids in the Eighties. Munich, Urban and Schwarzenberg, 1982

Ippoliti AF: Antacid therapy for duodenal and gastric ulcer: Experience in the United States. Scand J Gastroenterol 17(Suppl 75):82, 1982

Lewis JH: Treatment of gastric ulcer: What is old and what is new? Arch Intern Med 143(2):204, 1983

Morgan M: Control of intragastric pH and volume. Br J Anaesth 56:47, 1984

Peppercorn MA: Drug therapy of peptic ulcer disease. Compr Ther 9:47, 1983

Piper DW: Drugs for prevention of peptic ulcer recurrence. Drugs 26:439, 1983

Somerville KW, Langman MJ: Newer antisecretory agents for peptic ulcer. Drugs 25:315, 1983

Sontag SJ: Prostaglandins in peptic ulcer disease: An overview of current status and future directions. Drugs 32:445, 1986

Sucralfate for peptic ulcer—A reappraisal. Med Lett Drugs Ther 26:43, 1984

Todd B: Antiulcer preparations. Geriatr Nurs March/April:122, 1983

Walan A: Antacids and anticholinergics in the treatment of duodenal ulcer. Clin Gastroenterol 13(2):473, 1984

Weinstein WW: Treating peptic ulcer: Are you using all your options? Mod Med 53(5):44, 1985

Wilson DE (ed): Symposium on peptic ulcer disease. Drug Ther 13(7):53, 1983

SUMMARY. ANTACIDS AND ANTIULCER DRUGS

Drug	Preparations	Usual Dosage Range
Antacids	See Table 48-1	
Antacid Combinations	See Table 48-2	
Sucralfate	Tablets: 1 g	1 g four times a day on an empty stomach for 4 to 8 wk
Carafate		
Simethicone	Tablets: 50 mg, 60 mg, 95 mg	Tablets: 40 mg to 80 mg 4 times a day
Gas-X, Mylicon, Phazyme, Silain	Chewable tablets: 40 mg, 80 mg, 125 mg	Drops: 40 mg 4 times a day
	Drops: 40 mg/0.6 mL	
	Capsules: 125 mg	
Charcoal	Tablets: 325 mg, 650 mg	975 mg to 3.9 g 3 to 4 times a day
Charcocaps	Capsules: 260 mg	

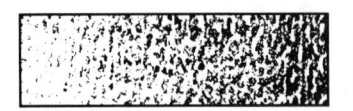

49 DIGESTANTS, GALLSTONE SOLUBILIZING AGENTS

Digestants are substances that assist the physiologic process of food digestion in the gastrointestinal (GI) tract. The major endogenous digestive enzymes, along with their source and action, are listed in Table 47-4, Chapter 47. The usefulness of most enzymes (e.g., amylase, lipase, protease, cellulose) as *exogenous* digestive aids is probably greatly overstated, inasmuch as symptoms of GI distress can rarely be attributed to an actual deficiency of endogenous digestive chemicals. Nevertheless, certain digestive substances, especially the pancreatic enzymes pancreatin and pancrelipase, have proved valuable as replacement therapy in elderly or debilitated persons or in persons with conditions such as GI surgery, achlorhydria, chronic pancreatitis, or gastric carcinoma, in whom there exists a definite lack of one or more of these digestive substances. In such cases, however, the deficient chemicals must be replaced in sufficient amounts to restore digestive activity, and it should be recognized that many commercially available products contain amounts *too small* to provide the required quantity of digestant. Thus, empiric use of combination or "shotgun" digestive products has no place in rational pharmacotherapy. Moreover, the inclusion of anticholinergics, barbiturates, or antacids in these formulations merely increases the likelihood of untoward reactions.

The digestive aids most frequently employed clinically may be grouped as follows:

- Gastric acidifiers (e.g., glutamic acid hydrochloride)
- Digestive enzymes (e.g., pepsin, pancreatin, pancrelipase)
- Bile salts and bile acids (e.g., dehydrocholic acid, ox bile extract)

Gastric hydrochloric acid deficiency (*achlorhydria*) can occur in association with various pathologic conditions such as pernicious anemia or gastric carcinoma, as well as in the absence of observable disease. Dilute solutions (10%) of hydrochloric acid were previously used to aid digestion in patients with achlorhydria and to relieve complaints such as belching, nausea, and epigastric distress. Today, glutamic acid hydrochloride is used as a source of hydrochloric acid, because it it available in capsule and tablet form and offers a safer and more convenient mode of therapy. However, glutamic acid does not yield as much free acid as does hydrochloric acid.

Pepsin is a proteolytic enzyme activated by gastric acid, and thus it is sometimes administered with glutamic acid to stimulate digestion. It is of doubtful benefit in most instances, because absolute lack of pepsin is relatively rare, except perhaps in gastric carcinoma and occasionally in pernicious anemia, and the acid deficiency is usually of far greater consequence. On the other hand, deficiency of pancreatic enzymes is a frequent occurrence, especially in cases of pancreatitis and duct obstruction, and of course following pancreatectomy. In these instances, replacement therapy with either pancreatin, a powdered concentrate of hog pancreas containing amylase, lipase, and protease activity, or pancrelipase, a more concentrated mixture of pancreatic enzymes of porcine origin, is indicated.

Natural bile contains a series of organic acids, secreted as sodium salts, that lower the surface tension of fat globules, breaking them into small droplets. Bile further aids fat digestion by stimulation of pancreatic secretions and activation of pancreatic lipase. Exogenous bile salts (e.g., ox bile extract) have occasionally been used as replacement therapy in patients with partial biliary obstruction or following removal of the gallbladder (cholecystectomy), but their effectiveness in this regard is subject to dispute. Bile salts also exhibit a choleretic action; that is, they stimulate the outflow of bile. Certain bile salts, especially the synthetic derivative dehydrocholic acid, markedly increase the output of a thin, watery bile and are termed *hydrocholeretics*. Dehydrocholic acid is used to facilitate flushing and drainage of partially obstructed bile ducts, thereby minimizing infections and preventing biliary calculi from lodging in the duct.

Several drugs that have become available in recent years can solubilize recently formed gallstones. They are indicated for the dissolution of radiolucent, noncalcified gallstones in patients in whom elective surgery may prove hazardous. These gallstone-solubilizing drugs are reviewed at the end of the chapter.

It should be *reemphasized* that many clinically available digestive products are multiple formulations containing digestive enzymes, bile extracts, or hydrochloric acid derivatives, frequently combined with anticholinergics, antiflatulents, antacids, or barbiturates. Not only is the content of these products often insufficient to provide the needed replacement in cases of deficiency states, but the digestants included in these formulations are frequently unnecessary and usually ineffective for the symptomatic treatment of simple digestive dysfunction, inasmuch as lack of endogenous digestive substances is only rarely the cause of GI distress.

BILE SALTS (CHOLERETICS)

Ox Bile Extract
Ox Bile Extract with Iron
Bilron

Bile salts are the dried extract of bile from cattle, the bile salt content approximating that of human bile. When combined with iron (Bilron), the complex is insoluble in an acid medium (e.g., the stomach). As the complex enters the small intestine, the iron dissociates and the bile salts become soluble and active.

MECHANISM

Lower the surface tension of fat globules, breaking them into smaller, more easily digestible particles by exposing a greater surface area to the enzymatic action of pancreatic lipases; exhibit a mild stimulating effect on GI smooth muscle; exert a choleretic action (i.e., increased flow of bile) following absorption; exhibit a mild laxative effect

USES

Symptomatic treatment of uncomplicated constipation
Replacement therapy in bile deficiency states (e.g., partial biliary obstruction, cholecystectomy)

NOTE

Conclusive evidence of a beneficial effect for bile salts in bile deficiency states is lacking

DOSAGE
150 mg to 600 mg one to three times a day during or after meals

SIGNIFICANT ADVERSE REACTIONS
Loose stools, nausea, cramping

CONTRAINDICATIONS
Complete biliary obstruction, severe jaundice. *Cautious use* in the presence of marked hepatic insufficiency (e.g., viral hepatitis, advanced cirrhosis), and when symptoms of appendicitis are present (e.g., abdominal pain, nausea, vomiting)

INTERACTIONS
Bile salts may enhance the absorption of fat-soluble vitamins (A, D, E, K)

HYDROCHOLERETICS

Dehydrocholic Acid
Atrocholin, Cholan-DH, Decholin
(CAN) Dycholium

Dehydrocholic acid, a semisynthetic derivative of cholic acid, is called a hydrocholeretic agent because its principal pharmacologic action is to increase the volume of dilute bile output without markedly altering the amount of solid bile constituents. Its major use is to facilitate biliary tract drainage. Hydrocholeretics are much less effective than natural bile salts or choleretics (such as ox bile extract) in emulsifying GI fats and in promoting fat absorption.

MECHANISM
Increases the volume of low-viscosity bile flow but does not change the amount of bile constituents

USES
Adjunctive treatment of chronic or recurrent biliary tract disorders (e.g., biliary dyskinesia, chronic partial biliary obstruction, noncalculous cholecystitis) to provide a flushing action
To facilitate prolonged drainage from biliary fistulas or T tubes
Postoperative management following cholecystectomy or surgery on the biliary tract to prevent occlusion or infection of the common bile duct (rarely used)
Temporary relief of constipation

DOSAGE
250 mg to 500 mg three times a day after meals

FATE
Absorbed from upper intestines, passes through the liver and is recycled in the intestinal tract by the bile ducts; excreted in the feces

SIGNIFICANT ADVERSE REACTIONS
Rare at recommended oral doses. Occasionally, mild diarrhea

CONTRAINDICATIONS
Jaundice, severe hepatitis, advanced cirrhosis, cholelithiasis, abdominal pain, vomiting, complete obstruction of the common or hepatic bile ducts or GI or urinary tract. *Cautious use* in patients with prostatic hypertrophy, acute hepatitis, acute yellow atrophy of the liver, partial obstruction of the GI or urinary tracts, history of asthma or allergies, and in children under 6 or in elderly persons

NURSING CONSIDERATIONS

Nursing Alert
- Question use of hydrocholeretics as diuretics or as adjuncts to diuretics, or when abdominal pain, nausea, or vomiting is present.

1. Suggest, as appropriate, simultaneous administration of bile salts during prolonged administration of a hydrochloretic or when bile is draining away from the intestinal tract to ensure adequate digestion and absorption of nutrients.
2. Note that dehydrocholic acid is available in combination with homatropine plus phenobarbital (Cholan HMB, G.B.S.). Use of the combination product is, however, rarely warranted.

GASTRIC ACIDIFIERS

Glutamic Acid HCL
Acidulin

Glutamic acid hydrochloride is a source of hydrochloric acid that aids digestion in conditions associated with reduced (hypoacidity) or absent (achlorhydria) gastric acid. It is used as a hydrochloride salt of glutamic acid in tablet or capsule form that releases hydrochloric acid in the stomach, thus minimizing oral mucosal irritation and damage to dental enamel.

MECHANISM
Facilitates conversion of pepsinogen to pepsin and provides optimal pH for action of pepsin; may stimulate pancreatic secretions and neutralize bicarbonates in gastrointestinal fluid, maintaining electrolyte balance; acidity may inhibit growth of putrefactive organisms in ingested food

USES
Replacement therapy to assist digestion in hydrochloric acid deficiency states (e.g., chronic gastritis, pernicious anemia, gastric carcinoma, primary achlorhydria, gastric resection)
Prevent growth of putrefactive microorganisms in ingested food

DOSAGE
1 to 3 capsules (340 mg) 3 times a day before meals

SIGNIFICANT ADVERSE REACTIONS
Occasional GI irritation; overdosage may lead to systemic acidosis

CONTRAINDICATIONS
Gastric hyperacidity states, peptic ulcer

INTERACTIONS
Glutamic acid may antagonize the antineoplastic action of vinblastine

NURSING CONSIDERATION
1. Assist with periodic assessment of acid-base status in patient on long-term or high-dosage therapy.

PATIENT EDUCATION
1. Instruct patient to prevent tablets or capsules from becoming wet because hydrochloric acid is released upon contact with water.

PANCREATIC ENZYMES

Pancreatin
Dizymes, Hi-Vegi-Lip

Pancrelipase
Cotazym, Creon Festal II, Ilozyme, Ku-Zyme HP, Pancrease, Viokase

Pancreatic enzyme concentrates of bovine or porcine origin containing lipase, protease, and amylase activity; aid in digestion and absorption of fats and carbohydrates. Pancrelipase has greater lipase activity than does pancreatin and can be used in lower doses to control steatorrhea (see Uses below).

MECHANISM
Provide enzymatic activity necessary to assist in the digestion of carbohydrates, fats, and proteins; exert their primary effects in the duodenum and upper jejunum

USES
Replacement therapy in pancreatic enzyme deficiency states, such as chronic pancreatitis or pancreatic insufficiency, steatorrhea of malabsorption syndrome, cystic fibrosis, postgastrectomy, or postpancreatectomy

In testing for pancreatic function, especially in pancreatic insufficiency due to chronic pancreatitis

DOSAGE
(Tablets, capsules, and powder packets of different manufacturers contain different amounts of lipase, protease, and amylase)

Pancreatin: Usually, 325 mg to 1000 mg (1 to 3 tablets) with meals or snacks; each milligram contains not less than 25 U amylase activity, 2 U lipase activity, and 25 U protease activity

Pancrelipase: 1 to 3 tablets or capsules *or* 1 or 2 powder packets before or with meals or snacks; each milligram contains not less than 100 U amylase activity, 24 U lipase activity, and 100 U protease activity

SIGNIFICANT ADVERSE REACTIONS
(Usually with high doses) Nausea, diarrhea, cramping, vomiting, anorexia, hypersensitivity reactions (sneezing, rash, lacrimation)

CONTRAINDICATIONS
Hypersensitivity to beef or pork products

INTERACTIONS
Pancreatic enzymes may retard the absorption of orally ingested iron

Availability of pancreatin in the duodenum may be enhanced by histamine$_2$ antagonists (see Chap. 14)

Antacids containing magnesium hydroxide or calcium carbonate may reduce the effects of the enzymes

NURSING CONSIDERATIONS
1. Rule out previous hypersensitivity to beef or pork products before administering pancreatic enzymes because they are derived from either bovine or porcine sources.
2. Help evaluate patient's response to drug by noting appearance of stools, monitoring weight, and checking results of periodically determined fecal fat and nitrogen.

PATIENT EDUCATION
1. Instruct patient to take drug with meals. Enteric-coated tablets should be swallowed whole. Powder or granules may be added to milk or water or sprinkled on food.
2. Refer patient for dietary consultation as needed to ensure that intake of starch, protein, and fat is balanced during therapy to minimize indigestion.
3. Inform patient that supplemental antacid may be used to control refractory steatorrhea. Antacid should not, however, be taken within 1 hour of pancreatic medication (see Interactions).

A large number of combination products containing different proportions of digestive enzymes, bile extracts, hydrocholeretics, and acidifiers as well as a myriad of other types of agents (e.g., anticholinergics, antacids, charcoal, barbiturates, simethicone) are available for symptomatic treatment of digestive disorders and for other GI dysfunctions. These combination products are rarely of clinical benefit, inasmuch as a GI disorder is seldom caused by a simultaneous overall deficiency of several substances. Specific deficiency states are more appropriately treated with the actual substance that is lacking rather than by employing a "shotgun" approach to therapy. Moreover, inclusion of many different drugs, especially barbiturates and anticholinergics in a single preparation, only serves to increase the likelihood of untoward reactions. Commercially available digestive combinations include, Donnazyme, Entozyme, Festalan, Kanulase, and Phazyme-PB.

GALLSTONE-SOLUBILIZING AGENTS

When cholesterol is present in bile in concentrations that exceed the capacity of bile acids and lecithin to solubilize it, crystals can precipitate and eventually coalesce into gallstones. Dissolution of these gallstones can now be effected in several ways by a number of drugs. The clinically available gallstone-solubilizing agents are considered individually below.

Chenodiol–Chenodeoxycholic Acid
Chenix

MECHANISM
Blocks hepatic synthesis of cholesterol and cholic acid, thereby reducing biliary cholesterol levels and gradually dissolving radiolucent cholesterol gallstones; drug has no apparent effect on radiopaque, calcified gallstones or on bile pigment stones; likelihood of stone dissolution decreases as the size and number of stones increase. Stones have recurred in approximately 50% of patients within 5 years. Retreatment with chenodiol has proved effective in dissolving newly reformed stones, but the long-term toxic effects of repeated therapy remain to be established.

USE
Treatment of patients with radiolucent gallstones in well opacified gallbladders, in whom surgery is not feasible owing to age or presence of systemic disease

DOSAGE
Initially 250 mg twice a day for 2 weeks; increase by 250 mg/day each week thereafter until the recommended dose (i.e., 13 mg/kg to 16 mg/kg/day) or the maximally tolerated dose is attained

NOTE
Doses less than 10 mg/kg/day are usually ineffective and may be associated with an *increased* risk that cholecystectomy will be required

FATE
Well absorbed orally but undergoes extensive first-pass hepatic clearance (see Chap. 2); converted in the colon to lithocholic acid, which is excreted largely (80%) in the feces; the remainder is absorbed and metabolized in the liver; in patients unable to form hepatic sulfate conjugates of lithocholic acid, liver toxicity can occur; fecal bile acids are increased three- to fourfold

COMMON SIDE EFFECTS
Diarrhea, elevated serum aminotransferase

SIGNIFICANT ADVERSE REACTIONS
Abdominal cramping, nausea, vomiting, anorexia, dyspepsia, flatulence, elevated serum cholesterol and HDL, and decreased white cell count

CONTRAINDICATIONS
Intrahepatic cholestasis, primary biliary cirrhosis, sclerosing cholangitis, radiopaque bile pigment stones, acute cholecystitis, gallstone pancreatitis, biliary GI fistula, and pregnancy

INTERACTIONS
Bile acid sequestering agents (cholestyramine, colestipol) and aluminum-based antacids may reduce absorption of chenodeoxycholic acid

Estrogens, oral contraceptives, clofibrate, and other lipid-lowering drugs may decrease the effectiveness of chenodeoxycholic acid by increasing biliary cholesterol secretion

NURSING CONSIDERATION

Nursing Alert
- Monitor results of serum aminotransferase determinations, which should be performed frequently during therapy. If SGPT levels rise to over three times the upper limit of normal, the drug should be discontinued. If levels increase to 1.5 to 3 times the limit, the drug should be stopped temporarily and resumed only after levels return to normal. Enzyme levels return to normal following drug discontinuation.

PATIENT EDUCATION
1. If a female patient becomes pregnant while taking the drug, supportively discuss the possibility of fetal damage. The drug is a potential teratogen and should not be used by a woman who is or is likely to become pregnant.
2. Inform patient that serum cholesterol levels are usually monitored at 4- to 6-month intervals because the drug should be discontinued if levels rise above the age-adjusted limit.
3. Instruct patient to report persistent or severe diarrhea. A temporary dosage reduction may be needed to alleviate it.
4. Inform patient that a prophylactic dosage has not been established. Stones have recurred on dosages as high as 500 mg/day; therefore, the drug is usually discontinued after stones have dissolved. Serial cholecystograms should be performed to monitor for recurrence, which occurs in approximately 50% of patients within 5 years.
5. Encourage patient to maintain low cholesterol, low carbohydrate diet following stone dissolution and to reduce weight to minimize stone recurrence.
6. Explain that the likelihood of successful therapy is greatly reduced if partial stone dissolution is not evident within 9 to 12 months. Treatment will probably be discontinued if there is no response after 15 to 18 months.

Monoctanoin
Moctanin
Monoctanoin is a semisynthetic esterified glycerol that acts as a solubilizing agent for cholesterol gallstones in the biliary tract. Treatment with monoctanoin results in complete stone dissolution in about one third of patients, especially those with single stones. Another one third of patients show reduction in stone size, while approximately one third of patients are not benefited.

MECHANISM
Acts as a solubilizing agent for cholesterol stones when perfused via the common bile duct; complete dissolution is most often achieved when a single stone is present

USE
Solubilization of radiolucent gallstones in the biliary tract following cholecystectomy, when other means of removal are inappropriate

DOSAGE
NOTE
Drug is administered as a continuous perfusion through a catheter inserted into the common bile duct or through a T-tube or nasobiliary tube.

3 mL to 5 mL per hour infused continuously for up to 10 days (average duration is 5 days); infusion solution should be maintained at body temperature (37°C)

FATE
Drug is readily hydrolyzed by pancreatic or other digestive lipases, and the resultant fatty acids are either absorbed and metabolized or excreted intact

COMMON SIDE EFFECTS
Abdominal pain or discomfort, nausea, vomiting, diarrhea, anorexia, fever

SIGNIFICANT ADVERSE REACTIONS
Indigestion, elevated serum amylase, bile shock, leukopenia, pruritus, fatigue, chills, diaphoresis, headache, allergic reactions, hypokalemia, metabolic acidosis, depression, and *rarely* acute pancreatitis, cholangiitis, and hematemesis

CONTRAINDICATIONS
Jaundice, biliary tract infection, acute pancreatitis, impaired hepatic function, recent duodenal ulcer, or jejunitis. *Cautious use* in pregnant or nursing women and in children

NURSING CONSIDERATIONS

Nursing Alerts
- Administer infusion with a positive pressure or peristaltic perfusion pump equipped with an overflow manometer to avoid complications associated with use of excessive pressure. Pressure should not exceed 15 cm H_2O.
- Monitor flow rate carefully. GI side effects usually worsen when rate is too rapid.
- Assess patient for GI side effects, particularly nausea and diarrhea. These effects must be controlled to prevent nutritional inadequacy and fluid/electrolyte imbalance.
- If GI side effects persist, consider interrupting the perfusion for 1 to 2 hours at mealtimes. Aspiration of the biliary tract may also relieve GI discomfort. Abdominal pain does not, however, appear to correlate with either dosage or perfusion rate.

1. Monitor patient for indications of ascending cholangiitis (elevated temperature, chills, severe right upper quadrant abdominal pain, jaundice). Notify physician if these occur.
2. Monitor patient for indications of leukopenia (decreased WBC, sore throat, fever, chills). Notify physician if these occur.

PATIENT EDUCATION
1. Explain to patient and family that therapy often continues for 10 or more days.
2. If treatment is to be administered at home, teach patient and family how to operate the infusion pump they will use in the home.

Ursodiol–Ursodeoxycholic Acid

Actigall

Ursodiol is a naturally occurring bile acid found in small quantities in normal human bile. The drug is used orally to dissolve radiolucent gallstones.

MECHANISM
Suppresses hepatic synthesis and secretion of cholesterol and inhibits intestinal absorption of cholesterol; ursodiol-rich bile solubilizes cholesterol by raising the concentration level at which saturation of cholesterol occurs; may also cause dispersion of cholesterol as liquid crystals in an aqueous medium; does not appear to significantly alter the secretion of bile acids or phospholipids into bile

USE
Facilitate dissolution of radiolucent, noncalcified gallbladder stones less than 20 mm in diameter in persons presenting an increased surgical risk or who decline surgery

DOSAGE
8 mg/kg/day to 10 mg/kg/day in 2 or 3 divided doses. Treatment generally requires months of therapy, and complete dissolution does not occur in all patients. Recurrence of stones within 5 years has occurred in 50% of patients

FATE
Well absorbed orally; extracted from the portal circulation by the liver, conjugated with glycine or taurine, and secreted into hepatic bile ducts; concentrated in the gallbladder and secreted into the duodenum via the cystic and common bile ducts; small amounts are found in the systemic circulation and excreted in the urine; following enterohepatic recirculation, most of a dose is eliminated in the feces

COMMON SIDE EFFECTS
Nausea, dyspepsia, metallic taste

SIGNIFICANT ADVERSE REACTIONS
Diarrhea, vomiting, abdominal pain, biliary pain, cholecystitis, stomatitis, flatulence, headache, fatigue, sleep disturbances, cough, anxiety, depression, arthralgia, myalgia, rash, pruritus, urticaria, dry skin, sweating

CONTRAINDICATIONS
Chronic liver disease, biliary obstruction, pancreatitis, acute cholecystitis, cholangiitis, bile acid allergy.

Ursodiol will not dissolve calcified cholesterol stones, radiopaque stones, or radiolucent bile pigment stones. *Cautious use* in persons with altered liver function values, in pregnant or nursing women, and in children

INTERACTIONS
Oral absorption of ursodiol may be impaired by aluminum-containing antacids, cholestyramine resin, and colestipol

Estrogens, oral contraceptives, and clofibrate may counteract the effectiveness of ursodiol by increasing the hepatic secretion of cholesterol

PATIENT EDUCATION
1. Instruct patient to report persistent or severe diarrhea. A temporary dosage reduction may be needed to alleviate it.
2. Inform patient that the drug is usually discontinued if stones have dissolved, but serial cholecystograms should be performed to monitor for recurrence, which occurs within 5 years in approximately 50% of patients.
3. Encourage patient to maintain low cholesterol, low carbohydrate diet following stone dissolution and to reduce weight to minimize stone recurrence.

Selected Bibliography
Hoffman AF: Gallstone dissolving drugs: New approach to an old disease. Drug Ther 12:57, 1982

Scherer P: New drugs of 1985 in theory and practice. Am J Nurs 86:407, 1986

Schoenfield LJ et al: Chenodiol (chenodeoxycholic acid) for dissolution of gallstones: The National Cooperative Gallstone Study. Ann Intern Med 95:257, 1981

SUMMARY. DIGESTANTS

Drug	Preparations	Usual Dosage Range
Bile Salts (Choleretics)		
Ox Bile Extract	Enteric-coated tablets: 325 mg	150 mg to 600 mg during or following each meal
Ox Bile Extract with Iron Bilron	Capsules: 150 mg, 300 mg with iron	
Hydrocholeretics		
Dehydrocholic Acid Atrocholin, Cholan-DH, Decholin	Tablets: 130 mg, 244 mg, 250 mg	250 mg to 500 mg 3 times a day after meals
Gastric Acidifiers		
Glutamic Acid Hydrochloride Acidulin	Capsules: 340 mg	1 to 2 capsules 3 times a day with meals
Pancreatic Enzymes		
Pancreatin Viokase	Tablets Powder containing different amounts of lipase, amylase, and protease	1 to 3 tablets or 0.75 g powder with meals
Pancrelipase Cotazym, Ilozyme Ku-Zyme HP, Pancrease	Tablets Capsules Powder packets containing various amounts of lipase, amylase, and protease	1 to 3 tablets or capsules, or 1 to 2 powder packets before meals or snacks
Gallstone Solubilizing Agents		
Chenodiol Chenix	Tablets: 250 mg	Initially, 250 mg twice a day for 2 weeks; increase by 250 mg/day once a week to maximally tolerated dose
Monoctanoin Moctanin	Infusion	3 mL to 5 mL/h infused continuously for up to 10 days into common bile duct
Ursodiol Actigall	Capsules: 300 mg	8 to 10 mg/kg/day in 2 or 3 divided doses

50 LAXATIVES

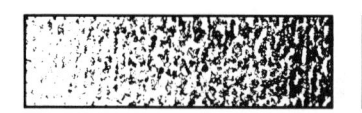

A laxative is an agent that facilitates evacuation of the bowel. The valid indications for use of such drugs are few, and laxatives are frequently misused and abused by a large number of persons suffering from constipation, a condition characterized by a reduced frequency of fecal elimination. Diagnosis of constipation is difficult because there is a tremendous variation in the "normal" frequency of bowel movements, estimated to range from as low as three per week to as high as three per day. Given this inherent variability, constipation cannot be characterized strictly in terms of bowel frequency but must be viewed in relation to previous bowel habits, presence of disease states, or to other drug therapy, diet, and other conditions.

Chronic simple constipation can frequently be relieved by proper diet, adequate fluid intake, and sufficient exercise; it does not usually require drug therapy. When indicated, laxative therapy should be short term (that is, 1 wk–2 wk) and should be discontinued once bowel regularity has returned. Prolonged use of laxative drugs should be strongly discouraged because regular use of most laxatives can lead to dependence on the drug rather than on the natural defecation reflex to achieve bowel movements. Persistent constipation is most often a result of improper diet, chronic disease states, prolonged laxative use, or a mental outlook or behavioral pattern adversely affecting bowel function. As such, drug therapy is usually ineffective and frequently harmful and should *not* be employed in lieu of determining and correcting the underlying cause of the dysfunction.

In contrast, *acute constipation* is often amenable to drug therapy, especially in those individuals who do not have a history of bowel irregularities. Certain laxative products (e.g., stimulants, saline, or osmotics) are also indicated for rapid lower bowel evacuation in preparation for radiographic or endoscopic examination of the intestinal tract or in cases of poisoning.

There are a variety of laxative products available that function by a number of different mechanisms. The choice of a laxative product is dependent on many factors, including speed and intensity of evacuation desired (e.g., chronic, mild constipation versus preradiologic intestinal flushing), presence of other disease states (e.g., cardiac impairment, anorectal disorders), or need for sodium restriction.

A classification of laxatives based upon their respective mechanisms of action is presented in Table 50-1. In general, bulk-producing agents (e.g., methylcellulose) are considered the safest and most "physiologic" type of laxative and are the preferred agents for short-term treatment of most types of mild constipation. Emollients or fecal softeners are likewise relatively safe and are widely used in conditions in which hard or dry stools might prove painful or dangerous, such as after rectal or anal surgery, or in the presence of hemorrhoids and other conditions in which straining is undesirable (e.g., heart disease, hernias).

The laxative products are discussed as a group, and are followed by a tabular listing of each product with nursing implications. It should be noted that in addition to the products reviewed here, several of the bile salts (see Chap. 49) have also been employed for the symptomatic treatment of mild, uncomplicated constipation, although their efficacy has been questioned.

LAXATIVES

Bisacodyl	Methylcellulose
Cascara sagrada	Mineral oil
Castor oil	Nondiastatic barley malt
Danthron	Phenolphthalein
Docusate calcium	Polycarbophil
Docusate potassium	Polyethylene glycol electrolyte solution
Docusate sodium	
Glycerin	Psyllium
Lactulose	Senna
Magnesium citrate	Sodium biphosphate
Magnesium hydroxide	Sodium phosphate
Magnesium sulfate	

MECHANISM
See Table 50-1.

USES
Short-term treatment of constipation
Evacuation of the lower intestinal tract in preparation for surgery or endoscopic or radiologic examination
Removal of toxic substances from the lower intestinal tract
Prevention of straining where such action is painful or hazardous (e.g., anorectal disorders, hernia, cardiac disease)
Management of constipation associated with irritable bowel syndrome (especially psyllium)

NOTE
Irritable bowel syndrome may be accompanied by diarrhea as well, in which case laxatives are inappropriate.

DOSAGE
See Table 50-2

FATE
(See Table 50-2 for specific information) Administered orally or rectally; systemic absorption is minimal in most cases; onset of action ranges from 5 to 10 minutes with many suppositories or rectal enemas, from 30 to 60 minutes with most oral products, and from 24 to 72 hours with some bulk-forming products; excreted largely unchanged in the feces, although a number of drugs may be partially metabolized upon systemic absorption and eliminated by the kidneys, often producing a colored urine

COMMON SIDE EFFECTS
(Incidence varies among different preparations) Excessive bowel activity, cramping, nausea, and unpleasant taste

SIGNIFICANT ADVERSE REACTIONS
(Not associated with all drugs and usually observed with excessive or prolonged use) Vomiting; profound diarrhea; perianal irritation; electrolyte imbalance (especially with saline/osmotic laxatives) resulting in weakness, fainting, dizziness, palpitations, and sweating; hypersensitivity reactions (especially with phenolphthalein); esophageal, intestinal, or rectal obstruction

Table 50-1
Classification of Laxatives

Bulk-Forming (e.g., Methylcellulose, Polycarbophil, Psyllium)

Cellulose derivatives that swell in intestinal fluid, stimulating peristalsis by retaining water in the stool; considered the safest and most physiologic type of laxative; each dose should be taken with sufficient water to minimize risk of intestinal or esophageal obstruction; onset of action is usually 12–24 h

Emollients/Fecal Softening (e.g., Docusate Sodium)

Anionic surfactants that increase the wetting efficiency of intestinal water, thus softening the fecal mass by facilitating mixture of aqueous and fatty substances; most useful in conditions in which straining is hazardous (e.g., heart disease, perianal disease, hypertension, hernia, rectal surgery); may require several days before an effect is seen

Lubricant (e.g., Mineral Oil)

Softens fecal matter by lubricating the intestinal mucosa, facilitating passage of the stool; may prevent absorption of fat-soluble vitamins and nutrients and delay gastric emptying; do *not* administer with meals; effects usually occur within 6–8 h

Saline/Osmotic (e.g., Magnesium Citrate, Sodium Phosphate, Polyethylene Glycolelectrolyte Solution, Lactulose)

Nonabsorbable cations (magnesium), anions (phosphate), or sugars (lactulose) that retain water in the intestinal lumen, thus mechanically stimulating peristalsis and altering stool consistency; action is rapid (0.5–2 h); should be used only for acute bowel evacuation, except for lactulose which may be administered in chronic constipation

Stimulant (e.g., Bisacodyl, Castor Oil, Phenolphthalein)

Increase intestinal propulsion by either a direct irritant effect on the mucosa or an activation of sensory nerve endings in intestinal smooth muscle; may produce excessive catharsis, leading to fluid and electrolyte disturbances; prolonged use can result in habituation and laxative dependency; onset of action is generally 6–8 h orally

Hyperosmolar (e.g., Glycerin)

Produce dehydration of exposed mucosal tissue, resulting in irritation and subsequent evacuation; laxative effect occurs within 30 min

---

(particularly with bulk laxatives); discoloration of urine or rectal muscosa, laxative dependence

CONTRAINDICATIONS

Presence of abdominal pain, nausea, vomiting, or other signs of acute appendicitis, diverticulitis, colitis, or regional enteritis; acute surgical abdomen, fecal impaction, intestinal obstruction or perforation, acute hepatitis, or late pregnancy

In addition, use of magnesium or potassium salts is contraindicated in patients with renal dysfunction, use of sodium salts is contraindicated in patients requiring sodium restriction, and use of emollients and mineral oil together is contraindicated altogether. *Cautious use* in persons with rectal bleeding, and in pregnant women or young children

> **NOTE**
> Bulk-forming laxatives should *not* be swallowed as a dry powder but should be taken in a large glass of water followed by a second glass; see Patient Education. Esophageal impaction could result from dry ingestion.

INTERACTIONS

Systemic absorption of mineral oil or danthron can be enhanced by emollient (i.e., fecal softening) laxatives

Mineral oil may impair the GI absorption of fat-soluble vitamins (A, D, E, K) or nutrients

Laxatives (particularly bulk-forming) may reduce absorption of other drugs present in the GI tract, either by chemically combining with them or by hastening their passage through the intestinal tract

Antacids, other alkaline substances, or histamine H_2 antagonists may prematurely dissolve the enteric coating on bisacodyl tablets, reducing the laxative action, and leading to gastric or duodenal stimulation

PATIENT EDUCATION

1. Stress the importance of adequate bulk and roughage (fiber) in the diet to minimize the occurrence and severity of constipation. Desirable foods include whole grain bread and cereal, raw and cooked vegetables, plums, and prunes. Adequate fluid intake is likewise important.
2. If constipation occurs only occasionally, suggest that patient include sufficient roughage in the diet, maintain adequate fluid intake, and undergo a normal exercise routine instead of relying on laxative drugs.
3. Help patient plan time of administration so that maximum effect occurs at the most convenient time (e.g., drug with a 6–8 h onset of action should be taken at bedtime for morning evacuation).
4. Instruct patient to take bulk laxatives in a large glass of water followed by a second glass of water to prevent esophageal impaction.
5. Instruct patient to notify primary health care provider immediately if rectal bleeding, severe abdominal pain, or a sudden change in bowel function occurs during therapy.
6. Explain that the cause of constipation should be ascertained and relieved; symptomatic treatment may mask an underlying disorder.
7. Inform patient that laxatives should not be used for more than 1 or 2 weeks without consulting primary health care provider. Dosage should be adjusted to provide sufficient but not excessive bowel activity, and the drug should be discontinued when bowel regularity is achieved. Dosage increases should be avoided if the product is ineffective because laxative dependence or electrolyte imbalance can develop.
8. Instruct patient to report signs of electrolyte imbalance, such as muscle cramping, weakness, or dizziness. Electrolytes should be monitored regularly during prolonged therapy.
9. Inform patient that certain laxatives (e.g., cascara, danthron, phenolphthalein, senna) may discolor urine (pink to red to yellow-brown) as well as rectal mucosa.
10. Instruct patient taking laxative product before endoscopic or radiologic examination to carefully follow instructions concerning timing of doses to achieve maximal bowel evacuation.
11. Inform parents that stimulant cathartics or laxative enemas should not be administered to children under 2 years of age.

(Text continued on page 513)

Table 50-2
Laxatives

Drug	Preparations	Usual Dosage Range	Nursing Implications
Bulk-Forming			
Methylcellulose Citrucel, Cologel	Liquid: 450 mg/5 mL Powder 2 g/tbsp	Adults: 5 mL to 20 mL *or* 1 tbsp of powder in 8 oz water 3 times/day with water Children: 1 tsp in 4 oz water 3 or 4 times a day	Used orally for constipation; also available in ophthalmic drops for relief of dry, irritated eyes and as an ocular lubricant for artificial eyes and contact lenses; oral doses should be taken with 1 or more glasses of water for each dose, and additional fluids are indicated throughout the day to prevent fecal impaction; sodium carboxymethylcellulose is available in capsule form with dioctyl sodium sulfosuccinate (Disoplex)
Nondiastatic Barley Malt Extract Maltsupex	Tablets: 750 mg Liquid Powder	*Tablets* Adults only: 4 tablets with meals and at bedtime 4 times a day with liquid *Powder/liquid* Adults: 2 tbsp twice a day for 3 to 4 days; then 1 to 2 tbsp at bedtime Children: 1 tbsp to 2 tbsp in milk 1 to 2 times a day	Useful in treating functional constipation in infants and children, as well as in adults, including those with laxative dependence; also may provide relief from itching in pruritis ani; use with caution in diabetic patients because preparations contain 14 g carbohydrates/tbsp and 0.6 g/tablet; mixes more easily with cold liquids when first stirred with a little hot water; available in combination with powdered psyllium seed as Syllamalt
Polycarbophil Calcium Fiber-Con, Mitrolan, Equalactin	Chewable tablets: (equivalent to 500 mg poly carbophil)	Adults: 2 tablets 4 times a day Children (6–12 yr): 1 tablet 1–3 times a day Children (3–6 yr): 1 tablet 1–2 times a day	A hydrophilic agent that is used for treating both diarrhea and constipation; claimed to restore a more normal moisture level and to provide bulk in the GI tract; as a laxative, retains free water in the lumen of the intestine; a full glass of water or other liquid should be taken with each dose; discontinue use after 1 wk if desired effects are not noted; also used for controlling simple diarrhea (see Chap. 51)
Psyllium Effersyllium, Konsyl, Metamucil, Serutan and other manufacturers (CAN) Karacil, Novomucilax	Powder Granules Flakes Chewable tablets containing different amounts of psyllium hemicellulose, psyllium hydrophillic muciloid, or psyllium seed husk powder	1 or 2 rounded teaspoons, *or* 1 packet of powder in a glass of liquid 1 to 3 times a day (check package instructions for individual dosage recommendations)	Natural products derived from the blond psyllium seed (*Plantago ovata*); available in several dosage forms, many containing dextrose as a dispersing agent; contact with water in GI tract produces a bland, nonirritating bulk that aids peristalsis; sodium content is negligible, except in effervescent mixes containing sodium bicarbonate; drug should be taken with adequate water to prevent esophageal, gastric, intestinal, or rectal obstruction; each dose should be followed by a second full glass of water; do not attempt to swallow dry; available in combination with barley malt extract (Syllamalt)

Continued

Table 50-2
Laxatives (continued)

Drug	Preparations	Usual Dosage Range	Nursing Implications
Emollient			
Docusate Calcium–Dioctyl Calcium Sulfosuccinate DC 240, Sulfolax, Surfak, Pro-Cal-Sof (CAN) PMS-Docusate Calcium	Capsules: 50 mg, 240 mg	Adults: 240 mg/day Children: 50 mg to 150 mg/day	Similar in action to docusate sodium (see below) but does not contain sodium, which may be hazardous in patients with hypertension, congestive heart failure, edema, impaired renal function, or in persons on sodium-restricted diets; do not use in combination with mineral oil, because drug may enhance systemic absorption of the oil; available in combination with phenolphthalein (Doxidan)
Docusate Sodium–Dioctyl Sodium Sulfosuccinate Colace, Doxinate, D-S-S, Modane Soft, and various other manufacturers (CAN) Laxagel, Regulex	Capsules: 50 mg, 60 mg, 100 mg, 240 mg, 250 mg, 300 mg Tablets: 50 mg, 100 mg Solution: 50 mg/mL Syrup: 50 mg/15 mL, 60 mg/15 mL Liquid: 150 mg/15 mL	Adults: 50 mg to 500 mg Children (6–12 yr): 40 mg–120 mg Children (3–6 yr): 20 mg–60 mg Children (under 3 yr): 10 mg–40 mg Larger doses may be given initially, then adjusted to optimal response	A surface-wetting agent that increases the wetting efficiency of intestinal water, thus facilitating the mixing of aqueous and fatty substances to soften the fecal mass for easier passage; effect on stools is apparent 1 to 3 days after first dose; does not exert a laxative action itself, but is mainly used as adjunctive treatment in constipation associated with hard, dry stools or in patients who should avoid straining (e.g., with cardiac disease, hernia, anorectal disorders); should not be used regularly by patients who must restrict sodium intake; may increase systemic absorption of mineral oil if given in combination; available in combination with casanthranol (e.g., Peri-Colace), senna concentrate (e.g., Senokot S, Senokap) phenophthalein (e.g., Correctol, Feen-a-Mint Pills, Unilax), sodium carboxymethylcellulose (e.g., Disoplex), and various other laxatives
Docusate Potassium–Dioctyl Potassium Sulfosuccinate Dialose, Diocto-K, Kasof	Capsules: 100 mg, 240 mg	100 mg to 300 mg/day with a full glass of water	*See* docusate sodium; may be used where sodium restriction is necessary; available in enema form with benzocaine and soft soap (Therevac) and in capsules combined with casanthranol (Dialose Plus)
Lubricants			
Mineral Oil Agoral Plain, Fleet Mineral Oil Enema, Kondremul Plain, Milkinol, Neo-Cultol, Zymenol	Liquid Jelly Emulsion: 50%, 55% Enema	*Oral* Adults: 5 mL to 30 mL at bedtime Children: 5 mL to 20 mL at bedtime *Rectal* Adults: 120 mL Children: 30 mL to 60 mL	Useful to maintain soft stools to avoid straining; coats fecal contents, preventing colonic absorption of water; probably not as effective or safe as emollients; may interfere with absorption of fat-soluble vitamins and nutrients, therefore administer on an empty stomach; do not use during pregnancy or with emollients; use

Continued

Table 50-2
Laxatives (continued)

Drug	Preparations	Usual Dosage Range	Nursing Implications
			of enema may avoid interference with nutrient absorption, but oil seepage from rectum can stain clothing; use *cautiously* in the very old, debilitated, or very young (under 2 yr), because danger of aspiration and possible development of lipid pneumonia is increased; emulsified preparations mask the objectionable consistency of plain oil and may be slightly more effective but tend to increase systemic absorption of oil and are significantly more expensive; avoid prolonged or excessive use; available in combination with docusate sodium (Liqui-Doss) phenolphthalein (Agoral, Kondremul with Phenolphthalein), cascara extract (Kondremul with Cascara), and magnesium hydroxide (Haley's M-O)
Saline/Osmotic			
Lactulose Cephulac, Cholac, Chronulac, Constilac, Constulose, Duphulac, Enulose (CAN) Acilac, Lactulax	Syrup: 10 g/15 mL with several other sugars	*Laxative:* 15 mL to 30 mL/day to a maximum of 60 mL/day *Portal–systemic encephalopathy* (Cephulac): 30 mL to 45 mL 3 to 4 times a day May also be given to comatose patient by means of retention enema as 300 mL in 700 mL of water or saline for acute hepatic coma; dosage is adjusted to minimize diarrhea and may be repeated every 4 to 6 h	A complex sugar that is not hydrolyzed in the GI tract, but enters the colon unchanged; there it is broken down primarily to lactic acid by colonic bacteria; this elevates the osmotic pressure, increasing stool water content and softening the fecal matter; may require 24 to 48 h to produce a bowel movement; use cautiously in pregnant or nursing women, in elderly or debilitated patients, and in diabetic patients; initial doses may produce flatulence and cramping; may be mixed with fruit juice or milk to improve palatability; reduces blood ammonia levels by 25% to 50% and is also used for prevention and treatment of portal–systemic encephalopathy, including the stages of hepatic precoma and coma; may be administered long-term for this indication, dosage is usually adjusted to produce 2 or 3 soft stools a day
Magnesium Citrate Citrate of Magnesia, Citroma, Citro-Nesia (CAN) Citro-Mag, National Laxative	Liquid	Adults: 200 mL to 250 mL (1 glass) at bedtime Children: 100 mL to 125 mL (½ glass) at bedtime	Chilling liquid improves the taste; do *not* use in patients with renal impairment; observe for signs of magnesium toxicity (thirst, drowsiness, dizziness); available in several bowel evacuation kits (Evac-Q-Kit, Evac-Q-Kwik, Tridrate Bowel Evacuant Kit)

Continued

Table 50-2
Laxatives (continued)

Drug	Preparations	Usual Dosage Range	Nursing Implications
Magnesium Hydroxide Milk of Magnesia, M.O.M.	Liquid: 78 mg/mL Concentrate: 233 mg/mL Tablets: 325 mg	Adults: 15 mL to 30 mL of regular liquid or 10 mL to 20 mL of concentrated liquid at bedtime Children: 0.5 mL/kg/dose of regular liquid	Recommended for short-term use only because accumulation of magnesium ions can result in serious toxicity (CNS or neuromuscular depression, fluid and electrolyte imbalances); tablets are less effective than liquid as a laxative; concentrated liquid (233 mg/mL) is lemon flavored to improve palatability; do *not* use in patients with renal impairment; also used as an antacid (see Chap. 48); available in emulsion form containing mineral oil (Haley's M-O)
Magnesium Sulfate Epsom salt	Granules	Adults: 10 g to 15 g in a glass of water or fruit juice Children: 5 g to 10 g in a glass of water	Administer in a flavored vehicle if necessary to mask the salty taste; effects are noted within several hours; infrequently used laxative
Polyethylene Glycol-Electrolyte Solution Colonite, CoLyte, GoLYTELY, OCL	Powder for oral solution: different amounts of electrolytes and PEG 3350.	Adults: 4 L of solution orally (240 mL every 10 min) prior to GI examination	Orally administered solution used to cleanse bowel prior to radiologic examination; contains PEG 3350, a nonabsorbable solution that acts as an osmotic agent in the intestines; electrolytes prevent any change in ion concentration following evacuation of bowel; transient bloating, nausea, and cramping may occur; patient should fast 3 to 4 h prior to ingestion of solution; first bowel movement occurs within 1 h after ingestion is complete; flavorings and other ingredients should not be added
Sodium Phosphate and Sodium Biphosphate Fleet Enema, Phospho-Soda	Solution: 1.8 g sodium phosphate and 4.8 g, sodium biphosphate per 10 mL Enema: 7 g sodium phosphate and 19 g sodium biphosphate per 118 mL	*Oral* Adults: 20 mL to 30 ml in ½ glass of water Children: 5 mL to 15 mL *Rectal* Adults: 118 mL Children: 60 mL	Indicated only for acute evacuation of the bowel (e.g., prior to rectal or bowel examinations); high sodium content (4.4 g/dose); available in packaged forms with bisacodyl tablets, suppositories, or enema (Fleet Barium Enema Prep Kits)
Stimulants **Bisacodyl** Bisco-Lax, Dacodyl, Deficol, Dulcolax, Fleet Bisacodyl, Theralax (CAN) Apo-Bisacodyl, Bisacolax, Laxit	Tablets: 5 mg Suppositories: 10 mg Enema: 10 mg/30 mL	*Oral* Adults: 10 mg–15 mg Children: 5 mg to 10 mg *Rectal (suppository)* Adults: 10 mg following each bowel movement Children: 5 mg *Rectal enema* 1 container (30 mL)	Increases peristalsis, probably by a direct effect on sensory nerve endings in colonic mucosa; used to relieve constipation and to evacuate the bowel before examination; onset of action is 6 to 10 h orally and 15 to 60 min after insertion of suppository; tablets should not be crushed or chewed, and milk or antacids should not be consumed within 1 h of the drug because they may prematurely dissolve the enteric coating

Continued

Table 50-2
Laxatives (continued)

Drug	Preparations	Usual Dosage Range	Nursing Implications
			on the tablet; rectal burning and itching may follow use of suppositories; no untoward systemic effects have been observed with either oral or rectal use; habituation can occur, with gradual loss of effectiveness
Bisacodyl Tannex Clysodrast	Powder packets: 1.5 mg bisacodyl and 2.5 g tannic acid per packet	Cleansing enema: 2.5 g in 1 L warm water Barium enema: 2.5 g to 5 g in 1 L barium suspension (maximum 4 packets in 72 h)	A nonabsorbable complex of bisacodyl and tannic acid used as a colonic evacuant; tannic acid is claimed to reduce intestinal secretions and when used with barium suspension, to improve the adherence of barium to intestinal walls; *contraindicated* in pregnant women and in children under 10 yr; tannic acid may be hepatotoxic if sufficient quantities are absorbed; use *cautiously* if multiple enemas are being administered and in elderly or debilitated patients
Cascara Sagrada	Tablets: 325 mg Aromatic fluid extract	1 to 2 tablets *or* 5 mL aromatic fluid extract at bedtime	Direct chemical irritant that increases propulsive movements in the colon; onset of action is 6 to 10 h; urine may be colored reddish to yellow brown, and rectal mucosa may become discolored; prolonged use should be avoided because habituation can result; available with phenolphthalein (Caroid tablets) or aloe (Nature's Remedy)
Castor Oil Alphamul, Emulsoil, Fleet Castor Oil, Kellogg's Castor Oil, Neoloid, Purge (CAN) Unisoil	Liquid or emulsion in several strengths	*Adults:* 15 mL to 60 mL *Children* Over 2 yr: 5 mL to 15 mL Under 2 yr: 1 mL to 5 mL (depending on strength of emulsion)	Natural product that is broken down in small intestine to glycerol and ricinoleic acid, a local irritant; stimulates intestinal activity, resulting in production of liquid stools; primarily used for prompt evacuation of bowel before radiologic examination or in cases of poisoning; onset is 2 to 6 h; do *not* use in pregnant women or in treating infestation with fat-soluble vermifuge, because systemic absorption may be increased
Danthron (CAN) Dorbane, Roydan	Tablets: 75 mg	75 mg to 150 mg with or 1 h after the evening meal	Synthetic irritant laxative that stimulates peristalsis in the large intestine; onset of action is approximately 6 to 10 h; administer in the evening for morning evacuation; do *not* use in nursing mothers (drug is excreted in breast milk); pink to brown discoloration of urine may occur; prolonged use may discolor rectal mucosa and cause liver damage; infrequently used

Continued

Table 50-2
Laxatives (continued)

Drug	Preparations	Usual Dosage Range	Nursing Implications
Phenolphthalein Alophen, Espotabs, Ex-Lax, Feen-A-Mint, Modane, and other manufacturers (CAN) Fructines-Vichy	Tablets: 60 mg, 90 mg, 130 mg Chewable tablets: 60 mg, 80 mg, 90 mg, 97.2 mg Wafers: 64.8 mg Liquid: 60 mg/5 mL, 65 mg/15 mL	60 mg to 194 mg at bedtime	Stimulant laxative similar to bisacodyl in most respects; onset of action is 6 to 8 h; may color urine red to yellow brown; effects may be prolonged for several days owing to enterohepatic circulation; allergic skin reactions can occur—drug should be discontinued at first sign of rash; some preparations are fruit or chocolate flavored—keep out of reach of children, because serious toxicity can result if large quantities are consumed; available in combination with docusate sodium (e.g., Colax, Correctol, Disolan), docusate calcium (Doxidan), mineral oil (e.g., Agoral, Kondremul w/Phenolphthalein), and Cascara (e.g., Caroid Laxative Tablets)
Senna Concentrate Genna, Gentlax B, Senexon, Senokot, Senna-Gen, Senolax, X-Prep	Tablets: 187 mg, 217 mg Granules: 326 mg/tsp Suppositories: 652 mg Syrup: 218 mg/5 mL	*Constipation* Adults: 2 tablets, 1 tsp granules, or 1 suppository at bedtime Children: ½ adult dose *Preradiographic bowel evacuation* 1 container liquid (75 mL) taken between 2 PM and 4 PM on day before examination	Natural product prepared from species of *Cassia*, having a similar but more potent laxative action than cascara; concentrate may provide a more uniform effect than other preparations, with less colic; onset of action is usually 6 to 12 h, but may require 24 h in some cases; may impart a yellow-brown to red color to the urine or feces
Senna Equivalent Black-Draught	Tablets: 600 mg Granules: 1.65 g/0.5 tsp	Adults: 2 tablets or ¼ tsp to ½ tsp granules with water	
Sennosides A&B—Calcium Salts Gentle Nature, Nytilax (CAN) Glysennid	Tablets: 12 mg, 20 mg	Adults: 1 to 2 tablets at bedtime Children: 1 tablet at bedtime	
Hyperosmolar			
Glycerin Fleet Babylax, Sani-Supp	Suppositories Liquid (4 mL/applicator)	1 suppository or 4 mL of liquid inserted high into the rectum	Produces dehydration of exposed mucosal tissue, leading to irritation and subsequent evacuation; laxative effect occurs within 15 to 30 min

Selected Bibliography

Aman RA: Treating the patient, not the constipation. Am J Nurs 80:1634, 1980

Binder HJ: Pharmacology of laxatives. Annu Rev Pharmacol Toxicol 17:355, 1977

Devroede G: Constipation: Mechanisms and management. In Sleisenger MH, Fordtran JS (eds): Gastrointestinal Disease, 2nd ed, p 288. Philadelphia, WB Saunders, 1983

Ewe K: Physiological basis of laxative action. Pharmacology 20(1):2, 1980

Gever LN: Lactulose: A crucial element in treating hepatic encephalopathy. Nursing '82 12(8):76, 1982

Thompson WG: Laxatives: Clinical pharmacology and rational use. Drugs 19(1):49, 1980

Wizwer PI: Management of constipation. A pratical approach. NARD J 106:77, 1984

ANTIDIARRHEAL DRUGS

Diarrhea, the passage of excessive, watery stools, is generally viewed as a *symptom* of an underlying pathologic condition rather than as a disease entity in itself. Distinction must be made, however, between acute and chronic diarrhea, because significant differences exist between the two conditions with respect to etiology, potential danger to the patient, and preferred treatment. *Acute diarrhea*, characterized by sudden onset of frequent, watery stools, often accompanied by fever, pain, vomiting, and weakness, may have several causes, including viral or bacterial infection, food or drug poisoning, or radiation exposure. The major danger of severe acute diarrhea is that it can quickly lead to dehydration and electrolyte imbalances, especially in infants and children. Fortunately, most episodes of acute diarrhea are self-limiting, that is, once the offending organisms, foods, or medications are removed, the symptoms soon subside.

Chronic diarrhea likewise may be related to any of a number of causative factors, such as secondary disease states (e.g., ulcerative colitis, diverticulitis, irritable colon, hyperthyroidism, gastric carcinoma), surgery (such as subtotal gastrectomy, vagotomy, ileal resection), or presence of excessive amounts of hormones, bile acids, or other substances in the GI tract. Chronic diarrhea may also be of psychogenic origin, a most difficult type to treat.

Whatever the type of diarrhea, every effort should be made to determine and remove the underlying cause of the distress. For example, diarrhea resulting from the presence of an infectious organism may best be treated by use of an appropriate antibiotic. Likewise, drug-induced diarrhea can often be corrected by simply discontinuing the offending drug. Successful treatment of secondary disease states associated with diarrhea usually reduces or eliminates the accompanying episodes of diarrhea. In those instances in which the cause of the diarrhea is not readily apparent or cannot be successfully eliminated by other means, use of antidiarrheal drugs for symptomatic relief should be considered on a short-term basis. In no instance, however, should the use of antidiarrheal agents be substituted for attempts to eradicate the cause of the condition, nor should these drugs be administered over prolonged periods except in unusual circumstances, because many of the more effective antidiarrheals have the potential to elicit a wide range of side effects in addition to becoming habituating.

The most effective antidiarrheal medications are the opiates (such as paregoric) and related opiate derivatives (e.g., difenoxin, diphenoxylate, loperamide): systemically acting agents that reduce intestinal hypermotility and slow peristalsis. Anticholinergics have also been used to reduce GI motility by impairing parasympathetic nerve stimulation to intestinal smooth muscle. Although these drugs are possibly effective in some forms of diarrhea, the dosages required to slow peristalsis effectively are quite high, the consequence being a wide range of unacceptable side effects. Anticholinergic drugs are reviewed in detail in Chapter 11 and are not discussed here.

Several locally acting drugs have been employed for the symptomatic relief of diarrhea, frequently in combination form. Among the pharmacologic products used in this way are adsorbents (kaolin, pectin, attapulgite), astringents (zinc phenolsulfonate), antacids (aluminum hydroxide, bismuth salts), and bacterial cultures (*Lactobacillus acidophilus*). These substances are relatively safe for normal use, but there is insufficient clinical evidence to establish their effectiveness for the intended purpose. Nevertheless, they are available without prescription and are widely used by the general public. Every product carries a warning against use for longer than 2 days, in the presence of high fever or in children under 3 years of age except upon physicians' orders.

Treatment of most types of diarrhea, with the possible exception of severe acute diarrhea in infants and children, is usually best carried out conservatively. One of the locally acting drug combinations (such as kaolin and pectin) is usually satisfactory for the symptomatic management of mild, episodic diarrhea. More intense acute diarrhea may require addition of one of the opiate derivatives plus the ingestion of large amounts of fluids or possibly electrolyte solutions (e.g., Lytren, Pedialyte—see Table 75-1) to prevent dehydration and electrolyte depletion. Persistent or recurrent diarrhea generally signifies an underlying pathologic condition that should be identified and corrected. Routine use of antidiarrheal drugs for extended periods should be confined to certain conditions (such as chronic inflammatory bowel disease, GI carcinoma, intestinal surgery, radiation therapy), undertaken only following careful examination, and closely supervised by a physician. Continuous self-use of antidiarrheal drug formulations by persons with mild, intermittent, or episodic diarrhea should be strongly discouraged, because the drug may not only elicit untoward reactions but can mask the symptoms of a more severe underlying disease.

The potent systemically active antidiarrheal drugs are reviewed individually, followed by a brief, general discussion of the principal locally acting antidiarrheal agents and a listing of commonly used antidiarrheal combination products.

SYSTEMIC ANTIDIARRHEALS

The systemic antidiarrheals comprise the opiates, principally camphorated tincture of opium (paregoric), anticholinergics, which are discussed in Chapter 11, and three opiate (meperidine) derivatives, difenoxin, diphenoxylate, and loperamide, which are claimed to have a lower incidence of CNS effects and less addiction liability than other opiates.

Difenoxin HCl with Atropine Sulfate
Motofen

Diphenoxylate HCl with Atropine Sulfate
Lomotil and other manufacturers

Difenoxin and diphenoxylate are structural analogs of meperidine with a rather low risk of dependence at normal doses, although typical opiate effects (such as euphoria) may occur with high doses. Prolonged ingestion can lead to habituation. These drugs are combined with a subtherapeutic amount of atropine to discourage deliberate abuse; excessive doses lead to a variety of atropine-induced adverse effects that are distinctly unpleasant (see Significant Adverse Reactions).

MECHANISM
Slow intestinal motility, probably by a direct inhibitory action on circular and longitudinal GI smooth muscle; may exert an antisecretory action as well; prolong intestinal transit time, increase viscosity and density of intestinal contents, and reduce daily fecal volume; little or no analgesic effect

USE
Adjunctive treatment of diarrhea

DOSAGE
Difenoxin
2 mg initially, then 1 mg after each loose stool or every 3 to 4 hours as needed; maximum dose is 8 mg/24 h
Diphenoxylate
Adults: 5 mg four times a day; reduce when symptoms are controlled
Children: Initially 0.3 mg to 0.4 mg/kg/day in divided doses. Average daily dosages:
2–5 yr: 4 mL (2 mg) three times a day
5–8 yr: 4 mL (2 mg) four times a day
8–12 yr: 4 mL (2 mg) five times a day

FATE
Drugs are well absorbed when taken orally; onset of action is 30 to 60 minutes. Diphenoxylate is quickly and extensively metabolized to diphenoxylic acid (difenoxin), the major active circulating metabolite. The plasma half-life of the parent drug is 2 to 3 hours, and the elimination half-life of difenoxin is 12 to 15 hours; difenoxin is metabolized to an inactive metabolite and both the parent drug and its metabolites are excreted in the feces (approximately 50%) and the urine

COMMON SIDE EFFECTS
Dry mouth, drowsiness, nausea, dizziness, headache

SIGNIFICANT ADVERSE REACTIONS
(Usually with large doses) Abdominal discomfort, vomiting, anorexia, restlessness, depression, malaise, numbness of extremities, pruritus, urticaria, angioneurotic edema, paralytic ileus, toxic megacolon, and respiratory depression

Atropine side effects are more common in children and include flushing, diminished secretions, hyperthermia, tachycardia, urinary retention, hypotonia, miosis, nystagmus, and blurred vision

CONTRAINDICATIONS
Diarrhea associated with organisms that can penetrate the intestinal mucosa, pseudomembranous colitis, obstructive jaundice, and in children under 2 years old. *Cautious use* in patients with cirrhosis or other advanced liver disease, ulcerative colitis, or glaucoma, in addiction-prone persons, and in pregnant or nursing women

INTERACTIONS
(See also Anticholinergics, Chap. 11)

Diphenoxylate and difenoxin may potentiate the depressant effects of barbiturates, alcohol, narcotics and other tranquilizers or sedatives
Concurrent use with MAO inhibitors may precipitate a hypertensive crisis

NURSING CONSIDERATIONS

Nursing Alerts
- Monitor patient, especially a young child, for signs of atropine overdosage (see atropine side effects under Significant Adverse Reactions). Notify primary health care provider if they occur because dosage should be reduced or drug should be discontinued.
- If overdosage occurs, observe patient for potential respiratory depression for at least 48 hours after last dose has been administered because respiratory depression may not occur for some time after overdosage. Naloxone (Narcan) is the drug of choice for reversing respiratory depression.
- Assess patient's abdomen frequently. Abdominal distention or pain is a possible indication of developing toxic megacolon, which is caused by delayed intestinal transit. The drug should be discontinued if these signs occur.

1. Assist to evaluate drug effects. Administration for acute diarrhea should be discontinued if clinical improvement is not noted within 48 hours.
2. With diphenoxylate (*not* difenoxin), follow proper procedures for handling a schedule V substance (see Chap. 8, Table 8-1).

PATIENT EDUCATION
1. Instruct patient taking liquid preparation to use only the calibrated dropper provided with the bottle.
2. Warn patient not to exceed recommended dosage because incidence of adverse effects greatly increase at high doses, and the danger of habituation is enhanced.
3. Instruct patient to avoid alcohol or other CNS depressants because an additive depressant effect can result.

Loperamide
Imodium, Imodium A-D

A structural analog of meperidine with a reduced risk of dependence at recommend doses, loperamide is similar to diphenoxylate and difenoxin in action but does not contain atropine, so anticholinergic side effects are eliminated. It is claimed to have less abuse potential than diphenoxylate, and opiatelike effects have not occurred with prolonged treatment. A liquid dosage form (Imodium A-D) is available over the counter.

MECHANISM
Slows intestinal motility and inhibits peristalsis by a direct depressant effect on intestinal smooth muscle; minimal action on the CNS at recommended dosage levels

USES
Control of acute nonspecific diarrhea and chronic diarrhea associated with inflammatory bowel disease
Reduction of volume of discharge from ileostomies

DOSAGE
Adults
Acute diarrhea: initially 4 mg, followed by 2 mg after each loose stool; maximum dose 16 mg/day
Chronic diarrhea: as above for acute diarrhea, then reduce to an

effective maintenance dose; usual dosage range 4 mg to 8 mg/day

Children (2–12 yr)
Acute diarrhea: 1 to 2 mg 2 to 3 times a day

FATE
Approximately 40% absorbed when taken orally; onset is 30 to 60 minutes, and duration is 4 to 5 hours; elimination half-life is about 10 to 12 hours; metabolized by the liver and excreted mainly in the feces as both unchanged drug and metabolites with small amounts in the urine

COMMON SIDE EFFECTS
(With prolonged therapy) Abdominal discomfort, drowsiness

SIGNIFICANT ADVERSE REACTIONS
Abdominal distention, constipation, dizziness, nausea, vomiting, skin rash, and CNS depression

CONTRAINDICATIONS
Patients in whom constipation should be avoided (e.g., severe cardiac disease, intestinal obstruction). *Cautious use* in persons with ulcerative colitis or hepatic dysfunction, in pregnant or nursing women, and in young children

INTERACTIONS
Loperamide may enhance the sedative effects of other CNS depressants (e.g., barbiturates, alcohol, narcotics, hypnotics)

NURSING CONSIDERATIONS
See difenoxin/diphenoxylate. In addition:
1. If clinical benefit is not obtained at a dosage of 16 mg/day for 10 days, question further administration because it is unlikely to be effective. However, drug may be continued as a supplement to diet or specific treatment (e.g., antibiotics).

PATIENT EDUCATION
See difenoxin/diphenoxylate.

Opium Tincture, Camphorated
Paregoric

Camphorated opium tincture contains 2 mg of morphine equivalent per 5 mL together with other ingredients (e.g., camphor, anise oil, benzoic acid) in 45% alcohol. Its antidiarrheal effectiveness is due to its morphine content. Opium tincture, camphorated, should not be confused with *opium tincture, deodorized,* which contains 25 times the morphine equivalency and should not be used for treating diarrhea (refer to the discussion of narcotics in Chap. 18).

MECHANISM
Decreases GI motility and peristalsis, reduces digestive secretions, and increases intestinal smooth muscle tone, thereby slowing passage of intestinal contents

USES
Treatment of acute diarrhea
Relief of abdominal cramping
Treatment of neonatal withdrawal syndrome (tremulousness, irritability, excessive crying, decreased sleeping time)

DOSAGE
Diarrhea; Cramping
Adults: 5 mL to 10 mL (2 mg–4 mg morphine equivalent) after loose bowel movements, up to 4 times a day
Children: 0.25 mL to 0.5 mL/kg up to 4 times a day
Neonatal Withdrawal Syndrome
Usually 4 to 6 drops every 3 to 6 hours; adjust dosage to control withdrawal symptoms; once stabilized, reduce dosage gradually over several weeks

COMMON SIDE EFFECTS
Drowsiness, lightheadedness

SIGNIFICANT ADVERSE REACTIONS
Allergic reactions (e.g., rash, urticaria, pruritus), vomiting, dizziness, sweating, constipation, and habituation

In addition, because the drug is a narcotic, large doses or prolonged administration can result in symptoms of narcotic overdosage (see Chap. 18 for other possible untoward reactions).

CONTRAINDICATIONS
Diarrhea resulting from poisoning. *Cautious use* in the presence of hepatic disease, prostatic hypertrophy, bronchial asthma and in persons with a history of drug dependence

INTERACTIONS
Paregoric can enhance the depressive effects of alcohol, barbiturates, tranquilizers, and other CNS depressants

NURSING CONSIDERATIONS
1. Monitor vital signs and intake and output during treatment of neonatal withdrawal syndrome.
2. During treatment of neonatal withdrawal syndrome, increase infant's intake of fluids and calories in proportion to severity of withdrawal symptoms (vomiting, diarrhea, sweating, increased motor activity).
3. Follow proper procedure for handling a Schedule III drug (see Chap. 8). Although small amounts of paregoric or powdered opium equivalent are contained in several OTC antidiarrheal preparations (see Table 51-1) that are either Schedule III or Schedule V products, paregoric alone is available only by prescription.

PATIENT EDUCATION
1. Suggest that drug be taken with water to facilitate passage through the GI tract.
2. Stress the importance of adhering closely to recommended dosage. Prolonged use or excessive doses may lead to habituation and dependence.
3. Discuss the need for adequate fluid replacement during periods of diarrhea to prevent dehydration and electrolyte imbalance.
4. Instruct patient to discontinue drug as soon as symptoms of diarrhea are controlled. Primary health care provider should be notified if diarrhea persists longer than 48 hours or if fever or abdominal pain develops.

LOCALLY ACTING ANTIDIARRHEALS

A large number of compounds exhibiting diverse pharmacologic effects have been employed in the treatment of diarrhea. Except for those drugs previously discussed in this chapter, most frequently used antidiarrheal agents are locally acting drugs; that is, they are primarily nonabsorbable chemicals that act within the lumen of the GI tract by a variety of mechanisms. The most commonly employed classes of locally acting antidiarrheal drugs are the adsorbents, antiseptics, and bacterial cultures, although astringents, antacids, bulk laxatives, digestive enzymes, and electrolytes have all been tried in the treatment of diarrhea. These locally acting agents, while essentially safe in recommended doses, have not been conclusively demonstrated to be clinically effective. Nevertheless, they are widely available without prescription, usually as combination products containing several different locally acting ingredients, and frequently including small amounts of paregoric or other opium equivalents. Because they are readily available and relatively safe, they are most often the initial agents tried in cases of occasional, uncomplicated diarrhea, and in many instances they provide sufficient relief. The warning that appears on every product should be heeded, however, and these agents should not be used for longer than 2 to 3 days, nor should they be used when high fever is present. Further, children under 3 years should be given these drugs only by prescription from a physician.

A general review of the pharmacology of the most frequently used locally acting antidiarrheals is presented here, followed by a listing of the ingredients of the commonly employed combination products in Table 51-1.

Table 51-1
Antidiarrheal Combination Products

Trade Name	Dosage Form	Opiate Derivative	Adsorbents/ Astringents	Anticholinergics	Other Ingredients
Amogel PG	Suspension	Powdered opium	Kaolin, pectin	Hyoscyamine, atropine, scopolamine	
Bacid	Capsules				*Lactobacillus acidophilus,* sodium carboxymethylcellulose
Corrective Mixture with Paregoric	Suspension	Paregoric	Bismuth subsalicylate, zinc sulfocarbolate, phenyl salicylate		
Devrom	Chewable tablets		Bismuth subgallate		
Diabismul	Tablets	Powdered opium	Bismuth subcarbonate, calcium carbonate		
Diabismul	Suspension	Opium	Kaolin, pectin		
Dia-Quel	Suspension	Opium tincture	Pectin	Homatropine	
Diar Aid	Tablets		Activated attapulgite, pectin		
Diasorb	Tablets Liquid		Activated attapulgite		
Donnagel	Suspension		Kaolin, pectin	Hyoscyamine, atropine, scopolamine	
Donnagel-PG	Suspension	Powdered opium	Kaolin, pectin	Hyoscyamine, atropine, scopolamine	
Infantol Pink	Liquid	Opium	Pectin, bismuth subsalicylate, zinc phenosulfonate		Extract Irish moss
Kaodene with Codeine	Suspension	Codeine phosphate	Kaolin, pectin, bismuth subsalicylate, sodium carboxy-methylcellulose		
Kaodene with Paregoric	Suspension	Anhydrous morphine	Kaolin, pectin, bismuth subsalicylate, sodium carboxymethylcellulose		
Kaodene Nonnarcotic	Suspension		Kaolin, pectin, bismuth subsalicylate, sodium carboxymethylcellulose		

Continued

Table 51-1
Antidiarrheal Combination Products (continued)

Trade Name	Dosage Form	Opiate Derivative	Adsorbents/Astringents	Anticholinergics	Other Ingredients
Kaopectate	Suspension Tablets		Kaolin, pectin Attapulgite		
Kao-tin	Suspension		Kaolin, pectin		
Kapectolin	Suspension		Kaolin, pectin		
Kapectolin Gel with Belladonna	Suspension		Kaolin, pectin	Hyoscyamine, atropine, scopolamine	
Kapectolin with Paregoric	Liquid	Paregoric	Kaolin, pectin		
Kapectolin PG	Suspension	Powdered opium	Kaolin, pectin	Hyoscyamine, atropine, scopolamine	
KBP/O	Capsules	Powdered opium	Kaolin, pectin, bismuth subcarbonate		
K-C	Suspension		Kaolin, pectin, bismuth subcarbonate		
K-P	Suspension		Kaolin, pectin		
K-Pek	Suspension		Kaolin, pectin		
Lactinex	Granules Tablets				*Lactobacillus bulgaricus, Lactobacillus acidophilus*
Mitrolan	Chewable tablets				Calcium polycarbophil
Parepectolin	Suspension	Opium	Kaolin, pectin		
PectoKay	Liquid		Kaolin, pectin		
Pepto-Bismol	Suspension Chewable tablets		Bismuth subsalicylate		
Quiagel	Suspension		Kaolin, pectin	Hyoscyamine, atropine, scopolamine	
Quiagel PG	Suspension	Powdered opium	Kaolin, pectin	Hyoscyamine, atropine, scopolamine	
Rheaban	Liquid Tablets		Colloidal activated attapulgite		
St. Joseph Antidiarrheal	Liquid		Activated attapulgite		

Adsorbents

The adsorbents are most frequently used for the treatment of mild diarrhea. Commercial products usually contain two or more adsorbents, frequently combined with small amounts of opium derivatives or anticholinergics, or both. The extent to which the adsorbents contribute to the overall antidiarrheal efficacy of such mixtures is a subject of controversy, however. These compounds have the ability to bind to their particle surface toxins, bacteria, and other irritants that may be present in the GI tract; in addition, some adsorbents (e.g., pectin) may also exert a soothing demulcent action on the mucosal surface of the irritated bowel. The adsorptive activity of these compounds is not selective for irritants or toxins, however, and they may also adsorb other drugs found in the intestinal tract at the same time. Thus, adsorbents can potentially interfere with the normal GI absorption of many drugs, and this possibility should be noted whenever an adsorbent substance is given to a patient receiving medications for other conditions.

The most frequently encountered adsorbents in commercial preparations are kaolin, pectin, activated attapulgite, and certain bismuth salts (e.g., subgallate, subsalicylate). Cholestyramine, an anion-exchange resin discussed in Chapter 33, has also been employed in some cases of severe diarrhea. It is thought to complex with bacterial toxins in the GI tract. Anion-exchange resins are not approved as antidiarrheal drugs, and their use in this manner is strictly experimental.

Antiseptics/Astringents

Drugs such as zinc phenolsulfonate, phenyl salicylate, and zinc sulfocarbolate are included in several proprietary antidiarrheal mixtures because of their astringent and reputed antiseptic action. It is doubtful whether inclusion of these substances significantly improves the antidiarrheal activity of the mixture.

Bacterial Cultures

Cultures of viable strains of *Lactobacillus acidophilus* and *Lactobacillus bulgaricus* have been used in the treatment of diarrhea resulting from a disruption of normal intestinal microorganism balance. Seeding the bowel with bacterial cultures is believed to reestablish the normal intestinal flora and suppress the growth of undesired microorganisms, thus improving those GI disturbances, including diarrhea, resulting from an altered intestinal flora. Although possibly effective in those cases of diarrhea induced by treatment with antibiotics that can upset the normal bacterial population of the GI tract, lactobacillus preparations are not recommended for most episodes of diarrhea, inasmuch as they are somewhat more costly than other locally acting drugs, and there is no conclusive evidence that modification of intestinal flora has a beneficial effect in acute diarrhea.

Other

Among the other types of locally acting products that have been used in the treatment of diarrhea are the bulk-producing laxatives or hydrophilic colloids (e.g., carboxymethylcellulose, polycarbophil, psyllium seed). The rationale behind this apparent paradoxical action is that these substances have the ability to absorb excess fecal fluid as they swell in the intestinal tract, thus aiding in the production of formed stools. Their suitability for most forms of diarrhea, however, remains speculative.

An important facet of the adjunctive treatment of persistent or severe, acute diarrhea is replenishment of fluid and electrolyte loss, especially in infants and young children. The parenteral fluids and electrolyte solutions available for this purpose are reviewed in Chapter 75.

Selected Bibliography

Anderson BJ: Tubefeeding: Is diarrhea inevitable? Am J Nurs 86:710F, 1986

Awouters CJ, Niemegeers E, Janssen PAJ: Pharmacology of antidiarrheal drugs. Annu Rev Pharmacol Toxicol 23:279, 1983

Black RE: The prophylaxis and therapy of secretory diarrhea. Med Clin North Am 66(3):621, 1982

Feldman M: Travelers' diarrhea. Am J Med Sci 288(3):136, 1984

Heel RC, Brogden RN, Speight TM, Avery GS: Loperamide: A review of its pharmacological properties and therapeutic efficacy in diarrhea. Drugs 15:33, 1978

Longe RL: Antidiarrheal and other gastrointestinal products. In: Handbook of Non-Prescription Drugs. Washington, DC, American Pharmaceutical Association, 1987, p 59

Satterwhite TK, DuPont HL: Infectious diarrhea in office practice. Med Clin North Am 67(1):203, 1983

Weiss BD: Travelers' diarrhea: Update 1983. Am Fam Physician 27:193, 1983

SUMMARY. ANTIDIARRHEAL DRUGS

Drug	Preparations	Usual Dosage Range
Difenoxin HCl with Atropine Sulfate Motofen	Tablets: 1 mg with 0.025 mg atropine sulfate	2 mg initially, then 1 mg every 3–4 h up to 8 mg/24 h
Diphenoxylate HCl with Atropine Sulfate Diphenatol, Lomotil, and other manufacturers	Tablets: 2.5 mg with 0.025 mg atropine sulfate Liquid: 2.5 mg/5 mL with 0.025 mg atropine/5 mL	*Adults:* 5 mg 4 times/day *Children:* 0.3 mg–0.4 mg/kg/day in divided doses 2–5 yr—4 mL (2 mg) 3 times/day 5–8 yr—4 mL (2 mg) 4 times/day 8–12 yr—4 mL (2 mg) 5 times/day
Loperamide Imodium, Imodium A-D	Capsules: 2 mg Liquid: 1 mg/5 mL	*Adults and children over 12 yr:* Initially 4 mg, followed by 2 mg after each loose stool to a maximum of 16 mg/day (usual maintenance dose 4 mg–8 mg a day) *Children:* (2–12yr): 1 mg–2 mg 2–3 times/day
Opium Tincture, Camphorated Paregoric	Liquid: 2 mg morphine equivalent per 5 mL	*Adults:* 5 mL–10 mL (2 mg–4 mg morphine equivalent) after each loose stool to a maximum of 4 times/day *Children:* 0.25 mL–0.5 mL/kg up to 4 times/day *Neonatal withdrawal syndrome:* 4–6 drops every 3–6 h; reduce gradually over several weeks
Locally Acting Antidiarrheals	See Table 51-1	

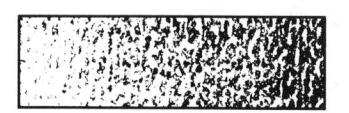

52 EMETICS AND ANTIEMETICS

Drugs having the ability to enhance vomiting reflex mechanisms, either through a peripheral (i.e., local gastric mucosal irritation) or central (i.e., stimulation of the medullary chemoreceptor trigger zone) action are termed *emetics*. They are used primarily to induce vomiting in cases of drug overdosage or poisoning with other types of chemicals or toxins.

Antiemetics are agents that reduce the hyperreactive vomiting reflex, largely by a central action, at the level of the vomiting center or chemoreceptor trigger zone (CTZ), or on the vestibular apparatus in the inner ear. The mechanisms that may be involved in eliciting the vomiting reflex are reviewed in Chapter 47.

EMETICS

Vomiting is an efficient means of removing unabsorbed drugs or toxins from the stomach; thus, emetics are frequently used in instances of drug overdosage or accidental ingestion of toxic chemicals or other substances. Prompt administration is essential in order to remove as much of the toxin as possible before significant amounts are absorbed into the system. Emetics generally should not be used, however, in certain types of poisoning—for example, with corrosive or caustic agents or petroleum products—because the expulsion of these substances by vomiting can severely irritate or damage the epithelium of the upper digestive tract. Likewise, patients who are comatose or semiconscious or who demonstrate hyperactive or convulsive activity should not receive emetics. Whenever possible, adjunctive drugs and other measures (e.g., materials for gastric lavage or suction, oxygen, specific antidotes to the common poisons) should be available and employed when necessary. Drug overdosage or chemical poisoning is a potentially serious problem, and everyone, especially parents, should have ready access to a poisoning chart giving explicit instructions for handling poisoning emergencies. The phone number of the closest poison prevention center should be posted, because speed of recognition and treatment is very often a critical factor for successful recovery.

Apomorphine
A synthetic derivative of morphine with a potent stimulant action on the CTZ, apomorphine also can, like other narcotics, depress several areas of the CNS, including the respiratory and vasomotor centers. However, its analgesic effects are not nearly equal to those of most other opiates. The degree of CNS depression noted with apomorphine is dose-dependent.

MECHANISM
Stimulates the CTZ, thus increasing activation of the medullary vomiting center and resulting in emesis; exhibits dopamine receptor–stimulating action, and may therefore reduce secretion of prolactin and alter central motor regulatory function (e.g., reduce akinesia or rigidity)

USE
Induction of vomiting

DOSAGE
Note: Drug is available as a *soluble* tablet (6 mg) that is dissolved in an appropriate vehicle and administered only once.
Adults: 5 mg SC (usual range 2 mg–10 mg)
Children: 0.05 mg/kg to 0.1 mg/kg SC

FATE
Onset of emesis is usually within 5 to 15 minutes; metabolized by the liver and excreted chiefly in the urine

COMMON SIDE EFFECTS
Sedation, nausea

SIGNIFICANT ADVERSE REACTIONS
Respiratory depression, orthostatic hypotension, dizziness, weakness, salivation, restlessness, tremors, and euphoria

Overdosage may cause violent vomiting, irregular respiration, cardiac depression, and vascular collapse

CONTRAINDICATIONS
Impending shock, poisoning with corrosives or petroleum products, overdosage with opiates, barbiturates, alcohol, or other CNS depressants, presence of seizure activity. *Cautious use* in persons with cardiac decompensation, epilepsy, following overdosage with digitalis drugs or convulsants, and in children and elderly or debilitated persons

INTERACTIONS
Apomorphine may enhance the effects of levodopa or bromocriptine

NURSING CONSIDERATIONS

Nursing Alerts
- Question use of apomorphine in cases of overdosage with CNS-depressant drugs (e.g., narcotics, hypnotics, alcohol) because it may lead to profound depression, coma, and possibly death.
- Have naloxone available for apomorphine overdose and atropine for cardiac depression as well as equipment for gastric lavage, suction, and respiratory assistance.
- Monitor vital signs for at least several hours after apomorphine injection because respiratory depression may develop slowly.

1. Dissolve drug, which is formulated as a soluble tablet, in an appropriate parenteral vehicle before administering. Protect solution from light and air.
2. Administer 200 mL to 300 mL of water or other liquid (smaller volumes in children) before injection to elicit a more efficient vomiting reaction.
3. Position patient on side to prevent aspiration of vomitus.
4. Discard solutions that are discolored or contain a precipitate.

Ipecac Syrup
An alkaloidal mixture containing principally emetine and cephaline, ipecac exerts its emetic effect by a direct irritant action on

the GI tract as well as a central action on the CTZ. Ipecac syrup is available in quantities up to 30 mL without prescription; larger sizes require a prescription.

> WARNING
> Ipecac must not be confused with *ipecac fluid extract*, which is 14 times more potent and can be fatal if given in the same dosage as the syrup

MECHANISM
Elicits emesis by a direct irritative action on the gastric mucosa and an activation of the CTZ; possesses an expectorant action, possibly by increasing bronchial secretions

USE
Induction of vomiting, primarily to remove unabsorbed drugs and poisons

DOSAGE
Adults and children over 1 yr: 15 mL syrup followed by one or two glasses of water; may be repeated in 20 to 30 minutes if vomiting has not occurred

Children under 1 yr: 5 mL to 10 mL followed by one half to one glass of water

FATE
Vomiting occurs within 15 to 30 minutes, and effects may persist for another 20 to 30 minutes

COMMON SIDE EFFECTS
Diarrhea, mild CNS depression

SIGNIFICANT ADVERSE REACTIONS
(Usually with large doses) Bloody diarrhea, myopathy, arrhythmias, cardiotoxicity, shock, and convulsions

CONTRAINDICATIONS
In semiconscious, unconscious or convulsing patients; shock; poisoning with corrosive or caustic substances, strychnine, petroleum distillates, or volatile oils. *Cautious use* in pregnant or nursing women

INTERACTIONS
Activated charcoal may absorb ipecac syrup, nullifying its emetic effect

NURSING CONSIDERATION

Nursing Alert
- Carefully distinguish ipecac syrup from ipecac fluid extract. The latter is 14 times stronger and can be fatal if ingested in the same amounts as the syrup.

PATIENT EDUCATION
1. Instruct patient not to take drug with milk or carbonated beverages, as they may reduce its effectiveness.
2. Advise patient to drink 200 mL to 300 mL of water after taking drug.
3. Instruct patient to contact a physician or emergency room immediately if vomiting does not occur within 20 minutes after the second dose because cardiotoxicity may occur from the amount of the alkaloid emetine that is absorbed.

ANTIEMETICS

The mechanisms involved in the vomiting reflex can involve several pathways and are outlined in detail in Chapter 47. To briefly review, the vomiting center in the medulla may be stimulated by the central trigger zone (CTZ), also in the medulla, by the vestibular nuclei via the labyrinthine apparatus in the inner ear, and also directly by GI irritation. Dopamine appears to be the major neurotransmitter in the CTZ, whereas acetylcholine is believed to be the neurotransmitter involved with impulse transmission along the labyrinthine pathway to the vomiting center.

A variety of drugs have been successfully employed for the prophylaxis and treatment of vomiting of diverse etiology. Although vomiting may have many causes (for example, drug or chemical poisoning, motion sickness, radiation exposure, bacterial or viral infection, pregnancy, endocrine disorders, neurological or psychic disturbances), most successful antiemetic drugs act mainly by inhibition of the CTZ or by depression of vestibular apparatus sensitivity in the inner ear. The major groups of drugs used to control nausea and vomiting are the phenothiazines, anticholinergics, antihistamines, and sedatives, along with a group of miscellaneous drugs, most of which also exhibit a central mechanism of action. These agents are listed in Table 52-1, with brief descriptions of their pharmacologic ef-

Table 52-1
Antiemetic Drugs

Phenothiazines (e.g., Chlorpromazine, Perphenazine, Prochlorperazine, Promethazine, Thiethylperazine)

Potent antiemetic drugs acting by inhibition of CTZ via a dopaminergic blocking action; primarily effective for drug-induced emesis and nausea and vomiting associated with surgery, anesthesia, radiation, carcinoma, and severe infections; little usefulness in motion sickness, because drugs do not affect the vestibular apparatus; possibility of numerous side effects (some serious); thus recommended for short-term use only; most drugs also used as antipsychotic agents (except thiethylperazine; see Chap. 22)

Antihistamines (e.g., Buclizine, Cyclizine, Dimenhydrinate, Meclizine)

Act by decreasing sensitivity of vestibular apparatus of inner ear, thus most effective in treating nausea and vomiting of motion sickness, Meniere's disease, or labyrinthitis; all elicit varying degrees of drowsiness and may have significant anticholinergic activity (see Chap. 14)

Anticholinergics (e.g., Scopolamine)

Depress the vestibular apparatus and inhibit cholinergic activation of the vomiting center; very effective in preventing motion sickness; high incidence of side effects limits oral usefulness, but scopolamine is also available as Transderm-Scop in the form of a circular, flat disk that adheres to the skin behind the ear and provides for a continuous steady rate of drug release over 3 days (5 $\mu g/h$) with minimal side effects (see Chap. 11)

Sedatives (e.g., Barbiturates, Hydroxyzine)

Decrease anxiety and possibly reduce excess stimulation of the vomiting center; largely ineffective and associated with a high incidence of drowsiness (see Chap. 20)

Miscellaneous (e.g., Benzquinamide, Diphenidol, Dronabinol, Nabilone, Trimethobenzamide)

Predominantly centrally acting antiemetics possessing several mechanisms of action; individual drugs are discussed in this chapter

fects. In addition, a variety of other drugs, predominantly local acting, have been used in the treatment of nausea and vomiting: antacids, adsorbents, antiflatulents, demulcents, and local anesthetics. The efficacy of most of these regionally acting antiemetic drugs is subject to considerable debate; nevertheless, the placebo effect of such medications cannot always be discounted, and their occasional use to settle an "upset stomach" is probably not harmful in the otherwise healthy patient.

Many clinically useful antiemetic drugs are considered elsewhere in this text. Thus, the phenothiazines, which are potent dopamine-blocking agents and therefore very effective against drug-induced emesis at the level of the CTZ, are discussed in Chapter 22. Antihistamines, which are primarily useful in preventing the nausea and vomiting of motion sickness, because they apparently reduce vestibular activation of the vomiting center, are reviewed in Chapter 14. Scopolamine, a highly effective antinauseant for motion sickness, is now frequently used as a transdermal patch, which provides a prolonged action (i.e., 3 days) and produces for fewer side effects than oral administration of the drug. Scopolamine is considered in Chapter 11.

A number of other drugs exhibiting an antiemetic action do not fit any of the above categories and therefore are reviewed individually in this chapter. One of these is metoclopramide, a drug with several GI indications, including antineoplastic drug–induced nausea and vomiting. In addition, dronabinol (the psychoactive principle in marijuana) and nabilone (a synthetic cannabinoid) have been demonstrated to be effective in controlling refractive cases of nausea and vomiting accompanying cancer chemotherapy; they are presented here as well.

Benzquinamide
Emete-Con

MECHANISM
Not established; believed to depress the CTZ and reduce activation of the vomiting center; possesses antihistaminic, anticholinergic, antiserotonin, and sedative action

USE
Prevention and treatment of nausea and vomiting associated with anesthesia or surgery

DOSAGE
IM: initially 50 mg at least 15 minutes before emergence from anesthesia; may be repeated in 1 hour, then at 3- to 4-hour intervals as needed
IV: 25 mg as a single dose administered at a rate of 1 mL/min; subsequent doses should be given IM

FATE
Rapidly absorbed from IM sites; onset of action within 15 minutes; duration is 2 to 4 hours; approximately one half of blood level is protein-bound; metabolized by the liver (elimination half-life is 45 min) and excreted in urine and feces, largely as metabolites

COMMON SIDE EFFECTS
Drowsiness, dry mouth

SIGNIFICANT ADVERSE REACTIONS
Autonomic: flushing, shivering, sweating, salivation, increased temperature, blurred vision, hiccups
CNS: restlessness, headache, excitement, fatigue, insomnia, weakness, tremors
Cardiovascular: hypotension, dizziness, atrial fibrillation, premature ventricular contractions (Sudden *hyper*tension may follow IV injection.)
GI: anorexia, nausea
Other: allergic reactions (rash, chills, fever, urticaria)

CONTRAINDICATIONS
Pregnant women and young children, IV injection in cardiac patients. *Cautious use* in elderly or debilitated patients and in persons with arrhythmias

INTERACTIONS
Markedly increased blood pressure may result from use of benzquinamide with other pressor agents
Benzquinamide may enhance the effects of other CNS depressants

NURSING CONSIDERATIONS

Nursing Alerts
- Seek clarification if prescribed IV for patient with cardiovascular disease because the danger of sudden hypertension or arrhythmias is high.
- Consider possible causes underlying nausea and vomiting because the drug may mask signs of overdosage with other drugs or prevent accurate diagnosis of conditions associated with nausea and vomiting (e.g., intestinal obstruction, carcinoma, brain tumors).

1. Expect to administer drug at least 15 minutes before anticipated awakening from anesthesia when it is used to control postoperative nausea and vomiting.
2. When giving IM, inject deeply into large muscle.
3. Reconstitute powder for injection with 2.2 mL sterile water for injection. This yields 2 mL of a solution containing 25 mg drug/mL that is stable for 14 days at room temperature.

Diphenidol
Vontrol

MECHANISM
Depresses excitability of vestibular apparatus and CTZ; exhibits relatively weak antihistaminic, anticholinergic, and CNS depressant activity

USES
Control of nausea and vomiting due to surgery, vestibular disturbances, infectious diseases, neoplasms, and radiation therapy
Treatment of vertigo due to Meniere's disease, labyrinthitis, or middle or inner ear surgery

DOSAGE
Adults: 25 mg to 50 mg every 4 hours orally
Children: 0.4 mg/lb (0.88 mg/kg) every 4 hours orally; maximum 2.5 mg/lb/day

FATE
Rapidly absorbed orally, onset of action is 30 to 60 minutes; metabolized in the liver and excreted largely by the kidney

COMMON SIDE EFFECTS
Drowsiness, indigestion, and dry mouth

SIGNIFICANT ADVERSE REACTIONS

> **WARNING**
> May cause confusion, disorientation, and hallucinations; use only in closely supervised persons and carefully weigh benefits versus risk

Malaise, depression, insomnia, dizziness, headache, skin rash, slight hypotension, and mild jaundice

CONTRAINDICATIONS

Anuria, IV administration in patients with sinus tachycardia, infants under 6 months or 50 lb, and pregnancy. *Cautious use* in patients with glaucoma, prostatic hypertrophy, obstructive lesions of the GI or urinary tracts, or hepatic disease, and in nursing mothers

INTERACTIONS

Additive CNS-depressant effects can occur in combination with other sedative or hypnotic drugs

NURSING CONSIDERATIONS

Nursing Alerts

- Administer only to hospitalized patient or one under close medical supervision because drug has caused auditory and visual hallucinations, disorientation, and confusion. The drug should be discontinued if such reactions occur (incidence about 0.5%; onset usually within 3 days after starting therapy; symptoms subside within several days after discontinuation of therapy).
- Consider possible causes underlying nausea and vomiting because drug may mask signs of drug overdosage or underlying pathology.

1. Provide frequent mouth care if patient is unable to take fluids for relief of dry mouth.

PATIENT EDUCATION

1. Warn patient that drowsiness can occur and may interfere with performance of tasks.

Dronabinol
Marinol
Nabilone
Cesamet

Dronabinol is delta-9-tetrahydrocannabinol (THC), the principal psychoactive substance found in *Cannabis sativa* or marijuana. *Nabilone* is a synthetic cannabinoid. These drugs are effective antiemetics, especially in controlling vomiting due to cancer chemotherapy, but their use should be reserved for those patients not helped by conventional antiemetic therapy, as they are capable of causing profound CNS effects. Cannabinoid administration has been associated with extreme mood changes (euphoria, anxiety, depression, panic, paranoia), altered states of reality, impaired memory, distorted perception, and hallucinations. In addition, tachycardia is noted frequently, and orthostatic hypotension and fainting have been reported. These drugs are highly addicting and are Schedule II controlled substances (see Chap. 8).

MECHANISM

Not completely established; may depress the vomiting mechanism in the brainstem; other nonrelated effects include increased heart rate, decreased blood pressure (mainly orthostatic), reduced body temperature, and profound CNS changes (see above)

USES

Treatment of nausea and vomiting due to cancer chemotherapy in patients who have not responded to more conventional antiemetic therapy

DOSAGE

Dronabinol

Initially, 5 mg/m^2 of body surface 1 to 3 hours prior to chemotherapy, then every 2 to 4 hours thereafter to a maximum of 6 doses/day; increase in 2.5-mg/m^2 increments, as needed, to a maximum of 15 mg/m^2

Nabilone

Initially, 1 mg to 2 mg twice a day, 1 to 3 hours before the antineoplastic drug is given; maximum dose is 6 mg/day

FATE

Oral absorption is adequate, although there is extensive first-pass hepatic metabolism, especially with dronabinol; peak plasma concentrations occur within 2 to 3 hours; within 72 hours, approximately one half of an oral dose is recovered in the feces, biliary excretion being the major route of elimination; smaller amounts are excreted in the urine; prolonged use may result in drug accumulation to toxic amounts

COMMON SIDE EFFECTS

Drowsiness, elation, giddiness, anxiety, dizziness, impaired thinking ability, decreased coordination, weakness, depression, memory impairment, ataxia. In addition, vertigo and dry mouth are common with nabilone

SIGNIFICANT ADVERSE REACTIONS

Paresthesias, visual distortions, confusion, disorientation, paranoia, tinnitus, nightmares, speech difficulty, flushing, sweating, tachycardia, hypotension, fainting, diarrhea, and muscle pain

CONTRAINDICATIONS

Treatment of nausea and vomiting due to causes other than cancer chemotherapy and in pregnant or nursing women. *Cautious use* in patients with hypertension, heart disease, depression, schizophrenia, or mania and in patients receiving other psychoactive drugs

INTERACTIONS

Enhanced CNS effects may occur with combined use of cannabinoids and alcohol, sedatives, hypnotics, or other psychotomimetic substances

NURSING CONSIDERATIONS

Nursing Alerts

- Ensure that patient will remain under close supervision of a responsible adult while using drug (inpatient therapy is recommended).
- Assess patient's mental and emotional status frequently. Cannabinoids induce some change in virtually all patients.
- If disturbing psychiatric symptoms occur, place patient in quiet environment and provide supportive measures, including reassurance. Such reactions, which occur more

> commonly with higher dosages, disappear spontaneously (within 24 hours with dronabinol; within 72 hours with nabilone) without specific therapy.
> - Monitor blood pressure and cardiac status of patient with hypertension or heart disease because hypotension, usually orthostatic, and tachycardia frequently occur.
> - Implement interventions to prevent injury resulting from CNS and systemic effects (see introductory section, Common Side Effects, and Significant Adverse Reactions) until reactions to drug are evident and thereafter as indicated.

1. Explore patient's feelings about taking a drug related to marijuana.
2. If psychotomimesis occurs, help patient explore his or her reactions to the experience. The patient may reject further use of cannabinoids.
3. With nabilone, institute interventions for dry mouth (see **Plan of Nursing Care** 4 in Chap. 14).
4. Use nonpharmacological nursing interventions for nausea and vomiting to augment the efficacy of antiemetic drugs used during cancer chemotherapy.
5. Follow procedures for administration of Schedule II substances (see Chap. 8).

PATIENT EDUCATION

1. Carefully prepare patient for the kinds of CNS reactions that may occur.
2. Caution patient not to drive or perform other potentially hazardous tasks because CNS functions are typically altered, and orthostatic hypotension may occur.
3. Warn patient that additive CNS depression occurs when cannabinoids are used in conjunction with other drugs that depress the CNS (see Interactions).
4. Inform patient that use with other substances that induce psychotomimesis (e.g., mixed opiate agonist–antagonists) may increase the likelihood of psychotic reactions.
5. Inform patient that conjunctival injection and increased heart rate are expected side effects. Dry mouth also occurs with nabilone.
6. If orthostatic hypotension occurs, teach patient control measures (see **Plan of Nursing Care** 8 in Chap. 31).

Metoclopramide

Maxolon, Clopra, Octamide, Reclomide, Reglan
(CAN) Emex, Maxeran

Metoclopramide is a smooth-muscle stimulant that acts largely on the upper GI tract. It increases gastric contractions and peristalsis of the duodenum and jejunum but relaxes the pyloric sphincter and duodenal bulb, thus accelerating gastric emptying and upper intestinal transit. Metoclopramide has little if any effect on colonic or gallbladder motility or on intestinal, biliary, or pancreatic secretions. It is used either orally or IV for a number of indications as listed below under Uses.

MECHANISM
Stimulates upper GI motility and decreases normal inhibitory tone, probably by blocking dopamine receptors and sensitizing tissues to the action of acetylcholine; action is not dependent on intact vagal innervation and can be reversed by anticholinergic drugs

USES
Symptomatic treatment of acute or chronic diabetic gastroparesis (gastric stasis). Symptoms of delayed gastric emptying, such as nausea, vomiting, anorexia, and abdominal fullness are progressively relieved over several weeks
Treatment of gastroesophageal reflux (short-term [i.e., 4–12 wk], course of therapy in patients who do not respond to conventional therapy)
Prevention of nausea and vomiting associated with cancer chemotherapy
Facilitation of small bowel intubation in patients in whom the tube does not pass the pylorus by conventional measures
Stimulation of gastric emptying and intestinal transit of barium where delayed emptying interferes with radiologic examination
Investigational uses include facilitation of lactation and symptomatic treatment of gastric ulcers, anorexia nervosa, and nausea and vomiting due to pregnancy or a variety of other causes

DOSAGE
Diabetic Gastroparesis
10 mg orally 30 minutes before each meal and at bedtime for 2 to 8 weeks; severe symptoms may necessitate IM or IV administration
Gastroesophageal Reflux
10 mg to 15 mg orally up to four times/day 30 minutes before meals and at bedtime *or* 20 mg as a single dose prior to the provoking situation
Chemotherapy-induced Emesis
Initially, 1 mg/kg to 2 mg/kg by slow infusion at least 30 minutes before beginning cancer chemotherapy; dose may be repeated every 2 hours for two doses, then every 3 hours for three doses; the higher dosage should be used when highly emetogenic antineoplastic drugs such as cisplatin or dacarbazine are used.
Small-bowel Intubation
Adults: 10 mg by slow IV injection (1–2 min)
Children 6 years to 14 years: 2.5 mg to 5 mg as above
Children under 6 years: 0.1 mg/kg as above

FATE
Onset of action is 1 to 2 minutes IV, 10 to 15 minutes IM, and 30 to 60 minutes orally; effects persist for 1 to 2 hours; protein binding is minimal; drug is primarily excreted in the urine (80% in 24 h) as both unchanged drug or metabolites; elimination half-life is 3 to 6 hours

COMMON SIDE EFFECTS
Drowsiness, fatigue, restlessness, nausea, diarrhea

SIGNIFICANT ADVERSE REACTIONS
CNS: extrapyramidal reactions, akathisia, dizziness, dystonia, anxiety, insomnia, headache, depression
Other: hypertension, tachycardia, myoclonus

CONTRAINDICATIONS
GI obstruction, perforation or hemorrhage, pheochromocytoma, and epilepsy. *Cautious use* in the presence of depression, diabetes, galactorrhea, or gynecomastia and in pregnant women or nursing mothers

INTERACTIONS
The action of metoclopramide can be antagonized by anticholinergics and narcotic analgesics
Metoclopramide may impair absorption of drugs from the stomach (e.g., digitalis glycosides, cimetidine) and increase ab-

sorption of drugs from the small intestine (e.g., acetaminophen, ethanol, tetracyclines, levodopa)

Increased sedation may be observed when metoclopramide is given with alcohol, barbiturates, narcotics, or other sedatives and hypnotics

Metoclopramide may alter insulin requirements by influencing the timing of food delivery to the intestines

NURSING CONSIDERATIONS

Nursing Alerts
- Ensure that baseline data are obtained for weight, vital signs, state of hydration, and for a diabetic patient, serum glucose before long-term therapy is initiated.
- Monitor patient for possible sodium retention and hypokalemia, particularly if congestive heart failure or cirrhosis is present.
- Be alert for development of extrapyramidal reactions, especially in children, young adults, or the elderly or when high dosages are used. Symptoms (e.g., restlessness, facial grimacing, involuntary movements), which occur both early and late in therapy, may take months to regress. If symptoms appear, notify the physician, discontinue the drug, and administer anticholinergic or antiparkinsonian drugs, as ordered, to control symptoms.
- Implement appropriate interventions to protect patient from injury because the drowsiness and dizziness that may occur following administration can last for several hours.

1. When giving IV push, inject slowly (1–2 min) to minimize restlessness and anxiety, which are often intense if injection is rapid. IV doses greater than 10 mg should be diluted and infused over 15 minutes.
2. During IV infusion, cover solution to protect it from light.
3. Note that, when used to facilitate small bowel intubation, the drug is usually given only when the small bowel tube has not passed the pylorus within 10 minutes with conventional maneuvers.

PATIENT EDUCATION
1. Warn patient to avoid driving or engaging in any other activity requiring alertness until drug effects are known because drowsiness is the most common side effect.

Phosphorated Carbohydrate Solution
Calm-X, Emetrol, Naus-A-Way, Nausetrol

These products are hyperosmolar solutions of different carbohydrates (e.g., sucrose, dextrose, levulose) with phosphoric acid. The phosphorated carbohydrate solutions are locally acting antiemetics available without prescription.

MECHANISM
Not established; probably exert a direct action on the wall of the GI tract, reducing smooth-muscle contraction

USE
Symptomatic relief of nausea and vomiting

DOSAGE
Acute vomiting (may be taken at 15-minute intervals until vomiting ceases)
Adults: 15 mL to 30 mL
Children: 5 mL to 10 mL
Regurgitation in infants: 5 mL to 10 mL, 10 to 15 minutes before each feeding
Morning sickness: 15 mL to 30 mL on arising and every 3 hours as needed
Motion sickness: 15 mL as needed

SIGNIFICANT ADVERSE REACTIONS
Diarrhea and abdominal pain with large doses

CONTRAINDICATIONS
Diabetes, hereditary fructose intolerance

PATIENT EDUCATION
1. Inform patient that drug is quite safe when taken as directed, is virtually free of side effects, and will not mask symptoms of underlying pathology.
2. Instruct patient not to dilute drug or ingest fluids immediately before or for at least 15 minutes after administration.
3. Advise patient to consult primary health care provider if symptoms are not relieved or recur following drug treatment.

Thiethylperazine
Torecan

A phenothiazine derivative used exclusively as an antiemetic–antivertigo agent, thiethylperazine is claimed to have less tranquilizing action than other phenothiazines.

MECHANISM
Not definitively established; probably exerts a direct depressant action on both the CTZ and vomiting center

USE
Symptomatic relief of nausea and vomiting

DOSAGE
Oral, rectal, IM: 10 mg to 30 mg/day in divided doses

FATE
Onset of action is 30 to 60 minutes with oral or rectal administration and 15 to 30 minutes following IM injection; metabolized in the liver and excreted both in the urine and feces

COMMON SIDE EFFECTS
Drowsiness

SIGNIFICANT ADVERSE REACTIONS
Headache, dizziness, blurred vision, restlessness, fever, altered taste perception, orthostatic hypotension, and cholestatic jaundice

See also Phenothiazines, Chapter 22, for other possible adverse reactions.

CONTRAINDICATIONS
Severe CNS depression, comatose states, IV administration, pregnancy, and in children under 12 years of age. *Cautious use* in patients with renal or hepatic disease, in nursing mothers, and following intracardiac or intracranial surgery

NURSING CONSIDERATION

Nursing Alert
- When giving IM, administer deeply into large muscle mass of recumbent patient. Keep patient in bed for at least 1 hour following injection to minimize orthostatic hypotension.

PATIENT EDUCATION
1. Urge caution in driving or performing hazardous tasks because drug can cause drowsiness, dizziness, and blurred vision.
2. Teach patient how to recognize and report extrapyramidal reactions (eye movements, difficulty speaking, unusual body movements, gait disturbances). If they should occur, dosage should be reduced or drug discontinued.

Trimethobenzamide
Tigan and other manufacturers

MECHANISM
Not established; may directly depress the CTZ and interfere with vestibular activation of the CTZ or the vomiting center; does not appear to block *direct* activation of the vomiting center; possesses weak antihistamine activity

USE
Symptomatic control of nausea and vomiting (combined with other antiemetics if vomiting is severe)

DOSAGE
Oral
Adults: 250 mg three or four times a day
Children: 100 mg to 200 mg three or four times a day
Rectal
Adults: 200 mg three or four times a day
Children: 100 mg to 200 mg three or four times a day
IM
Adults *only*: 200 mg three or four times a day

FATE
Onset of action following oral or rectal administration is 15 to 45 minutes, with duration of 3 to 4 hours; following IM injection, onset is 15 minutes and duration is 2 to 3 hours; metabolized in liver and excreted principally in the urine

SIGNIFICANT ADVERSE REACTIONS
Hypersensitivity reactions, hypotension (especially with IM use), blurred vision, depression, diarrhea, dizziness, drowsiness, jaundice, muscle cramping, and blood dyscrasias

In addition, during acute fever, gastroenteritis, dehydration, or electrolyte imbalance, drug has produced CNS reactions such as opisthotonos (tetanic spasm of back muscles), convulsions, extrapyramidal symptoms (rigidity, akathesia, tremor), and coma.

Following IM injection, redness, irritation, stinging, swelling, or burning at injection site

CONTRAINDICATIONS
Parenteral use in children; rectal administration in newborns, premature infants, or persons hypersensitive to benzocaine or other local anesthetics. *Cautious use* during acute febrile illnesses, in pregnant or nursing women, elderly or debilitated patients, and in persons receiving other centrally acting drugs.

INTERACTIONS
Additive depressant effects can occur with other CNS-depressant drugs (e.g., narcotics, alcohol, barbiturates)
Extrapyramidal reactions, convulsions, and other CNS disturbances may be enhanced if trimethobenzamide is given together with phenothiazines or barbiturates

NURSING CONSIDERATIONS

Nursing Alerts
- Observe patient for signs of CNS toxicity (e.g., disorientation, lethargy, tremors), particularly if patient is receiving other centrally acting drugs (e.g., phenothiazines, barbiturates, anticholinergics). Drug should be discontinued if signs occur.
- If signs of extrapyramidal reactions appear, ensure that they are carefully evaluated. They can be confused with symptoms of certain CNS disorders that may be responsible for the vomiting, such as encephalopathy or Reye's syndrome.
- Observe patient for abrupt onset of vomiting, confusion, lethargy, or irrational behavior, possible signs of Reye's syndrome (see Significant Adverse Reactions for salicylates, Chapter 19). Immediate medical attention is imperative if such symptoms occur. Although Reye's syndrome has not been *definitely* linked to trimethobenzamide and other antiemetic drugs, it has been associated with their use during febrile periods.
- Consider possible causes of nausea and vomiting because antiemetic drugs can mask symptoms of a more serious underlying disorder or impair diagnosis of a pathologic condition (e.g., appendicitis).

1. To minimize irritation and pain with IM injection, inject deeply into upper outer quadrant of gluteal region, and avoid escape of the solution along the injection route.
2. Monitor blood pressure following parenteral administration because hypotension can occur.
3. Do *not* administer IM in children of any age and do not use rectal suppositories in premature or full-term newborns.

PATIENT EDUCATION
1. Warn patient to use caution in performing hazardous tasks (driving, operating machinery) because drug may induce drowsiness, dizziness, and loss of orientation.
2. Instruct patient to report development of rash, itching, or other signs of hypersensitivity. Drug should be discontinued if they occur.

Selected Bibliography

Albibi R, McCallum RW: Metoclopramide: Pharmacology and clinical application. Ann Intern Med 98:86, 1983
Barbezat GO: The vomiting patient: The rational approach. Drugs 22:246, 1981
DiGregorio GJ, Froncillo RJ: Antiemetics. Am Fam Physician 26(1):200, 1982
Fiori JJ, Gralla RJ: Pharmacologic treatment of chemotherapy-induced nausea and vomiting. Cancer Invest 2(5):351, 1984
Frytak S, Moertel CG: Management of nausea and vomiting in the cancer patient. JAMA 245:393, 1981

Hanson SJ, McCallum RW: The diagnosis and treatment of nausea and vomiting. Prac Gastroenterol 9(3):22, 1985

Oderda GM, Korberly BH, Sohn CA: Emetic and antiemetic products. In: Handbook of Nonprescription Drugs. 8th ed, Washington, DC, American Pharmaceutical Association, 1987, p 99

Schulze-Delrieu R: Drug therapy: Metoclopramide. N Engl J Med 305:28, 1981

Wyman JB: The vomiting patient. Am Fam Physician 21:139, 1980

SUMMARY. EMETICS AND ANTIEMETICS

Drug	Preparations	Usual Dosage Range
Emetics		
Apomorphine	Soluble tablets: 6 mg	Adults: 5 mg SC (range 2 mg–10 mg) Children: 0.05 mg/kg–0.1 mg/kg *Do not repeat*
Ipecac Syrup	Syrup, containing 1½% or 2% alcohol	Adults: 15 mL followed by 200 mL–300 mL water Children (under 1 yr): 5 mL–10 mL followed by 20 mL water
Antiemetics		
Benzquinamide (Emete-Con)	Injection: 50 mg/vial	IM: initially 50 mg; repeat in 1 h, then at 3–4-h intervals as needed *IV:* 25 mg at a rate of 1 mL/min; do *not* readminister IV
Diphenidol Vontrol	Tablets: 25 mg	Adults: 25 mg–50 mg every 4 h Children: 0.4 mg/lb every 4 h
Dronabinol Marinol	Capsules: 2.5 mg, 5 mg, 10 mg	Initially, 5 mg/m² every 2–4 h (maximum 6 doses/day); increase in 2.5-mg/m² increments as needed
Nabilone Cesamet	Capsules: 1 mg	Initially, 1 mg–2 mg twice a day; maximum dose 6 mg/day
Metoclopramide Reglan and other manufacturers	Tablets: 5 mg, 10 mg Syrup: 5 mg/5 mL Injection: 5 mg/mL	*Oral* 10 mg–15 mg up to 4 times a day *IV injection* Adults: 10 mg Children: 2.5 mg–5 mg Infants: 0.1 mg/kg *IV infusion* Chemotherapy-induced emesis: 1 mg–2 mg/kg 30 min before chemotherapy; repeat every 2–3 h
Phosphorated Carbohydrate Solution Emetrol, Naus-A-Way, Nausetrol	Solution	Adults: 15 mL–30 mL Children: 5 mL–10 mL; repeat at 15-min intervals until vomiting ceases
Thiethylperazine Torecan	Tablets: 10 mg Suppositories: 10 mg Injection: 5 mg/mL	10 mg–30 mg/day in divided doses, orally, rectally, or IM
Trimethobenzamide Tigan and other manufacturers	Capsules: 100 mg, 250 mg Suppositories: 200 mg Pediatric suppositories: 100 mg Injection: 100 mg/mL	*Oral* Adults: 250 mg 3 or 4 times/day Children: 100 mg–200 mg 3 or 4 times/day *Rectal* Adults: 200 mg 3 or 4 times/day Children: 100 mg–200 mg 3 or 4 times/day *IM* Adults *only* 200 mg 3 or 4 times/day

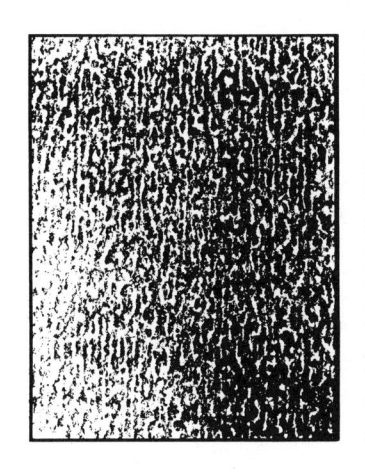

VII Drugs Acting on Respiratory Function

53 RESPIRATORY PHYSIOLOGY: A REVIEW

Normal metabolism requires the continual supply of oxygen (O_2) and removal of carbon dioxide (CO_2). The respiratory system functions in concert with the cardiovascular system to supply all body tissues with O_2 for cellular oxidative metabolism and to remove CO_2, a major metabolic waste product.

The respiratory system also plays a critical role in the regulation of acid–base balance, adjusting its activities rapidly to maintain a constant pH of the internal environment.

Respiration, which may be broadly defined as the exchange of gases (O_2 and CO_2) between a living organism and its external environment, consists of five interrelated phases that operate continuously:

- *Pulmonary ventilation:* the periodic flow of air into and out of the lungs
- *Pulmonary exchange of gases:* the diffusion of O_2 from the alveoli into the pulmonary capillaries and the diffusion of CO_2 out of the blood into the alveoli
- *Transport of gases:* the transport of O_2 by the blood from the lungs for distribution to all body tissues and the return of CO_2 from the tissues to the lungs for expiration
- *Blood–tissue exchange of gases:* the exchange of gases at the tissue level, with O_2 diffusing from the blood into the tissue cells and CO_2 diffusing from the cells into the blood
- *Cellular respiration:* the cellular utilization of O_2 for oxidative metabolism with the production of CO_2

ANATOMY/HISTOLOGY OVERVIEW

The respiratory system can be divided into two major functional divisions: the conducting division and the respiratory division.

CONDUCTING DIVISION

The components of the *conducting division* serve primarily as air conduits to the gas-exchanging areas of the lungs. During its passage through the upper segments of the conducting division, the air is filtered, warmed, and humidified. Components of the conducting division are the nose, pharynx, larynx, trachea, bronchi, bronchioles, and terminal bronchioles.

RESPIRATORY DIVISION

The respiratory bronchioles, alveolar ducts, alveolar sacs, and alveoli form the respiratory division of the lungs wherein the oxygen-rich, water-saturated air is exposed to the blood for gaseous exchange.

The Respiratory Tree

During *inspiration* the air passes through the nose (or mouth), pharynx, and larynx before entering the trachea. The trachea is structurally characterized by the presence of 16 to 20 C-shaped rings of hyaline cartilage (completed posteriorly by smooth muscle and connective tissue), which support the trachea and keep it patent. The tissue lining the trachea is pseudostratified ciliated epithelium with goblet cells. The trachea terminates in the thorax by dividing into two primary bronchi that pass to the roots of the lungs. The right bronchus is shorter, wider, and more vertical than the left and is therefore more likely to retain inhaled foreign particles.

Within the lungs, the primary bronchi undergo successive branching to form a treelike arrangement of smaller bronchi and bronchioles, often called the *bronchial tree.* The successive branching within the bronchial tree results in the formation of successively narrower tubes that collectively offer a greater total cross-sectional area of the lumina than the parent tubes.

The following histologic modifications occur with progressive branching:

1. The rings of cartilage are replaced by irregular plates of cartilage that gradually become smaller and finally disappear in the bronchioles.
2. As the amount of cartilage decreases the amount of smooth muscle progressively increases. The smooth muscle layer is crucial in determining the airway resistance because it governs the caliber of the bronchioles (which no longer have cartilage rings to maintain tubular patency).
3. The pseudostratified ciliated epithelium loses first its goblet cells and then its cilia, eventually thinning out to simple cuboidal epithelium in the terminal bronchioles.

Arising from the terminal bronchioles are the first components of the respiratory division—the *respiratory bronchioles*—whose free terminations open into *alveolar ducts.* The alveolar ducts communicate with spaces called *alveolar sacs,* which in turn open into a number of pocketlike expansions, the *alveoli.*

Histologically, the smooth muscle prominent in the latter segments of the conducting division is replaced by elastic connective tissue within the respiratory division.

The respiratory epithelium loses its cilia and thins out to a simple squamous configuration, thus allowing gaseous exchange to occur. Increasing vascularity and a greater cross-sectional surface area further promote efficient exchange of gases. It has been estimated that human lungs contain approximately 300 million alveoli and provide a total surface area of 70 m^2 for gaseous exchange.

The Lungs

All the components of the respiratory tract beyond the primary bronchi are contained within the lungs. The lungs are cone-shaped, paired structures located in the thoracic cavity, surrounded by a cagelike framework composed of the sternum, costal cartilage, ribs, and vertebrae. The muscular, dome-shaped diaphragm serves as the floor of the thoracic cage.

Blood vessels, lymphatics, nerves, and the bronchi enter the lungs at the *hilus* and form the root of the lung. The *parietal pleura,* which lines the thoracic cavity, and the *visceral pleura,* which covers the lung surface, are continuous serous membranes that reflect upon each other at the root of each lung. The potential space between these two membranes (the *pleural cavity*) contains a thin film of lubricating fluid that minimizes friction during respiratory movements.

The right lung contains three lobes and the left lung has two lobes, each of which is supplied by a *secondary* (or lobar) *bronchus.* Each lung is further subdivided into *bronchopulmonary segments* supplied by *tertiary* (or segmental) *bronchi.*

Each bronchopulmonary segment contains smaller anatomical units called *lobules,* supplied by a terminal bronchiole, arteriole, venule, and lymphatic vessel.

BLOOD SUPPLY

The pulmonary artery and its branches carry blood from the right ventricle of the heart to the respiratory tissue of the lung for oxygenation and removal of CO_2. *Venules,* arising from the vast network of pulmonary capillaries that surround the alveoli, collect oxygenated blood, which is then returned to the left atrium of the heart by the *pulmonary veins.*

Oxygenated blood reaches the visceral pleura and other portions of the lung through the *bronchial arteries* and their branches. Some *bronchial veins* empty into the superior vena cava through the azygos system, while others drain into the pulmonary veins.

In contrast to the systemic circulation, the pulmonary circulation is a low-pressure, low-resistance circuit.

NERVE SUPPLY

The bronchial tree is innervated by fibers from both divisions of the autonomic nervous system. Activation of parasympathetic (vagal) nerve fibers causes contraction of respiratory smooth muscle, whereas sympathetic stimulation brings about relaxation.

Autonomic nerves also supply pulmonary and bronchial blood vessels.

RESPIRATORY DEFENSE MECHANISMS

Large particulate matter inhaled through the *nares* (nostrils) is filtered by the coarse hairs lining the nasal vestibule. A blanket of mucus (secreted by goblet cells and mucous glands in the upper respiratory tract) traps dust and fine particulate matter. The mucus and entrapped materials are swept toward the mouth by ciliary movements. The cough reflex provides a more forceful mechanism for the expulsion of secretions and particulate matter from the respiratory tract.

Alveolar macrophages ("dust cells") provide a major defense against bacterial invasion of the lungs. These unique phagocytic cells migrate freely over the alveolar surface, engulfing and lysing bacteria and other particulate matter.

PULMONARY VENTILATION

Pulmonary ventilation operates on the principle that the pressure and volume of a closed cavity are inversely related. Therefore, if the volume of a closed cavity increases, the pressure within it will fall.

The lungs lie in separate airtight cavities within the thorax, surrounded by the pleura. The elastic recoil of the lungs tends to pull them away from the thoracic wall, creating a partial vacuum within the pleural cavity. The flow of air through the respiratory tract follows pressure gradients between the atmosphere and the lungs. Just before inspiration, the pressure inside the lungs (the *intrapulmonary pressure*) is equal to atmospheric pressure, whereas the pressure within the pleural cavity (the *intrapleural pressure*) is always below atmospheric.

Inspiration is an active process resulting from the expansion of the thorax. It is initiated by neural activity leading to the contraction of respiratory muscles. During normal quiet inspiration the contraction and descent of the *diaphragm* increases the vertical dimensions of the thoracic cavity, while contraction of the *external intercostal muscles* widens the thorax by elevating the ribs and sternum. The lungs expand as they follow the movements of the thoracic wall because the surface tension generated by the serous fluid in the pleural cavity causes the visceral and parietal pleura to adhere closely, much as two moist plates of glass resist separation.

As the lungs expand and the pulmonary volume increases, the intrapulmonary pressure falls below atmospheric, creating a pressure gradient that causes air to flow from the atmosphere through the conducting passageways into the lungs. As the lungs expand, elastic components of the lung stretch and develop tension.

Quiet expiration occurs passively through relaxation of the inspiratory muscles. As the diaphragm ascends and the ribs and sternum return to their resting positions, the size of the thoracic cavity decreases. As the thorax assumes its original size, the potential energy stored in the elastic elements of the lung is converted into kinetic energy. These events cause the intrapulmonary pressure to temporarily exceed the atmospheric pressure, thus reversing the flow of air.

Accessory muscles of respiration include the scalene and the pectoralis minor, which contract during forceful inspiration to further expand the thorax. During active, forceful expiration, coughing, and vomiting, the internal intercostal muscles contract to pull the ribs downward and inward, while the abdominal muscles contract to push the diaphragm upward.

Respiratory Compliance

Respiratory compliance, which may be defined as the lung volume change per unit of pressure, is a term often used to describe the ease with which the lungs may be inflated. Two major factors that affect respiratory compliance are surface tension and resistance to airflow.

SURFACE TENSION

Surface tension results from the forces of attraction between molecules on a fluid surface at a liquid–gas interface. The inner surface of the alveoli is coated with a thin film of fluid that exerts a surface tension tending to impair expansion of alveoli upon inspiration (and to favor collapse on expiration).

The surface tension and tendency for collapse are particularly great in the smaller alveoli. Normally, the alveolar septal (type II) cells secrete a lipoprotein *surfactant* that reduces the surface tension and lowers the resistance of the alveoli to expansion on inspiration. Pulmonary surfactant therefore increases respiratory compliance and reduces the work required for breathing.

A deficiency of pulmonary surfactant characterizes *respiratory distress syndrome* (also known as *hyaline membrane disease*), a condition often afflicting premature infants.

RESISTANCE TO AIRFLOW

Any obstruction or resistance to the flow of air would increase the force required to bring air into the alveoli. Airway resistance is encountered chiefly in the bronchi and bronchioles. It can be increased by the contraction of respiratory smooth muscle (*bronchoconstriction*) or by swelling of the respiratory mucosa (*mucosal edema*).

Reflex bronchoconstriction may follow mechanical or chemical stimulation of airway receptors. Parasympathetic stimulation, acetylcholine, and histamine cause bronchoconstriction. Sympathetic stimulation, epinephrine, and isoproterenol relax bronchiolar smooth muscle.

Bronchial asthma is a bronchospastic disease (frequently allergic in origin) characterized by great airway resistance. Major factors contributing to the heightened airway resistance are respiratory muscle spasm and mucosal edema leading to excessive accumulation of mucus.

The important mechanisms involved in bronchial constriction and relaxation are summarized in Figure 53-1.

Volumes of Air Exchanged

The amount of air exchanged during normal, quiet respiration (*eupnea*) varies with the age, sex, and size of the person. In the average adult the *tidal volume* (volume of air inspired or expired) is approximately 500 mL. The product of *tidal volume* and *respiratory rate* equals the *minute respiratory volume*, which represents the volume of air entering the lungs in 1 minute.

The most critical factor in the total process of pulmonary ventilation is *alveolar ventilation*. Alveolar ventilation (the volume of air that enters the alveoli per minute) is a fraction of the total ventilation because with each breath some air remains in the conducting passages and is therefore unavailable to the alveoli for gaseous exchange. The total internal volume of these conducting passages is termed *anatomic dead space*, estimated to be 150 mL. The *physiologic dead space*, which in normally functioning lungs is essentially equal to the anatomical dead space, is more variable (and larger) if nonfunctioning alveoli are present.

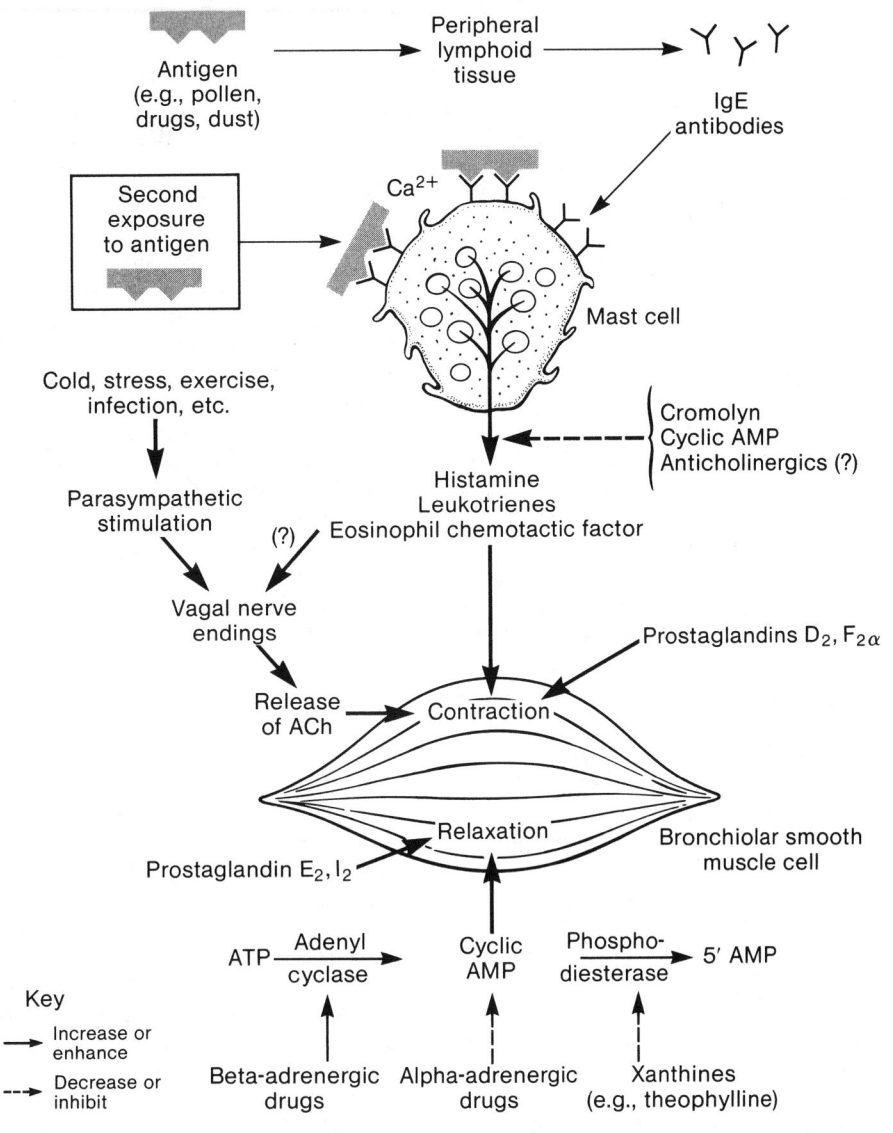

Figure 53–1 Factors regulating bronchiolar smooth muscle contraction and relaxation. On exposure to an antigen, lymphoid tissue forms IgE antibodies, which then attach to the surface of mast cells. Reexposure to antigen triggers an antigen–antibody reaction on the mast cell surface (termed *IgE bridging*), resulting in release of endogenous allergens from the mast cell, probably by way of increased calcium influx. The allergens elicit contraction of bronchiolar smooth muscle cells either by a direct action on the cells or by activating parasympathetic pathways.

EXCHANGE AND TRANSPORT OF RESPIRATORY GASES

In a mixture of gases (such as the atmosphere), the portion of the total pressure contributed by a particular gas in the mixture is termed the *partial pressure* or *tension*. The partial pressure exerted by each individual gas varies directly with its concentration in the mixture and with the total pressure of the mixture. For example, O_2, which makes up approximately 21% of atmospheric air, exerts a partial pressure (P_{O_2}) of 160 mm Hg under standard total atmospheric pressure of 760 mm Hg, that is, $0.21 \times 760 = 160$.

Atmospheric (inspired) air is composed predominantly of nitrogen and O_2 with very small amounts of CO_2, water vapor, and inert gases. Alveolar air differs from atmospheric air in composition because the inspired air becomes saturated with water vapor and mixed with old anatomical dead space air during its passage through the conducting components of the respiratory tract. *Alveolar* P_{O_2} is 100 mm Hg in contrast with the *atmospheric* P_{O_2} of 160 mm Hg.

The exchange of gases within the body occurs through diffusion, with each gas diffusing according to its partial pressure gradient. As shown in Figure 53-2, pressure gradients cause O_2 to diffuse from the alveoli into the blood, and from the blood into the tissues. The pressure gradients are reversed for CO_2, causing it to diffuse from the tissues into the blood and subsequently into the alveoli.

Within the alveoli, large volumes of water-saturated air are exposed to a vast volume of blood to effect efficient exchange of gases. Pulmonary venous blood is not maximally oxygenated because alveolar ventilation and perfusion are not uniform throughout the lung. During normal ventilation (in an upright person at rest) the lower (basal) segments of the lungs receive a relatively greater blood flow than the upper (apical) portions because of gravitational forces. Most respiratory disorders are characterized by even greater ventilation–perfusion inequalities. Possible pathologic causes of uneven ventilation include obstruction of airways (as in asthma), altered elasticity of airways (as in advanced emphysema), and reduced pulmonary expansion (as in atelectasis). Uneven capillary perfusion may result from shunts, embolization, and compression of pulmonary blood vessels.

During pulmonary exchange of gases, O_2 and CO_2 must diffuse across a functional respiratory membrane composed of (1) alveolar membrane, (2) interstitial fluid, (3) capillary endothelium and basement membrane, (4) plasma, and (5) erythrocyte (red blood cell) membrane.

The rate at which O_2 diffuses from the alveoli into the blood depends on (1) the partial pressure gradient for oxygen, (2) the total functional surface area of the alveolar and capillary membranes, (3) the thickness of the respiratory membrane, and (4) the ventilation–perfusion ratio.

The diffusion of a gas into a liquid medium, such as plasma, depends on the partial pressure gradient and the solubility of the gas in that fluid. Immediately upon entering the blood, the respiratory gases dissolve in the fluid portion of blood—the plasma (CO_2 is about 20 times more soluble in plasma than O_2).

Erythrocytes play an essential role in the transport of both O_2 and CO_2 because mere physical solution of these gases in blood plasma would not be adequate to meet even minimal body needs. The gas-carrying capacity of blood is greatly increased by rapidly reversible chemical reactions that remove O_2 and CO_2 from solution, thus steepening their gradients for diffusion.

Oxygen Transport

The amount of O_2 in the blood is essentially determined by three factors: (1) the amount of O_2 dissolved in the plasma, (2) the amount of *hemoglobin* (Hb) in the blood, and (3) the affinity of Hb for O_2.

Normally, the amount of O_2 physically dissolved in plasma is very small because of its low solubility in this fluid. Most (approximately 98%) of the O_2 in the blood is transported in combination with Hb, a conjugated protein present in erythrocytes. Hb contains four iron atoms, each of which can reversibly bind one molecule of oxygen. While the oxygenation of Hb occurs in a stepwise fashion, the overall process is generally represented by the simple equation:

$$\underset{\text{hemoglobin}}{HB} + \underset{\text{oxygen}}{O_2} \rightleftharpoons \underset{\text{oxyhemoglobin}}{HbO_2}$$

When fully saturated with the gas, each gram of Hb can hold 1.34 mL of O_2. At an average Hb concentration of 15 g per dL of blood, the O_2-carrying capacity of Hb is 20.1 volumes percent (15×1.34).

In arterial blood Hb is 97% saturated with O_2, whereas in venous blood the degree of saturation falls to 75%. The color of Hb reflects the degree of its saturation with O_2. HbO_2 is bright crimson, which explains the bright red color of arterial blood; reduced Hb is dark purple, imparting a port wine color to venous blood.

The affinity of Hb for O_2 is greatly affected by the P_{O_2}. When the P_{O_2} is high, as it is in the lungs, Hb binds large amounts of O_2 and becomes nearly saturated with it. In the tissue capillaries, where P_{O_2} is substantially lower, the affinity of Hb for O_2 is reduced, and O_2 is released for diffusion into the tissues.

The amount of O_2 in combination with Hb also depends upon the P_{CO_2}, pH, and temperature of the blood. Under conditions of increased P_{CO_2}, low pH (acidity), or elevated temperature of the blood, the amount of O_2 that binds to hemoglobin at any given P_{O_2} is diminished.

The reduced affinity of Hb for O_2 that occurs when blood pH falls is termed the *Bohr effect*. The pH of the blood falls as its CO_2 content increases because CO_2 combines with water to form carbonic acid (H_2CO_3), which rapidly dissociates into hydrogen (H^+) and bicarbonate ions (HCO_3^-), as shown below:

$$CO_2 + H_2O \rightleftharpoons H_2CO_3 \rightleftharpoons H^+ + HCO_3^-$$

Another metabolic factor that favors the dissociation of O_2 from Hb is 2,3 diphosphoglycerate (2,3 DPG), an organic phosphate present in erythrocytes that binds to Hb and decreases its affinity for O_2. Erythrocyte 2,3 DPG concentration increases during prolonged exercise, anemia, and in diseases marked by chronic hypoxia.

As the O_2 dissociates from Hb, it becomes available for diffusion into tissue cells. Metabolically active tissues tend to accumulate CO_2 and acidic metabolites and to undergo temperature elevation—conditions that favor O_2 dissociation from Hb and increase availability of O_2 to the tissue cells.

Carbon Dioxide Transport

CO_2, a principal end product of cellular metabolism, diffuses from the tissues into the blood for transport to the lungs (for elimination). It is transported by the blood in three forms as follows:

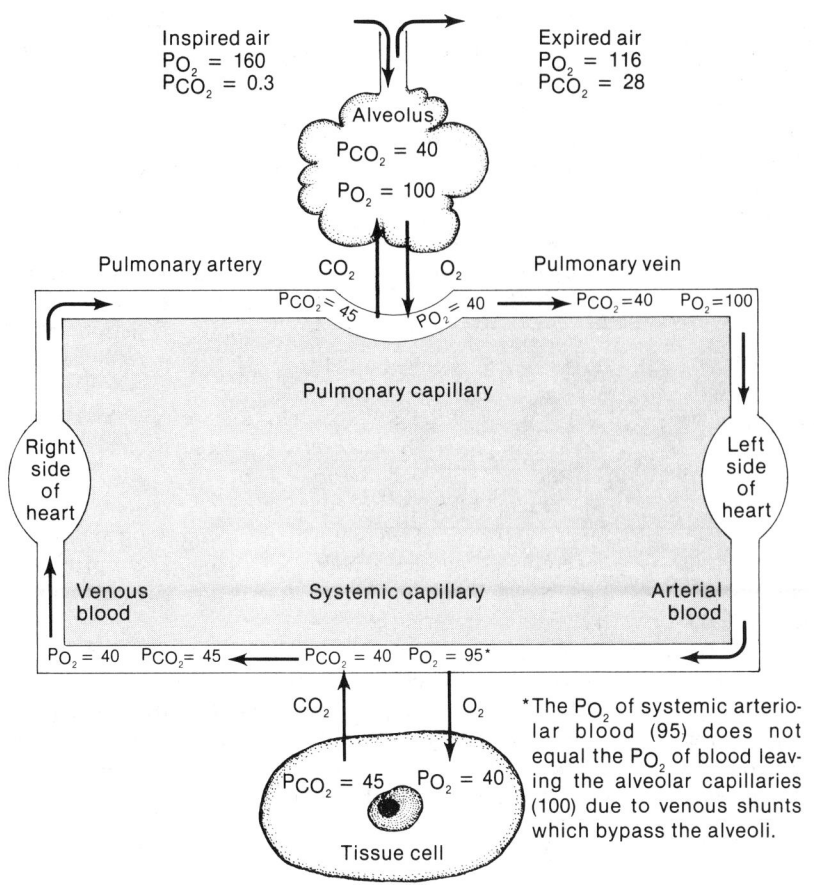

Figure 53-2 Gaseous exchange according to partial pressure gradients.

- *Dissolved* in the plasma
- As *carbamino compounds*
- As *bicarbonate ions*

CO_2 is highly soluble in plasma, and nearly 10% of the total CO_2 in the blood is carried in physical solution within the plasma.

Approximately 20% of blood CO_2 combines with *amino* groups of several blood proteins (principally Hb) to form *carbamino compounds.* Some of the CO_2 that diffuses from the plasma into the erythrocytes combines with Hb to form the compound *carbaminohemoglobin.* However, most of the CO_2 in the erythrocytes is readily hydrated in the presence of carbonic anhydrase enzyme, forming H_2CO_3. H_2CO_3 rapidly dissociates into H^+ and HCO_3^- ions. The H^+ ions are buffered, principally by Hb, while the HCO_3^- ions diffuse into the plasma. Electrochemical neutrality is maintained by the rapid diffusion of chloride (Cl^-) ions into the erythrocytes (the so-called *chloride shift*). Approximately 70% of the CO_2 in the blood is transported in the form of HCO_3^- ions.

REGULATION OF RESPIRATION

Neural Control of Respiration

The rhythmic pattern of normal respiration is maintained by the cyclic discharge of neurons located in the brainstem. Three bilateral interconnected respiratory "centers" (located in the medulla and pons) are generally recognized: the medullary center, the apneustic center, and the pneumotaxic center.

MEDULLARY RESPIRATORY CENTER

The *medullary respiratory center* consists of two anatomically intermingled but functionally distinct and reciprocally active aggregates of neurons: *inspiratory* neurons and *expiratory* neurons. The inspiratory neurons exhibit spontaneous bursts of activity during which the expiratory neurons are inhibited by the operation of oscillating negative feedback circuits.

Simultaneously, impulses originating in the inspiratory neurons travel along the phrenic and intercostal nerves to the diaphragm and external intercostal muscles, respectively, causing their contraction and the subsequent enlargement of the thorax, leading to inspiration. The medullary respiratory center receives afferent (sensory) input from central chemoreceptors, from several kinds of peripherally located receptors, and from higher brain centers (including the apneustic and pneumotaxic centers of the pons). The afferent input can modify the basic rhythmic discharge of the medullary respiratory neurons. For example, impulses originating in the cerebral cortex allow voluntary interruption of the normal breathing cycle for activities such as speaking, laughing, and breath-holding.

PONTINE RESPIRATORY CENTERS

The *pneumotaxic center,* located in the superior pons, inhibits inspiration and facilitates expiration by inhibiting both the apneustic center and the medullary inspiratory neurons directly.

The *apneustic center,* located in the reticular formation of the lower pons, provides tonic stimulation to the medullary inspiratory neurons, thereby facilitating and prolonging inspiration. The apneustic center is not necessary for the maintenance of a basic respiratory rhythm, and its level of activity can be modified (inhibited) by afferent input from the pneumotaxic center and from pulmonary stretch receptors.

Chemical Control of Respiration

The CO_2, O_2, and H^+ ion levels of the blood (and other body fluids) are of major importance in the control of respiration. CO_2 is the most potent physiological stimulant of respiration, exerting its effects chiefly through central chemoreceptors. It must be noted, however, that very high concentrations of CO_2 (in excess of 30% in inspired air) produce central nervous system (and respiratory) depression and may be lethal.

CENTRAL CHEMORECEPTORS

The ventral surface of the medulla contains chemosensitive cells that respond to elevations of CO_2 and H^+ ions in arterial blood and cerebrospinal fluid by stimulating the medullary respiratory center.

CO_2 readily diffuses from the blood plasma into the cerebrospinal fluid, where it combines with water to form H_2CO_3, which then dissociates into H^+ and HCO_3^- ions.

Because cerebrospinal fluid is not as well buffered as the blood, the H^+ ion concentration rises quickly, effectively stimulating the central chemoreceptors and thereby increasing pulmonary ventilation.

PERIPHERAL CHEMORECEPTORS

Located peripherally in the *carotid* and *aortic bodies* are chemoreceptors neurally connected to the medullary respiratory center by afferent glossopharyngeal and vagal nerve fibers.

These peripheral chemoreceptors are primarily sensitive to arterial O_2 levels, responding to lowered arterial P_{O_2} (*hypoxemia*) by stimulating respiration. They serve as an important emergency mechanism of respiratory stimulation in states of low O_2 intake.

Carotid and aortic chemoreceptors also respond to elevations in arterial P_{CO_2} and H^+ ion concentrations, mechanisms of importance in acidosis.

Reflex Regulation of Respiration

In addition to chemoreceptors, there are a number of peripheral receptors whose stimulation initiates reflex changes in respiration.

Sensory modalities such as pain, temperature, and touch affect respiration, with pain exerting a strong excitatory effect upon the medullary respiratory center.

Movements of joints, whether active or passive, stimulate respiration by way of afferent pathways originating in the proprioceptors of muscles, tendons, and joints. These pathways, which converge upon the respiratory center, augment pulmonary ventilation during exercise.

Sneezing and coughing are reflex, modified respiratory responses to irritants of the respiratory mucosa.

Inflation of the lungs stimulates pulmonary stretch receptors that lead to vagally mediated inhibition of inspiration. This "inflation reflex" (also termed the *vagal* or *Hering–Breuer reflex*) does not appear to be of great importance during normal respiration in humans.

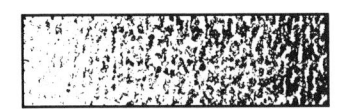

54 ANTITUSSIVES, EXPECTORANTS, AND MUCOLYTICS

Coughing is a protective mechanism initiated by chemical or mechanical stimulation of the tracheobronchial tree by which the body attempts to remove foreign particles or accumulated secretions from the respiratory tract. The cough reflex may be initiated by a number of factors, such as local inflammation of the bronchioles (e.g., smoking), mechanical or physical obstruction (e.g., foreign bodies, emboli), local or systemic disease states (e.g., pulmonary edema, bronchogenic carcinoma, or congestive heart failure), and emotional stress. To the extent that the cough is annoying or debilitating, proper drug therapy should be undertaken to eliminate the condition. Not all coughing is undesirable, however, and the productive type of cough that aids in removing excessive bronchiolar mucus in the form of sputum generally should not be suppressed. Of course, if the cough is secondary to some other disease, every effort should be made to identify and eliminate the underlying pathologic condition, such as pneumonia, bronchitis, or tuberculosis.

The most frequently employed drugs for the control of coughing may be divided into the antitussives and the expectorants. *Antitussives* are cough suppressants that may act centrally at the level of the "cough center" in the brainstem or peripherally at several sites along the tracheobronchial tree. Antitussives are primarily indicated in the treatment of annoying, dry, unproductive coughing, especially where it interferes with other functions (e.g., talking, sleeping) or leads to excessive weakness or progressive irritation.

Expectorants, in contrast, increase and liquefy bronchial secretions so that they can be more easily expelled. These drugs act either on the secretory glands of the respiratory tract or by irritation of the gastric mucosa, which reflexly increases respiratory secretions. They find their major clinical application in the treatment of obstructive pulmonary diseases associated with accumulation of excessive, tenacious mucus; they may reduce the viscosity of bronchial secretions, thus facilitating elimination. There is doubt, however, as to the efficacy of the usual amounts of expectorants found in over-the-counter cough formulations in reducing bronchial irritation or lessening the severity of nonproductive coughing. Exposure to humidified air and—especially adequate fluid intake—have proved as effective as most expectorants in relieving nonproductive coughing, liquefying thick, tenacious mucus, and facilitating removal of respiratory secretions.

Mucolytic agents also have the ability to liquefy mucus and thus facilitate its removal from the respiratory passages by normal physiologic processes such as ciliary action, bronchiolar peristalsis, and coughing, or through suction. Although numerous proteolytic enzymes and detergents have been tried as mucolytic agents, most exhibited undesirable side effects and were unsuitable for clinical use. The only currently available mucolytic drug is acetylcysteine, an amino acid derivative that disrupts the molecular structure of mucus. It is relatively nontoxic when used by inhalation for adjunctive therapy of a number of bronchoobstructive conditions resulting from excessive or highly viscous mucus.

ANTITUSSIVES

The antitussive drugs are used to reduce the frequency of dry, unproductive coughing, and most act to depress the cough reflex by a direct inhibition of the cough center in the medulla. Drugs possessing antitussive activity can be divided into two groups, the narcotic and the nonnarcotic cough suppressants. Although many opiate drugs possess a cough-suppressive action, most are deemed unsuitable for controlling simple coughing because they exhibit a significant danger of habituation and their use is associated with many undesirable side effects. Of the many opiates available, only codeine and hydrocodone are routinely used for the relief of coughing, and usually as a component of a combination product (see Table 54-1).

The nonnarcotic antitussives are a structurally diverse group of pharmacologic agents that possess both central and peripheral mechanisms of action. In most cases, they are nearly as effective as codeine, with perhaps a somewhat lower incidence of disturbing side effects. They are considered individually below.

Narcotic Antitussives

Codeine is the most commonly used narcotic antitussive because it is very effective in reducing the frequency of coughing but is less likely to depress respiration or lead to habituation than other narcotic agents. Although it is available in tablet form, it is most frequently administered as a component of liquid cough preparations, in which it may be combined with antihistamines, decongestants, expectorants, or analgesics (see Table 54-1).

Hydrocodone (dihydrocodeinone) is comparable to codeine in efficacy but may be somewhat more habituating. It is not available for use alone but like codeine, is found in a number of cough preparations in combination with expectorants, antihistamines, and decongestants. It is considered briefly in this chapter; however, the general information presented for codeine below applies to hydrocodone as well.

Codeine
(CAN) Paveral

MECHANISM
Suppresses cough reflex by a direct depressant effect on the cough center in the medulla

USES
Suppression of nonproductive coughing
Relief of mild to moderate pain, usually in combination with aspirin or acetaminophen (see Chap. 18)

DOSAGE
Adults: 10 mg to 20 mg every 4 to 6 hours; maximum 120 mg/day
Children 6 to 12 years: 5 mg to 10 mg every 4 to 6 hours; maximum 60 mg/day
Children 2 to 6 years: 2.5 mg to 5 mg every 4 to 6 hours; maximum 30 mg/day

FATE
Well absorbed when taken orally; onset of action is 15 to 30 minutes; duration of action is 3 to 4 hours; metabolized in the liver and excreted largely in the urine

Table 54-1
Representative Codeine-Containing Cough Preparations

Trade Names	Other Ingredients
Actifed with Codeine	pseudoephedrine, triprolidine
Ambenyl	bromodiphenhydramine
Cheracol	guaifenesin
Dimetane-DC	brompheniramine, phenylpropanolamine
Isoclor Expectorant	guaifenesin, pseudoephedrine
Naldecon-Cx	guaifenesin, phenylpropanolamine
Novahistine Expectorant	guaifenesin, pseudoephedrine
Nucofed	pseudoephedrine
Phenergan with Codeine	promethazine
Phenergan VC with Codeine	promethazine, phenylephrine
Robitussin A-C	guaifenesin
Terpin Hydrate with Codeine	terpin hydrate
Tussar-2	guaifenesin, chlorpheniramine, carbetapentane
Tussi-Organidin	iodinated glycerol

COMMON SIDE EFFECTS
(Frequent at *excessive* doses) Lightheadedness, dizziness, sedation, sweating, and nausea

SIGNIFICANT ADVERSE REACTIONS
GI: dry mouth, anorexia, vomiting, constipation, biliary spasm
CNS: euphoria, weakness, insomnia, headache, anxiety, fear, mood changes, disorientation, agitation, tremors, impaired physical performance, psychological dependence, delirium, hallucinations, coma, visual disturbances, respiratory and cardiovascular depression (especially with large doses)
Cardiovascular: flushing, tachycardia, palpitations, hypotension
Other: allergic reactions (rash, urticaria, pruritus, edema), urinary retention, decreased libido, impotence, flushing, tachycardia, palpitation, faintness, syncope, ureteral spasm

CONTRAINDICATIONS
Patients with known or suspected narcotic addiction. *Cautious use* in patients with asthma or other pulmonary diseases, cardiac disease (including arrhythmias), convulsive disorders, renal or hepatic impairment, prostatic hypertrophy, severe CNS depression, toxic psychoses, head injuries, intracranial lesions, hypothyroidism, or Addison's disease, and in alcoholics and pregnancy

INTERACTIONS
Profound sedation, hypotension, and respiratory depression may occur with combinations of codeine and other narcotics, sedatives, hypnotics, alcohol, phenothiazines, tricyclic antidepressants, general anesthetics, and other CNS depressants (see also Narcotic Analgesics, Chap. 18)

NURSING CONSIDERATIONS
See also nursing considerations related to opiate usage (Chapter 18) for those applicable to use of codeine as an antitussive.
1. Note that codeine alone in tablet form is a Schedule II drug, but codeine is most commonly used in combination with other agents in cough syrups. Depending upon the amount of codeine contained in the mixture, these combination antitussives may be Schedule III or Schedule V products. Follow proper procedures for handling controlled substances (see Chap. 8).

PATIENT EDUCATION
1. When syrup is used, instruct patient to take medication undiluted and *not* to drink water immediately afterwards.
2. Warn patient not to exceed recommended dosage because antitussive effect is not significantly enhanced, but untoward reactions and danger of habituation are increased.
3. Inform patient that drug may cause drowsiness, but that restlessness, anxiety, or nervousness sometimes occur instead, especially with large doses.
4. Suggest that patient drink large amounts of fluids (e.g., 2 L/day), which may help decrease the tenacity of bronchial secretions, and use a humidifier or vaporizer during the night.
5. Advise patient to use hard candy, gum, or throat lozenges to soothe pharyngeal mucosa irritated by constant coughing.

Hydrocodone
(CAN) Robidone

Hydrocodone (dihydrocodeinone) is a relatively weak analgesic and a strong antitussive found in combination with other agents such as expectorants and antihistamines in many cough formulations. It exhibits a relatively low degree of respiratory depression and physical dependence, although the likelihood of habituation appears to be greater than that of codeine. Commercial preparations containing hydrocodone include:

Entuss (with guaifenesin)
Hycodan (with homatropine)
Hycomine (with phenylpropanolamine)
Tussionex (with phenyltoloxamine)
Tussend (with pseudoephedrine and guaifenesin)

The recommended dosage for hydrocodone in these preparations is 5 mg up to four times a day. Refer to the preceding discussion of codeine for additional information regarding side effects, precautions, and interactions.

Nonnarcotic Antitussives

The principal nonnarcotic antitussive is dextromethorphan, which is reviewed in detail below. Other less frequently used nonnarcotic drugs are considered briefly.

Dextromethorphan

Benylin DM, Delsym, Hold, Pertussin, and other manufacturers
(CAN) Koffex, Robidex, Sedatuss

Dextromethorphan is the *d*-isomer of levorphanol, a codeine analog. It exhibits minimal CNS depressant action and has no analgesic effect, and its administration is unlikely to produce constipation or lead to tolerance. It is commonly found in over-the-counter cough formulations, frequently combined with antihistamines, decongestants, and expectorants. A 30-mg dose is approximately equivalent to 15 mg of codeine.

MECHANISM
Not conclusively established; appears to depress the cough center in the medulla

USES
Temporary relief of nonproductive coughing

DOSAGE
Lozenges/Syrup
Adults: 10 mg to 30 mg every 4 to 8 hours; maximum 120 mg/24 h
Children 6 to 12 years: 5 mg to 10 mg every 4 hours *or* 7.5 mg to 15 mg every 6 to 8 hours; maximum 60 mg/24 h
Children 2 to 6 years: 2.5 mg to 5 mg every 4 hours *or* 3.75 mg to 7.5 mg every 6 to 8 hours; maximum 30 mg/24 h
Controlled-Release Liquid (Delsym)
Adults: 60 mg twice a day
Children 6 to 12 years: 30 mg twice a day
Children 2 to 6 years: 15 mg twice a day

FATE
Onset of action is 15 to 30 minutes and antitussive effects persist 3 to 6 hours depending on the dose (up to 12 h with controlled release liquid)

SIGNIFICANT ADVERSE REACTIONS
Dizziness, GI distress, and drowsiness

CONTRAINDICATIONS
Patients taking MAO inhibitors (see Interactions, below). *Cautious use* in persons with chronic cough or cough associated with excessive secretions, chronic obstructive pulmonary disease, high fever, persistent headache, vomiting

INTERACTIONS
Combinations of dextromethorphan and MAO inhibitors can result in hyperpyrexia, muscular rigidity, and laryngospasm

NURSING CONSIDERATIONS
1. Note that the drug's antitussive activity is comparable to that of codeine, and, in therapeutic doses, the drug does not induce tolerance, hypnosis, respiratory depression, or analgesia. Also, constipation is much less frequent than with codeine.
2. Note that drug is available in throat lozenge form alone and combined with benzocaine (e.g., Formula 44 Cough Control Discs, Spec-T Sore Throat Cough Suppressant, Vick's Cough Silencers) for control of spasmodic coughing. Lozenges are not as effective as the syrup.

PATIENT EDUCATION
1. Instruct parents not to administer to children under 2 years of age except under medical supervision.
2. Instruct patient to take syrup undiluted to enhance its local effect.
3. Inform patient that increasing the dose increases the duration of action.
4. Advise patient to consult physician if coughing persists longer than 7 days with dextromethorphan or any other antitussive therapy.

Benzonatate

Tessalon Perles

Benzonatate is structurally related to tetracaine and exerts a local anesthetic action on stretch receptors in the respiratory passages, lungs, and pleural cavity. As a result, the activity of these receptors is suppressed and the cough reflex is dampened. The drug does not appear to alter the function of the respiratory center at recommended doses. It is used as capsules for relief of non-productive coughing, at a dosage of 100 mg three times a day; effects persist for 3 to 6 hours.

Adverse reactions may include sedation, dizziness, nasal congestion, constipation, nausea, GI upset, pruritus, skin eruptions, burning in the eyes, a "chilly" sensation, and numbness in the chest. Large doses can lead to CNS stimulation (restlessness, tremor, convulsions).

Benzonatate is contraindicated in persons who are allergic to tetracaine or related local anesthetics. The drug should be used *cautiously* in pregnant women or nursing mothers. Capsules should be swallowed whole and not chewed because release of the drug in the mouth can anesthetize the oral mucosa.

NURSING CONSIDERATIONS
1. If drug is used in patient who is vomiting, observe carefully for possible development of pneumonitis from aspiration.
2. Note that benzonatate is reportedly as effective as codeine in controlling nonproductive coughing and does not lead to habituation.

PATIENT EDUCATION
1. Instruct patient to swallow the capsule (perle) whole because release of drug in the mouth can produce temporary anesthesia in the oral mucosa.
2. Encourage patient to use interventions (e.g., adequate hydration, hard candy or gum, cessation of smoking, air humidification) that help control nonproductive coughing.

Diphenhydramine

Benylin and other manufacturers

Diphenhydramine is an antihistamine (see Chap 14) that is used as a syrup to control coughing due to colds or allergies. Oral dosage is 25 mg every 4 hours for adults, and 6.25 mg to 12.5 mg every 4 hours for children. The major side effect with diphenhydramine is drowsiness. The drug is also found in 25-mg and 50-mg strengths as the principal ingredient in over-the-counter sleep aids such as Nytol, Sleep-Eze 3, Sominex 2, Compoz, and Twilite.

EXPECTORANTS

Expectorants are claimed to facilitate removal of viscous mucus from the respiratory tree and to provide a soothing, demulcent action on the respiratory mucosa by stimulating secretion of a lubricating fluid. Although large doses of certain prescription-only expectorants (such as potassium iodide) may decrease the tenacity of mucus associated with chronic obstructive pulmonary disease, the efficacy of most nonprescription expectorants is subject to considerable debate. They are probably no more effective in providing relief of bronchial irritation or facilitating mucus liquefaction than high fluid intake, that is, 6 to 10 glasses/day, and humidification of the environment. There is little support for the claim that expectorants relieve dry, irritative coughing by increasing production of a soothing fluid any more than would be produced by use of a cough drop or throat lozenge. Therefore, their inclusion in cough/cold formulations containing antitussives, antihistamines, and decongestants among other medications apparently adds little to the overall therapeutic efficacy of such preparations.

On the other hand, adverse reactions are rare at usual therapeutic doses, the most frequent problem being GI distress. Thus the drugs are quite safe when taken as directed, and if patients believe the compounds are effective, it may be difficult to convince them otherwise.

Guaifenesin and several iodine-containing products are the most commonly employed expectorants and are discussed in detail. Other infrequently used expectorants are briefly considered.

Guaifenesin

Breonesin, Humibid, Robitussin, and other manufacturers—formerly known as glyceryl guaiacolate
(CAN) Balminil Expectorant, Resyl

MECHANISM
May increase output of respiratory tract fluid by reducing its adhesiveness and surface tension, thus facilitating removal of mucus; increased fluid flow is also claimed to soothe dry, irritated membranes, thereby relieving dry, hacking cough

USE
Symptomatic relief of dry, unproductive coughing associated with common respiratory disorders, such as colds, bronchitis, bronchial asthma (efficacy not conclusively established)

DOSAGE
Adults: 100 mg to 400 mg every 3 to 6 hours; maximum 1.2 g/day
Children 6 to 12 years: 100 mg to 200 mg every 4 hours maximum 600 mg/day
Children 2 to 6 years: 50 mg to 100 mg every 4 hours; maximum 300 mg/day

SIGNIFICANT ADVERSE REACTIONS
(Usually with large doses) Nausea, vomiting, GI distress, and drowsiness

CONTRAINDICATIONS
No absolute contraindications. *Cautious use* in persons with persistent cough, high fever, persistent headache, or rash

INTERACTIONS
Guaifenesin may decrease platelet aggregation, thus increasing the risk of bleeding with anticoagulants
Guaifenesin may cause a color interference with laboratory determinations of VMA and 5-HIAA

NURSING CONSIDERATION
1. Note that although drug is widely used alone or in combination with other cough suppressants, antihistamines, analgesics, and other drugs, convincing evidence that it is a clinically effective expectorant is lacking.

PATIENT EDUCATION
1. Encourage patient to employ adjunctive interventions (e.g., high fluid intake, humidification of room air) that facilitate liquefaction of mucus and relieve dry, nonproductive cough.

Iodine Products

Hydrogen Iodide
Hydriodic Acid
Iodinated Glycerol
Iophen, Organidin, R-Gen Elixir
Potassium Iodide
Pima and other manufacturers
Potassium Iodide/Niacinamide
Iodo-Niacin

Several iodine-containing preparations are used as expectorants, although their clinical efficacy is subject to doubt. In addition, they have the potential to cause a number of adverse reactions, and many persons display allergic reactions to iodine-containing drugs. Iodinated glycerol is claimed to be less irritating to the GI tract than other iodides but is probably less effective as well.

MECHANISM
Enhance secretion of respiratory fluid and decrease viscosity and tenacity of mucus; may also facilitate breakdown of fibrous material at inflammatory sites

USE
Adjunctive treatment of respiratory conditions associated with increased mucus, such as bronchitis, asthma, emphysema, and cystic fibrosis, and following surgery to help prevent atelectasis (efficacy not conclusively established)

DOSAGE
Potassium Iodide
Adults: 300 mg to 600 mg every 4 to 6 hours
Children: 150 mg to 300 mg every 4 to 6 hours
Hydrogen Iodide
Adults: 70 mg three to four times a day
Iodinated Glycerol
Adults: 60 mg four times a day
Children: Up to one half adult dosage based on weight
Potassium Iodide/Niacinamide
Adults: 2 tablets three times a day

FATE
Oral absorption is adequate; iodides are absorbed in conjunction with amino acids; attain high levels in gastric and salivary secretions; excretion is primarily by way of the kidney

COMMON SIDE EFFECTS
GI distress

SIGNIFICANT ADVERSE REACTIONS
Epigastric pain, sore throat, metallic taste, mucosal ulceration, sneezing, coryza, increased salivation, diarrhea, hypersensitivity reactions (arthralgia, fever, angioedema, lymph node enlargement, cutaneous bleeding, eosinophilia). Large doses may cause goiter, thyroid adenoma, or myxedema

CONTRAINDICATIONS
Hyperthyroidism, hyperkalemia, Addison's disease, kidney disease, sensitivity to iodides, tuberculosis, and acute bronchitis. *Cautious use* in persons with goiter, high fever, persistent cough, inflammatory bowel lesions, cystic fibrosis, acne, or dermatoses, and in pregnant women or nursing mothers

INTERACTIONS
The hypothyroid and goitrogenic effects of potassium iodide may be potentiated by lithium or other antithyroid drugs
Hyperkalemia can be intensified by potassium supplements or potassium-sparing diuretics

NURSING CONSIDERATIONS
See Chapter 40 for additional indications for iodide products.

Nursing Alert
- If enteric-coated tablets are administered, assess patient's abdomen often because small-bowel lesions resulting in obstruction, hemorrhage, and perforation have occurred. Dosage form should be discontinued immediately if abdominal pain or distention, vomiting, or GI bleeding occurs.

1. Seek clarification if prescription exceeds recommended dosage or iodide is administered for extensive period because prolonged use can lead to hypothyroidism and iodide-induced goiter.
2. If laboratory determinations of protein-bound iodine and 17-hydroxycorticosteroids are performed, interpret results cautiously. Iodide preparations may elevate values of the former and interfere with results of the latter.
3. Note that hydrogen iodide syrup (hydriodic acid) is an over-the-counter preparation. Other iodide expectorants are prescription drugs.

PATIENT EDUCATION
1. If a liquid drug form is used, instruct patient to dilute the preparation liberally with water or another vehicle before swallowing. Tablets should be taken with food or milk to minimize GI distress.
2. Encourage increased fluid intake, cessation of smoking, and use of humidifier to increase expectorant action of iodides.
3. Instruct patient to stop taking iodide if signs of iodism appear (e.g., skin rash, fever, sore throat, metallic taste, vomiting, epigastric pain, parotid gland swelling).

Ammonium Chloride
Ammonium chloride is used predominantly as a systemic and urinary acidifier to treat metabolic alkalosis, to correct chloride depletion and to assist in the urinary excretion of certain basic drugs. These indications are considered in Chapter 75. The drug has also been used as an expectorant and is found in a number of over-the-counter cough preparations, although its efficacy is subject to considerable doubt and its use in this manner should be discouraged.

The drug appears to exert an irritative action on the GI mucosa, leading to reflex stimulation of respiratory secretions. The average adult expectorant dose is 100 mg to 400 mg several times a day.

GI upset is common with oral administration of ammonium chloride. Large doses can cause metabolic acidosis, which is characterized by vomiting, thirst, weakness, lethargy, confusion, and hyperventilation. The drug must be used cautiously in persons with chronic heart disease.

The excretion of basic drugs (e.g., amphetamines, antidepressants, antihistamines, anti-anxiety agents, catecholamines, narcotic analgesics, quinidine, theophylline) may be enhanced by ammonium chloride, whereas the systemic actions of acidic drugs (e.g., barbiturates, clofibrate, mercurial diuretics, pyrazolones, salicylates, oral antidiabetics, thyroid hormones) may be potentiated by ammonium chloride, because their renal excretion may be retarded.

Terpin Hydrate
Terpin hydrate is used in liquid form to stimulate respiratory secretions, presumably by a direct action on respiratory tract secretory glands. The drug is occasionally used alone (85 mg every 3–4 h) for minor bronchial irritations but is most frequently employed in combination with codeine (85 mg/10 mg/5 mL) as terpin hydrate and codeine elixir for control of minor coughing. This preparation contains approximately 40% alcohol and may cause drowsiness. Gastric upset can occur, especially if it is given on an empty stomach. A glass of water should be taken after each dose to facilitate loosening of mucus.

MUCOLYTICS

Acetylcysteine
Mucomyst, Mucosol
(CAN) Airbron, Parvolex

Acetylcysteine may be administered by nebulization, using a face mask or mouthpiece, or if large volumes are required, by use of a tent or croupette. The drug may also be instilled directly into the bronchial tree *via* a tracheostomy tube or intratracheal cannula. However, when it is administered by an ordinary aerosol nebulizer, its effectiveness is compromised by its inability to penetrate deeply enough into the obstructed bronchiolar passages. Acetylcysteine is *not* indicated for routine use in bronchial asthmatic patients with mucus accumulation, because it is frequently irritating and may elicit reflex bronchospasm, further impairing the patient's respiratory function.

Prompt removal of the liquefied secretions is necessary following use of a mucolytic agent. When coughing is unsuccessful in eliminating the liquefied mucus, or in the case of elderly or debilitated patients who are unable to encourage productive coughing, the airway must be kept clear by mechanical suction.

Acetylcysteine may also be employed to prevent or to minimize hepatotoxicity associated with acetaminophen overdosage by blocking the formation of toxic metabolites. The drug is given orally for this indication, and the dosage is outlined below.

MECHANISM

Breaks disulfide linkages in the mucoprotein structure of mucus, thus lowering its viscosity; mucolytic activity increases with increasing pH and is optimal between pH 7 and 9. In acetaminophen overdosage, retards formation of a hepatotoxic metabolite by serving as an alternative substrate for conjugation of the metabolite

USES

Adjunctive therapy for the relief of abnormal, viscous mucus accumulation associated with a variety of chronic respiratory conditions, such as emphysema, asthmatic bronchitis, bronchiectasis, tuberculosis, or amyloidosis of the lung

Minimization of bronchiolar obstructive complications associated with tracheostomy, cystic fibrosis, atelectasis, surgery, anesthesia, or trauma

Facilitation of diagnostic bronchial studies

Prevention of hepatotoxicity due to acetaminophen overdosage

Investigational uses include ophthalmic administration for treatment of keratoconjunctivitis sicca (dry eye) and as an enema for treating bowel obstruction due to meconium ileus

DOSAGE

Nebulization (face mask, mouthpiece, tracheostomy): 1 mL to 10 mL (20% solution) *or* 2 mL to 20 mL (10% solution) every 2 to 6 hours; usual dose is 6 mL to 10 mL of 10% solution three to four times a day

Nebulization (tent, croupette): volume of 10% to 20% solution sufficient to maintain a *heavy* mist in the area for the desired time period

Direct instillation: 1 mL to 2 mL of 10% to 20% solution every 1 to 4 hours via a tracheostomy tube or tracheal cannula

Diagnostic bronchography: 1 mL to 2 mL (20% solution) *or* 2 mL to 4 mL (10% solution) by nebulization or direct instillation before diagnostic procedure

Antidote to acetaminophen overdosage (oral use: 20% is diluted with soft drinks to a final concentration of 5%; dilutions should be used within 1 hour; undiluted solutions may be kept refrigerated up to 96 hours) Initially, 140 mg/kg is given as a loading dose followed by 70 mg/kg every 4 hours thereafter for a total of 17 doses, *unless* an acetaminophen assay reveals a nontoxic plasma level

If the patient vomits within 1 hour of any dose, the dose should be repeated. Refer to the package instructions for further diluting and dosing instructions.

SIGNIFICANT ADVERSE REACTIONS

Nausea, vomiting, rhinorrhea, stomatitis, fever, tracheal and bronchial irritation, chest tightness, bronchospasm, and dermal eruptions

CONTRAINDICATIONS

No absolute contraindications. *Cautious use* in patients with bronchial asthma, and in elderly or debilitated patients with respiratory insufficiency

INTERACTIONS

Acetylcysteine is incompatible in solution with many antibiotics (e.g., tetracyclines, amphotericin B, sodium ampicillin, erythromycin) and should not be mixed in the same solution

NURSING CONSIDERATIONS

Nursing Alerts

- Closely observe asthmatic patient. Drug should be discontinued at first sign of bronchospasm. If necessary, a bronchodilator may be given by inhalation.
- Ensure that patient expectorates liquefied secretions. If coughing is inadequate, mucus may be aspirated mechanically.
- When used to prevent acetaminophen-induced hepatotoxicity, administer as soon as possible after ingestion of acetaminophen. Effectiveness is greatly reduced if given later than 18 hours after acetaminophen poisoning.

1. Use only nebulizers that have a compressed air source. Ordinary hand-held bulb nebulizers should not be used because output is too small and particle size of drug is too large.
2. Dilute nebulizing solution if indicated. The 20% solution may be diluted with sterile normal saline or sterile water for injection, whereas the 10% solution is usually used undiluted.
3. Ensure that patient clears airway by productive coughing before inhaling drug.
4. Prepare patient for the disagreeable, rotten egg–like odor that may be noticeable initially but will soon become less apparent.
5. Be prepared to assist patient if odor causes nausea or vomiting.
6. During prolonged nebulization, dilute the nebulizing solution to prevent extreme concentration, which might impair proper drug delivery.
7. Following use, wash patient's face, the mask, and the container with water because drug leaves a sticky coating.
8. Avoid contact of drug solution with rubber, iron, or copper because they can discolor solution and possibly reduce its potency.
9. Store unused portion of solution in refrigerator and use within 96 hours to minimize contamination. A light purple color may appear, but it does not impair drug's effectiveness.

COMBINATION COUGH MIXTURES

Although this chapter has dealt with individual antitussive and expectorant drugs, the most frequent use of these products is in combination cough mixtures. Such formulations may contain several other types of drugs in addition to an antitussive and an expectorant. The most commonly used of these additional agents are listed below, along with the rationale for their inclusion.

- *Analgesics*
  For example, aspirin, acetaminophen, sodium salicylate; used to provide relief of headache, fever, and muscle aches often accompanying an upper respiratory condition (see Chap. 19)

- *Anticholinergics*
  For example, atropine, belladonna alkaloids, methscopolamine; employed for their drying action on mucous membranes, thus are only beneficial in conditions characterized by excessive secretions (e.g., rhinorrhea); should be avoided in chronic obstructive pulmonary diseases (see Chap. 11)
- *Antihistamines*
  For example, chlorpheniramine, pyrilamine; provide symptomatic relief of running nose, sneezing, itching, watery eyes; may be effective in relieving chronic cough resulting from postnasal drip (e.g., allergic rhinitis, chronic sinusitis); exhibit an anticholinergic (drying) action, therefore should not be used in respiratory conditions characterized by excessive congestion; most have a sedative effect (see Chap. 14)
- *Bronchodilators*
  For example, ephedrine, theophylline; relax bronchiolar smooth muscle, thus are of greatest benefit in conditions characterized by excessive bronchiolar muscle tone (e.g., asthma) rather than mucus accumulation (see Chap. 55)
- *Decongestants*
  For example, phenylephrine, phenylpropanolamine, pseudoephedrine; used to reduce mucosal congestion by activating alpha-adrenergic receptor sites, thus eliciting vasoconstriction; probably not significantly effective and can lead to systemic side effects (e.g., hypertension; see Chap. 12)

The principal disadvantage of combination products is that the fixed dosage ratio of the ingredients precludes adjusting the dosage of each drug according to the needs of the patient. Moreover, the "shotgun" approach to drug therapy—inclusion of several different kinds of drugs in one preparation—is usually unnecessary from a therapeutic standpoint and most often simply increases the likelihood of untoward reactions without significantly improving the *desired* therapeutic effect. Finally, the cost of combination formulas is frequently in excess of the cost of the necessary individual ingredients used separately. Nevertheless, antitussive and expectorant combinations remain the most widely used over-the-counter preparations for the relief of cough, and it is essential that users of such medications be advised of the potential hazards inherent in the indiscriminate consumption of these readily available cough mixtures.

Selected Bibliography

Bailey BO: Acetaminophen hepatotoxicity and overdose. Am Fam Physician 22:83, 1980

Eigen H: The clinical evaluation of chronic cough. Pediatr Clin North Am 29:67, 1982

Kuhn JJ, Hendley JO, Adams KF, Clark JW, Gwaltney JM: Antitussive effect of guaifenesin in young adults with natural colds: Objective and subjective assessment. Chest 82:713, 1982

Mullan PA: Cough/cold preparations. Am Pharm 21:42, 1981

Prescott LF, Critchley J: The treatment of acetaminophen poisoning. Annu Rev Pharmacol Toxicol 23:87, 1983

Zanjanian MH: Expectorants and antitussive agents: Are they helpful? Ann Allergy 44:290, 1980

SUMMARY. ANTITUSSIVES, EXPECTORANTS, MUCOLYTICS

Drug	Preparations	Usual Dosage Range
Narcotic Antitussives		
Codeine	Tablets: 15 mg, 30 mg, 60 mg Liquid: several combinations with antihistamines, expectorants, etc.	*Adults:* 10 mg–20 mg every 4–6 h *Children (6–12 yr):* 5 mg–10 mg every 4–6 h *Children (2–6 yr):* 2.5 mg–5 mg every 4–6 h
Hydrocodone	Available in combination with expectorants and antihistamines in liquid cough formulations	5 mg up to 4 times/day
Nonnarcotic Antitussives		
Dextromethorphan Benylin DM, Delsym, Pertussin and other manufacturers	Syrup: 5 mg, 7.5 mg, 10 mg, 15 mg/5 mL Controlled-release liquid: 30 mg/5 mL Chewable tablets: 15 mg Lozenges: 5 mg Lozenges (with benzocaine): 2.5 mg, 5 mg, 10 mg	*Adults:* 10 mg–30 mg every 4–8 h *or* 60-mg controlled-release liquid twice a day *Children (6–12 yr):* 5 mg–10 mg every 4 h *or* 30-mg controlled-release liquid twice a day *Children (2–6 yr):* 2.5 mg–5 mg every 4 h *or* 15-mg controlled-release liquid twice a day
Benzonatate Tessalon Perles	Capsules (perles): 100 mg	100 mg 3 times a day (maximum 600 mg/day)
Diphenhydramine Benylin and other manufacturers	Syrup: 12.5 mg/5 mL, 13.3 mg/5 mL (see also Chap. 18)	*Adults:* 25 mg every 4 h *Children:* 6.25 mg–12.5 mg every 4 h

Continued

SUMMARY. ANTITUSSIVES, EXPECTORANTS, MUCOLYTICS (continued)

Drug	Preparations	Usual Dosage Range
Expectorants		
Guaifenesin Robitussin, Humibid, Breonesin, and other manufacturers	Tablets: 100 mg, 200 mg Capsules: 200 mg Sustained-release tablets: 600 mg Sustained-release capsules: 300 mg Syrup: 67 mg/5 mL, 100 mg/5 mL Liquid: 200 mg/5 mL	*Adults:* 100 mg–400 mg every 4–6 h *Children (6–12 yr):* 100 mg–200 mg every 4–6 h *Children (2–6 yr):* 50 mg–100 mg every 4 h
Hydrogen Iodide Hydriodic Acid	Syrup: 70 mg/5 mL	*Adults:* 5 mL in water 3–4 times/day *Children:* 1–10 drops in water 1–3 times/day
Iodinated Glycerol Organidin	Tablets: 30 mg Elixir: 60 mg/5 mL Solution (sugar-free): 50 mg/mL	*Adults:* 60 mg 4 times/day *Children:* Up to ½ adult dose based on weight
Potassium Iodide Pima and other manufacturers	Enteric-coated tablets: 300 mg Liquid: 500 mg/15 mL Saturated solution (SSKI): 1 g/mL Syrup: 325 mg/5 mL	*Adults:* 300 mg–600 mg every 4–6 h *Children:* 150 mg–300 mg every 4–6 h
Potassium Iodide–Niacinamide Hydroiodide Iodo-Niacin	Tablets: 135 mg potassium iodide and 25 mg niacinamide hydroiodide	*Adults:* 2 tablets 3 times/day *Children:* 1 tablet 3 times/day
Ammonium Chloride	Powder/crystals Tablets: 500 mg Enteric-coated tablets: 0.5 g, 1 g	*Expectorant* Adults: 100 mg–400 mg every 4 h *Urinary acidifier* 1 g 3 times/day
Terpin Hydrate	Elixir: 85 mg/5 mL	85 mg every 3–4 h
Mucolytics		
Acetylcysteine Mucomyst, Mucosol	Solution: 10%, 20%	*Nebulization:* 1 mL–10 mL (20%) or 2 mL–20 mL (10%) every 2–6 h *Direct instillation:* 1 mL–2 mL (10%–20%) every 1–4 h *Diagnostic procedures:* 1 mL–2 mL (20%) or 2 mL–4 mL (10%) before procedure *Acetaminophen overdose:* initially, 140 mg/kg *orally*, as a 5% solution; then, 70 mg/kg every 4 h for 17 doses

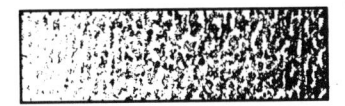

55 BRONCHODILATORS, ANTIASTHMATICS

Drugs capable of relaxing bronchiolar smooth muscle have their principal clinical application in three common respiratory disorders: bronchial asthma, chronic bronchitis, and emphysema. Although these three diseases differ in etiology and overall pathology, they share one important common characteristic, namely a reduced respiratory flow. The extent to which these *chronic obstructive pulmonary diseases* (COPDs) respond to bronchodilator therapy, however, is dependent in large measure on whether the increased resistance to airflow is primarily due to excessive bronchiolar smooth muscle tone, to the presence of mucus, or to obstructive lesions within the bronchiolar network. The mechanisms operative in the regulation of bronchiolar muscle tone are outlined in Chapter 53, Figure 53-1.

The most common of these COPDs is bronchial asthma, a bronchospastic disease characterized by increased airway resistance frequently manifested as coughing, wheezing, shortness of breath, and dyspnea.

Major factors contributing to the heightened airway resistance are respiratory muscle spasm, thickening of the respiratory mucosa related to edema, and excessive secretion of viscous mucus. Bronchospasm associated with asthma is frequently caused by increased responsiveness of bronchiolar smooth muscle to external stimuli such as dust and pollen, which trigger, by way of an antigen–antibody reaction, release of endogenous allergenic mediators (e.g., histamine, leukotrienes, eosinophil chemotactic factor) from mast cells (see Fig. 53-1). These substances then interact with bronchiolar smooth muscle cells to cause contraction. Asthma of this type is often termed *extrinsic asthma* or *atopic asthma*. It is commonly noted in younger persons and usually becomes progressively more severe. A second important mechanism contributing to bronchospasm is activation of parasympathetic reflex pathways, which appear to become hypersensitive in many persons with asthma. This reflex parasympathetic response triggers release of acetylcholine (ACh) from vagal nerve endings and may be elicited by the allergens extruded from the mast cells, although many other nonimmunologic factors, such as cold, stress, infection, or exercise, can also trigger an attack. ACh constricts bronchiolar smooth muscle cells, thereby narrowing the airways. This form of asthma has been termed intrinsic, and most attacks of this type can *not* be related to exposure to antigens. Because the increased airway resistance is muscular in origin, it frequently responds to systemic or local bronchodilators, and these drugs in fact represent the mainstay in the treatment of bronchial asthma.

Other chronic obstructive diseases of the respiratory tract may be related to excessive mucus accumulation within the tracheobronchial tree, as in chronic bronchitis or in loss of elasticity of terminal bronchiolar walls with an increase in dead air space, as occurs in emphysema. These latter conditions respond much less favorably to bronchodilator drugs, although the drugs are of some benefit as part of an overall regimen which may also include mucolytics and expectorants.

Distinction must be made between the therapeutic aims in treating acute versus chronic bronchospastic conditions. Sudden bronchial constriction, as seen during acute attacks of asthma, requires immediate and vigorous therapy and may be treated with epinephrine SC or IM, or, in less acute situations, one of the inhaled adrenergic bronchodilators. Intravenously administered aminophylline can also be useful in terminating acute asthmatic attacks. Maintenance therapy of the COPDs, on the other hand, is directed toward decreasing the overall tone and responsiveness of bronchiolar smooth muscle, which is usually considerably higher in the asthmatic person as compared with the nonasthmatic. Further, treatment is also intended to help keep the respiratory passages free of obstructions, thus reducing the incidence and severity of acute bronchospastic attacks. To accomplish these aims, a variety of pharmacologic agents are often employed, including oral or inhaled bronchodilators (e.g., aminophylline, beta-adrenergic agonists, anticholinergics), expectorants, mucolytics, corticosteroids, and cromolyn, an agent that has a prophylactic effect in certain asthmatic patients. In addition, persons with bronchospastic disorders should employ adjunctive measures such as adequate hydration, cessation of smoking, and avoidance of precipitating factors such as irritants, cold, and allergens to minimize the disturbing symptoms associated with these diseases and to avoid potentially dangerous complications.

The majority of drugs useful in bronchial asthma, such as xanthines, inhaled corticosteroids, ipratropium, and cromolyn, are considered in this chapter. However, the most widely used group of antiasthmatic agents are the adrenergic bronchodilators, which were reviewed in detail in Chapter 12. In addition, expectorants and mucolytics are sometimes employed adjunctively, and they are discussed in Chapter 54.

XANTHINE DERIVATIVES

Aminophylline   Oxtriphylline
Dyphylline   Theophylline

The methylated xanthine derivatives (methylxanthines) include theophylline, its soluble salts (e.g., aminophylline, oxtriphylline), and a chemically related derivative, dyphylline. These products are available in a number of different dosage forms. Theophylline itself has been used as an effective bronchodilator for over a quarter of a century, and many of the problems associated with its early use—GI upset, poor or erratic absorption—have been largely overcome by the synthesis of various theophylline salts as well as by the incorporation of theophylline into different dosage vehicles. Clinical efficacy is a direct function of theophylline plasma levels, and the desired therapeutic range has traditionally been given as 10 μg/mL to 20 μg/mL. Toxicity is common above 20 μg/mL, and recent studies indicate there is little additional bronchodilation above 10 μg/mL to 12 μg/mL. Thus, many clinicians are maintaining theophylline plasma levels at these lower values to reduce the incidence of adverse effects.

Principal reasons for the variation in theophylline plasma levels are:

- Variations in anhydrous theophylline content among different preparations
- Varying rates of absorption, metabolism, and elimination

- Altered availability of theophylline from different dosage forms
- Age and health status of the patient. A closer look at some of these factors is presented below.

Because of differences in anhydrous theophylline base content, the available salt preparations are not therapeutically equal on a weight basis, and equivalent doses of the theophylline products can differ by as much as 100%. Table 55-1 lists the percentage of theophylline base and approximate equivalent doses for each clinically available preparation. These differences become important if patients are transferred from one theophylline product to another, because the plasma concentration, and thus clinical efficacy, varies directly with the intake of *theophylline base*.

Oral absorption of theophylline appears to be related primarily to the dosage form. Although it was formerly believed to be poorly or erratically absorbed from the GI tract, most data indicate that theophylline is inherently well absorbed, tablet disintegration being the major rate-limiting step. Thus, oral liquids are the most rapidly absorbed form of theophylline, followed very closely by uncoated tablets, especially if they are chewed. In contrast, enteric-coated or sustained-release forms of the drug may be erratically or incompletely absorbed and can yield variable plasma levels. However, newer continuous-release formulations have provided more consistent serum drug levels for up to 12 hours and represent a major advance in the chronic treatment of asthma. They are especially useful for maintenance therapy during the night, when the duration of action of *inhaled* bronchodilators is often too short to provide nighttime control.

The presence of food generally has little effect on theophylline availability, although oral absorption may be somewhat slower when food is present than from an empty stomach. Rectal absorption in adults is generally considered to be slow and unreliable with suppositories but nearly equivalent to oral absorption when concentrated rectal solutions are used. IM administration yields effective serum levels about equal to those of oral dosing, although not quite so rapidly as with use of oral liquids.

Rates of metabolism and excretion of theophylline also vary widely. Hepatic metabolism is extensive (80%–90%), and the major metabolite is 3-methylxanthine, which exhibits approximately one third to one half the bronchodilator activity of theophylline itself. The plasma elimination half-life can range from 3 to 12 hours in adults and 1½ to 9 hours in children (see Fate). Decreased clearance is noted in patients with heart failure, liver dysfunction, respiratory infections, prolonged fever, obesity, and pulmonary edema, whereas smoking enhances plasma clearance. Children over 9 years of age generally respond to theophylline in a manner similar to adults, and should be given comparable doses. Younger children require higher infusion rates and larger oral doses of theophylline than adults to maintain effective plasma concentrations. However, some children are unusually sensitive to the CNS-stimulating effects of theophylline, and caution is recommended when administering this drug to pediatric patients.

Dosage must, of course, be individually adjusted and carefully titrated, and serum levels maintained in the range of 10 μg/mL to 20 μg/mL for optimal therapeutic effect. To achieve a rapid effect, an initial loading dose can be given, although many clinicians prefer to start at lower doses and gradually increase the dosage based upon the response. Dosage adjustments are usually made on the basis of clinical signs and careful monitoring of toxicity. Once the plasma levels have stabilized, they tend to remain constant so long as the dose and dosage form are kept consistent. Dosage intervals with immediate-release products are usually maintained at 6 hours in children and nonsmoking adults to provide stable blood levels, whereas sustained-release formulations may be given to nonsmokers every 12 hours. Smokers, however, may require sustained-release dosage forms every 8 hours owing to the increased rate of theophylline clearance. IV administration of aminophylline is usually accomplished by giving an initial loading dose over a 20- to 30-minute period, followed by a continuous maintenance infusion (see Dosage, below).

Owing to the difficulties in individualizing theophylline dosage, the use of fixed-combination bronchodilator products (e.g., theophylline, ephedrine, sedatives, or expectorants) should be strongly discouraged. Although frequently employed, such combination formulations do not allow the dosage flexibility necessary in bronchodilator therapy, and they may increase the overall incidence of untoward reactions. Moreover, inclusion of barbiturates in these preparations may enhance the

Table 55-1
Theophylline Content of Xanthine Derivatives

Preparation	Percent Theophylline Base	Equivalent Dosage
Theophylline, anhydrous	100%	100 mg
Aminophylline anhydrous	86%	115 mg
Aminophylline dihydrate	79%	127 mg
Dyphylline	a	a
Oxtriphylline	64%	156 mg
Theophylline sodium glycinate	49%	204 mg

[a] A derivative of theophylline that is *not* metabolized to theophylline in vivo; approximately one tenth as potent as theophylline.

hepatic metabolism of theophylline, necessitating use of larger doses to maintain steady-state blood levels. Ephedrine, another frequent inclusion in such formulations, may potentiate the CNS-excitatory action of the methylxanthines.

MECHANISM
Not completely established; appear to competitively antagonize the action of adenosine at its receptors, diminishing its bronchoconstrictive action; other postulated mechanisms include prostaglandin antagonism, stimulation of endogenous catecholamine release and an agonistic action at beta$_2$ receptors in the bronchioles. Also believed to inhibit the enzyme phosphodiesterase, thus increasing levels of cyclic AMP, a bronchodilator; this latter action, however, is negligible at therapeutic plasma levels; other actions include myocardial stimulation, mild diuresis, CNS excitation, increased respiration and gastric acid secretion, glycogenolysis, lipolysis, and release of epinephrine from the adrenal medulla

USES
Symptomatic relief or prevention of bronchial asthma and bronchospasm associated with chronic bronchitis, emphysema, and other obstructive pulmonary diseases

Treatment of bradycardia and apnea in premature infants (investigational use only)

DOSAGE
Highly individual and adjusted on the basis of theophylline serum levels (optimal range 10µg–20 µg/mL); following doses are for *anhydrous theophylline*—refer to Table 55-1 for conversion factors.

Acute Therapy (patients *not* receiving theophylline)

Adults: 6 mg/kg as a loading dose, then 3 mg/kg every 6 hours for 2 doses, then 3 mg/kg every 8 hours

Older adults: 6 mg/kg as a loading dose, then 2 mg/kg every 6 for 2 doses, then 2 mg/kg every 8 hours

Adults with congestive heart failure: 6 mg/kg as a loading dose, then 2 mg/kg every 8 hours for 2 doses, then 1 mg to 2 mg/kg every 12 hours

Children 9 to 16 years and adult smokers: 6 mg/kg as a loading dose, then 3 mg/kg every 4 hours for three doses, then 3 mg/kg every 6 hours

Children under 9 years: 6 mg/kg as a loading dose, then 4 mg/kg every 4 hours for three doses, then 4 mg/kg every 6 hours

Acute Therapy (patients currently receiving theophylline)

Initially 2.5 mg/kg; subsequent doses based on serum theophylline levels; each 0.5 mg/kg will raise the serum theophylline concentration approximately 1.0 µg/mL

Prolonged Therapy

Initially 16 mg/kg/day or 400 mg/day (whichever is less) in divided doses every 6 to 8 hours; increase in approximately 25% increments at 2- to 3-day intervals, if tolerated, until optimal response or maximum dose is attained; maximum doses are the following:

Adults: 13 mg/kg/day, or 900 mg
Children 12 to 16 years: 18 mg/kg/day
Children 9 to 12 years: 20 mg/kg/day
Children under 9 years: 24 mg/kg/day

See Table 55-2 for recommended dosage schedules for individual preparations.

FATE
Well absorbed orally, except for enteric-coated and some sustained-release dosage forms; rectal absorption from suppositories is slow and unreliable but concentrated rectal solutions yield good absorption; peak effects differ among preparations and dosage forms, ranging from 1 hour with most liquids to 10 hours with sustained-release tablets and capsules; plasma elimination half-life of theophylline averages 7 to 9 hours in adult nonsmokers, 4 to 5 hours in adult smokers, and 3 to 5 hours in children; decreased plasma clearance occurs in patients with congestive heart failure, liver dysfunction, pulmonary edema, cor pulmonale, respiratory infections, and in alcoholism; metabolized in the liver to several metabolites, which are excreted largely in the urine; less than 15% of the drug is eliminated unchanged

COMMON SIDE EFFECTS
GI upset, nausea, nervousness, urinary frequency

SIGNIFICANT ADVERSE REACTIONS
GI: vomiting, hematemesis, diarrhea, intestinal bleeding, activation of ulcer pain

CNS: restlessness, dizziness, insomnia, muscle twitching, headache, reflex hyperexcitability, depression, speech difficulties, tonic or clonic convulsions

Cardiovascular: palpitations, tachycardia, flushing, hypotension, extrasystoles, circulatory failure

Renal: diuresis, dehydration, proteinuria

Other: tachypnea, respiratory arrest, fever, hyperglycemia, rectal irritation and strictures with use of suppositories

Rapid IV injection can result in flushing, palpitations, dizziness, hyperventilation, hypotension, and anginalike pain.

CONTRAINDICATIONS
Severe peptic ulcer, active gastritis, and in patients in whom myocardial stimulation might prove dangerous. *Cautious use* in patients with acute cardiac disease, renal or hepatic disease, severe hypoxemia, hypertension, myocardial damage, congestive heart failure, glaucoma, hyperthyroidism, diabetes, prostatic hypertrophy; in pregnant or nursing mothers, and in children and alcoholics

INTERACTIONS
Xanthines may increase the CNS stimulation seen with amphetamines, ephedrine, and other sympathomimetic drugs

Increased theophylline plasma levels (decreased clearance) may occur with use of cimetidine, allopurinol, influenza virus vaccine, oral contraceptives, erythromycin, clindamycin, lincomycin, and troleandomycin

The effects of theophylline may be decreased by nicotine, marijuana, aminoglutethimide, and phenobarbital due to hepatic enzyme induction

Xanthines can increase the excretion of lithium and phenytoin, and decrease their effectiveness

Xanthines and beta-adrenergic blocking agents may be mutually antagonistic

Xanthines can enhance the diuretic action of other types of diuretics

The toxicity of digitalis glycosides may be increased by xanthines

Tachycardia can result when xanthines are given together with reserpine

Table 55-2
Xanthine Bronchodilators

Drug	Preparations	Usual Dosage Range	Nursing Implications
Aminophylline Amoline, Phyllocontin, Somophyllin, Truphylline (CAN) Corophyllin, Palaron	Tablets: 100 mg, 200 mg Timed-release tablets: 225 mg Liquid (alcohol-free): 315 mg/15 mL Suppositories: 250 mg, 500 mg Rectal solution: 300 mg/5mL Injection (IV): 250 mg/10 mL, 500 mg/20 mL Injection (IM): 500 mg/2 mL Injection (with 0.45% sodium chloride): 100 mg/100 mL, 200 mg/100 mL	*Oral* Adults: 500 mg initially, then 200 mg–300 mg every 6–8 h Children: 7.5 mg/kg initially, then 5 mg/kg–6 mg/kg every 6–8 h *Timed-release tablets* Adults and children 12 and over: 1–2 tablets every 8–12 h before meals and at bedtime *Rectal solutions* Adults: 300 mg 1–3 times/day *or* 450 mg twice a day Children: 5 mg/kg every 6–8 h *Suppositories* Adults: 500 mg 1–2 times a day Children: 7 mg/kg *IM* Adults: 500 mg *IV* Initially: 6-mg/kg loading dose at a rate not exceeding 25 mg/min For continuous infusion: rates (mg/kg/h) are as follows: |	0–12 h	>12 h
---	---	---
Nonsmoking adults	0.7	0.5
Smoking adults and children 9–16 yr	1.0	0.8
Children 6 mo–9 yr	1.2	1.0
Older patients	0.6	0.3
Patients with congestive heart failure	0.5	0.1–0.2		Ethylenediamine salt of theophylline with similar pharmacologic properties; only xanthine derivative used IV for acute attacks of bronchial asthma; sensitivity reactions and dermatitis have occurred, especially with parenteral use; suppositories may produce rectal irritation; IM injections are very painful and should be avoided if possible; use only diluted solutions (25 mg/mL) for IV injection and warm to room temperature; inject very slowly (maximum 25 mg/min) to avoid cardiovascular disturbances, and closely monitor vital signs during infusion. Timed-release tablets are *not* recommended in children under 12; drug is incompatible in IV fluids with ascorbic acid, chlorpromazine, corticotropin, dimenhydrinate, hydralazine, hydroxyzine, insulin, meperidine, methadone, morphine, oxytetracycline, penicillin G potassium, phenobarbital, phenytoin, prochlorperazine, promethazine, tetracycline, and vancomycin
Dyphylline Dilor, Dyflex, Lufylin, Neothylline (CAN) Protophylline	Tablets: 200 mg, 400 mg Elixir: 100 mg/15 mL, 160 mg/15 mL Injection (IM): 250 mg/mL	*Oral* Adults: up to 15 mg/kg every 6 h depending on response Children: 4.4 mg–6.6 mg/kg/day in divided doses *IM* Adults only: 250 mg–500 mg	A chemically related derivative of theophylline that is *not* metabolized to theophylline in vivo; equivalent to approximately 70% theophylline by molecular weight ratio; claimed to produce less GI upset and fewer overall side effects, but blood levels and activity are somewhat lower than theophylline; peak plasma levels occur in 1 h; short half-life (2 h) requires frequent dosing to maintain effective blood levels; inject drug *slowly* IM and aspirate to avoid inadvertent IV injection; excreted essentially unchanged in the urine; specific dyphylline blood levels must be used to monitor therapy; serum *theophylline* levels are *not* indicative of dyphylline levels
Oxtriphylline Choledyl (CAN) Apo-Oxtriphylline, Chophylline, Novotriphyl	Tablets: 100 mg, 200 mg Sustained-release tablets: 400 mg, 600 mg Elixir: 100 mg/5 mL Syrup: 50 mg/5 mL (pediatric)	Adults: 200 mg 4 times a day *or* 400 mg–600 mg sustained action tablets every 12 h Children: 3.6 mg/kg 4 times a day (100 mg/60 lb)	Choline salt of theophylline containing 64% theophylline; claimed to be more uniformly absorbed and more stable than theophylline and to pro-

Continued

Table 55-2
Xanthine Bronchodilators (continued)

Drug	Preparations	Usual Dosage Range	Nursing Implications
			duce less GI distress and tolerance; regular tablets are partially enteric coated, which delays onset but not completeness of absorption
Theophylline Aerolate, Bronkodyl, Elixophyllin, Slo-Phyllin, Somophyllin, Theo-Dur and other manufacturers (CAN) Pulmophylline, PMS Theophylline	Tablet: 100 mg, 125 mg, 200 mg, 225 mg, 250 mg, 300 mg Timed-release tablets: 100 mg, 200 mg, 250 mg, 260 mg, 300 mg, 400 mg, 450 mg, 500 mg Capsules: 100 mg, 200 mg, 250 mg Timed-release capsules: 50 mg, 60 mg, 65 mg, 100 mg, 125 mg, 130 mg, 200 mg, 250 mg, 260 mg, 300 mg Encapsulated powder (Theo-Dur Sprinkle): 50 mg, 75 mg, 125 mg, 200 mg Elixir: 80 mg/15 mL, 150 mg/15 mL Liquid (alcohol-free): 80 mg/15 mL, 150 mg/15 mL, 160 mg/15 mL Syrup (alcohol-free): 80 mg/15 mL, 150 mg/15 mL Suspension: 100 mg/5 mL	*Oral* Adults: 100 mg–250 mg every 6 h *or* 1–2 timed-release preparations every 8–12 h Children: 4 mg/kg to 6 mg/kg every 6 h (see Dosage under general discussion of xanthines)	Standard xanthine derivative widely used as a bronchodilator; available in several dosage forms, allowing flexibility in dosing; sustained-release preparations provide for gradual release of active drug so that they may be given every 8–12 h depending on formulation; a 24-h timed-release preparation is available (Theo-24), but plasma levels may not remain constant for the entire time; liquid formulations may be hydro-alcoholic elixirs or alcohol-free syrups or suspensions; aqueous solutions provide similar serum levels as alcoholic elixirs but lack CNS-depressant effects and are better tasting; some timed-release products may exhibit unpredictable absorption; found in many combination products with ephedrine, sedatives, or expectorants; fixed-combination preparations do not allow individual dosage adjustments that are often necessary to obtain optimal action
Theophylline Sodium Glycinate Synophylate	Elixir: 330 mg/15 mL	Adults: 330 mg–660 mg every 6–8 h Children (6–12 yr): 220 mg–330 mg every 6–8 h Children (under 6 yr): 55 mg–165 mg every 6–8 h	Mixture of sodium theophylline and glycine containing 47% theophylline; claimed to elicit fewer adverse GI effects; infrequently used preparation

Concurrent use of theophylline and tetracyclines may result in an increased incidence of GI side effects

Dosage requirements for nondepolarizing muscle relaxants (e.g., pancuronium) may be increased by concurrent use of theophylline

Antacids can retard the *rate* of absorption of orally administered theophylline, but *not* the overall extent

An increased likelihood of cardiac arrhythmias is associated with concurrent use of theophylline and halothane

NURSING CONSIDERATIONS
See Plan of Nursing Care 11 in this chapter. In addition:

Nursing Alerts
- Observe patient for early signs of possible overdose (see Significant Adverse Reactions). Notify physician if they occur.

- With IV infusion, monitor vital signs and observe closely for development of untoward reactions such as hypotension, arrhythmias, or convulsions, which may be the *initial* signs of toxicity.

1. Question use of liquid formulation containing alcohol because alcohol is *not* necessary for absorption and may be potentially harmful, especially in younger patient.
2. Because IM injection is usually quite painful, advocate use of another route of administration when appropriate.
3. If suppositories are used, insert before meals and keep patient recumbent for 15 to 20 minutes or until defecation reflex subsides. Because rectal absorption is much faster in children than in adults, suppositories should be used very cautiously in children.
4. Assist with evaluation of drug efficacy. Dosage adjustments should be made carefully on the basis of clinical response (e.g., respiratory function, pulse rate, urine output) and

PLAN OF NURSING CARE 11
PATIENTS TREATED WITH METHYLXANTHINE (XANTHINE) BRONCHODILATORS

Nursing Diagnosis: Potential Complication: CNS toxicity secondary to therapy with xanthine drugs
Goal: Patient will incur minimal CNS toxicity related to therapy with xanthine drugs

Intervention	Rationale	Expected Outcome
Administer drug at equally spaced intervals throughout the day (24 h). Monitor results of serum theophylline level determinations.	Unequal intervals of administration cause great fluctuations in serum levels. Because xanthine metabolism varies in individuals, monitoring of serum level and patient response prevents toxicity. Therapeutic range is 10 µg to 20 µg/mL.	Serum drug levels will remain stable. High serum drug levels will be noted.
Monitor patient, especially child, for indications of CNS toxicity, such as insomnia, nervousness, restlessness, headache, and irritability.	Xanthines stimulate the CNS. Children are more susceptible than adults to CNS effects. Severe toxicity may lead to hyperreflexia, muscle twitching, convulsions, and coma.	Indications of CNS toxicity will be detected promptly.
Report indications of CNS toxicity to drug prescriber.	If CNS stimulation is excessive, dosage should be reduced or different xanthine preparation should be used.	Patient will be treated for CNS toxicity.
Minimize environmental stimuli as needed (e.g., noise, number of interruptions to implement nursing care, number of visitors and frequency of visits and phone calls).	A restful environment can limit drug-induced CNS effects by eliminating unnecessary additional stimulation.	Patient's environment will be restful.
Instruct patient to limit intake of beverages that contain caffeine (coffee, tea, cocoa, colas, and many other commercial soft drinks).	Caffeine is a xanthine. Excessive intake of caffeine-containing beverages increases CNS stimulation.	Patient will acknowledge benefit of limited caffeine intake.
Warn patient to avoid other CNS stimulants (e.g., ephedrine, amphetamines) and OTC drugs that contain xanthines.	Other CNS stimulants add to CNS effects of xanthines.	Patient will state types of drugs to avoid.
Teach patient how to recognize and report CNS effects of xanthines.	CNS reactions may herald toxicity, thereby necessitating dosage reduction or change to another xanthine preparation.	Patient will describe drugs' CNS effects and what to do if they occur.
Administer drug at equally spaced intervals throughout the day (24 h). Monitor results of serum theophylline level determinations.	Unequal intervals of administration cause great fluctuations in serum levels. Because xanthine metabolism varies in individuals, monitoring of serum level and patient response prevents toxicity. Therapeutic range is 10 µg to 20 µg/mL.	Serum drug levels will remain stable. High serum drug levels will be noted.
Monitor pulse and blood pressure for tachycardia and hypotension.	Xanthines exert positive inotropic, chronotropic, and dromotropic actions by stimulating beta$_1$ adrenergic receptors. They also dilate peripheral blood vessels.	Signs of cardiac toxicity will be detected promptly.
Report indications of myocardial toxicity to drug prescriber.	Dosage should be reduced or another xanthine preparation used if toxicity occurs.	Patient's cardiac toxicity will be treated.
If hypotension occurs, keep patient in bed until drug effects wear off.	Hypotension may be pronounced in some patients.	Hypotension will not result in injury to patient.
When administering drug IV: 1. Use infusion control device and microdrip infusion set 2. Monitor vital signs every 15 minutes until stable 3. Record intake and output	Xanthines have a low therapeutic index. Very high serum levels from rapid IV administration have resulted in flushing, profound hypotension, dysrhythmias, and cardiac arrest.	IV xanthines will be administered slowly to patient. Adverse effects of IV infusion will be detected promptly.
Teach patient how to recognize and report cardiac effects of xanthines.	Cardiac effects should be reported to prescriber, as they may represent toxicity.	Patient will explain how to recognize and report drug's cardiac effects.
Teach patient how to prevent injuries that can result from dizziness.	Dizziness may occur, especially in the elderly.	Patient will state safety measures to use if dizziness occurs.

Continued

PLAN OF NURSING CARE 11
PATIENTS TREATED WITH METHYLXANTHINE (XANTHINE) BRONCHODILATORS (continued)
Potential Complication: Cardiac toxicity secondary to therapy with xanthine drugs
Goal: Patient will incur minimal cardiac toxicity related to therapy with xanthine drugs.

Intervention	Rationale	Expected Outcome
Instruct patient to limit intake of beverages that contain caffeine (coffee, tea, cocoa, colas, and many other commercial soft drinks).	Caffeine is a xanthine. Excessive intake of caffeine-containing beverages increases myocardial stimulation.	Patient will acknowledge benefit of limited caffeine intake.

See also **Plan of Nursing Care 1** in Chap. 4 and **Plan of Nursing Care 2** in Chap. 7.

---

plasma levels, if possible. When blood is difficult to obtain, saliva levels (approximately 60% of simultaneous plasma levels) may be used.
5. When one xanthine preparation is used instead of another, expect appropriate dosage adjustments to be based on content of theophylline base (see Table 55-1).
6. Carefully check compatabilities before mixing with any other drugs in solution because many incompatibilities exist (see Nursing Implications for aminophylline in Table 55-2).

PATIENT EDUCATION
1. Instruct patient to take oral preparation with a full glass of water and with food, if necessary, to minimize GI upset.
2. Warn patient not to chew or crush enteric-coated or sustained-release formulation because premature release of drug or release of excessive amounts of drug may result.
3. Instruct patient to avoid indiscriminate use of OTC preparations containing medications that can alter respiratory function (e.g., adrenergics, expectorants, antitussives).
4. Inform patient that cigarette smoking may shorten the drug's duration of action, necessitating dosage adjustment (see Dosage).
5. To improve respiratory function, recommend use of adjunctive measures such as adequate fluid intake, humidification of room air, breathing exercises, postural drainage to remove secretions, and avoidance of smoking, irritants, and cold weather.
6. Explain that charcoal-broiled foods may increase theophylline elimination.
7. Recommend moderation in consumption of caffeine-containing beverages (e.g., coffee, tea, cocoa, soft drinks) because large amounts may increase the side effects of theophylline.

INHALED CORTICOSTEROIDS

Beclomethasone   Dexamethasone
Flunisolide   Triamcinolone

Several corticosteroids are available for inhalation in the treatment of steroid-dependent bronchial asthma. These agents are synthetic steroids with glucocorticoid activity, and the basic pharmacology of glucocorticoids is reviewed in detail in Chapter 43. This discussion is limited to their application in treating bronchial asthma, and a listing of the drugs, with recommended doses and pertinent remarks, is given in Table 55-3.

Inhaled corticosteroids are indicated for the control of bronchial asthma in patients who are either presently receiving such therapy systemically or whose condition is inadequately controlled with a nonsteroid regimen. These drugs are generally *not* necessary for relief of bronchial asthma, which can be adequately managed by bronchodilators, or in patients who require corticosteroid therapy only on an infrequent basis. Moreover, they are *not* suitable for control of acute bronchospastic episodes. The advantage of inhaled corticosteroid therapy over systemic therapy is a reduced incidence of adverse effects. Most common side effects with these drugs are throat irritation, coughing, dry mouth, and hoarseness. Oral and pharyngeal fungal infections have occurred but respond promptly to discontinuation of medication and appropriate antifungal medication. An inhaled bronchodilator should be administered several minutes prior to inhalation of the steroid to enhance its penetration into the lungs. Following inhalation, the mouth should be rinsed with water or mouthwash to reduce the likelihood of dry mouth or hoarseness.

Asthmatic patients transferred from systemic to inhaled corticosteroids are at risk for adrenal insufficiency, and deaths have occurred. Chronic systemic steroid therapy suppresses hypothalamic–pituitary–adrenal (HPA) function through a negative feedback mechanism. However, systemic steroid levels remain high owing to the presence of the exogenously administered steroid. Following withdrawal of systemic steroids, many months are often required for HPA function to return to normal, and the inhaled steroid can no longer supply the high plasma concentrations of exogenous steroid. During this period (i.e., while patients are being transferred from systemic steroid to inhaled steroid and for several months thereafter), symptoms of adrenal insufficiency can occur if a sudden demand is made on adrenal function, such as with trauma, stress, severe infection, or surgery. Thus, during periods of stress or in the event of an acute asthmatic attack, patients receiving only inhaled corticosteroids should *immediately* resume systemic steroid treatment and contact their physician for further instructions. Although the inhaled steroid is usually sufficient to control asthmatic symptoms during transfer periods, it can *not* provide the systemic steroid necessary in these emergencies.

Transfer from systemic to inhaled steroid must be accomplished gradually. The aerosol should be initiated while the patient is still receiving normal maintenance doses of systemic

Table 55-3
Inhaled Corticosteroids Used in Bronchial Asthma

Drug	Preparations	Usual Dosage Range	Nursing Implications
Beclomethasone Beclovent, Vanceril	Aerosol: each activation delivers approximately 42 µg	Adults: 2 inhalations 3 or 4 times a day up to 20 inhalations/day in severe asthma Children: 1 to 2 inhalations 3 or 4 times a day up to 10 inhalations a day	Systemic absorption is rapid, and drug and metabolites are eliminated primarily in the feces; improvement in symptoms is noted in 1 to 4 wk; not recommended in children under 6 yr
Dexamethasone Decadron	Aerosol: each activation releases 84 µg dexamethasone	Adults: 3 inhalations 3 or 4 times a day (maximum 3/dose and 12/day) Children: 2 inhalations 3 to 4 times a day (maximum 2/dose and 8/day)	Dosage is gradually reduced when a favorable response is noted; aerolized particles dissolve rapidly in bronchial secretions; systemic absorption is about 50% (higher with larger dosages or more frequent inhalation)
Flunisolide AeroBid (CAN) Bronalide, Rhinalar	Aerosol: each activation delivers approximately 250 µg	Adults: 2 inhalations twice a day (maximum 4 inhalations twice a day) Children (6–15 yr): 2 inhalations twice a day	Systemic absorption is approximately 40%; rapidly and extensively metabolized during first-pass through the liver; half-life is about 2 h; *not* recommended in children under 6 yr
Triamcinolone Azmacort	Aerosol: each activation delivers approximately 100 µg	Adults: 2 inhalations 3 or 4 times a day (maximum 16 inhalations/day) Children (6–15 yr): 1 or 2 inhalations 3 or 4 times a day (maximum 12 inhalations/day)	Drug disappears rapidly from the lungs; blood levels are maximum in 1 to 2 h; the major route of elimination is the feces; *not* recommended in children under 6 yr; improvement is usually noted within 1 to 2 wk

steroids. After 1 week, the systemic steroid dosage should be reduced gradually at 1- to 2-week intervals while the patient is observed for signs of adrenal insufficiency. The importance of a slow rate of withdrawal cannot be overemphasized.

NURSING CONSIDERATION

Nursing Alert
- If patient is being transferred from systemic to inhaled corticosteroid therapy, during, and for at least several months after, withdrawal of systemic corticosteroids, monitor patient for signs (hypotension and weight loss) and symptoms (e.g., weakness, fatigue, depression, light-headedness, muscle or joint discomfort, nausea and vomiting) of adrenal insufficiency, particularly during periods of increased stress, such as trauma, severe infection, or surgery (see explanation above). If these occur, usually the dosage of systemic steroid is temporarily increased and the withdrawal schedule is slowed.

PATIENT EDUCATION
1. If an inhaled bronchodilator is also prescribed, explain importance of inhaling bronchodilator several minutes *prior to* inhalation of corticosteroid (see explanation above).
2. Teach patient correct technique for use of particular inhaler (directions are included with package inserts). Nasal and oral inhalation products are *not* to be used interchangeably.
3. Explain that proper administration is required to ensure that drug is adequately absorbed.
4. Explain that regular use at prescribed intervals is essential to therapeutic effectiveness.
5. Ensure that patient understands that inhaled corticosteroids are not intended to provide immediate relief of acute symptoms. If the patient is not receiving simultaneous systemic steroids, pulmonary function does not usually improve until after 1 to 4 weeks of therapy.
6. Warn patient not to exceed prescribed dosage. If symptoms do not improve within several weeks, the physician should be notified.
7. Instruct patient to rinse mouth and gargle with warm water after each inhalation to remove residual medication. This may delay or minimize the occurrence of dry mouth, hoarseness, and oral fungal infections.
8. Teach patient how to recognize and report indications of oral or pharyngeal candidiasis (e.g., oropharyngeal soreness, presence of white patches or red splotches on oral membranes).
9. Reassure patient that oral or pharyngeal fungal infections usually respond promptly to appropriate therapy (discontinuation of inhaled corticosteroid, antifungal medication) when they occur.
10. Caution patient not to discontinue medication sud-

denly without appropriate consultation. After prolonged usage, if inhaled corticosteroids need to be discontinued, they should be terminated gradually under medical supervision.

ANTICHOLINERGICS

Anticholinergic agents are effective bronchodilators, and the naturally occurring belladonna alkaloids (e.g., atropine) have been used for hundreds of years in treating bronchial asthma. Unfortunately, the wide range of side effects associated with *systemic* anticholingeric drugs greatly limits their usefulness in the management of bronchoconstrictive disorders. However, the clarification of the role played by the parasympathetic nervous system in intrinsic (i.e., nonallergic) forms of asthma has brought about a resurgence of interest in cholinergic antagonists as potential therapeutic agents for treating bronchial asthma. These mechanisms are outlined in the introductory section of the chapter.

Ipratropium
Atrovent

MECHANISM

Ipratropium is a quaternary ammonium compound that, following oral inhalation, exerts an anticholinergic action in the bronchioles to prevent the increase in cyclic GMP resulting from parasympathetic nerve activation. Thus, drug blocks the contraction of bronchiolar smooth muscle and the increase in mucus secretion resulting from increased vagal (i.e., parasympathetic) activity. In addition, it may inhibit acetylcholine-induced release of allergenic mediators from the mast cells; interpatient variation in the bronchial response to ipratropium appears to be substantial

USES

Treatment of bronchospasm associated with chronic obstructive lung diseases, such as asthma, chronic bronchitis, or emphysema

DOSAGE

2 inhalations (delivering 18 μg each) 4 times a day, to a maximum of 12 inhalations within 24 hours

FATE

Much of an inhaled dose is swallowed, and is eliminated in the feces; systemic absorption is minimal because of the quaternary configuration of the drug, which lowers its lipid solubility; bronchodilation begins within minutes and reaches maximum within 30 to 60 minutes; duration is 4 to 6 hours; elimination half-life is about 2 hours following inhalation

COMMON SIDE EFFECTS

Coughing, dryness of the oropharynx, gastric upset, nervousness

SIGNIFICANT ADVERSE REACTIONS

Headache, dizziness, palpitations, skin rash, blurred vision; rarely, tachycardia, drowsiness, coordination difficulties, itching, constipation, tremor, paresthesias, and mucosal ulceration

CONTRAINDICATIONS

Treatment of acute bronchospastic episodes. *Cautious* use in patients with narrow-angle glaucoma, prostatic hypertrophy, or bladder neck obstruction, and in in pregnant women, nursing mothers, and young children

PATIENT EDUCATION
1. Teach patient correct procedure for using inhaler (directions are on package insert). Treatment failure is often due to improper administration. If patient has difficulty mastering technique, extenders are available for metered dose inhalers.
2. Inform patient that rinsing mouth after each treatment may help to relieve bitter taste and dry mouth.

In addition to ipratropium, an inhaled dosage form of atropine sulfate may also be useful in preventing broncial spasm, although systemic side effects are more likely with atropine because of its greater systemic absorption. *Dey-Dose Atropine Sulfate* is administered by a nebulizer three to four times a day, 0.025 mg/kg of atropine sulfate diluted with 3 mL to 5 mL of saline provides bronchodilation without significant changes in heart rate or salivation. Bronchodilator activity varies inversely with the degree of preexisting airway obstruction and appears to be more marked on large airways compared to smaller airways. The effects of atropine are largely additive to those of inhaled beta agonists. Systemic absorption of atropine can occur, and doses greater than 2.5 mg are likely to cause increased side effects with little improvement in clinical efficacy. Adverse reactions include dry mouth, flushing, blurred vision, headache, tachycardia, slurred speech, and confusion.

ASTHMA PROPHYLACTIC AGENT

Cromolyn Sodium
Intal
(CAN) Fivent

An adjunctive agent for the management of severe bronchial asthma, cromolyn may decrease the severity of the clinical symptoms of asthma, reduce the requirements for concomitant drug therapy, or both. It is strictly a prophylactic drug and possesses no intrinsic bronchodilator, antihistaminic, or anti-inflammatory activity. It is of no value in the treatment of acute asthmatic attacks. The drug is available for oral inhalation as powder-containing capsules, a solution for nebulization, and an aerosol spray; no significant difference in effectiveness has been demonstrated between these three dosage forms, although the aerosol appears to be the most patient-accepted dosage form. Cromolyn is also marketed as a *nasal* spray (Nasalcrom) for treatment of chronic allergic rhinitis and as *ophthalmic* drops (Opticrom) for treatment of allergic ocular disorders such as allergic keratoconjunctivitis or vernal keratitis. These latter two dosage forms are considered briefly following the discussion of the orally inhaled form of cromolyn.

MECHANISM

Stabilizes the mast cell membrane, thereby inhibiting the release of endogenous allergens such as histamine and leukotrienes from mast cells that normally occurs following exposure to specific antigens.

USES

Prophylactic management of severe, perennial bronchial asthma (reduces severity of symptoms or bronchodilator drug dosage requirements). Improvement is usually noted within 4 weeks

Prevention of exercise-induced bronchospasm

Symptomatic control of chronic allergic rhinitis (Nasalcrom) or ocular allergies (Opticrom)—see below

Investigational uses include treatment of food allergies, systemic mastocytosis, eczema, dermatitis, urticaria pigmentosa, chronic urticaria, hay fever, and postexercise bronchospasm

DOSAGE

20 mg inhaled four times a day; capsules are placed into inhaler (Spinhaler) and powder is administered according to package directions; nebulizer solution is administered using a power-assisted nebulizer equipped with a suitable face mask. (*Note:* hand-operated nebulizers are not suitable)

Prevention of exercise-induced bronchospasm: 10 mg inhaled 30 minutes to 60 minutes prior to exercise

FATE

Approximately 8% to 10% of dose is absorbed by the lungs following inhalation, then rapidly excreted unchanged in the bile and urine; remainder of dose is either exhaled or swallowed and then excreted in the feces (GI absorption is poor); elimination half-life is 80 to 90 minutes

COMMON SIDE EFFECTS

Cough, nasal congestion, pharyngeal irritation,

SIGNIFICANT ADVERSE REACTIONS

Lacrimation, parotid gland swelling, wheezing, rash, urticaria, angioedema, dysuria, urinary frequency, joint swelling, dizziness; *rarely,* hoarseness, myalgia, vertigo, photosensitivity, peripheral neuritis, nephrosis, anemia, exfoliative dermatitis, vasculitis, pericarditis, eosinophilia, and anaphylactic reactions

CONTRAINDICATIONS

Children under 5 years; to abort an acute asthmatic attack. *Cautious use* in persons with impaired renal or hepatic function, and in pregnancy or lactation

NURSING CONSIDERATIONS

Nursing Alerts

- Observe for abatement of an acute attack, clearance of the airway, and ability of patient to inhale adequately. Cromolyn therapy should be initiated only after these conditions have been met. An inhaled bronchodilator may be prescribed for use before each dose of cromolyn to aid penetration into lungs.
- Once patient is stabilized on cromolyn, be alert for worsening of symptoms as attempts are made to reduce dosage to lowest effective level. Symptomatic therapy should be provided as necessary.
- If a steroid-dependent asthmatic patient improves with cromolyn, and appropriate gradual reduction of the corticosteroid dosage is undertaken, closely observe patient for deterioration of condition or symptoms of adrenal insufficiency (see beclomethasone, Chap. 43). Steroid therapy may need to be reinstituted during periods of stress or loss of respiratory control.

1. To ensure sufficient penetration, administer inhalant solution only with a power-operated nebulizer with an adequate flow rate and suitable face mask. Do *not* use a hand-operated nebulizer.
2. Assist with evaluation of drug efficacy. Patient's drug regimen should be reevaluated if no improvement is noted after 4 weeks of cromolyn therapy.

PATIENT EDUCATION

1. Instruct patient to clear airway of as much mucus as possible before inhalation.
2. Teach patient correct procedure for administering powdered capsular form of drug. Instruct patient to follow package instructions carefully, not to swallow capsules, and to avoid exhaling moisture into the capsule inhaler (because drug is in a powder form, moisture may cause particle clumping, which can interfere with proper administration).
3. Instruct patient to avoid inhaling drug during acute asthmatic attacks because it may be irritating to respiratory passages, thus worsening symptoms.
4. Inform patient that cromolyn therapy should not be abruptly discontinued except under professional care because asthma may be exacerbated.

Cromolyn Intranasal

Nasalcrom

(CAN) Nalcrom

Cromolyn is also available as a nasal spray for the management of symptoms of allergic rhinitis. Repeated inhalation of the drug is believed to decrease the occurrence and severity of attacks of allergic rhinitis. One spray is administered into each nostril three to six times a day using the inhaler supplied with the drug cartridge. Side effects are rare and the drug is well tolerated, although there are occasional reports of sneezing and nasal stinging or burning. Headaches, bad taste in the mouth, and epistaxis occur rarely. Nasal passages should be cleared by blowing prior to inhalation. Effects should become apparent within several weeks; however, antihistamines or decongestants will probably be required during this initial period. The need for these drugs should diminish with continued use of intranasal cromolyn.

Cromolyn Ophthalmic

Opticrom 4%

Cromolyn is also used as a 4% solution in the eye for the treatment of allergic ocular disorders. Itching, redness, tearing, or discharge usually diminishes within several days, but treatment is often continued for up to 6 weeks. Dosage is 1 to 2 drops in each eye four to six times a day at regular intervals. Most frequent side effect is a transient stinging or burning on instillation. Other infrequent reactions are ocular irritation; dryness; watery, puffy eyes; and styes. Soft contact lenses should not be worn during treatment, but may be reinserted within a few hours after discontinuation of the drug. Corticosteroids may be used concomitantly.

Selected Bibliography

Au WY, Dutt AK, DeSoyza N: Theophylline kinetics in chronic obstructive airway disease in the elderly. Clin Pharmacol Ther 37:472, 1985

Bukowskyj M: Theophylline: An overview. Ration Drug Ther 22(1):1, 1988

Burton AJ: Asthma inhalation devices: What do we know? Br Med J 288:1650, June 2, 1984

Corticosteroid aerosols for asthma. Med Lett Drugs Ther 27:5, 1985

Dwyer JM: A pharmacological approach to the management of asthma. Nat Drug Ther 18(10):1, 1984

Flenley DC: New drugs in respiratory disorders. Br Med J 266:995, 1983

Fredholm BB, Persson CG: Xanthine derivatives as adenosine receptor antagonists. Eur J Pharmacol 81:673, 1982

Gillilland JL: Asthma Rx: Which drug for which patient? Mod Med 54(3):106, 1986

Gross NJ: Ipratropium, bromide: First of a new class of bronchodilators. IM 8(6):242, 1987

Henney HR et al: Knowledge of nurses and respiratory therapists about using cannister nebulizers. Am J Hosp Pharm 41:2402, Nov 1984

Kirilloff LH, Tibbals SC: Drugs for asthma—A complete guide. Am J Nurs 83(1):55, 1983

Lynch JP: Bronchoconstriction: Drugs that help patients breathe easier. Mod Med 53(1):104, 1985

McDonald G: A home program for patients with chronic lung disease. Nurs Clin North Am 16(2):259, 1981

Morris H: Pharmacology of corticosteroids in asthma. In Middleton E, Reed C, Ellis E (eds): Allergy—Principles and Practice. St. Louis, CV Mosby, 1983

Owens GR: A strategy for the diagnosis and management of asthma. Mod Med 56:84, 1988

Owens GR: New concepts in bronchodilator therapy. Am Fam Physician 352:218, 1986

Petty TL: Drug strategies for airflow obstruction. Am J Nurs 87:180, 1987

Rall TW: Evolution of the mechanism of action of methylxanthines: From calcium mobilizers to antagonists of adenosine receptors. Pharmacologist 24:277, 1982

Shapiro GG, Konic P: Cromolyn sodium: A review. Pharmacotherapy 5:156, 1985

Sustained-release theophylline. Med Lett Drugs Ther 26:1, 1984

Todd B: Precautions in using bronchodilators. Geriatr Nurs Sept/Oct 328, 1984

Wang VA, Dworetzky M: How to manage the asthmatic patient. Drug Ther 13(9):79, 1983

Weissman G: The eicosanoids of asthma. N Engl J Med 308:454, 1983

Wickland S (ed): 24-Hour theophylline—Who can use it? Nurse's drug alert. Am J Nurs 85(4):428, 1985

SUMMARY. BRONCHODILATORS, ANTIASTHMATICS

Drug	Preparations	Usual Dosage Range
Xanthine Derivatives	See Table 55-2	
Inhaled Corticosteroids	See Table 55-3	
Ipratropium Atrovent	Aerosol: 18 μg per actuation	2 inhalations 4 times/day (maximum 12 inhalations/24 h)
Cromolyn Sodium Intal	Capsules: (for inhalation): 20 mg Solution (for nebulizer): 20 mg/2 mL Aerosol: 800 μg per actuation	20 mg inhaled 4 times/day Exercise-induced bronchospasm: 10 mg inhaled 30–60 min before exercise
Cromolyn Sodium, Intranasal Nasalcrom	Nasal spray: 5.2 mg per actuation	1 spray each nostril 3–5 times/day
Cromolyn, Ophthalmic Opticrom 4%	Ophthalmic solution: 4%	1–2 drops each eye 4–6 times/day

VIII

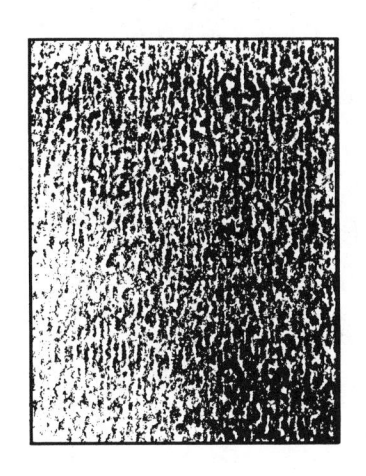

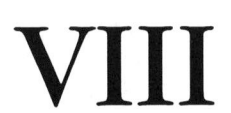

Antiinfective and Chemotherapeutic Agents

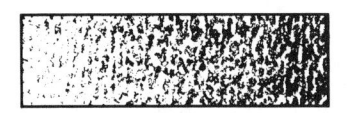

ANTIINFECTIVE THERAPY: GENERAL CONSIDERATIONS

Drugs used for the treatment of infectious diseases may be termed *antibiotics, antiinfectives, antimicrobials,* or *chemotherapeutic agents.* Although these terms are often used interchangeably, the first three, that is, antibiotics, antiinfectives, and antimicrobials, are properly used to describe those drugs commonly employed for the treatment of infections. The designation *chemotherapeutic agent* has come to be more closely associated with those drugs used in the treatment of cancer.

Antibiotics are strictly defined as *natural* substances produced by microorganisms and capable of inhibiting the growth of other microorganisms. Little distinction is made, however, between those substances having a natural origin and those with a synthetic origin. In fact, the term *semisynthetic* is often applied to the product of a chemical alteration of a naturally derived antiinfective compound.

Although the use of substances extracted from soil, plants, or living organisms to kill other organisms has been described for centuries, the modern age of chemotherapy had its origin in the late 1930s and early 1940s with the introduction of sulfonamides and penicillins, respectively. Since that time, a variety of antimicrobial agents with differing mechanisms of action, spectrum, and profile of side effects have become available. Consequently, overall morbidity and mortality caused by infectious diseases has steadily diminished. Nevertheless, the search for newer antiinfective drugs continues unabated, because some infectious diseases still have not been completely eradicated, while other newer diseases are just beginning to appear. In addition, the treatment of some previously susceptible microorganisms by currently available antimicrobial drugs is becoming more difficult because increasing numbers of resistant strains are emerging. Although many different antibiotics are now available to the clinician, enabling a wide range of bacterial infections to be treated successfully, no single agent yet represents the "ideal" antimicrobial drug in terms of spectrum of action, efficacy, safety, and cost.

CLASSIFICATION

Several different characteristics may be used to classify the currently available antimicrobial drugs. However, no single classification is sufficient to completely categorize a particular drug; rather, complete description of any agent requires reference to a number of these characteristics. The most commonly used classifying characteristics are spectrum of activity, antimicrobial activity, and mechanism of action.

Spectrum of Activity

A broad classification of antibiotics divides them according to the range of their antimicrobial activity into broad spectrum and narrow spectrum. Broad-spectrum antibiotics exert their effects against a number of different types of bacteria and other microorganisms. Tetracyclines are, for example, active against a wide range of both gram-positive and gram-negative bacteria, as well as several other categories of microorganisms, such as *Rickettsia, Chlamydia,* and *Mycoplasma* species. Generally, if an agent is effective against both gram-positive and gram-negative organisms, it is referred to as *broad spectrum,* although some broad-spectrum antibiotics are active against a much wider range of organisms than others.

Antibacterial drugs that primarily affect only one group of microorganisms are termed *narrow-spectrum* antibiotics. For example, penicillin G affects only gram-positive bacteria and *Neisseria* at normal therapeutic dosages and therefore is considered narrow spectrum. It is worth noting here, however, that spectrum of activity does *not* necessarily correlate with antimicrobial effectiveness. In fact, because of excessive use and subsequent emergence of resistant strains, many broad-spectrum antibiotics are much less active against many microorganisms than the more selective narrow-spectrum drugs.

Antimicrobial Activity

Antimicrobial agents may also be categorized on the basis of their antibacterial activity as either bacteriostatic or bactericidal. *Bacteriostatic* drugs (e.g., tetracyclines, sulfonamides) suppress the growth of microorganisms without actually killing existing microbes. The invading microorganisms are removed by the host defense mechanisms. *Bactericidal* drugs (such as the penicillins), on the other hand, are capable of directly destroying organisms, especially those in an active state of replication. Theoretically, bactericidal drugs are more desirable from a therapeutic standpoint, but it is important to recognize that their lethal action on microorganisms is dependent on their being present in sufficient concentrations. In subtherapeutic doses, bactericidal drugs are merely bacteriostatic, and conversely, at very high doses some bacteriostatic drugs may exert a bactericidal action. Nevertheless, even the most potent bactericidal drugs is usually incapable of totally eliminating an infection without intervention of the patient's own natural defense mechanisms, such as antibody production, phagocytosis, and leukocyte proliferation. Impaired defense mechanisms can result from disease states (neoplasms, diabetes, hematologic disorders) or drugs (e.g., antineoplastics, corticosteroids) and can severely compromise the action of antimicrobial drugs.

Mechanism of Action

Antimicrobial agents exhibit several different mechanisms of action and may also be categorized on this basis. Most antibiotics exert their effects on microorganisms in one of five ways: (1) by inhibiting synthesis of the bacterial cell wall, (2) by altering cell membrane function, (3) by inhibiting protein synthesis, (4) by inhibiting metabolism of nucleic acid, or (5) by interfering with intermediate cell metabolism.

INHIBITION OF BACTERIAL CELL WALL SYNTHESIS

Examples of drugs employing this mechanism are the penicillins, cephalosporins, and bacitracin. Unlike animal cells, bacteria possess a *rigid* cell wall composed of macromolecules cross-linked by peptide chains. This arrangement maintains the shape of the cell and prevents cell rupture, because most bacteria have a high internal osmotic pressure. Thus, the viability of these bacterial cells depends on the integrity of the cell wall. Drugs acting by inhibiting cell wall synthesis do so by interfering with different steps in the assembly of the peptide chains that impart rigidity to the wall. The weakened cell wall can then no longer support the internal pressure and the cells undergo lysis and disintegrate. Drugs acting in this manner are bactericidal.

ALTERATION IN CELL MEMBRANE FUNCTION

Drugs that alter bacterial cell membrane function include amphotericin, nystatin, and the polymyxins. The semipermeable bacterial cell membrane (located between the cell wall and cytoplasm) helps control the internal environment of the cell by functioning as a selective barrier to extrusion of cell constituents and nutrients. Disruption of this membrane by antibiotics alters its permeability, allowing escape of proteins, nucleotides, sugars, amino acids, and so on, resulting in damage to the cell and ultimately in cellular death. Drugs acting in this manner may be either bacteriostatic or bactericidal depending on the drug, dosage, and organism.

INHIBITION OF PROTEIN SYNTHESIS

The aminoglycosides, erythromycin, and the tetracyclines are among the drugs that inhibit protein synthesis. Certain antibiotics can interfere with ribosomal-mediated protein synthesis in bacterial cells without affecting normal mammalian cells. It is believed that this occurs because the composition of the ribosomes in bacterial cells is different. Antibiotics may disrupt bacterial protein synthesis at several stages; for example, by binding to the ribosomes, blocking attachment of transfer RNA, causing a misreading of the genetic code, interfering with attachment of amino acids to the developing peptide chain, or tying up essential cofactors such as calcium, magnesium, or iron. Drugs inhibiting protein synthesis may be either bactericidal or bacteriostatic.

INHIBITION OF NUCLEIC ACID METABOLISM

Nalidixic acid, rifampin, and trimethoprim are examples of drugs that inhibit metabolism of nucleic acid. Although most agents interfering with nucleic acid metabolism are used as antineoplastic drugs, a few antibacterial compounds act in this manner as well. Nalidixic acid inhibits DNA synthesis, rifampin interferes with DNA-dependent RNA synthesis, and trimethoprim can inhibit dihydrofolate reductase, an enzyme essential for production of tetrahydrofolic acid, an intermediate in the formation of DNA. These drugs are bacteriostatic.

INTERFERENCE WITH INTERMEDIATE CELL METABOLISM

The sulfonamides are a widely used class of drugs that interfere with bacterial cell metabolism. All bacteria require dihydrofolic acid for production of nucleic acids; however, certain bacteria cannot assimilate preformed dihydrofolic acid but must synthesize it themselves from precursors within the cell. An essential precursor is paraaminobenzoic acid (PABA) and because sulfonamides are close structural analogs of PABA, they compete with it for active sites within bacterial cells, impairing synthesis of dihydrofolic acid and thus cell replication. Sulfonamides are bacteriostatic at normal dose levels.

SELECTION OF APPROPRIATE DRUG

Several important considerations go into the choice of a suitable antimicrobial drug for use in a particular patient. The most important of these factors are examined below.

Necessity of Therapy

Even before deciding which antibiotic should be prescribed, the clinician must determine whether antibiotic therapy is necessary at all. Many infectious conditions do not require systemic antimicrobial therapy, and the patient's status and the location and severity of the infection should be carefully assessed before antibiotic therapy is undertaken. Unfortunately, overprescribing of antibiotics, especially in children with "colds" or "flu," occurs to a significant extent and is responsible for an undue number of untoward reactions as well as increased development of resistant strains of microorganisms. Likewise, indiscriminate medication of children by parents with "refillable" antibiotics has contributed to the reduced effectiveness of these drugs in many infectious conditions. Although antibiotics occupy a deservedly important place in pharmacotherapy, they are indeed frequently misused, usually to the detriment of the patient.

Identification of the Pathogen

Accurate determination of the infecting organism or organisms is the cornerstone of safe and effective antimicrobial therapy. Appropriate antiinfective therapy is best accomplished by bacteriologic culture of the infected material (sputum, pus, urine), subsequent isolation and identification of the pathogen, and selection of an antibiotic known to be effective against the offending organism. It is always desirable to have the results of bacterial culturing before initiating antimicrobial treatment, but this is not always practical or feasible. For example, in acute, life-threatening infections (such as septicemia, peritonitis, pneumonia), a delay in initiating treatment of 24 to 48 hours while awaiting results of culture testing can prove fatal and cannot be justified. In these situations, as well as others requiring immediate antibiotic therapy, the initial choice of an antibiotic should be made on the basis of a patient history, physical examination, clinical symptoms, and, most especially, an awareness on the part of the clinician as to what microorganisms are *likely* to be present considering the site of infection and the circumstances under which it developed. In some cases, the probable organism can be determined by the attending physician by performing a simple Gram stain on smears of exudate from the infected area. However, proper bacteriologic culturing is essential for *accurate* diagnosis of the infecting pathogen, and it should be ordered as soon as possible. Once the microbiological information has been obtained, definitive antimicrobial therapy can be initiated. The physician will either continue with the antibiotic prescribed initially if appropriate or change to one that is more active or more selective against the bacterial species shown to be present.

Sensitivity Testing

Because many common microorganisms exhibit varying degrees of antibacterial resistance, once a pathogen has been identified by bacteriologic culturing, the *sensitivity* of the infecting organism to different antimicrobial drugs is often determined. Sensitivity testing, however, is not always necessary, because some microorganisms are uniformly susceptible to certain antibiotics. For example, *Pneumococcus,* group A beta-hemolytic *Streptococcus, Clostrida,* and *Treponema pallidum* respond predictably to penicillin G. Conversely, *Staphylococcus aureus, Streptococcus viridans,* and several gram-negative bacilli (such as *Escherichia coli, Pseudomonas aeruginosa, Klebsiella pneumoniae, Salmonella, Shigella, Hemophilus influenzae*) exhibit varying degrees of resistance to different antibiotics and should be tested for susceptibility in vitro.

The most widely used procedure for sensitivity testing is the Kirby-Bauer or disk diffusion method, in which paper disks containing known amounts of different antibiotics are placed on an agar surface that has been swabbed with bacteria isolated from the patient. After an 18-hour incubation, the size of the clear zone of inhibition around each disk is a measure of the activity of each antibiotic to inhibit the growth of the particular microorganism. Although useful as an index of microbial susceptibility to various antibiotics, the disk method of sensitivity testing measures only growth inhibition and thus is an indication of bacteriostatic activity only. In addition, there are several false-positive reactions to cephalosporins with this method, including enterococci, *Shigella*, and methicillin-resistant *Staphylococcus*.

If *bactericidal* action is essential (as for bacterial endocarditis), demonstration of sensitivity by the disk method is meaningless. In these situations, more reliable tube dilution sensitivity testing may be employed to determine both the minimum inhibitory concentration (i.e., lowest concentration of drug that prevents visible growth after 24 hours) and the minimum bactericidal concentration (i.e., lowest concentration that sterilizes the medium) of an antibiotic against a particular organism. There is frequently a discrepancy between in vitro results and clinical response, owing to a number of factors such as pH, temperature, and the ability of the drug to reach the site of infection. Demonstration of in vitro bacterial susceptibility does not guarantee clinical success but merely provides another parameter on which to base selection of an antimicrobial agent.

Location of the Infection

Generally, once the offending pathogen has been identified and its susceptibility ascertained, an appropriate choice of an antimicrobial agent can be made. However, consideration must also be given to the location of the infection when choosing an antibiotic. The distribution of an antibacterial drug in the body is an important determinant of its ultimate efficacy. Although the concentration of an antimicrobial agent in the body is usually defined in terms of blood or plasma levels, the critical concentration is that which is achieved in the infected tissues themselves. Plasma levels often do *not* accurately reflect tissue levels, and in spite of high plasma concentrations, some drugs may not attain sufficient tissue concentrations at the desired site of action. It is difficult to generalize about the distribution of antibiotics, because the attainment of adequate levels in infected tissue is dependent on a multitude of factors such as dosage and route of administration, protein binding, lipid solubility, presence of tissue fluid or abscesses, pH, site of infection, causative organism, and others. For example, drugs used in meningitis must be able to readily penetrate the CNS (meninges). Drugs excreted largely unchanged in the urine are quite effective in urinary tract infections (provided they are active at a pH of 5 to 6) even though they may exhibit very low plasma levels.

There are, of course, other factors that can influence the choice of an antibiotic; these include severity of the infection, a previous hypersensitivity or serious adverse reaction to a particular drug, patient acceptance of parenteral administration, and cost of the drug. Although proper selection of antimicrobial agents can lead to quick eradication of most infections with minimal adverse effects or complications, injudicious use of antibiotics may ultimately prove harmful to the patient. The decision to initiate antibacterial therapy must be based on careful assessment of the patient and the choice of drugs determined by accurate bacteriologic and sensitivity testing whenever possible. Antibiotic therapy in the absence of proper culturing should be undertaken only with those drugs most likely to be effective against the *suspected* pathogen. It should then be modified if necessary as soon as the culture and sensitivity test results are known. Further, adequate dosage and duration of therapy are essential to ensuring complete drug efficacy. These factors are considered next.

DOSAGE AND DURATION OF THERAPY

The dosage of an antiinfective drug should always be high enough and duration of treatment long enough to provide effective drug concentrations in infected tissues for a suitable period. As indicated earlier, blood levels of the antibiotic do not always reflect tissue concentrations at the infection site; nonetheless, they are frequently used as a guide to determine if proper dosage is being administered. Despite the importance of maintaining treatment long enough to completely eradicate the microorganism, antibiotics are sometimes discontinued too early. The consequence may be either reinfection with the same organism or emergence of mutant strains resistant to the drug being used.

Although different infections require different treatment durations, oral antimicrobial therapy of most common respiratory and urinary infections should be continued for a minimum of 7 to 10 days. Patients may decide to discontinue antimicrobial drugs as soon as the overt symptoms (e.g., fever, sore throat, painful urination) of their disease subside. For this reason, they should be carefully instructed to continue the drugs for at least 48 to 72 hours after symptoms disappear to ensure that the pathogen is completely eliminated. Follow-up cultures are also desirable to confirm the effectiveness of therapy.

More severe infections, such as endocarditis and staphylococcal pneumonia, generally require parenteral administration of higher doses of antibiotics and for longer periods than the more common infections, which can be treated orally. Large doses of antimicrobial drugs may also be necessary in debilitated patients or in patients with disease or drug-impaired defense mechanisms.

In infections characterized by the presence of purulent exudates or large abscesses, drainage of these areas is often necessary; antibiotics frequently are unable to penetrate these infected lesions sufficiently to eradicate the large quantity of pathogens at these sites. Similarly, patients with urinary infections associated with the presence of renal stones will continue to suffer recurrent infections despite the use of antibiotics unless the stones are removed. It is important to recognize that no antibiotic alone can be expected to completely control every infection, and appropriate adjunctive measures are frequently necessary to treat certain types of infections. Additional supportive measures that may be undertaken to facilitate recovery from severe infections include correction of electrolyte or acid–base disturbances, support of respiration, use of antipyretic drugs such as acetaminophen to reduce elevated temperature, and maintenance of an adequate nutritional status.

PROPHYLACTIC USE OF ANTIBIOTICS

The use of antimicrobial drugs to prevent rather than treat infections is a controversial area of antiinfective therapy. Although doubtless effective in certain situations, antiinfective prophylaxis is without proven value in many conditions and may in fact be detrimental in certain instances. There is general agreement that successful chemoprophylaxis is most often attained when a *single* drug known to be effective against a specific pathogen is used to prevent invasion of that pathogen before it has a chance to become established. Some generally accepted indications for antimicrobial prophylaxis are as follows:

- *Penicillin G:* for prophylaxis of group A streptococcal infection in patients with rheumatic heart disease, recurrent cellulitis in lymphedema, and subacute bacterial endocarditis
- *Rifampin or minocycline:* prophylaxis of meningococcal meningitis
- *Isoniazid:* prophylaxis of tuberculosis
- *Doxycycline:* prevention of "traveler's diarrhea"
- *Chloroquine:* prevention of malaria
- *Amantadine:* prevention of influenza A
- *Trimethoprim plus sulfmethoxazole:* prophylaxis of recurrent urinary tract infections and *Pneumocystis carinii* pneumonia
- *Cefazolin or metronidazole:* perioperatively for surgical prophylaxis in "contaminated surgery" such as colonic resection or vaginal hysterectomy

In contrast, conclusive evidence is lacking on the effectiveness of antibiotics used prophylactically in patients with chronic obstructive pulmonary disease; in patients undergoing urologic, dental, or neurologic surgical procedures; and in patients with acute pancreatitis. Finally, chemoprophylaxis is considered to be ineffective in preventing (1) secondary bacterial infection in "common colds," influenza, or other viral diseases; (2) urinary infections in the presence of stones, obstruction, or indwelling urinary catheters; (3) recurring herpes simplex ulcers of the mouth; (4) secondary infections in burn patients; and (5) infections associated with prolonged use of corticosteroids, immunosuppressants, or antineoplastic drugs.

A major danger of chemoprophylaxis is the development of superinfections with drug-resistant strains, the incidence of which is closely related to the duration of exposure to the antibiotic. Therefore, short-term prophylaxis is preferred wherever possible, and antimicrobial drugs used for surgical prophylaxis generally should be given no more than 48 hours preoperatively and 4 to 6 hours postoperatively. Prolonged use of prophylactic antibiotics, as in rheumatic fever, endocarditis, or chronic bronchitis, must be continually monitored and patients closely observed for signs of a developing superinfection (diarrhea, glossitis, perianal or vaginal itching).

Other disadvantages to antimicrobial chemoprophylaxis include an increased incidence of allergic reactions and diarrhea, and frequently a substantially higher cost to the patient.

COMBINED ANTIMICROBIAL THERAPY

Although most infections can be treated adequately with a single antiinfective agent, simultaneous administration of two or more antimicrobial agents is justifiable under certain circumstances. When combination antimicrobial therapy is indicated, it should be accomplished by administration of two or more *individual* drugs whose doses can be titrated independently to provide an optimal effect. The once widespread use of "fixed-dose" antibiotic combinations has essentially been eliminated by the removal of most of these combinations from the market, on the grounds that many contained subtherapeutic amounts of antibiotic drugs, were often ineffective, and favored emergence of resistant bacterial populations.

The primary indications for combination antiinfective therapy are described below.

Treatment of Mixed Bacterial Infections

Some infections (e.g., peritonitis, urinary infections, otitis media) may be complicated by the presence of two, or possibly more, microorganisms possessing different antimicrobial susceptibility. Although broad-spectrum antibiotics are occasionally successful when used alone in such infections, combination therapy is frequently necessary to ensure complete eradication of all pathogens present in mixed infections. Sensitivity testing is essential in such cases.

Initial Treatment of Severe Infections Whose Causative Agent Is Unknown

Before the results of bacteriologic culturing in an unknown infection are obtained, combination therapy is occasionally undertaken to ensure that the widest range of possible organisms is covered. Such treatment, of course, should be modified as necessary as soon as culture and sensitivity data are available.

Postponement of the Emergence of Resistant Strains

Development of resistance to antibiotic agents is often delayed (but not necessarily prevented) when a sensitive pathogen is exposed to two drugs simultaneously. This is particularly apparent with the combined use of two or more antitubercular drugs (e.g., isoniazid, rifampin) or combinations of carbenicillin and gentamicin or tobramycin for severe pseudomonal infections.

Enhancement of Antibacterial Activity

Increased antibacterial activity compared with that of each drug alone is frequently observed with simultaneous use of two antibiotics. This synergistic effect is noted, for example, with an extended spectrum penicillin and an aminoglycoside for pseudomonal infections, with isoniazid and ethambutol in treating tuberculosis, with tetracycline and streptomycin in treating brucellosis or glanders, and with amphotericin B and flucytosine in treating certain systemic fungal infections.

A relatively new combination is the use of a penicillin such as ampicillin or ticarcillin with clavulanic acid, an inhibitor of beta-lactamase enzyme (see below under Resistance). Clavulanic acid prevents the destruction of the penicillin by the beta-lactamase enzymes secreted by certain microorganisms (e.g., staphylococci, *H. influenzae*), thus allowing successful eradication of the microbe by the penicillin drug. Preventing enzymatic destruction can expand the usefulness of certain antibiotics previously ineffective against beta-lactamase–producing organisms.

Reduction of Toxicity

In certain instances, combined antimicrobial therapy is used to reduce the untoward effects of one or more antibacterial agents, especially in cases where the individual drugs are each administered in reduced doses. On the other hand, the addition of a second drug to the regimen, especially at full dosage, can *increase* the likelihood of adverse effects compared to that seen with a single drug. Again, a knowledge of the potential toxicities of the antiinfective drugs is essential in maximizing the therapeutic effects while minimizing the potential for untoward reactions.

As indicated, combination antiinfective drug therapy can result in undesirable effects, reduced clinical effectiveness, and superinfections. For example, combined use of two or more aminoglycosides can increase the incidence of ototoxicity and nephrotoxicity above that observed with each drug alone. Therefore, other than those circumstances outlined above where combination antimicrobial therapy has proved beneficial, use of more than one carefully selected antiinfective drug to treat a particular infectious condition should be avoided.

ADVERSE EFFECTS OF ANTIMICROBIAL DRUGS

A wide range of adverse reactions have been reported with the several classes of drugs used in the treatment of infections, and these are reviewed in detail in the individual chapters dealing with each group of drugs. The most frequently encountered untoward reactions with antibiotics are considered briefly here.

Hypersensitivity Reactions

Both acute and delayed allergic responses have occurred with a number of antimicrobial drugs, most frequently with the penicillins and sulfonamides. These may range from mild dermatologic manifestations such as skin rash, itching, and urticaria, to severe anaphylactic reactions, which have proved fatal in a number of instances. The importance of obtaining a careful patient history before administration of an antimicrobial agent known to be associated with hypersensitivity reactions cannot be overemphasized.

Organ Toxicity

Several classes of antibiotics are known to exert selective toxic effects upon certain structures or organs of the body. For example, aminoglycosides and vancomycin cause both renal and eighth cranial nerve damage. Amphotericin B and polymyxins, among others, impair kidney function while lincomycin and clindamycin often induce severe diarrhea and colitis. Tetracyclines may damage teeth, nails, or bones, and rifampin and the estolate salt of erythromycin can be hepatotoxic.

Superinfection

Development of secondary infections is a potentially serious problem connected with antibiotic usage. It is most often associated with prolonged antiinfective therapy, insufficient drug dosage, impaired host defense mechanisms, concurrent therapy with immunosuppressive drugs, or a combination of these factors. Pathogens frequently responsible for secondary infections include *Pseudomonas, Proteus, Candida,* and drug-resistant staphylococci and fungi. These organisms may be especially difficult to eradicate because they often represent strains resistant to conventional antimicrobial agents. Although superinfection can theoretically occur anywhere in the body, it is found most commonly in the GI tract and may be manifested by diarrhea, glossitis, stomatitis, "furry" tongue, and perineal irritation. Prompt recognition of a secondary infection is critical to its effective management. Therapy is best accomplished by discontinuing the initial antibiotic, culturing the infected area, and administering an antimicrobial drug shown by sensitivity testing to be effective against the new organism.

Resistance

Bacteria are susceptible to eradication by some antiinfective drugs but not others. The phenomenon whereby certain organisms are unaffected by a particular antimicrobial agent is called *resistance.* Bacterial resistance may be broadly categorized as either natural or acquired. *Natural resistance* is genetically determined and may be characteristic of either an entire species or only certain strains within a species. It is not a significant therapeutic problem, inasmuch as the resistance is usually to a particular mechanism of antimicrobial action, and there are usually other antibiotics with different mechanisms of action to which the organism is susceptible. *Acquired resistance,* on the other hand, can develop in previously susceptible pathogens for a number of reasons and is a major clinical problem with many antiinfective drugs. Development of bacterial resistance has severely limited the usefulness of many antibiotics in certain infections.

Unfortunately, the more an antimicrobial agent is employed in clinical practice, the greater the likelihood that resistant strains of once susceptible bacteria will develop. This further underscores the importance of sensitivity testing whenever there is doubt about the susceptibility of an infecting microorganism to a chosen antibiotic. Complicating the picture is the problem of *cross-resistance,* that is, not only the resistance of a certain bacteria to all members of a particular antibiotic group (e.g., penicillins, tetracyclines, sulfonamides) but resistance to other chemically related drugs (e.g., penicillins and cephalosporins) or in some cases to chemically unrelated drugs (e.g., erythromycin and lincomycin). Microbial resistance has presented a serious dilemma in many hospitals where a variety of antiinfective agents must be used to control the many types of infections frequently encountered in this setting. Hospital-acquired infections are referred to as *nosocomial* infections. In these situations, secondary infections occur to a significant extent, and these are often caused, as already indicated, by strains or mutants of pathogens resistant to conventional therapy. Control of these nosocomial infections is therefore often difficult. Of particular concern in this regard are infections caused by methicillin-resistant *Staphylococcus aureus* (MRSA), an extremely difficult infection to control.

Microorganisms can develop resistance to antiinfective drugs in a number of ways, the most important of which are:

- Elaboration of enzymes (e.g., beta-lactamases such as penicillinases or cephalosporinases) that destroy the drug
- Decreased permeability of the microbial cell membrane to certain antibiotics (e.g., tetracyclines, aminoglycosides,

(Text continued on page 566)

PLAN OF NURSING CARE 12
PATIENTS TREATED WITH ANTIBACTERIAL DRUGS

Potential Complication: Hypersensitivity reaction secondary to antibacterial drug therapy
Goal: Patient will either avoid or be treated promptly for an allergic reaction to an antibacterial drug.

Intervention	Rationale	Expected Outcome
Prior to initiating antibacterial drug therapy: 1. Carefully determine whether patient has history of allergic disorders (asthma, hives, hayfever, eczema)	Patients with a history of allergic disorders are at risk for allergic reactions to antibacterial drugs.	Patient will reveal any history of allergy.
2. Ascertain previous reactions to antibacterial agents in general and to particular drug prescribed	A detailed medication history may reveal allergy to prescribed drug or to agent closely related to prescribed drug.	Patient will describe previous reactions to antibacterial drugs.
3. Assist with sensitivity (skin) testing, as needed	Skin testing helps rule out suspected or highly probable allergy to a drug before the drug is prescribed.	Patient's reaction to drug will be determined.
4. Tell patient the name of prescribed drug	Telling the patient the name of the drug before administering it creates one last opportunity for the patient who is allergic to the drug to communicate this information.	Patient with known allergy to drug will so indicate.
Ensure that antihistamines, epinephrine, aminophylline, corticosteroids, oxygen, and emergency equipment are on hand to treat hypersensitivity reactions.	Antihistamines and epinephrine lessen the effects of vasoactive mediators of the allergic response. Epinephrine also relieves bronchoconstriction, as does aminophylline. Corticosteroids reduce effects of the inflammatory response, such as edema and tissue injury.	Drugs and equipment needed to treat an allergic reaction will be readily available.
Withhold drug and seek clarification before initiating therapy with a penicillin or cephalosporin if patient has known allergy to any penicillin drug.	Cross-allergies may occur between drugs within the same chemically related class or between drugs in different chemically related classes. Penicillins and cephalosporins are closely related drug classes. Because cross-sensitization may occur between them (incidence is about 10%), use of cephalosporins for patients with acute penicillin allergies entails some risk.	Patient will not receive drug that might cause allergic reaction.
Monitor patient for development of allergic reaction for at least half hour after administration (especially parenteral) of antibacterial drug, particularly penicillin.	Allergic reactions can occur with any antibacterial agent, especially with parenteral administration. More people are allergic to penicillin than to any other drug, and of all classes of antibacterial drugs, penicillins most often cause acute anaphylaxis.	An allergic reaction will be detected promptly.
With any route of administration, including topical, monitor patient for indications of an allergic reaction, which may be immediate or delayed for up to several weeks: 1. Mild reactions include rash, urticaria, angioedema, fever, and eosinophilia 2. Severe reactions include anaphylaxis, serum sickness, and Stevens–Johnson syndrome.	The patient may develop an allergy to a drug at any time and without any history of previous exposure to the drug.	Indications of an allergic reaction will be detected promptly.
If allergic reaction occurs, discontinue administration of drug immediately, notify drug prescriber, and institute interventions appropriate to nature and severity of reaction.	The drug causing the allergy must be discontinued as quickly as possible to control the reaction.	Patient will be treated promptly for allergic reaction.
Teach patient signs and symptoms of allergic reaction.	The patient should be able to recognize an allergic reaction in order to take appropriate action.	Patient will state signs and symptoms of allergic reaction.
Instruct patient to discontinue drug immediately and to notify drug prescriber if signs of allergic reaction occur.	The patient needs to know what to do if an allergic reaction occurs.	Patient will explain what to do if signs of allergic reaction occur.
Instruct patient with known allergy to carry medical alert information at all times.	Medical alert information helps avert treatment with a drug to which patient is allergic.	Patient will acknowledge value of medical alert information.

Continued

PLAN OF NURSING CARE 12
PATIENTS TREATED WITH ANTIBACTERIAL DRUGS (continued)
Potential Complication: Superinfection secondary to antibacterial drug therapy
Goal: Patient will either avoid or be treated promptly for a superinfection resulting from antibacterial drug therapy.

Intervention	Rationale	Expected Outcome
Assess risk factors for development of superinfection during antibacterial drug therapy according to the following information: 1. Dosage of drug 2. Antimicrobial spectrum of drug 3. Length of drug therapy 4. Number and type of drugs used concurrently	Superinfections develop in about 2% of patients treated with antibacterial drugs. The risk increases when (1) large doses are used, (2) broad-spectrum drugs are prescribed (they widely suppress normal microbial flora), (3) therapy is prolonged, and (4) several drugs are administered simultaneously.	Patient's degree of risk for developing superinfection will be noted.
Monitor patient for indications of superinfection, particularly if a tetracycline is used: abdominal cramping, severe or prolonged diarrhea (especially with use of a cephalosporin), foul-smelling stools, dysuria, foul-smelling urine, recurrent fever, stomatitis, glossitis, white patches on oral mucosa, black or "furry" tongue, vaginal discharge, or severe perineal itching.	Antibacterial agents may reduce the body's normal microbial flora, sometimes causing other, drug-resistant microorganisms to overgrow. The sinuses, mouth, respiratory tract, intestines, genitourinary tract, vagina, or skin may be affected. *Tetracyclines* are more likely to induce superinfections than any other class of antimicrobials; monilial infections are particularly prevalent. *Cephalosporins* sometimes permit a microbe that causes pseudomembranous colitis to proliferate.	Indications of superinfection will be detected promptly.
If drug therapy is prolonged, be prepared to obtain cultures of upper respiratory tract and feces.	With cultures, it is possible to determine changes in bacterial flora that may subsequently be responsible for secondary infection.	Cultures will be obtained from appropriate areas of patient's body.
Notify drug prescriber if indications of superinfection occur.	If a superinfection develops, the antibacterial drug should be discontinued or replaced with another drug to which the organism causing the primary infection is sensitive. The area of the secondary infection should be cultured, and a drug effective against the organism causing the secondary infection may be prescribed.	Patient will be treated for superinfection.
Teach patient mouth, skin, and perineal hygiene measures that help prevent development of superinfection.	Appropriate hygiene helps prevent introduction of microorganisms into susceptible body locations and may help control overgrowth of endogenous microbes.	Patient will state hygiene measures that help deter superinfection.
Teach patient how to recognize and report signs and symptoms of superinfection (see above).	The patient should report possible indications of superinfection to drug prescriber.	Patient will explain how to recognize and report symptoms of superinfection.

Nursing Diagnosis: Knowledge Deficit related to antibacterial drug therapy
Goal: Patient will possess the knowledge and skills to implement antibacterial drug regimen and related actions.

Intervention	Rationale	Expected Outcome
See also **Plans of Nursing Care 1 and 2** in Chapters 4 and 7, respectively.		
As appropriate, explain that antibacterial agents are ineffective against viral infections.	Patients often receive, or expect to receive, antibacterial drugs for colds, flu, or other viral infections.	Patient will acknowledge ineffectiveness of antibacterial drugs in viral infections.
Ensure that patient understands importance of complying with prescribed drug regimen, especially: 1. Completing the full course of therapy (usually at least 7–10 days) 2. Maintaining the prescribed dosage	Patients often discontinue drug therapy before an infection is eradicated because their symptoms have abated. The infection may then relapse or drug resistance may develop. Group A beta-hemolytic streptococcal infection should	Patient will express importance of complying with drug regimen.

Continued

PLAN OF NURSING CARE 12
PATIENTS TREATED WITH ANTIBACTERIAL DRUGS (continued)
Nursing Diagnosis: Knowledge Deficit related to antibacterial drug therapy
Goal: Patient will possess the knowledge and skills to implement antibacterial drug regimen and related actions.

Intervention	Rationale	Expected Outcome
3. Spacing administration times appropriately	be treated for *at least* 10 days to prevent development of acute glomerulonephritis or rheumatic fever. Treatment of all infections should be continued for at least 48 h after symptoms disappear or evidence of bacterial presence is lacking. Adequate dosage and evenly spaced intervals of administration are necessary to maintaining therapeutic blood levels.	
Instruct patient to take oral preparation with a full glass of water on an empty stomach (1–2 h before or 2–3 h after meals) unless otherwise directed. Some drugs (e.g., cephalosporins) may have to be taken with food if GI upset occurs.	Food either decreases or delays absorption of many antibacterial drugs; other antibacterials are acid-labile (destroyed by gastric acid). GI absorption improves when drugs such as these are taken on an empty stomach.	Patient will explain when and how to take drug in relation to food and fluid intake.
Instruct patient to discard leftover medication and to avoid giving drugs to others.	Residual drugs from old prescriptions are probably no longer potent, and they are unlikely to be appropriate for another person.	Patient will explain what to do with leftover medication.
As appropriate, instruct patient to store reconstituted oral liquid formulation in cool place (refrigerator) and to discard contents after period indicated on bottle (usually 10–14 days).	Many antibacterial solutions or suspensions rapidly lose their effectiveness at room temperature and are potent for only a limited period after reconstitution.	Patient will explain storage and disposal of oral liquid drug.
Discuss the importance of adjunctive measures in treatment of infection, such as the following: 1. Adequate nutrition, fluid intake, and rest 2. Prevention of spread of infection	These factors enhance host defenses, improve the effectiveness of antibacterial drugs, and help prevent further infection.	Patient will verbalize importance of adjunctive measures in treatment of infection.

chloramphenicol) that depend upon penetration into the bacteria for their effectiveness
- Development of altered binding sites (e.g., loss of specific ribosomal proteins) within the bacterial cell for certain antibiotic drugs (e.g., aminoglycosides, erythromycins) that normally interrupt ribosomal function by chemically binding to ribosomal proteins
- Development of altered enzymatic or metabolic pathways that either entirely bypass the reaction inhibited by the antimicrobial drug or that become less susceptible to interruption by antibiotic drugs such as sulfonamides
- Production by bacteria of a direct antibiotic drug antagonist (e.g., PABA versus sulfonamides)

In many cases, the emergence of resistant bacterial strains has necessitated the use of less effective and more toxic antimicrobial agents to treat an infection formerly controlled by a more desirable drug. Moreover, the increasing numbers of antiinfective drugs proving ineffective against certain infectious organisms (e.g., staphylococci, gram-negative bacilli) have raised the specter of some diseases eventually becoming largely uncontrollable by the currently available antibiotic drugs. To minimize this possibility, it is essential that antimicrobial drugs be used sensibly and that only those drugs necessary to eliminate the organisms known to be present should be prescribed.

ANTIBIOTICS IN RENAL FAILURE

Kidney function is a major determinant of the response to many antimicrobial drugs. Drugs eliminated principally by the kidney are potentially more hazardous when employed at normal doses in the patient with renal impairment, because the slowed elimination leads to serum levels being more elevated for longer periods. Therefore, clinicians should be aware of the mode of excretion of any antiinfective agent they administer. Further, renal function should be determined not only before administration of an antiinfective agent that is cleared by the kidney but throughout the course of therapy as well, particularly if the course of treatment is prolonged. Antibiotics eliminated largely by the kidneys include the penicillins, cephalosporins, aminoglycosides, polymyxins, vancomycin, trimethoprim–sulfamethoxazole, and most tetracyclines. The penicillins and cephalosporins are relatively nontoxic even at high plasma levels and therefore can be used safely in the presence of limited renal dysfunction. The tetracyclines are cleared by the kidney at varying rates, and those derivatives with extended half-lives (except doxycycline) should not be used when renal function is impaired. The aminoglycosides, polymyxins, and vancomycin will accumulate rapidly when kidney function is reduced;

thus, the dosage or frequency of administration of these drugs must be reduced in the patient with renal impairment. Moreover, these latter drugs are themselves nephrotoxic and thus can elicit or aggravate renal failure, further reducing their own excretion. It is unfortunate that patients with renal failure are often subject to precisely those infections (e.g., gram-negative bacilli) that are usually most responsive to nephrotoxic drugs such as aminoglycosides, thus setting up a potentially vicious cycle. Nevertheless, there are a number of effective antimicrobial agents that may be employed with reasonable safety in patients with kidney impairment, provided that the appropriate dosage adjustments are undertaken. The excretion patterns and related cautions to be observed with the use of each class of antibiotic drugs are noted in the discussions of individual drugs in succeeding chapters.

DRUGS OF CHOICE FOR SPECIFIC INFECTIONS

The selection of an individual antimicrobial agent as a drug of choice for a particular infection is sometimes subject to debate, and opinions often change as new drugs become available or resistant strains of previously susceptible organisms emerge. Nevertheless, some agreement does exist on the first-line drugs for a number of common infections, providing sensitivity tests have confirmed pathogen susceptibility. Although it is by no means definitive, Table 56-1 outlines recommended drugs of choice as well as alternative drugs for the treatment of infections resulting from a number of microorganisms. It also lists the type of organism and the most

(*Text continued on page 572*)

Table 56-1
Antimicrobial Drugs of Choice for Common Infections

Organism	Classification	Representative Clinical Illnesses	Drugs of First Choice	Alternative Drugs
Acinetobacter (*Mima, Herellea*) species	Gram-negative bacilli	Bacteremia, endocarditis, meningitis, urethritis	imipenem	amikacin, gentamicin, tobramycin, netilmicin, doxycycline, minocycline, carbenicillin, ticarcillin, mezlocillin, piperacillin, azlocillin
Actinomyces israelli	Actinomycetes	Actinomycosis	penicillin G	tetracycline, erythromycin
Alcaligenes faecalis	Gram-negative bacilli	Urinary infections, wound infections	chloramphenicol, tetracycline	colistimethate, polymyxin B, gentamicin, kanamycin
Aspergillus	Fungi	Systemic fungal infections, (e.g., skin, lung, bone)	amphotericin B	flucytosine
Bacillus anthracis	Gram-positive bacilli	Anthrax, pneumonia, meningitis	penicillin G	erythromycin, tetracycline, cephalosporins (first generation)
Bacteroides (several strains)	Gram-negative bacilli	Bacteremia, brain and lung abscesses, genital infections, pulmonary infections, endocarditis	penicillin G (oropharyngeal strains) clindamycin, metronidazole, (GI strains, endocarditis)	tetracycline, piperacillin, mezlocillin, azlocillin, chloramphenicol, cefoxitin, cefotetan, metronidazole, imipenem
Blastomyces dermatidis	Fungi	Blastomycosis	amphotericin B	hydroxystilbamidine, ketoconazole
Bordetella pertussis	Gram-negative bacilli	Whooping cough	erythromycin	ampicillin, tetracycline, trimethoprim–sulfamethoxazole
Borrelia recurrentis	Spirochetes	Relapsing fever	tetracycline	penicillin G
Branhamella catarrhalis	Gram-negative cocci	Respiratory infections, sinusitus, otitis media	amoxicillin-clavulanic acid	cefuroxime, cefotaxime, ceftizoxime, tetracycline, trimethoprim–sulfamethoxazole
Brucella	Gram-negative bacilli	Brucellosis	tetracycline with or without streptomycin	chloramphenicol (with or without streptomycin), trimethoprim–sulfamethoxazole

Continued

Table 56-1
Antimicrobial Drugs of Choice for Common Infections (continued)

Organism	Classification	Representative Clinical Illnesses	Drugs of First Choice	Alternative Drugs
Calymmato-bacterium granulomatis	Gram-negative bacilli	Granuloma inguinale	tetracycline	streptomycin
Candida (several species)	Fungi	Local and systemic fungal infections	Systemic: amphotericin B (with or without flucytosine) Gastrointestinal: oral nystatin Local: miconazole, clotrimazole, nystatin	Systemic: flucytosine *alone*
Chlamydia psittaci	Chlamydiae	Psittacosis, ornithosis	tetracycline	chloramphenicol
Chlamydia trachomatis	Chlamydiae	Inclusion conjunctivitis	erythromycin	tetracycline, sulfonamide
		Pneumonia	erythromycin	sulfonamide
		Trachoma	tetracycline	sulfonamide
		Urethritis	tetracycline	erythromycin
		Lymphogranuloma venereum	tetracycline	erythromycin, sulfonamide
Clostridium difficile	Gram-positive bacilli	Pseudomembranous colitis (antibiotic associated)	vancomycin	metronidazole
Clostridium perfringens	Gram-positive bacilli	Gas gangrene	penicillin G	chloramphenicol, metronidazole, clindamycin, tetracycline
Clostridium tetani	Gram-positive bacilli	Tetanus	penicillin G	tetracycline, cephalosporins
Coccidioides immitis	Fungi	Systemic fungal infections	amphotericin B	miconazole, ketoconazole
Corynebacterium diphtheriae	Gram-positive bacilli	Laryngitis, pharyngitis, pneumonia, tracheitis	erythromycin	cephalosporin (first generation), penicillin G
Cryptococcus neoformans	Fungi	Systemic fungal infections	amphotericin B, (with or without flucytosine)	ketoconazole, miconazole
Dermatophytes (tinea)	Fungi	Infections of the skin, hair, and nails	clotrimazole, miconazole	Oral: griseofulvin Topical: tolnaftate, haloprogin
Enterobacteriaceae (*Aerobacter aerogenes*)	Gram-negative bacilli	Urinary infections, bacteremia, wound infections	third-generation cephalosporins	amikacin, gentamicin, tobramycin, mezlocillin, piperacillin, azlocillin, aztreonam, netilmicin, imipenem, carbenicillin, ciprofloxacin, ticarcillin, amdinocillin
Escherichia coli	Gram-negative bacilli	Urinary infections, bacteremia, meningitis, gastroenteritis	ampicillin, with or without gentamicin, tobramycin *or* amikacin	aztreonam, carbenicillin, mezlocillin, piperacillin, azlocillin, cephalosporin (third generation) amdinocillin, norfloxacin, ticarcillin, netilmicin, kanamycin, imipenem, trimethoprim-sulfamethozazole, ciprofloxacin
Francisella tularensis	Gram-negative bacilli	Tularemia	streptomycin, gentamicin	tetracycline, chloramphenicol
Hemophilus ducreyi	Gram-negative bacilli	Chancroid	ceftriaxone, erythromycin	trimethoprim–sulfamethoxazole

Continued

Table 56-1
Antimicrobial Drugs of Choice for Common Infections (continued)

Organism	Classification	Representative Clinical Illnesses	Drugs of First Choice	Alternative Drugs
Hemophilus influenzae	Gram-negative bacilli	Pharyngitis, pneumonia, meningitis, otitis media, tracheobronchitis, epiglottiditis	Life-threatening—cefotaxime, ceftriaxone Other infections—ampicillin, amoxicillin	aztreonam, trimethoprim–sulfamethoxazole, cefuroxime, amoxicillin–clavulanic acid, tetracycline, cefuroxime, cefaclor, sulfonamide, cefaclor
Hemophilus vaginalis (*Gardnerella*)	Gram-negative bacilli	Vaginal infections	metronidazole	ampicillin
Herpes simplex	Virus	Keratitis	Topical: acyclovir, trifluridine	Topical: idoxuridine, vidarabine
		Encephalitis	acyclovir	vidarabine
Histoplasma capsulatum	Fungi	Pneumonia, meningitis, skin, lung, and bone lesions	amphotericin B	ketoconazole
Influenza A	Virus	Influenza	amantadine (prophylaxis)	
Klebsiella pneumoniae	Gram-negative bacilli	Pneumonia, urinary and biliary infections, osteomyelitis	cephalosporin	gentamicin, tobramycin, aztreonam, imipenem, mezlocillin, piperacillin, azlocillin, amikacin, netilmicin, tetracycline, amdinocillin, trimethoprim–sulfamethoxazole, chloramphenicol, ciprofloxacin, norfloxacin
Legionella pneumophila	Gram-negative bacilli	Legionnaires' disease	erythromycin (with or without rifampin)	trimethoprim–sulfamethoxazole
Leptospira	Spirochetes	Meningitis, Weil's disease	penicillin G	tetracycline
Leptotrichia buccalis	Gram-negative bacilli	Vincent's infection	penicillin G	tetracycline, clindamycin
Listeria monocytogenes	Gram-positive bacilli	Bacteremia, meningitis, endocarditis, recurrent abortion	ampicillin (with or without gentamicin)	erythromycin, trimethoprim–sulfamethoxazole
Mucor	Fungi	Systemic fungal infections	amphotericin B	
Mycobacterium (atypical)	Acid-fast bacilli	Lymphadenitis, pulmonary lesions	isoniazid with rifampin (with or without ethambutol)	erthromycin, cycloserine, ethionamide
Mycobacterium leprae	Acid-fast bacilli	Leprosy	dapsone with rifampin	ethionamide
Mycobacterium tuberculosis	Acid-fast bacilli	Pulmonary, renal, meningeal, or other tuberculosis infections	isoniazid with rifampin	streptomycin, pyrazinamide, ethambutol, cycloserine, ethionamide, kanamycin
Mycoplasma hominis	Mycoplasmas	Nonspecific urethritis, septicemia	clindamycin, tetracycline	erthromycin, chloramphenicol, gentamicin
Mycoplasma pneumoniae	Mycoplasmas	Atypical viral pneumonia	erythromycin, tetracycline	
Neisseria gonorrhoeae	Gram-negative cocci	Gonorrhea, meningitis, urethritis, vaginitis, endocarditis, arthritis	ceftriaxone	penicillin G, amoxicillin, spectinomycin, cefoxitin, trimethoprim-sulfamethoxazole, ciprofloxacin

Continued

Table 56-1
Antimicrobial Drugs of Choice for Common Infections (continued)

Organism	Classification	Representative Clinical Illnesses	Drugs of First Choice	Alternative Drugs
Neisseria meningitidis	Gram-negative cocci	Meningitis, bacteremia	penicillin G, rifampin (carrier state)	chloramphenicol, cefuroxime, cefotaxime, ceftizoxime, trimethoprim–sulfamethoxazole
Nocardia	Actinomycetes	Pulmonary lesions, brain abscess	trisulfapyrimidines (with or without minocycline or ampicillin)	trimethoprim–sulfamethoxazole, amikacin, cycloserine
Pasteurella multocida	Gram-negative bacilli	Bacteremia, meningitis	penicillin G	tetracycline, cephalosporin, amoxicillin–clavulanic acid
Pneumocystis carinii	Protozoan	Pneumonia in immunologically compromised patients	trimethoprim–sulfmethoxazole	pentamidine, dapsone
Proteus mirabilis	Gram-negative bacilli	Urinary and other infections	ampicillin	aztreonam, carbenicillin, ticarcillin, amikacin, gentamicin, tobramycin, mezlocillin, azlocillin, piperacillin, norfloxacin, ciprofloxacin, cephalosporin
Proteus (other species, indole positive)	Gram-negative bacilli	Urinary and other infections	cefotaxime, ceftizoxime, ceftriaxone	carbenicillin, ticarcillin, mezlocillin, azlocillin, piperacillin, gentamicin, tobramycin, amikacin, norfloxacin, ciprofloxacin, aztreonam, tetracycline, imipenem, chloramphenicol
Providencia stuartii	Gram-negative bacilli	Urinary and other infections	cefotaxime, ceftizoxime, ceftriaxone	gentamicin, tobramycin, amikacin, carbenicillin, ticarcillin, mezlocillin, azlocillin, imipenem, chloramphenicol, aztreonam
Pseudomonas aeruginosa	Gram-negative bacilli	Urinary and other infections (e.g., respiratory, skin)	Antipseudomonal penicillins (e.g., mezlocillin, azlocillin, piperacillin) with an aminoglycoside (such as gentamicin, amikacin, or tobramycin)	Aminoglycoside (e.g., amikacin, gentamicin, tobramycin, netilmicin) with a third generation cephalosporin (e.g., cefoperazone, cefotaxime, ceftizoxime), aztreonam, norfloxacin, ciprofloxacin, imipenem
Pseudomonas mallei	Gram-negative bacilli	Glanders	streptomycin with tetracycline	streptomycin with chloramphenicol
Pseudomonas pseudomallei	Gram-negative bacilli	Melioidosis	trimethoprim–sulfamethoxazole	sulfonamide, tetracycline (with or without chloramphenicol)
Rickettsia (several species)	Rickettsiae	Rocky Mountain spotted fever, typhus, Q fever, tick-bite fever	tetracycline	chloramphenicol

Continued

Table 56-1
Antimicrobial Drugs of Choice for Common Infections (continued)

Organism	Classification	Representative Clinical Illnesses	Drugs of First Choice	Alternative Drugs
Salmonella typhi	Gram-negative bacilli	Typhoid fever	chloramphenicol	ampicillin, amoxicillin, ciprofloxacin, trimethoprim–sulfamethoxazole
Salmonella (other species)	Gram-negative bacilli	Paratyphoid fever, gastroenteritis, bacteremia	ampicillin, amoxicillin	chloramphenicol, trimethoprim–sulfamethoxazole, ciprofloxacin, cefotaxime
Serratia	Gram-negative bacilli	Several systemic infections (usually secondary to immunosuppressive therapy)	cefotaxime, ceftizoxime, ceftriaxone	aztreonam, imipenem, trimethoprim–sulfamethoxazole ciprofloxacin, carbenicillin, ticarcillin, mezlocillin, azlocillin, piperacillin, gentamicin, amikacin, netilmicin
Shigella	Gram-negative bacilli	Acute gastroenteritis	trimethoprim–sulfamethoxazole	ciprofloxacin, ampicillin, tetracycline
Spirillum minus	Gram-negative bacilli	Rat-bite fever	penicillin G	tetracycline, streptomycin
Sporothrix schenckii	Fungi	Sporotrichosis	amphotericin B	potassium iodide (for cutaneous form *only*)
Staphylococcus aureus	Gram-positive cocci	Pneumonia, meningitis, endocarditis, bacteremia, abscesses, osteomyelitis	*Nonpenicillinase-producing:* penicillin G or V *Penicillinase-producing:* penicillinase-resistant penicillin, imipenem *Methicillin-resistant:* vancomycin (with or without gentamycin or rifampin)	cephalosporin, clindamycin, vancomycin, imipenem, amoxicillin plus clavulanic acid, ciprofloxacin, trimethoprim–sulfamethoxazole
Streptobacillus moniliformis	Gram-negative bacilli	Rat-bite fever, Haverhill fever, bacteremia	penicillin G	tetracycline, streptomycin
Streptococcus (anaerobic species)	Gram-positive cocci	Bacteremia, endocarditis, peritonitis, brain abscess	penicillin G	clindamycin, vancomycin, cephalosporins
Streptococcus bovis	Gram-positive cocci	Urinary infections, endocarditis, bacteremia, meningitis	penicillin G (with or without gentamicin)	cephalosporin, vancomycin
Streptococcus faecalis (enterococcus group)	Gram-positive cocci	Endocarditis, septicemia, meningitis, severe systemic infection	ampicillin or penicillin G with gentamicin or tobramycin	vancomycin with gentamicin, imipenem
		Urinary infections	ampicillin, amoxicillin	nitrofurantoin, norfloxacin, ciprofloxacin
Streptococcus (Diplococcus) pneumoniae	Gram-positive cocci	Pneumonia, meningitis, endocarditis, arthritis	penicillin G or V	erythromycin, cephalosporin, (first generation), chloramphenicol, ciprofloxacin, vancomycin
Streptococcus pyogenes (Groups A, C, G)	Gram-positive cocci	Several infections	penicillin G or V	erythromycin, cephalosporin, vancomycin (bacteremia), ciprofloxacin

Continued

Table 56-1
Antimicrobial Drugs of Choice for Common Infections (continued)

Organism	Classification	Representative Clinical Illnesses	Drugs of First Choice	Alternative Drugs
Streptococcus pyogenes (Group B)	Gram-positive cocci	Several infections	penicillin G, ampicillin	erythromycin, imipenem, cephalosporins, vancomycin
Streptococcus (viridans group)	Gram-positive cocci	Urinary infections, dental infections, endocarditis, meningitis, bacteremia	penicillin G (with or without gentamicin)	cephalosporin, vancomycin
Treponema pallidum	Spirochetes	Syphilis	penicillin G	tetracycline, erythromycin
Treponema pertenue	Spirochetes	Yaws	penicillin G	tetracycline
Vibrio cholerae	Gram-negative bacilli	Cholera	tetracycline	trimethoprim–sulfamethoxazole, chloramphenicol, erythromycin
Yersinia (Pasteurella) pestis	Gram-negative bacilli	Plague	streptomycin (with or without tetracycline)	tetracycline, chloramphenicol, gentamicin

common illnesses associated with it. The recommendations made in Table 56-1 represent a distillate of several sources and are presented *only as a guide* to aid the clinician in choosing an appropriate antibiotic. They are *not* intended as a substitute for careful sensitivity testing, and the drug ultimately used to treat a specific infectious state should be chosen on the basis of as much laboratory and clinical data as can be obtained.

Selected Bibliography

Antimicrobial prophylaxis for surgery. Med Lett Drugs Ther 25:113, 1983

Burnakis TG: Surgical antimicrobial prophylaxis: Principles and guidelines. Pharmacotherapy 4:248, 1984

Calderwood SB, Moellering RC: Principles of anti-infective therapy, In Stein JH (ed): Internal Medicine. p. 1139. Boston, Little, Brown & Co, 1983

Choice of antimicrobial drugs. Med Lett 30:33, 1988

Coleman DL, Horwitz RI, Andriole VT: Association between serum inhibitory and bactericidal concentrations and therapeutic outcome in bacterial endocarditis. Am J Med 73:260, 1982

Cunha BA, Ristuccia AM: Adverse effects of antibiotics. Heart Lung 13:465, 1984

Gleckman RA, Gants NM (eds): Infections in the Elderly. Boston, Little, Brown & Co, 1983

Johnston JB, Davidson MR: Use of a mini-infuser syringe pump for the self-administration of IV antibiotics in the home. NITA 7:381, 1984

Mandell GL, Douglas RG, Bennett JE (eds): Principles and Practice of Infectious Diseases, 2nd ed. New York, John Wiley & Sons, 1985

Neuman M (ed): Useful and harmful interactions of antibiotics. Boca Raton, CRC Press, 1985

Pratt WB, Fekety RF: The antimicrobial drugs. New York, Oxford University Press, 1986

Prevention of bacterial endocarditis. Med Lett Drugs Ther 26:3, 1984

Ristuccia AM, Cunha BA (eds): Antimicrobial Therapy. New York, Raven Press, 1984

Root RK, Sande MA (eds): New Dimensions in Antimicrobial Therapy. New York, Churchill Livingstone, 1984

Sanford JP: Guide to Antimicrobial Therapy. Bethesda, MD, Sanford, 1983

Snavely SR, Hodges GR: The neurotoxicity of antibacterial agents. Ann Intern Med 101:92, 1984

Washington AE: Update on treatment recommendations for gonococcal infections. Rev Infect Dis 4(Suppl):5758, 1982

Yoos L: Factors influencing maternal compliance to antibiotic regimens. Pediatr Nurs 10:141, 1984

57 SULFONAMIDES

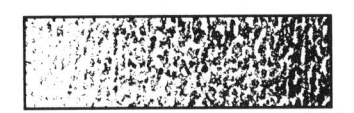

Sulfonamides were the first group of systemic antimicrobial agents to be effective when used clinically and were the mainstay of antiinfective therapy before the introduction of the penicillins in the 1940s. Sulfonamides are bacteriostatic against a broad spectrum of both gram-positive and gram-negative organisms, but their use has declined somewhat in recent years with the introduction of more potent and, in some cases, more specific antibacterial drugs. Nonetheless, they remain valuable therapeutic agents in certain infectious conditions, most notably acute urinary tract infections, because the high solubility in urine of certain derivatives allows them to reach effective concentrations without danger of kidney damage.

Significant differences exist among the sulfonamide drugs in their rates of absorption, metabolism, and excretion, and these differences are important with regard to the indications, efficacy, and toxicity of the different compounds. Based upon such differences, the sulfonamides may be categorized into several groups; such a classification is presented in Table 57-1. Among the systemic agents, the short-acting compounds are rapidly absorbed and quickly eliminated by the kidney. Sulfamethoxazole, an intermediate-acting sulfonamide, is somewhat more slowly absorbed and excreted than the short-acting drugs, and thus it may be used twice a day rather than four to six times a day, possibly improving dosing compliance.

Although most systemic sulfonamide use is by oral ingestion, sulfisoxazole is available for injection. Parenteral use of sulfonamides should be undertaken only where oral administration is impractical (as in a comatose patient) and is best accomplished by slow IV injection. The solutions are highly alkaline and irritating, and the drug may precipitate out of solution.

Locally acting sulfonamides may be employed in several ways. Sulfasalazine is administered orally for the treatment of ulcerative colitis. The compound is split by the action of intestinal microflora into sulfapyridine and 5-aminosalicylate, the latter agent accumulating in significant amounts in the colon, where it may exert an antiinflammatory action. Five-aminosalicylic acid is also available alone as Mesalamine, a suspension enema also used for ulcerative colitis (see Chap. 78). Other indications for use of locally acting sulfonamides are eye and vaginal infections (sulfacetamide, sulfathiazole, sulfisoxazole) and prevention and treatment of sepsis in second- and third-degree burns (mafenide, silver sulfadiazine). Topical application of sulfonamides occasionally elicits allergic hypersensitivity reactions and local ocular irritation.

A major deterrent to the continuing use of sulfonamides has been the emergence of resistant strains of microorganisms that were once sensitive to the action of these drugs (e.g., gonococci, beta-hemolytic streptococci, meningococci, coliform organisms). Development of sulfonamide resistance in these organisms has been greatly abetted by the previous widespread prophylactic use of the drugs in subtherapeutic doses for the attempted control of gonorrhea, upper respiratory infections, and urinary infections. Among the major causes of increased sulfonamide resistance among microorganisms are production of excessive amounts of para-aminobenzoic acid (PABA) by the bacteria (PABA is an essential component of folic acid synthesis necessary for cell growth and is competitively antagonized by sulfonamides); enhanced destruction of the sulfonamide molecule by the microorganism; or development of alternative metabolic pathways for handling essential amino acids (see Chap. 56). Acquired bacterial resistance plays a major role in therapeutic failures with sulfonamides, and the clinical usefulness of these agents, despite their relatively low cost, is rather limited. Cross-resistance between sulfonamides is very common as well. The principal indications for sulfonamides are listed under Uses in the discussion that follows, and their usefulness in certain infections is also documented in Chapter 56, Table 56-1.

SULFONAMIDES

Mafenide	Sulfamethoxazole
Sulfacetamide	Sulfapyridine
Sulfacytine	Sulfasalazine
Sulfadiazine	Sulfisoxazole
Sulfamethizole	Multiple sulfonamides

The sulfonamides, with the exception of those drugs used in the treatment of severe burns, are reviewed as a group and then are listed in Table 57-2. Mafenide and silver sulfadiazine are then discussed individually, as is trimethoprim-sulfamethoxazole, a synergistic combination of two antibacterial agents, one a sulfonamide, used in both acute and chronic urinary tract infections as well as for several other indications including treatment of pneumocystis pneumonia in AIDS patients. Resistance has been shown to develop more slowly to this combination than to either drug alone. The sulfonamide discussion focuses principally on the systemic effects of the drugs, with mention being made of specific points pertaining to their local application wherever necessary.

MECHANISM
Bacteriostatic at normal doses; interfere with bacterial cell synthesis of folic acid, an essential precursor of nucleic acids, by competitively antagonizing PABA; by preventing PABA utilization, bacterial cell replication is halted

USES
(*See also* Table 57-2 for specific indications for each drug.)

Acute, recurrent, or chronic urinary tract infections in the absence of obstruction. Acute infections generally respond to a single sulfonamide drug, usually sulfisoxazole or sulfamethoxazole; recurrent infections or infections complicated by obstruction or bacteremia are less effectively controlled by a sulfonamide alone and usually require adjunctive therapy.
Chancroid
Trachoma
Nocardiosis
Toxoplasmosis (with pyrimethamine)
Acute otitis media due to *Hemophilus influenzae* (with penicillin or erythromycin); also, prophylaxis of recurrent otitis media (sulfisoxazole)
Adjunctive therapy of malaria (chloroquine-resistant strains of *Plasmodium falciparum*)

Table 57-1
Sulfonamides

Systemic

Short Acting
sulfacytine
sulfadiazine
sulfamerazine
sulfamethazine
sulfamethizole
sulfisoxazole

Intermediate Acting
sulfamethoxazole
sulfapyridine

Local

Intestinal
sulfasalazine

Ophthalmic
sulfacetamide
sulfisoxazole

Vaginal
sulfabenzamide
sulfacetamide
sulfathiazole
sulfisoxazole

Topical
mafenide
silver sulfadiazine

Prophylaxis and treatment of sulfonamide-sensitive group A strains of meningococcal menigitis or hemophilus meningitis (with streptomycin)

Prophylaxis of recurrent rheumatic fever (sulfadiazine *only*)

Conjunctivitis and superficial eye infections (sulfacetamide, sulfisoxazole)

Hemophilus vaginalis vaginitis (sulfabenzamide, sulfacetamide, sulfathiazole, sulfisoxazole)

Ulcerative colitis (sulfasalazine)

Dermatitis herpetiformis (sulfapyridine only)

DOSAGE
See Table 57-2

FATE
Orally administered sulfonamides, except for those designed for their local effects in the bowel, are readily absorbed from the GI tract; absorption from other sites, such as the skin or vagina, is more variable and unreliable. Drugs distribute widely in the body and may be found in cerebrospinal, pleural, peritoneal, synovial, ocular, and placental as well as other body fluids. Protein binding is variable (20%–90%). Duration of action is largely dependent on the rate of metabolism and renal excretion; drugs are metabolized in the liver by several pathways, one of which, acetylation, can occur at varying rates. "Slow acetylators" have an increased risk of drug accumulation and subsequent toxicity. Eliminated in the urine as both unchanged drug and metabolic products, glomerular filtration playing the major role in excretion. Urinary solubility of sulfonamides is pH dependent; alkalinization of the urine favors excretion (increases ionization of molecule and solubility of drug) and reduces danger of crystallization in the urinary fluid.

Some derivatives (e.g., sulfacytine, sulfadiazine, sulfisoxazole) are readily absorbed and quickly excreted and must be given up to six times a day to maintain adequate plasma concentrations. Sulfamethoxazole is somewhat more slowly absorbed and excreted and is given less frequently (two to three times a day). Sulfasalazine, an orally administered drug, is only very slightly absorbed and is excreted largely in the feces

COMMON SIDE EFFECTS
GI distress (nausea, abdominal discomfort)

SIGNIFICANT ADVERSE REACTIONS
(Incidence differs depending on drug)

GI: vomiting, diarrhea, anorexia, stomatitis, pancreatitis, jaundice, hepatitis, impaired folic acid absorption

CNS: headache, drowsiness, dizziness, insomnia, vertigo, tinnitus, ataxia, depression, convulsions, hallucinations, peripheral neuritis, hearing loss, psychosis

Renal: proteinuria, albuminuria, hematuria, oliguria, anuria, crystalluria, nephrotic syndrome

Hematologic: petechiae, hemolytic or macrocytic anemia, blood dyscrasias, hypoprothrombinemia, methemoglobinemia, purpura

Allergic hypersensitivity: pruritus, urticaria, photosensitivity, arthralgia, periorbital edema, erythema multiforme, exfoliative dermatitis, serum sickness, anaphylactic reactions, myocarditis

Other: fever, chills, malaise, alopecia, cyanosis, goiter, diuresis, hypoglycemia, reduction in sperm count, periarteritis nodosum, lupuslike syndrome

|| *WARNING*
Sulfonamides given to pregnant women near term or to neonates may cause a serious disorder known as kernicterus (see Interactions). ||

CONTRAINDICATIONS
Advanced kidney disease, near term of pregnancy or during the nursing period, porphyria, in infants less than 2 months of age (except for treating congenital toxoplasmosis), group A beta-hemolytic streptococcal infections (drugs will not eradicate organisms), hypersensitivity to sulfonylurea antidiabetics or thiazide diuretics

In addition, sulfasalazine is contraindicated in intestinal or urinary obstruction, in children under 2 years, and in patients with salicylate allergy. *Cautious use* in persons with liver or kidney dysfunction, blood dyscrasias, a history of allergic reactions, bronchial asthma, or a glucose-6-phosphate dehydrogenase deficiency (hemolytic anemia can occur); also in persons receiving anticoagulant or antiplatelet drugs, because increased bleeding can occur

INTERACTIONS
Because of competition for protein-binding sites, sulfonamides may potentiate or be potentiated by other protein-bound drugs (e.g., oral anticoagulants, oral hypoglycemics, methotrexate, phenytoin, salicylates, antiinflammatory agents, sulfinpyrazone, probenecid, and barbiturates)

Effects of sulfonamides may be impaired by local anesthetics that are metabolized to PABA, for example, chloroprocaine, procaine, and tetracaine

Sulfonamides can displace bilirubin from plasma protein binding sites, possibly resulting in kernicterus (abnormal pigmentation of gray matter of CNS by bilirubin, leading to neuronal degeneration and, frequently, death) in premature and newborn infants

Incidence of crystalluria with sulfonamides can be increased by paraldehyde, methenamine, or urinary acidifiers (e.g., ammonium chloride)

Antacids and possibly mineral oil may decrease the effects of sulfonamides by impairing absorption

Sulfasalazine can reduce the bioavailability of digoxin and can retard the absorption of folic acid

Concurrent use of sulfonamides may reduce oral contraceptive efficacy and increase the incidence of breakthrough bleeding

Tolbutamide and methotrexate may increase sulfonamide

plasma levels by competing for renal tubular excretory mechanisms

The effects of tolbutamide, chlorpropamide, and phenytoin may be potentiated by sulfonamides through inhibition of their hepatic metabolism

NURSING CONSIDERATIONS

See also Table 57-2 and **Plan of Nursing Care** 12 in Chapter 56.

Nursing Alerts

- Monitor results of blood counts and urinalyses as well as liver and kidney function tests, which should be performed during extended therapy. Renal complications occur much less frequently with the more soluble sulfonamides (sulfisoxazole, sulfamethiazole).
- Monitor intake–output ratio and observe for symptoms of possible renal impairment (renal colic, oliguria, hematuria).
- Closely observe patient for appearance of severe headache, rhinitis, urticaria, conjunctivitis, stomatitis, or rash because these may signal early development of Stevens–Johnson syndrome (*severe* erythema multiforme), which is occasionally fatal. If symptoms occur, drug should be discontinued immediately.

1. Cleanse wound thoroughly before applying a topical sulfonamide because the drug may be inactivated in the presence of pus, blood, or cell breakdown products.
2. Assist with evaluation of drug efficacy. In vitro sulfonamide sensitivity tests are not always reliable. Data should be correlated with bacteriologic studies as well as clinical response.
3. Be alert for signs of increased systemic absorption of the "insoluble" sulfonamide sulfasalazine following oral administration in patient with extensive ulceration of the colon.

PATIENT EDUCATION

See also **Plan of Nursing Care** 12 in Chapter 56.

1. As appropriate, teach patient how to test urine pH before taking a longer-acting sulfonamide. If necessary, sodium bicarbonate may be used to alkalinize urine sufficiently to ensure drug solubility, and patient should take drug with liberal amount of fluids to prevent crystalluria (urinary output should be at least 1500 mL/day).
2. Caution patient to be aware of early signs of possible developing hematologic toxicity (sore throat, fever, mucosal ulceration, malaise, pallor, jaundice) and to discontinue the drug and consult physician if they occur.
3. Instruct patient taking drug for prolonged time to notify prescriber of any unusual bleeding because hypoprothrombinemia and bleeding tendencies (due to decreased synthesis of vitamin K by intestinal microflora) can occur.
4. Explain that patient should avoid prolonged exposure to sunlight or ultraviolet light because photosensitization can occur.
5. Warn patient applying sulfonamide topically to discontinue drug at first sign of local irritation or other allergic reaction.
6. Instruct patient to minimize use of OTC preparations during sulfonamide therapy because some vitamin combinations and analgesic mixtures contain PABA, which can reduce sulfonamide effectiveness.
7. Inform diabetic patient that dosage of antidiabetic agent may need to be adjusted. Serum glucose level should be monitored, and patient should be aware that sulfonamides can produce false-positive urinary glucose tests using Benedict's method.
8. Teach patient measures that help prevent recurrence of urinary tract infections.

(*Text continued on page 578*)

Table 57-2
Sulfonamides

Drug	Preparations	Usual Dosage Range	Nursing Implicatons
Sulfacetamide Ak-Sulf, Bleph-10, Cetamide, Isopto Cetamide, Opthacet, Sebizon Lotion, Sodium Sulamyd, Sulf-10, Sulfair-15, Sulten-10 (CAN) Minims; Sulfex	Ophthalmic drops: 10%, 15%, 30% Ophthalmic ointment: 10% Lotion: 10%	Drops: 1 to 2 drops every 1 h to 4 h as condition dictates Ointment: small amount in conjunctival sac 2 to 4 times/day Lotion: apply 2 to 4 times/day for bacterial infections or at bedtime for seborrheic dermatitis	Ophthalmic drops or ointment are indicated for treatment of conjunctivitis, corneal ulcers, superficial ocular infections and as adjunctive therapy with systemic sulfonamides for trachoma; lotion is used for seborrheic dermatitis and cutaneous bacterial infections with susceptible organisms; solutions are incompatible with silver preparations; nonsusceptible organisms may proliferate with use of sulfacetamide; drug may be inactivated by PABA produced by purulent exudates; ophthalmic ointment may impair corneal healing; 30% drops may be irritating upon application; do *not* use if ophthalmic solution

Continued

Table 57-2
Sulfonamides (continued)

Drug	Preparations	Usual Dosage Range	Nursing Implicatons
			is dark brown; discontinue drug if signs of hypersensitivity develop; apply topical lotion cautiously to abraded or denuded skin areas; available with phenylephrine as ophthalmic solution (Vasosulf) and combined with sulfathiazole and sulfabenzamide as vaginal creme and vaginal tablets (Sultrin, Triple Sulfa, Sulfa-Gyn, Trysul)
Sulfacytine Renoquid	Tablets: 250 mg	Adults: 500 mg initially, then 250 mg 4 times/day for 10 days	Short-acting sulfonamide not recommended in children under 14 years of age; used *only* for treatment of urinary tract infections
Sulfadiazine Microsulfon	Tablets: 500 mg	Adults: 2 g to 4 g initially, then 2 g to 4 g/day in 3 to 6 divided doses Children: 75 mg/kg initially, followed by 150 mg/kg/day in 4 to 6 divided doses (maximum 6 g/day) Rheumatic fever prophylaxis: 0.5 g to 1 g once daily	Short-acting sulfonamide infrequently used, as drug is poorly soluble in acid urine and danger of nephrotoxicity exists; high urine volume must be maintained; component of triple sulfa formulations with sulfamerazine and sulfamethazine; combination claimed to reduce chance of crystalluria; alkalinization of urine is also recommended when drug is used
Sulfamethizole Proklar, Thiosulfil Forte	Tablets: 500 mg	Adults: 0.5 g to 1 g 3 or 4 times/day Children: 30 mg to 45 mg/kg/day in 4 divided doses	Short-acting sulfonamide principally used for acute and chronic urinary infections; highly bound to plasma proteins; use with caution with other protein-bound drugs; rapidly excreted in urine, mostly in active form; drug may impart an orange-yellow color to urine or skin; available in combination with phenazopyridine (Thiosulfil-A) and oxytetracycline (Urobiotic)
Sulfamethoxazole Gamazole, Gantanol, Urobak (CAN) Apo-Sulfamethoxazole	Tablets: 500 mg, 1000 mg Suspension: 500 mg/5 mL	Adults: 2 g initially, followed by 1 g 2 or 3 times/day Children: 50 mg to 60 mg/kg initially, then 25 mg to 30 mg/kg morning and night (maximum 75 mg/kg/day)	Intermediate-acting sulfonamide similar to sulfisoxazole but with somewhat slower oral absorption and urinary excretion; used twice a day in most cases to prevent accumulation; available in combination with trimethoprim (Bactrim, Septra; *see* separate discussion) and phenazopyridine (Azo Gantanol), the latter drug serving as a urinary analgesic for relief of dysuria associated with urinary tract infection
Sulfapyridine (CAN) Dagenan	Tablets: 500 mg	Adults: 500 mg 4 times/day until improvement is noted, then reduce by 500 mg/day at 3-day intervals to effective maintenance level	Intermediate-acting agent used in the treatment of dermatitis herpetiformis (recurrent, inflammatory skin disease, herpetic in nature, characterized by erythema, vesicles, and pustules); slowly absorbed

Continued

Table 57-2
Sulfonamides (continued)

Drug	Preparations	Usual Dosage Range	Nursing Implicatons
			from GI tract (peak levels in 6–8 h); excreted both as intact drug and conjugated metabolites, largely within 3 to 4 days; administer with sufficient fluids to prevent crystalluria
Sulfasalazine Azaline, Azulfidine, S.A.S.-500 (CAN) PMS Sulfasalazine, Salazopyrin	Tablets: 500 mg Enteric-coated tablets (EN-Tabs): 500 mg Suspension: 250 mg/5 mL	Adults: 1 g to 2 g/day in divided doses initially; usual maintenance dosage is 500 mg 4 times/day Children: 40 mg to 60 mg/kg/day in 3 to 6 divided doses initially, followed by 30 mg/kg/day in 4 divided doses	Locally acting sulfonamide used orally in the treatment of mild to moderate ulcerative colitis; hydrolyzed in intestinal tract to sulfapyridine (antibacterial) and 5-aminosalicylic acid (antiinflammatory); systemic absorption of parent drug and hydrolysis products are variable (increased in the presence of severe ulceration); frequently induces GI intolerance; if noted early in therapy, space daily dosage more evenly or use enteric-coated tablets; note that enteric-coated tablets have passed through GI tract without disintegrating, if this occurs, discontinue therapy; if GI distress is observed after several days of therapy, reduce dosage or stop drug for 5 to 7 days, then resume at a lower dosage; drug is often continued at reduced levels even when clinical symptoms, including diarrhea, are controlled; dosage and duration of therapy are primarily governed by endoscopic evaluation; if diarrhea recurs, increase dosage to previously effective level; infertility has been reported in men; withdrawal of drug reverses this effect; advise patient that drug may impart an orange-yellow color to skin and to alkaline urine; sulfasalazine may impair absorption of folic acid
Sulfisoxazole Gantrisin, Gulfasin, Lipo Gantrisin (CAN) Apo-Sulfisoxazole, Novosoxazole	Tablets: 500 mg Syrup: 500 mg/5 mL (chocolate) Pediatric suspension: 500 mg/5 mL (raspberry) Emulsion (Lipo Gantrisin): 1 g/5 mL in homogenized vegetable oil (long acting) Ophthalmic drops: 4% Ophthalmic ointment: 4%	*Oral* (except emulsion, see Nursing Implications) Adults: 2 g to 4 g initially, then 4 g to 8 g/day in 4 to 6 divided doses Children: 150 mg/kg/day in 4 to 6 divided doses (initial dose is 1/2 the 24-h dose) *Ophthalmic* 1 to 2 drops every 1 to 4 h as condition warrants or small amount of ointment 3 or 4 times/day	Short-acting sulfonamide used orally, and locally (eye) for a number of bacterial infections; peak blood levels occur within 3 to 4 h following oral administration; highly protein bound but rapidly excreted in the urine (95% within 24 h); emulsion (Lipo Gantrisin) is long acting and is administered every 12 h (adults 4 g–5 g; children 60 mg–75 mg/kg); *see* sulfacetamide for remarks concerning ophthalmic and vaginal application; available in combination with phenazopyridine (e.g., as Azo Gantrisin), which provides an

Continued

Table 57-2
Sulfonamides (continued)

Drug	Preparations	Usual Dosage Range	Nursing Implicatons
			analgesic effect for relief of dysuria associated with urinary infections, or erythromycin (as Pediazole), used for acute otitis media in children caused by *Hemophilus influenzae*
Multiple Sulfonamides Neotrizine, Sul-Trio MM, Terfonyl, Triple Sulfa	Tablets: 162 mg *or* 167 mg each of sulfadiazine, sulfamerazine, and sulfamethazine Suspension: 167 mg each of sulfadiazine, sulfamerazine, and sulfamethazine per 5 mL	Adults: 2 g to 4 g initially, then 2 g to 4 g/day in 4 to 6 divided doses Children: 75 mg/kg initially, then 150 mg/kg/day in 4 to 6 divided doses	A combination of three short-acting sulfonamides that provides the therapeutic effect of the total sulfonamide content, but reduces the risk of precipitation in the kidneys because the solubility of each sulfonamide is independent of the others; infrequently used preparation, because other equally effective and more soluble sulfonamides are available (e.g., sulfisoxazole)

Mafenide
Sulfamylon

A topical sulfonamide used to retard invasion of avascular burn sites by a variety of gram-positive and gram-negative organisms, mafenide is effective against proliferation of *Pseudomonas aeruginosa* and certain strains of anaerobes, even in the presence of pus and serum, and its activity is not altered by changes in pH. It facilitates spontaneous healing of deep, partial-thickness burns.

MECHANISM
See general discussion of sulfonamides

USE
Adjunctive therapy to prevent sepsis in second- and third-degree burns

DOSAGE
Applied aseptically twice a day over burned surface to a depth of 1 mm to 2 mm; should be reapplied whenever necessary to maintain continuous covering of area; continue application until healing is well along or skin is ready for grafting

FATE
Diffuses through devascularized areas and is quickly absorbed from burn surface, with peak plasma concentrations in 2 to 4 hours; rapidly metabolized and eliminated by the kidney

COMMON SIDE EFFECTS
Pain, burning, or stinging at application site

SIGNIFICANT ADVERSE REACTIONS
(Often difficult to distinguish between adverse drug reactions and secondary effects of burn) Bleeding of skin, allergic reactions (rash, itching, surface edema, urticaria, erythema, eosinophilia); rarely, hyperventilation, acidosis, excoriation of new skin, fungal colonization of wound area, and superinfections

CONTRAINDICATIONS
No absolute contraindications. *Cautious use* in patients with acute renal failure, pulmonary infection, or impaired respiratory function, history of sulfonamide allergy (cross-sensitivity has *not* been demonstrated), and in pregnant women

NURSING CONSIDERATIONS

Nursing Alerts
- Monitor acid–base balance, especially in patient with extensive burns or one who exhibits pulmonary or renal dysfunction, because the drug and its metabolite inhibit carbonic anhydrase and may cause metabolic acidosis.
- Assess patient for early signs of developing acidosis (e.g., nausea, vomiting, abdominal pain, weakness, diarrhea, disorientation), and inform physician if they occur.
- Be alert for appearance of allergic reaction (rash, itching, urticaria). If one occurs, it may be necessary to discontinue drug temporarily.

1. Advocate appropriate prescription of an analgesic if drug application results in significantly increased pain, and administer analgesic sufficiently far ahead of sulfonamide use to ensure that maximum analgesia is in effect when topical drug is applied.
2. Cleanse and debride wound area before applying mafenide. Although a dressing is not required, if patient needs one, use only a thin layer.
3. When feasible, bathe patient daily, preferably by whirlpool, to facilitate burn débridement.

Silver Sulfadiazine
Flint SSD, Silvadene

A condensation product of silver nitrate with sulfadiazine, silver sulfadiazine possesses broad antimicrobial activity and is bactericidal against a number of both gram-positive and gram-negative bacteria as well as yeasts. It is used topically to prevent invasion as well as to *eradicate* sensitive microorganisms from burns. Does not affect electrolyte or acid-base balance, and application is less painful than mafenide.

MECHANISM
Not completely established; appears to exert its bactericidal effect on bacterial cell membranes and cell wall; sulfadiazine is released in body tissues, and may produce a bacteriostatic action by usual means, that is, antagonism of PABA

USE
Prevention and treatment of sepsis in second- and third-degree burns

DOSAGE
Apply aseptically one or two times a day to a thickness of 1 mm to 2 mm; reapply as necessary to maintain continuous covering until healing has occurred

FATE
Hydrolyzed to a silver salt, which is poorly absorbed systemically, and sulfadiazine, which may attain significant plasma levels

COMMON SIDE EFFECTS
Burning at application site

SIGNIFICANT ADVERSE REACTIONS
Rash, itching, pain, interstitial nephritis (rare); also, because sulfadiazine may be absorbed in significant amounts, see general discussion of sulfonamides for possible systemic adverse effects

CONTRAINDICATIONS
Pregnancy at term, premature infants, and infants under 2 months of age. *Cautious use* in patients with a history of sulfonamide hypersensitivity, impaired renal or hepatic function, or glucose-6-phosphate dehydrogenase deficiency (danger of hemolysis), and during pregnancy

INTERACTION
Silver may inactivate topically applied proteolytic enzymes

NURSING CONSIDERATIONS
See mafenide. In addition:

> **Nursing Alert**
> - Monitor results of determinations of serum and urine sulfonamide levels, and check results of kidney function tests, all of which should be obtained during long-term treatment of burns involving large areas because continuous silver sulfadiazine absorption may cause the systemic sulfonamide concentration to approach toxic level.

1. Use cream only if it retains its white color. Discard if darkened.
2. Note that silver sulfadiazine, unlike mafenide, is bactericidal as well as bacteriostatic, and it does not appear to alter acid–base balance significantly.

Trimethoprim–Sulfamethoxazole (Co-Trimoxazole)
Bactrim, Septra, and other manufacturers

A synergistic combination of antimicrobial drugs that interfere with two sequential steps in an essential enzymatic reaction necessary for bacterial multiplication. Consequently, clinical efficacy is enhanced and development of resistance is significantly reduced when compared to the use of either agent alone. Its antibacterial spectrum includes common urinary pathogens (except *Pseudomonas aeruginosa*) and middle ear pathogens, as well as several organisms associated with respiratory conditions such as acute bronchitis and pneumonitis.

A severe form of pneumonitis due to *Pneumocystis carinii* can occur in immunocompromised persons such as those receiving cancer chemotherapy, other immunosuppressant drugs, or those afflicted with AIDS. This opportunistic infection is difficult to eradicate, and trimethoprim–sulfamethoxazole has now become a favored drug in treating this serious disease.

MECHANISM
Sulfamethoxazole inhibits synthesis of dihydrofolic acid by competitive antagonism of PABA; trimethoprim inhibits the dihydrofolate reductase enzyme, thus blocking production of tetrahydrofolic acid from folic acid; thus, two consecutive steps in the synthesis of essential proteins and nucleic acids in many bacteria are impaired

USES
Recurrent or chronic urinary tract infections due to susceptible organisms (i.e., *Escherichia coli, Klebsiella-Enterobacter, Proteus mirabilis, Proteus vulgaris, Proteus morgani*)
  Initial episodes of uncomplicated acute urinary tract infections should be treated with a *single* agent (e.g., a sulfonamide or cephalosporin) rather than this combination
Acute otitis media in children over 2 years of age due to susceptible strains of *Hemophilus influenzae* (including ampicillin- and amoxicillin-resistant strains) or *Streptococcus pneumoniae*
Acute exacerbations of chronic bronchitis in adults due to susceptible strains of *H. influenzae* or *S. pneumoniae*
Enteritis due to susceptible strains of *Shigella*
Pneumocystis carinii pneumonitis in children and adults immunosuppressed by cancer chemotherapy or other immunosuppressive therapy or suffering from AIDS (drug of choice)
Treatment of *Nocardia asteroides* infections (usually for 6–12 mo)
Investigational uses include treatment of cholera, salmonella type infections, melioidosis, brucellosis, chancroid, penicillinase-producing *Neisseria gonorrhoeae*, and for prophylaxis of traveler's diarrhea

DOSAGE
(Dosage ratios given refer to the amount of trimethoprim/sulfamethoxazole [TMP/SMZ] in the preparation)

Urinary infections, bronchitis, shigellosis, otitis media; prostatitis
  Adults and children weighing 40 kg or more: 160 mg TMP/800 mg SMZ every 12 hours for 10 to 14 days (7 days in shigellosis)
  Children under 40 kg: 8 mg TMP/kg/day and 40 mg SMZ/kg/day in two divided doses every 12 hours for 10 days (5 days in shigellosis)

Severe urinary infections or shigellosis
  8 mg to 10 mg/kg/day (trimethoprim equivalent) by IV infusion in two to four divided doses for up to 14 days in urinary infections and 5 days in shigellosis

Prevention of recurrent urinary infections in females:
    40 mg TMP/200 mg SMZ daily at bedtime or 80 mg/400 mg two to three times a week

Pneumocystis carinii *pneumonitis:*
    Adults and children: 20 mg TMP/kg/day and 100 mg SMZ/kg/day, orally or by IV infusion in equally divided doses every 6 hours for 14 days

Chancroid:
    160 mg TMP/800 mg SMZ orally twice daily for a minimum of 7 days

Penicillinase-producing Neisseria gonorrhoeae
    Pharyngeal infection: 9 tablets (80 mg TMP/400 mg SMZ) in a single dose daily for 5 days

When administering IV, give slowly over 60 to 90 minutes. Do *not* give IM. Infusion solution (5-mL ampule) is diluted with 125 mL of 5% dextrose in water, and the dilution should not be mixed with other drugs or solutions.

FATE

Rapidly absorbed when taken orally; peak serum levels occur in 1 hour with trimethoprim and 4 hours with sulfamethoxazole; half-lives for both drugs are 10 hours with oral administration and 11 to 13 hours with IV infusion; ratio for trimethoprim to sulfamethoxazole in the blood is 1:20; approximately 45% of trimethoprim and 70% of sulfamethoxazole are protein-bound; widely distributed in the body, including cerebrospinal fluid; excreted primarily by kidneys; urine concentrations are significantly higher than serum concentrations

COMMON SIDE EFFECTS

Nausea, diarrhea, rash, mild thrombocytopenia

SIGNIFICANT ADVERSE REACTIONS

GI: vomiting, abdominal pain, glossitis, stomatitis, pancreatitis
CNS: Headache, tinnitus, vertigo, fatigue, insomnia, muscle weakness, ataxia, convulsions, peripheral neuritis, depression, hallucinations
Allergic/hypersensitivity: pruritus, urticaria, periorbital edema, generalized skin eruptions, photosensitivity, arthralgia, myocarditis, anaphylactic reactions, serum sickness, erythema multiforme, Stevens–Johnson syndrome, epidermal necrolysis
Hematologic: blood dyscrasias, purpura, hemolytic anemia, hypoprothrombinemia, methemoglobinemia
Other: chills, fever, oliguria, anuria, lupuslike syndrome, goiter, diuresis, hypoglycemia, periarteritis nodosa, jaundice, hepatitis

IV use at high doses or for prolonged periods may result in bone marrow depression.

> **NOTE**
> Patients with AIDS frequently react adversely when trimethoprim–sulfamethoxazole is administered to treat pneumocystis pneumonia. Fever, rash, malaise, and pancytopenia are common occurrences

CONTRAINDICATIONS

Pregnancy, in nursing mothers or infants less than 2 months of age, streptococcal pharyngitis, megaloblastic anemia due to folate deficiency. *Cautious use* in patients with reduced hepatic function, folate deficiency, bronchial asthma, severe allergy, or glucose-6-phosphate dehydrogenase deficiency; the drug should *not* be used to treat streptococcal pharyngitis because it will neither eradicate the organism nor prevent complications

INTERACTIONS

See Interactions under general sulfonamide monograph earlier in this chapter and under trimethoprim in Chap. 64

NURSING CONSIDERATIONS

See sulfonamides (this chapter) and trimethoprim (Chap. 64). In addition:

Nursing Alerts

- If patient has AIDS, observe for development of fever, rash, and malaise, common adverse reactions in AIDS patients.
- If patient has AIDS, monitor results of complete blood cell counts, and observe patient for development of symptoms of pancytopenia, which often occurs in patients with AIDS.

PATIENT EDUCATION

See sulfonamides (this chapter) and trimethoprim (Chap. 64). In addition:
1. As supportively as possible, prepare patient with AIDS for the possibility of adverse reactions, which occur frequently when TMP-SMZ is used to treat *Pneumocystis carinii* pneumonitis in patients with AIDS.

Selected Bibliography

Abshagen D: Topical agents and emergency care for minor burn injuries. J Emerg Nurs 10:325, 1984

Harrison HN: Pharmacology of sulfadiazine silver. Arch Surg 114:281, 1979

Hughes WT: Trimethoprim-sulfamethoxazole. Pediatr Clin North Am 30:27, 1983

Keys TF: Urinary tract infection: New perspectives on diagnosis and treatment. Mod Med 54(6):34, 1986

Patel RB, Welling PG: Clinical pharmacokinetics of co-trimoxazole (trimethoprim-sulfamethoxazole). Clin Pharmacokin 5:405, 1980

Robertson KE, et al: Burn care: The first crucial days. Am J Nurs 85:30, 1985

Robin RH, Swartz MN: Trimethoprim-sulfamethoxazole. N Engl J Med 303:426, 1980

Sattler FR, Remington JR: Intravenous trimethoprim-sulfamethoxazole therapy for Pneumocystis carinii pneumonia. Arch Intern Med 143:1709, 1983

Stamm WE: Prevention of urinary tract infections. Am J Med 76:146, 1984

Wharton M, et al: Prospective randomized trial of trimethoprim-sulfamethoxazole versus pentamidine for Pneumocystis carinii pneumonia in the acquired immunodeficiency syndrome. Annu Rev Respir Dis 129:1, 1984

Wormser GP, Keusch GT, Rennie CH: Cotrimoxazole (trimethoprim-sulfamethoxazole): An updated review of its antibacterial activity and clinical efficacy. Drugs 24:459, 1982

SUMMARY. SULFONAMIDES

Drug	Preparations	Usual Dosage Range
Systemic, Ophthalmic, and Vaginal Drugs	*See* Table 57-2	
Mafenide Sulfamylon	Cream: 85 mg/g	Apply twice a day to burn area to a thickness of 1 mm to 2 mm; reapply as necessitated by patient's activity to ensure continuous covering
Silver Sulfadiazine Flint SSD, Silvadene	Cream: 10 mg/g	Apply 1 or 2 times a day to burn to a thickness of 1 mm to 2 mm; reapply as needed to maintain continuous covering
Trimethoprim–Sulfamethoxazole Bactrim, Septra, and other manufacturers	Tablets: 80 mg/400 mg, 160 mg/800 mg Suspension: 40 mg/200 mg per 5 mL Pediatric suspension (flavored): 40 mg/200 mg per 5 mL Infusion solution: 80 mg/400 mg per 5 mL	*Urinary infections, bronchitis, shigellosis, otitis media* Adults and children weighing 40 kg or more: 160 mg/800 mg every 8 to 12 h Children weighing under 40 kg: 8 mg per kg/40 mg per kg every 24 h in 2 divided doses *Pneumocystis carinii pneumonitis:* Adults: 20 mg/kg/100 mg/kg per day orally or IV in equally divided doses every 6 h for 14 days *Chancroid:* 160 mg/800 mg every 12 h for 7 days *Penicillinase-producing* Neisseria gonorrhoeae: 9 tablets (80 mg/400 mg) in a single daily dose for 5 days

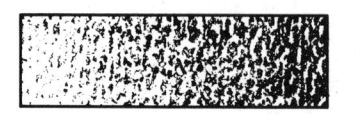

58 PENICILLINS, CARBAPENEMS, MONOBACTAMS

Several groups of antiinfective agents possessing a similar beta-lactam ring structure are considered in this chapter. The penicillin group of antibiotics includes natural extracts from several strains of the *Penicillium* mold and a number of semisynthetic derivatives. The carbapenems are represented by imipenem, a thienamycin antibiotic produced by *Streptomyces cattleya*, whereas the monobactams are represented by aztreonam, a monocyclic beta-lactam isolated from *Chromobacterium violaceum*.

PENICILLINS

Of the many natural products isolated from the fermentation medium used to culture *Penicillium*, penicillin G exhibits the greatest antimicrobial activity and is the only natural penicillin in current use. Penicillin G, however, possesses several undesirable characteristics, such as instability in gastric acid, susceptibility to inactivation by penicillinase enzyme, rapid renal excretion, and a relatively narrow antimicrobial spectrum of action. Some of these problems have been at least partially eliminated in many of the newer semisynthetic penicillin derivatives. These drugs have been prepared by incorporating specific precursors into the mold cultures (e.g., penicillin V) or, more commonly, by chemically replacing a side chain on the 6-aminopenicillanic nucleus, as in ampicillin. Although these chemically modified derivatives of penicillin G each possess distinct advantages in certain aspects, it must be recognized that none of these agents represents the "ideal" penicillin in terms of activity and toxicity. In fact, penicillin G, by virtue of its good antibacterial activity, minimal toxicity, and low cost is still the preferred drug for a number of infections due to susceptible organisms, especially the more common gram-positive cocci such as streptococci, gonococci, and meningococci.

Many penicillin derivatives are available, differing principally in stability in gastric acid, resistance to inactivation by penicillinase (a beta-lactamase enzyme produced by many bacteria, which can destroy the activity of penicillin), degree of protein binding, and spectrum of antimicrobial activity. The important characteristics of the various penicillins are outlined in Table 58-1. The usefulness of these derivatives in treating specific bacterial infections may be ascertained by reference to Chapter 56, Table 56-1, which presents a listing of the preferred antimicrobial drugs for treating a number of microorganisms.

Penicillins exert their antibacterial effects by blocking biosynthesis of cell wall mucopeptide, rendering the bacteria osmotically unstable and thus unable to survive. Penicillins, in adequate concentrations, are bactericidal, and are most effective when active bacterial cell multiplication is occurring. Moreover, the penicillins are virtually nontoxic toward human cells, inasmuch as these cells do not have rigid walls like those of bacteria but merely a limiting cytoplasmic membrane. The greater activity of most penicillins toward gram-positive organisms than toward gram-negative organisms is due to the higher proportion of mucopeptide in the cell walls of gram-positive bacteria and their higher internal osmotic pressure. Unlike the activity of some other antibiotics, such as sulfonamides, that of the penicillins is not inhibited by blood, pus, or other tissue breakdown products.

The major untoward reaction associated with use of the penicillins is hypersensitivity. This can range from mild skin rash and contact dermatitis to severe allergic reactions, including exfoliative dermatitis, serum sickness, and anaphylaxis. The incidence of allergic reactions to penicillin is higher in patients with previously demonstrated hypersensitivity to multiple allergens or a history of hay fever or asthma, and the drugs should be used with extreme caution in such persons. No single penicillin derivative is safer in this respect than any other. Penicillin-sensitive patients can also exhibit *cross*-sensitivity to certain other antibacterial agents, notably cephalosporins, and caution must be exercised in using any of these drugs in patients sensitive to any of the others.

Bacterial resistance to the penicillins is variable. Despite extensive clinical use of penicillin for over 25 years, some species of bacteria have remained uniformly susceptible (e.g., *Diplococcus pneumoniae*, *Neisseria meningitidis*) whereas other species have developed progressively increasing resistance. This variability in development of resistance may be explained in part by the fact that there are several mechanisms responsible for resistance to penicillins. Most commonly, resistance occurs because some bacteria (such as staphylococci) can synthesize beta-lactamase enzymes, such as penicillinase, which convert the drugs to inactive products. Such bacteria would display resistance to penicillins susceptible to enzyme activity, but not to penicillinase-resistant derivatives (see Table 58-1). On the other hand, certain bacteria may develop resistance to all penicillins, possibly because their cell surfaces have become impermeable to the drugs or because they have developed alternative metabolic pathways that avoid steps sensitive to the action of the drugs.

The penicillin drugs may be categorized into several classes based on their respective characteristics, such as spectrum of activity, resistance to penicillinase, and source (see Chap. 56). The major groups of penicillin drugs are briefly described below.

Natural Products

PENICILLIN G
First penicillin in extensive clinical use; still considered a first-line drug against most gram-positive bacteria (except penicillinase-producing staphylococci) when given by IM injection. Virtually nontoxic to human cells, thus can be given safely in large amounts. Widely distributed in the body, especially following IM injections, and rapidly bactericidal. Low cost. Major disadvantages are irregular oral absorption, destruction by gastric acid, inactivation by penicillinase enzyme, and rather narrow antimicrobial spectrum of action. Effects may be prolonged by parenteral (IM) use of benzathine or procaine salts of penicillin G, repository forms of the drug producing lower serum blood levels but longer duration of action.

Semisynthetic Derivatives

PENICILLIN V
Semisynthetic analog of penicillin G with similar spectrum of activity. More completely absorbed orally than penicillin G and

Table 58-1
Penicillins—General Characteristics

Drug	Routes of Administration	Oral Absorption	Protein Binding	Acid Stable	Penicillinase Resistant	Remarks
Amdinocillin	IV, IM	NA	5%–10%	NA	Yes	Structurally unique penicillinase-resistant drug active against *E. coli, Klebsiella* sp., *Enterobacter* sp.; not effective vs gram-positive organisms; synergistic with other beta-lactam drugs, because mechanism is different
Amoxicillin	Oral	Excellent	20%–25%	Yes	No	Similar to ampicillin but better absorbed, thus giving more rapid and higher serum levels
Ampicillin	Oral, IV, IM	Good	20%–25%	Yes	No	Broad spectrum; effective against many gram-negative organisms, but no real advantage over penicillin G for most gram-positive infections
Azlocillin	IV	NA	20%–40%	NA	No	Broad spectrum; good effectiveness against *Pseudomonas* and most other gram-negative bacilli
Bacampicillin	Oral	Excellent	20%–25%	Yes	No	Rapidly hydrolyzed to ampicillin during GI absorption; peak ampicillin blood levels 3 times those obtained with ampicillin itself
Carbenicillin	Oral, IV, IM	Good	50%	Yes	No	Broad spectrum with high activity against most strains of *Pseudomonas*; less active than ampicillin against gram-positive bacteria
Cloxacillin	Oral	Good	95%	Yes	Yes	Effective against penicillinase-producing staphylococci as well as most other gram-positive organisms
Cyclacillin	Oral	Excellent	20%	Yes	No	Broad spectrum but somewhat less active than ampicillin despite higher peak blood levels
Dicloxacillin	Oral	Good	95%–98%	Yes	Yes	Similar to but slightly more active than cloxacillin or oxacillin
Methicillin	IV, IM	NA	40%–50%	NA	Yes	Parenteral antibiotic active against penicillinase-producing staphylococci but less effective than penicillin G against most other gram-positive infections
Mezlocillin	IV, IM	NA	20%–40%	NA	No	Broad spectrum; highly active against *Enterobacter*; good activity *versus* most other gram-negative organisms
Nafcillin	Oral, IV, IM	Fair	90%	Yes	Yes	Highly resistant to penicillinase but erratically absorbed orally; good activity against gram-positive organisms
Oxacillin	Oral, IV, IM	Good	90%–95%	Yes	Yes	Similar to cloxacillin; most effective when given parenterally
Penicillin G	Oral, IV, IM	Poor	50%–60%	No	No	Highly active against gram-positive bacteria; much less active against gram-negative organisms
Penicillin V	Oral	Good	80%–90%	Yes	No	Similar to penicillin G; much more reliably absorbed but less potent
Piperacillin	IV, IM	NA	20%–40%	NA	No	Broad spectrum; very effective against *Pseudomonas* and *Enterobacter*; uniformly active against gram-negative bacilli
Ticarcillin	IV, IM	NA	45%–50%	NA	No	Broad spectrum, including *Pseudomonas, Serratia, Citrobacter*; effective only parenterally

NA, not applicable.

not destroyed by gastric acid, thus yielding three to five times higher blood levels. Preferred over penicillin G for oral therapy of mild infections of the throat, upper respiratory tract, or soft tissues caused by non-penicillinase-producing staphylococci and other gram-positive cocci, but ineffective for gonorrhea. Used only orally, therefore not indicated during *acute* stages of serious infections with susceptible organisms, because these usually require parenteral penicillin G. Potassium salt is the preferred form, because it is better absorbed than plain penicillin V.

PENICILLINASE-RESISTANT PENICILLINS (CLOXACILLIN, DICLOXACILLIN, METHICILLIN, NAFCILLIN, OXACILLIN)

Resistant to inactivation by penicillinase and used in the treatment of infections due to penicillinase-producing *Staphylococcus aureus*. Cloxacillin or dicloxacillin is indicated for oral use, because these drugs are acid stable and well absorbed, although their GI absorption is reduced by food. Parenteral methicillin, nafcillin, or oxacillin should be employed in serious infections. Less effective than penicillin G against *non*-penicillinase-producing staphylococci and other gram-positive organisms. Inactive against gram-negative organisms.

BROAD-SPECTRUM PENICILLINS (AMOXICILLIN, AMPICILLIN, BACAMPICILLIN, CYCLACILLIN)

Effective against a range of both gram-positive and gram-negative organisms. No real advantage over the less costly penicillin G or V in treating most gram-positive infections, but significantly more active against many gram-negative organisms, especially *Hemophilus influenzae, Escherichia coli, Proteus mirabilis, Salmonella,* and *Shigella*. Thus, frequently employed as initial drugs where the identity of the microorganism has not been determined, for example, urinary infections, respiratory infections such as sinusitis or bronchitis, and otitis media. Drugs are not resistant to penicillinase enzyme, but are acid stable.

EXTENDED-SPECTRUM [ANTIPSEUDOMONAL] PENICILLINS (AZLOCILLIN, CARBENICILLIN, MEZLOCILLIN, PIPERACILLIN, TICARCILLIN)

Wide antimicrobial spectrum, including *Pseudomonas* and many other gram-negative bacilli resistant to the broad spectrum penicillins. In addition to the organisms listed under Broad-Spectrum Penicillins, above, these agents are *also* effective against *Pseudomonas*, several *Proteus* species, *Acinetobacter, Enterobacter,* and *Serratia*. In addition, azlocillin, mezlocillin, and piperacillin also demonstrate in vitro activity against *Klebsiella* and *Citrobacter* and contain less than one half the sodium content of carbenicillin and ticarcillin. Their activity is nearly comparable to that of the aminoglycosides, but they are considerably less toxic. Extended-spectrum penicillins are not penicillinase-resistant.

AMIDINOPENICILLIN (AMDINOCILLIN)

Good activity against *E. coli, Klebsiella, Enterobacter, Serratia, Salmonella,* and *Shigella. Not* active, however, against gram-positive organisms or anaerobes; binds to different proteins than other penicillins and thus has a synergistic effect with other beta-lactam drugs; action is primarily bacteriostatic, although drug attains high levels in urinary tract, which provide a bactericidal action.

Discussion of the penicillins focuses on these agents as a group, inasmuch as the basic pharmacology and toxicology of all derivatives are identical. Drugs are listed in Table 58-2, where appropriate dosages and individual characteristics are given.

Penicillins

Amdinocillin	Methicillin
Amoxicillin	Mezlocillin
Ampicillin	Nafcillin
Azlocillin	Oxacillin
Bacampicillin	Penicillin G
Carbenicillin	Penicillin V
Cloxacillin	Piperacillin
Cyclacillin	Ticarcillin
Dicloxacillin	

MECHANISM

Bind to cellular receptor proteins and inhibit the action of enzymes necessary for formation of cell wall peptidoglycans, substances necessary for rigidity of the bacterial cell wall; thus, cells become osmotically unstable and the high internal pressure causes swelling and lysis of the bacterial cells; most penicillins bind to proteins 1B$_s$ and 3; however amdinocillin binds to protein 2 and is synergistic with other penicillins; gram-positive microorganisms possess much larger amounts of peptidoglycan in their cell walls than gram-negative organisms, and these walls are up to fifty times thicker. The greater susceptibility of some gram-positive organisms to penicillins compared to gram-negative organisms is related to several factors, including the relative amounts of cell wall peptidoglycans, increased affinity of cellular receptors for the drugs, and higher internal osmotic pressure, which causes rupture of the cells as the cell wall is weakened; in adequate concentrations, penicillins are bactericidal and most effective during active cellular multiplication; lower concentrations may produce only bacteriostatic activity

USE

(See Chap. 56, Table 56-1, for specific indications for different penicillins in various infections; see also Table 58-2)
Treatment of infections due to organisms sensitive to normal serum levels of the drugs

DOSAGE
See Table 58-2

FATE

Oral absorption ranges from excellent (amoxicillin, bacampicillin, cyclacillin) to fair-to-poor (nafcillin, penicillin G); most other orally effective derivatives are reasonably well absorbed. Peak serum levels occur within 1 to 2 hours after oral administration. Following IM injection, most drugs yield rapid and high serum levels, except for the procaine and benzathine salts of penicillin G, which provide lower blood levels but more prolonged effects. Drugs diffuse readily into most body tissues, and tissue levels equal serum levels at most sites except the CNS and the eye where significant penetration occurs only when the meninges are inflamed. All derivatives are protein-bound to varying degrees (5% with amdinocillin to 98% with dicloxacillin). Penicillin V and oxacillin are the only derivatives metabolized to any extent; others are rapidly excreted largely unchanged in the urine. Elimination half-life is less than 1 hour for most drugs, slightly longer for ampicillin and amoxicillin. Also secreted into the bile, which is only a minor route of elimination for all drugs except nafcillin and oxacillin, which are excreted in significant amounts in the bile

COMMON SIDE-EFFECTS

Allergic reactions (e.g., skin rash, urticaria, itching), especially in patients with a history of allergies

SIGNIFICANT ADVERSE REACTIONS

(Most adverse reactions are rare and are usually only seen with large doses. Hypersensitivity reactions, however, can occur with small doses of any penicillin derivative)

Hypersensitivity: severe reactions (wheezing, laryngeal edema, macropapular rash, serum sickness, exfoliative dermatitis, erythema multiforme, arthralgia, prostration, anaphylaxis)

GI: nausea, vomiting, epigastric distress, glossitis, stomatitis, dry mouth, abnormal taste, "hairy" tongue, diarrhea, flatulence, enterocolitis (due to secondary microbial overgrowth), abdominal pain, GI bleeding

Electrolyte: hypokalemia (extended-spectrum penicillins), hypernatremia (especially carbenicillin, ticarcillin)

Renal-hepatic: interstitial nephritis (most frequently with methicillin), glomerulonephritis, cholestatic hepatitis

CNS: neurotoxicity (irritability, lethargy, hallucinations, seizures), anxiety, confusion, agitation, depression

Hematologic: blood dyscrasias, bone marrow depression, hemolytic anemia, hemorrhagic manifestations associated with abnormalities of coagulation tests

Other: pain and irritation at injection site, phlebitis, oral and rectal candidiasis, overgrowth of nonsusceptible organisms, vaginitis, neuropathy, sciatic neuritis

CONTRAINDICATIONS

History of previous hypersensitivity to any penicillin. *Cautious use* in nursing mothers and in patients with asthma, hay fever, history of any allergy, or renal impairment; always skin test for allergenicity if doubt exists

> **WARNING**
> Care must be taken to avoid inadvertent intravascular injection because severe neurovascular damage has occurred, including necrosis and sloughing at the injection site, and gangrene. Repeated IM injections into the anterolateral thigh have resulted in development of fibrosis and localized tissue atrophy. IV injection can result in thrombophlebitis, neuromuscular excitability, and convulsions

INTERACTIONS

Concurrent use of *bacteriostatic* antibiotics (e.g., tetracyclines, erythromycin) may diminish the effectiveness of penicillins by slowing the rate of bacterial growth, because penicillins are most effective during rapid multiplication

Probenecid prolongs blood levels of penicillins by blocking their elimination by renal tubular secretion

Highly protein-bound penicillins, for example, cloxacillin, dicloxacillin, nafcillin, and oxacillin, can be potentiated by other highly protein-bound drugs (e.g., oral anticoagulants, antiinflammatory agents)

Antacids and other alkalinizing agents as well as colestipol and cholestyramine can inhibit the action of oral penicillins by impairing absorption

Increased incidence of skin rash can occur with combined use of ampicillin and allopurinol

The effectiveness of oral contraceptives may be reduced by ampicillin or penicillin V

Penicillins mixed in solution with an aminoglycoside may inactivate the aminoglycoside

High doses of IV penicillins (especially carbenicillin) may increase the risk of bleeding in patients receiving heparin or oral anticoagulants

Use of penicillin and chloramphenicol together may reduce the effectiveness of penicillin and slow the elimination of chloramphenicol

Extended-spectrum penicillins may be synergistic with aminoglycosides against certain gram-negative organisms, such as *Pseudomonas, Providencia,* and enterococci

NURSING CONSIDERATIONS

See **Plan of Nursing Care 12 Antibacterial Drugs** in Chapter 56 and Table 58-2. In addition:

Nursing Alerts

- In suspected staphylococcal infections, because there are a number of resistant strains, be sure that appropriate, correctly timed culture and sensitivity tests are performed to ensure that the proper antibiotic is prescribed. Penicillinase-resistant penicillins are commonly used as *initial* therapy for any suspected staphylococcal infection until culture and sensitivity results are known. However, some strains of staphylococci capable of producing serious disease and death are resistant to penicillinase-resistant penicillins.

- Use particular care in aspirating syringe prior to injecting a penicillin IM because intravascular administration may result in severe neurovascular damage, including gangrene and paralysis (see *Warning* above). Injection into or near a nerve may cause permanent neurologic damage.

- Assist with evaluation of drug efficacy. If desired clinical response does not occur within 24 to 48 hours with oral administration, consideration should be given to adding or substituting a parenteral penicillin. *Oral* preparations are contraindicated in patient who is vomiting or who has intestinal hypermotility, gastric dilitation, or cardiac spasm.

- During prolonged therapy, periodically assess renal, hepatic, and hematopoietic function, especially in small children or if large doses are used.

- When large doses of nafcillin or one of the extended-spectrum penicillins are administered, be alert for possible development of coagulation test abnormalities associated with bleeding tendencies. Upon drug withdrawal, bleeding should cease, and test results should revert to normal.

- During prolonged infusion or repeated IV administration of the sodium or potassium salts of penicillins, monitor results of serum electrolyte determinations, which should be performed, because high-dose IV therapy with these salts can lead to electrolyte overload.

1. When giving drug IV, dilute according to manufacturer's directions, and closely observe patient for signs of thrombophlebitis because IV administration can be irritating.
2. When giving IM, inject into body of a large muscle mass (e.g., gluteus), and do *not* massage site after injection. Sites should be rotated.

(Text continued on page 595)

Table 58-2
Penicillins

Drug	Preparations	Usual Dosage Range	Nursing Implications
Amdinocillin Coactin	Powder for injection: 500-mg, 1-g vials	Adults: 60 mg/kg/day in divided doses by IM injection or IV infusion over 15–30 min *In combination* with other beta-lactam antibiotics or in patients with renal impairment, reduce dose to 40 mg/kg/day in divided doses	Chemically unique penicillin primarily used in serious urinary tract infections caused by susceptible strains of *E. coli, Klebsiella* sp. and *Enterobacter* sp.; synergistic with other beta-lactam antibiotics owing to different mechanisms of action (see general discussion under Mechanism); penicillinase-resistant and minimally protein bound; *no* demonstrated activity against gram-positive organisms or anaerobes; when used in combination with another antiinfective drug, administer by separate means; may be given IM into a large muscle mass
Amoxicillin Amoxil, Larotid, Polymox, Trimox, Utimox, Wymox (CAN) Apo-Amoxi, Novamoxin	Capsules: 250 mg, 500 mg Chewable tablets: 125 mg, 250 mg Powder for oral suspension: 125 mg/5 mL 250 mg/5 mL Drops: 50 mg/mL	*General indications* Adults and children over 20 kg: 250 mg–500 mg every 8 h Children under 20 kg: 20 mg–40 mg/kg/day in divided doses every 8 h *Uncomplicated gonorrhea (adults)* 3 g with 1 g oral probenecid as a single dose *Disseminated gonococcal infection* As above, followed by 500 mg oral amoxicillin 4 times/day for 7–10 days *Pelvic inflammatory disease* As above, followed by 100 mg oral doxycycline twice daily for 14 days	Broad spectrum acid-stable penicillin rapidly and completely absorbed from the GI tract; absorption is not significantly affected by food; activity similar to ampicillin but less effective against *Shigella*; widely used in acute otitis media due to *Hemophilus*, although resistant strains are emerging; also effective against *E. coli, Proteus, Neisseria gonorrhoeae*, streptococci, pneumococci, and non-penicillinase-producing staphylococci; less likely to disturb GI flora than ampicillin; often used as initial therapy before culture and sensitivity tests because of broad spectrum of action; no more effective than penicillin G or V against susceptible gram-positive organisms; available in combination with potassium clavulanate as Augmentin (see below)
Amoxicillin and Potassium Clavulanate Augmentin	Tablets: 250 mg, 500 mg with 125 mg clavulanic acid (as potassium salt) Chewable tablets: 125 mg, 250 mg with 31.25 mg and 62.5 mg clavulanic acid (as potassium salt), respectively Powder for suspension: 125 mg/5 mL (with 31.25 mg clavulanic acid) and 250 mg/5 mL (with 62.5 mg clavulanic acid)	Dosage is given as amoxicillin equivalent) Adults: 250 mg–500 mg every 8 h Children: 20 mg/kg/day–40 mg/kg/day in divided doses every 8 h *Pelvic inflammatory disease* 500 mg 3 times a day for 10 days with doxycycline, 100 mg twice a day	Contains the potassium salt of clavulanic acid, a beta-lactam that inactivates beta-lactamase enzymes that destroy amoxicillin; combination serves to protect amoxicillin from degradation by beta-lactamase enzymes produced by certain bacteria, thereby extending the spectrum of action of amoxicillin to include organisms normally resistant to the drug (e.g., *Klebsiella*, beta-lactamase-producing strains of *Hemophilus, E. coli*, and staphylococci)
Ampicillin Amcill, Omnipen, Polycillin, Principen, Totacillin, and other manufacturers	Capsules: 250 mg, 500 mg Capsules with probenecid: 389 mg/111 mg Powder for oral suspension:	*Respiratory and soft tissue infections* Adults and children over 40 kg Oral: 250 mg every 6 h	Broad-spectrum penicillin widely used in respiratory, GI, urinary, and soft tissue infections including otitis media,

Continued

Table 58-2
Penicillins (continued)

Drug	Preparations	Usual Dosage Range	Nursing Implications
Ampicillin (cont'd) (CAN) Ampicin, Ampilean, Apo-Ampi	125 mg/5 mL, 250 mg/5 mL, 500 mg/5 mL Drops: 100 mg/mL Oral suspension with probenecid: 3.5 g/1 g Powder for injection: 125 mg, 250-mg, 500-mg, 1-g, 2-g, 10-g vials	IM, IV: 250 mg–500 mg every 6 h Children under 40 kg Oral: 50 mg/kg/day in divided doses IM, IV: 25 mg–50 mg/kg/day in divided doses *GI and urinary infections* Adults and children over 40 kg Oral, IM, IV: 500 mg every 6 h Children under 40 kg Oral: 100 mg/kg/day in divided doses IM, IV: 50 mg/kg/day in divided doses *Bacterial meningitis and septicemia* Adults and children: 150 mg–200 mg/kg/day in divided doses every 3–4 h; begin with IV administration, then continue with IM *Gonorrheal urethritis* 3.5 g with 1 g probenecid orally or 500 mg IM every 8 h–12 h *Gonorrhea* 3.5 g with 1 g probenecid orally as single dose *Disseminated gonococcal infection* As above, followed by 500 mg oral ampicillin 4 times/day for 7 days *Pelvic inflammatory disease* As above, followed by 100 mg oral doxycycline twice a day for 14 days *Prevention of bacterial endocarditis* 1 g IM or IV plus gentamicin 1.5 mg/kg; give initial doses 30–60 min prior to procedure and then 2 additional doses ever 8 h thereafter	septicemia, and bacterial meningitis; skin rash can occur, especially in patients with mononucleosis or hyperuricemia; parenteral form should be used only for severe infections or in patients unable to take oral medications; treatment should be continued 48–72 h after symptoms have disappeared; administer on an empty stomach to enhance GI absorption; during extended therapy (e.g., chronic urinary infections), frequent bacteriologic tests should be performed and sufficient doses must be given; clinical and bacteriologic follow-up should be maintained for several months after cessation of therapy; use only freshly prepared solutions for parenteral administration, dilute according to package directions with suitable diluent, and use within 1 h after preparation; available with sulbactam sodium as Unasyn (see below)
Ampicillin and Sulbactam Sodium Unasyn	Powder for injection: 1 g ampicillin/0.5 g sulbactam; 2 g ampicillin/1 g sulbactam	(Dosage given in ampicillin equivalents) 1 g–2 g ampicillin IV or IM every 6 h (maximum 4 g/day); reduce frequency of dosing in patients with renal impairment	Sulbactam inhibits a wide range of beta-lactamases found in many microorganisms, thereby extending the spectrum of action of ampicillin to include many bacteria normally resistant to it (e.g., beta-lactamase-producing strains of *E. coli, Klebsiella, Enterobacter, Proteus, Bacteroides,* and *Staph. aureus*); pain at injection site occurs frequently; both drugs are eliminated largely unchanged in the urine—*caution* in renal impairment
Azlocillin Azlin	Powder for injection: 2-g, 3-g, 4-g vials	*Urinary infections* IV *only*: 100 mg–200 mg/kg/day (2 g–3 g every 6 h) *Serious systemic infections* 200 mg–300 mg/kg/day in 4–6 divided doses (3 g every 4 h)	Extended spectrum antipseudomonal penicillin used either by slow IV injection (over 5–10 min) or by IV infusion (30 min); very effective *in vitro* against *Pseudomonas,*

Continued

Table 58-2
Penicillins (continued)

Drug	Preparations	Usual Dosage Range	Nursing Implications
Azlocillin (cont'd)		*Life-threatening infections* Up to 350 mg/kg/day (4 g every 4 h)	*Proteus*, *Salmonella*, and *Acinetobacter*; rapid IV administration has elicited transient chest discomfort; contains 2.17 mEq/g of sodium, less than one half the amount in carbenicillin or ticarcillin; dosage should be reduced in patients with significant renal impairment; synergistic with aminoglycosides against pseudomonal infections but must be administered in a separate syringe; solutions are stable at room temperature for 24 h; to minimize venous irritation, do *not* use solutions more concentrated than 10%; bile levels of drug are 10 to 15 times greater than serum levels—*danger* in biliary obstruction; drug may depress serum uric acid level; in immunosuppressed patients, azlocillin is combined with a cephalosporin or aminoglycoside
Bacampicillin Spectrobid (CAN) Penglobe	Tablets: 400 mg Powder for oral suspension: 125 mg/5 mL	*Upper respiratory, urinary and skin infections* Adults: 400 mg–800 mg every 12 h Children: 25 mg–50 mg/kg/day in 2 equally divided doses *Lower respiratory infections* 800 mg every 12 h *Gonorrhea* 1.6 g with 1 g probenecid as a single dose	Rapidly hydrolyzed to ampicillin during GI absorption; each tablet equivalent to 280 mg ampicillin; more completely absorbed than ampicillin, yielding effective serum levels for up to 12 h; much more costly than ampicillin; *see* ampicillin for additional remarks; do *not* administer with disulfiram (see Chap. 78)
Carbenicillin disodium Geopen (CAN) Pyopen	Powder for injection: 1-g, 2-g, 5-g, 10-g, 20-g, 30-g piggyback units or bulk packages	*Urinary infections* Adults: 200 mg/kg/day IV drip *or* 1 g–2 g IM or IV every 6 h Children: 50 mg–200 mg/kg/day IM *or* IV in divided doses *Soft tissue or respiratory infections, septicemia* Adults: 15 g–40 g daily IV in divided doses *or* by continuous drip Children: 250 mg–500 mg/kg/day IM or IV in divided doses (maximum dose 40 g/day) *Gonorrhea* 1 g probenecid orally followed in 1 h by 4 g carbenicillin IM *Presence of renal insufficiency* (creatinine clearance less than 5 ml/min): 2 g IV every 8–12 h	Extended-spectrum penicillin especially effective against many gram-negative organisms, such as *Pseudomonas*, *Proteus*, *Escherichia*, *Salmonella*, and *Enterobacter* as well as anaerobes; most *Klebsiella*, *Shigella* and *Acinetobacter* are resistant; attains very high levels in urine when given IM or IV; synergistic with aminoglycosides against *Pseudomonas*; may elicit increased bleeding tendencies associated with abnormal coagulation tests; be alert for signs of hemorrhage (bruising, petechiae); fairly high in sodium content; monitor serum electrolytes during extended administration; use very cautiously in patients with impaired renal function; IV therapy is recommended for serious urinary or systemic infections; IM injections should not exceed 2 g/dose; reconstitute solutions according to

Continued

Table 58-2
Penicillins (continued)

Drug	Preparations	Usual Dosage Range	Nursing Implications
			package directions and discard unused solutions after 24 h at room temperature (72 h in refrigerator); do *not* mix carbenicillin and gentamicin together in the same IV fluid—administer separately
Carbenicillin Indanyl Sodium Geocillin	Tablets: 382 mg	382 mg–764 mg 4 times a day	Indanyl ester of carbenicillin, suitable for oral use; indicated mainly for acute and chronic upper and lower urinary tract infections and prostatitus due to *Escherichia coli, Proteus, Pseudomonas, Enterobacter,* and Enterococcus; readily absorbed orally and hydrolyzed to carbenicillin, which is rapidly excreted in the urine, attaining high levels
Cloxacillin Cloxapen, Tegopen (CAN) Apo-Cloxi, Bactopen, Novocloxin, Orbenin	Capsules: 250 mg, 500 mg Powder for oral solution: 125 mg/5 mL	Adults: 250 mg–1 g every 6 h Children: 50 mg–100 mg/kg/day in divided doses every 6 h	Penicillinase-resistant penicillin principally used to treat infections caused by penicillinase-producing staphylococci; may also be used to initiate therapy in patients in whom a staphylococcal infection is suspected; somewhat less effective than penicillin G against most other gram-positive cocci; best absorbed from an empty stomach; highly protein-bound
Cyclacillin Cyclapen-W	Tablets: 250 mg, 500 mg Powder for oral suspension: 125 mg/5 mL, 250 mg/5 mL	Adults: 250 mg–500 mg 4 times a day in equally spaced doses Children: 125 mg–250 mg 3–4 times a day in equally spaced doses	Broad-spectrum agent, rapidly and completely absorbed when taken orally; peak serum levels within 30 min; rapidly excreted in the urine; dosage frequency must be reduced in renal impairment; indicated for treatment of bronchitis, pneumonia, upper respiratory infections, urinary infections, and otitis media due to susceptible organisms; *not* used in children under 2 mo; somewhat lower incidence of skin rash and diarrhea than with ampicillin or amoxicillin; should not be used for infections caused by *Escherichia coli* or *Proteus mirabilis* other than urinary tract
Dicloxacillin Dicloxacil, Dycill, Dynapen, Pathocil	Capsules: 125 mg, 250 mg, 500 mg Powder for oral suspension: 62.5 mg/5 mL	Adults and children over 40 kg: 125 mg–250 mg every 6 h, up to 4 g/day Children under 40 kg: 12.5 mg–25 mg/kg/day in divided doses every 6 h	Penicillinase-resistant penicillin similar to cloxacillin and oxacillin, but producing slightly higher plasma levels than equivalent doses of other related penicillins; do *not* use in neonates; *see* Cloxacillin
Methicillin Staphcillin	Powder for injection: 1-g, 4-g, 6-g, 10-g vials	Adults: IM or IV infusion 4 g–12 g/day in divided doses every 4–6 h Children: 100–300 mg/kg/day in divided doses every 4–6 h	Penicillinase-resistant penicillin with same uses as cloxacillin but used by injection *only*; considerably less active than penicillin G against streptococci and pneumococci;

Continued

Table 58-2
Penicillins (continued)

Drug	Preparations	Usual Dosage Range	Nursing Implications
Methicillin (cont'd)		Infants: 50–150 mg/kg/day in divided doses every 6–12 h	well tolerated by deep IM injection, slow IV injection, or continuous IV infusion; observe injection sites for signs of irritation, inflammation, or hypersensitivity; be alert for development of drug-induced febrile reactions with IV administration; drug has produced interstitial nephritis within 2–4 wk of start of therapy—observe for early indications (e.g., cloudy urine, oliguria, spiking fever) and discontinue drug; methicillin is *incompatible* in solution with a wide range of drugs—do *not* mix with other drugs, including antibiotics but administer separately; carefully follow instructions on container when diluting powder for injection; higher concentrations (10 mg–30 mg/mL) are stable for 8 h at room temperature, but weaker dilutions (2 mg/mL) are only stable for 4 h
Mezlocillin Mezlin	Powder for injection: 1-g, 2-g, 3-g, 4-g vials or infusion bottles	Adults IV: 1.5 g–4 g every 4–6 h depending on the severity of infection (life-threatening infections—4 g every 4 h) IM: 1.5 g–2 g every 6 h *Acute gonococcal urethritis:* 1 g–2 g, as a single IV or IM injection, together with 1 g probenecid orally *Prevention of postoperative infection in contaminated surgery:* 4 g IV 1 h before surgery, and again 6 and 12 h after surgery Children IV, IM: 75 mg/kg every 6–8 h (neonates every 12 h)	Extended-spectrum penicillin similar in activity to piperacillin but somewhat less effective against *Pseudomonas;* may be used with an aminoglycoside or cephalosporin in severe infections for which the causative agent is unknown; do *not* inject more than 2 g IM and give slowly (15 sec) well into the body of a large muscle mass; inject IV over a period of 3–5 min (concentration of drug in solution should not exceed 10% to minimize venous irritation); IV infusion should be given over 30 min; follow package directions for mixing and diluting, for dosage reductions in patients with impaired renal function (based on creatinine clearance), and for compatibility and stability data; low sodium content (1.85 mEq/g)
Nafcillin Nafcil, Nalipen, Unipen	Capsules: 250 mg Tablets: 500 mg Powder for oral solution: 250 mg/5 mL Powder for injection: 500-mg, 1-g, 2-g, 4-g, 10-g vials	Adults *Oral:* 250 mg–1000 mg every 4–6 h depending on severity of infection IM: 500 mg every 4–6 h IV: 500 mg–1000 mg every 4 h Children *Oral:* 50 mg/kg/day in 4 divided doses *Scarlet fever/pneumonia:* 25 mg/kg/day in 4 divided doses	Penicillinase-resistant penicillin with same indications as cloxacillin; oral absorption is inferior to that of other similar penicillins; major route of elimination is by way of the bile; parenteral therapy is indicated initially in severe infections—change to oral therapy should be made as condition warrants; not as ac-

Continued

Table 58-2
Penicillins (continued)

Drug	Preparations	Usual Dosage Range	Nursing Implications
		Neonates IM: 10 mg/kg twice a day	tive as penicillin G against non-penicillin-producing organisms; for IV use, dilute powder in 15 mL–30 mL sterile water for injection or sodium chloride injection and inject over 5–10 min; avoid extravasation because tissue necrosis can occur; reconstitute solution for IM injection with sterile or bacteriostatic water for injection; administer immediately by deep intragluteal injection; solution may be kept refrigerated for up to 48 h
Oxacillin Bactocil, Prostaphlin	Capsules: 250 mg, 500 mg Powder for oral solution: 250 mg/5 mL Powder for injection: 250-mg, 500-mg, 1-g, 2-g, 4-g, 10-g vials	Adults and children over 40 kg Oral: 500 mg–1000 mg every 4–6 h for a minimum of 7 days depending on severity of infection IM, IV: 250 mg–1000 mg every 4–6 h depending on severity of infection Children under 40 kg Oral: 50 mg–100 mg/kg/day in divided doses IM, IV: 50 mg–100 mg/kg/day in divided doses	Penicillinase-resistant drug similar in most respects to cloxacillin and dicloxacillin but slightly less potent orally; in serious infections, parenteral therapy is indicated, because oral absorption may be unreliable; following initial control of infection, oral therapy may then be substituted; drug should be taken on an empty stomach; solutions for IM or IV use should be prepared by diluting powder with sterile water for injection or sodium chloride injection; discard unused IM injection after 3 days at room temperature or 7 days with refrigeration; consult package for suitable diluents for IV infusion solutions; at concentrations of 0.5-mg to 40-mg/mL dilutions are stable for approximately 6–8 h at room temperature—adjust rate of infusion to deliver intended drug dose within this time; transient elevations in serum enzymes (SGOT, SGPT, LDH) may occur with oxacillin
Penicillin G, Potassium or Sodium Pentids, Pfizerpen G, and other manufacturers (CAN) Crystapen, Megacillin, Novopen G, P-50	Tablets: 200,000 U, 250,000 U, 400,000 U, 500,000 U, 800,000 U Powder for oral solution: 200,000 U/5 mL, 400,000 U/5 mL Powder for injection: 200,000 U/vial, 500,000 U/vial; 1-, 5-, 10-, 20-million U/vial (400,000 units = 250 mg)	Adults and children over 12 Oral: 200,000 U–500,000 U every 6–8 h for at least 10 days IM, IV: 300,000 U–8 million U daily (some severe infections, e.g., meningococcal meningitis, gram-negative bacteremia, clostridial infections may require up to 20–30 million U/day) Children under 12 Oral: 25,000 U–90,000 U/kg/day in 3–6 divided doses IM, IV: 300,000 U–1.2 million U/day in divided doses (up to 10 million U/day may be required)	Natural penicillin preparation derived from the *Pencillium* mold; considered drug of choice for treating infections due to susceptible organisms (see Chap. 56); rapid-acting, inexpensive, and very effective against many gram-positive cocci and anaerobes, but destroyed by gastric acid and penicillinase—administer orally on an empty stomach; refrigerate reconstituted oral solution and discard within 14 days; do *not* use oral penicillin G as prophylaxis for genitourinary instrumentation or surgery, lower intestinal surgery, sigmoidoscopy, or

Continued

Table 58-2
Penicillins (continued)

Drug	Preparations	Usual Dosage Range	Nursing Implications
			childbirth; IM is the preferred parenteral route; keep injection volume small and inject deeply into a large muscle mass; maximal plasma concentrations are attained within 30–60 min; doses exceeding 10 million U/day must be given by IV infusion *only*; administer large doses slowly because electrolyte overload may occur depending on which salt is used; use extreme caution in renal insufficiency—half-life (normally 30 min) increases to 10 h in patients with anuria; perform periodic serum electrolyte determinations during high-dosage therapy and be alert for symptoms of hyperkalemia (hyperreflexia, convulsions, arrhythmias) when using potassium salts
Penicillin G, Benzathine Bicillin, Permapen (CAN) Megacillin	Tablets: 200,000 U Injection: 300,000 U/ml, 600,000 U/mL 1.2 million U/dose, 2.4 million U/dose	Adults and children over 12 Oral: 400,000 U–600,000 U every 4–6 h IM: 1,200,000 U as a single injection *Syphilis (early):* 2.4 million U as a single dose *Syphilis (of more than 1 yr duration):* 2.4 million U IM/wk for 3 wk Children under 12 Oral: 25,000 U–90,000 U/kg/day in 3–6 divided doses IM: 600,000 U–1,200,000 U depending on weight *Prophylaxis of rheumatic fever:* 200,000 U orally twice a day, 1.2 million U IM once a month, *or* 600,000 U IM every 2 wk	Benzathine salt of penicillin G providing a slowly absorbed and hence long-acting dosage form; oral preparations are less effective than IM forms owing to unpredictable GI absorption; use a large-gauge needle for administration, inject deeply into a large muscle, and do *not* massage injection site; not for IV or SC use; when high sustained serum levels of penicillin are desired, use aqueous penicillin G, because benzathine salt provides fairly low serum concentrations; in small children, divide dose between two injection sites if necessary
Penicillin G, Procaine Crysticillin A.S., Duracillin A.S., Pfizerpen-AS, Wycillin (CAN) Ayercillin	Injection: 300,000 U/mL, 500,000 U/mL Injection: 300,000 U; 600,000 U; 1.2-, 2.4-million U per unit dose	600,000 U–1.2 million U every 1–3 days *Gonorrheal infections:* 1 g probenecid followed in 30 minutes by 4.8 million U divided into 2 doses and injected at different sites	Long-acting form of penicillin G, similar to benzathine penicillin G in most respects; indicated in moderately severe infections due to organisms (e.g., pneumococci, streptococci) sensitive to persistent low serum levels of penicillin G; may also be effective in treating syphilis, acute pelvic inflammatory disease, diphtheria, anthrax, Vincent's gingivitis, and for perioperative prophylaxis against bacterial endocarditis; given only IM; contains procaine, which provides for slow release and absorption of penicillin; may be allergenic; procaine may impart a local anesthetic effect, making injections less painful than ben-

Continued

Table 58-2
Penicillins (continued)

Drug	Preparations	Usual Dosage Range	Nursing Implications
			zathine preparation; single-dose therapy for gonorrhea has elicited anxiety, confusion, depression, hallucinations, seizures, and extreme weakness; also available in a combination package with probenecid tablets, which delay the excretion of penicillin G
Penicillin G, Benzathine and Procaine Bicillin C-R	Injection: 150,000 U/150,000 U; 300,000 U/300,000 U, and 900,000 U/300,000 U per mL each, respectively, benzathine and procaine penicillin G	*Streptococcal infections* Adults: 2.4 million U IM Children 30–60 lb: 900,000–1.2 million U IM Children under 30 lb: 600,000 U IM *Pneumococcal infections:* 600,000 U in children *or* 1.2 million U in adults every 2–3 days until patient is afebrile for 48 h	Combination of long-acting forms of penicillin G, used to treat moderate to severe streptococcal and pneumococcal infections of the upper respiratory tract, skin and soft tissues and also erysipelas; only administered IM; not effective against streptococcal group D; do *not* use in sexually transmitted diseases; *see* benzathine penicillin G and procaine penicillin G
Penicillin V; Penicillin V, Potassium Pen-Vee K, V-Cillin K, and other manufacturers (CAN) Apo-Pen-VK, Novopen-VK	Tablets: 125 mg, 250 mg, 500 mg Powder for oral suspension; 125 mg/5 mL, 250 mg/5 mL Powder for oral solution (potassium salt): 125 mg/5 mL, 250 mg/5 mL	Adults: 125 mg–500 mg every 6–8 h depending on severity of infection Children: 25 mg–50 mg/kg/day in 3–6 divided doses *Prevention of bacterial endocarditis* Adults: 2 g, 30–60 min prior to procedure, then 500 mg every 6 h for 8 doses Children: 1 g, 30–60 min prior to procedure, then 250 mg every 6 h for 8 doses	Phenoxymethyl derivative of penicillin G, with identical range of activity but more resistant to inactivation by gastric acid, hence better absorbed, yielding 2–5 times higher blood levels; potassium salt is preferred owing to better overall GI absorption; used orally only for mild infections of the throat, respiratory tract or soft tissues; also useful to prevent bacterial endocarditis in patients with rheumatic or acquired valvular heart disease about to undergo surgery or dental procedures; not indicated as initial therapy when parenteral penicillins are necessary (e.g., in severe infections); highly bound to plasma proteins; rapidly excreted in the urine; effective when given with food, but blood levels are higher if administered on an empty stomach
Piperacillin Pipracil	Powder for injection: 2-g, 3-g, 4-g vials or infusion bottles; 40 g per bulk vial	Adults: 3–4 g every 4–6 h over 20–30 min (maximum 24 g/day) *Uncomplicated gonorrheal infection:* 2 g IM in a single dose with 1 g probenecid ½ h before injection *Prophylaxis during surgery:* 2 g IV just prior to surgery, 2 g during or immediately following surgery and 2 g 6–12 h following surgery	Extended-spectrum penicillin, used IM or IV for treatment of a variety of gram-positive and gram-negative infections; similar to mezlocillin in spectrum of activity and efficacy; synergistic with aminoglycosides against *Pseudomonas aeruginosa*, but do *not* mix in the same bottle; sodium content (1.88 mEq/g) is lower than that of carbenicillin or ticarcillin; reduce dosage in patients with renal impairment according to creatinine

Continued

Table 58-2
Penicillins (continued)

Drug	Preparations	Usual Dosage Range	Nursing Implications
Piperacillin (cont'd)			clearance values; *not* recommended for use in children under 12; maximum adult daily dosage is 24 g; do not inject more than 2 g at any one IM injection site; refer to package insert for mixing, diluting, and storage instructions; solutions are stable for 24 h at room temperature, and up to 1 wk refrigerated
Ticarcillin Ticar	Powder for injection: 1-g, 3-g, 6-g vials; 20-g, 30-g bulk vials	Adults and children over 40 kg IV infusion: 150 mg–300 mg/kg/day in divided doses every 3–6 h IV, IM injection: 1 g every 6 h Children under 40 kg IV infusion: 150 mg–300 mg/kg/day in divided doses every 4–6 h IV, IM injection: 50 mg–100 mg/kg/day in divided doses every 6–8 h Neonates under 7 days: 150–225 mg/kg/day in divided doses every 8–12 h by IM injection or IV infusion for 7 days Neonates over 7 days: 225–300 mg/kg/day in divided doses every 8 h by IM injection *or* IV infusion	Extended-spectrum penicillin, not absorbed when taken orally; similar in activity to carbenicillin but more active against most strains of *Pseudomonas*; synergistic with gentamicin and tobramycin against *Pseudomonas* organisms; high in sodium content, therefore monitor serum electrolytes during prolonged therapy and use with *caution* in sodium-restricted patients; IM injections should not exceed 2 g/dose; children weighing more than 40 kg should receive the adult dose; administer IM deeply into large muscle mass; discard IM solutions after 24 h at room temperature or 72 h if refrigerated; inject slowly IV to avoid vein irritation; reduce dosage according to package instructions in patients with renal insufficiency based on creatinine clearance; do *not* mix ticarcillin and gentamicin or tobramycin in same solution because latter drugs may be inactivated
Ticarcillin and potassium clavulanate Timentin	Powder for injection: 3 g ticarcillin and 0.1 g clavulanic acid (as potassium salt) per vial	Adults: 3.1 g ticarcillin/0.1 g clavulanic acid every 4–6 h by IV infusion Children (over 12): 200 mg/kg/day to 300 mg/kg/day (ticarcillin content) in divided doses every 4–6 h	Combination of ticarcillin and potassium salt of clavulanic acid which protects ticarcillin from destruction by beta-lactamase enzymes produced by certain bacteria, thereby extending its spectrum of action; use in children under age 12 has not been established; dosage must be reduced in presence of renal impairment; solutions are stable up to 6 h at room temperature and up to 72 h if refrigerated; drug is reconstituted for infusion with either sterile water for injection or sodium chloride injection

3. Interpret results of the following laboratory tests cautiously because indicated penicillins may cause the alterations noted: urine glucose using Clinitest (false positive with ampicillin), serum uric acid (decreased with azlocillin), serum proteins (false positive with azlocillin or mezlocillin), plasma estrogens (decreased with ampicillin), Coombs' test (positive with IV carbenicillin or piperacillin).

PATIENT EDUCATION

See **Plan of Nursing Care 12, Antibacterial Drugs,** in Chapter 56. In addition:
1. Inform patient for whom either penicillin V, bacampicillin, or amoxicillin has been prescribed that the drug may be taken with meals to reduce GI distress. These drugs apparently are not significantly affected by the presence of food.

CARBAPENEMS

Imipenem–Cilastatin

Primaxin

Imipenem is a beta-lactam that is structurally different from the penicillins and cephalosporins but possesses a similar mechanism of action. It is effective against a wide range of gram-positive, gram-negative, and anaerobic microorganisms and is useful in treating serious infections due to a variety of bacteria resistant to many other antimicrobial drugs. It may be useful as a *single agent* in infections that would ordinarily require multiple anti-infective drug therapy. The drug is as effective as aminoglycosides or third generation cephalosporins for severe gram-negative infections. Imipenem is rapidly hydrolyzed by an enzyme in the proximal renal tubules resulting in urinary drug levels that are very low and are probably inadequate for an antibacterial action. This problem has been overcome by the addition to the formulation of cilastatin, which is an inhibitor of the renal enzyme that destroys imipenem.

MECHANISM

Penetrates gram-positive and gram-negative bacterial cells and binds avidly to penicillin-binding proteins 1B and 2, thus interfering with synthesis of peptidoglycan and subsequent cell wall formation; highly resistant to destruction by beta-lactamase enzymes; inhibits more than 90% of the clinically important pathogens, the notable exceptions being *Pseudomonas maltophilia; Streptococcus faecium;* groups A, C, and G streptococci; and methicillin-resistant staphylococci

USES

Treatment of serious infections due to most common pathogens, except those mentioned under Mechanism above

> NOTE
> Many infections resistant to antibiotics such as penicillins, cephalosporins, or aminoglycosides have responded to treatment with imipenem

DOSAGE

250 mg to 1 g every 6 to 8 hours by IV infusion (30 min), depending on severity of infection; maximum daily dose is 4 g

FATE

Plasma half-life is about 1 hour and plasma levels decline to 1 µg/mL or less within 4 to 6 hours; about 20% protein bound. If administered alone, is rapidly metabolized in the kidneys by a dihydropeptidase enzyme; this metabolism is markedly slowed by cilastatin. Approximately 75% of a dose appears in the urine within 10 hours after administration

COMMON SIDE EFFECTS

Nausea, diarrhea, thrombophlebitis (approximately 3%)

SIGNIFICANT ADVERSE REACTIONS

GI: vomiting, colitis, abdominal pain, glossitis, gastroenteritis
CNS: fever, dizziness, fatigue, confusion, headache, paresthesia, seizures, somnolence, myoclonus, vertigo, encephalopathy
Cardiovascular: tachycardia, palpitations, hypotension
Allergic/dermatologic: skin rash, pruritus, urticaria, flushing, candidiasis, erythema multiforme
Respiratory: dyspnea, chest discomfort, hyperventilation, cyanosis
Other: tinnitus, transient hearing loss, polyarthralgia, weakness, oliguria, polyuria, sweating, pain at injection site, venous induration

Altered laboratory values include:

Increased: SGOT, SGPT, alkaline phosphatase, LDH, bilirubin, BUN, creatinine, potassium, chloride, eosinophils, basophils, lymphocytes, monocytes
Decreased: sodium, platelets, hemoglobin, hematocrit, neutrophils

CONTRAINDICATIONS

No absolute contraindications. *Cautious use* in patients with a history of seizure disorders, thrombophlebitis, renal impairment, or allergic reactions, and in pregnant women or nursing mothers

INTERACTIONS

No reported Interactions. Refer to the Interactions under Penicillins (this chapter) and Cephalosporins (Chap. 59) for *possible* interactions, because the drug is also a beta-lactam

NURSING CONSIDERATION

See **Plan of Nursing Care 12, Antibacterial Drugs,** in Chapter 56. See also penicillins.

PATIENT EDUCATION

See **Plan of Nursing Care 12, Antibacterial Drugs,** in Chapter 56. See also penicillins.

MONOBACTAMS

Aztreonam

Azactam

The monobactam group of antiinfective agents are a relatively new class of drugs that differ from other beta-lactams in that they have a monocyclic rather than a bicyclic nucleus. Aztreonam is the first of the clinically available monobactams. It possesses a wide spectrum of action against gram-negative aerobic pathogens but is inactive against gram-positive organisms or anaerobes.

MECHANISM

Binds to penicillin-binding protein 3, thus inhibiting bacterial cell wall synthesis; highly resistant to beta-lactamase enzymes; bactericidal toward gram-negative aerobic pathogens, including *Pseudomonas aeruginosa, E. coli, Enterobacter, Klebsiella, Proteus mirabilis, Serratia,* and *Hemophilus;* antibacterial efficacy is maintained over a pH range of 6 to 8; synergistic with aminoglycosides against many gram-negative aerobic bacilli

USES

Treatment of infections resulting from susceptible strains of the above-named organisms; responsive diseases include urinary tract, lower respiratory tract, intraabdominal, gynecologic, skin and soft tissue infections and septicemia

NOTE
Aztreonam is usually given initially with another antimicrobial agent in seriously ill patients because it is largely ineffective against gram-positive organisms and anaerobic organisms

DOSAGE

Urinary tract infections: 500 mg to 1 g IV or IM every 8 to 12 hours

Other infections: 1 g to 2 g IV or IM every 6 to 12 hours

NOTE
In patients with impaired renal function (i.e., creatinine clearance between 10 and 30 mL/min), administer an initial loading dose of 1 g to 2 g, then reduce subsequent doses by one half

FATE

Following IM injection, peak serum levels occur within 1 hour; serum half-life is 1.5 to 2 hours in patients with normal renal function; approximately 70% of an IV or IM dose is recovered in the urine within 8 hours; smaller amounts are found in the feces; serum protein binding is approximately 50% and single doses given 8 hours apart do not appear to result in cumulation of drug in the body

COMMON SIDE EFFECTS

Swelling or discomfort at IM injection site, phlebitis with IV administration, nausea, diarrhea, mild skin rash

SIGNIFICANT ADVERSE REACTIONS

Vomiting, confusion, headache, weakness, paresthesia, insomnia, abdominal cramping, hypotension, tinnitus, altered taste, nasal congestion, urticaria, petechiae, muscular aching, fever, malaise, breast tenderness, blood dyscrasias, jaundice, and hepatitis; alterations in liver function enzymes, prothrombin and partial thromboplastin times, serum creatinine, and a positive direct Coombs' test have also been reported during aztreonam treatment

CONTRAINDICATIONS

No absolute contraindications. *Cautious use* in patients with liver or kidney dysfunction or previous hypersensitivity to beta-lactam antiinfectives and in pregnant or nursing women

INTERACTIONS

Beta-lactamase inducing antibiotics (e.g., cefoxitin, imipenem) should not be used concurrently with aztreonam, because they may reduce its effectiveness against beta-lactamase secreting gram-negative aerobes

Aztreonam is incompatible in solution with nafcillin, cephradine, and metronidazole.

NURSING CONSIDERATIONS

See **Plan of Nursing Care 12, Antibacterial Drugs,** in Chapter 56. See also penicillins.

PATIENT EDUCATION

See **Plan of Nursing Care 12, Antibacterial Drugs,** in Chapter 56. See also penicillins.

Selected Bibliography

Bauk NV, Kammer RB: Hematologic complications associated with beta-lactam antibiotics. Rev Infect Dis 5(Suppl 7):5380, 1983

Brooks GF, Barriere SL: Clinical use of the new beta-lactam antimicrobial drugs. Ann Intern Med 98:530, 1983

Cleeland R, Squires E: Enhanced activity of beta-lactam antibiotics with amdinocillin. Am J Med 75(Suppl):21, 1983

Donowitz GR, Mandell GL: Drug therapy: Beta-lactam antibiotics. N Engl J Med 318:419 and 490, 1988

Eliopoulos GM, Moellering RC: Azlocillin, mezlocillin and piperacillin: New broad-spectrum penicillins. Ann Intern Med 79:755, 1982

Goldstein E, Lipman M: Appropriate use of the newer penicillins and cephalosporins. Mod Med 56:102, 1988

Landis BJ, Dunn L: Adverse toxic reaction to aqueous procaine penicillin G. Nurs Pract 9(11):36, 1984

McCloskey WW, Jeffrey LP: Drug stop: Newer beta-lactam antimicrobials. J Neurosurg Nurs 17:210, 1985

Mills J: A guide to using the newer penicillins and beta-lactam antibiotics. Mod Med 55:46, 1987

Neu HC: The in vitro activity human pharmacology and clinical effectiveness of new beta-lactam antibiotics. Annu Rev Pharmacol Toxicol 22:599, 1982

Neu HC: Structure-activity relations of new β-lactam compounds and in-vitro activity against common bacteria. Rev Infect Dis 5(Suppl 2):5319, 1983

Neu HC: Penicillins. In Mandell GL, Douglas RG, Bennett JE (eds): Principles and Practice of Infectious Diseases, 2nd ed, p 166. New York, John Wiley & Sons, 1985

Neu HC, Reeves DS, Leigh DA: Azlocillin—An antipseudomonas penicillin. J Antimicrob Chemother 11(Suppl B):1, 1983

Parry MF, Pancoast SJ: Antipseudomonal penicillins. In Ristuccia AM, Cunha BA (eds): Antimicrobial Therapy, p 197. New York, Raven Press, 1984

Root RK, Sande MA (eds): Contemporary Issues in Infectious Diseases. Vol. I, New Dimensions in Antimicrobial Therapy. New York, Churchill Livingstone, 1984

Sykes RB, Bonner DP: Discovery and development of the monobactams. Rev Infect Dis 7(Suppl 4):S579, 1985

Symposium. An international review of amdinocillin: A new beta lactam antibiotic. Am J Med 75:1, 1983

SUMMARY. PENICILLINS, CARBAPENEMS, MONOBACTAMS

Drug	Preparations	Usual Dosage Range
Penicillins	*See* Table 58-2	
Imipenem-Cilastatin Primaxin	Powder for injection: 250 mg, 500 mg per vial or infusion bottle	250 mg–1 g every 6–8 h by IV infusion over 30 min (maximum 4 g/day)
Aztreonam Azactam	Powder for injection: 500 mg, 1 g, 2 g per vial or infusion bottle	500 mg to 2 g IV or IM every 6–12 h depending on severity of infection

59 CEPHALOSPORINS

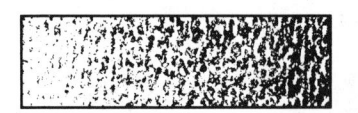

The cephalosporins are a large group of semisynthetic antibiotics mostly derived from cephalosporin C, a natural product of the fungus *Cephalosporium acremonium*. In addition to the several cephalosporin C derivatives, cefoxitin and cefotetan (semisynthetic derivatives of cephamycin C) and moxalactam (a beta-lactam) are also viewed as cephalosporins because of their structural and pharmacologic similarities to the other derivatives.

Cephalosporins are divided into first-, second- and third-generation drugs. As outlined in Table 59-1, differences among the three groups are primarily noted in their antibacterial spectrum of action. Activity against gram-negative bacilli *increases* from first- to third-generation drugs, as does efficacy against resistant organisms as well as drug cost. Conversely, efficacy against gram-positive organisms is greatest with the first-generation drugs and progressively *decreases* through the second- and third-generation compounds. The organisms susceptible to each of the three groups of cephalosporins are also indicated in Table 59-1. Within each group of drugs, the individual agents differ primarily in their pharmacokinetic properties, such as oral versus parenteral efficacy, half-life, protein binding, and principal route of excretion. Some of these differences are also presented in Table 59-1.

Cephalosporin antibiotics are usually bactericidal against most gram-positive cocci (except enterococci, which are unaffected by any drug except possibly cefoperazone) and many gram-negative bacilli. In general, the older, first-generation drugs are the most effective against staphylococci and streptococci, whereas the newer, second- and third-generation drugs display increased activity against the gram-negative enterobacteria. However, although widely prescribed, cephalosporins are recognized as drugs of choice for only a few infections, owing primarily to the availability of more specific, more effective, or less costly alternatives.

Cephalosporins (especially cefazolin) are indicated for surgical prophylaxis, and for treatment of gram-positive infections (except enterococci) in patients allergic to penicillin. However, cross-allergenicity exists between the penicillins and the cephalosporins (estimated incidence is 5%–15%), so caution is indicated when cephalosporins are given to patients with a history of penicillin allergy.

Second- and third-generation drugs should be viewed as alternative choices *only* for treating common gram-positive infections, because they are less effective than first-generation agents and significantly more expensive as well. More specific, more active, and less costly alternatives (e.g., penicillins, erythromycins) should be considered.

Many gram-negative bacilli are susceptible to the second- and third-generation cephalosporins (see Table 59-1), so these drugs are frequently used in respiratory, genitourinary, skin, and soft-tissue infections caused by a variety of gram-negative microorganisms. In addition, the third-generation drugs display differing degrees of activity against *Pseudomonas, Serratia*, and possibly *Salmonella* and *Acinetobacter* and are often employed in combination with or as alternatives to the more toxic (however more effective) aminoglycosides. Cefoxitin, as well as the third-generation drugs, are variably active against *Bacteroides fragilis*, but this activity is not so great or so predictable as with other noncephalosporin drugs. Moreover, many gram-negative bacilli develop resistance to the cephalosporins, greatly restricting their usefulness in many infections.

Most first-generation drugs are susceptible to inactivation by beta-lactamase (i.e., cephalosporinase) enzymes. Second-generation agents (except cefamandole) and all third-generation cephalosporins display greater resistance to enzymatic inactivation, including that of the cephalosporinases produced by many gram-negative pathogens, such as *Pseudomonas, Hemophilus, Acinetobacter, Neisseria*, and some strains of *Bacteroides*.

Compared to many other antibacterial drugs, cephalosporins are relatively nontoxic. The most commonly occurring adverse reactions are allergic in nature and include rash, urticaria, fever, angioedema, and occasionally serum sickness, eosinophilia, and anaphylaxis (for additional untoward reactions, refer to the general discussion of cephalosporins that follows).

A major factor in the selection of cephalosporins is their cost. Parenterally administered cephalosporins are among the most expensive antibiotics in use today, and their cost increases substantially as their spectrum broadens. Thus, second-generation drugs are approximately twice as expensive as first-generation drugs, while third-generation drugs can exceed the cost of first-generation drugs by a factor of four or five. It becomes cost imperative, then, to use the least expensive cephalosporin that is effective against the microorganisms shown to be present. Empiric therapy with third-generation cephalosporins is a frightfully expensive undertaking, and considerable justification should be established for this procedure, such as the presence of severe ototoxicity or nephrotoxicity that would contradict the use of aminoglycosides.

The cephalosporins are considered here as a group. Individual drugs are then listed in Table 59-2, together with specific information pertaining to each drug. In addition, reference should be made to Table 56-1, Chapter 56, for the recommended indications for the cephalosporins.

CEPHALOSPORINS

Cefaclor	Cefoxitin
Cefadroxil	Ceftazidime
Cefamandole	Ceftizoxime
Cefazolin	Ceftriaxone
Cefixime	Cefuroxime
Cefonicid	Cephalexin
Cefoperazone	Cephalothin
Ceforanide	Cephapirin
Cefotaxime	Cephradine
Cefotetan	Moxalactam

MECHANISM
Inhibit mucopeptide synthesis in the bacterial cell wall, resulting in a defective, osmotically unstable wall; may be bactericidal

Table 59-1
Cephalosporins: Pharmacokinetics and Bacterial Spectrum of Action

Drug	Routes of Administration	% Protein Binding	Plasma Half-Life (min)	Urinary Excretion (% Unchanged)	Sodium Content (mEq/g)	Susceptible Microorganisms[a]
First Generation						
Cefaclor	Oral	25	40–50	60–80		Staphylococci
Cefadroxil	Oral	20	70–80	90–95		Streptococci (including beta-hemolytic),
Cephalexin	Oral	10–15	30–50	80–100		*Escherichia coli,*
Cephradine	Oral, IM, IV	10–15	45–60	80–90	6.0	*Hemophilus influenzae* (except cefadroxil),
Cephapirin	IM, IV	40–50	20–40	50–75	2.4	*Klebsiella, Proteus mirabilis*
Cephalothin	IM, IV	65–75	30–60	50–75	2.8	
Cefazolin	IM, IV	75–85	90–120	75–100	2	
Second Generation						
Cefamandole	IM, IV	65–75	30–60	60–80	3.3	All the above, plus: *Neisseria gonorrhoeae* (except cefamandole), *Proteus morganii* (except cefonicid, ceforanide, cefixime), *Proteus vulgaris,* (except cefonicid, ceforanide), *Providencia* (except cefonicid, cefamandole), *Enterobacter* (except cefoxitin), *Citrobacter* (except cefoxitin, cefamandole), *Neisseria meningitidis* (cefuroxine only), *Clostridium, Peptococcus, Peptostreptococcus, Bacteroides fragilis* (cefoxitin only), *Fusobacterium* (except cefoxitin), *Salmonella* (cefuroxime only), *Shigella* (cefuroxime only)
Cefonicid	IM, IV	95–98	240–300	99	2.7	
Cefoxitin	IM, IV	65–75	30–60	90–100	2.3	
Cefuroxime	Oral, IM, IV	40–50	60–120	70–95	2.4	
Ceforanide	IM, IV	80	150–180	80–95	0	
Third Generation						
Cefotaxime	IM, IV	30–50	60–70	50–60	2.2	All the above, plus: *Pseudomonas aeruginosa* (except cefotetan, cefixime), *Serratia, Acinetobacter* (ceftizoxime, ceftriaxone, cefoperazone, ceftazidime only), *Eubacterium* (cefoperazone, moxalactam, ceftizoxime only), *Clostridium difficile* (cefoperazone, cefotetan only)
Ceftizoxime	IM, IV	30	100–120	75–80	2.6	
Cefoperazone	IM, IV	80–90	100–150	20–25	1.5	
Moxalactam	IM, IV	45–55	120–210	70–90	3.8	
Ceftriaxone	IM, IV	85–95	350–500	30–60	3.6	
Cefotetan	IM, IV	80–90	180–270	50–80	3.5	
Ceftazidime	IM, IV	5–15	100–120	80–90	2.3	
Cefixime	Oral	60–70	180–240	50		

[a] Susceptibility may vary with individual members of the group, and in some cases has only been demonstrated in vitro.

or bacteriostatic depending on dosage, tissue concentrations of drug, organism susceptibility, and rate of bacterial replication; most effective against rapidly growing organisms

USES

Alternatives to penicillins for treatment of infections of the respiratory tract, skin and soft tissues, genitourinary tract, middle ear, and bloodstream caused by susceptible organisms (see Chap. 56, Table 56-1, and Table 59-1 for susceptible microorganisms)

Surgical prophylaxis when expanded gram-negative activity is desired, in procedures where there is a significant risk of contamination (e.g., GI surgery, cholecystectomy, vaginal hysterectomy); usually first-generation drugs (e.g., cefazolin)

Treatment of serious *Klebsiella* infections, frequently in conjunction with an aminoglycoside

Treatment of meningitis caused by gram-negative enteric bacteria

Adjunctive treatment (with an aminoglycoside) of bacteremia of unknown origin in debilitated or immunosuppressed patients

Adjunctive therapy in septicemia, acute endocarditis, meningitis, and bone and joint infections

DOSAGE
See Table 59-2

FATE
Oral drugs are well absorbed from GI tract, but absorption may be delayed by food. Absorption from IM sites is good. Peak blood levels are attained rapidly (usually 30-60 min). Half-lives are given in Table 59-1. Cephalosporins are distributed extensively, but only cefuroxime and the third-generation drugs diffuse into the cerebrospinal fluid, especially when the meninges are inflamed. Penetration into bone is variable. Drugs readily cross placental barrier and are secreted into milk of nursing mothers. Most derivatives (except cefotaxime, cephalothin, ceftriaxone, and cephapirin) are not appreciably metabolized and are excreted largely unchanged in the urine. Cefoperazone, however, is eliminated predominantly in the bile; ceftriaxone and cefotaxime are also found in appreciable amounts in the bile.

COMMON SIDE EFFECTS
Nausea and diarrhea with oral administration, hypersensitivity reactions in persons with a history of allergy

SIGNIFICANT ADVERSE REACTIONS
(Most reactions occur more commonly with large doses or during prolonged therapy.)

GI: anorexia, abdominal pain, dyspepsia, heartburn, vomiting, severe diarrhea, oral candidiasis, glossitis, GI bleeding, enterocolitis

Allergic/hypersensitivity: urticaria, pruritus, skin rash, fever, chills, serum sickness, eosinophilia, angioedema, exfoliative dermatitis, anaphylactic reactions

Hematologic: neutropenia, leukopenia, thrombocytopenia, agranulocytosis, hemolytic anemia, bleeding due to hypoprothrombinemia, positive direct Coombs' test

Genitourinary: dysuria, elevated BUN, proteinuria, hematuria, vaginal discharge, candidal vaginitis, genitoanal pruritus, genital candidiasis

Hepatic: elevated SGOT, SGPT, bilirubin, alkaline phosphatase and LDH levels; hepatitis (rare)

Other: headache, weakness, dizziness, dyspnea, paresthesia, candidal overgrowth, hepatomegaly; IM administration may cause pain, induration, tenderness, fever, and tissue sloughing

> **WARNING**
> Coagulation abnormalities associated with bleeding episodes, some of a severe nature, have occurred with use of several cephalosporins, including cefamandole, cefoperazone, and especially moxalactam

CONTRAINDICATIONS
No absolute contraindications. *Cautious use* in patients with a history of allergies, asthma, hay fever, penicillin sensitivity (see introductory comments), or impaired renal function, and in small children, during pregnancy, and in nursing mothers.

In addition, cefoperazone, ceftriaxone, and cefotaxime should be given cautiously to persons with impaired liver function, as they are excreted in the bile.

INTERACTIONS
Use of bacteriostatic antibiotics (e.g., tetracyclines, erythromycins) may reduce cephalosporin effectiveness, especially in acute infections where the organisms are proliferating rapidly

The nephrotoxic effects of cephalosporins may be augmented by aminoglycosides, colistin, vancomycin, polymyxin B, ethacrynic acid, furosemide, bumetanide, probenecid, and sulfinpyrazone

Cephalosporins are incompatible in parenteral mixtures with tetracyclines, erythromycins, calcium chloride, and magnesium salts

Probenecid may increase and prolong cephalosporin plasma levels (except moxalactam) by inhibiting renal tubular secretion of the drugs

Alcohol may elicit a disulfiram-like reaction (see Chap. 78) with cefamandole, cefoperazone, cefotetan, or moxalactam

NURSING CONSIDERATIONS
See **Plan of Nursing Care 12: Antibacterial Drugs** in Chapter 56. See Table 59-2 for specific information on each drug. In addition:

Nursing Alerts
- Monitor results of prothrombin times because cephalosporins (especially moxalactam, cefamandole, and cefoperazone) can interfere with hemostasis by decreasing availability of vitamin K and interfering with normal platelet function. Smallest effective doses should be used to minimize effect on platelet function, and supplemental vitamin K (10 mg/wk) should be prescribed if necessary.
- Monitor results of hematologic, renal, and hepatic function tests, which should be performed periodically (i.e., every 3-6 mo) during prolonged therapy.
- Observe for signs of diminished renal function (e.g., decreased urine output, proteinuria, elevated BUN or serum creatinine) because nephrotoxity may occur.
- Monitor results of electrolyte determinations during prolonged infusion because sodium overload can occur with drugs that contain significant amounts of sodium (see Table 59-1).

1. When giving IM, inject deeply into large muscle. In patient with bacteremia, septicemia, or other severe infection, IV administration is preferable.
2. When giving IV infusion, use small needle, inject into large vein, and alternate infusion sites to minimize danger of phlebitis.
3. When both cephalosporin and aminoglycoside solutions are prescribed, administer them separately.
4. Interpret results of the following laboratory tests cautiously because cephalosporins may cause false readings: urinary glucose using Benedict's or Fehling's solution or Clinitest tablets, urinary protein with acid and denaturization-precipitation tests, urinary 17-ketosteroids, and positive direct Coombs' test.

(*Text continued on page 608*)

Table 59-2
Cephalosporins

Drug	Preparations	Usual Dosage Range	Nursing Implications
First Generation			
Cefaclor Ceclor	Capsules: 250 mg, 500 mg Oral suspension: 125 mg/5 mL, 187 mg/5 mL, 250 mg/5 mL, 375 mg/5 mL	Adults: 250 mg–500 mg every 8 h (maximum 4 g/day) Children: 20 mg–40 mg/kg/day in divided doses every 8 h (maximum 1 g/day)	Orally effective, short-acting cephalosporin used in respiratory, urinary, skin, and soft-tissue infections and otitis media; classified as second-generation but spectrum resembles first generation; a single 2-g dose has been used in acute, uncomplicated urinary tract infections; be alert for onset of skin rash, fever, polyarthritis and erythema multiforme within 1–2 wk—corticosteroids and antihistamines may be used to treat symptoms, which usually resolve within several days
Cefadroxil Duricef, Ultracef, and other manufacturers	Capsules: 500 mg Tablets: 1 g Oral suspension: 125 mg/5 mL, 250 mg/5 mL, 500 mg/5 mL	Adults: 1 g–2 g/day in a single or divided doses Children: 30 mg/kg/day in divided doses every 12 h	Orally effective drug used principally to treat urinary tract infections due to *Escherichia coli*, *Proteus mirabilis*, or *Klebsiella*; also used in staphylococcal and streptococcal infections of skin, pharynx, and tonsils; not metabolized to any extent and excreted essentially intact in the urine; oral absorption is not significantly affected by food; adjust dosage according to package instructions in patients with renal impairment
Cefazolin Ancef, Kefzol, Zolicef	Powder for injection: 250 mg, 500 mg, 1 g, 5 g, 10 g, 20 g per vial	Adults: 250 mg–1.5 g IV *or* IM every 6–12 h depending on severity of infection (maximum 12 g/day) Children: 25 mg–100 mg/kg/day in 3 or 4 divided doses *Acute uncomplicated urinary tract infections:* 1 g/12 h *Perioperative prophylaxis:* 1 g ½–1 h before surgery, 0.5 g–1 g during surgery of 2 h or longer, then 0.5 g–1 g every 6–8 h for 24 h after surgery	Parenteral cephalosporin similar to cephalothin but claimed to be less irritating and less nephrotoxic; used in treatment of respiratory, urinary, and biliary tract infections, skin and soft tissue infections, septicemia, bone and joint infections, and endocarditis; also indicated as alternative therapy for gonorrhea in pregnant patients allergic to penicillin; widely used perioperatively to reduce risk of infection following certain surgical procedures; highly protein bound; do *not* use in children under 1 mo; follow manufacturer's recommendations for dosing in renal impairment; pain on injection is infrequent; diluted solutions are stable for 24 h at room temperature and 96 h under refrigeration; hemiparesis has occurred following large doses
Cephalexin Keflex, Keflet, Keftab, and other manufacturers (CAN) Ceporex, Novolexin	Capsules: 250 mg, 500 mg Tablets: 250 mg, 500 mg, 1 g Oral suspension: 125 mg/5 mL, 250 mg/5 mL	Adults: 250 mg–500 mg every 6 h (maximum dose is 4 g/day) Children: 25 mg–100 mg/kg/day	Orally effective cephalosporin indicated for respiratory, urinary, skin, bone, and soft-tissue infections, and otitis media in

Continued

Table 59-2
Cephalosporins (continued)

Drug	Preparations	Usual Dosage Range	Nursing Implications
Cephalexin (cont'd)	Pediatric drops: 100 mg/mL	in 4 divided doses depending on severity of infection	penicillin-sensitive patients; due to susceptible organisms (*see* Table 59-1); some staphylococci are resistant; stable in gastric acid, well absorbed, and only slightly protein-bound; if doses greater than 4 g/day are necessary, parenteral cephalosporins should be used; refrigerate oral suspension and discard unused portion in 14 days
Cephalothin Keflin (CAN) Ceporacin	Powder for injection: 1 g, 2 g, 20 g/vial Injection: 1 g, 2 g per 50 ml vial	Adults: 500 mg–1000 mg IM *or* IV injection every 4–6 h (up to 2 g every 4 h IV in life-threatening infections) Children: 80 mg–160 mg/kg/day IM in divided doses *Perioperative prophylaxis* Adults: 1 g–2 g IM *or* IV ½–1 h before surgery, during surgery as needed, and every 6 h following surgery for 24 h Children: 20 mg/kg–30 mg/kg following the above schedule	Prototype cephalosporin used to treat respiratory, GI, urinary, skin, bone, joint, and soft-tissue infections as well as septicemia and meningitis (see Table 59-1); not effective against *Pseudomonas, Serratia,* indole-positive *Proteus* or *Enterococcus*; may be employed perioperatively to reduce incidence of certain infections in high-risk situations (e.g., vaginal hysterectomy, intestinal or colorectal surgery, open heart surgery, cholecystectomy, prosthetic arthroplasty); IM injection often elicits pain, induration, and sloughing; IV administration may lead to phlebitis or other inflammatory reactions; may be added to peritoneal dialysis fluid in concentrations up to 6 mg/100 mL and instilled throughout the dialysis procedure; owing to short half-life (30–45 min), initial perioperative dose should be given just before start of surgery and readministered at appropriate intervals throughout procedure to maintain sufficient blood levels; prophylactic use should be discontinued within 24 h following surgery; maintenance dose must be reduced according to creatinine clearance in patients with impaired renal function; solutions are stable for 12–24 h at room temperature and 96 h under refrigeration; slight darkening does not affect potency
Cephapirin Cefadyl	Powder for injection: 500 mg, 1 g, 2 g, 4 g, 20 g per vial	Adults: 500 mg–1000 mg IM *or* IV every 4–6 h (up to 12 g/day IV in serious infections) Children: 40 mg–80 mg/kg/day IM in divided doses *Perioperative prophylaxis:* 1 g–2 g IM *or* IV ½–1 h before surgery, during surgery if needed, and every 6 h after surgery for 24 h	Parenteral cephalosporin similar to cephalothin in action but causing less tissue irritation; clinical evidence of renal damage has not been reported; jaundice has occurred; do *not* use in children under 3 mo; dilutions are stable for 24 h at room temperature and up to 10 days with refrigera-

Continued

Table 59-2
Cephalosporins (continued)

Drug	Preparations	Usual Dosage Range	Nursing Implications
			tion; check package instructions for compatibility with other infusion solutions
Cephradine Anspor, Velosef and other manufacturers	Capsules: 250 mg, 500 mg Oral suspension: 125 mg/5 mL, 250 mg/5 mL Powder for injection: 250 mg, 500 mg; 1 g, 2 g per vial or infusion bottle	*Oral* Adults: 250 mg–500 mg every 6 h *or* 1 g every 12 h Children (over 9 mo): 25 mg–100 mg/kg/day in divided doses every 6–12 h (maximum 4 g/day) *IV, IM* Adults: 500 mg–1000 mg 4 times/day (maximum 8 g/day) Children (over 12 mo): 50 mg–100 mg/kg/day in 4 divided doses *Perioperative prophylaxis* 1 g IV *or* IM 30–40 min before surgery, then 1 g every 4–6 h thereafter up to 24 h *Cesarean section* 1 g IV when cord is clamped, then again at 6 and 12 h	Available in both oral and parenteral dosage forms; oral preparations are primarily used as follow-up therapy to parenteral treatment; may be given without regard to meals because drug is acid-stable; excreted largely unchanged in urine, mostly within 6 h, thus is effective in urinary infections due to susceptible organisms; very slightly protein-bound; following reconstitution, IM or direct IV solutions should be used within 2 h at room temperature; continuous IV solutions retain potency for 10 h at room temperature, infusion solution should be replaced at that time; do *not* combine cephradine solutions with those of other antibiotics; doses smaller than those indicated should not be used; persistent infections may require several weeks of therapy
Second Generation			
Cefamandole Mandol	Powder for injection: 500 mg, 1 g, 2 g, 10 g per vial	Adults: 500 mg–1000 mg IM *or* IV every 4–8 h (up to 2 g/4 hr in severe infections) Children: 50 mg–100 mg/kg/day in divided doses every 4–8 h *Perioperative prophylaxis* Adults: 1 g–2 g IM *or* IV 1 h prior to incision, then 1 g–2 g every 6 h for 24–48 h Children: 50 mg–100 mg/kg/day in equally divided doses according to above schedule	Parenteral cephalosporin indicated for infections of the respiratory or urinary tracts and skin, for surgical prophylaxis, and for septicemia and peritonitis caused by susceptible organisms; effective against anaerobic organisms (*Clostridium, Peptococcus*), indole-positive *Proteus* and some strains of *Bacteroides fragilis*; also used in combination with an aminoglycoside for gram-positive or gram-negative sepsis (danger of nephrotoxicity, *see* Interactions); reduce dosage as indicated in package insert in patients with renal impairment—may cause acute tubular necrosis; bleeding episodes have occurred—monitor prothrombin time and platelet count; jaundice has been noted in some patients; do *not* mix with aminoglycoside in same container; dilute drug solution as instructed with appropriate diluent; reconstituted cefamandole is stable for 24 h at room temperature and 96 h under refrigeration; IV dosage can be up to 12 g/day depending on severity of infection (e.g., bacterial septicemia)

Continued

Table 59-2
Cephalosporins (continued)

Drug	Preparations	Usual Dosage Range	Nursing Implications
Cefonicid Monocid	Powder for injection: 500 mg, 1 g, 10 g per vial	Adults: 0.5 g–1 g IM *or* slow IV injection once every 24 h (maximum dose is 2 g once daily) *Perioperative prophylaxis* Adults: 1 g given 1 h prior to incision, then 1 g once daily for 48 h	Long-acting cephalosporin given once daily for respiratory, urinary, skin, bone, and joint infections, and septicemia; not active against *Pseudomonas, Serratia, Enterococcus, Acinetobacter*, and most strains of *B. fragilis*; may cause pain on injection; doses larger than 1 g should be divided and given at two different IM sites; reduce dosage in patients with impaired renal function according to package directions; dilutions are stable for 24 h at room temperature and 72 h if refrigerated
Ceforanide Precef	Powder for injection: 500 mg, 1 g per vial	Adults: 0.5 g–1 g IM or IV every 12 h Children: 20–40 mg/kg/day in equally divided doses every 12 h *Perioperative prophylaxis* 0.5 g–1 g IM or IV 1 h prior to start of surgery; intraoperative administration is not necessary	Long-acting parenteral cephalosporin given twice a day for respiratory, urinary, and skin and soft-tissue infections due to staphylococci, streptococci, *Klebsiella, Hemophilus, E. coli, Proteus mirabilis*, also effective in bone and joint infections and endocarditis caused by staphylococci, septicemia due to staphylococci, streptococci, or *E. coli*, and for perioperative prophylaxis, active against *Enterobacter, Citrobacter*, and *Providencia*; reduce dosage in renal impairment; elevated creatinine phosphokinase has occurred following IM injection; contains no sodium
Cefoxitin Mefoxin	Powder for injection: 1 g, 2 g, 10 g per vial or infusion bottle	Adults: 1 g–2 g every 6 h–8 h IV *or* IM (maximum is 12 g/day) Children: 80–160 mg/kg/day in 4–6 divided doses; maximum 12 g/day *Gonorrhea* (see Nursing Implications): 2 g IM with 1 g probenecid *Disseminated gonorrhea:* 1 g IV 4 times/day for at least 7 days *Acute pelvic inflammatory disease:* 2 g IV 4 times/day with 100 mg doxycycline IV twice a day for at least 4 days; continue 100 mg doxycycline, orally, twice a day for an additional 10–14 days *Perioperative prophylaxis:* 2 g IV or IM ½–1 h before surgery and every 6 h thereafter for up to 24 h	Effective against a variety of organisms susceptible to first-generation cephalosporins as well as anaerobic organisms, indole-positive *Proteus, Bacteroides fragilis,* and some gram-negative bacteria resistant to other cephalosporins and broad-spectrum penicillins; may reduce incidence of postoperative infections in patients undergoing surgical procedures that are classified as potentially contaminated (e.g., GI surgery, vaginal hysterectomy); also indicated for penicillinase-producing *Neisseria gonorrheae* resistant to spectinomycin and for acute pelvic inflammatory disease; highly resistant to beta-lactamase; reconstituted solutions maintain potency for 24 h at room temperature, 1 wk under refrigeration, and up to 26 wk frozen; dry material may darken with time but potency is not affected; frequently painful upon IM

Continued

Table 59-2
Cephalosporins (continued)

Drug	Preparations	Usual Dosage Range	Nursing Implications
Cefuroxime Kefurox, Zinacef **Cefuroxime axetil** Ceftin	Powder for injection: 750 mg, 1.5 g, 7.5 g per vial Tablets: 125 mg, 250 mg, 500 mg	*Oral* Adults and children over 12: 125 mg–500 mg every 12 h depending on severity of infection Children (under 12): 125 mg every 12 h *Parenteral* Adults: 2.25 g–6 g/day IM or IV in divided doses every 6–8 h (maximum dose is 9 g/day in bacterial meningitis) Children (over 3 mo): 50 mg–100 mg/kg/day in divided doses every 6–8 h *Uncomplicated gonorrhea:* 1.5 g IM as a single dose with 1 g oral probenecid *Perioperative prophylaxis:* 1.5 g IV just prior to surgery, then 750 mg IV *or* IM every 8 h for 24 h *Bacterial meningitis (children):* 200 mg–240 mg/kg/day IV in divided doses every 6–8 h; reduce to 100 mg/kg/day IV upon improvement	injection; follow package directions for dosing patients with renal impairment Unlike other first- and second-generation drugs, attains significant concentrations in the cerebrospinal fluid, especially if the meninges are inflamed; effective against many gram-negative bacilli, including *Enterobacter* and *Citrobacter* (some strains, however, are resistant); oral treatment indicated for upper and lower respiratory tract, urinary, skin and soft-tissue infections and otitis media due to susceptible organisms (see Table 59-1); administer single 1.5-g IM dose for gonorrhea at two different sites; dosage is reduced according to package instructions, in patients with renal dysfunction; inject slowly (3–5 min) IV or infuse either intermittently or continuously; do *not* mix with aminoglycosides; powder and solutions may darken with time, but potency of solution is unaffected for 24 h at room temperature and 48 h refrigerated
Third Generation **Cefoperazone** Cefobid	Powder for injection: 1 g, 2 g per vial	Adults: 2 g–4 g/day IM *or* IV in equally divided doses every 12 h; up to 16 g/day has been given by constant infusion in severe infections	Cephalosporin with an extensive spectrum of action; used in respiratory, intraabdominal, and urogenital infections, bacterial septicemia, and infections of the skin and associated structures; highly protein-bound; extensively excreted in the bile, do *not* exceed 4 g/day in patients with hepatic disease or biliary obstruction; no dosage adjustment is required in the presence of renal failure; long half-life requires only twice-a-day dosing, although more frequent administration can be used in severe infections; highly resistant to beta-lactamase enzymes produced by most gram-negative pathogens; pseudomembranous colitis has occurred—be alert for development of diarrhea; symptoms of hepatitis have been reported; may interfere with hemostasis resulting in bleeding—supplemental vitamin K (10 mg/wk) reduces likelihood of bleeding

Continued

Table 59-2
Cephalosporins (continued)

Drug	Preparations	Usual Dosage Range	Nursing Implications
Cefotaxime Claforan	Powder for injection: 1 g, 2 g, 10 g per vial	Adults: 1 g–2 g every 6–12 h IV *or* IM (maximum dose 12 g/day) Children: 50 mg–180 mg/kg/day in 4–6 divided doses *Perioperative prophylaxis:* 1 g IV *or* IM 30–90 min before surgery, then 1 g within 2 h following surgery *Gonorrhea:* 1 g IM as a single injection *Disseminated gonorrhea:* 500 mg IV 4 times/day for at least 7 days	Parenteral cephalosporin used in the treatment of serious infections of the abdomen, lower respiratory tract, urinary tract, skin, and genital tract; also indicated as a surgical prophylactic agent and for penicillinase-producing *Neisseria gonorrhoeae* infections resistant to spectinomycin; many strains of *Pseudomonas* and enterococci are resistant; most common adverse reactions are pain, tenderness, and inflammation at injection site; reduce dosage according to package instructions in patients with renal impairment; does not appear to be nephrotoxic; may be used concurrently with an aminoglycoside, but *do not* mix in same syringe; drug and metabolite attain high concentration in the bile
Cefotetan Cefotan	Powder for injection: 1 g, 2 g, 10 g per vial	Adults: 1 g–2 g IV *or* IM every 12 h for 5–10 days (maximum 3 g every 12 h in life-threatening infections) *Perioperative prophylaxis:* 1 g–2 g IV 30–60 min before surgery	Long-acting parenteral cephamycin effective against most common organisms *except Pseudomonas* and *Acinetobacter*; highly resistant to beta-lactamases; use cautiously in persons with bleeding tendencies because drug may interfere with hemostasis; may produce acute alcohol intolerance; reconstituted solutions retain potency for 24 h at room temperature, 96 h refrigerated, and at least 1 wk frozen; do not refreeze; dosage reduction in patients with renal failures based on creatinine clearance
Ceftazidime Fortaz, Tazicef, Tazidime (CAN) Magnacef	Powder for injection: 500 mg, 1 g, 2 g, 6 g per vial or infusion pack	Adults: Usually 1 g–2 g IV *or* IM every 8–12 h Children: 30 mg–50 mg/kg IV every 8 h (neonates every 12 h) *Urinary infections:* 250 mg–500 mg every 8–12 h *Pseudomonal lung infection in cystic fibrosis patients:* 30 mg–50 mg/kg IV every 8 h to a maximum of 6 g/day *Dialysis:* 1-g loading dose followed by 1 g after each hemodialysis period	Very broad-spectrum cephalosporin used for a variety of infections (respiratory, urinary, bone, skin, gynecologic, intra-abdominal CNS, septicemia); good activity against *Pseudomonas* but poorly active vs *Bacteroides fragilis*; protein binding is minimal; very stable in the presence of beta-lactamases; administer separately from aminoglycosides
Ceftizoxime Cefizox	Powder for injection: 1 g, 2 g, 10 g per vial Injection: 1 g/50 mL, 2 g/50 mL	Adults: 1 g–2 g IM *or* IV every 8–12 h (maximum dose is 12 g/day) Children: 50 mg/kg every 6–8 h (see Nursing Implications) *Uncomplicated gonorrhea:* 1 g IM as a single dose	Broad-spectrum drug used in a variety of infections due to both gram-positive and gram-negative organisms; long half-life allows twice daily dosing in less severe infections, but serious infections require ad-

Continued

Table 59-2
Cephalosporins (continued)

Drug	Preparations	Usual Dosage Range	Nursing Implications
			ministration every 8 h; stable *against* beta-lactamase enzymes and only slightly (30%) protein-bound; may be active against some microorganisms that have developed resistance to other cephalosporins; dosage must be reduced in patients with impaired renal function; may be injected directly IV (3–5 min) *or* given by intermittent or continuous infusion; reconstitute powder in sterile water for injection; stable for 8 h at room temperature and 48 h if refrigerated; may result in elevations in SGOT, SGPT, CPK in children
Ceftriaxone Rocephin	Powder for injection: 250 mg, 500 mg, 1 g, 2 g, 10 g per vial	Adults: 1 g–2 g daily in a single or two divided doses IM *or* IV (maximum 4 g/day) Children: 50 mg–75 mg/kg/day in divided doses every 12 h *Meningitis:* 100 mg/kg/day in divided doses IV every 12 h following a loading dose of 75 mg/kg *Uncomplicated gonorrhea:* 250 mg as a single IM dose *Surgical prophylaxis:* 1 g IM *or* IV ½–2 h before surgery	Very long-acting cephalosporin usually given once daily (except for meningitis); stable against beta-lactamase enzymes; highly protein-bound; excreted in both the urine and the bile; may alter prothrombin time; casts in urine have occurred during therapy; dosage adjustment is seldom necessary in patients with renal or hepatic impairment; solutions should *not* be mixed with other antimicrobial drugs owing to incompatability
Moxalactam Moxam	Powder for injection: 1 g, 2 g, 10 g per vial	Adults: 500 mg–2 g IV *or* IM every 8–12 h for most mild to moderate infections; serious or life-threatening infections— up to 4 g every 8 h Children: 50 mg/kg every 6–8 h Infants: 50 mg/kg every 6 h Neonates: 50 mg/kg every 8–12 h	Long-acting cephalosporin, highly resistant to inactivation by beta-lactamases; indicated in lower respiratory, urinary, intraabdominal, CNS (penetrates blood–brain barrier), skin, bone, and joint infections due to susceptible organisms; effective against many strains of *Pseudomonas* but high doses are necessary and other therapy (e.g., aminoglycosides) should be instituted if a clinical response does not occur promptly; may be given concomitantly with an aminoglycoside; probenecid does *not* alter the elimination of moxalactam; hypoprothrombinemia and increased bleeding tendency has been reported; monitor bleeding time (especially if dose exceeds 4 g/day) and observe for signs of bleeding; discontinue drug or provide supplemental vitamin K (10 mg/wk); IV administration of moxalactam is preferred for more serious infections, i.e., slow injection (3–5 min) or infusion; reconstituted solution is

Continued

Table 59-2
Cephalosporins (continued)

Drug	Preparations	Usual Dosage Range	Nursing Implications
Moxalactam (cont'd)			stable for 90 h if stored under refrigeration; can cause a disulfiram-like reaction in patients who drink alcohol (see Chap. 78)
Cefixime Suprax	Tablets: 200 mg, 400 mg Powder for oral suspension: 100 mg/5 mL	Adults: 400 mg/day in a single or 2 divided doses Children under 12: 4 mg/kg every 12 h	Orally effective drug used in urinary tract infections, otitis media, pharyngitis and acute and chronic bronchitis; *not* active vs. *staphylococci, Proteus morganii, Pseudomonas aeruginosa Acinetobacter sp.* or *Salmonella* typhi; suspension yields higher peak blood levels than tablet; reduce dose if creatinine clearance is less than 60 mL/min

Selected Bibliography

Bank NV, Kammer RB: Hematologic complications associated with beta-lactam antibiotics. Rev Infect Dis 5(Suppl 2):380, 1983

Baumgartner J, Glauser MP: Single daily dose treatment of severe refractory infections with ceftriaxone. Arch Intern Med 143:1868, 1983

Bertino JS, Speck WT: The cephalosporin antibiotics. Pediatr Clin North Am 30:17, 1983

Byrd HJ, Fischer RG: Cephalosporins: A brief overview of three generations. Pediatr Nurs 9:330, 1983

Ceftriaxone sodium (Rocephin). Med Lett Drugs Ther 27:37, 1985

Donowitz GR, Mandell GL: Drug therapy: Beta-lactam antibiotics. N Engl J Med 318:419, 490, 1988

Garzone P, Lyon J, Yu VL: Third-generation and investigational cephalosporins, Parts I and II. Drug Intell Clin Pharm 17:507, 615, 1983

Goldstein E, Lipman M: Appropriate use of the newer penicillins and cephalosporins. Mod Med 56:102, 1988

Klein JO, Neu HC: Empiric therapy for bacterial infections: Evaluation of cefoperazone. Rev Infect Dis 5:S1, 1983

Mandell GL: Cephalosporins. In Mandell GL, Douglas RG, Bennett JE (eds): Principles and Practice of Infectious Diseases, 2nd ed, p 180. New York, John Wiley & Sons, 1985

McCloskey WW, Jeffrey LP: Drugstop: New beta-lactam antimicrobials. J Neurosurg Nurs 17:210, 1985

Mullaney DT, John JF: Cefotaxime therapy. Arch Intern Med 143:1705, 1983

Neu HC: Advances in cephalosporin therapy. Am J Med 79(Suppl 2A):114, 1985

Neu HC: New beta-lactamase-stable cephalosporins. Ann Intern Med 97:408, 1982

Neu HC: Clinical uses of cephalosporins. Lancet 1:252, 1982

Phillips I, Wise R, Leigh DA: Cefotetan: A new cephamycin. J Antimicrob Chemother 11(Suppl B):1, 1983

Polk R: Moxalactam (Moxam). Drug Intell Clin Pharm 16:104, 1982

Quintiliana R, et al: Cephalosporins: An overview. In Ristuccia AM, Cunha BA (eds): Anti-microbial Therapy, p 289. New York, Raven Press, 1984

Schumacher GE: Pharmacokinetic and microbiologic evaluation of dosage regimens for newer cephalosporins and penicillins. Clin Pharm 2:448, 1983

Smith BR, LeFrock JL: Cefuroxime: Antimicrobial activity, pharmacology and clinical efficacy. Ther Drug Monit 5:149, 1983

Sykes RB, Bush K: Interaction of new cephalosporins with beta lactamases and beta-lactamase-producing gram negative bacilli. Rev Infect Dis 5:S356, 1983

Thompson RL, Wright AJ: Cephalosporin antibiotics. Mayo Clin Proc 58:79, 1983

Weitekamp MR, Aber RC: Prolonged bleeding times and bleeding diathesis associated with moxalactam administration. JAMA 249:69, 1983

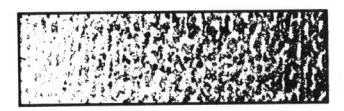

60 TETRACYCLINES, QUINOLONES

The *tetracycline* group of antibiotics is composed of a number of naturally derived and semisynthetic compounds possessing similar pharmacologic properties. The *quinolone* derivatives encompass several agents that are selectively used for urinary tract infections as well as newer agents that possess a very broad spectrum of action in treating systemic infections.

TETRACYCLINES

Tetracyclines are bacteriostatic anti-infective agents that exhibit a broad spectrum of activity, but because of their extensive and often indiscriminate use in past years, their current clinical usefulness has been restricted by the emergence of a number of resistant bacterial strains. Many previously sensitive staphylococcal, streptococcal, pneumococcal, and other gram-positive organisms are now largely resistant to the tetracyclines, and in vitro laboratory susceptibility tests are necessary to determine the usefulness of a given tetracycline in a particular patient.

Although essentially alike in their antimicrobial activity, the tetracyclines differ in some of their pharmacokinetic properties, and these differences are indicated in Table 60-1. Oral absorption is variable and erratic, and except for doxycycline and minocycline, may be reduced by elevated gastric pH and the presence of food or polyvalent cations such as iron, calcium, magnesium, and aluminum. Plasma protein binding varies among the derivatives. Tetracyclines diffuse readily into most body tissues, attaining highest concentrations in the lungs, liver, kidney, spleen, bone marrow, and lymph. Penetration of the drugs into the CNS is largely determined by their lipid solubility, minocycline and doxycycline being the most lipophilic derivatives and thus best able to enter the CNS. In addition, minocycline attains high levels in saliva, making it useful in eliminating meningococci from the nasopharynx of carriers. (see Uses).

The drugs cross the placental barrier and concentrations in the fetal circulation may reach as high as 70% of the maternal circulation. Owing to the high affinity of tetracyclines for calcium, the development of any fetal tissue undergoing active calcification (e.g., bone, teeth) may be impaired by the presence of tetracyclines. Likewise, prolonged use of tetracyclines during the entire period of tooth development (fourth fetal month through the eighth year of life) may cause inadequate calcium deposition and discoloration of both deciduous and permanent teeth. Therefore, these drugs should be avoided if possible during pregnancy and lactation (because they are secreted in breast milk), and in children under 8 years of age.

With the exception of minocycline, the other tetracyclines are not metabolized to an appreciable extent. Except for minocycline and doxycycline these drugs are excreted largely in the urine. Doxycycline is secreted into the intestinal lumen and is eliminated in the feces. Minocycline and its metabolites are found in both the urine and feces, but renal clearance is quite low. The percentage of unchanged drug eliminated by the kidneys varies widely among the different derivatives (see Table 60-1). Drugs having a high renal clearance (e.g., oxytetracycline, tetracycline) are more effective in treating urinary tract infections than drugs with low renal clearances, but they may be more dangerous in the presence of renal impairment because of accumulation of drug in the body.

The systemic tetracyclines can be divided arbitrarily into two broad groups on the basis of their serum half-lives. Tetracycline and oxytetracycline are considered short-acting drugs, having half-lives of 6 to 10 hours. The remaining derivatives possess half-lives of approximately 10 to 20 hours and thus exhibit a longer duration of action. There is no convincing evidence, however, that one derivative is significantly more effective than any other for most susceptible infections. The more completely absorbed, longer acting drugs (i.e., doxycycline, minocycline) require less frequent administration (twice a day versus three or four times a day) than the other derivatives, and thus may improve patient compliance; however, they are considerably more expensive, and minocycline is associated with a high incidence of vestibular disturbances (e.g., dizziness, ataxia, lightheadedness). Because doxycycline and minocycline are not appreciably excreted by the kidney, they are the preferred tetracyclines for use in patients with renal impairment.

As noted previously, the emergence of resistant strains has severely limited the clinical application of the tetracyclines. Currently they are considered first-choice drugs for only the following infections: cholera, brucellosis, granuloma inguinale, melioidosis, chlamydial infections (ornithosis, psittacosis, trachoma, urethritis, cervicitis, lymphogranuloma venereum), *Mycoplasma pneumoniae* infections, rickettsial infections (Rocky Mountain spotted fever, endemic typhus, tick-bite fever, typhus, Q fever), relapsing fever, Lyme disease, and gonorrhea and syphilis in penicillin-sensitive patients. Tetracyclines are also indicated as alternative drugs for a number of gram-positive and gram-negative infections (see Chap. 56, Table 56-1), although sensitivity tests are necessary to confirm susceptibility. Although active in vitro against many gram-positive cocci, tetracyclines should not be used to treat staphylococcal, group A beta-hemolytic streptococcal or *Streptococcus pneumoniae* infections because of the occurrence of many resistant strains. Oral tetracyclines have been used as adjunctive therapy for severe acne, because they reduce the amount of free fatty acids in acne lesions as well as decreasing the population of *Proprionibacterium acnes* in sebaceous glands. Topical application of tetracycline solution or meclocycline cream is also effective in the treatment of acne vulgaris lesions, although the mechanism is not well established. Both oral and topical tetracyclines may be employed for treatment of inclusion conjunctivitis. Finally, doxycycline appears to be useful in preventing "travelers' diarrhea" caused by *Escherichia coli*, and minocycline can be used to treat asymptomatic carriers of *Neisseria meningitidis*.

Tetracyclines

Chlortetracycline	Methacycline
Demeclocycline	Minocycline
Doxycycline	Oxytetracycline
Meclocycline	Tetracycline

The following discussion considers the tetracyclines as a group. Individual members of the class are then listed in Table 60-2.

Table 60-1
Characteristics of Tetracyclines

Drug	Routes of Administration	Approximate Oral Absorption (%)	Protein Binding (%)	Plasma Half-life	Major Route of Elimination	Unchanged Drug Excreted in the Urine (%)
Chlortetracycline	Ophthalmic Topical					
Demeclocycline	Oral	60–70	50–80	10 h–16 h	Kidney	40–50
Doxycycline	Oral, IV	90–95 [a]	60–90	12 h–24 h	Feces	30–40
Meclocycline	Topical					
Methacycline	Oral	30–60	75–90	12 h–16 h	Kidney	40–50
Minocycline	Oral, IV	95–100 [a]	60–75	12 h–20 h	Kidney/feces (metabolites)	5–10
Oxytetracycline	Oral, IV, IM	50–60	20–30	6 h–10 h	Kidney	50–70
Tetracycline	Oral, IV, IM Ophthalmic Topical	70–80	20–60	6 h–10 h	Kidney	60–70

[a] Absorption is not significantly decreased by the presence of food, dairy products, or antacids.

MECHANISM
Bacteriostatic at recommended doses against a range of gram-positive and gram-negative organisms; inhibit protein synthesis in microbial cells by binding to 30S ribosomes, thereby blocking binding of transfer RNA to the messenger RNA–ribosome complex; may also inhibit replication of DNA on the cell membrane at high doses

USES
Treatment of infections due to susceptible organisms (see above introduction and also Chap. 56, Table 56-1)
Adjunctive therapy for severe acne or inclusion conjunctivitis (oral or topical tetracycline)
Adjunctive therapy (with amebicides) in the treatment of acute intestinal amebiasis
Treatment of uncomplicated urethral, endocervical, or rectal infections in adults caused by *Chlamydia trachomatis*
Alternative therapy for gonorrhea or syphilis in penicillin-sensitive patients
Treatment of early (stage I and II) Lyme disease
Elimination of meningococci from the nasopharynx of asymptomatic carriers of *Neisseria meningitidis* (oral minocycline only)
Investigational uses include:
  Prevention of travelers' diarrhea due to enterotoxic *Escherichia coli* (doxycycline)
  Management of chronic inappropriate antidiuretic hormone secretion (demeclocycline)
  Alternative to sulfonamides in treatment of nocardiosis (minocycline)
  Sclerosing agent (by chest tube) in malignant pleural effusion (tetracycline)
  Treatment of acute pelvic inflammatory disease (PID)

DOSAGE
See Table 60-2

FATE
Oral absorption of the tetracyclines is variable and incomplete; the percentage of the oral dose absorbed ranges from as low as 30% (methacycline) to nearly 100% (minocycline) but rises as the dosage is increased. Absorption is greater in the fasting state, except for doxycycline and minocycline which should be taken with food. Oral absorption of tetracyclines is reduced in the presence of milk or dairy products, calcium, magnesium, aluminum, and iron probably owing to chelation (see under Interactions). Distribution of tetracyclines is variable; most derivatives are widely distributed in the body, except for the CNS, where only highly lipophilic derivatives (e.g., doxycycline, minocycline) attain appreciable levels. Minocycline is also highly concentrated in saliva and tears. Plasma half-lives vary from 6 to 24 hours (see Table 60-1), and extent of protein binding differs considerably among the different drugs. Other than minocycline, the drugs are not metabolized to a significant extent. Doxycycline and minocycline and its metabolites are excreted largely in the feces whereas other derivatives are eliminated primarily by the kidneys, a considerable amount as unchanged drug. Thus, dosage reduction may be necessary in patients with renal impairment.

COMMON SIDE EFFECTS
Diarrhea, nausea, anorexia, vestibular disturbances (minocycline only), photosensitivity (especially with demeclocycline)

SIGNIFICANT ADVERSE REACTIONS
GI: stomatitis, glossitis, sore throat, dysphagia, vomiting, enterocolitis, steatorrhea, inflammation in the anogenital region, esophageal ulceration
Dermatologic: macropapular and erythematous rash, exfoliative dermatitis
Hypersensitivity: fever, urticaria, angioedema, headache, impaired vision, papilledema, pericarditis, anaphylaxis, exacerbation of systemic lupus erythematosus
Hematologic: hemolytic anemia, eosinophilia, neutropenia, thrombocytopenia, leukopenia, leukocytosis
Other: increased BUN, hepatic toxicity (large doses), permanent discoloration of teeth, enamel hypoplasia, impaired calcification of bony structures, increased intracranial pressure and bulging fontanels in young infants, nephrogenic diabetes

insipidus (demeclocycline only), irritation at IM injection sites, thrombophlebitis with IV administration, overgrowth of nonsusceptible organisms

WARNING

Outdated tetracycline products are potentially nephrotoxic, and use has resulted in development of the Fanconi syndrome, characterized by nausea, vomiting, polyuria, polydipsia, proteinuria, glycosuria, and acidosis. Symptoms disappear within several weeks after cessation of therapy

CONTRAINDICATIONS
Severe renal or liver impairment (except doxycycline), pregnancy, in nursing mothers, and in children under 8 years of age (unless no other drugs are effective for a particular infection). *Cautious use* in the presence of renal dysfunction

INTERACTIONS
Oral absorption of tetracyclines (except doxycycline and minocycline) may be impaired by the presence of food, dairy products, antacids, iron, or other polyvalent cations (e.g., calcium, magnesium, aluminum), and alkali (e.g., sodium bicarbonate)

Because they are bacteriostatic, tetracyclines can reduce the effectiveness of penicillins and other bactericidal antibiotics

The action of doxycycline may be shortened by barbiturates, other sedative–hypnotics, phenytoin, and carbamazepine because of hepatic enzyme induction

Elevation of BUN can occur with combined tetracycline–diuretic use

Tetracycline may enhance the effects of oral anticoagulants by interfering with synthesis of vitamin K by intestinal microorganisms

Plasma levels of digoxin and lithium can be increased by tetracyclines

Tetracyclines may enhance methoxyflurane-induced nephrotoxicity

The effects of oral contraceptives may be reduced by tetracyclines, possibly resulting in breakthrough bleeding or pregnancy

Theophylline and tetracyclines can result in increased GI side effects

Cimetidine may decrease the oral absorption of tetracyclines

NURSING CONSIDERATIONS

See **Plan of Nursing Care 12, Antibacterial Drugs,** in Chapter 56. *See* Table 60-2 for specific information on each drug. In addition:

Nursing Alerts

- Observe patient with renal impairment for vomiting, azotemia, acidosis, weight loss, or dehydration. The drug should be discontinued if these symptoms occur.
- When drug is administered IV, monitor results of liver and kidney function tests, which should be obtained frequently. IV administration should be prescribed very cautiously in the presence of renal dysfunction or pregnancy, and dosage should not exceed 2 g/day because high-dosage IV tetracycline therapy has been associated with liver failure and death.
- Assess indicators of renal, hepatic, and hematopoietic function at regular intervals.
- If diarrhea occurs, determine whether it is related to the drug (first few days of therapy) or an intestinal superinfection (later in therapy and often more intense).

1. When giving IM, question patient about lidocaine allergy (IM preparations contain lidocaine). Inject deeply into body of large muscle.
2. Administer IV at a slow rate, and observe infusion site for redness or swelling because prolonged IV administration can cause thrombophlebitis.
3. Interpret results of laboratory tests cautiously because tetracyclines may increase serum levels of creatinine, urea nitrogen, bilirubin, alkaline phosphatase, SGPT, and SGOT and urinary levels of catecholamines and protein. Hemoglobin and platelet values may be decreased, and urine glucose may be false positive with Clinitest or false negative with Clinistix or TesTape.

PATIENT EDUCATION

See **Plan of Nursing Care 12, Antibacterial Drugs,** in Chapter 56. *See* Table 60-2 for specific information on each drug. In addition:

1. Suggest that patient take drug with small quantities of food (except that high in calcium) if nausea, GI distress, or diarrhea occurs, as this should not significantly impair efficacy. Food does not appreciably alter absorption of doxycycline or minocycline.
2. Instruct patient to avoid using antacids, antidiarrheals, milk or other dairy products, and calcium-containing foods while taking a tetracycline because these substances significantly impair oral tetracycline absorption.
3. Warn patient not to use outdated or stale tetracycline products because the incidence of nephrotoxicity is much higher than with fresh preparations. Tetracyclines readily decompose, frequently to toxic products, with age or exposure to excessive light, heat, or humidity.
4. Instruct patient to avoid prolonged contact with direct sunlight or other ultraviolet light during therapy, especially with demeclocycline, to prevent photosensitization. The drug should be discontinued if skin discomfort or allergic reaction persists.

QUINOLONES

The quinolones are a group of structurally similar anti-infectives that exhibit a variety of actions against many different microorganisms. The older derivatives, nalidixic acid and cinoxacin, are primarily used in treating acute urinary tract infections due to common gram-negative pathogens. Newer agents, such as norfloxacin and ciprofloxacin, have an extended spectrum of action which includes gram-positive organisms as well as the more serious gram-negative organisms such as *Pseudomonas* and gram-negative aerobic bacteria. Norfloxacin is indicated for severe or resistant urinary infections, whereas ciprofloxacin is an extremely broad-spectrum agent that is used to treat serious *systemic* infections. The quinolone antibiotics are reviewed individually below.

Cinoxacin

Cinobac

MECHANISM
Inhibits DNA replication in susceptible bacteria within the range of urinary pH; bactericidal at normal dosage levels and is

(Text continued on page 614)

Table 60-2
Tetracyclines

Drug	Preparations	Usual Dosage Range	Nursing Implications
Chlortetracycline Aureomycin	Ophthalmic ointment: 1% Topical ointment: 3%	Ophthalmic: place small amount of ointment into lower conjunctival sac every 3 h as needed Topical: apply small amount every 3 h–6 h as needed	Tetracycline derivative not given systemically and infrequently used topically due to risk of sensitization; be alert for appearance of allergic reactions and discontinue drug; ophthalmic ointment may retard corneal healing; topical use should be supplemented by appropriate systemic antibiotics
Demeclocycline Declomycin	Tablets: 150 mg, 300 mg Capsules: 150 mg	Adults: 150 mg 4 times a day or 300 mg twice a day Children: 3 mg–6 mg/lb (6.6 mg–13.2 mg/kg) divided into 2–4 daily doses *Gonorrhea in penicillin-sensitive patients:* 600 mg initially, followed by 300 mg every 12 h for 5 days *Uncomplicated chlamydial infections:* 300 mg 4 times/day for at least 7 days	Orally effective tetracycline that is slowly excreted in part because of enterohepatic circulation; among tetracyclines, produces highest incidence of photosensitivity reactions; may precipitate diabetes insipidus–like syndrome (polyuria, polydipsia, weakness) on prolonged therapy—syndrome is caused by interference with action of vasopressin (ADH) on the kidneys, is dose-dependent, and is reversible upon discontinuation of drug; intake–output ratio should be monitored routinely
Doxycycline Doxychel, Vibramycin, Vibra Tabs and other manufacturers	Tablets: 50 mg, 100 mg Capsules: 50 mg, 100 mg Slow-release capsules (coated pellets): 100 mg Powder for oral suspension: 25 mg/5 mL Syrup: 50/5 mL Powder for injection: 100 mg/vial, 200 mg/vial	*Oral* Adults: 200 mg in 2 divided doses initially, followed by 100 mg/day in single *or* 2 divided doses; severe infections require 100 mg every 12 h Children: 2 mg/lb (4.4 mg/kg) in divided doses the first day; then 1 mg–2 mg/lb (2.2 mg–4.4 mg/kg) as a single dose or 2 divided doses each day. *Gonococcal infections:* Following a single dose of penicillin or cephalosporin, 100 mg twice a day for 7 days; for patients allergic to penicillin and cephalosporins—100 mg twice a day for 7 days *Syphilis:* 300 mg/day orally or IV for at least 10 days *Uncomplicated chlamydial infections:* 100 mg twice a day for at least 7 days *Acute pelvic inflammatory disease:* 100 mg twice a day for 10–14 days following a single dose of amoxicillin, cefoxitin, or ceftriaxone *Prevention of "traveler's diarrhea" (investigational):* 100 mg/day as a single dose *IV infusion* Adults: 200 mg the first day; then 100 mg–200 mg/day in 1–2 infusions	Semisynthetic tetracycline that is well absorbed orally, exhibits a prolonged duration of action, and is slowly excreted, primarily in the feces; may be used safely in patients with renal impairment; IV infusion is *not* recommended in children under 8 yr of age; oral absorption is not significantly affected by food or milk—drug has low affinity for calcium; low incidence of photosensitivity; duration of IV infusion varies with the dose, and ranges from 1–4 h; minimum infusion time for 100 mg of a 0.5 mg/mL solution is 1 h; therapy should be continued for at least 24–48 h after symptoms have subsided; follow package instructions for preparation and storage of IV infusion solutions; do *not* inject solutions IM or SC and avoid extravasation, because solutions are irritating

Continued

Table 60-2
Tetracyclines (continued)

Drug	Preparations	Usual Dosage Range	Nursing Implications
		Children 8 yr and older: 2 mg/lb (4.4 mg/kg) first day in 1–2 infusions; then 1 mg–2 mg/lb (2.2 mg–4.4 mg/kg) in 1–2 infusions each day	
Oxytetracycline E.P. Mycin, Terramycin, Uri-Tet	Capsules: 250 mg IM injection: 50 mg/mL, 125 mg/mL (with 2% lidocaine) Powder for injection: 250 mg, 500 mg per vial	*Oral* Adults: 1 g–2 g/day in 2–4 equally divided doses Children: 10 mg–20 mg/lb/day (22 mg–44 mg/kg/day) in 2–4 equally divided doses *IM* Adults: 250 mg/day in a single dose or 300 mg/day in divided doses every 8–12 h Children: 15 mg–25 mg/kg/day in divided doses every 8–12 hours (maximum 250 mg/day) *IV* Adults: 250 mg–500 mg every 12 h (maximum 2 g/day) Children: 12 mg/kg/day in 2 divided doses (range 10 mg–20 mg/kg/day)	Naturally derived tetracycline with actions similar to tetracycline itself; oral absorption is incomplete, half-life is 6–10 h, and protein binding is minimal; renal clearance is highest of all tetracyclines, thus drug may be more effective than other derivatives in urinary infections; use with *caution* in presence of renal impairment, because drug may accumulate rapidly; IM solution contains 2% lidocaine—do *not* inject IV; use only injection marked "IV" for IV administration; reconstituted solutions for injection are stable for 48 h with refrigeration
Tetracycline Achromycin, Panmycin, Sumycin, and other manufacturers (CAN) Apo-Tetra, Neo-Tetrine, Novotetra	Capsules: 100 mg, 250 mg, 500 mg Tablets: 250 mg, 500 mg Syrup: 125 mg/5 mL Powder for IM injection: 100 mg/vial, 250 mg/vial with 2% procaine Powder for IV injection: 250 mg/vial, 500 mg/vial Ophthalmic drops: 1% Ophthalmic ointment: 1% Topical ointment: 3% Topical solution: 2.2 mg/mL	*Oral* Adults: 1 g–2 g/day in 2–4 equal doses Children: 25 mg–50 mg/kg/day in 2–4 equal doses *Gonorrhea:* 1.5 g initially; then 0.5 g every 6 h for 5–7 days *Syphilis:* 30 g–40 g in equally divided doses over 10–15 days *Chlamydial infections:* 500 mg 4 times/day for at least 7 days *Acne:* 1 g/day initially (maintenance 125 mg–500 mg/day) *IM* Adults: 250 mg/day in a single dose *or* 300 mg/day in divided doses every 8–12 h (maximum 800 mg/day) Children: 15 mg–25 mg/kg/day in divided doses every 8–12 h *IV* Adults: 250 mg–500 mg every 12 h (maximum 2 g/day) Children: 10 mg–20 mg/kg/day in 2 divided doses *Ophthalmic* 1–2 drops or small amount of ointment in affected eye 2–4 times a day *Topical* Apply 2–4 times a day	Semisynthetic tetracycline produced from chlortetracycline or obtained naturally; most widely used and least expensive of the tetracyclines; used orally, parenterally, or locally; topical application may result in hypersensitivity reactions—discontinue drug at first sign of allergic response; ophthalmic use may retard corneal healing; IM injections contain procaine and are *not* suitable for IV administration; injection of IM solution into subcutaneous layer may cause pain and induration; do *not* dilute injectable solutions with calcium-containing diluents because precipitate can form; reconstituted solutions stable for 12 h at room temperature
Meclocycline Meclan	Cream: 1%	Apply twice a day in generous amounts until skin is thoroughly wet	Locally acting tetracycline that is not absorbed to a significant extent; used in the treatment of mild to moderate acne vulgaris; avoid contact with eyes, nose, or mouth;

Continued

Table 60-2
Tetracyclines (continued)

Drug	Preparations	Usual Dosage Range	Nursing Implications
Meclocycline (cont'd)			may produce skin irritation; slight yellowing of the skin can occur but may be removed by washing; cosmetics may be applied in the usual manner during treatment; formaldehyde is a component of the vehicle—*caution* in persons allergic to this substance
Methacycline Rondomycin	Capsules: 150 mg, 300 mg	Adults: 600 mg/day in 2–4 divided doses Children: 3 mg–6 mg/lb/day (6.6 mg–13.2 mg/kg/day) in 2–4 divided doses *Gonorrhea:* 900 mg initially, then 300 mg 4 times/day to a total of 5.4 g *Syphilis:* 18 g–24 g in equally divided doses over 10–15 days	Semisynthetic, orally effective tetracycline; incompletely absorbed orally; highly bound to plasma proteins; excreted largely in urine; use with *caution* in presence of renal impairment; similar to tetracycline in most other respects, and significantly more expensive
Minocycline Minocin	Capsules: 50 mg, 100 mg Tablets: 50 mg, 100 mg Syrup: 50 mg/5 mL Powder for injection: 100 mg/vial	*Oral* Adults: 200 mg initially, then 100 mg every 12 h *or* 50 mg 4 times a day Children (over 8 yr): 4 mg/kg initially; then 2 mg/kg every 12 h *Gonorrhea:* 200 mg initially then 100 mg every 12 h for a minimum of 5 days *Syphilis:* 100 mg every 12 h for 10–15 days *Meningococcal carrier state:* 100 mg every 12 h for 5 days *Chlamydial infections:* 100 mg twice a day for at least 7 days *IV injection* Adults: 200 mg initially then 100 mg every 12 h (maximum 400 mg/day) Children: 4 mg/kg initially, then 2 mg/kg every 12 h	Semisynthetic tetracycline that is almost completely absorbed orally; very lipid soluble and possesses a long half-life (up to 20 h); low renal clearance; oral absorption is not appreciably altered by food or dairy products; only tetracycline drug metabolized to any extent; photosensitivity occurs rarely; vestibular side effects are *very common* (lightheadedness, dizziness, vertigo)—therefore, urge caution in driving or operating machinery; indicated in treatment of asymptomatic carriers of *Neisseria meningitidis* to eliminate organism from nasopharynx; *not* recommended for treatment of meningococcal infection; also used in treatment of nocardiosis; IV solutions are stable at room temperature for 24 h; may result in blue-gray skin pigmentation

active against most strains of *Escherichia coli, Klebsiella* species, *Enterobacter* species, and *Proteus* species; not effective, however, against *Pseudomonas,* staphylococci, or enterococci; bacterial resistance occurs in less than 5% of patients given recommended doses

USES
Treatment of initial and recurrent urinary tract infections resulting from susceptible organisms (see above)

DOSAGE
1 g daily in 2 to 4 divided doses; continue for 7 to 14 days; reduce dosage in the presence of impaired renal function

FATE
Rapidly absorbed from the GI tract; peak serum concentrations occur within 1 to 2 hours, and detectable levels persist for 10 to 12 hours; food decreases peak serum levels by about one fourth but does not alter the total amount absorbed. The drug is excreted almost entirely in the urine, 60% as unaltered drug and the remainder as metabolites; approximately 97% of an oral dose is excreted in the urine within 24 hours. Drug is 60% to 80% protein bound; serum half-life is 1 to 2 hours with normal renal function but increases markedly in the presence of impaired renal function

COMMON SIDE EFFECTS
Nausea, abdominal cramping

SIGNIFICANT ADVERSE REACTIONS
GI: anorexia, vomiting, diarrhea
CNS: headache, tinnitus, photophobia, insomnia, dizziness, tingling sensation, nervousness, confusion
Hypersensitivity: rash, pruritus, urticaria, edema
Other: altered BUN, SGOT, SGPT, serum creatinine, and alkaline phosphatase

CONTRAINDICATIONS
Anuria, in pregnant women and prepubertal children (cartilage erosion has occurred). *Cautious use* in persons with reduced renal or hepatic function and in nursing mothers

INTERACTIONS
Probenecid blocks tubular secretion of cinoxacin, reducing its elimination rate in the urine and increasing its half-life and serum concentration

The rate of cinoxacin excretion may be slowed by acidification and enhanced by alkalinization of the urine

NURSING CONSIDERATIONS
See **Plan of Nursing Care 12, Antibacterial Drugs,** in Chapter 56. In addition:

Nursing Alerts
- If patient has renal disease, monitor intake and output. Notify drug prescriber if input exceeds output.
- If patient has history of renal or liver impairment, ensure that appropriate laboratory tests (e.g., BUN, serum creatinine, liver enzymes, alkaline phosphatase) are obtained and evaluated before initiating drug administration. These tests should be repeated at the conclusion of therapy.

PATIENT EDUCATION
See **Plan of Nursing Care 12, Antibacterial Drugs,** in Chapter 56. In addition:
1. Suggest that patient take drug with food if GI distress occurs.

Nalidixic Acid
Neg Gram

MECHANISM
Bactericidal over the entire urinary pH range against most gram-negative bacteria causing urinary infections; probably acts by inhibiting DNA polymerization and may impair RNA synthesis as well; exhibits good activity against *Proteus* species, *Escherichia coli*, *Enterobacter*, and *Klebsiella*; ineffective against *Pseudomonas*; resistance has developed in some cases

USES
Treatment of urinary tract infections caused by susceptible organisms (see above); disk susceptibility testing should be performed; see Chapter 56

DOSAGE
Adults: initially 1 g four times a day for 2 weeks; reduce to 2 g/day in divided doses for prolonged therapy
Children over 3 months: initially 55 mg/kg/day in four divided doses for at least 2 weeks; maintenance dose is 33 mg/kg/day

FATE
Rapidly absorbed orally; peak serum levels occur in 1 to 2 hours; highly (90%–95%) protein-bound in plasma; partially metabolized in the liver and rapidly excreted by the kidneys both as unchanged drug and several metabolites; plasma half-life is 1 to 3 hours when renal function is normal; hydroxynalidixic acid, an active metabolite, represents 85% of the biologically active drug in the urine

COMMON SIDE EFFECTS
Nausea, diarrhea, abdominal distress

SIGNIFICANT ADVERSE REACTIONS
CNS: drowsiness, dizziness, weakness, headache, vertigo, visual disturbances (e.g., difficulty in focusing, double vision, altered color perception); convulsions and toxic psychosis with large doses
Infants and children may experience increased intracranial pressure, papilledema, severe headache, and bulging anterior fontanel
Allergic: rash, pruritus, urticaria, angioedema, eosinophilia, arthralgia, photosensitivity reactions, anaphylactic reaction (rare)
Other: (rare) GI bleeding, cholestasis, paresthesias, metabolic acidosis, blood dyscrasias, glucose-6-phosphate dehydrogenase deficiency

CONTRAINDICATIONS
History of convulsive disorders, early pregnancy, and in infants under 3 months. *Cautious use* in patients with liver disease, epilepsy, cerebral arteriosclerosis, severe renal failure, and in young children, because cartilage erosion can occur in weight-bearing joints

INTERACTIONS
Nalidixic acid may potentiate the action of other strongly protein-bound drugs (e.g., oral anticoagulants, phenytoin, oral hypoglycemics, antiinflammatory agents)
Nitrofurantoin may inhibit the antibacterial activity of nalidixic acid
Urinary acidifiers can potentiate the antibacterial activity of nalidixic acid by reducing its urinary excretion *rate*
Antacids may impair GI absorption of nalidixic acid, reducing its *activity*
Cross-resistance has occurred between nalidixic acid and cinoxacin

NURSING CONSIDERATIONS
1. Ensure that prescribed disk sensitivity tests have been performed before therapy is initiated. If clinical response is unsatisfactory or relapse occurs, culture and sensitivity tests should be repeated because resistance can develop within 48 hours, especially if dosage is inadequate.
2. Interpret results of urine glucose tests cautiously because nalidixic acid can yield a false-positive reaction with Benedict's or Fehling's solution or Clinitest tablets. TesTape or Clinistix can still be used reliably. Urinary 17-ketosteroids may also be falsely elevated.

PATIENT EDUCATION
1. Suggest that patient take drug with food or milk if GI intolerance occurs.
2. Warn patient to use caution in driving or operating other machinery because drowsiness and dizziness can occur.
3. Instruct patient to avoid excessive exposure to sunlight. The drug should be discontinued if photosensitivity reactions occur.

4. Teach family how to recognize and report the development of CNS reactions (irritability, headache, vomiting, excitement, drowsiness, vertigo, bulging of anterior fontanel in children), which are especially likely to occur in an infant, a child, or an elderly patient. Such reactions often occur rapidly and are usually reversible shortly after discontinuation of the drug.
5. Instruct patient to report any visual disturbances immediately. These usually disappear quickly with a reduction in dosage.
6. Inform patient that periodic blood counts and liver function tests are recommended during prolonged (usually longer than 2 wk) therapy.

Norfloxacin

Noroxin

Norfloxacin is a synthetic fluoroquinolone antiinfective possessing in-vitro activity against a broad spectrum of gram-positive and gram-negative organisms. The drug is bactericidal against many organisms, including gram-negative aerobic bacteria and *Pseudomonas aeruginosa*. Its action is generally limited to the urinary tract, bile, and gut.

MECHANISM

Inhibits bacterial DNA synthesis; the fluorine atom provides increased potency against gram-negative organisms; drug is bactericidal; resistance is rare; not active against obligate anaerobes

USES

Treatment of uncomplicated or complicated urinary tract infections caused by susceptible strains of *E. coli, Klebsiella pneumoniae, Proteus* species, *Enterobacter, Pseudomonas aeruginosa, Citrobacter freundii, Staphylococcus aureus,* and group D streptococci

DOSAGE

400 mg twice daily for 7 to 10 days; reduce dosage to 400 mg once daily if creatinine clearance is less than 30 mL/min

FATE

Oral absorption is incomplete (30%–40%) but generally rapid following single doses; peak plasma levels occur in approximately 1 hour; plasma half-life is 3 to 4 hours, and steady-state plasma levels are attained within 2 days; serum protein binding is minimal (10%–15%); eliminated both as unchanged drug and metabolites in both the urine and feces

COMMON SIDE EFFECTS

Nausea, headache, dizziness

SIGNIFICANT ADVERSE REACTIONS

Rash, fatigue, depression, insomnia, abdominal pain, constipation, flatulence, heartburn, dry mouth, fever, visual disturbances, vomiting, and elevated BUN, serum creatinine, and LDH. Eosinophilia and elevated SGPT, SGOT, and alkaline phosphatase have also been reported during therapy.

CONTRAINDICATIONS

In pregnant women or young children. *Cautious use* in patients with impaired renal function, predisposition to or a history of seizures, and in nursing mothers

INTERACTIONS

Probenecid can reduce the urinary excretion of norfloxacin during concomitant administration

Concurrent use of nitrofurantoin can impair the antibacterial activity of norfloxacin

Antacids may reduce the oral absorption of norfloxacin

NURSING CONSIDERATIONS

See **Plan of Nursing Care 12, Antibacterial Drugs,** in Chapter 56. In addition:

Nursing Alert

- If patient has renal or hepatic impairment or is likely to be on extended therapy, ensure that appropriate laboratory tests (e.g., CBC with differential, BUN, serum creatinine, liver enzymes, alkaline phosphatase) are performed prior to initiating drug administration and periodically as needed thereafter.

PATIENT EDUCATION

See **Plan of Nursing Care 12, Antibacterial Drugs,** in Chapter 56. In addition:

1. Instruct patient to take drug either 1 hour before or 2 hours after meals with a full glass of water to maximize absorption.
2. Instruct patient taking antacid to take it 2 or more hours after norfloxacin to avoid interfering with norfloxacin absorption.
3. Suggest that patient take drug with small amount of nondairy food if GI distress occurs.
4. Encourage patient to increase fluid intake to 2500 mL to 3000 mL per day during therapy to minimize the risk of crystalluria, a rare but serious side effect.
5. Warn patient to exercise caution in driving or performing tasks requiring mental alertness until response to drug is known, because dizziness may occur.
6. Teach patient how to prevent falls if dizziness occurs.
7. Inform patient that headaches sometimes occur, often transiently, and may be treated with mild analgesics.
8. Instruct patient to report fever, rash, sore throat, or fatigue immediately because hematologic abnormalities can occur.

Ciprofloxacin

Cipro

Ciprofloxacin is an orally effective synthetic fluoroquinolone antiinfective that exerts a bactericidal action against a wide range of gram-positive and gram-negative organisms. Unlike its structurally related analog norfloxacin, however, it is useful not only in treating urinary infections but also in treating respiratory, skin, soft tissue, bone and joint infections due to organisms resistant to most other broad-spectrum antiinfectives.

MECHANISM

Interferes with DNA gyrase, an enzyme necessary for synthesis of bacterial DNA; possesses additive antibacterial action with beta-lactams, aminoglycosides, metronidazole, and other broad-spectrum agents; among the few resistant organisms are *Streptococcus fecalis, Mycobacterium tuberculosis,* and *Chlamydia trachomatis*

USES

Treatment of infections caused by most bacterial microorganisms *except* those listed above

DOSAGE
250 mg to 750 mg every 12 hours depending on type and severity of infection; usual duration is 7 to 14 days, but may be longer in bone or joint infections

FATE
Oral absorption is rapid and complete; first pass metabolism is minimal; food delays rate of absorption but not total amount absorbed; peak serum levels attained within 1 to 2 hours after dosing; serum protein binding is minimal (20%–30%); approximately one half of an oral dose is excreted in urine as unchanged drug; up to one third of an oral dose is recovered in the feces within 5 days; plasma half-life in patients with normal renal function is about 4 hours; urinary excretion is virtually complete within 24 hours

COMMON SIDE EFFECTS
Nausea, diarrhea, vomiting, abdominal discomfort, headache, skin rash

SIGNIFICANT ADVERSE REACTIONS
CNS: dizziness, restlessness, insomnia, nightmares, irritability, tremors, weakness, convulsions, depression
GI: dysphagia, oral candidiasis, intestinal bleeding
Cardiovascular: palpitations, ventricular ectopy, hypertension, angina
Respiratory: epistaxis, laryngeal edema, hiccoughs, dyspnea, bronchospasm
Allergic/dermatologic: pruritus, urticaria, photosensitivity, flushing, angioedema, hyperpigmentation
Other: blurred vision, diplopia, tinnitus, altered taste perception, joint or back pain, polyuria, urinary retention, vaginitis, nephritis

CONTRAINDICATIONS
No absolute contraindications. *Cautious use* in patients with CNS disorders, in young children, and in pregnant or nursing women

INTERACTIONS
Antacids may decrease the oral absorption of ciprofloxacin
Increased serum levels of ciprofloxacin may occur if probenecid is administered concurrently
Plasma concentrations of theophylline may be elevated if given together with ciprofloxacin

NURSING CONSIDERATION
See **Plan of Nursing Care 12, Antibacterial Drugs,** in Chapter 56. In addition:

Nursing Alert
- Monitor results of liver function tests (i.e., SGPT, SGOT, LDH, alkaline phosphatase, serum bilirubin) because elevations may occur during therapy.

PATIENT EDUCATION
See **Plan of Nursing Care 12, Antibacterial Drugs,** in Chapter 56. In addition:
1. Inform patient that drug may be taken with food if GI distress occurs. Although food delays rate of drug absorption, it does not affect total amount absorbed.
2. Instruct patient taking antacid to take it 2 or more hours after ciprofloxacin to avoid interfering with ciprofloxacin absorption.
3. Encourage patient to maintain high fluid intake during therapy to minimize the risk of crystalluria.
4. Warn patient to exercise caution in driving or performing tasks requiring mental alertness until response to drug is known because dizziness may occur.
5. Instruct patient and family to observe for and report signs of CNS stimulation (see Significant Adverse Reactions) and reassure them that, if any of these infrequent effects occur, they are reversible.

Selected Bibliography
Banza M, Schiefe RJ: Antimicrobial spectrum, pharmacology and therapeutic use of antibiotics. 1. Tetracyclines. Am J Hosp Pharm 34:49, 1977

Chopra I, Howe TG: Bacterial resistance to the tetracyclines. Microbiol Rev 42:707, 1978

Elmore MF, Rogge JD: Tetracycline-induced pancreatitis. Gastroenterology 81:1134, 1981

Hooper DC, Wolfson JS: The fluoroquinolones: Pharmacology, clinical uses and toxicities in humans. Antimicrob Agents Chemother 28:716, 1985

Muytjens HL, vanderRos-vandeRepe J, van Veldhuizen G: Comparative activities of ciprofloxacin, norfloxacin, pipemidic acid and nalidixic acid. Antimicrob Agents Chemother 24:302, 1983

Neu HC (ed): Ciprofloxacin: A major advance in quinolone chemotherapy. A symposium. Am J Med 82(Suppl 4A):1, 1987

Norrby SR, Jonsson M: Antibacterial activity of norfloxacin. Antimicrob Agents Chemother 23:15, 1982

Ory EM: The tetracyclines. In Kagan BM (ed): Antimicrobial Therapy, 3rd ed, p 117. Philadelphia, WB Saunders, 1980

Scavone JM, Gleckman RA, Fraser DG: Cinoxacin: Mechanisms of action, spectrum of activity, pharmacokinetics, adverse reactions and therapeutic indications. Pharmacotherapeutics 2:266, 1982

Standiford HC: The tetracyclines and chloramphenicol. In Mandell GL, Douglas RG, Bennett JE (eds): Principles and Practice of Infectious Diseases, 2nd ed, p 206. New York, John Wiley & Sons, 1985

Winckler K: Tetracycline ulcers of the oesophagus: Endoscopy, histology and roentgenology in two cases and a review of the literature. Endoscopy 13:225, 1981

SUMMARY. TETRACYCLINES, QUINOLONES

Drug	Preparations	Usual Dosage Range
Tetracyclines	*See* Table 60-2	
Quinolones		
Cinoxacin Cinobac	Capsules: 250 mg, 500 mg	1 g daily in 2 to 4 divided doses for 7 days to 14 days
Nalidixic Acid Neg Gram	Tablets: 250 mg, 500 mg, 1 g Oral suspension: 250 mg/5 mL	*Adults:* 1 g 4 times/day for 2 weeks, then 2 g/day in divided doses *Children:* 55 mg/kg/day in 4 divided doses for 2 weeks, then 33 mg/kg/day
Norfloxacin Noroxin	Tablets: 400 mg	400 mg twice daily for 7 days to 10 days
Ciprofloxacin Cipro	Tablets: 250 mg, 500 mg, 750 mg	250 mg to 750 mg every 12 hours for 7 days to 14 days

61 ERYTHROMYCINS

The *erythromycins* are members of the macrolide group of antibiotics, so named because the chemical structure of the compounds consists of a large lactone ring to which one or more sugars are attached. Erythromycin itself as a base is an orally effective antibiotic originally isolated from a strain of *Streptomyces erythreus*. Although erythromycin base is a biologically active form, it is unstable in gastric acid and thus must be formulated in an enteric-coated preparation for oral administration. Absorption of enteric-coated products is occasionally less than adequate, however, and blood levels may not reach sufficient concentrations. Therefore, to avoid destruction of the drug by gastric juices while maintaining good oral absorption, erythromycin has also been formulated in several salts (estolate, ethylsuccinate, stearate), all of which are largely acid-stable and yield biologically effective plasma levels of free erythromycin base. The strength of erythromycin products is expressed in terms of base equivalents. Thus, 400 mg of the ethylsuccinate salt provides serum levels of free erythromycin equivalent to those resulting from administration of 250 mg of erythromycin base or the stearate or estolate salts. Two other soluble salts of erythromycin (gluceptate, lactobionate) are available for IV use and are indicated mainly in severe infections where high serum levels of the drug are required immediately. The other clinically available macrolide antibiotic is *troleandomycin*, an agent resembling erythromycin in both structure and pharmacologic activity, but somewhat less effective and more toxic and hence infrequently used. It is discussed briefly at the end of the chapter.

Erythromycins inhibit protein synthesis and are bacteriostatic at normal therapeutic doses, although they may be bactericidal against certain organisms at high concentrations. Their antibacterial spectrum of action is similar to that of the penicillins, being most effective against certain gram-positive cocci, such as staphylococci, streptococci, enterococci, and pneumococci. Although used principally as *alternatives* to penicillin in treating susceptible organisms, the erythromycins may be considered the drugs of choice against the following organisms: *Bordetella pertussis* (whooping cough), *Corynebacterium diphtheriae*, *Legionella pneumophila* (Legionnaires' disease), *Mycoplasma pneumoniae* (atypical viral pneumonia), and strains of *Chlamydia trachomatis* causing pneumonia and inclusion conjunctivitis (refer to Chap. 56, Table 56-1, for a listing of the organisms for which erythromycin is considered an alternative drug).

Microbial resistance has become a problem with use of the erythromycins and is especially frequent in staphylococci. Prolonged use of erythromycin in staphylococcal infections is almost invariably associated with the emergence of resistance, and alternative drugs should be used in treating severe staphylococcal infections. Erythromycin-resistant streptococci and pneumococci are likewise developing with increasing frequency. Although cross-resistance is not a significant problem between erythromycin and most other antibiotics, it has been reported with lincomycin and clindamycin and is virtually complete among all the members of the macrolides. Gram-negative organisms are largely impermeable to erythromycin and are usually resistant to the drug unless their cell walls are altered.

As noted earlier, erythromycin is used as the free base as well as several salts, and the several preparations are available for oral, IV, topical, and ophthalmic administration. Absorption of the base and the stearate preparations are impaired by the presence of food, and these drugs should be administered on an empty stomach, if possible. Conversely, absorption of the estolate and ethylsuccinate salts are either unaffected or enhanced by the presence of food. However, the estolate and ethylsuccinate salts have been associated with cholestatic hepatitis, especially in adults, and must be used with caution in the presence of liver disease. Still, erythromycins are relatively safe antibiotics, the most frequently reported side effects being GI distress such as nausea, diarrhea, and abdominal cramping.

Following a general discussion of erythromycin, the several salts, their doses and dosage forms, and pertinent comments are presented in Table 61-1. The other macrolide antibiotic, troleandomycin, is then reviewed at the end of the chapter.

Erythromycins

Erythromycin base	Erythromycin lacto-
Erythromycin estolate	bionate
Erythromycin ethylsuccinate	Erythromycin stea-
Erythromycin gluceptate	rate

MECHANISM
Inhibit bacterial protein synthesis by attaching to 50S ribosomal subunits of sensitive microorganisms, thereby blocking binding of tRNA to donor site; do not affect nucleic acid synthesis nor act on the cell wall; the non-ionized form of the drug penetrates bacterial cells most efficiently, thus the antimicrobial activity of erythromycin is increased in an alkaline pH, as the drug exists predominantly in the un-ionized form in such an environment

USES
Treatment of respiratory infections caused by susceptible organisms, such as the following: *Mycoplasma pneumoniae* (drug of choice), *Legionella pneumophila* (drug of choice), *Streptococcus pneumoniae*, group A beta-hemolytic *Streptococcus* (in penicillin-sensitive patients), and *Bordetella pertussis*

Treatment of acute skin and soft-tissue infections due to *Staphylococcus aureus* (resistance is commonly encountered)

Prophylaxis of subacute bacterial endocarditis and recurrence of acute rheumatic fever in penicillin-sensitive patients

Treatment of *Neisseria gonorrhoeae* (gonorrhea) and *Treponema pallidum* (syphilis) in penicillin- and tetracycline-sensitive patients

Treatment of chlamydial infections (e.g., uncomplicated urethritis, endocervicitis, conjunctivitis, pneumonia) in tetracycline-sensitive patients

Treatment of *Campylobacter jejuni* gastroenteritis

Treatment of respiratory and middle ear infections due to *Hemophilus influenzae* (in conjunction with sulfonamides)

Adjunctive treatment of *Corynebacterium* infections (with antitoxin)

Topical control of mild to moderate acne vulgaris
Reduction of wound complications when given with neomycin prior to colorectal surgery

DOSAGE

See Table 61-1

FATE

Oral absorption is generally good, but base and stearate absorption may be impaired by food, and these preparations should be given on an empty stomach; base is destroyed by gastric acid, thus is formulated in enteric-coated tablets or capsules; drug diffuses readily into most body tissues (except CNS, unless meninges are inflamed) and passes through the placental barrier, although fetal blood levels remain rather low; one of only a few antibiotics to attain high levels in prostatic fluid; peak serum levels occur in 1 to 4 hours with oral use; drug is approximately 70% protein-bound; concentrated in the liver and excreted in active form primarily in the bile; less than 5% of an oral dose and 15% of an IV dose is excreted in the urine

COMMON SIDE EFFECTS

Abdominal discomfort (cramping, nausea, diarrhea, and anorexia)

SIGNIFICANT ADVERSE REACTIONS

Vomiting, allergic reactions (rash, urticaria, fever, eosinophilia, anaphylaxis); reversible hearing loss; superinfections by nonsusceptible organisms; cholestatic hepatitis (primarily from estolate and ethylsuccinate salt); pain, irritation, or phlebitis with IV injection; impaired hearing with IV infusion of lactobionate or gluceptate salts (4 g/day or more)

CONTRAINDICATIONS

Estolate and ethylsuccinate salt in preexisting liver disease. *Cautious use* in patients with impaired liver function or history of allergic disorders, and in pregnant or nursing women

INTERACTIONS

The activity of erythromycins may be enhanced by urinary alkalinizers (e.g., sodium bicarbonate, acetazolamide) and decreased by urinary acidifiers (e.g., ammonium chloride, citric acid beverages)

The effects of lincomycin and clindamycin may be antagonized by erythromycin, which competes for ribosomal binding sites

Tetracyclines and cephalothin are incompatible with erythromycin in parenteral mixtures

Erythromycin can elevate serum digoxin levels in a small percentage of patients who metabolize digoxin in the GI tract by slowing its metabolism in the gut

Erythromycins can increase serum levels of theophylline, carbamazepine and cyclosporine by reducing their clearance

Erythromycin, being primarily bacteriostatic, may impair the antimicrobial activity of penicillins or other bactericidal antibiotics

The effects of oral anticoagulants may be increased by erythromycins

NURSING CONSIDERATIONS

See **Plan of Nursing Care 12, Antibacterial Drugs,** in Chapter 56. See Table 61-1 for information on specific drugs. In addition:

> **Nursing Alerts**
> - Monitor results of hepatic function tests, which should be performed regularly during prolonged (i.e., several weeks) therapy.
> - Assess patient carefully for early signs of hepatic dysfunction (malaise, nausea, vomiting, cramping, fever). Jaundice (dark urine, pale stools, pruritus, yellow skin or sclerae) may or may not occur. Withhold drug and notify prescriber immediately if these signs occur.

1. When giving IM, inject deeply into large muscle mass because injection can cause considerable pain. Rotate injection sites, and administer no more than 600 mg at a single site.
2. When administering IV, use only dilute solutions, and closely observe patient for signs of phlebitis.
3. Cleanse affected area of skin before application of topical solution or ointment unless directed otherwise. Keep topical preparations away from eyes, nose, mouth, and other mucous membranes.
4. Interpret certain laboratory test results cautiously because erythromycins can elevate serum levels of SGPT, SGOT, and alkaline phosphatase, decrease serum levels of glucose and cholesterol, and give false elevations of urinary catecholamines and 17-ketosteroids.
5. Note that 400 mg of erythromycin ethylsuccinate produces the same free erythromycin serum levels as 250 mg of the base, stearate, or estolate.

PATIENT EDUCATION

See **Plan of Nursing Care 12, Antibacterial Drugs,** in Chapter 56. In addition:
1. Instruct patient to avoid fruit juice or other acidic beverages when taking drug. Estolate and ethylsuccinate salts may be taken without regard for meals.
2. Instruct patient to swallow enteric-coated tablets whole.

Troleandomycin

Tao

A semisynthetic derivative of oleandomycin, troleandomycin is a macrolide antibiotic obtained from *Streptomyces antibioticus*. It is similar to erythromycin in activity but somewhat less effective and more toxic, hence its clinical usefulness is limited. Troleandomycin is generally effective in eradicating streptococci from the nasopharynx.

MECHANISM

Inhibits protein synthesis in susceptible bacteria

USES

Treatment of upper respiratory infections due to susceptible strains of *Diplococcus pneumoniae* and *Streptococcus pyogenes* (alternative therapy *only*)

DOSAGE

Adults: 250 mg to 500 mg four times a day
Children: 125 mg to 250 mg every 6 hours

FATE

Well absorbed orally; widely distributed in the body, including the CNS; metabolized in the liver and excreted in the bile and urine

Table 61-1
Erythromycins

Drug	Preparations	Usual Dosage Range	Nursing Implications
Erythromycin Base Ak-Mycin, E-Mycin, Ery-Tab, Eryc Ilotycin, PCE, Robimycin (CAN) Apo-Erythro Base, Novorythro Base	Enteric-coated tablets: 250 mg, 333 mg, 500 mg Film-coated tablets: 250 mg, 500 mg Capsules (enteric-coated pellets): 125 mg, 250 mg Ointment: 2% Ophthalmic ointment: 0.5%	*Oral* Adults: 250 mg–500 mg every 6–12 h up to 4 g/day for severe infections Children: 30 mg/kg–50 mg/kg/day in 3–4 divided doses, up to 100 mg/kg/day *Legionnaires' disease:* 1 g–4 g daily in divided doses *Pertussis:* 40 mg–50 mg/kg/day in divided doses for 5–15 days *Sexually transmitted diseases* (syphilis, gonorrhea, nongonococcal urethritis, chancroid, lymphogranuloma): 500 mg 4 times a day for at least 7–10 days (up to 30 days for syphilis) *Ophthalmic* Prevention of neonatal conjunctivitis: Apply 2–3 times a day *Topical* Apply to skin or eye 2–4 times/day as necessary	Free-base form of erythromycin, which is acid-labile and thus administered orally in enteric-coated form; absorption is variable depending upon product used; should be administered on an empty stomach if possible; do not break or crush enteric-coated tablets; ophthalmic ointment may retard corneal healing; be alert for hypersensitivity reactions with topical application
Erythromycin Base, Topical Solution Akne-Mycin, A/T/S, C-Solve, Erycette, Eryderm, Erymax, E-Solve-2, ETS-2%, Staticin, T-Stat	Topical solution: 1.5%, 2%	Apply morning and evening to areas usually affected by acne	Alcohol solution of erythromycin base used in the treatment of acne vulgaris; avoid contact with eyes, nose, mouth, or other mucous membranes; use *cautiously* with other topical acne treatment, because severe irritation can occur; most common side effect is excessive drying of treated area; erythema, pruritus, burning, and desquamation have also been reported; wash, rinse, and dry area to be treated before application
Erythromycin Estolate Ilosone (CAN) Novorythro estolate	Tablets: 500 mg Chewable tablets: 125 mg, 250 mg Capsules: 125 mg, 250 mg Drops: 100 mg/mL Suspension: 125 mg/5 mL, 250 mg/5 mL	Adults: 250 mg every 6 h (*or* 500 mg every 12 h) up to 4 g/day Children: 30 mg/kg–50 mg/kg/day orally in divided doses, up to 100 mg/kg/day *Syphilis:* 20 g over 10 days in divided doses	Ester salt of erythromycin that is acid-stable, well absorbed in the presence of food, and yields higher and more sustained blood levels than other derivatives; may produce hepatotoxicity—thus be alert for early signs of liver dysfunction (vomiting, malaise, cramping, right upper quadrant pain, fever, jaundice), and discontinue drug; symptoms usually occur with 1–2 wk of continuous therapy and are reversible upon discontinuation of medication; not indicated for prolonged administration (e.g., acne, prophylaxis or rheumatic fever) or for treatment of syphilitic infections in pregnant women;

Continued

Table 61-1
Erythromycins (continued)

Drug	Preparations	Usual Dosage Range	Nursing Implications
			regular tablets should be swallowed whole; liquid should be kept refrigerated and unused portion discarded after 14 days
Erythromycin Ethylsuccinate E.E.S., E-Mycin E, EryPed, Pediamycin, Wyamycin-E (CAN) Apo-Erythro-ES	Film-coated tablets: 400 mg Chewable tablets: 200 mg Drops: 100 mg/2.5 mL Suspension: 200 mg/5 mL, 400 mg/5 mL Powder for suspension: 200 mg/5 mL, 400 mg/5 mL	Adults: 400 mg every 6 h, up to 4 g/day for severe infections Children: 30 mg/kg–50 mg/kg/day up to 100 mg/kg/day *Syphilis:* 48 g–64 g over 10 days in divided doses	Acid-stable salt of erythromycin that is reliably absorbed from the GI tract; requires a higher dose (i.e., 400 mg vs 250 mg) than other oral salts to yield comparable blood levels of erythromycin base, the active form; oral liquids are stable for 14 days with refrigeration; reconstituted powder is stable for 10 days
Erythromycin Gluceptate Ilotycin Gluceptate	Powder for injection: 250 mg, 500 mg, 1 g in 30-mL vials	Adults and children: 15 mg/kg–20 mg/kg/day by continuous (preferred) *or* intermittent infusion; up to 4 g/day can be used in severe infections *Acute pelvic inflammatory disease due to* Neisseria gonorrhoeae: 500 mg every 6 h for 3 days, followed by 250 mg oral erythromycin every 6 h for 7 days	Soluble salt of erythromycin indicated in severe infections requiring immediate high serum levels or when oral administration is not possible or feasible; may produce pain, irritation, and possibly phlebitis upon administration; solution is prepared initially by adding sterile water for injection to the vial according to package directions and shaking until dissolved; *no* preservatives should be used; reconstituted solution should be stored in refrigerator and used within 7 days; intermittent infusion is performed by administering 250 mg–500 mg in 100 mL–250 mL of sodium chloride injection or 5% dextrose over 30–60 min 4 times a day; initial solution may be added to sodium chloride injection or 5% dextrose in water to give 1 g/L for slow IV infusion; pH of diluted solution should be kept between 6 and 8; do *not* give by IV push because irritation is common; high dosages have resulted in alterations in liver function—periodic hepatic function tests are required during prolonged therapy
Erythromycin Lactobionate Erythrocin Lactobionate-IV	Powder for injection: 500 mg/vial, 1 g/vial Piggyback single dose vial: 500 mg/vial when reconstituted	Adults and children: 15 mg/kg–20 mg/kg/day by continuous (preferred) *or* intermittent infusion; up to 4 g/day may be given in severe infections *Acute pelvic inflammatory disease:* See erythromycin gluceptate, above	Soluble salt of erythromycin used in a similar manner as the gluceptate salt; see gluceptate for mixing and diluting instructions; IV infusion of 4 g/day or more has caused reversible hearing loss; *do not exceed this dosage;* intermittent IV administration is accomplished by giving ¼ the daily dose over 30–60 min

Continued

Table 61-1
Erythromycins (continued)

Drug	Preparations	Usual Dosage Range	Nursing Implications
			every 6 h by slow injection of 250 mg–500 mg in 100 mL–250 mL of sodium chloride or 5% dextrose; IV therapy should be replaced by oral therapy as soon as is feasible
Erythromycin Stearate Eramycin, Erypar, Erythrocin, Wyamycin-S (CAN) Apo-Erythro-S, Novorythro Stearate	Film-coated tablets: 250 mg, 500 mg	Adults: 250 mg every 6 h (*or* 500 mg every 12 h) up to 4 g/day in divided doses Children: 30 mg/kg–50 mg/kg/day in divided doses 4 times a day, up to 100 mg/kg/day *Syphilis:* 30 g–40 g in divided doses over 10–15 days	Acid-stable salt of erythromycin claimed to be the most completely and reliably absorbed of all the derivatives when taken on an empty stomach; may be associated with a slightly higher incidence of allergic reactions than other forms of erythromycin

COMMON SIDE EFFECTS
Abdominal discomfort and cramping

SIGNIFICANT ADVERSE REACTIONS
Nausea, vomiting, diarrhea, allergic reactions (rash, fever, pruritus, urticaria, anaphylaxis), overgrowth of nonsusceptible organisms, and cholestatic hepatitis

CONTRAINDICATIONS
Liver impairment

INTERACTIONS
Combined use of ergotamine and troleandomycin can induce ischemic reactions
Troleandomycin may elevate serum levels of theophylline, carbamazepine, and corticosteroids if used concurrently
Concomitant use of troleandomycin and oral contraceptives can cause cholestatic jaundice

NURSING CONSIDERATIONS
See erythromycin.

PATIENT EDUCATION
See erythromycin.

Selected Bibliography

Anders BJ, Laver BA, Paisley JW, Reller LB: Double-blind placebo controlled trial of erythromycin for treatment of campylobacter enteritis. Lancet 1:131, 1982

Bernstein G, Davis J, Katcher M: Prophylaxis of neonatal conjunctivitis. Clin Pediatr 21:545, 1982

Istre GR, Welch DF, Marks MI, Moyer N: Susceptibility of group A beta-hemolytic Streptococcus isolates to penicillin and erythromycin. Antimicrob Agents Chemother 20:244, 1981

Karmody CS, Weinstein L: Reversible sensorineural hearing loss with intravenous erythromycin lactobionate. Ann Otol Rhinol Laryngol 86:9, 1977

May DC, Jarboe CH, Ellenburg DT, Roe EJ, Karibo J: The effects of erythromycin on theophylline elimination in normal males. J Clin Pharmacol 22:125, 1982

Meade RH: Antimicrobial spectrum, pharmacology and therapeutic use of erythromycin and its derivatives. Am J Hosp Pharm 36:1185, 1979

Sasso SC: Erythromycin for eye prophylaxis. Matern Child Nurs 9:417, 1984

Steigbigel NH: Erythromycin, lincomycin and clindamycin. In Mandell GL, Douglas RG, Bennett JE (eds): Principles and Practice of Infectious Diseases, 2nd ed, p 224. New York, John Wiley & Sons, 1985

SUMMARY. ERYTHROMYCINS–TROLEANDOMYCIN

Drug	Preparations	Usual Dosage Range
Erythromycins	See Table 61-1	
Troleandomycin Tao	Capsules: 250 mg	Adults: 250 mg to 500 mg 4 times/day Children: 125 mg to 250 mg every 6 h

62 AMINOGLYCOSIDES

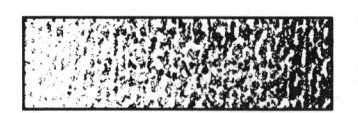

The aminoglycosides are a group of broad-spectrum bactericidal antibiotics that exhibit similar pharmacologic, antimicrobial, and toxicologic properties. Their principal use is in the treatment of serious systemic gram-negative infections caused by *Pseudomonas, Proteus, Klebsiella, Enterobacter, Serratia,* and *Escherichia* species. Aminoglycoside treatment of infections due to other organisms, both gram-negative and gram-positive is generally reserved for those instances in which less toxic agents have failed. The major limitation to the routine use of aminoglycoside antibiotics is their potential for eliciting serious untoward reactions, most notably ototoxicity (both auditory and vestibular) and nephrotoxicity. Toxicity can develop even with conventional therapeutic doses, especially in patients with impaired renal function. It is also commonly encountered with prolonged or high dosage therapy. Adverse effects are considered in more detail below. Because of the narrow margin between efficacy and toxicity with aminoglycosides, serum concentrations should be monitored frequently in critically ill patients and in persons with renal impairment. Peak serum concentrations are determined 30 minutes after completion of IV infusion or 1 hour after IM injection. Minimum (i.e., trough) levels are taken immediately prior to the next dosing. Peak levels are used as an indication of drug activity, whereas excessive trough levels serve to indicate drug cumulation and possible toxicity.

Absorption of aminoglycosides from the GI tract is negligible, and the drugs must be administered parenterally for treatment of systemic infections. Several aminoglycosides may also be given orally for localized intraintestinal infections or as adjunctive therapy in the treatment of hepatic coma. Some drugs are also applied topically to the eye, skin, or mucous membranes for treatment of superficial infections due to susceptible organisms. Thus, despite similar chemical and pharmacologic properties, the aminoglycosides do *not* share similar modes of administration or clinical indications. Table 62-1 lists the routes of administration for each of the aminoglycosides, as well as their major antimicrobial spectrum of action. Although the aminoglycosides are active against a variety of gram-positive organisms, they are rarely used clinically against these organisms because more effective, less toxic antibacterial agents are available. As indicated above, their principal application is in treating severe systemic infections caused by a number of gram-negative aerobic bacilli (see Table 62-1).

Of the available aminoglycosides, gentamicin, tobramycin amikacin, and netilmicin are the most often used derivatives and are virtually interchangeable in the treatment of most infections caused by *Acinetobacter, Enterobacter, Escherichia coli, Klebsiella pneumoniae, Proteus* species, *Pseudomonas aeruginosa, Providencia,* and *Serratia.* In many instances a synergistic action is obtained against these organisms when an extended-spectrum penicillin (such as carbenicillin or ticarcillin) or a third-generation cephalosporin (such as cefoperazone or ceftizoxime) is obtained with one of these aminoglycosides. Streptomycin is the agent of choice for treating infections due to *Francisella tularensis* (tularemia), *Pseudomonas mallei* (melioidosis), and *Yersinia pestis* (plague) and may also be useful in treating tuberculosis (see Chap. 66). Orally administered neomycin has been used for preoperative bowel sterilization, relief of *E. coli*–induced diarrhea, and as adjunctive therapy for hepatic coma. Kanamycin has a somewhat more limited spectrum of action than other aminoglycosides, and its use has declined in recent years.

The aminoglycosides are also employed as alternative agents against a wide variety of organisms as outlined in Chapter 56, Table 56-1.

Resistance to aminoglycosides is becoming more prevalent as their use increases. Resistant strains of *Enterobacter, Klebsiella, Proteus, Pseudomonas,* and *Serratia* have appeared in many hospitals in which the aminoglycosides are widely used. This resistance can occur in a number of ways, the most common being decreased penetration of the drug into the bacterial cell, a deficiency of the ribosomal receptor (see Mechanism), or increased enzymatic destruction of the drug. The newer derivatives (amikacin, netilmicin) may still be effective, however, against certain organisms that have become resistant to the action of the older agents such as kanamycin, tobramycin, and gentamicin. In addition, amikacin is not degraded by most aminoglycoside-inactivating enzymes that affect other derivatives, and thus it may be useful against enzyme-producing organisms resistant to the other systemic aminoglycosides. Nevertheless, culture and sensitivity tests should be performed to determine the susceptibility of an infecting organism to a particular aminoglycoside.

The possibility of serious adverse reactions is a major limitation to the routine use of the aminoglycosides. All derivatives exhibit essentially the same range of toxic effects, although some effects occur less frequently with some of the newer agents. Foremost among the untoward reactions seen with aminoglycoside use is ototoxicity, which can involve both the auditory and vestibular functions of the eighth cranial nerve. The risk is greatest in patients with renal impairment or preexisting hearing loss, and although the incidence of ototoxicity is generally related to the dosage and duration of treatment, it has occasionally occurred with normal therapeutic dosages. Patients should be observed closely for early signs of impending toxicity (tinnitus, vertigo, high-frequency deafness), and the dosage lowered or the drug discontinued to prevent irreversible deafness. Vestibular toxicity is more common with gentamicin and streptomycin, whereas auditory toxicity is more prevalent with kanamycin, neomycin, amikacin, and netilmicin. The relative ototoxicity of aminoglycosides is neomycin > streptomycin, kanamycin > amikacin, gentamicin, tobramycin, netilmicin.

Because aminoglycosides are eliminated almost entirely by the kidneys, they may accumulate in patients with compromised renal function. Moreover, the drug's own toxic effects may further reduce the organ's ability to excrete nitrogenous wastes. The result is increased nitrogen retention (i.e., elevated BUN or serum creatinine), frequently accompanied by oliguria, proteinuria, azotemia, and the presence of red and white cell casts in the urine. Because renal tubular damage is usually reversible if detected early enough, careful monitoring of renal function and serum creatinine levels is essential during prolonged aminoglycoside therapy, especially in the patient with preexisting renal dysfunction. Decreased creatinine clearance necessitates a reduction in drug dosage or an increase in dosing intervals, or both; the presence of casts in the urine suggests that hydration of the patient should be increased; the appear-

Table 62-1
Administration and Antimicrobial Spectrum of Aminoglycosides

Drug	Routes of Administration	Plasma Half-Life (h)	Principal Antimicrobial Spectrum of Action[a]
Amikacin	IM, IV	2–3	1, 2, 3, 7, 10, 11, 12, 15
Gentamicin	IM, IV, intrathecal, ophthalmic, topical	1–4	2, 3, 7, 10, 12, 13, 14, 15
Kanamycin	IM, IV, intraperitoneal, aerosol, oral	2–4	1, 3, 6, 7, 9, 10, 13, 14, 15
Neomycin	Ophthalmic, topical, oral	2–3	3, 7, 10, 12
Netilmicin	IM, IV	2–3	1, 2, 3, 7, 10, 12, 13, 14, 15
Streptomycin	IM	2–3	3, 4, 5, 6, 7, 8, 10, 16, 17
Tobramycin	IM, IV, ophthalmic	2–3	2, 3, 7, 10, 11, 12, 15

Organisms

1. *Acinetobacter* species
2. *Citrobacter freundii*
3. *Escherichia coli*
4. *Francisella tularensis*
5. *Hemophilus ducreyi*
6. *Hemophilus influenzae*
7. *Klebsiella–Enterobacter–Serratia* species
8. *Mycobacterium tuberculosis*
9. *Neisseria gonorrhoeae*
10. *Proteus* species
11. *Providencia* species
12. *Pseudomonas aeruginosa*
13. *Salmonella* species
14. *Shigella* species
15. *Staphylococcus* species
16. *Streptococcus* (group D)
17. *Yersinia pestis*

[a] Does *not* necessarily indicate drug of choice; see Chapter 56, Table 56-1.

---

ance of symptomatic azotemia or a progressive decrease in urine output is usually an indication to discontinue the drug. It should be noted, however, that when patients are well hydrated and kidney function is normal, the risk of nephrotoxicity with aminoglycosides is comparatively *low* provided dosage limits are not exceeded. The relative nephrotoxicity of these agents is approximately neomycin > amikacin, gentamicin, kanamycin, netilmicin > tobramycin > streptomycin.

Interference with neuromuscular transmission, possibly leading to respiratory depression or paralysis, has occurred with the aminoglycosides, especially when given either simultaneously with or shortly after general anesthetics or muscle relaxants. Reversal of aminoglycoside-induced neuromuscular blockade, characterized by apnea and muscle paralysis, may be accomplished with either neostigmine or calcium salts.

Inasmuch as the different aminoglycosides share the same properties, they are considered as a group. Characteristics of individual drugs are then presented in Table 62-2. The discussion focuses primarily on the parenteral use of the drugs, with references to their oral and topical application where appropriate.

Aminoglycosides

Amikacin	Netilmicin
Gentamicin	Streptomycin
Kanamycin	Tobramycin
Neomycin	

MECHANISM
Inhibit protein synthesis in the bacterial cell; bind to the 30S ribosomal subunit, causing a misreading of the genetic code and thus formation of improper peptide sequences in the protein chain. Drugs are more active in an alkaline medium; thus, their efficacy against urinary pathogens can be increased by alkalinization of the urine

USES
(See Tables 56-1 and 62-1 for susceptible organisms)

Treatment of severe gram-negative infections of the GI, respiratory or urinary tracts, CNS, skin, bone, and soft tissues due to susceptible organisms (parenteral use only)

Suppression of intestinal bacteria (kanamycin or neomycin orally)

Adjunctive therapy of hepatic coma to reduce concentration of ammonia-forming bacteria in the GI tract (kanamycin, neomycin, or paromomycin orally)

Treatment of superficial infections of the eye, skin, or mucous membranes due to susceptible organisms (gentamicin or tobramycin)

Treatment of severe diarrhea due to *Escherichia coli* (neomycin orally)

DOSAGE
See Table 62-2

FATE
Not appreciably absorbed from the GI tract; absorption following IM injection is rapid; peak blood levels occur in 1 to 2 hours; plasma half-life is 1 to 4 hours with normal kidney function but may be longer in infants (5–8 h), in elderly persons, or in patients with renal impairment (up to 96 h); widely distributed in the body, except for the CNS (unless meninges are inflamed); drugs are not significantly protein-bound; serum levels in febrile patients are generally lower than those in afebrile patients given the same dosage, and half-lives are shorter; not metabolized to a significant extent, but eliminated largely unchanged

by the kidneys following parenteral injection (up to 98% of a single IV dose is excreted within 24 h); orally administered drugs are excreted almost completely in the feces; drugs have a narrow margin between the therapeutic and toxic serum levels

COMMON SIDE EFFECTS
Oral: nausea, diarrhea
Parenteral: headache, tinnitus, dizziness (especially at high doses)
Topical: hypersensitivity reactions (especially with neomycin)

SIGNIFICANT ADVERSE REACTIONS
Oral
Malabsorption syndrome (i.e., decreased absorption of vitamins, minerals, electrolytes, fats), steatorrhea, anorexia, stomatitis, salivation
Parenteral
CNS: ototoxicity (vertigo, ataxia, impaired hearing, irreversible deafness), confusion, disorientation, lethargy, depression, visual disturbances, amblyopia, nystagmus, optic neuritis, numbness and paresthesias, muscle twitching, tremor, convulsions
Renal: proteinuria, oliguria, azotemia, red and white cell casts in urine, elevated BUN and serum creatinine
Allergic/hypersensitivity: rash, pruritus, urticaria, alopecia, laryngeal edema, fever, exfoliative dermatitis, anaphylaxis
Hematologic: agranulocytosis, leukopenia, thrombocytopenia, eosinophilia, pancytopenia, anemia
Hepatic: increased serum transaminase and bilirubin, hepatomegaly, hepatic necrosis
Other: palpitations, myocarditis, splenomegaly, arthralgia, hypotension, pulmonary fibrosis, superinfections, muscle weakness, respiratory depression, pain and irritation with IM injection
Topical
Burning, itching, urticaria, erythema, photosensitivity, macropapular dermatitis

CONTRAINDICATIONS
Oral use in patients with bowel obstruction, long-term parenteral therapy in patients with renal impairment, and concurrent administration with other ototoxic or nephrotoxic drugs (see Interactions). *Cautious use* in persons with neuromuscular disorders or those taking skeletal muscle relaxants and in children, elderly patients, and pregnant or nursing women

INTERACTIONS
Concurrent use of aminoglycosides and amphotericin, bacitracin, cephalothin, colistimethate, polymyxin, or vancomycin can increase the incidence of nephrotoxicity
The ototoxic effects of the aminoglycosides can be enhanced by potent diuretics such as ethacrynic acid, bumetanide, furosemide, and mannitol
Dimenhydrinate, meclizine, cyclizine, and other antivertigo drugs may mask the ototoxic effects of aminoglycosides
Aminoglycosides can enhance the muscle-relaxing effects of neuromuscular blocking agents and general anesthetics, possibly leading to respiratory depression
Aminoglycosides exert a synergistic effect with antipseudomonal penicillins (e.g., carbenicillin, ticarcillin, piperacillin, mezlocillin, azlocillin) against *Pseudomonas* infections at normal concentrations; however, high concentrations of the penicillins may inhibit the antibacterial activity of aminoglycosides
Orally administered neomycin and possibly other aminoglycosides may decrease the absorption of digoxin, penicillin V, and vitamin B_{12}

NURSING CONSIDERATIONS
See **Plan Of Nursing Care 12, Antibacterial Drugs,** in Chapter 56. See Table 62-2 for information on specific drugs. In addition:

Nursing Alerts
- Assess vestibular and auditory function before, at regular intervals during, and for 3 to 4 weeks after therapy, *particularly* if patient's kidney function is impaired or treatment is prolonged, and closely observe patient for evidence of dizziness, tinnitus, vertigo, ataxia, nystagmus, or hearing loss at high frequencies. Aminoglycosides can cause serious ototoxicity, even in normal therapeutic doses, especially if renal function is impaired, and onset of hearing loss may be delayed
- Assess status of kidney function before initiating therapy, monitor intake–output ratio during therapy, and monitor BUN and serum creatinine values as guides to dosage adjustments. Decreased urinary output and urinary creatinine levels and increased BUN or serum creatinine levels, signs of possible nephrotoxicity, are indications for dosage reduction or discontinuation of therapy. The likelihood of both ototoxicity and nephrotoxicity increases with extended therapy.
- Monitor results of trough drug-level determinations, which should be obtained at regular intervals. Dosage should be adjusted as necessary to prevent drug accumulation.
- Avoid concurrent or sequential administration of other potentially ototoxic or nephrotoxic drugs (see Interactions).
- Keep patient well hydrated to prevent renal tubular irritation. If signs of renal irritation are noted (red or white cells, albumin, or casts in urine), increase fluid intake (i.e., 2000–3000 mL/day) to prevent further damage.
- If an oral drug is administered to a patient with ulcerative lesions of the bowel, observe patient for signs of renal toxicity because systemic absorption may be enhanced, thus increasing nephrotoxicity.
- When giving IV, infuse slowly to minimize possibility of severe neuromuscular blockade and subsequent development of apnea.

1. When giving IM, inject deeply into large muscle mass, observe for signs of irritation, and rotate injection sites.
2. Use only ophthalmic preparations (ophthalmic ointment or drops) in the eye. Do not apply topical neomycin or gentamicin ointment to the eyes or to external ear canal if eardrum is perforated.
3. Consult package instructions for appropriate dosage modification if patient's renal function is impaired. Parameters used to determine proper dosage adjustment include trough serum levels of aminoglycoside and creatinine clearance.
4. Use solutions as soon as possible after reconstituting because drugs are relatively unstable in solution. Check manufacturer's instructions for stability data.

(Text continued on page 630)

Table 62-2
Aminoglycosides

Drug	Preparations	Usual Dosage Range	Nursing Implications
Amikacin Amikin	Injection: 100 mg/2 mL; 500 mg/2 mL; 1 g/4 mL	*IM, IV* Adults and older children: 15 mg/kg/day in 2–3 divided doses (maximum 1.5 g/day) *Urinary tract infections:* 250 mg IM twice a day *Neonatal sepsis:* Initially 10 mg/kg, followed by 7.5 mg/kg every 12 h	Semisynthetic aminoglycoside derived from kanamycin, exhibiting a similar spectrum of action; *not* degraded by most aminoglycoside-inactivating enzymes, therefore may be effective against organisms resistant to other derivatives; amikacin resistance is emerging, however, as its use increases; duration of treatment should be 7–10 days—longer therapy necessitates daily monitoring of renal and auditory function; if a clinical response does *not* occur within 5 days, stop drug and reevaluate; may be used in uncomplicated urinary tract infections (dose: 250 mg IM twice a day) due to organisms not susceptible to other, less toxic agents; urine should be examined during treatment for the presence of protein, blood cells, or casts; maintain high degree of hydration to minimize renal irritation; solution for IV use is prepared by adding contents of 500-mg vial to 200 mL of appropriate diluent (see package instructions) and administered over a 30–60-min period (1–2 h for neonates); do *not* premix with other drugs; stable for extended period at room temperature
Gentamicin Garamycin, Genoptic, Gentacidin, Gentafair, GentAK, Jenamicin (CAN) Alcomicin, Cidomycin	Injection: 10 mg/mL, 40 mg/mL Piggyback injection: 60 mg/dose, 80 mg/dose, 100 mg/dose Intrathecal injection: 2 mg/mL Ophthalmic drops: 0.3% Ophthalmic ointment: 0.3% Topical ointment: 0.1% Topical cream: 0.1%	*IM, IV* Adults: 3 mg/kg–5 mg/kg/day in 3–4 divided doses Children: 6 mg/kg–7.5 mg/kg/day in 3 divided doses Infants and neonates: 7.5 mg/kg/day in 3 divided doses Premature infants and neonates (less than 1 wk): 5 mg/kg/day in 2 equal doses *Intrathecal* Adults: 4 mg–8 mg/day in a single dose Children and infants (over 3 mo): 1 mg–2 mg once/day *Ophthalmic* 1 or 2 drops or small amount of ophthalmic ointment 2–4 times/day *Topical* Apply sparingly to affected area 3–4 times/day	Broad-spectrum aminoglycoside obtained from an *Actinomyces* organism; drug of choice against several gram-negative organisms (see Chap. 56, Table 56-1), synergistic with extended-spectrum penicillins against *Pseudomonas* infections; may be used in combination with a penicillin or cephalosporin in treating serious unknown infections before sensitivity testing; also used with antistaphylococcal penicillins for treatment of staphylococcal endocarditis; generally given IM but may be used IV in patients with septicemia, shock, congestive heart failure, severe burns, or hematologic disorders; do *not* mix with other drugs before injection; intrathecal administration is used as an adjunct to systemic administration in serious CNS infections (e.g., meningitis, ventriculitis) due to *Pseudomonas* species; topi-

Continued

Table 62-2
Aminoglycosides (continued)

Drug	Preparations	Usual Dosage Range	Nursing Implications
			cal application is used to treat superficial infections of the skin and mucous membranes due to susceptible organisms; photosensitivity reactions have occurred following topical use; systemic toxicity can result from application to large abraded areas of skin; use *cautiously* on burns or large wounds
Kanamycin Kantrex, Klebcil (CAN) Anamid	Injection: 500 mg/2 mL; 1 g/3 mL Pediatric injection: 75 mg/2 mL Capsules: 500 mg	*IM* Adults and children: 7.5 mg/kg every 12 h (maximum 1.5 g/day) *IV* Up to 15 mg/kg/day in 2–3 divided doses infused over a 30–60-min period *Intraperitoneal* 500 mg/20 mL sterile distilled water instilled into peritoneal cavity through a wound catheter *Aerosol* 250 mg (1 mL) diluted with 3 mL saline 2 to 4 times/day, using a nebulizer *Oral* *Suppression of intestinal bacteria:* 1 g every hour for 4 h, then 1 g every 6 h for 36–72 h *Hepatic coma:* 8 g–12 g/day in divided doses	Aminoglycoside derived from a species of *Streptomyces*; similar in activity to neomycin but not as toxic; effective against many common gram-negative organisms (except *Pseudomonas*) but not considered drug of choice for any infection; used mainly as alternative to gentamicin or tobramycin; occasionally used as adjunctive therapy of *Mycobacterium tuberculosis*; inject deeply IM and rotate sites; discontinue drug if a clinical response does not occur within 5 days; prepare IV solutions by adding 500 mg to 200 mL, *or* 1 g to 400 mL, of sterile diluent, and infuse over 30–60 min 2–3 times a day; do *not* mix dilution with other drug solutions; solution in vials may darken on shelf with no loss of potency, intraperitoneal instillation should be postponed until patient has recovered from effects of anesthesia and muscle relaxants (danger of respiratory depression and muscle paralysis); may be used as an irrigating solution (0.25%) in abscess cavities, peritoneal, ventricular, or pleural spaces; when used orally, be alert for malabsorption syndrome (e.g., increased fecal fat) or secondary bacterial or fungal infections (e.g., diarrhea, stomatitis); use with caution orally in patients with GI ulceration, because enhanced systemic absorption can occur; nausea, vomiting, and diarrhea are common with oral ingestion
Neomycin Mycifradin, Myciguent	Tablets: 500 mg Oral solution: 125 mg/5 mL Topical ointment: 0.5% Topical cream: 0.5%	*Oral* *Preoperative bowel preparation:* 88 mg/kg (40 mg/lb) in 6 equally divided doses every 4 h before surgery or 1 g every	Broad-spectrum antibiotic obtained from a species of *Streptomyces*; similar in action to kanamycin but is the most potent neuromuscular blocker

Continued

Table 62-2
Aminoglycosides (continued)

Drug	Preparations	Usual Dosage Range	Nursing Implications
		hour for 4 doses, then 1 g every 4 h for the next 20 h *Hepatic coma* Adults: 4 g–12 g/day in divided doses Children: 50 mg–100 mg/kg/day in divided doses *Infectious diarrhea:* 50 mg/kg/day in divided doses for 2–3 days *Topical* Apply 2–4 times a day	and reportedly the most toxic of all aminoglycosides; many organisms exhibit moderate to marked resistance against neomycin; principal indications for oral neomycin are severe diarrhea due to *Escherichia coli* and preoperative bowel sterilization in conjunction with a low-residue diet; a saline cathartic is administered before first dose of neomycin; may interfere with absorption of other drugs (e.g., digitalis glycosides, methotrexate, penicillins; see Interactions); nausea and diarrhea are fairly common with oral administration; widest application is topically, either alone or more commonly with bacitracin and polymyxin (e.g., Neosporin, Mycitracin, Neo-Polycin) for superficial infections of eye, skin, and mucous membranes; hypersensitivity reactions are common with topical application; discontinue drug if irritation, redness, or itching occurs; do *not* use over large body surface areas or if skin is broken or abraded, because increased systemic absorption and toxicity can occur
Netilmicin Netromycin	Injection: 100 mg/mL	*IM, IV* Adults: 3 mg/kg–6.5 mg/kg/day in divided doses every 8–12 h Children: 5.5 mg/kg–8 mg/kg/day in divided doses every 8–12 h Neonates: 4 mg/kg–6 mg/kg/day in divided doses every 12 h	Semisynthetic derivative similar to gentamicin in activity but somewhat less effective against *Pseudomonas;* may be slightly less nephrotoxic and ototoxic than other aminoglycosides; used in serious staphylococcal infections where penicillins are contraindicated and in suspected or confirmed gram-negative infections; usual duration of treatment is 7–14 days—for longer therapy, carefully monitor renal, auditory, and vestibular functions; follow package instructions for dosage adjustment in the presence of impaired renal function
Streptomycin Streptomycin	Powder for injection: 1 g/vial, 5 g/vial Injection: 400 mg/vial	*IM use only* *Tuberculosis:* 1 g/day, together with other antitubercular drugs (e.g., isoniazid, ethambutol, rifampin); may reduce to 1 g 2–3 times a week as condition improves *Tularemia:* 1 g–2 g/day in divided doses for 7–10 days	Aminoglycoside isolated from a species of *Streptomyces;* fairly high toxicity and rapid development of resistance limits its usefulness to those infections not controlled by other less toxic drugs, except in tularemia, plague, and melioidosis, where it is the

Continued

Table 62-2
Aminoglycosides (continued)

Drug	Preparations	Usual Dosage Range	Nursing Implications
		Plague: 2 g–4 g/day in divided doses *Bacterial endocarditis:* 0.5 g–1 g twice a day for 2 wk with a penicillin *Prophylaxis of bacterial endocarditis in patients undergoing intestinal or urinary tract surgery:* 1 g IM ½–1 h before surgery in combination with 2 million U penicillin G *or* 1 g ampicillin IM *or* IV *Other infections:* 1 g–4 g/day in divided doses depending on severity of infection *Children:* 20 mg–40 mg/kg/day in divided doses every 6–12 h	drug of choice, and tuberculosis, where it is commonly used in combination with several other tuberculostatic agents; (see Chap. 66); total treatment period for tuberculosis is a minimum of 1 yr; also indicated for prophylaxis of bacterial endocarditis in high-risk patients undergoing respiratory, gastrointestinal, or genitourinary surgery or instrumentation, in combination with penicillin G or ampicillin; most frequent adverse effect is vestibular toxicity; observe for headache, vomiting, dizziness, difficulty in reading, or ataxia and consult physician; incidence of nephrotoxicity is lowest of all aminoglycosides, but use with caution in renal impairment and perform frequent determinations of serum drug concentration; adequate hydration is important, especially during prolonged therapy (e.g., tuberculosis therapy); commercially available IM solutions contain a preservative and should *not* be injected IV or SC; solution may darken during storage but potency is not affected

Continued

PATIENT EDUCATION

See **Plan of Nursing Care 12, Antibacterial Drugs,** in Chapter 56. In addition:

1. Explain to patient that treatment may be prolonged if infection is severe or complicated. Bacterial resistance to aminoglycosides develops slowly, with the exception of streptomycin, to which resistance can develop very rapidly (see Chap. 66).
2. Warn patient to report immediately any ringing in the ears, decreased hearing acuity, dizziness, or unsteady gait, possible signs of ototoxicity.

Selected Bibliography

Betts RF et al: Five year surveillance of aminoglycoside usage in a university hospital. Ann Intern Med 100:219, 1984

Blumer JL, Reed MD: Clinical pharmacology of aminoglycoside antibiotics in pediatrics. Pediatr Clin North Am 30:195, 1983

Bryan LE: Mechanisms of action of aminoglycosides antibiotics. In Root RK, Sande MA (eds): Contemporary Issues in Infectious Diseases, Vol. 1: New Dimensions in Antimicrobial Therapy, p 1. New York, Churchill Livingstone, 1984

Edson RS, Keys TF: The aminoglycosides. Mayo Clin Proc 58:99, 1983

Gever LN: Parenteral aminoglycosides: Administering them safely. Nursing 84 14(3):90, 1984

Langslet J, Habel ML: The aminoglycoside antibiotics. Am J Nurs 81:1144, 1981

Lerner AM et al: Randomized controlled trial of the comparative efficacy, auditory toxicity and nephrotoxicity of tobramycin and netilmicin. Lancet 1:1123, 1983

Lietman PS: Aminoglycosides and spectinomycin: Aminocyclitols. In Mandell GL, Douglas RG, Bennett JE (eds): Principles and Practice of Infectious Diseases, 2nd ed, p 192. New York, John Wiley & Sons, 1985

Lietman PS, Smith CR: Aminoglycoside nephrotoxicity in humans. J Infect Dis 5(Suppl 2):284, 1983

Moore RD, Smith CR, Lietman PS: Risk factors for the development of auditory toxicity in patients receiving aminoglycosides. J Infect Dis 149:23, 1984

Neu HC: New antibiotics: Areas of appropriate use. J Infect Dis 155:403, 1987

Shannon K, Phillips I: Mechanisms of resistance to amino-

Table 62-2
Aminoglycosides (continued)

Drug	Preparations	Usual Dosage Range	Nursing Implications
Tobramycin Nebcin, Tobrex	Injection: 40 mg/mL, 60 mg/1.5 mL Pediatric injection: 20 mg/2 mL Powder for injection: 30 mg/mL, 40 mg/mL when reconstituted Ophthalmic solution: 0.3% Ophthalmic ointment: 3 mg/g	*IM, IV* Adults: 3 mg/kg–5 mg/kg/day in 3–4 equally divided doses depending on severity of infection Children: 6 mg/kg–7.5 mg/kg/day in 3–4 equally divided doses Neonates (1 wk or less): up to 4 mg/kg/day in 2 equal doses every 12 h *Ophthalmic* 1–2 drops or ½-inch ribbon of ointment every 4 h; in severe infections 2 drops every hour until improvement is noted	Aminoglycoside antibiotic with pharmacologic properties, indications, and overall toxicity similar to gentamicin; somewhat lower incidence of vestibular toxicity has been reported; do *not* exceed 5 mg/kg/day unless serum levels are monitored; prolonged serum concentrations above 12 μg/mL should be avoided; urine should be observed for presence of protein, cells, and casts; follow package directions for dosage reduction in patients with renal impairment—reduced doses may be based upon creatinine clearance or serum creatinine; IV dose should be diluted to 50 mL–100 mL for adults (and proportionately less for children) with sodium chloride or 5% dextrose injection and infused over 20–60 min; do *not* premix with other drugs but administer separately; usual duration of treatment is 7–10 days; in severe or complicated infections, a longer course of therapy may be necessary; auditory, vestibular, and renal function should be monitored frequently during prolonged therapy; local allergic reactions have occurred with eye drops or eye ointment

glycosides in clinical isolates. J Antimicrob Chemother 9:91, 1982

Silverblatt FJ: Pathogenesis of nephrotoxicity of cephalosporins and aminoglycosides: A review of current concepts. Rev Infect Dis 4(Suppl):360, 1982

Smith CR, Lietman PS: Effect of furosemide on aminoglycoside-induced nephrotoxicity and auditory toxicity in humans. Antimicrob Agents Chemother 23:133, 1983

Whelton A, Neu HC (eds): The Aminoglycosides: Microbiology, Clinical Use and Toxicity. New York, Marcel Dekker, 1982

63 POLYPEPTIDES

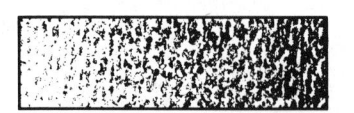

The polypeptide group of antibiotics comprises polymyxin B, colistin (polymyxin E), the methanesulfonate salt of colistin (colistimethate), and bacitracin. The first three of these drugs are commonly termed the *polymyxins,* and while certain similarities exist between these agents and bacitracin, significant differences are noted as well.

The polymyxins, a group of strongly basic polypeptides obtained from *Bacillus polymyxa* and variants, are designated as polymyxins A, B, C, D, and E. Of these, only polymyxins B and E are employed clinically, because the remaining derivatives are too toxic for human use.

The polymyxins are bactericidal, primarily against gram-negative bacilli such as *Pseudomonas, Escherichia coli, Klebsiella, Enterobacter, Salmonella,* and Shigella. However, most strains of *Proteus* and *Neisseria* and virtually all gram-positive organisms are unaffected by the polymyxins. These drugs exert their antibacterial action by disrupting the bacterial cell membrane, thus allowing cell constituents to escape. The drugs are not absorbed orally, and following parenteral administration they do not reach the CNS (unless given intrathecally), the joints, or the eye in appreciable amounts. Excretion is by the kidney (except orally administered colistin); thus cumulation toxicity can occur in the presence of renal impairment. The polymyxins are used systemically for severe infections only, especially of the urinary tract, caused by susceptible gram-negative organisms not sensitive to other less toxic antimicrobial drugs. They find their widest application for topical treatment of skin and mucous membrane infections (including the eye and ear), especially if *Pseudomonas* is the offending pathogen. Principal adverse effects are of two major types, neurotoxicity and nephrotoxicity, and the incidence and severity of these untoward reactions severely limit the systemic usefulness of the polymyxins to all but very severe infections.

Polymyxin B is available as an injection, as a powder for preparing ophthalmic drops, and in several combination products (e.g., with neomycin, bacitracin, and corticosteroids) for ophthalmic or otic use. Colistin sulfate (polymyxin E) can be used either as an oral suspension for control of diarrhea and gastroenteritis or in combination with hydrocortisone and neomycin as ear drops (ColyMycin S Otic). Colistimethate, as a powder for injection, may be administered either IV or IM for serious systemic or urinary infections, particularly when caused by *Pseudomonas.* Because there are many differences among these three polymyxin preparations, they are considered individually in this chapter.

Bacitracin is a mixture of several polypeptides isolated from a strain of *Bacillus subtilis,* the major constituent being bacitracin A. This antibiotic appears to inhibit bacterial cell wall formation and is bactericidal against a variety of gram-positive bacteria as well as a few gram-negative organisms. The drug is available for IM injection and as a topical and ophthalmic ointment. Because of its potential for serious toxicity, however, it is used parenterally *only* for treatment of staphylococcal pneumonia or empyema in infants. Bacitracin is most often used topically, alone or in combination with neomycin and polymyxin, for treatment of cutaneous or ocular infections, because it is highly effective against susceptible organisms and rarely causes hypersensitivity reactions. Kidney damage is a major danger with parenteral use of bacitracin, and renal function must be closely monitored during therapy.

Bacitracin

AK-Tracin, Baciguent

MECHANISM

Not completely established; probably acts by inhibiting bacterial cell wall synthesis and may alter cell membrane permeability as well; bactericidal at therapeutic doses; spectrum of action in vitro is similar to that of penicillin G; systemic use is virtually obsolete because parenteral administration is highly nephrotoxic

USES

Treatment of superficial infections of the skin, mucous membrane, and eye due to susceptible organisms (topical use *only*)

Treatment of antibiotic-induced pseudomembranous colitis caused by *Clostridium difficile* (investigational use for *orally* administered bacitracin)

Treatment of infants with pneumonia and empyema caused by staphylococci (rarely used)

DOSAGE

IM

Infants under 2.5 kg: 900 U/kg/day in two or three divided doses
Infants over 2.5 kg: 1000 U/kg/day in two or three divided doses
Topical: apply two or three times a day to affected area
Ophthalmic: apply to lower conjuctival sac several times a day

FATE

Rapidly absorbed from IM injection site; distributed widely in the body, duration of action is 6 to 8 hours with single IM doses; excreted largely in the urine; absorption from topical sites is minimal

COMMON SIDE EFFECTS

Pain and irritation at IM injection site

SIGNIFICANT ADVERSE REACTIONS

WARNING
Bacitracin (IM) can result in renal failure due to glomerular injury or tubular necrosis. Use only when indicated (see Uses), monitor renal function daily, and maintain adequate fluid intake

Renal: proteinuria, azotemia, urinary frequency, oliguria, hematuria, increased BUN, uremia, renal failure
Other: neuromuscular weakness, hypersensitivity reactions (rash, urticaria, hypotension), nausea, vomiting, tinnitus, diarrhea, altered taste sensations, allergic contact dermatitis (with topical use). With ophthalmic use—ocular burning, stinging, and irritation

CONTRAINDICATIONS

Severe renal impairment; intraocular use in patients with viral or fungal infections. *Cautious use* in persons with myasthenia gravis or a history of allergic reactions

INTERACTIONS

Nephrotoxic effects of bacitracin may be additive to those of other antibiotics having similar toxicity, for example, aminoglycosides, polymyxins, vancomycin

Bacitracin can enhance or prolong the muscle-relaxing effects of neuromuscular blocking agents and anesthetics, or other drugs with neuromuscular blocking actions, that is, aminoglycosides, procainamide, succinylcholine

NURSING CONSIDERATIONS

See **Plan of Nursing Care 12, Antibacterial Drugs,** in Chapter 56. In addition:

Nursing Alerts

- When drug is used IM, monitor results of renal function tests, which should be performed prior to initiation of therapy and daily throughout the course of treatment; closely monitor urinary output, maintain fluid intake at a sufficient level to avoid renal toxicity, and ensure that patient is under constant supervision during treatment (see Significant Adverse Reactions).
- Assess patient's renal status for early indications of dysfunction (hematuria, proteinuria, oliguria, polyuria, elevated BUN). Discontinue drug immediately if signs appear.

1. Dissolve drug in sodium chloride injection containing 2% procaine hydrochloride because IM injections are painful.
2. Refrigerate bacitracin solutions (stable up to 1 wk) because they are rapidly inactivated at room temperature.

Colistimethate

Coly-Mycin M

MECHANISM

Disrupts the bacterial cell membrane, probably through a surface action, thus allowing escape of cell constituents

USE

Treatment of acute or chronic infections due to sensitive strains of certain gram-negative organisms, especially *Pseudomonas aeruginosa, Escherichia coli, Klebsiella pneumoniae,* and *Enterobacter aerogenes* (not effective against *Proteus* or *Neisseria*)

DOSAGE

Adults and children: 2.5 mg/kg to 5 mg/kg/day, IM or IV, in two to four divided doses (maximum 5 mg/kg/day in patients with normal renal function).

IV administration may be by direct injection (one half daily dose over 3–5 min every 12 h) or by infusion (one half dose over 3–5 min, then 5 mg–6 mg/h starting 1–2 h after initial injection)

FATE

Absorption from IM sites is good; blood levels are maximum 1 hour to 2 hours after IM injection; serum half-life is 2 to 3 hours; does not enter CNS, even if meninges are inflamed; excreted primarily in the urine, mostly within 18 to 24 hours

COMMON SIDE EFFECTS

Pain at IM injection site

SIGNIFICANT ADVERSE REACTIONS

Renal: decreased urine output, increased BUN, proteinuria, azotemia, renal failure

Neurologic: paresthesias; numbness in the extremities; visual, auditory, or speech disturbances; dizziness; ataxia

Allergic/hypersensitivity: pruritus, urticaria, drug fever, dermatoses

Other: neuromuscular blockade (muscle weakness, respiratory depression or paralysis), GI upset, agranulocytosis, superinfections

CONTRAINDICATIONS

Severe renal failure. *Cautious use* in patients with myasthenia gravis, renal impairment, or in persons receiving muscle relaxants or potentially nephrotoxic drugs (e.g., aminoglycosides, vancomycin)

INTERACTIONS

Additive nephrotoxic effects can result from concurrent use of colistimethate and other drugs that impair renal function (e.g., aminoglycosides, vancomycin)

Extreme muscle weakness and muscle paralysis can occur if colistimethate is administered with several anesthetics, neuromuscular blocking agents, aminoglycosides, or other drugs having a neuromuscular blocking action

NURSING CONSIDERATIONS

See **Plan of Nursing Care 12, Antibacterial Drugs,** in Chapter 56. In addition:

Nursing Alerts

- Have appropriate resuscitative equipment and drugs available, and observe patient closely for signs of respiratory distress (dyspnea, chest pain, restlessness) because respiratory arrest has occurred following injection.
- Seek clarification if dosage exceeds 5 mg/kg/day, even if patient's renal function is normal, because overdosage can result in neuromuscular blockade and renal insufficiency (see Significant Adverse Reactions).
- Assess patient for changes in visual, auditory, or verbal function or development of drowsiness, dizziness, or paresthesias, early signs of possible neurologic toxicity.
- Ensure that prescribed baseline renal function tests are obtained before therapy is initiated. During therapy, be alert for changes in urinary output or elevations in BUN, serum creatinine, or plasma drug levels, possible indications of renal toxicity.

1. When giving IM, inject deeply into large muscle, and rotate injection sites. Injection may be painful.
2. Discard unused portion of IM drug solution 7 days after reconstitution. Solution may be stored at room temperature.
3. Prepare IV infusion solution with appropriate diluent according to package instructions; use within 24 hours.

Colistin Sulfate

Coly-Mycin S

MECHANISM

Disrupts bacterial cell membrane, causing loss of cellular constituents; bactericidal against most gram-negative enteric pathogens, except *Proteus*

USES

Control of diarrhea in infants and children due to susceptible strains of enteropathogenic *Escherichia coli* (oral suspension)

Treatment of gastroenteritis due to *Shigella* organisms (oral suspension)

Treatment of superficial infections of the ear canal (combination with neomycin and hydrocortisone as Coly-Mycin S Otic)

DOSAGE

Oral: adults and children—5 mg/kg to 15 mg/kg/day in three divided doses; higher doses may be required in severe infections

Otic: three or four drops into external ear canal three or four times a day

FATE

Not absorbed to a significant extent from the GI tract; excreted in the feces

SIGNIFICANT ADVERSE REACTIONS

Rare at recommended doses; superinfection can occur with prolonged use

CONTRAINDICATIONS

(Topical use) Fungal or viral infections of the ear, herpes simplex, vaccinia, varicella. *Cautious use* orally in patients with preexisting renal damage

INTERACTIONS

See Bacitracin for *potential* drug interactions; actual incidence is minimal, because drug is not absorbed systemically

NURSING CONSIDERATIONS

Nursing Alert
- Be alert for signs of possible renal toxicity, especially if large doses are employed or azotemia is present, because slight systemic absorption may occur in some instances.

1. Reconstitute powder for oral suspension with distilled water. Store in refrigerator; discard unused portion after 2 weeks.
2. Clean and dry external ear canal before instillation of drops.
3. If patient has perforated eardrum or chronic otitis media, question use of otic solution. It should be used very cautiously with such patients because it contains neomycin, which is ototoxic.

Polymyxin B Sulfate
Aerosporin

MECHANISM
Disrupts the lipoprotein cell membrane of susceptible bacteria, resulting in leakage of cellular constituents and cell death; bactericidal against most gram-negative bacilli, except *Proteus*; gram-positive bacteria and gram-negative cocci are resistant.

USES
Treatment of acute infections due to susceptible strains of *Pseudomonas aeruginosa* (IM, IV) *Note:* treatment of choice for pseudomonal meningitis given intrathecally

Alternative treatment of severe infections of the blood, meninges, or urinary tract due to *Escherichia coli, Klebsiella pneumoniae, Enterobacter aerogenes,* or *Hemophilus influenzae* when less toxic drugs are ineffective (IM, IV)

Treatment of superficial infections of the eye, ear, mucous membranes, or skin due to susceptible organisms (topical combination products containing polymyxin B)

DOSAGE

IV infusion
Adults and children: 15,000 U/kg/day to 25,000 U/kg/day; infusions may be given every 12 hours
Infants: Up to 40,000 U/kg/day

IM
Adults and children: 25,000 U/kg/day to 30,000 U/kg/day, divided and given at 4- to 6-hour intervals
Infants: up to 40,000 U/kg/day

Intrathecal (e.g., in pseudomonal meningitis)
Adults and children over 2 years: 50,000 U once daily for 3 to 4 days; then 50,000 U every other day for at least 2 weeks after cultures of the cerebrospinal fluid are negative and its glucose content has returned to normal
Children under 2 years: 20,000 U once daily for 3 to 4 days; then 25,000 U every other day

Bladder irrigation (Neosporin G.U. Irrigant—polysporin plus neomycin)
Add 1 mL irrigant to 1 L isotonic saline solution; infuse by catheter at a rate of 1 L/24 h *continuously*; if urine output exceeds 2 L/day, increase flow rate to 2 L/24 h

Ophthalmic
One or two drops in affected eye several times a day, as necessary

Topical
Apply several times a day to affected area

FATE
Not significantly absorbed from the GI tract or mucous membranes; peak plasma concentrations are reached within 2 hours after IM injection; plasma half-life is 4 to 6 hours; active blood levels are low, because drug loses up to one half its activity in the serum; activity levels are higher in infants and children than in adults; diffusion into many tissues is poor, and drug does not enter CNS unless given intrathecally; slowly excreted by the kidneys, largely in unchanged form

COMMON SIDE EFFECTS
Pain on IM injection

SIGNIFICANT ADVERSE REACTIONS

WARNING
Nephrotoxicity and neurotoxicity can occur, especially with IM or intrathecal administration. Administer only to hospitalized patients and provide constant supervision

Renal: proteinuria, hematuria, azotemia, cellular casts, increasing blood levels of drug without increases in dosage
Neurologic: flushing, paresthesias, drowsiness, dizziness, neuromuscular blockade (muscle weakness, respiratory depression, apnea)
Hypersensitivity/allergic: pruritus, dermatoses, urticaria, drug fever, local burning or irritation with topical application

Other: meningeal irritation (headache, stiff neck, fever) with intrathecal administration, thrombophlebitis with IV infusion, GI disturbances, overgrowth of nonsusceptible organisms

CONTRAINDICATIONS
Severe renal impairment, concurrent use of other nephrotoxic or neurotoxic drugs (e.g., bacitracin, aminoglycosides, colistimethate). *Cautious use* in persons with neurologic disorders and in pregnant or nursing women

INTERACTIONS
Concurrent use of polymyxin and other nephrotoxic drugs (e.g., aminoglycosides, vancomycin, bacitracin, colistimethate) may increase the danger of kidney damage

Use of polymyxin with neuromuscular blocking agents, general anesthetics, or aminoglycosides can lead to extreme muscle weakness and respiratory paralysis

NURSING CONSIDERATIONS
See **Plan of Nursing Care 12, Antibacterial Drugs,** in Chapter 56. In addition:

Nursing Alerts
- Ensure that patient receiving drug IM or intrathecally is under constant professional supervision. The drug should be administered IM or intrathecally *only* to patients who are hospitalized (see Significant Adverse Reactions).
- Have appropriate resuscitative equipment and drugs available, and observe patient closely for signs of neuromuscular blockade (dyspnea, shortness of breath, muscle weakness). If these occur, the drug should be discontinued and symptoms treated as necessary.
- Assess patient's neurologic status frequently for symptoms of neurotoxicity (irritability, dizziness, paresthesias, numbness, blurred vision). These can usually be eliminated by a dosage reduction.
- Ensure that prescribed baseline renal function tests are obtained before therapy is initiated. Renal toxicity usually occurs within several days after treatment is started. During therapy, be alert for reductions in urinary output or elevations in BUN, serum creatinine, plasma drug levels, or urinary proteins. The drug should be discontinued if these occur.

- Advocate route of administration other than IM, as appropriate, because IM injection may be extremely painful, especially in infants and children.

1. Plan with patient to ensure that daily fluid intake is maintained at a level sufficient to produce urine output of at least 1500 mL/day.
2. Reconstitute drug with the following diluents:
   IM: Sterile water for injection or sterile physiologic saline, *or* 1% procaine hydrochloride solution
   IV: 5% dextrose in water
   Intrathecal: Sterile physiologic saline
   Ophthalmic drops: Sterile physiologic saline *or* sterile distilled water
3. Store reconstituted parenteral solution under refrigeration. Discard unused portion after 72 hours.
4. Ear drops should be warmed before instilling into auditory canal, but avoid heating beyond body temperature because potency may be diminished.
5. Note that polymyxin is available as an ophthalmic solution or ointment with neomycin (Statrol), bacitracin (Polysporin), oxytetracycline (Terramycin), neomycin plus bacitracin (Neosporin Ophthalmic, Ak-Spore), and neomycin plus a corticosteroid (Corticosporin Ophthalmic, Maxitrol).
6. Note that polymyxin is available as an otic solution or suspension with hydrocortisone (Pyocidin—Otic Solution) and hydrocortisone plus neomycin (Cortisporin Otic, Otocort) for treatment of superficial ear infections.
7. Note that polymyxin is not available *alone* for topical application, but it is found in combination with several other antibiotics in many different ointments, aerosols, and powders.
8. Note that polymyxin and neomycin are available as a genitourinary irrigant solution (Neosporin G. U. Irrigant) for use with catheter systems, permitting continuous irrigation of the urinary bladder. The solution contains 40 mg of neomycin and 200,000 U of polymyxin B sulfate per mL.

Selected Bibliography
Chang TW et al: Bacitracin treatment of antibiotic-associated colitis and diarrhea caused by *Clostridum difficile* toxin. Gastroenterology 78:1584, 1980

Davis SD: Polymyxins, colistin, Vancomycin and bacitracin. In Kagan BM (ed): Antimicrobial Therapy, 3rd ed. Philadelphia, WB Saunders, p 77

Petersdorf RG: Colistin—A reappraisal. JAMA 183:123, 1963

SUMMARY. POLYPEPTIDES

Drug	Preparations	Usual Dosage Range
Bacitracin Baciguent	Injection: 10,000 U/vial, 50,000 U/vial Ophthalmic ointment: 500 U/g Topical ointment: 500 U/g	*IM* 900 U/kg to 1000 U/kg/day in 2 to 3 divided doses *Topical* Apply 2 to 3 times a day *Ophthalmic* Apply to lower conjunctival sac several times a day

Continued

SUMMARY. POLYPEPTIDES (continued)

Drug	Preparations	Usual Dosage Range
Colistimethate Coly-Mycin M **Colistin Sulfate** Coly-Mycin S	Powder for injection: 150 mg/vial Oral suspension: 25 mg/5 mL Otic suspension: 3 mg/mL with neomycin and hydrocortisone	Adults and children: 2.5 mg/kg to 5 mg/kg/day IM *or* IV in 2 to 4 divided doses *Oral* 5 mg/kg to 15 mg/kg/day in 3 divided doses *Otic* 3 to 4 drops into ear canal 3 to 4 times a day
Polymyxin B Sulfate Aerosporin	Injection: 500,000 U/vial Powder for ophthalmic drops: 500,000 U (50 mg)/vial Otic solution: 10,000 U/mL	*IV infusion* (every 12 h) 15,000 U/kg to 25,000 U/kg/day Infants: up to 40,000 U/kg/day *IM* 25,000 U/kg to 30,000 U/kg/day divided and given every 4 hours to 6 hours Infants: up to 40,000 U/kg/day *Intrathecal* Adults and children over 2 years: 50,000 U once daily for 3 days to 4 days, then 50,000 U every other day Children under 2 years: 20,000 U once daily for 3 days to 4 days, then 25,000 U every other day *Ophthalmic* 1 to 2 drops several times/day *Topical* Apply several times a day to affected area

64 URINARY ANTIINFECTIVES

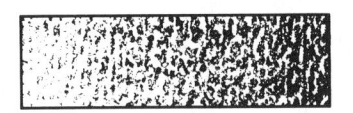

Although the term *urinary antiinfective* refers theoretically to any drug capable of eradicating pathogens present in the urinary tract, it is generally applied only to those agents specific for urinary infections by virtue of their lack of significant *systemic* antibacterial action. Thus, while other antimicrobial drugs, such as broad-spectrum penicillins, cephalosporins, tetracyclines, sulfonamides, aminoglycosides, and polypeptides, have all been employed successfully in the treatment of urinary tract infections, they are not considered specific urinary antiinfectives because most attain significant plasma levels throughout the body and can therefore be used to treat a number of systemic infections as well. The drugs considered to be selective urinary antiinfectives are cinoxacin, methenamine, nalidixic acid, nitrofurantoin, norfloxacin, and trimethoprim. Cinoxacin, nalidixic acid and norfloxacin are members of the quinolone group of antiinfectives and are discussed with other quinolones in Chapter 60. The remaining urinary antiinfectives are considered here.

Although specific for urinary infections by virtue of their rapid elimination in the urine and their lack of significant systemic antimicrobial activity, these agents are usually not considered drugs of choice for acute uncomplicated urinary tract infections, inasmuch as they are often less effective against many common urinary pathogens than sulfonamides, broad-spectrum penicillins, or cephalosporins. The urinary antiinfectives are most often reserved for those persons who are either intolerant of or unresponsive to one of the first-line drugs. Urinary antiinfectives are also of value for the control of *chronic* urinary infections due to organisms that have developed resistance to commonly used antibiotics. For example, low doses of nitrofurantoin, administered once a day at bedtime, have been used successfully for long-term prophylaxis in chronic urinary infections. Likewise, trimethoprim–sulfamethoxazole and methenamine have also been employed in treating chronic urinary infections.

Perhaps the most troublesome situation is the chronic urinary infection that often complicates an anatomic or physiological abnormality such as urinary stones, urethral strictures, or prostate enlargement. Treatment of these conditions requires prolonged therapy with a urinary antiinfective capable of interfering with bacterial growth without favoring emergence of resistant organisms. The drugs most commonly employed for chronic urinary conditions are trimethoprim–sulfamethoxazole (see Chap. 57), nitrofurantoin, and methenamine. Of course, surgical intervention is often necessary when a blockage or some other anatomic lesion is present.

The fact that urinary antiinfectives generally do not attain effective antibacterial blood levels does not mean that they are free of systemic toxic effects. On the contrary, with the exception of methenamine, the other agents in this group all have the potential to elicit serious untoward reactions, and their use should be accorded the same respect as any other antimicrobial drug.

Patients receiving a urinary antiinfective drug should be advised to continue taking the prescribed dose for the recommended period (usually 10–14 days), even though the symptoms of the infection, such as low back pain, burning on urination, or fever, have disappeared. *Complete* eradication of the infecting organism, not simply symptomatic relief, is the goal of urinary chemotherapy, because relapses and reinfection are major problems in the treatment of urinary infections. A *relapse*, the result of failure to eliminate completely the original pathogen from the urinary system with the initial course of therapy, is usually due to insufficient dose or duration of therapy, or both. *Recurring infections* are frequently noted some time after successful recovery from an initial attack and are often caused by microorganisms different from those responsible for the initial infection. These may include resistant forms that have emerged during the first course of therapy.

In addition to the urinary antiinfectives mentioned, several other drugs may be employed in urinary infections. Methylene blue, a dye, is a weak germicide and is occasionally used orally as a mild urinary antiseptic. Phenazopyridine, another dye, is excreted in the urine following oral ingestion and exerts a mild analgesic effect. It is used to relieve irritation and pain in conjunction with an appropriate antiinfective. Acetohydroxamic acid (AHA) inhibits the urease-mediated hydrolysis of urea and the subsequent production of ammonia in urine infected with urea-splitting organisms. It is indicated as adjunctive therapy in chronic urea-splitting urinary infections. The foregoing drugs are considered in this chapter along with the urinary antiinfectives.

Methenamine

Methenamine is a urinary antibacterial agent whose action depends on its hydrolysis to ammonia and formaldehyde in an acidic urine. Formaldehyde is bactericidal against a variety of gram-positive and gram-negative organisms (see Mechanism below). Methenamine is used in the form of an acid salt (hippurate or mandelate), which helps maintain a low urinary pH. Characteristics of the two methenamine salts are presented in Table 64-1.

MECHANISM
In an acid urine (pH 5.5 or lower), drug is hydrolyzed to form ammonia and formaldehyde, the latter being bactericidal; acid liberated from the salt (i.e., mandelic or hippuric) may also exert a weak antibacterial action; susceptible organisms include *Escherichia coli*, staphylococci, and enterococci. *Enterobacter aerogenes* is resistant, as are *Pseudomonas* and *Proteus* species, the latter two being urea-splitting organisms that can raise urinary pH above the effective level; bacteria do *not* appear to develop resistance to formaldehyde, which is therefore well suited for treating chronic infections

USES
Treatment of chronic bacteriuria associated with cystitis, pyelonephritis, or other chronic urinary conditions
Adjunctive treatment of patients with anatomic abnormalities of the urinary tract

DOSAGE
See Table 64-1

FATE
Readily absorbed orally; excreted largely unchanged (75%–90%) in the urine within 24 hours; formation of formaldehyde is dependent on urinary pH, level of methenamine, and

length of time urine is retained in the bladder; peak formaldehyde concentrations occur at a urine pH of 5.5 or less; a level of 25 µg/mL or greater is necessary for antimicrobial activity; peak urinary formaldehyde levels occur within 2 to 6 hours; steady-state levels are attained within 2 to 3 days with regular dosing

COMMON SIDE EFFECTS
GI upset with large doses

SIGNIFICANT ADVERSE REACTIONS
Cramping, vomiting, diarrhea, stomatitis, anorexia, urinary frequency or urgency, bladder irritation, dysuria, proteinuria, hematuria, hypersensitivity reactions (rash, pruritus), and abdominal pain

CONTRAINDICATIONS
Renal insufficiency, severe hepatic disease (because ammonia is liberated), and severe dehydration. *Cautious use* in pregnant women or nursing mothers, and in patients with gout, because methenamine salts may cause precipitation of urate crystals in the urine

INTERACTIONS
Sulfonamides can form insoluble precipitates with formaldehyde in the urine
Effectiveness of methenamine can be reduced by drugs that raise urinary pH, for example, sodium bicarbonate, acetazolamide, thiazide diuretics
Methenamine salts may increase the urinary excretion of amphetamines, lowering their activity

NURSING CONSIDERATIONS
See **Plan of Nursing Care 12, Antibacterial Drugs,** in Chapter 56. In addition:

1. Monitor intake and output to ensure that normal levels are maintained.
2. Interpret results of the following urine tests cautiously because methenamine can interfere with them: catecholamines, 17-hydroxycorticosteroids, estriol, and 5-hydroxyindoleacetic acid (5-HIAA), a serotonin metabolite.
3. Note that bacteria and fungi do *not* develop resistance to formaldehyde, making methenamine suitable for long-term prophylaxis in chronic infections. It is *not,* however, suitable for prevention of urinary tract infections in patients with indwelling catheters because the bladder does not retain the drug long enough to form sufficient levels of formaldehyde, and it should not be used alone for acute infections or infections with renal parenchymal involvement associated with systemic symptoms.
4. Note that methenamine is available in many combination products with anticholinergics, urinary acidifiers, methylene blue, and salicylates.

PATIENT EDUCATION
See **Plan of Nursing Care 12, Antibacterial Drugs,** in Chapter 56. In addition:
1. Tell patient to take drug with food to minimize GI distress.
2. Instruct patient to drink adequate fluids (8–10 glasses/day) but to avoid *excessive* hydration because increased urinary flow can reduce the amount of free formaldehyde in urine.
3. Teach patient how to monitor urinary pH with Nitrazine paper (see Chap. 76). Supplementary acidification (e.g., ascorbic acid [vitamin C], 4–12 g/day in divided doses) may be prescribed for PRN use if urine pH exceeds 5.5.
4. Instruct patient to inform drug prescriber if painful urination occurs because large drug doses (8 g/day for several weeks) can cause bladder irritation, painful urination, and hematuria, which are indications for reducing drug dosage and acidifying urine.
5. Tell patient to avoid excessive intake of alkalinizing foods such as milk or citrus fruits.
6. Inform patient with liver dysfunction who is undergoing prolonged therapy that periodic liver function studies are recommended.

Methylene Blue
Urolene Blue

MECHANISM
Exerts a weak germicidal action; is primarily bacteriostatic; high concentrations convert the ferrous iron of reduced hemoglobin to the ferric state, resulting in formation of methemoglobin; this latter action is the basis for its use as an antidote in cyanide poisoning, because methemoglobin competes with cytochrome oxidase, a vital enzyme, for the cyanide ion, leading to formation of cyanmethemoglobin and the resulting preservation of cytochrome oxidase

USES
Symptomatic treatment of cystitis and urethritis (infrequent use)
Treatment of idiopathic and drug-induced methemoglobinemia and as an antidote for cyanide poisoning (IV)
Investigational uses include treatment of oxalate urinary tract calculi and diagnostic confirmation of rupture of amniotic membranes

DOSAGE
Oral: 55 mg to 130 mg 3 times/day
IV: 1 mg/kg to 2 mg/kg injected over several minutes

COMMON SIDE EFFECTS
Discoloration of the urine

SIGNIFICANT ADVERSE REACTIONS
Nausea, vomiting, diarrhea, bladder irritation; large doses can cause abdominal pain, fever, dizziness, headache, sweating, confusion and cyanosis

CONTRAINDICATIONS
Renal insufficiency, intraspinal injection. *Cautious use* in patients with glucose-6-phosphate dehydrogenase deficiency, anemia, and decreased hemoglobin levels; IV use with caution in persons with cardiovascular disease

PATIENT EDUCATION
1. Instruct patient to take oral drug after meals with a full glass of water.
2. Inform patient that drug may discolor urine and possibly the stool blue-green.

Table 64-1
Methenamine Derivatives

Drug	Preparations	Usual Dosage Range	Nursing Implications
Methenamine Hippurate Hiprex, Urex	Tablets: 1 g	Adults: 1 g twice a day Children (6–12 yr): 0.5 g–1 g twice a day	Effective in lower daily doses than mandelate salt; safe use in early pregnancy has not been established; may transiently elevate serum transaminase levels; periodic liver function tests are indicated
Methenamine Mandelate Mandameth, Mandelamine (CAN) Sterine	Tablets: 0.5 g, 1 g Enteric-coated tablets: 0.5 g, 1 g Oral suspension: 0.25 g/5 mL Suspension forte: 0.5 g/5 mL Granules: 1 g/packet	Adults: 1 g 4 times a day Children (6–12 yr): 0.5 g 4 times a day Children under 6 yr: 0.25 g/30 lb 4 times a day	Most commonly used methenamine salt; enteric-coated tablets are claimed to lower incidence of GI upset; oral suspensions have a vegetable oil base; use cautiously in elderly or debilitated patients because of danger of aspiration (lipid) pneumonia; granules are orange flavored

Nitrofurantoin

Furadantin, Furalan, Furan, Furanite, Nitrofan
(CAN) Apo-Nitrofurantoin, Nephronex, Novofuran

Nitrofurantoin Macrocrystals

Macrodantin

A synthetic nitrofuran derivative, nitrofurantoin is a specific urinary antibacterial agent effective against a range of gram-positive and gram-negative organisms. The macrocrystalline dosage form is most often preferred, since it causes less GI distress than the normal oral dosage forms.

MECHANISM
Bacteriostatic in low concentrations and bactericidal in higher concentrations; probable mechanism is interference with carbohydrate metabolism by inhibition of acetyl coenzyme A; may also impair bacterial cell wall formation; most effective against *Escherichia coli*, *Klebsiella*, *Enterobacter*, and *Citrobacter* species, group B streptococci, enterococci, and staphylococci; some strains of *Enterobacter* and *Klebsiella* are resistant, as are most strains of *Proteus*, *Serratia*, and *Acinetobacter*; *Pseudomonas* is highly resistant; acquired resistance of susceptible organisms is minimal

USES
Treatment of urinary tract infections due to susceptible organisms (see above)
antiinfect against recurrent bacteriuria (Macrodantin—small dose)

DOSAGE
Oral
Adults: 50 mg to 100 mg four times a day for 10 to 14 days; long-term therapy 50 mg to 100 mg once daily at bedtime
Children (over 3 mo): 5 mg/kg to 7 mg/kg/day in 4 divided doses
Prophylaxis of recurrent infections (Macrodantin): 50 mg daily at bedtime for at least 6 months

FATE
Well absorbed orally (macrocrystalline form is absorbed more slowly than other oral forms but causes less GI distress); absorption is *enhanced* by ingestion of food; therapeutic serum and tissue levels are not attained, except in the urinary tract; plasma half-life is 15 to 30 minutes; approximately one half of a dose is rapidly inactivated in body tissues and excreted in the urine and bile, the remainder is eliminated unchanged in the urine; activity is increased in an acid urine

COMMON SIDE EFFECTS
Nausea, anorexia, vomiting

SIGNIFICANT ADVERSE REACTIONS
GI: diarrhea, abdominal pain, pancreatitis, parotitis
Pulmonary: chills, cough, chest pain, dyspnea, pulmonary infiltration with consolidation or pleural effusion, diffuse interstitial pneumonitis or fibrosis (with prolonged therapy)
Dermatologic: rash, pruritus, urticaria, angioedema, alopecia; *rarely,* exfoliative dermatitis, erythema multiforme
Hematologic: hemolytic anemia, megaloblastic anemia, leukopenia, granulocytopenia, eosinophilia, thrombocytopenia, agranulocytosis
Allergic: drug fever, asthmatic attack, cholestatic jaundice, arthralgia, anaphylaxis
Neurologic: dizziness, paresthesias, headache, drowsiness, nystagmus, peripheral neuropathy
Other: Hypotension, myalgia, superinfections, tooth staining from oral suspension

CONTRAINDICATIONS
Anuria, oliguria, significant renal impairment (creatinine clearance less than 40 mL/min) and pregnancy at term; in infants under 3 months (possibility of hemolytic anemia due to immature enzyme systems). *Cautious use* in the presence of anemia, antiinfectchronic lung disease, vitamin B deficiency, electrolyte imbalances, hepatic disease, glucose-6-phosphate dehydrogenase deficiency, and in pregnant or nursing women

INTERACTIONS

Nitrofurantoin can antagonize the action of nalidixic acid

Acidifying agents (e.g., ammonium chloride, ascorbic acid) may potentiate nitrofurantoin, whereas alkalinizing agents (e.g., acetazolamide, sodium bicarbonate) can reduce its effectiveness

Probenecid reduces the renal clearance of nitrofurantoin, and may increase its toxicity

Antacids can reduce the effectiveness of nitrofurantoin by impairing its GI absorption

Anticholinergics, other GI antispasmodic drugs, and food may increase GI absorption of nitrofurantoin by prolonging gastric emptying time

NURSING CONSIDERATIONS

See **Plan of Nursing Care 12, Antibacterial Drugs,** in Chapter 56. In addition:

Nursing Alerts

- Observe carefully for development of acute pulmonary sensitivity reaction during early days (up to 3 wk) of therapy. Common symptoms are fever, chills, cough, dyspnea, chest pain, and eosinophilia. Discontinuation of drug usually results in rapid resolution of symptoms.
- During prolonged therapy, be alert for insidious development of subacute or chronic pulmonary reactions (cough, malaise, dyspnea on exertion, x-ray findings of diffuse pneumonitis or pulmonary fibrosis). Early recognition is important in preventing serious pulmonary impairment.
- Monitor results of hematologic evaluations and liver function tests, which should be performed periodically during extended therapy because hemolytic anemia and hepatitis have occurred.
- Monitor intake–output, and assess patient for signs of renal impairment (oliguria, anuria, creatinine clearance below 40 mL/min). If these are present, therapy should be terminated to minimize risk of serious toxicity.
- Assess patient for signs of urinary tract superinfection, which, during nitrofurantoin therapy, is most commonly caused by *Pseudomonas*.

1. Expect parenteral form of nitrofurantoin to be used only in patients with clinically significant urinary infection to whom oral dosage forms cannot be given.
2. Administer oral drug with meals or milk to reduce GI distress and possibly to improve absorption. Use of macrocrystalline dosage form further minimizes GI upset.
3. Protect drug from strong light to prevent darkening and possible loss of potency.
4. Interpret results of the following laboratory tests cautiously because nitrofurantoin may cause them to be false positive: serum glucose, bilirubin, alkaline phosphatase, and BUN.

PATIENT EDUCATION

1. Instruct patient to note and report development of early neurologic symptoms (numbness, paresthesias, muscle weakness). If these occur, the drug should be discontinued to prevent severe and possibly irreversible peripheral neuropathy.
2. Inform patient that drug may impart a harmless brownish color to urine.
3. Instruct patient to rinse mouth thoroughly after using oral suspension to prevent staining of the teeth.

Trimethoprim

Proloprim, Trimpex

A synthetic antibacterial agent, trimethoprim has demonstrated activity against common urinary tract pathogens, *except Pseudomonas aeruginosa.*

MECHANISM

Blocks production of tetrahydrofolic acid by reversible inhibition of dihydrofolate reductase, thus interfering with synthesis of proteins and nucleic acids in susceptible bacteria; acts synergistically with sulfonamides (see trimethoprim–sulfamethoxazole, Chap. 57)

USE

Treatment of initial episodes of uncomplicated urinary tract infections due to susceptible strains of *Escherichia coli, Proteus mirabilis, Klebsiella pneumoniae, Enterobacter* species, and coagulase-negative *Staphylococcus* species

DOSAGE

Adults and children (over 12 yr): 100 mg every 12 hours for 10 days, or 200 mg once daily

FATE

Rapidly absorbed orally; peak serum levels occur in 1 to 4 hours; half-life is 8 to 10 hours; about half is protein-bound in plasma; excreted in the urine; largely as unmetabolized drug, 50% to 60% of an oral dose within 24 hours

COMMON SIDE EFFECT

Pruritic rash

SIGNIFICANT ADVERSE REACTIONS

GI: epigastric distress, nausea, vomiting, glossitis
Dermatologic: macropapular or morbilliform rash, exfoliative dermatitis
Hematologic: thrombocytopenia, leukopenia, neutropenia, megaloblastic anemia, methemoglobinemia
Other: fever; elevations in BUN, serum creatinine, serum transaminase, and bilirubin

CONTRAINDICATIONS

Megaloblastic anemia due to folate deficiency, severe renal impairment (creatinine clearance below 15 mL/min). *Cautious use* in patients with liver impairment, reduced renal function, folate deficiency, and in pregnant or nursing women

INTERACTIONS

Trimethoprim may potentiate the action of oral anticoagulants and possibly phenytoin owing to impairment of hepatic metabolism

NURSING CONSIDERATIONS

Nursing Alert

- Monitor results of complete blood counts, which should be performed during prolonged therapy. If signs of bone marrow depression are noted (thrombocytopenia, leukopenia, megaloblastic anemia), the drug should be discontinued, and 3 mg to 6 mg of leucovorin should be administered IM daily for 3 days to restore normal hematopoiesis.

1. Ensure that prescribed culture and sensitivity tests are performed to determine susceptibility of the pathogens to

trimethoprim, but therapy can be initiated before obtaining results.
2. Note that trimethoprim is available in combination with sulfamethoxazole (Bactrim, Septra) for treatment of both acute and chronic urinary infections, acute otitis media, acute exacerbations of chronic bronchitis, and enteritis (see Chap. 57).

PATIENT EDUCATION
1. Instruct patient to note appearance of skin rash, a common side effect, which usually appears 7 to 14 days after initiation of therapy. Symptoms usually disappear following discontinuation of drug.
2. Instruct patient to note appearance of signs of possible blood dyscrasias (sore throat, fever, bruising, mucosal ulceration, pallor) and to notify drug prescriber immediately if these occur.

URINARY ANALGESIC

Phenazopyridine

Pyridium, and other manufacturers
(CAN) Phenazo, Pyronium

Phenazopyridine is an azo dye that is excreted in the urine, where it exerts a mild analgesic action. It is usually given in combination with a urinary antiinfective, most often a sulfonamide.

MECHANISM
Not established; may exert a local anesthetic effect on mucosal membranes

USES
Symptomatic relief of pain, burning, irritation, and urinary urgency or frequency resulting from lower urinary tract infections, trauma, surgery, or endoscopic procedures

DOSAGE
Adults: 200 mg three times a day
Children 6 to 12 years: 100 mg three times a day

FATE
Adequately absorbed orally; partially metabolized, but mainly excreted unchanged in the urine

SIGNIFICANT ADVERSE REACTIONS
(Rare) GI distress, hemolytic anemia, methemoglobinemia, renal or hepatic damage

CONTRAINDICATIONS
Renal insufficiency, uremia, and chronic glomerulonephritis

NURSING CONSIDERATIONS
1. Help evaluate the appropriateness of phenazopyridine use. Drug-induced relief of symptoms could delay recognition, diagnosis, and proper treatment of underlying pathology.
2. If phenazopyridine is discontinued as soon as discomfort is relieved, ensure that any accompanying antiinfective is continued for the duration of time prescribed.
3. Interpret laboratory test results based on urinary colorimetric procedures cautiously because the drug can interfere with them.
4. Note that phenazopyridine is available in fixed combination with sulfamethizole (Thiosulfil-A), sulfamethoxazole (Azo Gantanol), and sulfisoxazole (Azo Gantrisin).

PATIENT EDUCATION
1. Inform patient that drug may produce a reddish orange discoloration of urine, which can stain fabrics.
2. Instruct patient to observe for appearance of yellowish tinge to sclerae or skin, a possible indication of reduced renal excretion and accumulation toxicity. If this occurs, the drug prescriber should be notified immediately.

UREASE INHIBITOR

Acetohydroxamic Acid

Lithostat

Acetohydroxamic acid is used to enhance the effectiveness of antimicrobial agents used to treat chronic urinary infections resulting from urea-splitting organisms.

MECHANISM
Inhibits the bacterial enzyme urease, thus retarding hydrolysis of urea to ammonia in the presence of urea-splitting organisms; decreased ammonia levels and reduced pH enhance the action of antimicrobial agents and improve the cure rate; the drug does not acidify the urine directly, nor does it possess an antibacterial action

USES
Adjunctive treatment of urinary infections due to urea-splitting organisms (*not* indicated in place of appropriate antimicrobial therapy)

DOSAGE
Adults: 250 mg three to four times/day to a maximum of 12 mg/kg/day
Children: 10 mg/kg/day, initially, in divided doses; titrated to desired response

FATE
Well absorbed orally; peak blood levels occur within 1 hour; plasma half-life is approximately 5 to 10 hours in patients with normal renal function and is prolonged in persons with impaired renal function; one third to two thirds of a dose, which constitutes the active fraction of the drug, is excreted unchanged in the urine

COMMON SIDE EFFECTS
Headache (30%); anxiety, nervousness, mild tremor, depression, nausea, vomiting, anorexia, malaise (20%); reticulocytosis (5%)

SIGNIFICANT ADVERSE REACTIONS
Hemolytic anemia, superficial phlebitis, palpitations, nonpruritic skin rash, alopecia, teratogenicity

CONTRAINDICATIONS
Decreased renal function (serum creatinine greater than 2.5 mg %), urinary infections due to *non*-urease-producing organisms, pregnancy, and females not using contraceptive methods. *Cautious use* in patients with anemia, blood dyscrasias, bone marrow depression, thrombophlebitis, skin rash, depression, and in nursing mothers

INTERACTIONS
Alcohol has produced a rash in the presence of acetohydroxamic acid

Acetohydroxamic acid can reduce oral absorption of iron by forming a chelate with the metal

NURSING CONSIDERATIONS

Nursing Alerts

- Monitor results of complete blood counts, which should be performed 2 weeks after beginning therapy and every 3 months thereafter. If reticulocyte count is greater than 6%, dosage should be reduced. Most patients develop a *mild* reticulosis, but hemolytic anemia occurs in about 30% of patients, usually accompanied by nausea, vomiting, anorexia, and malaise.
- Carefully assess patient with renal impairment for signs of overdose because drug is eliminated primarily by the kidneys.

PATIENT EDUCATION

1. Warn women of childbearing potential receiving the drug to use appropriate contraceptive measures because the drug may cause fetal damage.
2. Inform patient that headache is very common during the first 48 to 72 hours of treatment, but that it usually disappears spontaneously. Mild analgesics may be used, if necessary.
3. Warn patient that alcohol ingestion during therapy often results in development of a nonpruritic macular skin rash, which may range from mild and transient to severe.
4. Inform patient taking oral iron supplement that iron absorption is impaired by acetohydroxyamic acid. If iron is necessary, parenteral iron is recommended.
5. As indicated, prepare patient, supportively and with reassurance, for the possibility that treatment may be lengthy because it must continue until the urea-splitting organism is eradicated.

Selected Bibliography

Andriole VT: Urinary tract agents: Nalidixic acid, oxolinic acid, cinoxacin, nitrofurantoin and methenamine. In Mandell GL, Douglas RG, Bennett JE (eds): Principles and Practice of Infectious Diseases, 2nd ed, p 244. New York, John Wiley & Sons, 1985

Black M, Robin L, Schatz N: Nitrofurantoin-induced chronic active hepatitis. Ann Intern Med 92:62, 1980

Bushby SR, Hitchings GH: Trimethoprim, a sulfonamide potentiator. Br J Pharmacol Chemother 33:72, 1968

Gleckman R, Alvarez S, Jouvert DW, Matthews SJ: Drug therapy reviews: Methenamine mandelate and methenamine hippurate. Am J Hosp Pharm 36:1509, 1979

Hamilton-Miller JM, Brumfitt W: Methenamine and its salts as urinary antiseptics. Invest Urol 14:287, 1977

Holmberg L, Boman G, Bottiger LE, Eriksson BA, Spross R, Wessling A: Adverse reactions to nitrofurantoin. Am J Med 69:733, 1980

Spielberg SP, Gordon GB: Nitrofurantoin cytotoxicity. J Clin Invest 67:37, 1981

Stamm WE: Prevention of urinary tract infections. Am J Med 76:148, 1984

SUMMARY. URINARY ANTI-INFECTIVES AND ANALGESICS

Drug	Preparations	Usual Dosage Range
Anti-infectives		
Methenamine	*See* Table 64-1	
Methylene Blue Urolene Blue	Tablets: 55 mg, 65 mg Injection: 10 mg/mL	*Oral:* 55 mg–130 mg 3 times/day *IV:* 1 mg/kg–2 mg/kg over several minutes
Nitrofurantoin Furadantin, Furalan, Furan, Furanite, Nitrofan	Tablets: 50 mg, 100 mg Capsules: 50 mg, 100 mg Oral suspension: 25 mg/5 mL	*Oral* Adults: 50 mg–100 mg 4 times a day (Chronic 50 mg–100 mg once daily)
Nitrofurantoin Macrocrystals Macrodantin	Capsules—25 mg, 50 mg, 100 mg	Children: 5 mg/kg–7 mg/kg/day in 4 divided doses Prophylaxis: 50 mg (Macrodantin) daily for 6 mo
Trimethoprim Proloprim, Trimpex	Tablets: 100 mg, 200 mg	100 mg every 12 h for 10 days *or* 200 mg once daily
Analgesics		
Phenazopyridine Pyridium and other manufacturers	Tablets: 100 mg, 200 mg	Adults: 200 mg 3 times/day Children: 100 mg 3 times/day
Urease Inhibitor		
Acetohydroxamic Acid Lithostat	Tablets: 250 mg	Adults: 250 mg 3–4 times/day to a maximum of 1.5 g/day Children: initially, 10 mg/kg/day; titrate as necessary

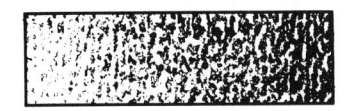

65 MISCELLANEOUS ANTIBIOTICS

A number of antimicrobial drugs in current clinical use cannot be precisely categorized according to their chemical structure or biologic activity. These drugs are most conveniently grouped under a miscellaneous heading and are reviewed here individually.

Chloramphenicol

Ak-Chlor, Chloracol, Chlorofair, Chloromycetin, Chloroptic, Ophthochlor

(CAN) Fenicol, Minims, Nova Phenicol, Pentamycetin

Chloramphenicol is a synthetic, broad-spectrum, bacteriostatic antibiotic effective against a wide range of gram-positive and gram-negative bacteria, rickettsiae, and chlamydiae. Its potential for eliciting serious toxicity, however, largely restricts its systemic use to *severe* infections in which other, less toxic drugs are ineffective or contraindicated. The drug is also commonly employed locally in the eye for treating superficial ocular infections and in the ear for infections of the external auditory canal. Currently, it is considered to be the drug of choice for acute *Salmonella typhi* infections (typhoid fever), but it should not be used for routine treatment of the typhoid "carrier state." Other organisms against which it is quite active are *Hemophilus influenzae*, *Bacteroides fragilis*, other *Salmonella* species, *Rickettsiae*, the lymphogranuloma–psittacosis group, and various gram-negative bacteria causing bacteremia or meningitis. The major danger associated with chloramphenicol is bone marrow depression, and fatal blood dyscrasias have occurred following both short-term and long-term use. Frequent blood studies are therefore essential during its administration. Other untoward reactions noted with chloramphenicol are neurotoxicity and the gray syndrome in newborns (see Adverse Reactions). Although it is a valuable antiinfective for certain severe infections, chloramphenicol should never be used for minor infections (e.g., colds, flu, throat infections) or as a prophylactic agent.

MECHANISM
Binds to the 50S ribosomal subunits of bacteria, preventing binding of tRNA to the ribosome; inhibits synthesis of bacterial protein by cellular ribosomes; bacteriostatic at normal concentrations

USES
Treatment of acute infections caused by *Salmonella typhi* (drug of choice)
Alternative treatment of severe infections due to susceptible organisms for which less toxic drugs are ineffective or contraindicated (see Chap. 56, Table 56-1. Principal indications include *Hemophilus influenzae* meningitis, pneumococcal or meningococcal meningitis in penicillin-sensitive patients, *Bacteroides fragilis* infections, and rickettsial infections in tetracycline-sensitive patients.
Adjunctive therapy in cystic fibrosis regimens
Superficial infections of the skin, eye, and external auditory canal due to susceptible microorganisms (topical application only)

DOSAGE
Oral, IV
Adults and children: 50 mg/kg/day in divided doses every 6 hours (maximum 100 mg/kg/day)
Newborns and infants with immature metabolic processes: 25 mg/kg/day in four equally divided doses
Topical
Apply several times a day to affected area
Ophthalmic
One or two drops or small amount of ointment to infected eye two to four times a day
Otic
Two to three drops three times a day

FATE
Rapidly absorbed orally; peak serum levels occur in 1 to 2 hours; distribution is variable—highest concentrations occur in the liver and kidney, while lowest amounts are found in the brain and cerebrospinal fluid (about one half the levels in the blood); approximately 50% to 60% protein-bound; elimination half-life is 3 to 4 hours; metabolized by the liver and excreted in the urine, largely as glucuronic acid conjugate, with small amounts (8%–12%) of unchanged drug; minor quantities of active drug are found in the bile and feces; readily crosses placental barrier and appears in breast milk

COMMON SIDE EFFECTS
GI distress

SIGNIFICANT ADVERSE REACTIONS

> **WARNING**
> Serious and potentially fatal blood dyscrasias (e.g., aplastic anemia, thrombocytopenia, granulocytopenia) have occurred with both short-term and prolonged use of chloramphenicol. Thus, it should be employed only in severe infections unresponsive to other, less hazardous antibiotics, and careful blood studies should be performed at least every 2 days during therapy. A dose-related *reversible* type of bone marrow depression may occur during treatment. It is readily detectable by blood studies, and responds promptly to discontinuation of the drug. An *irreversible* type of bone marrow depression leading to aplastic anemia which may terminate in leukemia with a high mortality rate has also been reported (1:25,000–40,000) but does not appear to be dose-related. It may occur weeks or even months following therapy and is characterized by bone marrow aplasia or hypoplasia. Most important, it is not readily predictable by routine blood studies performed *during* treatment. Follow-up blood tests and close observation of the patient are necessary.

Hematologic: blood dyscrasias (leukopenia, reduction in erythrocytes, granulocytopenia, hypoplastic anemia, thrombocytopenia, aplastic anemia)
Neurologic: headache, confusion, depression, delirium, optic and peripheral neuritis
Allergic/Hypersensitivity: fever, rash, urticaria, angioedema, anaphylaxis; itching or burning with topical application

GI: vomiting, glossitis, stomatitis, diarrhea, enterocolitis (rare)
Other: jaundice, superinfections, *gray syndrome* in premature infants and newborns (abdominal distention, emesis, pallid cyanosis, vasomotor collapse, irregular respiration, hypothermia; occurs in 3 or 4 days, usually after initiation of high-dosage therapy within the first 48 h of life and can be fatal)

CONTRAINDICATIONS

Treatment of trivial infections (colds, flu, sore throat), prophylactic use, infections other than those indicated as susceptible by testing, and concurrent therapy with other bone marrow depressive drugs. *Cautious use* in patients with renal or hepatic impairment, glucose-6-phosphate dehydrogenase deficiency, acute intermittent porphyria; in infants and in pregnant or nursing women

Repeated courses of therapy should be avoided; do not extend treatment longer than the time required to effect a cure with little risk of relapse (e.g., a normal temperature for 48 h)

INTERACTIONS

Chloramphenicol can inhibit the metabolism of oral anticoagulants, oral hypoglycemics, cyclophosphamide, barbiturates, and phenytoin, thus potentiating their effects

Chloramphenicol may inhibit the hematinic activity of vitamin B$_{12}$, folic acid, and iron

The bactericidal action of other antibiotics (e.g., penicillins) may be reduced by chloramphenicol

Chloramphenicol can interfere with the immune response to diphtheria and tetanus toxoids

Concomitant administration of acetaminophen may elevate serum levels of chloramphenicol

A disulfiram-like reaction to alcohol may occur with use of chloramphenicol (see Chap. 78)

NURSING CONSIDERATIONS

See **Plan of Nursing Care 12, Antibacterial Drugs,** in Chapter 56. In addition:

Nursing Alert

(See *Warning* under Significant Adverse Reactions).
- Monitor results of blood studies (differential, leukocyte, and reticulocyte counts), which should be performed before initiation of therapy (baseline), at 48-hour intervals during therapy, and periodically for *several months* after termination. The drug should be discontinued immediately if any abnormality is noted.

1. Monitor blood glucose of diabetic patients receiving oral hypoglycemic agent and prothrombin time of patients receiving oral anticoagulant drug during chloramphenicol therapy because loss of control may occur.
2. Note that chloramphenicol *base* solution is used by IV infusion in adults only, whereas the *sodium succinate salt* may be given by slow (1–2 min) IV injection to both adults and children (it is largely ineffective IM). Oral dosage should be substituted as soon as possible.

PATIENT EDUCATION

1. Instruct patient to notify drug prescriber immediately if any signs of blood dyscrasias are noted (fever, sore throat, bruising or bleeding, fatigue), even after drug has been discontinued.
2. Instruct patient to report any visual disturbances. If they occur, the drug should be discontinued to minimize the danger of optic neuritis.

Clindamycin
Lincomycin

Clindamycin and lincomycin are two chemically related, primarily bacteriostatic antibiotics frequently termed *lincosamides*. They exhibit antibacterial activity similar to but not identical to that of the erythromycins. Lincomycin and its chlorine-substituted derivative clindamycin are effective against most of the common gram-positive pathogens, particularly *Staphylococcus, Streptococcus, Corynebacterium,* and *Nocardia,* as well as many anaerobic organisms, such as *Bacteroides, Actinomyces, Propionibacterium, Peptococcus,* and most strains of *Clostridium* (except *Clostridium difficile*). In contrast, most gram-negative organisms are resistant. Because of their toxic potential, however, lincomycin and clindamycin are usually recommended only for treatment of serious anaerobic infections for which penicillin or erythromycin is ineffective or inappropriate (e.g., when penicillin hypersensitivity is present). The major dangers associated with use of clindamycin and lincomycin are related to the GI tract and include persistent profuse diarrhea, severe abdominal cramping, and pseudomembranous colitis. These effects, although most frequent with systemic use, have occurred upon topical application of clindamycin as well. Clindamycin is generally regarded as the preferred drug of the two for systemic use, because it is better absorbed orally, has a somewhat broader spectrum of action, including *Bacteroides fragilis,* and is reported to elicit fewer GI side effects. In addition, clindamycin is commonly used as a topical solution for the management of acne, since it exhibits good activity against *Propionibacterium,* the causative agent found in acne lesions.

Although the two drugs are sufficiently alike in their pharmacologic properties to be discussed together, some important differences do exist. These are noted whenever appropriate in the following discussion as well as in Table 65-1.

MECHANISM

Interfere with protein synthesis in susceptible organisms by binding to the 50S subunits of bacterial ribosomes; resistance, possibly related to chromosomal alterations develops slowly; possess neuromuscular blocking activity; both drugs are active against most common gram-positive pathogens; clindamycin demonstrates a slightly wider range of action against anaerobic gram-positive organisms (e.g., *Actinomyces, Peptococcus, Clostridia,* microaerophilic streptococci) and anaerobic gram-negative bacilli (e.g., *Bacteroides, Fusobacterium*)

USES

Alternative therapy for serious streptococcal, pneumococcal, or staphylococcal infections in patients in whom penicillins and erythromycins are ineffective or inappropriate

Alternative treatment of serious infections due to anaerobic organisms, such as *Bacteroides, Fusobacterium, Peptococcus,* or *Actinomyces* species, in penicillin-sensitive patients (clindamycin is most effective)

Treatment of acne (topical application of clindamycin solution)

Treatment of acute pelvic inflammatory disease, e.g., endometritis, pelvic cellulitis, nongonococcal tubo-ovarian abscess

DOSAGE

See Table 65-1

FATE
Oral absorption is rapid and virtually complete (90%) for clindamycin, whereas only about 20% to 30% of an oral dose of lincomycin is absorbed. Food markedly impairs absorption of lincomycin but not clindamycin. Peak plasma levels occur within 45 minutes with oral clindamycin and 2 to 4 hours with oral lincomycin. IM injection yields peak serum levels within 30 minutes with lincomycin and 1 to 3 hours with clindamycin. Plasma half-lives are 2 to 3 hours for clindamycin and 4 to 6 hours for lincomycin. Both drugs are widely distributed in the body and are approximately 70% protein-bound. Effective antibacterial blood levels are maintained for 6 to 8 hours after oral administration, and up to 12 hours following IM injection or IV infusion; excreted in the urine, bile, and feces, primarily (90%) as inactive metabolites. Most of a dose of clindamycin is metabolized in the liver and excreted in the urine and bile. Less than 15% is eliminated unchanged by the kidneys. Lincomycin is partially metabolized in the liver and excreted both in the urine and the feces

COMMON SIDE EFFECTS
Nausea, diarrhea, skin rash

SIGNIFICANT ADVERSE REACTIONS

> **WARNING**
> Severe persistent diarrhea and pseudomembranous colitis, occasionally fatal, have occurred with these drugs. The colitis is probably due to toxins secreted by resistant strains of *Clostridium difficile*. Do *not* use for minor infections, and discontinue drug if diarrhea, bloody stools, severe abdominal pain, or high fever occurs. Vancomycin, 2 g/day administered orally in divided doses, may be effective for *Clostridium difficile*-induced colitis (see Vancomycin—this chapter)

GI: vomiting, persistent or severe diarrhea, abdominal pain, glossitis, esophagitis, stomatitis, acute enterocolitis, or pseudomembranous colitis (occasionally fatal)
Hypersensitivity: urticaria, angioedema, serum sickness, erythema multiforme (rare), Stevens–Johnson syndrome (rare), exfoliative dermatitis (rare)
Hematologic: eosinophilia, infrequent blood dyscrasias (neutropenia, leukopenia, thrombocytopenia, agranulocytosis, aplastic anemia)
Cardiovascular: hypotension (parenteral injection), cardiopulmonary arrest following IV injection
Other: vaginitis, pruritus ani, jaundice, abnormal liver function tests, tinnitus, vertigo, pain or induration on IM injection; topical application of clindamycin can result in contact dermatitis, skin dryness, oily skin, facial swelling, stinging sensation, gram-negative folliculitis

CONTRAINDICATIONS
Minor systemic bacterial or viral infections or meningitis, pregnancy, liver disease; in nursing mothers and in neonates. *Cautious use* in patients with mild liver impairment, history of GI disease, asthma or other allergic diseases, or renal dysfunction; and in elderly or debilitated persons

INTERACTIONS
The activity of clindamycin and lincomycin may be antagonized by concurrent use of erythromycin or chloramphenicol

Clindamycin and lincomycin can enhance the action of neuromuscular blocking drugs
Use of antiperistaltic drugs such as opiates, loperamide, and diphenoxylate may prolong or aggravate the diarrhea observed with clindamycin and lincomycin
The oral absorption of clindamycin and lincomycin can be impaired by kaolin, pectin, other antidiarrheal medications, and cyclamates

NURSING CONSIDERATIONS
See **Plan of Nursing Care 12, Antibacterial Drugs**, in Chapter 56. In addition:

Nursing Alerts
(See *Warning* under Significant Adverse Reactions)
- Monitor bowel function. Diarrhea is a common side effect of clindamycin or lincomycin, although it may not indicate GI superinfection with a resistant organism, as it usually does.
- Question prescription of a systemic antiperistaltic drug such as an opiate, diphenoxylate, or loperamide, for a patient experiencing drug-induced diarrhea because it may aggravate the condition. Fluid and electrolyte supplementation is indicated. Corticosteroids may help relieve colitis.

1. Expect dosage to be reduced by 50% to 75% in the presence of impaired renal function.
2. Interpret serum levels of SGOT, SGPT, and alkaline phosphatase cautiously because these drugs may increase them. Platelet counts may be decreased.

PATIENT EDUCATION
1. Explain to patient that clindamycin may be taken with meals because its absorption is largely unaffected by food. The same is not true of lincomycin.
2. Stress the importance of immediately informing drug prescriber if abdominal cramps, prolonged, excessive diarrhea, or bloody stools develop. This may occur after just a few days of therapy. If such symptoms appear, the drug should be discontinued, and endoscopic examination of the large bowel should be performed.
3. Inform patient that periodic blood studies and liver and kidney function tests are recommended during prolonged therapy.

Clofazimine
Lamprene
Clofazimine is an antibacterial and anti-inflammatory leprostatic drug that is slowly bactericidal toward *Mycobacterium leprae* or Hansen's bacillus. The drug is deposited in tissues upon systemic absorption, and pigmentation (pink to brownish-black) usually occurs on the skin, conjunctivae, on other tissues, and in urine. Clearing of the discoloration occurs gradually on drug withdrawal.

MECHANISM
Not completely established; drug binds preferentially to mycobacterial DNA and can inhibit growth of the organism; its anti-inflammatory effects are useful for controlling erythema nodosum leprosum reactions

Table 65-1
Clindamycin–Lincomycin

Drug	Preparations	Usual Dosage Range	Nursing Implications
Clindamycin Cleocin (CAN) Dalacin C	Capsules: 75 mg, 150 mg, 300 mg Granules for suspension: 75 mg/5 mL Injection: 150 mg/mL, 300 mg/2 mL, 600 mg/4 mL, 900 mg/6 mL Topical solution: 10 mg/mL (Cleocin-T) Lotion: 10 mg/mL	*Oral* Adults: 150 mg–450 mg every 6 h depending on severity of infection Children: 8 mg/kg–12 mg/kg/day in 3–4 divided doses (up to 25 mg/kg/day in severe infections) *IM, IV* Adults: 600 mg–2700 mg/day in 2–4 equally divided doses depending on severity of infection Children over 1 mo: 15 mg/kg–40 mg/kg/day in 3–4 equal doses depending on severity of infection *or* 350 mg–450 mg M^2/day *Acute pelvic inflammatory disease* 600 mg IV every 6 h *plus* gentamicin or tobramycin (2 mg/kg initially, followed by 1.5 mg/kg 3 times/day for 4 days). Continue clindamycin orally (450 mg 4 times/day for at least 7–10 days) *Topical* Apply thin film to affected area twice a day	Do *not* use in children under 1 mo; minimum recommended oral dose in children weighing 10 kg or less is 37.5 mg 3 times a day; do *not* refrigerate reconstituted granules because mixture may thicken and become difficult to pour; solution is stable for 2 wk at room temperature; use parenteral therapy initially in children to treat anaerobic infections; follow with oral administration when appropriate; in severe infections children should receive no less than 300 mg a day parenterally, regardless of body weight; adults may be given up to 4.8 g a day IV in life-threatening infections; single IM injections of more than 600 mg are *not* recommended; do *not* give more than 1200 mg an hour by IV infusion; physically incompatible with ampicillin, phenytoin, aminophylline, barbiturates, calcium gluconate, and magnesium sulfate; applied topically to acne vulgaris lesions; alcohol base may be irritating to sensitive surfaces (eye, mucous membranes, wounds)
Lincomycin Lincocin	Capsules: 250 mg, 500 mg Injection: 300 mg/mL	*Oral* Adults: 500 mg 3–4 times a day Children over 1 mo: 30 mg/kg–60 mg/kg/day in 3–4 divided doses *IM* Adults: 600 mg every 12–24 h Children over 1 mo: 10 mg/kg every 12–24 h *IV infusion* Adults: 600 mg–1 g every 8–12 h Children over 1 mo: 10 mg/kg–20 mg/kg/day in divided doses *Subconjunctival injection* 0.25 mL (75 mg)	Do *not* use in children under 1 mo; administer orally on an empty stomach; IM injections should be made deeply and slowly to minimize pain; severe cardiopulmonary reactions have occurred when drug has been given IV at higher than recommended doses or rates; in life-threatening situations, daily IV doses of up to 8 g have been used; dilute 1 g lincomycin in 100 mL of a compatible infusion solution (see package insert) and infuse over a period of not less than 1 h; repeat as often as needed to a maximum of 8 g a day; subconjunctival injection results in effective ocular fluid levels of antibiotics for 5 h; drug is incompatible with novobiocin and kanamycin, as well as phenytoin sodium and protein hydrolysates

USES
Treatment of leprosy including dapsone-resistant leprosy and lepromatous leprosy complicated by erythema nodosum leprosum. (Drug is generally administered in combination with one or more other antileprosy drugs, such as dapsone or rifampin)

DOSAGE
100 mg daily in combination with one or more other antileprosy drugs for 3 years, followed by 100 mg clofazimine alone thereafter

FATE
Absorption is variable and can range from about 45% to 65% of an oral dose; highly lipophilic and is deposited primarily in fatty tissue and in the reticuloendothelial system; drug is retained by the body for long periods; half-life with repeated dosage is at least 60 to 70 days; some drug is eliminated in the feces, probably by biliary excretion

COMMON SIDE EFFECTS
Discoloration of the skin, urine, feces, and other bodily fluids; GI distress, dryness of the skin

SIGNIFICANT ADVERSE REACTIONS
GI: bleeding, constipation, weight loss, bowel obstruction, hepatitis, jaundice, enteritis, enlarged liver
CNS: dizziness, drowsiness, fatigue, depression, neuralgia, taste alteration
Skin: rash, pruritus, phototoxicity, acneiform eruptions, monilial cheilosis
Ocular: dryness, itching, or burning of the eyes
Other: cystitis, anemia, edema, fever, bone pain, lymphadenopathy, reduced vision, splenic infarction, thromboembolism, vascular pain, elevated serum albumin, bilirubin and SGOT, eosinophilia, hypokalemia

CONTRAINDICATIONS
No absolute contraindications. *Cautious use* in persons with serious GI disorders, and in pregnant or nursing women

PATIENT EDUCATION
1. Instruct patient to take drug with meals to minimize GI distress.
2. Tell patient to report symptoms of GI irritation (abdominal cramping, nausea, vomiting, diarrhea) because dosage may need to be reduced.
3. Stress the importance of adhering to prescribed drug regimen (see **Plan of Nursing Care 2, Compliance,** in Chapter 7).
4. Warn patient not to operate hazardous equipment until reaction to drug is known because dizziness and drowsiness, which are usually dosage-related, may occur.
5. Explain to patient that, within a few weeks after treatment is initiated, the drug usually causes skin, conjunctivae, tears, sweat, sputum, urine, or feces to turn reddish-brown (incidence is 75%–90%). Skin discoloration may persist for months or even years after therapy is terminated. Provide appropriate support and reassurance.
6. Teach patient interventions to alleviate dry skin and thickened, scaling scalp. Hydration and lubrication are usually adequate, but patient should also be instructed to use soap sparingly, to avoid applying it directly to dry skin, and to thoroughly rinse it off skin.
7. Inform patient that artificial tears or other appropriate eye drops may be used if eyes feel dry or burn.
8. Teach patient to increase fluid and dietary fiber intake to prevent constipation.
9. Instruct patient to promptly report symptoms suggestive of crystalline drug deposition (e.g., bone or joint pain, GI bleeding, reduced vision). Although usually reversible, these reactions may linger (months to years), and they may necessitate long-term corticosteroid therapy.

Dapsone
(CAN) Avlosulfon

Sulfones, of which the sole clinically available representative is dapsone, are chemical analogs of the sulfonamides that are used in the treatment of all forms of leprosy (Hansen's disease). Although clinical benefit is often noted within a few months, the more severe skin lesions characteristic of the disease may require several years for complete resolution. Because of its high potential for toxicity, dapsone is usually used only for the treatment of leprosy, although it has been shown to be effective in the treatment of dermatitis herpetiformis and relapsing polychondritis, and for prophylaxis of malaria.

MECHANISM
Not completely established; may interfere with essential components of bacterial nutrition; also possesses immunosuppressant action and may inhibit certain bacterial enzymes

USES
Treatment of leprosy (except in cases of proven dapsone resistance)
Treatment of dermatitis herpetiformis
Management of relapsing polychondritis (investigational use only)
Prophylaxis of malaria (investigational use only)

DOSAGE
Leprosy
Adults: 50 mg to 100 mg per day
Children: ¼ to ½ adult dose
Therapy is usually continued for many years
Dermatitis Herpetiformis
Initially 50 mg/day; increase gradually until desired effect (usual dosage range 50 mg to 300 mg daily); reduce to maintenance level when skin lesions have cleared

FATE
Slowly and completely absorbed orally; peak plasma concentrations occur in 4 to 8 hours; dapsone is 70% to 90% protein-bound; well distributed in the body; metabolized in the liver by acetylation and slowly excreted in the urine (70%–85%) as both unchanged drug and metabolites; plasma half-life averages 25 to 30 hours

COMMON SIDE EFFECTS
Anorexia, pallor, skin rash, back or leg pain

Hemolysis is common at dosages above 100 mg/day, "sulfone syndrome" is common during the *first year* of therapy (fever, malaise, joint swelling, epistaxis, orchitis, tender skin)

SIGNIFICANT ADVERSE REACTIONS
Dermatologic: dermatitis, phototoxicity, drug-induced lupus erythematosus
Hematologic: hemolytic anemia, leukopenia, granulocytopenia, agranulocytosis
GI: nausea, vomiting
CNS: headache, paresthesias, tinnitus, insomnia, vertigo, psychotic reactions (rare)
Other: muscle weakness, drug fever, methemoglobinemia, blurred vision, hematuria, albuminuria, nephrotic syndrome, renal papillary necrosis, liver damage, motor neuropathy, infertility, infectious mononucleosis–like syndrome

CONTRAINDICATIONS
Advanced renal amyloidosis. *Cautious use* in patients with anemia, liver or kidney disease, glucose-6-phosphate dehydrogenase deficiency, or hypersensitivity to sulfonamides; and in pregnant or nursing women

INTERACTIONS
Probenecid inhibits the renal tubular secretion of dapsone, thus elevating its plasma level
Rifampin and barbiturates can reduce the effects of dapsone by increasing hepatic microsomal enzyme activity
The leprostatic effects of dapsone can be antagonized by para-aminobenzoic acid (PABA)

NURSING CONSIDERATIONS
See **Plan of Nursing Care 12, Antibacterial Drugs,** in Chapter 56. In addition:

Nursing Alerts
- Monitor patient for indications of possible blood dyscrasias (fever, sore throat, bruising, malaise). Blood counts should be performed at frequent intervals, and the drug should be discontinued if blood picture is abnormal or if signs of severe anemia are present.
- Assess hepatic function at regular intervals, and note early signs of developing hepatotoxicity (anorexia, vomiting, abdominal pain, light colored stools). Evidence of liver impairment mandates immediate drug withdrawal.

1. Provide appropriate emotional support because the patient with leprosy often has to deal with severe surface disfigurement.

PATIENT EDUCATION
1. Instruct patient to take drug with food to minimize GI distress.
2. Stress the importance of adhering to prescribed dosage regimen (See **Plan of Nursing Care 2, Compliance,** in Chapter 7).
3. As appropriate, explain that, because bacterial resistance can develop when sulfones are used alone, rifampin or ethionamide is frequently prescribed for concurrent use during initial months of therapy. In most cases, sulfone therapy must be continued for several years, occasionally for a lifetime in severe, complicated forms of leprosy.
4. Inform patient that drug needs to be temporarily discontinued if hypersensitivity develops, but that it can be resumed at a low dosage after the reaction has subsided.

Furazolidone
Furoxone
Furazolidone is a synthetic nitrofuran with both antibacterial and antiprotozoal activity. It is effective against many common GI pathogens, such as *Escherichia coli, Salmonella, Shigella, Enterobacter aerogenes, Proteus, Vibrio cholerae,* and staphylococci, as well as the protozoan *Giardia lamblia.* Furazolidone is poorly absorbed orally, and its action is largely restricted to the GI tract

MECHANISM
Interferes with several bacterial enzyme systems; development of resistance is minimal; does not alter normal bowel flora nor lead to fungal overgrowth; possesses an MAO-inhibitory action if used for longer than 4 to 5 days, which is probably due to accumulation of a metabolite, 2-hydroxyethylhydrazine

USES
Treatment of bacterial or protozoal diarrhea and enteritis due to susceptible organisms

DOSAGE
Adults: 100 mg four times a day
Children 5 years and over: 25 mg to 50 mg four times a day
Children 1 through 4 years: 17 mg to 25 mg four times a day
Children under 1 year: 8 mg to 17 mg four times a day (maximal daily dose 8.8 mg/kg/day)

FATE
Oral absorption is minimal; drug is metabolized in the intestine and excreted largely in the feces; approximately 5% is eliminated in the urine, along with colored metabolites, which may color the urine brown

COMMON SIDE EFFECTS
Nausea, anorexia

SIGNIFICANT ADVERSE REACTIONS
Vomiting, headache, malaise, hypersensitivity reactions (fever, skin rash, urticaria, arthralgia), hypotension, hypoglycemia, reversible intravascular hemolysis, disulfiram-like reaction to alcohol (see Chap. 78)

CONTRAINDICATIONS
In infants under 1 month; concurrent use of alcohol, other drugs having an MAO-inhibitory action, sympathomimetic amines, or tyramine-containing foods (see MAO Inhibitors, Chap. 24). *Cautious use* in persons with diabetes or glucose-6-phosphate dehydrogenase deficiency; and in pregnant or nursing women

INTERACTIONS
Alcohol may elicit a mild disulfiram-like reaction (flushing, hyperthermia, sweating, dyspnea, tachycardia, palpitations) in the presence of furazolidone
Hypertension can result from concurrent use of furazolidone with other MAO inhibitors, sympathomimetic amines, or tyramine-containing foods (see Patient Education)
The actions of sedatives, narcotics, and other CNS depressants can be enhanced by furazolidone, leading to hypotension and excessive drowsiness
A toxic psychosis can result from concurrent use of furazolidone and a tricyclic antidepressant

The antihypertensive effectiveness of guanethidine may be reduced by furazolidone

Furazolidone may potentiate the hypoglycemic effect of insulin and sulfonylurea antidiabetic drugs

Concurrent use of furazolidone and meperidine may lead to sudden development of hypertension, restlessness, agitation, seizures, and coma

NURSING CONSIDERATION

Nursing Alert
- Assess patient for signs of dehydration or electrolyte depletion (hypotension, "sunken" eyes, irregular pulse, cramping) during episodes of diarrhea. Notify drug prescriber if signs occur.

PATIENT EDUCATION

1. Counsel patient to adhere to recommended dosing regimen and to inform drug prescriber if diarrhea persists longer than 5 days or worsens. If clinical response is not satisfactory after 7 days, drug should be discontinued.
2. Caution patient to avoid alcohol during treatment and for at least 4 days following therapy to prevent development of a disulfiram-like reaction.
3. During extended therapy (i.e., longer than 5 days), instruct patient to limit or avoid foods high in tyramine (e.g., unpasteurized cheese, beer, wine, broad beans, yeast, and fermented products) to minimize the danger of a hypertensive reaction due to the MAO inhibitory action of furazolidone.
4. Warn patient to avoid OTC drugs unless specifically prescribed. Hypertension can occur if furazolidone and products containing vasopressor agents are used concurrently.
5. Inform patient that drug may cause urine to turn brown, a harmless effect.
6. Instruct patient to report weakness, faintness, or dizziness, possible signs of hypotension or hypoglycemia. Dosage adjustment may be necessary.
7. Advise diabetic patient that blood sugar needs to be monitored closely because hypoglycemia may occur, in which case the dosage of antidiabetic medication may need to be adjusted.

Hydroxystilbamidine

An antifungal, antiprotozoal agent, hydroxystilbamidine is active against *Leishmania donovani* and *Blastomyces dermatitidis* and is useful in the treatment of visceral leishmaniasis (kala-azar), American mucocutaneous leishmaniasis, and North American blastomycosis, although the rate of relapse in North American blastomycosis is very high.

MECHANISM
Combines with bacterial ribonucleic acid, perhaps disrupting normal bacterial cell replication

USES
Treatment of visceral leishmaniasis (kala-azar) and American mucocutaneous leishmaniasis

Alternate treatment of North American blastomycosis

DOSAGE
Adults: 225 mg/day IV as a single dose infused over 2 to 3 hours
Children: 3 mg/kg to 4.5 mg/kg/day IV infused over 2 to 3 hours

FATE
Drug is stored in body tissues and slowly released; excretion is by way of the urine and bile

COMMON SIDE EFFECTS
Anorexia, nausea, malaise, diarrhea

SIGNIFICANT ADVERSE REACTIONS
Headache, dizziness, drowsiness, paresthesias, pruritus, chills, fever, rash, arthralgia, leukopenia, thrombophlebitis, hypotension, tachycardia, hepatitis, and renal insufficiency

CONTRAINDICATIONS
No absolute contraindications. *Cautious use* in patients with liver or kidney disease and in pregnant women

NURSING CONSIDERATIONS

Nursing Alerts
- Infuse drug slowly because hypotension, tachycardia, dyspnea, and anaphylaxis are more common with rapid administration.
- Monitor results of liver and kidney function studies, which should be performed before, and at regular intervals during, therapy.

1. Expect total course of therapy to be divided into two treatment periods, with an intervening rest period, because clinical effects persist for some time after drug is discontinued.
2. Prepare fresh solution for each injection, and protect from heat and light to avoid rapid decomposition.
3. Be prepared to give IM, if necessary. Although IV is preferred route of administration, the drug can be given IM, but injection is painful.

Nitrofurazone

Furacin

A synthetic nitrofuran, nitrofurazone exhibits a broad antibacterial spectrum of action. It is used topically to prevent infection in burns or skin grafts.

MECHANISM
Inhibits function of enzymes necessary for carbohydrate metabolism in bacteria; bactericidal against both aerobic and anaerobic organisms, although some strains of *Pseudomonas* and *Proteus* are resistant; virtually nontoxic to human cells

USES
Adjunctive therapy to prevent bacterial contamination of second-degree or third-degree burns or skin grafts

NOTE
Not for treatment of minor burns, wounds, or skin infections, because effectiveness has not been demonstrated in these conditions

DOSAGE
Soluble dressing or cream: apply directly to lesion or place on sterile gauze; reapply once daily or every few days as necessary

SIGNIFICANT ADVERSE REACTIONS
Contact dermatitis, irritation, and superinfections

CONTRAINDICATIONS

No absolute contraindications. *Cautious use* in patients with a glucose-6-phosphate dehydrogenase deficiency (danger of hemolytic anemia if significant systemic absorption occurs), marked renal impairment; and in pregnant women

NURSING CONSIDERATIONS

1. Observe for signs of allergic hypersensitivity (itching, burning, swelling, rash), and discontinue drug if these occur.
2. Apply only to affected area. Protect surrounding skin with petrolatum or zinc oxide.
3. Autoclave gauze only once. Solutions used to impregnate gauze may become discolored upon autoclaving or exposure to light, but this does not affect drug potency.

Novobiocin

Albamycin

A bacteriostatic antibiotic effective against certain gram-positive cocci, especially *Staphylococcus aureus* and some strains of *Proteus vulgaris*, novobiocin is infrequently used because resistance usually develops rapidly and there is a high incidence of hypersensitivity reactions (such as urticaria, dermatitis) associated with it. Blood dyscrasias and hepatic dysfunction have also occurred.

MECHANISM

Not completely established; inhibits protein and nucleic acid synthesis and interrupts bacterial cell wall synthesis; may also alter stability of cell membrane by complexing with magnesium within the bacterial cell

USES

Treatment of serious infections due to susceptible strains of *Staphylococcus aureus* or *Proteus* species in patients unresponsive or sensitive to other, less toxic antibiotics, such as penicillins, cephalosporins, tetracyclines, or erythromycin

DOSAGE

Adults: 250 mg every 6 hours or 500 mg every 12 hours (maximum 1 g every 12 h)
Children: 15 mg/kg to 45 mg/kg/day in divided doses every 6 to 12 hours depending on severity of infection

FATE

Well absorbed orally; peak plasma levels occur within 2 hours; highly (90%–95%) bound to plasma proteins; diffuses poorly into most body tissues; excreted primarily in the bile and feces

COMMON SIDE EFFECTS

Hypersensitivity reactions (urticarial, erythematous, maculopapular, or scarlatiniform rash)

SIGNIFICANT ADVERSE REACTIONS

Erythema multiforme (rare), liver dysfunction, jaundice, nausea, vomiting, diarrhea, intestinal hemorrhage, alopecia, and blood dyscrasias (leukopenia, eosinophilia, anemia, pancytopenia, agranulocytosis, thrombocytopenia)

CONTRAINDICATIONS

In newborn or premature infants. *Cautious use* in patients with hepatic disease or history of allergic reactions and in pregnant or nursing women

NURSING CONSIDERATIONS

Nursing Alert

- Monitor results of hepatic function studies, which should be performed periodically during treatment. Therapy should be terminated if signs of liver disease are noted (e.g., elevated serum bilirubin).

1. Expect to administer another antibiotic concurrently. Because resistance to novobiocin emerges rapidly, it is rarely used alone. It may be given with penicillin because cross-resistance has not been demonstrated.
2. Question use for minor infections or for infections caused by organisms other than those with demonstrated sensitivity to novobiocin.

PATIENT EDUCATION

1. Teach patient how to recognize and report hypersensitivity reactions (rash, urticaria, fever). Drug should be discontinued if reactions cannot be managed by usual measures.
2. Inform patient that routine blood studies are recommended, and teach patient how to recognize and report early signs of possible blood dyscrasias (fever, sore throat, bruising, or bleeding). Patient should discontinue therapy if signs occur.
3. Instruct patient to note and report any yellowing of skin or eyes or abdominal pain, signs of possible liver disease.

Pentamidine

Pentam 300, Nebu Pent

Pentamidine is a diamidine antiprotozoal agent that is effective against several protozoa and fungi. It is used for both the prevention and treatment of pneumocystis pneumonia (due to *Pneumocystis carinii*), a serious, opportunistic respiratory infection occurring frequently in immunocompromised patients, such as patients with acquired immune deficiency syndrome (AIDS). Pentamidine is an alternative drug to trimethoprim-sulfamethoxazole (see Chap. 57) and is available for injection or oral inhalation.

MECHANISM

Exact mechanism of action has not been established; drug may interfere with nuclear metabolism and inhibit the synthesis of DNA, RNA, proteins, and phospholipids

USES

Alternative treatment of *Pneumocystis carinii* pneumonia (IV, IM)
Prevention of *Pneumocystis carinii* pneumonia in high-risk HIV-infected patients
Treatment of trypanosomiasis and visceral leishmaniasis (investigational uses)

DOSAGE

Injection:
4 mg/kg once daily for 14 days; given by IV infusion or deep IM injection
Aerosol:
300 mg once every 4 weeks administered via a nebulizer

FATE

Well absorbed from IM injection sites but exists in the bloodstream only temporarily, because it is extensively bound to tissues; approximately one third of a dose is excreted unchanged by the kidneys within 6 hours; the remainder is very slowly eliminated over several weeks; drug does not enter the CNS in appreciable amounts. Plasma concentrations following aerosol administration are low

COMMON SIDE EFFECTS

Injection:
Elevated serum creatinine and liver function tests, nausea, anorexia, fever, hypotension, rash, hypoglycemia, sterile abscess or pain at IM injection site

Aerosol:
Metallic taste, shortness of breath, anorexia, fatigue, cough, dizziness, rash, pharyngitis, nausea, chills, vomiting, bronchospasm

SIGNIFICANT ADVERSE REACTIONS

Confusion, hallucinations, anemia, neuralgia, hyperkalemia, phlebitis, thrombocytopenia, acute renal failure, hypocalcemia, ventricular tachycardia, arrhythmias, and Stevens–Johnson syndrome

Too-rapid IV administration can result in headache, dizziness, tachycardia, vomiting and possibly fainting.

> NOTE
> The incidence of adverse reactions is significantly higher in patients with AIDS receiving pentamidine than in patients with other conditions

CONTRAINDICATIONS

No absolute contraindications. *Cautious use* in persons with hypotension; hypoglycemia; hypocalcemia; leukopenia; thrombocytopenia; anemia, renal or hepatic disease; arrhythmias; and in pregnant women

NURSING CONSIDERATIONS

Nursing Alerts

- When giving IM, inject into large muscle mass, rotate sites, and apply warm compresses to site. Because injection is painful and may cause sterile abscesses, intermittent IV infusion is preferred route of administration.
- Before IV infusion, prepare patient for confinement to bed in supine position. Keep patient supine during infusion.
- Monitor blood pressure at least every 15 minutes during IV infusion, every ½ hour for 2 hours after infusion is terminated, and every 4 hours thereafter until stable because sudden, severe hypotension may develop.
- During infusion, ensure that emergency equipment and drugs, including vasopressors, are on hand to treat hypotension.
- Monitor temperature, and institute measures to control, as needed. Although fever is a symptom of the illness, it may rapidly rise as high as 40°C (104°F) shortly after drug infusion.
- After infusion, when patient is not dizzy and blood pressure is stable, help patient out of bed and protect from injury until all potentially hazardous reactions have subsided.
- Monitor results of BUN and serum creatinine determinations, measure and record intake and output, and assess for edema because acute renal failure may occur. If signs of impending dysfunction appear, dosage should be adjusted.
- Check patient's pulse at least twice daily to detect arrhythmias because cardiac function may be affected.
- Monitor results of liver function tests because hepatic dysfunction may occur.
- Assess patient for signs of hypoglycemia. Blood glucose can be monitored with finger stick methods. If hypoglycemia occurs, increased food intake (5–6 small meals/day) may control the problem.
- Prior to initiating pentamidine prophylaxis, assess symptomatic patients to exclude the presence of *active* pneumocystis pneumonia. The dose of aerosolized pentamidine is insufficient to treat acute pneumocystis pneumonia.

1. Routinely rotate IV sites and assess frequently for pain, redness, and swelling because phlebitis may occur.
2. Implement other interventions for patient with AIDS (e.g., protect from infection, provide emotional support, promote adequate nutrition, prevent transmission of HIV virus to others).
3. Instruct patients who experience bronchospasm or cough with aerosolized pentamidine to use an inhaled bronchodilator prior to each pentamidine dose.
4. Note that the safety and efficacy of the inhalant solution in children has not been established.

Spectinomycin

Trobicin

An antibiotic related to the aminoglycosides, spectinomycin is used IM for alternative treatment of gonorrhea in patients hypersensitive to penicillins, or for eradication of organisms resistant to penicillins.

MECHANISM

Inhibits protein synthesis in the bacterial cell at the 30s ribosomal subunit; bacteriostatic at normal doses; active against most strains of *Neisseria gonorrhoeae*; not effective against *Treponema* (syphilis)

USES

Treatment of acute gonorrheal urethritis, proctitis, and cervicitis due to susceptible strains of *Neisseria gonorrhoeae* (usually in patients sensitive to penicillins or tetracyclines or when organisms are resistant to these drugs)

DOSAGE

Adults and children over 100 lb: usually 2 g (5 mL) IM in a single dose; in areas where antibiotic resistance is known to be present, 4 g (10 mL) divided into two equal parts and injected at different sites

Children under 100 lb (safety has *not* been established): 40 mg/kg IM

FATE

Absorption from IM injection site is rapid; serum levels peak in 1 to 2 hours and effective levels are still present at 8 hours; not significantly protein-bound; excreted by the kidneys in a biologically active form

COMMON SIDE EFFECTS
Irritation and soreness at injection site

SIGNIFICANT ADVERSE REACTIONS
Urticaria, fever, dizziness, nausea, chills, insomnia, and reduced urine output

Multiple doses have elicited decreases in hemoglobin and hematocrit and creatinine clearance, and elevations in BUN, alkaline phosphatase, and SGPT

CONTRAINDICATIONS
Treatment of pharyngeal infections due to *Neisseria gonorrhoeae*. *Cautious use* in persons with a history of allergies, in infants and young children, and in pregnant or nursing women

NURSING CONSIDERATIONS
1. Expect person known to have recently been exposed to gonorrhea to be treated the same as one proven to have gonorrhea by culture.
2. Using a 20-gauge needle, inject IM deeply into upper outer quadrant of buttocks. Administer no more than 5 mL per injection.
3. Reconstitute powder for injection with accompanying diluent, and mix thoroughly. Use within 24 hours.

PATIENT EDUCATION
1. Explain the need for a serologic test for syphilis, which should be performed at the time of diagnosis and again after 3 months (the drug may mask or delay symptoms of incubating syphilis).

Vancomycin
Lyphocin, Vancocin, Vancoled

Vancomycin is a bactericidal glycopeptide antibiotic active against many gram-positive organisms, such as streptococci, staphylococci (including penicillinase-producing), *Clostridium difficile, Corynebacterium,* and *Listeria*. In addition, it appears to be bacteriostatic against enterococci. The potential for serious toxicity, however, limits its systemic usefulness to treatment of life-threatening infections in patients allergic or unresponsive to less toxic antibacterial drugs. It may be administered orally for treatment of staphylococcal enterocolitis and antibiotic-induced pseudomembranous colitis (for which it is generally considered to be the drug of choice), because it is poorly absorbed from the GI tract.

MECHANISM
Inhibits bacterial cell wall synthesis by binding to precursors of the cell wall, such as the D-alanyl-D-alanine portion of the precursor units; drug may also inhibit bacterial RNA synthesis and damage bacterial cytoplasmic membranes. There appears to be no cross-resistance between vancomycin and any other antibiotic

USES
Treatment of serious staphylococcal infections (e.g., endocarditis, septicemia, pneumonia, osteomyelitis) in patients who cannot tolerate or who do not respond to penicillins, cephalosporins, or other less toxic antibiotics

Treatment of staphylococcal enterocolitis (oral use only)

Treatment of antibiotic-induced (e.g., clindamycin, lincomycin) pseudomembranous colitis caused by *Clostridium difficile*

DOSAGE
Oral, IV (Slow Infusion)

Adults: 500 mg every 6 hours *or* 1 g every 12 hours

Children: 44 mg/kg/day in divided doses (maximum 2 g/day)

Prevention of bacterial endocarditis in penicillin-allergic patients undergoing dental procedures or upper respiratory tract surgery:

Adults: 1 g IV infused over 30 to 60 minutes ½ to 1 hour before surgery; then oral erythromycin 500 mg every 6 hours for 8 doses

Children: 20 mg/kg IV infused over 30 to 60 minutes as above; then 10 mg/kg oral erythromycin every 6 hours for 8 doses

Prevention of bacterial endocarditis in penicillin-allergic patients undergoing GI or genitourinary surgery:

Adults: 1 g IV infused over 60 minutes *plus* 1.5 mg/kg gentamicin IM or IV concurrently 1 hour prior to procedure

Children less than 27 kg: 20 mg/kg IV slowly over 1 hour *and* 2 mg/kg gentamicin IM or IV concurrently 1 hour prior to procedure

Oral Only

Pseudomembranous colitis:

Adults: 500 mg to 2 g every 6 to 8 hours for 7 to 10 days

FATE
Poorly absorbed orally, although measurable plasma levels have occurred following oral use in treating colitis; IV administration yields rapid attainment of effective serum levels; half-life is 4 to 8 hours in adults and 2 to 3 hours in children; half-life increases in renal failure; widely distributed in the body but does not readily cross the blood–brain barrier; penetrates into pleural, pericardial, ascitic, and synovial fluid in the presence of inflammation; approximately 80% of injected drug is excreted by the kidneys

COMMON SIDE EFFECTS
Nausea with oral administration

SIGNIFICANT ADVERSE REACTIONS
(Parenteral administration) "Red neck" syndrome (fever, chills, erythema of the neck and back, paresthesias—usually seen with too-rapid injection); macular rash, urticaria, eosinophilia, ototoxicity, (tinnitus, hearing loss); nephrotoxicity, anaphylactoid reactions, pain and thrombophlebitis with IV injection, superinfections, dyspnea, wheezing, pruritus, hypotension, phlebitis, elevated serum creatinine or BUN, and thrombocytopenia

CONTRAINDICATIONS
Concurrent use with other ototoxic or nephrotoxic drugs (see Interactions). *Cautious use* in patients with renal impairment, hearing disturbances and in neonates, elderly persons, and pregnant or nursing women

INTERACTIONS
Increased ototoxicity and nephrotoxicity can result from concurrent use of vancomycin with aminoglycosides, polymyxin B, colistin, amphotericin B, cisplatin, bumetanide, furosemide, and ethacrynic acid

The action of vancomycin may be antagonized by concurrent use of bacteriostatic antibiotics, for example, tetracyclines, erythromycins

Antivertigo and antinausea drugs (e.g., meclizine, dimenhydrinate, promethazine) may mask the ototoxic effects of vancomycin

NURSING CONSIDERATIONS

Nursing Alerts
- Monitor results of hematologic studies, urinalyses, and liver and kidney function tests, which should be performed periodically on any patient receiving the drug.
- Assess patient for signs of possible nephrotoxicity (oliguria, proteinuria, urinary casts), and notify drug prescriber immediately if these occur.
- Ensure that serial tests of auditory function and vancomycin serum levels, which should be performed on any patient with borderline renal function and on elderly persons, are obtained as prescribed.

1. Seek clarification if prescribed orally for systemic infection because drug is poorly absorbed from GI tract.
2. To prepare oral solution, dilute contents of one vial (500 mg) in 30 mL water and administer by mouth or by nasogastric tube.
3. For *intermittent* IV infusion, dilute powder for injection with 10 mL sterile water for injection, then add to 100 mL to 200 mL infusion solution. Infuse over 20 to 30 minutes every 6 hours. Drug should be administered IV by intermittent infusion if possible.
4. If *continuous* IV infusion is necessary, dilute 1 g to 2 g powder in sufficient vehicle and administer by slow IV drip over 24 hours.
5. Closely observe IV infusion site for signs of extravasation, which can cause severe irritation and necrosis.

PATIENT EDUCATION

1. Instruct patient to report tinnitus or other auditory disturbances *immediately* because drug must be discontinued to prevent deafness, which may progress despite cessation of therapy.
2. When administering IV, instruct patient to report any pain in extremity used for infusion, and closely observe extremity for signs of thrombophlebitis. The risk of thrombophlebitis can be reduced by mixing drug with 200 mL or more of glucose or saline solution.

Selected Bibliography

Bullock WE: Mycobacterium leprae (leprosy). In Mandell GL, Douglas RG, Bennett JE (eds): Principles and Practice of Infectious Disease, 2nd ed, p 1406. New York, John Wiley & Sons, 1985

Cunha BA, Ristuccia AM: Clinical usefulness of vancomycin. Clin Pharm 2:417, 1983

Dhawan VK, Thadepalli H: Clindamycin: A review of fifteen years of experience. Rev Infect Dis 4:1133, 1982

Farber BF, Moellering RC: Retrospective study of the toxicity of preparations of vancomycin from 1974 to 1981. Antimicrob Agents Chemother 23:138, 1983

Feder HM, Osler C, Maderazo FG: Chloramphenicol: A review of its use in clinical practice. Rev Infect Dis 3:479, 1981

Fekety R: Vancomycin. Med Clin North Am 66:175, 1982

Goa KL, Campoli-Richards DM: Pentamidine isethionate: A review of its antiprotozoal activity, pharmacokinetic properties and therapeutic use in *Pneumocystis carinii* pneumonia. Drugs 33:242, 1987

Jacobson RR: The treatment of leprosy (Hansen's disease). Hosp Formulary 17:1076, 1982

Kueers A: Good antimicrobial prescribing: Chloramphenicol, erythromycin, vancomycin, tetracyclines. Lancet 2:425, 1982

McHenry MC, Gavan TL: Vancomycin. Pediatr Clin North Am 30:31, 1983

Powell DA, Nahata MC: Chloramphenicol: A new perspective on an old drug. Drug Intell Clin Pharm 16:295, 1982

Sands M, Kron MA, Brown RB: Pentamidine: A review. Rev Infect Dis 7:625, 1985

Schietinger H: A home care plan for AIDS. Am J Nurs 86:1021, 1986

Sharpe SM: Pentamidine and hypoglycemia. Ann Intern Med 99:128, 1983

Smith AL, Weber A: Pharmacology of chloramphenicol. Pediatr Clin North Am 30:209, 1983

Steigbigel NH: Erythromycin, lincomycin and clindamycin. In Mandell GL, Douglas RG, Bennett JE (eds): Principles and Practice of Infectious Diseases, 2nd ed, p 224. New York, John Wiley & Sons, 1985

World Health Organization (WHO) Study Group: Chemotherapy of leprosy for control programs. WHO Technical Report, Series No. 675, WHO, Geneva, 1982, p 7

SUMMARY. MISCELLANEOUS ANTIBIOTICS

Drug	Preparations	Usual Dosage Range
Chloramphenicol Ak-Chlor, Chloracol, Chlorofair, Chloromycetin, Chloroptic, I-Chlor, Ophthochlor, and other manufacturers	Capsules: 250 mg, 500 mg Oral suspension: 150 mg/5 mL Injection (sodium succinate): 100 mg/mL Ophthalmic drops: 0.5% Powder for ophthalmic solution: 25 mg/vial Ophthalmic ointment: 10 mg/g Otic solution: 0.5% Topical cream: 1%	*Oral, IV* Adults and children: 50 mg/kg/day in divided doses (maximum 100 mg/kg/day) Newborns: 25 mg/kg/day in 4 equally divided doses *Topical* Apply several times a day *Ophthalmic* 1–2 drops or a small amount of ointment in affected eye 2–4 times a day *Otic* 2–3 drops 3 times a day

Continued

SUMMARY. MISCELLANEOUS ANTIBIOTICS (continued)

Drug	Preparations	Usual Dosage Range
Clindamycin Cleocin	*See* Table 65-1	
Lincomycin Lincocin	*See* Table 65-1	
Clofazimine Lamprene	Capsules: 50 mg, 100 mg	100 mg daily for at least 3 yr
Dapsone	Tablets: 25 mg, 100 mg	*Leprosy* Adults: 50 mg–100 mg/day Children: ¼–½ adult dose *Dermatitis herpetiformis* Initially 50 mg/day; increase gradually until desired effect (usual range 50 mg–300 mg daily)
Furazolidone Furoxone	Tablets: 100 mg Liquid: 50 mg/15 mL	Adults: 100 mg 4 times a day Children 5 yr and over: 25 mg–50 mg 4 times a day Children 1 through 5 yr: 17 mg–25 mg 4 times a day Children under 1 yr: 8 mg–17 mg 4 times a day
Hydroxystilbamidine	Powder for injection: 225 mg/20 mL	Adults: 225 mg/day, infused over 2–3 h Children: 3 mg/kg–4.5 mg/kg/day, infused over 2–3 h
Nitrofurazone Furacin, Furazyme	Soluble dressing: 0.2% Topical cream: 0.2% Topical solution: 0.2%	Apply directly to lesions or place on sterile gauze; reapply daily or several times a week
Novobiocin Albamycin	Capsules: 250 mg	Adults: 250 mg every 6 h *or* 500 mg every 12 h (maximum 2 g/day) Children: 15 mg/kg–45 mg/kg/day dependent on severity of infection
Pentamidine Pentam 300, NebuPent	Powder for injection: 300 mg/vial Aerosol: 300 mg/vial	Injection: 4 mg/kg by IV infusion *or* IM injection once daily for 14 days Aerosol: 300 mg once every 4 wk via nebulizer
Spectinomycin Trobicin	Powder for injection: 2 g with 3.2 mL diluent *or* 4 g with 6.2 mL diluent (400 mg/mL when reconstituted)	2 g (5 mL) IM in a single dose; if resistance is known to be present, 4 g (10 mL) IM in 2 equally divided doses at different sites
Vancomycin Lyphocin, Vancocin, Vancoled, Vancor	Powder for injection: 500 mg/vial, 1 g/vial Powder for oral solution: 1 g, 10 g Capsules: 125 mg, 250 mg	*Oral, IV* Adults: 500 mg every 6 h *or* 1 g every 12 h Children: 44 mg/kg/day in divided doses (maximum 2 g/day) Prevention of bacterial endocarditis: *See* text Pseudomembranous colitis: 500 mg–2 g orally every 6–8 h for 7–10 days

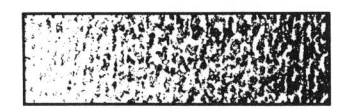

66 ANTITUBERCULAR AGENTS

Tuberculosis, an infection caused by *Mycobacterium tuberculosis*, is most commonly confined to the lungs and is characterized by severe inflammation, tissue necrosis, and frequently by the development of open cavities, all of which can impair pulmonary function. In some cases, the offending pathogen gains access to the blood or lymph, and the infection may spread to other body tissues as well. Transmission of the disease is usually by inhalation of droplets of cough from infected persons.

Current drug therapy for tuberculosis is very effective, provided strict patient compliance can be ensured, but it may be complex, difficult, and prolonged. Infections tend to be chronic, and the microorganisms can exhibit extended periods of inactivity, making complete eradication difficult. The pathogen rapidly develops resistance to single-drug antitubercular therapy and, perhaps even more serious, increasing numbers of bacterial strains are proving resistant to some multiple-drug regimens. To minimize the emergence of resistant strains, therefore, antitubercular agents are almost always administered as combinations of two or three drugs. Moreover, combination therapy allows use of lower doses of each individual drug than would be required if each were used alone, thereby reducing the likelihood of adverse effects.

Antitubercular drugs vary markedly both in efficacy and toxicity and may be divided into first-line drugs and second-line drugs on the basis of these differences. The first-line drugs are almost always used to initiate treatment of a newly diagnosed infection, inasmuch as they are the most dependable and least toxic agents when employed in low- to moderate-dose combination therapy. Second-line drugs, in contrast, are often less effective and usually more toxic than the first-line drugs, and thus they are reserved for treatment of resistant infections. Classification of the available antitubercular drugs in this text is as follows:

First-line drugs	*Second-line drugs*
ethambutol	aminosalicylic acid and salts
isoniazid (INH)	capreomycin
rifampin	cycloserine
streptomycin	ethionamide
	pyrazinamide

Some references, however, group the antitubercular agents into three categories—that is, primary (isoniazid, rifampin), secondary (ethambutol, pyrazinamide, streptomycin), and tertiary (aminosalicylic acid, capreomycin, cycloserine, ethionamide).

Treatment of an active case of tuberculosis is almost always initiated with isoniazid (INH), the most active antitubercular drug, usually in combination with rifampin, both given in single daily doses. Clinical effectiveness (i.e., cessation of *Mycobacterium tuberculosis* growth in culture of sputum) is usually demonstrated within one month with this regimen. However, approximately one fourth of patients treated with this regimen show laboratory evidence of impaired liver function, although only about 5% of them develop symptoms (nausea, anorexia, vomiting, jaundice). The drug regimen should be discontinued if these symptoms persist.

Other treatment regimens used successfully are

- INH–rifampin for 20 weeks followed by INH–ethambutol for 12 months
- INH-streptomycin-ethambutol initially, followed by INH–ethambutol for 18 to 24 months
- INH-ethambutol–rifampin for 2 to 3 months, then INH-ethambutol for 18 to 24 months.

Although para-aminosalicylic acid (PAS) was formerly widely used with INH, it is poorly tolerated by many patients, and the GI distress caused by the large doses that are required reduced patient compliance. PAS is still a valuable adjunctive drug, but as indicated above, it has been replaced in many INH drug regimens by ethambutol or rifampin. Streptomycin is likewise an effective antitubercular drug but must be given only in combination with other drugs such as INH, PAS, ethambutol, and rifampin, because resistance develops rapidly. It is used principally for extensive pulmonary or disseminated tuberculosis. The second-line drugs, because of their toxicity, are indicated only where treatment with the first-line drugs has failed. In addition, pyrazinamide is only effective for approximately two months and should not be continued for longer periods of time.

Because there are numerous differences among the clinically available antitubercular drugs, they are considered individually in alphabetical order.

Para-aminosalicylate Sodium (PAS)

P.A.S. Sodium, Teebacin,
(CAN) Nemasol

The sodium salt of PAS contains 73% aminosalicylic acid equivalent and 10.9% sodium. It is used *in combination with* isoniazid, rifampin, and/or streptomycin to delay the emergence of bacterial resistance to these first-line antitubercular drugs. PAS should *never* be used as the sole therapeutic agent in treating tuberculosis.

MECHANISM
Inhibits mycobacterial folic acid synthesis by competing with enzyme systems for incorporation of para-aminobenzoic acid (PABA)

USE
Adjunctive treatment of tuberculosis in combination with isoniazid, rifampin, and/or streptomycin to delay development of resistance

DOSAGE
Adults: 14 g to 16 g/day in two to three divided doses
Children: 275 mg/kg to 420 mg/kg/day in three to four divided doses

FATE
Well absorbed orally; widely distributed, concentrating in pleural tissue; half-life is about 1 hour; rapidly excreted in the urine, 80% to 90% within 8 to 10 hours, as both intact drug and metabolites

COMMON SIDE EFFECTS
GI distress, nausea, anorexia, diarrhea

SIGNIFICANT ADVERSE REACTIONS
GI: vomiting, abdominal pain, epigastric burning, ulceration, gastric hemorrhage

Hypersensitivity: fever, skin rash, malaise, joint pain, mononucleosis-like syndrome, jaundice, hepatitis, pancreatitis
Hematologic: leukopenia, agranulocytosis, thrombocytopenia, hemolytic anemia
Other: goiter, hypokalemia, acidosis, vasculitis, Löffler's syndrome (fever, cough, dyspnea), encephalopathy, crystalluria

CONTRAINDICATIONS
Salicylate hypersensitivity. *Cautious use* in persons with impaired renal or hepatic function, gastric ulcer, congestive heart failure and other situations requiring sodium restriction; goiter; or hematologic abnormalities

INTERACTIONS
PAS plasma levels may be increased by probenecid, salicylates, or sulfinpyrazone

PAS may decrease absorption of rifampin, folic acid, and vitamin B$_{12}$

PAS may increase INH plasma levels by reducing its rate of metabolism

Urinary acidifiers (e.g., ammonium chloride, ascorbic acid) increase the possibility of PAS crystalluria

PAS may potentiate the action of oral anticoagulants

NURSING CONSIDERATION
1. Interpret results of the following urine tests cautiously because the drug may interfere with them: protein, urobilinogen, vanillylmandelic acid (VMA), and glucose determinations with copper sulfate reagents (Clinitest tablets).

PATIENT EDUCATION
1. Instruct patient to take drug with food to minimize GI upset. Suggest use of sugar-free gum or candy to eliminate the sour or bitter aftertaste that sometimes ensues.
2. If powder is used, instruct patient to take it dissolved in water (the sodium salt of PAS is freely soluble in water). Powder is available in preweighed packets and in bulk containers.
3. Teach patient how to recognize and report indications of hypersensitivity (e.g., skin eruptions, fever, malaise, fatigue, pruritus, joint pain). If these appear, all drugs should be discontinued, if necessary, to prevent development of liver or kidney damage or pancreatitis. Therapy may be resumed with low doses once symptoms have abated, but patient should be observed closely.
4. Instruct patient to notify physician if fever, sore throat, unusual bleeding or bruising, or skin eruptions occur, because these may indicate a developing blood dyscrasia.
5. Instruct patient not to use tablets or solutions (made from powder) that have turned brown or purple because discoloration indicates deterioration of drug.
6. Warn patient to protect drug from heat and moisture because it is very unstable. Solutions of drug should be used within 24 hours.
7. Instruct patient to avoid excessive intake of cranberry or prune juice because they tend to acidify urine, which increases the danger of crystalluria.

Capreomycin
Capastat
Capreomycin is a polypeptide antibiotic used in combination with other appropriate drugs as an alternative antitubercular agent when the first-line drugs are ineffective. Capreomycin is both ototoxic and nephrotoxic and must be administered cautiously.

MECHANISM
Not established; bacteriostatic against human strains of *Mycobacterium tuberculosis;* exhibits a neuromuscular blocking action in large doses; no cross-resistance with other tuberculostatic drugs

USE
Adjunctive therapy of pulmonary tuberculosis in patients intolerant of or resistant to first-line drug regimens (i.e., INH, ethambutol, rifampin, streptomycin)

DOSAGE
IM only: 1 g/day for 60 to 120 days, followed by 1 g two to three times a week (maximum 20 mg/kg/day)

FATE
Not appreciably absorbed when administered orally; peak serum levels in 1 to 2 hours following IM injection; excreted essentially unchanged in the urine, 50% within 12 hours

COMMON SIDE EFFECTS
Elevated BUN and nonprotein nitrogen (NPN), subclinical hearing loss (5–10 dB), and eosinophilia (with daily injections)

SIGNIFICANT ADVERSE REACTIONS
Hematuria, proteinuria, abnormal urinary sediment, renal tubular necrosis, tinnitus, vertigo, anorexia, clinically apparent hearing loss, leukocytosis, leukopenia, abnormal liver function tests, pain and induration of IM injection site, urticaria, maculopapular skin rash, hypokalemia

CONTRAINDICATIONS
Concurrent administration with streptomycin or other ototoxic drugs (e.g., aminoglycosides, polymyxin, colistin); severe renal impairment. *Cautious use* in patients with renal or hepatic dysfunction, auditory impairment, history of allergies; in children and during pregnancy

INTERACTIONS
Capreomycin may enhance the muscle-relaxing action of neuromuscular blocking agents, polypeptide antibiotics, aminoglycosides, and general anesthetics

The potential for nephrotoxicity is increased by combined use of capreomycin with aminoglycosides, cephalothin, high-ceiling diuretics, polymyxins, and vancomycin

Ototoxic effects of capreomycin can be potentiated by aminoglycosides, ethacrynic acid, furosemide, and vancomycin

NURSING CONSIDERATIONS

Nursing Alert
- Monitor intake and output and check urine samples and laboratory findings for indications of renal toxicity (e.g., hematuria; urinalysis showing casts, red cells, white cells, or protein; BUN above 30 mg/dL). If these appear, drug should be discontinued to prevent serious kidney damage. Renal function tests should be performed regularly during therapy.

1. Inject IM deeply into large muscle, and observe for inflammation and bleeding.
2. Employ interventions to maximize compliance with drug regimen (see **Plan of Nursing Care 2, Compliance,** in Chapter 7). Because therapy for tuberculosis usually continues for 18 to 24 months, orally administered drugs should be substituted as soon as feasible to improve patient compliance.
3. Prepare solution by dissolving powder for injection in 2 mL of sodium chloride injection or sterile water for injection. Complete dissolution may require 2 to 3 minutes of mixing. Solution may darken over time, without affecting potency. Store for 48 hours at room temperature or up to 14 days under refrigeration.

PATIENT EDUCATION
1. Explain implications of drug's ototoxicity. Patient should understand that any sign of hearing impairment or vertigo must be promptly reported to appropriate person because drug needs to be discontinued immediately to prevent development of serious ear disorders. Also, audiometric and vestibular function tests should be performed periodically during therapy.
2. Teach patient how to recognize and report symptoms of potassium deficiency (e.g., paresthesias, muscle cramping, palpitations), and explain that serum potassium levels are usually checked frequently because hypokalemia may occur during prolonged therapy.

Cycloserine

Seromycin

A broad-spectrum antibiotic, cycloserine is effective against a variety of gram-positive and gram-negative bacteria as well as *Mycobacterium tuberculosis*. A second-line drug in the treatment of tuberculosis, it can also be used for acute urinary tract infections unresponsive to commonly employed drugs. Major untoward reactions are CNS toxicity (e.g., convulsions, psychosis, depression) and allergic reactions.

MECHANISM
Inhibits cell wall synthesis in susceptible bacteria by antagonizing D-alanine, an essential factor in bacterial cell wall synthesis; bactericidal at usual therapeutic doses

USES
Alternative treatment of active tuberculosis in conjunction with other tuberculostatic drugs when first-line therapy has failed

Alternative treatment of acute urinary tract infections, especially those due to *Enterobacter* and *Escherichia coli*, only where other antimicrobial agents are ineffective and the infecting organism has demonstrated sensitivity to cycloserine

DOSAGE
Oral: initially 250 mg twice a day for 2 weeks; maintenance dose is 500 mg to 1000 mg/day in divided doses as necessary; do not exceed 1 g/day

FATE
Well absorbed orally; peak plasma levels attained in 3 to 4 hours; widely distributed, including the CNS; half-life is 10 hours; excreted primarily in the urine, both as active drug and metabolites

SIGNIFICANT ADVERSE REACTIONS
Neurotoxicity (*dose-related*; symptoms include vertigo, paresthesias, irritability, headache, aggression, hyperreflexia, drowsiness, tremor, dysarthria, confusion, disorientation, loss of memory, convulsions, localized clonic seizures, psychoses, suicidal tendencies, coma)

Other adverse reactions are skin rash, allergic dermatitis, photosensitivity, elevated serum transaminase, vitamin B_{12} or folic acid deficiency, megaloblastic anemia.

CONTRAINDICATIONS
Epilepsy, severe anxiety, psychoses, excessive alcohol consumption, depression, and severe renal insufficiency. *Cautious use* in persons with liver or kidney impairment, in young children, and in pregnant women

INTERACTIONS
Cycloserine can potentiate the effects of MAO inhibitors and phenytoin

Ethionamide, isoniazid, and alcohol can enhance the neurotoxic effects of cycloserine

Cycloserine can increase the excretion of the B-complex vitamins

NURSING CONSIDERATIONS

Nursing Alert
● Be prepared to administer oxygen, artificial respiration, IV fluids, vasopressors, and anticonvulsants in case convulsions or other manifestations of CNS toxicity occur. Because CNS toxicity is related to serum drug levels, high dosage (greater than 500 mg/day) or inadequate renal clearance predisposes to neurotoxicity.

1. Monitor results of hematologic, renal excretion, liver function, and serum drug level studies, which should be performed periodically during therapy. Serum drug level should be determined at least weekly if patient is receiving large doses or exhibits reduced renal function. Dosage should be adjusted if serum level exceeds 30 µg/mL or if renal impairment as indicated by creatinine clearance develops (see package instructions).

PATIENT EDUCATION
1. Emphasize the importance of informing drug prescriber immediately if symptoms of allergic dermatitis or CNS toxicity occur (see Significant Adverse Reactions) because dosage should be reduced or drug discontinued to avoid more serious untoward reactions. Anticonvulsants, pyridoxine, or sedatives may be effective in controlling CNS toxicity.
2. Warn patient to exercise caution in driving or performing hazardous tasks because drowsiness, dizziness, and confusion may occur.
3. Instruct patient to avoid excessive alcohol consumption because this increases risk of convulsions.

Ethambutol

Myambutol
(CAN) Etibi

A synthetic orally administered tuberculostatic drug effective against actively dividing mycobacteria, ethambutol is a first-line drug for treatment of pulmonary tuberculosis. It is most often used in combination with INH—with or without rifampin or streptomycin, depending on the severity of the condition—because it is somewhat less active alone than other first-line drugs. Previously unexposed microorganisms are uniformly sensitive to ethambutol, but resistance does develop in a stepwise manner. Ethambutol may have adverse effects on visual acuity, thus monthly eye examinations are recommended during therapy.

MECHANISM
Inhibits protein synthesis and impairs cellular metabolism, thus blocking multiplication of bacterial cells; does not exhibit cross-resistance with other agents

USES
Treatment of pulmonary tuberculosis, usually in combination with INH and possibly rifampin or streptomycin

DOSAGE
Initial treatment: 15 mg/kg as a single oral dose every 24 hours with INH
Retreatment: (patients having previous antituberculosis treatment) 25 mg/kg as a single oral dose every 24 hours with at least one other antitubercular drug to which the organism is susceptible; decrease to 15 mg/kg after 60 days

FATE
Readily absorbed from GI tract; absorption unaffected by the presence of food; peak serum level occurs in 2 to 4 hours; no accumulation has been reported in patients with normal kidney function; approximately 50% excreted unchanged in the urine, 20% to 25% eliminated unchanged in the feces and remainder excreted as metabolites in the urine

SIGNIFICANT ADVERSE REACTIONS
CNS: decreased visual acuity due to optic neuritis (e.g., altered color perception, blurred vision), fever, malaise, headache, dizziness, confusion, disorientation, paresthesias, hallucinations
GI: abdominal pain, GI upset, vomiting, anorexia
Allergic/hypersensitivity: pruritus, dermatitis, joint pain, anaphylactic reactions
Other: elevated serum uric acid, acute gout, transient impairment of liver function, epidermal necrolysis, thrombocytopenia

CONTRAINDICATIONS
Optic neuritis; in children under 12 years of age. *Cautious use* in patients with hepatic or renal dysfunction, hyperuricemia, or history of acute gout; during pregnancy

INTERACTIONS
Ethambutol may reduce the effectiveness of uricosuric drugs such as probenecid and sulfinpyrazone
Aluminum-containing antacids may impair oral absorption of myambutol

NURSING CONSIDERATIONS

Nursing Alert
- Ensure that visual function is tested before therapy is initiated. It should be retested periodically during treatment (monthly if drug is administered in high dosages).

1. Expect dosage to be reduced in patient with impaired renal function. Dosage should be based upon desired serum level of drug (e.g., 2 µg–5 µg/mL).
2. Interpret SGPT, SGOT, and serum uric acid findings cautiously because drug can increase levels.

PATIENT EDUCATION
1. Instruct patient to take drug with food to minimize GI upset.
2. Warn patient to report promptly any change in visual acuity or color perception because the drug should be discontinued. Inform patient that recovery from these symptoms may take several weeks to several months. Effects are generally reversible, but in rare cases they may be prolonged or permanent.

Ethionamide
Trecator-SC

MECHANISM
Not established; probably similar to that of isoniazid; may inhibit peptide synthesis in mycobacterial cells

USE
Alternative therapy of active tuberculosis in combination with other effective antitubercular drugs when treatment with first-line drugs (INH, ethambutol, rifampin, streptomycin) has failed

DOSAGE
Adults: 0.5 g to 1 g/day in divided doses with at least one other antitubercular drug and pyridoxine (50 mg/day)—see below
Children: optimum dosage is not established; 4 mg/kg to 5 mg/kg every 8 hours has been suggested

FATE
Well absorbed orally and distributed widely in the body, including the CNS; peak serum levels attained in 3 to 4 hours; excreted largely in the urine, almost entirely as metabolites

COMMON SIDE EFFECTS
GI upset (nausea, vomiting, cramping), salivation, metallic taste, stomatitis, diarrhea, anorexia, drowsiness, asthenia

SIGNIFICANT ADVERSE REACTIONS
Neurotoxicity: blurred vision, diplopia, optic neuritis, peripheral neuritis, olfactory disturbances, dizziness, headache, restlessness, tremors, convulsions, psychosis
GI: hepatitis, jaundice
Other: orthostatic hypotension, impotence, gynecomastia, acne, skin rash, alopecia, pellagra-like syndrome, thrombocytopenia

CONTRAINDICATIONS
Severe hepatic dysfunction. *Cautious use* in patients with diabetes mellitus, liver or renal impairment, in children, and during pregnancy (fetal damage has been reported in experimental animals)

INTERACTIONS
Ethionamide can enhance the neurotoxicity of cycloserine and may intensify the adverse effects of other tuberculostatic agents

Ethionamide may increase the neurotoxic effects of alcohol

Ethionamide may potentiate the hypotensive effects (especially orthostatic) of antihypertensive drugs

Ethionamide may interfere with the management of diabetes by hypoglycemic drugs

NURSING CONSIDERATION
1. Ensure that serum transaminase (SGOT, SGPT) is measured before therapy is initiated. It should also be determined at 2 to 4-week intervals throughout therapy.

PATIENT EDUCATION
1. Instruct patient to take drug with food to minimize GI upset.
2. Caution patient to avoid excessive use of alcohol to minimize danger of neurotoxicity.
3. Instruct diabetic patient to carefully monitor blood sugar because management of diabetes mellitus may be more difficult. Dosage of hypoglycemic drugs should be adjusted on the basis of blood glucose determinations.
4. Explain that 50 mg per day of vitamin B_6 may be prescribed during therapy (when used with isoniazid, ethionamide may contribute to isoniazid-induced pyridoxine deficiency).

Isoniazid (INH)
Laniazid, Nydrazid, Teebaconin
(CAN) Isotamine, PMS Isoniazid

A first-line drug of choice for most cases of active tuberculosis, isoniazid (INH) is usually prescribed in combination with ethambutol or rifampin, or both, to delay the emergence of resistant strains. It is also indicated for prophylactic use in high-risk patients, such as household members of infected persons or persons with positive tuberculin skin test reactions. A major danger associated with INH is severe and sometimes fatal hepatitis. The risk of developing hepatitis increases with advancing age (see Significant Adverse Reactions).

MECHANISM
Not completely established; drug is bactericidal; may interfere with biosynthesis of lipids, proteins, and nucleic acid in susceptible organisms; resistance frequently develops rapidly when INH is used alone; can antagonize the activity of vitamin B_6

USES
Treatment of all forms of active tuberculosis due to susceptible organisms, usually in combination with other tuberculostatic drugs

Prophylaxis in high-risk patients such as household members or close associates of actively infected individuals or persons evidencing positive tuberculin skin test reactions in the absence of positive bacteriologic findings; also used in persons under 35 (especially children under 7 yr) with positive skin test reactions, patients with hematologic diseases (e.g., leukemia, Hodgkin's disease) or diabetes, persons undergoing immunosuppressive therapy or prolonged treatment with corticosteroids, and following a gastrectomy

DOSAGE
Active Tuberculosis
Adults: 5 mg/kg/day in a single dose (maximum 300 mg/day)
Children: 10 mg/kg to 20 mg/kg/day in a single dose (maximum 500 mg/day)

Prophylaxis
Adults: 300 mg/day in a single dose for 1 year
Children: 10 mg/kg/day in a single dose for 1 year

Note: Pyridoxine (vitamin B_6) is given concurrently with INH at a dosage of 15 mg to 50 mg a day (see Nursing Considerations)

FATE
Completely absorbed from the GI tract; absorption is reduced by food; peak blood levels in 1 hour to 2 hours, declining to 50% or less within 6 hours; widely distributed in the body including cerebrospinal, pleural, and ascitic tissues; less than one half is excreted unchanged in the urine—most of the remainder is acetylated or hydrolyzed by the liver and metabolites are removed by the kidneys; rate of acetylation is genetically determined and may be slow (in approximately 50% of Blacks and Caucasians) or rapid (rest of Blacks and Caucasians, Orientals, and Eskimos); rate of acetylation does *not* alter clinical efficacy of INH but may influence toxicity (i.e., slow acetylators are more prone to elevated blood levels and increased toxic reactions, including peripheral neuropathies; rapid acetylators are more likely to develop hepatitis); liver disease can prolong clearance of INH

COMMON SIDE EFFECTS
Paresthesias, peripheral neuropathy (especially in malnourished, diabetic, or alcoholic persons), and mild hepatic dysfunction (transient elevation of serum transaminase)

SIGNIFICANT ADVERSE REACTIONS
CNS: optic neuritis, toxic encephalopathy, memory impairment, toxic psychosis, convulsions
GI: nausea, vomiting, epigastric distress
Hepatic: bilirubinemia, bilirubinuria, jaundice, severe (occasionally fatal) hepatitis
Hematologic: hemolytic or aplastic anemia, agranulocytosis, eosinophilia, thrombocytopenia
Allergic/hypersensitivity: fever, skin rashes (morbilliform, maculopapular, purpuric, exfoliative), vasculitis, lymphadenopathy
Other: vitamin B_6 deficiency, hyperglycemia, metabolic acidosis, gynecomastia, pellagra, rheumatoid or systemic lupus-like symptoms, irritation at IM injection site

CONTRAINDICATIONS
Acute liver disease, previous adverse reaction with isoniazid. *Cautious use* in patients with chronic liver disease, renal dysfunction, diabetes, convulsive disorders, psychoses, a history of allergic reactions; in alcoholics and in pregnant or nursing women

INTERACTIONS
INH can increase serum levels of phenytoin by reducing its metabolism

The efficacy of INH may be reduced when given concurrently with corticosteroids

Alcohol increases the risk of INH-induced hepatitis

INH can potentiate the pharmacologic and toxicologic effects of carbamazepine and benzodiazepine antianxiety agents

Antacids reduce GI absorption of INH if they are given together

Disulfiram and INH can impair coordination and elicit behavioral changes

Concurrent use of INH and rifampin may increase the likelihood of hepatotoxicity, whereas combined use of INH and cycloserine can increase CNS toxicity

INH may exhibit MAO-inhibitory activity and can potentiate sympathomimetic amines, leading to increased blood pressure

INH has been reported to potentiate anesthetics, anticoagulants, anticonvulsants, hypoglycemics, antihypertensives, antiparkinsonian agents, anticholinergics, antidepressants, narcotics, and sedatives, although the clinical importance of these potential interactions has not been definitely established

NURSING CONSIDERATIONS

Nursing Alerts

- Assess patient carefully for indications of hepatic dysfunction (anorexia, malaise, nausea, vomiting, darkening of urine, paresthesias, jaundice). Drug should be discontinued immediately if these occur. Monthly liver function tests should be performed during therapy.
- Observe for development of hypersensitivity reactions. Drug should be discontinued if these occur. If therapy is reinstituted, very small doses should be used, and drug should be withdrawn immediately if hypersensitivity recurs.

1. Expect to administer IM only if oral route is unavailable or impractical. Inform patient that IM injection may be irritating or painful.
2. Expect supplemental vitamin B_6 (10 mg–100 mg/day) to be prescribed to minimize neurotoxic effects, especially in malnourished or diabetic patient or slow acetylator of INH (see Fate). INH is available in fixed combinations with vitamin B_6 (100 mg INH/5 mg vitamin B_6; 100 mg/10 mg; and 300 mg/30 mg) as Teebaconin and Vitamin B_6 and P-I-N Forte.
3. Note that INH is available in fixed combinations with rifampin as Rifamate or Rimactane/INH Dual Pack.

PATIENT EDUCATION

1. Instruct patient to take drug on an empty stomach, if possible, and to avoid simultaneous administration of antacids. Food may be taken to minimize GI irritation, but it will slow drug absorption
2. Stress the importance of adhering to dosage regimen (see **Plan of Nursing Care 2, Compliance,** in Chapter 7). Because adverse effects, especially hepato- and neurotoxicity, are more prevalent at higher doses, recommended dosages should not be exceeded. Conversely, consequences of skipping doses or discontinuing therapy without prescriber knowledge may also be serious because insufficient dosage permits resistant strains to emerge, and relapse rates are high if treatment is terminated prematurely.
3. Urge patient to reduce intake of alcohol to minimize risk of hepatitis.
4. Instruct patient to obtain periodic ophthalmic examinations during therapy and to notify drug prescriber if visual disturbances occur.
5. Instruct diabetic patient to monitor blood sugar carefully. Dosage of hypoglycemic medication should be adjusted as needed to maintain control because INH can elevate blood sugar *or* potentiate the action of hypoglycemic drugs.

Pyrazinamide

(CAN) PMS Pyrazinamide, Tebrazid

Pyrazinamide is a second-line tuberculostatic agent, used only in combination with primary drugs (INH, ethambutol, rifampin, streptomycin) in resistant patients or for short-term therapy before pulmonary surgery in advanced cases to minimize further spread of infection. Principal adverse effects are hepatotoxicity (the incidence of which ranges from 2%–20% and is dependent on the dosage) and hyperuricemia.

MECHANISM

Not established; primarily bacteriostatic, possibly by interfering with protein synthesis; active only at slightly acidic pH

USE

Adjunctive therapy of tuberculosis in combination with other first-line drugs in patients in whom these primary agents are ineffective

DOSAGE

20 mg/kg to 35 mg/kg/day in three or four divided doses (maximum dose 3 g/day)

FATE

Readily absorbed orally; peak serum levels in 2 hours; half-life is 9 to 10 hours; widely distributed in the body, partially metabolized by the liver and excreted in the urine primarily (70%) as metabolites with some unchanged drug

SIGNIFICANT ADVERSE REACTIONS

Hepatic dysfunction (fever, anorexia, malaise, hepatomegaly, abdominal tenderness, splenomegaly, jaundice, yellow atrophy of the liver), GI distress, arthralgia, anemia, dysuria, urinary retention, hyperuricemia, acute gout, skin rash, urticaria, and photosensitivity

CONTRAINDICATIONS

Severe liver damage; in children. *Cautious use* in patients with a history of gout or hyperuricemia, diabetes mellitus, impaired renal function, peptic ulcer, acute intermittent porphyria; and in alcoholics

INTERACTIONS

Pyrazinamide can interfere with the uricosuric action of probenecid and sulfinpyrazone

Pyrazinamide may alter the dosage requirements for insulin or oral hypoglycemic drugs in diabetics

NURSING CONSIDERATIONS

Nursing Alerts

- Assess patient frequently for signs of liver dysfunction (see Significant Adverse Reactions). Drug should be discontinued immediately if signs appear. Liver function tests should be performed before initiation of therapy and every 2 to 4 weeks during therapy. Effects of hepatotoxicity can range from an asymptomatic abnormality of liver cell function to severe jaundice and fulminating acute yellow atrophy.
- Ensure that prescribed serum uric acid determinations are obtained before and during treatment.

PATIENT EDUCATION
1. Instruct patient to report development of pain in toes, ankle, heel, or other joints to appropriate person.
2. Inform diabetic patient that dosage of hypoglycemic medication may need to be adjusted to maintain stable blood glucose levels because pyrazinamide can affect control of diabetes.

Streptomycin

An aminoglycoside antibiotic effective against *Mycobacterium tuberculosis,* streptomycin is considered a primary drug. It is most often used in combination with INH, rifampin, or ethambutol for control of more severe infections. Resistance develops rapidly, hence combination therapy is necessary to maintain effectiveness. It is administered IM only, thus patient compliance during prolonged therapy may be poor. The principal danger associated with use of streptomycin is ototoxicity, both vestibular and auditory, and patients receiving the drug must be observed carefully. Streptomycin has been reviewed previously in Chapter 62, and only the dosage regimen for use in tuberculosis is given here.

DOSAGE

Usual regimen is 1 g streptomycin IM with an appropriate dose of additional antitubercular drugs, such as INH, ethambutol, or rifampin; reduce streptomycin dosage to 1 g two or three times a week as symptoms improve

Use smaller doses in the elderly or in patients with impaired renal function

NURSING CONSIDERATIONS
See Chapter 62.

PATIENT EDUCATION
See Chapter 62.

Rifampin

Rifadin, Rimactane
(CAN) Rofact

A derivative of the antibiotic rifamycin B, rifampin is a first-line bacteriostatic antitubercular drug. It is most often used in combination with INH and ethambutol, because resistance develops rapidly if it is given alone. The drug should be taken on an uninterrupted schedule, because intermittent therapy is associated with a higher incidence of adverse reactions, especially involving the liver and kidneys.

MECHANISM

Inhibits DNA-dependent RNA polymerase activity in bacterial cells, thus interfering with nucleic acid synthesis; active against a number of gram-positive and gram-negative organisms; no apparent cross-resistance with other antitubercular drugs

USES

Treatment of pulmonary tuberculosis in conjunction with at least one other tuberculostatic drug (e.g., INH, ethambutol)

Treatment of asymptomatic carriers of *Neisseria meningitidis* to eliminate meningococci from the nasopharynx (*not* indicated for meningococcal infections)

Investigational uses include treatment of staphylococcal infections, Legionnaire's disease not responsive to erythromycin, gram-negative bacteremia in infancy, leprosy (with dapsone), and prophylaxis of *Hemophilus* meningitis

DOSAGE
Pulmonary Tuberculosis
Adults: 600 mg/day in a single oral dose
Children over 5 years: 10 mg/kg to 20 mg/kg day in a single dose
Meningococcal Carriers
Adults: 600 mg/day for 4 consecutive days
Children over 5 years: 10 mg/kg to 20 mg/kg/day for 4 consecutive days

FATE

Oral absorption is nearly complete; peak blood levels vary widely and occur between 1 and 4 hours; 70% to 80% protein-bound; metabolized in the liver and excreted both in the feces (via bile) and to a lesser extent in the urine as both free drug and deacetylated metabolites; half-life varies from 1.5 to 5 hours but is progressively shortened during the initial weeks of therapy because microsomal enzyme induction accelerates the drug's metabolism

COMMON SIDE EFFECTS

Elevation of liver enzymes, rash, mild GI distress, flu-like syndrome at high doses (fever, chills, myalgia, and occasionally eosinophilia, thrombocytopenia, and hemolytic anemia)

SIGNIFICANT ADVERSE REACTIONS

GI: anorexia, vomiting, diarrhea, cramping, flatulence, sore mouth, pancreatitis, pseudomembranous colitis

CNS: headache, drowsiness, fatigue, dizziness, ataxia, confusion, visual disturbances, muscle weakness, generalized numbness, hearing disturbances

Allergic/hypersensitively: pruritus, urticaria, rash, acneiform lesions, fever

Hepatic/renal: abnormal liver function tests (elevated BUN, serum bilirubin, serum transaminase, alkaline phosphatase), hepatitis, hemoglobinuria, hematuria, proteinuria, renal insufficiency, acute renal failure

Hematologic: transient leukopenia, thrombocytopenia, decreased hemoglobin, hemolytic anemia, eosinophilia

Other: conjunctivitis, elevated serum uric acid, menstrual irregularities, osteomalacia, myopathy

CONTRAINDICATIONS

Not to be given on an *intermittent* dosage schedule (increased incidence of adverse reactions). *Cautious use* in persons with hepatic or renal disease or a history of alcoholism; in pregnant women and in children under 5 years of age

INTERACTIONS

Rifampin induces microsomal enzymes and thus may decrease the effects of other drugs metabolized by these liver enzymes, for example, oral anticoagulants, estrogens, progestins, metoprolol, propranolol, quinidine, clofibrate, corticosteroids, oral hypoglycemics, and methadone

PAS administered concurrently can impair GI absorption of rifampin and can reduce rifampin serum levels

The action of rifampin can be potentiated by probenecid or isoniazid, which compete for hepatic uptake

Concomitant use of rifampin and alcohol may increase the incidence of hepatotoxicity

NURSING CONSIDERATION
1. Because rifampin can interfere with standard assays for serum folate and vitamin B_{12}, notify laboratory of drug use if these determinations are required because alternative testing methods must be used.

PATIENT EDUCATION

1. Instruct patient to take drug on an empty stomach, if possible, because food may delay absorption and reduce peak serum concentration.
2. Stress the importance of taking drug on a continual basis because interruptions in therapy may increase the likelihood of adverse reactions (see **Plan of Nursing Care 2, Compliance,** in Chapter 7).
3. Instruct patient to report development of flulike symptoms (fever, chills, headache, muscle aches) because they may signal impending hepatorenal dysfunction, especially if drug has been used intermittently.
4. Teach patient how to recognize and immediately report appearance of jaundicelike symptoms (yellowing of skin or sclerae, pruritus, darkened urine, light-colored stools). Liver function must be evaluated periodically during therapy.
5. Warn patient to note occurrence of sore throat, unusual bleeding or bruising, or excessive weakness, indications of possible blood dyscrasias, and to inform prescriber immediately if they occur. Hematologic studies should be performed.
6. Inform patient that drug may impart a harmless red-orange color to urine, feces, saliva, sputum, sweat, and tears. Inform premenopausal female that menstrual irregularities may occur.
7. With woman using oral contraceptive, discuss use of alternative contraceptive methods during rifampin therapy because effectiveness of oral contraceptives may be reduced.

Selected Bibliography

American Thoracic Society: Treatment of tuberculosis and tuberculosis infection in adults and children. Annu Rev Resp Dis 134:355, 1986

Bullock WE: Rifampin in the treatment of leprosy. Rev Infect Dis 5(suppl 3):606, 1983

Centers for Disease Control: Primary resistance to antituberculosis drugs. Ann Intern Med 32:521, 1983

Coleman DA: TB: The disease that's not dead yet. RN 47(9):48, 1984

DesPrez RM, Goodwin RA: Mycobacterium tuberculosis. In (Mandell GL, Douglas RG, Bennett JR (eds): Principles and Practice of Infectious Diseases, 2nd ed, p 1383. New York, John Wiley & Sons, 1985

Drugs for tuberculosis. Med Lett Drugs Therap 24:17, 1982

Farr B, Mandell GL: Rifampin. Med Clin North Am 66:157, 1982

Glassroth J, Robins AG, Snider DE: Tuberculosis in the 1980's. N Engl J Med 302(26):1441, 1980

Grosset J, Leventis S: Adverse effects of rifampin. Rev Infect Dis 5(Suppl 3):S440, 1983

Hauser M, Baier H: Interactions of isoniazid with foods. Drug Intell Clin Pharm 16:617, 1982

Mangione RA, Souse RB: Antimicrobial management of pulmonary tuberculosis. Pharm Times 50:74, 1984

Mitchinson DA: The action of antituberculosis drugs in short course chemotherapy. Tubercle 66:219, 1985

Pilhev JA, DeSalvo MD, Koch O: Liver alterations in antituberculosis regimens containing pyrazinamide. Chest 80:720, 1981

Reed MD, Blumer JL: Clinical pharmacology of antitubercular drugs. Pediatr Clin North Am 30:177, 1983

Snider DE et al: Standard therapy for tuberculosis. Chest 87(Suppl 2): 117, 1985

Van Scoy RE, Wilkowske CJ: Antituberculous agents. Mayo Clin Proc 58:233, 1983

Wehrli W: Rifampin: Mechanisms of action and resistance. Rev Infect Dis 5(Suppl 3):S407, 1983

SUMMARY. ANTITUBERCULAR DRUGS

Drug	Preparations	Usual Dosage Range
Para-aminosalicylate Sodium P.A.S. Sodium, Teebacin	Tablets: 0.5 g, 1 g Powder	Adults: 14 g–16 g/day in 2–3 divided doses Children: 275 mg/kg–420 mg/kg/day in 3–4 divided doses
Capreomycin Capastat	Powder for injection: 1 g/5 mL	1 g/day IM for 60–120 days, then 1 g 2–3 times a week
Cycloserine Seromycin	Capsules: 250 mg	250 mg twice a day for 2 weeks, then 500 mg–1000 mg/day in divided doses
Ethambutol Myambutol	Tablets: 100 mg, 400 mg	Initially: 15 mg/kg/day as a single dose Retreatment: 25 mg/kg/day as a single oral dose
Ethionamide Trecator-SC	Tablets: 250 mg	Adults: 0.5 g–1 g/day in divided doses
Isoniazid (INH) Laniazid, Nydrazid, Teebaconin	Tablets: 50 mg, 100 mg, 300 mg Syrup: 50 mg/5 mL Injection: 100 mg/mL Powder	*Treatment* Adults: 5 mg/kg/day in a single dose (maximum 300 mg a day) Children: 10 mg–20 mg/kg/day in a single dose (maximum 500 mg a day) *Prophylaxis* Adults: 300 mg/day in a single dose Children: 10 mg/kg/day in a single dose

Continued

SUMMARY. ANTITUBERCULAR DRUGS (continued)

Drug	Preparations	Usual Dosage Range
Pyrazinamide Pyrazinamide	Tablets: 500 mg	20 mg–35 mg/kg/day in 3–4 divided doses (maximum 3 g/day)
Streptomycin Streptomycin	Injection: 1 g, 5 g	1 g IM with an appropriate dose of INH, rifampin, or ethambutol
Rifampin Rifadin, Rimactane	Capsules: 150 mg, 300 mg	*Tuberculosis* Adults: 600 mg/day in a single dose Children: 10 mg/kg–20 mg/kg/day in a single dose *Meningococcal carrier state* Adults: 600 mg/day for 4 consecutive days Children: 10 mg–20 mg/kg/day for 4 consecutive days

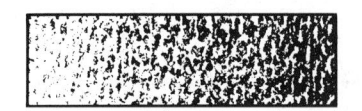

67 ANTIMALARIAL AGENTS

Malaria is a parasitic disease that is still prevalent in many areas of the world, especially Southeast Asia, Africa, and Central and South America. Four species of the protozoan Plasmodium can cause malaria in humans, and these are described briefly below.

- *Plasmodium falciparum:* causes malignant tertian (MT) malaria, a severe, often fulminating infection that may progress to a fatal outcome if not treated quickly and vigorously; prompt therapy is usually highly successful, however, and relapses generally do not occur, but inadequate treatment can lead to periodic outbreaks due to multiplication of parasites persisting in the blood
- *Plasmodium vivax:* causes benign tertian (BT) malaria, a less severe disease than that produced by the *Plasmodium falciparum* strain, having a low mortality but characterized by periodic relapses that may continue for years if untreated
- *Plasmodium malariae:* causes quartan malaria; so named because the attacks of chills and high fever recur every 4 days rather than every 3 days as in the tertian form of the disease; outbreaks tend to appear in localized regions of the tropics; clinical signs may remain dormant for many years, and relapses do occur, but less frequently than with the *Plasmodium vivax* organism
- *Plasmodium ovale:* causes ovale tertian malaria, a rare form of relapsing malaria similar to but milder and more readily cured than the vivax infection

Malaria is usually transmitted to humans by the bite of the female Anopheles mosquito, which deposits the infective sporozoites, formed in the blood of the mosquito by the union of male and female gametocytes, into the human. The sporozoites localize in the liver, where they form primary tissue schizonts. These then grow and multiply into merozoites. This is the pre-erythrocytic or symptom-free stage of the infection. When mature, the merozoites are released from the liver and invade the erythrocytes (red blood cells) to begin the blood-cycle phase of the infection. Young parasites in the red blood cell, termed *trophozoites,* grow and divide into mature schizonts, also known as *blood merozoites.* Periodically, the blood merozoites burst from the ruptured cells and invade a new group of erythrocytes, beginning the process anew. This periodic (every 3–4 days) rupturing of infected erythrocytes is responsible for the characteristic fever and chills that accompany acute attacks of malaria.

Another phase of the plasmodial life cycle, which occurs in infections caused by *P. vivax, P. ovale,* and possibly *P. malariae,* is termed the exoerythrocytic cycle. Following the release of most of the mature merozoites from the liver, some parasites in the merozoite stage of these three forms of *Plasmodium* remain in the liver and continue to multiply in liver cells for extended periods. Relapses developing months or even years following the initial infection can then occur as new merozoites are released from the liver cells to reinvade erythrocytes. Thus, malarial attacks can occur for several years unless these exoerythrocytic forms are eradicated during the primary treatment phase.

Finally, some of the merozoites that invade erythrocytes do not undergo the above-described process of *asexual* reproduction but instead differentiate into male and female gametocytes. Upon ingestion into a female mosquito (i.e., when the mosquito draws blood from an infected human by a bite), sexual fertilization of the female gametocyte by the male gametocyte occurs in the gut of the mosquito, giving rise to new infective sporozoites.

Drug therapy of malaria may be directed either toward prevention of infection, suppression of clinical symptoms, treatment of acute attacks, or prevention of relapses.

- *Prevention of infection:* Drugs that kill the malarial organisms during their pre-erythrocytic (exoerythrocytic) stages are termed *causal prophylactics;* however, no drug is currently available that can *selectively* destroy sporozoites at therapeutic levels that are considered safe. Prophylaxis of malaria is best accomplished by mosquito control.
- *Suppression of clinical symptoms:* Inhibition of the erythrocytic stage of the cycle can prevent development of clinical symptoms in an infected individual. Several antimalarial drugs (i.e., chloroquine, hydroxychloroquine, pyrimethamine) act in this manner, but acute attacks can occur when therapy is discontinued if exoerythrocytic forms of the organism are still present.
- *Treatment of acute attacks:* Interruption of erythrocytic parasite multiplication can terminate the symptoms of an acute malarial attack, and drugs acting in this way are termed *schizonticides.* The 4-aminoquinolines are generally considered drugs of choice in this case, but they do not completely eliminate the parasite from the body; hence the possibility of relapse exists, especially with the *vivax* strains.
- *Prevention of relapse:* Drugs that eradicate the exoerythrocytic parasites (secondary tissue forms) can prevent relapse infections, and such treatment is sometimes referred to as a *radical cure.* The only currently available drug producing a radical cure in vivax malaria is primaquine, which is usually given in combination with a drug (e.g., chloroquine) that suppresses the erythrocyte cycle as well.

Combination suppressive therapy and radical cure (e.g., with chloroquine and primaquine) is widely employed in travelers to areas in which malaria is endemic. Therapy is begun before arrival and repeated at weekly intervals during and for at least 2 months after return from the malarial region to ensure that in the event infection occurs, clinical symptoms are suppressed and any secondary tissue forms are eradicated.

Prophylaxis may also be accomplished by use of the combination product sulfadoxine and pyrimethamine (Fansidar) beginning 1 to 2 days before exposure to an endemic area, continuing during the stay and then for 4 to 6 weeks following departure.

An increasingly prevalent problem in treating malaria is the extent of acquired resistance that has developed to many antimalarial drugs. The most serious problem with resistance appears to be with *P. falciparum,* because this species is responsible for the large majority of cases of malaria and most of the human mortality associated with the disease. Resistance of *P. falciparum* to chloroquine, a mainstay in the treatment of malaria for many years, is increasing dramatically throughout the world, and there is increasing resistance to pyrimethamine–sulfadoxine, a combination considered to be the preferred alternative to chloroquine for prophylaxis of falciparum malaria.

Owing to the many differences among them, the available antimalarial drugs are considered individually here.

4-Aminoquinolines

Chloroquine
Hydroxychloroquine

The 4-aminoquinolines are synthetic drugs that are particularly active against the erythrocytic forms of *Plasmodium vivax* and *Plasmodium malariae* and against most forms of *Plasmodium falciparum*. Because they are ineffective against the exoerythrocytic forms, they do not prevent initial infection nor do they prevent relapses in infected persons. Their principal indications are as suppressive agents in vivax or malariae malaria and for terminating acute attacks of all types of malaria. The two drugs are reviewed together, then listed individually in Table 67-1.

MECHANISM
Not entirely known; appear to complex with DNA molecules of the parasite, thereby inhibiting RNA replication and subsequent nucleic acid synthesis; may also exert an amebicidal action and may exhibit anti-inflammatory activity as well

USES
Suppression and treatment of acute attacks of malaria due to *Plasmodium vivax*, *Plasmodium malariae*, *Plasmodium ovale*, and susceptible strains of *Plasmodium falciparum*

Treatment of extraintestinal amebiasis (chloroquine, see Chap. 69)

Treatment of systemic lupus erythematosus and rheumatoid arthritis (investigational use for hydroxychloroquine—see Table 67-1)

DOSAGE
See Table 67-1

FATE
Rapidly and completely absorbed orally; widely distributed in the body, attaining high concentrations in many tissues; approximately 50% protein bound; partially metabolized in the liver and slowly excreted by the kidneys; urinary elimination is enhanced by acidification of the urine; tissue levels are detectable for months and occasionally years, especially after termination of prolonged therapy

COMMON SIDE EFFECTS
Mild and transient headaches, GI distress, pruritus, visual disturbances (blurring, difficulty in focusing)

SIGNIFICANT ADVERSE REACTIONS
(Usually seen with prolonged high-dosage therapy)

CNS: corneal edema or opacity, retinal changes, scotomata, optic atrophy, vertigo, tinnitus, impaired hearing, fatigue, psychic stimulation, convulsions, psychotic episodes

Cardiovascular: hypotension, ECG changes (T wave inversion, widening of the QRS complex)

Dermatologic: skin eruptions, pruritus, alopecia, dermatoses, skin and mucosal pigmentary changes

Hematologic: blood dyscrasias

Other: vomiting, diarrhea, stomach pain, anorexia, neuromyopathy, muscle weakness

CONTRAINDICATIONS
Retinal damage, visual field changes, pregnancy, prolonged therapy in children, patients receiving bone marrow depressants or hemolytic drugs. *Cautious use* in patients with neurologic or hepatic disease, glucose-6-phosphate dehydrogenase deficiency, blood disorders, psoriasis, porphyria, severe GI disorders, or alcoholism; in infants or small children; and in pregnant or nursing women

INTERACTIONS
Liver toxicity may be increased by combined use of other known hepatotoxic drugs

Gold compounds, anti-inflammatory drugs, and other agents known to cause drug sensitization and dermatitis may increase the dermatologic side effects of the 4-aminoquinolines

Excretion of the 4-aminoquinolines may be enhanced by urinary acidifiers (e.g., ammonium chloride) and reduced by urinary alkalinizers (e.g., sodium bicarbonate)

The action of antipsoriatic drugs may be antagonized by the 4-aminoquinolines, and a severe psoriatic attack can be precipitated

MAO inhibitors can increase the toxicity of 4-aminoquinolines by impairing their hepatic inactivation

The GI absorption of 4-aminoquinolines may be decreased by concurrent administration of kaolin or magnesium trisilicate

NURSING CONSIDERATIONS

Nursing Alerts
- Monitor results of blood counts, which should be obtained regularly during therapy. Drug should be discontinued if any severe abnormality is detected.
- Seek clarification if more than 5 mg/kg IM is prescribed as a single dose for a child because children are very susceptible to adverse reactions.

PATIENT EDUCATION
1. Explain that weekly suppressive treatment is started at least 2 weeks before anticipated exposure and continued for at least 8 weeks after leaving endemic area. The drug should be taken on the same day each week.
2. Instruct patient to take oral drug with meals to minimize GI irritation.
3. Instruct patient to obtain baseline and periodic ophthalmologic examinations during and following prolonged therapy and to promptly report any visual disturbances because retinal damage is frequently irreversible and may progress even after therapy has been terminated.
4. Warn patient to be alert for and to report development of muscular weakness or impaired reflexes, especially during prolonged therapy. Treatment should be discontinued if these develop.
5. Instruct patient to observe for appearance of dermatologic reactions (rash, pruritus, pigmentary changes) and to notify drug prescriber if any occur because dosage should be lowered or an alternative drug should be employed.
6. Inform patient that drug may harmlessly discolor urine yellow-brown.
7. Inform patient that certain strains of *Plasmodium falciparum* are resistant to 4-aminoquinolines and may require treatment with quinine or other appropriate antimalarial drugs.

Table 67-1
4-Aminoquinolines

Drug	Preparations	Usual Dosage Range	Nursing Implications
Chloroquine Aralen	Tablets (phosphate): 250 mg, 500 mg (equivalent to 150 mg, 300 mg of base) Injection (hydrochloride): 50 mg/mL (equivalent to 40 mg/mL base)	**Treatment of acute attack** *Adults* Oral: 600 mg (base) initially followed by 300 mg (base) 6 h, 24 h, and 48 h later IM: 160 mg–200 mg (base) initially; repeat in 6 h; (maximum 800 mg base/24 h) *Children* Oral: 10 mg/kg (base) initially, followed by 5 mg/kg (base) 6 h, 24 h, and 48 h later IM: 5 mg/kg (base) initially; repeat in 6 h (maximum 10 mg/kg base in a 24-h period) **Suppression (oral only)** *Adults* 300 mg (base) once weekly, beginning 2 wk before exposure; continue for 6–8 wk after leaving endemic area *Children* 5 mg/kg (base) weekly as for adults **Treatment of amebiasis** Oral: 600 mg (base) daily for 2 days, then 300 mg (base) daily for 2–3 wk IM: 160 mg–200 mg (base) injected daily for 10–12 days	Indicated for treatment of acute attacks and suppressive therapy of all forms of malaria; also used with an amebicide for treatment of extraintestinal amebiasis (see Chap. 69); for radical cure of vivax malaria, should be combined with primaquine; parenteral therapy should be terminated and oral therapy initiated as soon as possible; children and infants are very susceptible to adverse effects from parenteral chloroquine; do *not* exceed 5 mg/kg base for any single injection in young children; may be used for treating symptoms of rheumatoid arthritis (150 mg of base in a single daily dose) but hydroxychloroquine is preferred
Hydroxychloroquine Sulfate Plaquenil	Tablets: 200 mg (equivalent to 155 mg base)	**Treatment of acute attack** *Adults* 620 mg (base) initially, followed by 310 mg (base) 6 h, 24 h, and 48 h later *Children* 10 mg/kg (base) initially, followed by 5 mg/kg (base) 6 h, 24 h, and 48 h later **Suppression** *Adults and children* 5 mg/kg (base) once weekly beginning 2 wk before exposure (maximum 310 mg base per week); continue for 6–8 wk after leaving endemic area **Rheumatoid arthritis** Initially 400 mg–600 mg/day in a single dose; reduce to 200 mg–400 mg/day when optimum response is observed **Lupus erythematosus** Initially 400 mg once or twice a day; continue for weeks or months, but reduce to 200 mg–400 mg/day when possible	Used for suppression and treatment of all forms of susceptible malaria and for treatment of rheumatoid arthritis and systemic lupus erythematosus; children's dose should never exceed adult dose; radical cure of vivax and malariae malaria requires concomitant therapy with primaquine; several weeks may be required to demonstrate an effect in rheumatoid arthritis; safe use in juvenile arthritis has not been established

Primaquine Phosphate
Primaquine

Primaquine phosphate is a synthetic 8-aminoquinoline derivative that eliminates the tissue or exoerythrocytic forms of the organism, thereby preventing relapse of vivax malaria. Primaquine is not effective alone during an acute attack but is administered in combination with chloroquine or hydroxychloroquine, which destroy the blood or erythrocytic forms.

MECHANISM
Not completely established; appears to produce mitochondrial swelling in parasitic cells, thereby disrupting energy metabolism and impairing protein synthesis; prevents development of blood (erythrocytic) forms of vivax malaria; also active against gametocytes of Plasmodium falciparum

USE
Prevention of relapse (radical cure) of vivax malaria

DOSAGE
Adults: 26.3 mg (equivalent to 15 mg base) daily for 14 days, *or* 79 mg (45 mg base) once a week for 8 weeks
Children: 0.3 mg (base)/kg/day for 14 days *or* 0.9 mg (base)/kg/wk for 8 weeks

FATE
Well absorbed orally; plasma levels are maximum within 2 to 3 hours but fall rapidly thereafter; relatively low levels are found in the lung, liver, heart, skeletal muscles, or brain; rapidly and completely metabolized and excreted largely in the urine; metabolism is impaired by quinacrine (see Interaction)

COMMON SIDE EFFECTS
Epigastric distress

SIGNIFICANT ADVERSE REACTIONS
(Usually with large doses)
Nausea, vomiting, abdominal cramping, headache, impaired visual accommodation, pruritus, granulocytopenia, leukopenia, hemolytic anemia, and methemoglobinemia

CONTRAINDICATIONS
In patients receiving quinacrine (see Interaction), acutely ill patients; rheumatoid arthritis, lupus erythematosus, granulocytopenia, concurrent therapy with potentially hemolytic drugs or bone marrow depressants. *Cautious use* in pregnant women

INTERACTIONS
Quinacrine can potentiate the toxicity of primaquine, presumably by impairing its metabolism

NURSING CONSIDERATIONS

Nursing Alerts
- Assess patient for signs of developing hemolytic anemia (darkened urine, fall in hemoglobin or erythrocyte count, chills, fever, precordial pain). Dark-skinned persons are particularly susceptible to hemolytic anemia owing to a congenital deficiency of erythrocyte glucose-6-phosphate dehydrogenase. Drug should be discontinued if hemolytic anemia occurs.
- Monitor results of blood cell counts and hemoglobin determinations, which should be performed regularly during therapy. Recommended dosages should not be exceeded.

1. Note that primaquine (45 mg base) is available in fixed combination with chloroquine (300 mg base) as Aralen Phosphate with Primaquine Phosphate for prophylaxis of malaria in areas where the disease is endemic. Adult dosage is one tablet weekly during exposure and for 8 weeks after leaving endemic area.

PATIENT EDUCATION
1. Instruct patient to take drug with meals to minimize gastric irritation.
2. Explain to patient with parasitized red cells or one treated for acute attack of vivax malaria that chloroquine should be taken concurrently with primaquine to destroy the erythrocytic parasites.

Pyrimethamine
Daraprim

A folic acid antagonist that interferes with development of fertilized gametes in the mosquito, pyrimethamine is used for prophylaxis of malaria due to susceptible strains. Its slow onset of action reduces its usefulness in treating acute attacks. Commonly given with a fast-acting schizonticide such as chloroquine to provide both transmission control and suppressive (*not* radical) cure.

MECHANISM
Selectively inhibits the enzyme dihydrofolate reductase in protozoal cells, thereby blocking conversion of dihydrofolic acid to tetrahydrofolic acid, an essential step in protozoal cell metabolism; reduces sporogony (i.e., reproduction of spores) in the mosquito but does not destroy gametocytes; plasmodial resistance can develop rapidly when pyrimethamine is used alone

USES
Prophylaxis of malaria due to susceptible strains of *Plasmodia* (usually in combination with a 4-aminoquinoline during acute attacks)
Treatment of toxoplasmosis, in combination with a sulfonamide

DOSAGE
Prophylaxis
Adults and children over 10 years: 25 mg once a week
Children 4 years through 9 years: 12.5 mg once a week
Children under 4 years: 6.25 mg (*or* 0.5 mg/kg) once a week
(Drug is given for at least 10 weeks after leaving the exposure area)
Treatment of Acute Attacks
With a rapid-acting schizonticide, for example chloroquine: 25 mg/day for 2 days, then 12.5 mg to 25 mg/wk
Toxoplasmosis
Adults: 50 mg to 75 mg/day with 1 g to 4 g/day of a sulfapyrimidine for 1 to 3 weeks; reduce dose by one half and continue for another 4 to 5 weeks
Children: 1 mg/kg/day in two divided doses with appropriate dose of a sulfonamide for 2 to 4 days; reduce by one half and continue for 30 days

FATE
Well absorbed orally; plasma half-life is about 4 days, but effective levels are maintained for up to 2 weeks; excreted mainly in the urine, slowly over a period of several weeks

COMMON SIDE EFFECTS
Gastric upset, skin rash

SIGNIFICANT ADVERSE REACTIONS
(Usually with larger doses, as used for toxoplasmosis) Anorexia, vomiting, atrophic glossitis, megaloblastic anemia, leukopenia, thrombocytopenia, pancytopenia, hemolytic anemia in patients with a glucose-6-phosphate dehydrogenase deficiency, convulsions with overdosage

CONTRAINDICATIONS
No absolute contraindications. *Cautious use* in patients with convulsive disorders or glucose-6-phosphate dehydrogenase deficiency, and in pregnant women

INTERACTIONS
The action of pyrimethamine can be impaired by folic acid or para-aminobenzoic acid (PABA)

Pyrimethamine can increase quinine blood levels by competing for protein-binding sites

NURSING CONSIDERATION

Nursing Alert
- Monitor patient treated for toxoplasmosis very closely because the dose used is 10 to 20 times the dosage used for malaria, and it approaches the toxic level. Recommended dosage for malaria suppression should not be exceeded because incidence of untoward reactions is significantly higher at elevated dosage levels.

PATIENT EDUCATION
1. Instruct patient to take drug with food to minimize stomach upset.
2. Caution patient to report signs of possible developing blood dyscrasia immediately (fever, sore throat, mucosal ulceration, bruising or bleeding).
3. Explain that weekly blood counts (including platelet counts) are required during high-dosage therapy because the drug should be discontinued if hematologic abnormalities occur. Folinic acid (leucovorin) may be given (3 mg–9 mg IM daily for 3 days) to return depressed platelet or white blood cell count to normal.

Sulfadoxine and Pyrimethamine
Fansidar

A fixed combination of sulfadoxine (500 mg) and pyrimethamine (25 mg) is available for prophylaxis of malaria and for treatment of susceptible strains of *Plasmodia* resistant to chloroquine.

MECHANISM
The two drugs block sequential enzymatic steps involved in the biosynthesis of folinic acid, a necessary intermediate in the parasitic cellular synthesis of purines, pyrimidines, and certain amino acids. Thus, protein and nucleic acid production is impaired in the plasmodial organisms

USES
Treatment of *Plasmodium falciparum* malaria in chloroquine-resistant cases

Prophylaxis of malaria in travelers to areas where chloroquine-resistant *P. falciparum* is endemic

DOSAGE
Acute attacks

Adults: 2 to 3 tablets (500 mg/25 mg) as a single dose, either alone or in sequence with quinine or primaquine, followed by primaquine for 2 weeks to prevent relapse

Children: 1/2 to 2 tablets, according to age, given as outlined for adults

Prophylaxis

Once a week or once every two weeks, according to the schedule below; give first dose 1 to 2 days before entering endemic area, continue during the stay, and then for 4 to 6 weeks following return

	Weekly	Biweekly
Adults	1 tablet	2 tablets
Children (9 yr–14 yr)	3/4 tablet	1 1/2 tablet
Children (4 yr–8 yr)	1/2 tablet	1 tablet
Children (under 4 yr)	1/4 tablet	1/2 tablet

NOTE
If folate deficiency develops during therapy, discontinue drug and administer folinic acid (Leucovorin), 3 mg to 9 mg/day IM for 3 days or longer to restore depressed platelet or white cell count

FATE
Both drugs are well absorbed orally; peak serum concentrations are attained in 2 to 8 hours; elimination half-life is prolonged, averaging 7 days for sulfadoxine and 4.5 days for pyrimethamine

SIGNIFICANT ADVERSE REACTIONS
See sulfonamides (Chap. 57) and pyrimethamine (this chapter)

NOTE
Although all adverse reactions reported for the sulfonamides and pyrimethamine are *theoretically* possible with Fansidar, not all have been documented thus far for this combination drug.

Rarely, toxic epidermal necrolysis, Stevens–Johnson syndrome, leukopenia, fulminant hepatic necrosis

CONTRAINDICATIONS
Megaloblastic anemia due to folate deficiency; sulfonamide hypersensitivity; pregnancy, and lactation; in infants less than 2 months of age. *Cautious use* in patients with renal or hepatic impairment, folate deficiency, severe allergy, or bronchial asthma

INTERACTIONS
See sulfonamides (Chap. 57) and pyrimethamine (this chapter)

PATIENT EDUCATION
See also discussion of individual drugs.
1. Help patient develop plan to maintain adequate fluid intake to prevent crystalluria or stone formation.

2. Instruct patient to notify drug prescriber at first sign of fever, sore throat, abnormal bruising, pallor, jaundice, rash, pruritus, pharyngitis, or glossitis, possible indications of developing toxicity.
3. Because leukopenia may occur, explain to patient receiving prophylactic treatment for 2 months or longer that drug will be discontinued if the count of any formed blood element is significantly reduced or if active bacterial or fungal infection develops.
4. Encourage woman with childbearing potential to practice contraception during therapy.

Quinacrine

Atabrine

Although quinacrine is an effective antimalarial, its use in malaria has been supplanted largely by more active and less toxic drugs. It has been used for both treatment and suppression of malaria, inasmuch as it destroys both erythrocytic forms of vivax, falciparum, and quartan malaria as well as gametocytes of vivax and quartan malaria. Quinacrine is ineffective, however, against falciparum gametocytes and all sporozoites. The drug may also be used in the treatment of tapeworm infestations and giardiasis, and this application is considered in Chapter 68.

MECHANISM

Not completely established; may interfere with nucleic acid synthesis by blocking DNA replication and interfering with transcription of RNA

USES

Treatment and suppression of susceptible strains of *Plasmodia*
Treatment of giardiasis and cestodiasis (tapeworm infestations; see Chap. 68)

DOSAGE

Treatment of Malaria
Adults: 200 mg (with 1 g sodium bicarbonate) every 6 hours for five doses, then 100 mg three times a day for 6 days
Children: 100 mg to 200 mg three times a day the first day, then 100 mg one or two times a day for 6 days

Suppression of Malaria
Adults: 100 mg/day for 1 to 3 months
Children: 50 mg/day for 1 to 3 months

FATE

Readily absorbed from GI tract; maximum plasma levels occur in 1 to 3 hours; highly protein-bound; widely distributed in the body and binds to many tissues; slowly excreted by the kidneys, and cumulation of drug in the body is gradual

COMMON SIDE EFFECTS

Nausea, abdominal cramping, diarrhea, headache, dizziness, and yellowing of the urine, skin, and nails

SIGNIFICANT ADVERSE REACTIONS

GI: vomiting
Dermatologic: skin eruptions, contact dermatitis, exfoliative dermatitis
CNS: nervousness, vertigo, irritability, insomnia, emotional changes, nightmares, transient psychosis, convulsions (rare)
Hematologic: (rare) aplastic anemia, agranulocytosis, bone marrow depression
Other: hepatitis, corneal edema or deposits

CONTRAINDICATIONS

Psoriasis, porphyria, and combined use with primaquine (see Interactions). *Cautious use* in patients with hepatic or renal disease, alcoholism, history of psychosis, glucose-6-phosphate dehydrogenase deficiency, during pregnancy, and in small children and patients over 60

INTERACTIONS

Quinacrine increases the toxicity of primaquine and may potentiate the effects of other hepatotoxic drugs
Quinacrine may produce a disulfiram-like reaction with alcohol (see Chap. 78)
The anticoagulant effects of heparin, an acidic drug, may be antagonized by quinacrine, a basic drug
The adverse effects of quinacrine can be potentiated by MAO inhibitors, which reduce its hepatic metabolism
Urinary alkalinizers can increase the effects of quinacrine by delaying its urinary excretion

PATIENT EDUCATION

1. Inform patient that drug should be taken daily for at least 1 to 2 months to effect suppression of malaria.
2. Instruct patient and family to be alert for signs of CNS toxicity (emotional instability, insomnia, irritability, vertigo) and to notify drug prescriber if they occur because dosage should be reduced or drug should be discontinued.
3. Caution patient that periodic blood counts may be required during prolonged therapy and that the drug will be discontinued if any significant abnormality is detected.
4. Instruct patient to promptly report onset of any visual changes and to obtain ophthalmologic examinations at regular intervals during prolonged treatment.

Quinine Sulfate

Legatrin, Quinamm, Quine, Quiphile, Strema
(CAN) Novoquinine

A natural alkaloid from the bark of the cinchona tree, quinine is an effective antimalarial drug that has been largely replaced by more active and less toxic drugs. However, it is used in conjunction with pyrimethamine and sulfadiazine or tetracycline for treatment of *Plasmodia* resistant to other antimalarials, especially chloroquine-resistant falciparum strains. Owing to its skeletal-muscle relaxant effects, it is also occasionally used for relief of nocturnal leg cramps.

MECHANISM

Not completely established; may inhibit protein synthesis in malarial organisms by complexing with parasite DNA and may interfere with cellular metabolism; suppresses oxygen uptake and carbohydrate metabolism of *Plasmodia*; actively schizonticidal for all forms of malaria and gametocidal for *Plasmodium vivax* and *Plasmodium malariae* strains; also possesses an analgesic, antipyretic, skeletal-muscle relaxant, oxytocic, and hypoprothrombinemic action; exerts muscle-relaxing action by increasing refractory period of muscle cells, decreasing excitability of the motor end plate, and altering distribution of calcium within the muscle fiber

USES

Adjunctive treatment of chloroquine-resistant falciparum malaria, along with pyrimethamine and sulfadiazine or tetracycline and in combination with other antimalarials for radical cure of relapsing vivax malaria

Relief of nocturnal leg cramps

DOSAGE
Malaria
Adults: 650 mg every 8 hours for 10 to 14 days
Children: 25 mg/kg/day in divided doses every 8 for 10 days to 14 days
Leg Cramps
260 mg to 300 mg at bedtime

FATE
Rapidly absorbed orally; peak plasma levels occur in 1 hour to 3 hours; highly (70%–80%) protein-bound; widely distributed in the body, except to the CNS; metabolized by the liver and excreted in the urine, largely as metabolites with some (10%) unchanged drug

COMMON SIDE-EFFECTS
Cinchonism (tinnitus, headache, dizziness, GI upset, visual disturbances)—frequently seen at full therapeutic doses

SIGNIFICANT ADVERSE REACTIONS
CNS: temporary deafness, fever, apprehension, restlessness, excitement, confusion, delirium, syncope, hypothermia, convulsions
Ophthalmic: photophobia, amblyopia, scotomata, diplopia, mydriasis, altered color perception, optic atrophy
GI: vomiting, stomach cramps, diarrhea
Allergic/hypersensitivity: rash, pruritus, flushing, urticaria, facial edema, asthmatic-like reaction
Hematologic: hypoprothrombinemia, hemolytic anemia, thrombocytopenia, agranulocytosis
Other (usually observed with very large doses): hypotension, respiratory depression, muscle paralysis

CONTRAINDICATIONS
Pregnancy, myasthenia gravis, glucose-6-phosphate dehydrogenase deficiency, tinnitus, and optic neuritis. *Cautious use* in patients with cardiac arrhythmias (quinine has cardiovascular actions similar to quinidine), angina, renal impairment, or a history of allergic reactions; and in nursing mothers

INTERACTIONS
Pyrimethamine may increase blood levels of quinine, possibly leading to toxic effects

Quinine can enhance the effects of skeletal-muscle relaxants and increase their respiratory depressant action

Quinine may potentiate the effects of oral anticoagulants through its hypoprothrombinemic action

The urinary excretion of quinine can be reduced by urinary alkalinizers (e.g., sodium bicarbonate, acetazolamide)

Aluminum-containing antacids can delay or reduce the oral absorption of quinine

Owing to its similarity to quinidine, quinine may increase plasma levels of digoxin and digitoxin if given concurrently, as has been documented for quinidine

NURSING CONSIDERATION
1. In interpreting laboratory test results, be aware that quinine may interfere with 17-hydroxycorticosteroid determinations and may cause elevated 17-ketogenic steroid values.

PATIENT EDUCATION
1. Instruct patient to take drug with food and to avoid breaking the capsule because the drug powder tastes very bitter.
2. Advise patient to exercise caution in driving or operating other machinery because blurred vision or dizziness may occur.
3. Teach patient how to recognize and report symptoms of cinchonism (tinnitus, dizziness, visual disturbances, headache, GI distress), and inform patient that dosage will be reduced or drug will be discontinued if symptoms occur. Effects usually disappear quickly when drug is stopped.

Selected Bibliography

Bruce-Chwatt LJ et al: Chemotherapy of Malaria, 2nd ed, World Health Organization, 1986

Cohen S (ed): Malaria. A symposium. Br Med Bull 38:115, 1982

Davidson DE, Ager AL, Brown JL et al: New tissue schizonticidal antimalarial drugs. Bull WHO 59:463, 1981

Drugs for parasitic infections. Med Lett Drugs Ther 26:27, 1984

Ellis CJ, Chiodini PL: The treatment of falciparum malaria. J Antimicrob Chemother 13:311, 1984

Fitch CD: Mode of action of antimalarial drugs. In Malaria and the Red Cell, p 222. Ciba Foundation Symposium 94. London, Pitman, 1983

Goldsmith RS, Heyneman D (eds): Tropical Medicine, and Parasitology. Appleton and Lange, 1988

Olansky AJ: Antimalarials and ophthalmologic safety. J Am Acad Dermatol 6:19, 1982

Wyler DJ: Malaria: Resurgence, resistance, and research. N Engl J Med 308:875 and 934 (2 parts), 1983

Wyler DJ: Plasmodium species (Malaria). In Mandell GL, Douglas RG, Bennett JE (eds): Principles and Practice of Infectious Diseases, 2nd ed, p 1514. John Wiley & Sons, New York, 1985

SUMMARY. ANTIMALARIAL AGENTS

Drug	Preparations	Usual Dosage Range
4-Aminoquinolines	*See* Table 67-1	
Primaquine Primaquine	Tablets: 26.3 mg (equivalent to 15 mg base)	Adults: 26.3 mg daily for 14 days *or* 79 mg once a week for 8 wk Children: 0.3 mg (base)/kg/day for 14 days *or* 0.9 mg (base)/kg/wk for 8 wk
Pyrimethamine Daraprim	Tablets: 25 mg	*Prophylaxis* Adults: 25 mg once a week Children: 6.25 mg–12.5 mg once a week *Acute attacks* 25 mg/day for 2 days with a rapid-acting schizonticide, then 12.5 mg–25 mg/wk *Toxoplasmosis* Adults: 50 mg–75 mg/day for 1–3 wk, then one half dose for another 4–5 wk Children: 1 mg/kg/day for 2–4 days; then one half dose for another 30 days (given with an appropriate sulfonamide)
Sulfadoxine and Pyrimethamine Fansidar	Tablets: 500 mg sulfadoxine/25 mg pyrimethamine	*Acute attacks* Adults: 2–3 tablets as a single dose followed by primaquine for 2 wk Children: ½–2 tablets, as outlined for adults *Prophylaxis* Adults: 1 tablet/wk *or* 2 tablets every other week during and for 4–6 wk following exposure Children: ¼–¾ tablet/wk *or* ½–1½ tablets every other week during and for 4–6 wk following exposure
Quinacrine Atabrine	Tablets: 100 mg	*Treatment* Adults: 200 mg with 1 g sodium bicarbonate every 6 h for 5 doses, then 100 mg 3 times a day for 6 days Children: 100 mg–200 mg 3 times a day first day, then 100 mg 1–2 times a day for 6 days *Suppression* Adults: 100 mg/day Children: 50 mg/day
Quinine Legatrin, Quinamm, Quine, Quiphile, Strema	Capsules: 130 mg, 195 mg, 200 mg, 300 mg, 325 mg Tablets: 260 mg, 325 mg Suspension: 110 mg/5 mL	*Malaria* Adults: 650 mg every 8 h for 10–14 days Children: 25 mg/kg/day in divided doses every 8 h for 10–14 days *Leg cramps* 260 mg–300 mg at bedtime

ANTHELMINTICS

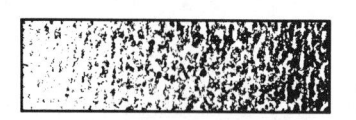

Anthelmintics are drugs used to facilitate the expulsion from the body of parasitic worms or helminths. Helminthiasis or worm infection is the most common disease in the world today. While endemic in many tropical countries, helminthiasis is by no means limited to these areas but is found in increasing numbers in many temperate climates as well. Poor living conditions, inadequate sanitation, lack of careful hygiene, and malnutrition are major contributory factors to the high incidence of helminthiasis in underdeveloped countries.

Helminthic infections are caused by two principal types of worms, roundworms (nematodes) and flatworms (cestodes, trematodes). Table 68-1 lists the major species of each type of worm and the drugs that are most effective against each helminth. Most nematodal infections are confined to the intestinal tract and include parasites such as roundworms, pinworms, whipworms, hookworms, and threadworms. However, tissue-invading nematodes such as filarial worms and pork roundworms (trichinella) can enter body organs, including the heart, liver, lungs, skeletal muscle, and CNS, in which case eradication is often quite difficult and more serious sequelae can ensue.

Cestodal infestations can occur with several types of tapeworms, the most common being the beef tapeworm (*Taenia saginata*). These infections are usually localized in the GI tract, although larvae of the pork tapeworm (*Taenia solium*) can occasionally gain access to the systemic circulation, resulting in inflammatory and granulomatous reactions in other organs (e.g., cysticercosis).

Tissue-invading trematodes or blood flukes are responsible for a chronic infection termed *schistosomiasis*, or bilharziasis, which is widespread throughout Africa and parts of South America. Complications may range from minor conditions such as rash, itching, or headache to severe damage to vital organs. Other trematodes include the lung, liver, and intestinal flukes.

Accurate diagnosis of the invading helminth is essential for the successful treatment of the infestation, because many anthelmintic drugs are highly specific for a particular infection. Diagnosis is usually accomplished by obtaining a stool specimen or removing worms from the outer anal area with cellophane tape. Once the type of worm involved has been determined, selection of an appropriate anthelmintic drug can be made. Although a large number of different kinds of chemicals have been used in the past for treating the different types of worm infestations, they have been replaced by fewer but more effective and less toxic agents. Most of these newer anthelmintic drugs are not appreciably absorbed following oral administration, and thus they attain high levels in the GI tract while systemic toxicity is largely avoided. Another advantage of certain of the newer drugs (mebendazole, thiabendazole, praziquantel) is that they have a broad spectrum of action and thus are effective against several types of helminths. These drugs are particularly valuable in mixed infections or when the diagnosis is uncertain.

An important aspect of successful anthelmintic therapy is proper patient education with regard to personal hygiene. Because many worms are primarily transmitted by transfer of eggs (ova) via hands, food, or contaminated articles such as toilet paper, towels, clothes, or sheets, it is imperative that patients be instructed in the necessary procedures for minimizing spread of the infection. Important measures that should be stressed are careful washing of hands following each bowel movement; daily or more frequent changes of underwear, towels, and bedding; and avoidance of scratching of the perianal area. Nail biting should also be strongly discouraged. Diagnosis of pinworm infection in one family member makes it imperative that all other family members be tested as well, because this infection commonly affects an entire family.

The principal drugs used to treat nematodal and cestodal infections (see Table 68-1) are discussed in detail in this chapter. Other anthelmintic drugs, such as niridazole, bithional, metrifonate, stibocaptate, and suramin, are used principally for certain filarial or trematodal infections and are currently available only upon request from the Parasitic Disease Drug Service of the Centers for Disease Control. These agents are reviewed briefly in Table 68-2. Still other drugs that are occasionally used in certain helminthic infections (e.g., emetine, chloroquine, paromomycin) have additional therapeutic actions as well and are reviewed elsewhere in this book.

Antimony Compounds

Antimony compounds were major antischistosomal drugs for many years, but they are seldom used today because of their toxicity and the availability of other more effective drugs. Antimony potassium tartrate (tartar emetic) is a highly effective drug for the treatment of most schistosomal infections, but because of its high toxicity (e.g., dizziness, vomiting, tachycardia, arrhythmias, renal damage, blood dyscrasias), and the necessity for IV administration, it is now seldom employed. Antimony sodium dimercaptosuccinate (stibocaptate) is an alternative drug in the treatment of schistosomal infections (see Table 68-1) and is available as Astiban from the Centers for Disease Control in Atlanta. Stibocaptate is stable in solution, can be administered IM, and is considerably less toxic than antimony potassium tartrate. The dose of stibocaptate is 40 mg/kg for *Schistosoma haematobium* and *Schistosoma mansoni* infections and 50 mg/kg for *Schistosoma japonicum* infections. The total dosage is divided into 5 equal parts given once a week for 5 weeks. The course of therapy can be repeated in 2 months if necessary.

Diethylcarbamazine
Hetrazan

MECHANISM

Appears to immobilize small worms (microfilaria), increasing their susceptibility to phagocytosis by fixed tissue macrophages; does not appear to alter phagocytosis in the bloodstream; considered the drug of choice for filarial infections

USES

Treatment of filarial worm infections (Bancroft's filariasis, loiasis, onchocerciasis)
Treatment of roundworm infections (ascariasis)
Treatment of tropical eosinophilia

DOSAGE
Filarial Worm Infections
2 mg/kg orally three times a day for 3 to 4 weeks

Table 68-1
Helminthiasis Classification and Treatment

Class of Helminth	Disorder	Suggested Drugs of Choice Primary	Secondary
Nematodes			
Roundworm *Ascaris lumbricoides*	Ascariasis	mebendazole, pyrantel pamoate	piperazine, thiabendazole, diethylcarbamazine
Hookworm *Necator americanus* *Ancylostoma duodenale*	Uncinariasis	mebendazole	pyrantel pamoate, thiabendazole
Whipworm *Trichuris trichiura*	Trichuriasis	mebendazole	thiabendazole
Threadworm *Strongyloides stercoralis*	Strongyloidiasis	thiabendazole	mebendazole
Cutaneous larva migrans *Ancylostoma braziliense*	Creeping eruption	thiabendazole	
Capillary worm *Capillaria philippinensis*	Capillariasis	mebendazole	thiabendazole
Pinworm *Enterobius vermicularis*	Enterobiasis	mebendazole, pyrantel pamoate	thiabendazole, piperazine
Pork roundworm *Trichinella spiralis*	Trichiniasis, trichinosis	corticosteroids	thiabendazole, mebendazole
Filarial worms *Wuchereria bancrofti* *Brugia malayi* *Loa loa* *Onchocerca volvulus*	Filariasis Filariasis Loiasis Onchocerciasis	diethylcarbamazine diethylcarbamazine diethylcarbamazine diethylcarbamazine and suramin[a]	mebendazole
Guinea worm *Dracunculus medinensis*	Dracunculiasis	niridazole,[a] metronidazole	mebendazole, thiabendazole
Rat lungworm *Angiostrongylus cantonensis*	Angiostrongyliasis	thiabendazole	mebendazole
Cestodes			
Tapeworms Beef *Taenia saginata*	Taeniasis	niclosamide	praziquantel
Pork *Taenia solium*	Taeniasis	niclosamide, praziquantel	paromomycin, mebendazole
Fish *Diphyllobothrium latum*	Diphyllobothriasis	niclosamide	dichlorophen, praziquantel, paromomycin
Dwarf *Hymenolepsis nana*	Hymenolepiasis	niclosamide, praziquantel	mebendazole, paromomycin
Trematodes			
Blood flukes *Schistosoma haematobium* *Schistosoma mansoni*	Schistosomiasis (Bilharziasis) Schistosomiasis	praziquantel, metrifonate praziquantel, oxamniquine	niridazole,[a] stibocaptate[a] niridazole,[a] stibocaptate[a]
Blood flukes *Schistosoma japonicum* *Schistosoma mekongi*	Schistosomiasis Schistosomiasis	praziquantel, niridazole[a] praziquantel	stibocaptate[a] niridazole[a]
Lung flukes *Paragonimus westermani*	Paragonimiasis	praziquantel	chloroquine, bithionol[a]
Liver flukes *Opisthorchis viverrini* *Fasciola hepatica* *Clonorchis sinensis*	Opisthorchiasis Fascioliasis Clonorchiasis	praziquantel praziquantel, bithionol[a] praziquantel	mebendazole metronidazole, emetine mebendazole
Intestinal fluke *Fasciolopsis buski*	Fasciolopsiasis	niclosamide, praziquantel	tetrachloroethylene, hexylresorcinol

[a] Available only by request from the Parasitic Disease Drug Service, Centers for Disease Control, Atlanta, GA 30333.

NOTE

Above dosage can be given for 3 to 5 days to treat large numbers of patients known to harbor microfilariae, as a public health measure.

Roundworm Infections

Adults: 13 mg/kg/day in a single dose for 7 days

Children: 6 mg/kg to 10 mg/kg 3 times a day for 7 days to 10 days)

Tropical Eosinophilia

13 mg/kg/day for 4 to 7 days

FATE

Well absorbed orally; peak blood levels occur in 3 to 4 hours; widely distributed in the body; excreted primarily in the urine, both as metabolites and unchanged drug

COMMON SIDE EFFECTS

Headache, weakness, lassitude, malaise, nausea, joint pain, and leukocytosis

In patients with onchocerciasis, facial edema, pruritus of the eyes, and skin rash are common.

SIGNIFICANT ADVERSE REACTIONS

Vomiting, skin rash, lymphadenopathy, tachycardia, visual disturbances, GI upset, abdominal pain, anorexia, fever, and severe allergic reactions due to release of helminthic proteins

CONTRAINDICATIONS

No absolute contraindications. *Cautious use* in persons with a history of allergic reactions and in debilitated or malnourished patients

NURSING CONSIDERATIONS

Nursing Alert

- Monitor patient for development of allergic reactions, especially during treatment for onchocerciasis. Have antihistamines, epinephrine, and corticosteroids available in case of severe allergic response. Oral antihistamines may be given during the first several days of therapy to reduce the incidence of allergic reactions.

1. Note that when diethylcarbamazine is used to treat onchocerciasis, it is usually combined with suramin to kill the adult worms as well as the microfilaria.

PATIENT EDUCATION

1. Teach patient personal hygiene measures that help minimize the danger of reinfection.

Mebendazole

Vermox

MECHANISM

Blocks uptake and utilization of glucose by worms, thereby depleting endogenous glycogen, reducing energy supply below that necessary for survival; worms are cleared from the GI tract over several days

USES

Treatment of single or mixed whipworm, pinworm, roundworm, and hookworm infestations

Alternative therapy for trichinosis, onchocerciasis, taeniasis, and infestation with liver flukes

DOSAGE

Whipworm, Hookworm, Roundworm

Adults and children: 100 mg twice a day for 3 consecutive days; if necessary repeat in 2 weeks

Pinworm

Adults and children: 100 mg as single dose

FATE

Only 5% to 10% of an oral dose is absorbed; approximately 2% of an administered dose is excreted in the urine, both as unchanged drug and a metabolite; the remainder is excreted in the feces

SIGNIFICANT ADVERSE REACTIONS

(Usually with massive infections) Abdominal pain, nausea, vomiting, and diarrhea due to expulsion of worms; fever; neutropenia (high doses)

CONTRAINDICATIONS

Pregnancy. *Cautious use* in children under 2 years of age

NURSING CONSIDERATIONS

1. Expect a second course of therapy to be initiated if patient is not cured 3 weeks after initial treatment.
2. Note that fasting or post-treatment purging is not required with mebendazole.

PATIENT EDUCATION

1. Inform patient that tablets may be chewed, swallowed whole, or crushed and mixed with food.

Niclosamide

Niclocide

MECHANISM

Inhibits oxidative phosphorylation in the mitochondria of cestodal parasites and may also stimulate ATPase; the head (scolex) and proximal segments of the worm are killed on contact, and the parasite is released from its attachment on the intestinal wall; the partially digested worms are then expelled in the feces; drug does not appear to produce any hematologic, renal, or hepatic abnormalities

USE

Treatment of cestodal (tapeworm) infections—see Table 68-1 (drug of choice)

DOSAGE

(Tablets are thoroughly chewed and swallowed with a little water)

Taenia/Diphyllobothrium Infections

Adults: 2 g in a single dose

Children: 1.0 g to 1.5 g in a single dose depending on weight

NOTE

In the treatment of *pork* tapeworm infections, a purgative *must be given* within 1 to 2 hours after niclosamide, because the lethal action of the drug is against the adult worm but not the ova, which can be liberated into the lumen of the gut. Subsequently, they may be absorbed and may invade other tissues, (muscles, liver, lung, brain), leading to a condition termed *cysticercosis,* which can produce muscle pain, weakness, nervousness, convulsions, and paralysis.

Table 68-2
Anthelmintic Drugs Available by Request to Centers for Disease Control[a]

Drug	Principal Indications	Preparation	Usual Dosage Range	Remarks
Bithionol Actamer, Bitin, Lorothidol	Lung fluke (*Paragonimus*) and liver fluke (*Fasciola*) infections	Powder	30 mg/kg–50 mg/kg orally in 2 or 3 divided doses on alternate days for 10 to 15 days	Alternative drug for treating lung fluke infections; GI side effects are common; use with *caution* in children under 8 years of age
Metrifonate Bilarcil	Schistosomiasis	Tablet: 100 mg	7.5 mg/kg–10 mg/kg as a single dose; repeat twice at 2-week intervals	One of the drugs of choice for *Schistosoma haematobium* infections; *not* effective against *S. mansoni* or *S. japonicum*; well tolerated; minimal side effects
Niridazole Ambilhar	Schistosomiasis, guinea worm infections	Tablets: 100 mg, 500 mg	25 mg/kg/day orally in 2 or 3 divided doses for 7 days	Primary drug for *Schistosoma japonicum* infections and alternative drug for other schistosomal infections; high incidence of side effects (70%), especially GI and allergic; CNS toxicity can occur, especially at high doses; patients must be hospitalized; generally contraindicated in cardiac, liver, or renal disease, hypertension, epilepsy, psychiatric disorders, GI ulceration, or hemorrhage
Stibocaptate Astiban	Schistosomiasis	Powder for injection: 0.5 g/vial (5 mL saline added to prepare a 10% solution)	40 mg/kg–50 mg/kg total dose divided into 5 injections given at weekly intervals	Highly effective in treating schistosomal infections; antimony-containing compound with high incidence of side effects but less toxic than antimony potassium tartrate; do *not* use in the presence of bacterial or viral infections, hepatic, renal, or cardiac insufficiency, or anemia
Suramin Antrypol, Bayer 205, Belganyl, Germanin, Moranyl, Naganol, Naphuride	Onchocerciasis (filarial worm infection), African trypanosomiasis (sleeping sickness)	Powder for injection: 0.5 g/vial, 1 g/vial	1 g by *slow* IV injection weekly for 4 to 7 weeks	Used to eradicate adult filariae of *Onchocerca volvulus* following treatment with diethylcarbamazine to eliminate microfilariae; also effective in early stages of African trypanosomiasis before CNS involvement; proteinuria can occur; avoid extravasation because severe pain can result

[a] Parasitic Disease Drug Service, Bureau of Epidemiology, Centers for Disease Control, Atlanta, GA 30333.

Hymenolepis Nana (Dwarf Tapeworm) Infections

Adults: 2 g as a single dose daily for 7 days

Children 75 lb and over: 1.5 g the first day, then 1 g daily for 6 days

Children under 75 lb: 1.0 g the first day, then 0.5 g daily for 6 days

FATE

Not absorbed from the GI tract, excreted in the feces

COMMON SIDE EFFECTS

Nausea, vomiting, anorexia, diarrhea

SIGNIFICANT ADVERSE REACTIONS

GI: constipation, rectal irritation or bleeding
CNS: headache, drowsiness, dizziness
Dermatologic: skin rash
Other: fever, oral irritation, bad taste in mouth, sweating, palpitations, weakness, backache, irritability, alopecia

CONTRAINDICATIONS

No absolute contraindications. *Cautious use* in pregnant or nursing women and in children under 2

NURSING CONSIDERATION

1. If *Taenia* or *Diphyllobothrium* segments or ova are still present in the stool 7 days after treatment, expect treatment to be repeated. A negative stool for at least 3 months is the criterion for cure.

PATIENT EDUCATION

1. Instruct patient to take tablets following a light meal (e.g., breakfast). For young children, tablets may be crushed and mixed with a little water to form a paste.
2. Advise patient to use a mild laxative, if needed, to relieve constipation.
3. With patient treated for *Hymenolepis* infection, emphasize the importance of continuing treatment for the entire 7 days, as recommended, to ensure complete destruction of both mature and larval stages of the worm.

Oxamniquine

Vansil

MECHANISM

Not completely established; may cause a shift in worms from the mesentery to the liver, where they die; appears to be more toxic to male schistosomes than to females, but surviving female worms no longer lay eggs

USE

Treatment of all stages (acute, subacute, chronic) of *Schistosoma mansoni* infections

DOSAGE

Adults: 12 mg/kg to 15 mg/kg as a single oral dose

Children under 30 kg: 20 mg/kg in two divided doses with a 2 to 8-hour interval between doses

FATE

Readily absorbed orally; peak serum concentration in 1 to 2 hours; plasma half-life is about 1 to 3 hours; extensively metabolized and excreted in the urine, largely as inactive metabolites

COMMON SIDE EFFECTS

Drowsiness, dizziness

SIGNIFICANT ADVERSE REACTIONS

Headache, anorexia, abdominal pain, nausea, vomiting, urticaria, liver enzyme elevations, and rarely, convulsions

CONTRAINDICATIONS

No absolute contraindications. *Cautious use* in patients with a history of convulsive disorders and in pregnant or nursing women

PATIENT EDUCATION

1. Instruct patient to take drug with food to improve tolerance.
2. Urge patient to exercise caution in performing hazardous tasks because drug causes drowsiness and dizziness in about a third of patients.
3. Inform patient that drug may color urine a harmless orange-red.

Piperazine

Vermizine,
(CAN) Entacyl

MECHANISM

Produces flaccid paralysis in worms, possibly by blocking acetylcholine, resulting in expulsion of the helminths by normal peristaltic movement

USE

Alternative treatment of roundworm and pinworm infestations

DOSAGE

Roundworm

Adults: 3.5 g once daily for 2 days

Children: 75 mg/kg/day as a single dose for 2 days; may repeat in 1 week in severe infections; if repeat therapy is impractical or for mass therapy as a public health measure, 150 mg/kg may be given in a single dose

Pinworm

Adults and children: 65 mg/kg/day for 7 consecutive days (maximum daily dose 2.5 g)

FATE

Oral absorption is variable; a portion of the absorbed drug is metabolized and excreted in the urine; remainder is eliminated in the feces or urine as unchanged drug

SIGNIFICANT ADVERSE REACTIONS

(Usually with high doses)

GI: nausea, vomiting, diarrhea, abdominal cramping
CNS: headache, vertigo, muscular weakness, hyporeflexia, blurred vision, paresthesias, tremors, choreiform movements, convulsions, impaired memory, EEG abnormalities, worsening of epileptic seizures
Allergic/hypersensitivity: fever, urticaria, arthralgia, purpura, lacrimation, eczematous skin eruptions, rhinorrhea, bronchospasm, erythema multiforme

CONTRAINDICATIONS

Renal or hepatic impairment, convulsive disorders. *Cautious use* in patients with anemia, severe malnutrition, or neurologic disorders, and in pregnant women

INTERACTION

Piperazine may increase the severity of extrapyramidal reactions caused by phenothiazine administration

NURSING CONSIDERATIONS

1. Note that dietary restrictions, enemas, or laxatives are not required.
2. Note that piperazine is available as the citrate salt but is converted to the hexahydrate in solution. Dosage is therefore given in hexahydrate equivalents.

PATIENT EDUCATION

1. Explain the importance of adhering to prescribed dosage regimen. If recommended dose or duration of therapy is exceeded, potential for neurotoxicity is increased, especially in children.
2. Teach patient how to recognize and report CNS, GI, and hypersensitivity reactions.
3. Teach patient interventions to prevent spread of infection or reinfection (e.g., careful hand washing; daily changes of underwear, towels, and bedding; bathing; proper disposal of fecal matter) because pinworm infection is easily transmitted.

Praziquantel

Biltricide

Praziquantel is an anthelmintic that exhibits a rather broad spectrum of activity and a low overall incidence of serious adverse effects. It is considered a first-line drug in schistosomal infections, and it is also active against other trematodes as well as cestodes (see Table 68-1). In addition, praziquantel may also be useful in the treatment of cysticercosis, a serious complication of cestodal infections in which the larvae of *Taenia* invade other organs of the body, leading to fatigue, muscle pain, weakness, nervousness, and possibly convulsions or general paralysis.

MECHANISM

Increases cell membrane permeability of susceptible worms, altering intracellular calcium and leading to paralysis; also produces vacuolization and subsequent disintegration of the surface tegumentum of the parasite, leading to death of the schistosomal organism

USES

Treatment of schistosomal infections (i.e., *S. haematobium, S. mansoni, S. japonicum*)—drug of choice
Treatment of lung, liver, and intestinal flukes—drug of choice
Alternative treatment of cestodal (tapeworm) infections

DOSAGE

Schistosomiasis
20 mg/kg 3 times a day for 1 day, at intervals of 4 to 6 hours; may repeat in 2 to 3 months
Cestodal infections
10 mg/kg to 25 mg/kg as a single dose followed by a purgative in 2 hours
Tissue stage: 50 mg/kg in 3 divided doses daily for 14 days

FATE

Rapidly and almost completely (80%) absorbed orally; peak serum levels occur within 1 to 3 hours; metabolized in the liver and excreted largely by the kidneys

COMMON SIDE EFFECTS

Headache, dizziness, anorexia

SIGNIFICANT ADVERSE REACTIONS

Abdominal discomfort, elevated liver enzymes, fever, urticaria, pruritus, diarrhea, arthralgia, myalgia (more frequent in heavily infected patients and those receiving high doses)

CONTRAINDICATIONS

Ocular cysticercosis (parasite destruction may cause irreparable lesions). *Cautious use* in pregnant or nursing women and in children under 4 years of age

NURSING CONSIDERATION

1. Note that when schistosomiasis or another trematodal infection is associated with cysticercosis, the patient should be hospitalized.

PATIENT EDUCATION

1. Instruct patient to swallow tablet whole with a little liquid, preferably during a meal. Tablets are bitter and can cause gagging or vomiting if chewed or kept in the mouth too long.
2. Advise patient to exercise caution in driving or operating other machinery because drowsiness or dizziness can occur.

Pyrantel Pamoate

Antiminth, Reese's Pinworm

MECHANISM

Paralyzes worms, probably by a depolarizing neuromuscular blocking action that may result from inhibition of cholinesterase enzyme; thus, worms are expelled by peristalsis

USE

Treatment of roundworm and pinworm infections

DOSAGE

Adults and children: 11 mg/kg in a single dose (1 mL suspension/10 lb of body weight; maximum dose 1 g)

FATE

Poorly absorbed orally; plasma levels are maximum in 1 to 3 hours but are quite low; metabolized in the liver; greater than 50% of an oral dose is excreted unchanged in the feces and less than 7% in the urine as both unchanged drug and metabolites

COMMON SIDE EFFECTS

Anorexia, nausea, abdominal cramping

SIGNIFICANT ADVERSE REACTIONS

GI: vomiting, diarrhea, tenesmus, elevated SGOT (transient)
CNS: headache, dizziness, drowsiness, insomnia
Allergic/hypersensitivity: rash, fever

CONTRAINDICATIONS

No absolute contraindications. *Cautious use* in patients with liver dysfunction, in pregnant women, and in children under 2 years of age

PATIENT EDUCATION

1. Inform patient that drug may be taken without regard to presence of food or time of day and that use of a laxative is not necessary.
2. Stress the importance of meticulous hygiene for complete eradication of the parasites because pinform infection is readily transmitted from person to person.

Quinacrine
Atabrine

Quinacrine may occasionally be employed as an alternative drug in the management of tapeworm infections, but it has largely been replaced by other more effective, less toxic agents such as niclosamide, praziquantel, or mebendazole. It apparently acts by causing the head of the worm to detach from the intestinal wall; the worm is then expelled by use of a purgative. Because rather high doses of quinacrine are required to treat tapeworm infections, side effects are common. Nausea and vomiting are frequently produced by the drug, as well as dizziness, headache, abdominal cramping, and signs of CNS stimulation (e.g., anxiety, restlessness, confusion, aggression, and psychotic behavior). Treatment with quinacrine is best carried out in the hospital.

Dosage depends on the type of parasite present and is usually administered in divided amounts. For treating beef, pork, or fish tapeworm, adults are given four doses of 200 mg each, 10 minutes apart, together with 600 mg of sodium bicarbonate with each dose. Children are given a total dose of 400 mg to 600 mg in three to four divided doses at 10-minute intervals, together with 300 mg sodium bicarbonate with each dose. A saline purge is administered 1 to 2 hours later to remove the worm from the intestinal tract. The expelled worm is stained yellow.

Quinacrine is also indicated for the treatment of giardiasis, an intestinal protozoal infection caused by the flagellated protozoan *Giardia lamblia*. This disease is the most common protozoal infection in developed countries and is transmitted by cysts in contaminated food or water. Travelers or campers are particularly at risk, as are persons living in crowded, unhygienic conditions. Diagnosis of giardiasis is made by identification of cysts or active trophozoites in fecal specimens. Because most infected individuals are largely asymptomatic, the disease is difficult to recognize and treat.

Adult dosage for quinacrine in giardiasis is 100 mg three times a day for 5 to 7 days. Children are given 7 mg/kg/day in three divided doses after meals for 5 days. A repeat course may be given 2 weeks later if necessary.

Quinacrine has also been employed in the treatment of malaria, and this application is discussed in Chapter 67.

Thiabendazole
Mintezol

MECHANISM

Not established; broad-spectrum anthelmintic that also possesses anti-inflammatory and analgesic activities; appears to enhance T-cell function; may interfere with enzyme systems in helminths; suppresses egg and larval production by *Trichinella spiralis* (pork roundworm) and reduces fever and eosinophilia; it is a first-line drug against threadworm infections and cutaneous larva migrans, but despite its broad spectrum of activity, it is not recommended as first choice in other nematodal infections

USES

Treatment of threadworm (*Strongyloides*) and rat lungworm (*Angiostrongylus*) infections—drug of choice
Treatment of cutaneous larva migrans (creeping eruption)—drug of choice
Alternative treatment of pinworm, whipworm, hookworm, roundworm, and guinea worm infections
Symptomatic treatment of invasive trichinosis

DOSAGE

Usual dosage schedule is 2 doses per day for 2 successive days

Adults and children under 150 lb: 10 mg/lb per dose
Adults and children over 150 lb: 1.5 g per dose

Maximum daily dose is 3 g

FATE

Well absorbed orally; peak plasma levels occur in 1 to 2 hours; metabolized in the liver and excreted largely (90%) within 24 hours in the urine

COMMON SIDE EFFECTS

Anorexia, nausea, vomiting, dizziness

SIGNIFICANT ADVERSE REACTIONS

GI: diarrhea, epigastric distress, cramping, perianal rash
CNS: lethargy, drowsiness, giddiness, headache, tinnitus, irritability, blurred vision, numbness
Allergic/hypersensitivity: pruritus, fever, flushing, chills, angioedema, erythema multiforme, lymphadenopathy, anaphylaxis
Renal/hepatic: enuresis, malodor of the urine, crystalluria, hematuria, cholestasis, jaundice, parenchymal liver damage, elevated SGOT
Other: hypotension, bradycardia, hyperglycemia, leukopenia

CONTRAINDICATIONS

No absolute contraindications. *Cautious use* in patients with impaired kidney or liver function, anemia, or malnutrition, and in pregnant or nursing women

NURSING CONSIDERATIONS

Nursing Alert

- Observe patient for development of hypersensitivity reactions (fever, chills, skin rash). If any appear, the drug should be discontinued. Fatalities have occurred from severe erythema multiforme (Stevens–Johnson syndrome).

1. Note that dietary restrictions, laxatives, and enemas are not necessary.

PATIENT EDUCATION

1. Instruct patient to chew tablets well. Drug is best taken after meals.
2. Warn patient to avoid performing hazardous tasks during therapy because dizziness, drowsiness, and other CNS side effects may occur.

Selected Bibliography

Anderson RM, May RM: Population dynamics of human helminth infections: Control by chemotherapy. Nature 297:557, 1982

Andrews P, Thomas H, Pohlke R, Seubert J: Praziquantel. Med Res Rev 3:147, 1983

Barrett-Connor E: Drugs for treatment of parasitic infection. Med Clin North Am 66:245, 1982

Cook, JA: Schistosome infection in humans: Perspectives and recent findings. Ann Intern Med 97:740, 1982

Drugs for parasitic infections. Med Lett Drugs Ther 30:15, 1988

Henley M, Sears JR: Pinworms: A persistent pediatric problem. Matern Child Nurs 10:111, 1985

Keusch GT: Anthelmintic therapy: The worm has turned. Drug Ther 12(8):213, 1982

Pearson RD, Guerrant RL: Praziquantel: A major advance in anthelmintic therapy. Ann Intern Med 99:195, 1983

Pearson RD, Hewlett EL: Niclosamide therapy for tapeworm infections. Ann Intern Med 102:550, 1985

Sinniah B, Sinniah D: The anthelmintic effect of pyrantel pamoate, oxantel-pyrantel pamoate, levamisole and mebendazole in the treatment of intestinal nematodes. Ann Trop Med Parasitol 75:315, 1981

Sotelo J et al: Therapy of parenchymal brain cysticercosis with praziquantel. N Engl J Med 310:1001, 1984

Storchler D: Chemotherapy of human intestinal helminthiasis: A review, with particular reference to community treatment. Adv Pharmacol Chemother 19:129, 1982

Van den Bossche H, Rochette F, Horig C: Mebendazole and related anthelmintics. Adv Pharmacol Chemother 19:67, 1982

Van den Bossche H, Thienpont D, Janssens, PG (eds): Chemotherapy of gastrointestinal helminths. Berlin, Springer-Verlag, 1985

Warren KS, Mahmoud AA (eds): Tropical and Geographical Medicine. New York, McGraw-Hill, 1984

World Health Organization: WHO Scientific Working Group on the Biochemistry and Chemotherapy of Schistosomiasis, p 1. Geneva, WHO, 1984

Xiao S, Catto BA, Webster LT: Effects of praziquantel on different stages of *Schistosoma mansoni*, in vitro and in vivo. J Infect Dis 151:1130, 1985

SUMMARY. ANTHELMINTIC DRUGS

Drug	Preparations	Usual Dosage Range
Diethylcarbamazine Hetrazan	Tablets: 50 mg	*Filariasis* 2 mg/kg 3 times a day for 3 to 4 wk *Ascariasis* 13 mg/kg/day for 7 days *or* 6 mg/kg to 10 mg/kg 3 times a day for 7 days *Tropical eosinophilia* 13 mg/kg/day for 4 to 7 days
Mebendazole Vermox	Chewable tablets: 100 mg	*Pinworm* 100 mg as a single dose *Whipworm, hookworm, roundworm* 100 mg twice a day for 3 days; repeat in 3 weeks if necessary
Niclosamide Niclocide	Chewable tablets: 500 mg	*Taenia/Diphyllobothrium* Adults: 2 g (single dose) Children: 1.0 g to 1.5 g (single dose) depending on weight *Hymenolepsis* Adults: 2 g/day for 7 days Children: 1.0 g to 1.5 g the first day, then 0.5 g to 1.0 g daily for 6 days
Oxamniquine Vansil	Capsules: 250 mg	Adults: 12 mg to 15 mg/kg as a single dose Children (under 30 kg): 20 mg/kg in 2 divided doses 2 to 8 h apart
Piperazine Antepar, Vermizine	Tablets: 250 mg hexahydrate equivalent Syrup: 500 mg/5 mL hexahydrate equivalent	*Roundworm* Adults: 3.5 g/day for 2 days Children: 75 mg/kg/day for 2 days—may repeat in 1 wk in severe infections; alternatively, 150 mg/kg as a single dose (less effective) *Pinworm* Adults and children: 65 mg/kg/day for 7 days
Praziquantel Biltricide	Tablets: 600 mg	*Schistosomiasis* 20 mg/kg 3 times a day for 1 day, at 4- to 6-h intervals *Cestodal infections* 10 to 25 mg/kg as a single dose

Continued

SUMMARY. ANTHELMINTIC DRUGS (continued)

Drug	Preparations	Usual Dosage Range
Pyrantel Pamoate Antiminth, Reese's Pinworm	Suspension: 50 mg/mL Liquid: 144 mg/mL	11 mg/kg as a single dose (maximum 1 g)
Quinacrine Atabrine	Tablets: 100 mg	200 mg orally every 10 min for 4 doses with 600 mg sodium bicarbonate; follow in 1 to 2 h with a saline purgative
Thiabendazole Mintezol	Chewable tablets: 500 mg Suspension: 500 mg/5 mL	Under 150 lb: 10 mg/lb per dose Over 150 lb: 1.5 g per dose; 2 doses per day for 2 successive days

69 AMEBICIDES

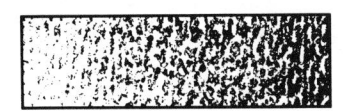

The term *amebiasis* refers to infection with the organism *Entamoeba histolytica*, a protozoan that usually invades the lower intestinal tract but may be found in the liver, lungs, brain, and other organs as well. Amebiasis affects approximately 10% of the world's population, is endemic in many tropical regions, and is present in many people in the United States, especially those exposed to poor sanitary conditions.

The disease can be manifested in one of several ways as follows:

- *Asymptomatic intestinal amebiasis:* presence of the organism in the intestinal tract without evidence of clinical symptoms; treatment is indicated because these patients are at risk for developing GI pathology and can serve as carriers, spreading the infection to other less resistant persons
- *Symptomatic intestinal amebiasis:* presence of overt clinical symptoms ranging from mild manifestations (such as diarrhea, cramping, and flatulence) to severe dysentery with accompanying bloody diarrhea, vomiting, fever, and dehydration. Intestinal mucosal scarring and ulceration can promote systemic absorption of the protozoa, leading to the third stage of the disease, extraintestinal amebiasis
- *Extraintestinal amebiasis:* presence of organisms in other body organs, most commonly the liver and lungs; may result in liver necrosis, amebic hepatitis, lung abscesses, and empyema; organisms can also invade the heart, causing pericarditis, and the CNS, leading to brain abscesses

The drugs used in the treatment of amebiasis can be characterized on the basis of their predominant site of action. That is, some agents (e.g., iodoquinol, carbarsone, diloxanide) are active only against organisms present in the lumen of the intestine, whereas others (e.g., emetine, chloroquine) are effective against parasites found in the bowel wall and other tissues. Still other drugs (e.g., metronidazole) are claimed to affect both intestinal and extraintestinal protozoa. To better understand the rationale for the use of a particular drug in the different stages of amebiasis, it is helpful to briefly review the two-stage life cycle of *Entamoeba histolytica*.

The organism is transmitted from person to person via ingestion of amebic cysts, a form in which the protozoa are extremely resistant to destruction outside the body. The cysts are likewise unaffected by gastric juice, and they pass intact to the small intestine where some develop into motile trophozoites that can invade the intestinal mucosa, be absorbed systemically, and find their way to other organs in the body. The remaining cysts are excreted intact, and they can thus continue the reinfective cycle in another person.

Interruption of this cycle can be accomplished in several ways. Most drugs for treating amebiasis are amebicidal, either directly killing or inhibiting the growth and maturation of the trophozoites, whereas some drugs exhibit a cystocidal action. Because most of the currently effective amebicides have the potential to elicit serious untoward reactions, their use should be undertaken only upon a definitive diagnosis of *Entamoeba histolytica* as the causative agent, and patients must be closely observed during therapy for development of adverse reactions.

There is lack of general agreement about the preferred drug regimens for treating the several forms of amebiasis.

Luminal amebicides (iodoquinol, carbarsone, diloxanide) are used principally in the treatment of asymptomatic or mild intestinal forms of amebiasis. In addition, they are frequently given together with a systemic or mixed amebicide to completely eradicate an infection.

Systemic amebicides (dehydroemetine, chloroquine) are useful in invasive forms of amebiasis such as amebic dysentery or hepatic abscesses. They are infrequently used today, however, because the preferred drug in most cases of symptomatic intestinal or systemic amebiasis is metronidazole, a *mixed* amebicide effective against both intestinal and systemic forms of the disease.

However, metronidazole has been demonstrated to be carcinogenic in mice and rats, and some clinicians feel that it should be reserved for use in severe acute intestinal amebiasis with hepatic abscesses. In treating symptomatic intestinal or systemic amebiasis, metronidozole is usually used together with the luminal drugs diloxanide or iodoquinol, because metronidazole is well absorbed and may fail to reach effective amebicidal levels in the large intestine. Emetine is also active against both intestinal and extraintestinal organisms but is a potentially dangerous drug and must be administered parenterally in a hospital setting under close supervision.

Other drugs that may be effective in intestinal forms of amebiasis are the antibiotics tetracycline, erythromycin, and paromomycin. Of these, however, only paromomycin is sometimes used as an alternative drug in chronic intestinal amebiasis, usually in conjunction with one or more other luminal amebicides.

It should be noted that dehydroemetine and diloxanide are not available for general use in the United States but may be obtained by request from the Parasitic Disease Drug Service of the Centers for Disease Control. They are briefly discussed in Table 69-1. Interestingly, diloxanide alone is viewed by many as the drug of choice for eradication of microorganisms from asymptomatic carriers of the disease, and it is also considered as a primary drug for treatment of milder intestinal infections, sometimes combined with iodoquinol.

The amebicides are discussed individually in this chapter. Several drugs used in amebiasis (e.g., paromomycin, chloroquine) are also effective in other disease states and have been reviewed elsewhere. Only those aspects of their pharmacology related to the treatment of amebic infections are considered here.

Carbarsone

Carbarsone

Carbarsone is an organic arsenical compound containing approximately 30% arsenic. The drug is amebicidal and can eradicate cysts by destroying trophozoites. It is rarely used today in treating intestinal amebiasis (and is not effective in systemic forms) because it is more toxic than the other available drugs. Adverse effects with carbarsone include nausea, diarrhea, abdominal cramping, weight loss, sore throat, skin rash, pruritus, icterus, mucosal ulceration, hepatitis, neuritis, visual disturbances, polyuria, edema, splenomegaly, liver necrosis, exfoliative dermatitis, and kidney damage.

Carbarsone is contraindicated in persons with liver or kidney diseases, amebic hepatitis, and contracted visual fields. The drug is given in a dosage of 250 mg two to three times a day for

10 days; if a repeat course of therapy is needed, 10 to 14 days' rest must be allowed between treatment courses to prevent cumulation toxicity.

Chloroquine
Aralen

Primarily employed as an antimalarial drug, chloroquine is also effective in the treatment of amebic liver abscesses (often with emetine), because chloroquine localizes in the liver in a concentration several hundred times greater than in the plasma. The drug is largely ineffective against intestinal organisms because it is rapidly absorbed; therefore it is always given either in combination with or following other drugs active against intestinal amebiasis. When used in hepatic amebiasis, chloroquine may also be combined with metronidazole or diloxanide or both to ensure that all protozoa are eradicated. Chloroquine is discussed fully in Chapter 67 and only information pertinent to its use in amebiasis is presented here.

USES
Treatment of extraintestinal amebiasis, in combination with other amebicides active against intestinal forms

DOSAGE
Oral: (phosphate salt) 1 g/day for 2 days, then 500 mg/day for at least 2 weeks to 3 weeks
IM: (hydrochloride salt) 200 mg to 250 mg/day for 10 days to 12 days; oral therapy should be substituted as soon as possible
Children: maximum single dose is 5 mg (base)/kg

Emetine
Emetine

Emetine is a potent amebicide effective against both intestinal and extraintestinal tissue parasites. Its use is restricted to severe cases of amebic dysentery and amebic hepatitis or liver abscesses, inasmuch as the drug can cause serious untoward reactions related to cumulative toxicity as well as a wide range of milder adverse effects. The close structural analog dehydroemetine is available as Mebadin from the Centers for Disease Control in Atlanta; it is equally effective and may be somewhat less toxic (see Table 69-1).

MECHANISM
Exerts a direct lethal action on trophozoites, probably blocking protein synthesis by interfering with attachment of tRNA to the ribosomes; much more effective against motile forms than against cysts; exhibits some anticholinergic and antiadrenergic action; may depress cardiac conduction and contraction; ECG changes have occurred

USES
Symptomatic treatment of acute amebic dysentery or acute episodes of chronic amebic dysentery, in combination with other amebicides
Treatment of amebic hepatitis and amebic abscesses in other tissues, in combination with an amebicide effective against intestinal parasites
Alternative treatment of balantidiasis, fascioliasis, and paragonimiasis

DOSAGE
(Deep SC injection is preferred; may be given IM)
Acute Amebic Dysentery
65 mg/day SC or IM for 3 days to 5 days, in a single or two divided doses
Amebic Hepatitis or Abscesses
65 mg/day SC or IM for 10 days
Children (under 8 yr): maximum 10 mg/day
Children (over 8 yr): maximum 20 mg/day

NOTE
Do not extend therapy beyond 10 days or exceed a total dose of 650 mg in adults, because cumulative toxicity can occur. Do not repeat a course of therapy until 6 to 8 weeks have elapsed

FATE
Well absorbed from SC or IM injection sites; widely distributed in the body (e.g., kidney, spleen, lungs), highest concentrations being found in the liver; excreted very slowly by the kidneys, some drug still present in the body 60 days after administration; danger of cumulative toxicity is appreciable

COMMON SIDE EFFECTS
Pain, tenderness, stiffness, and local muscle weakness at injection sites; nausea, diarrhea, abdominal pain, dizziness, fainting

SIGNIFICANT ADVERSE REACTIONS
GI: vomiting
Cardiovascular: hypotension, tachycardia, precordial pain, cardiac dilatation, ECG abnormalities (T wave inversion, QT prolongation), gallop rhythm, dyspnea, congestive heart failure, and arrhythmias
Neuromuscular: muscle stiffness and weakness, tremors
Dermatologic: urticarial, eczematous, or purpuric skin lesions

CONTRAINDICATIONS
Organic heart or kidney disease; pregnancy; in children (except those with severe dysentery not controlled by other amebicides) and persons receiving a course of emetine therapy within the previous 2 months; IV injection of the drug. *Cautious use* in persons with liver disease, ECG abnormalities; in nursing mothers and in elderly or debilitated persons

NURSING CONSIDERATIONS

Nursing Alerts
- During therapy and for several days thereafter, confine patient to bed and observe very carefully. Monitor pulse and blood pressure several times a day. Drug should be discontinued if tachycardia, marked drop in blood pressure, neuromuscular symptoms, muscle weakness, or severe GI symptoms occur.
- Notify drug prescriber if fatigability or listlessness occurs, or if patient experiences muscle stiffness, pain, or tenderness, especially in the neck or upper extremities, because these are often early signs of more serious neuromuscular toxicity. Drug should be discontinued.
- Monitor results of ECG, which should be obtained before initiating therapy, after the fifth dose, upon completion of treatment, and again 1 week later. Although ECG changes are common and are not an absolute indication for discon-

tinuing therapy, the patient must be carefully observed for additional complications (e.g., dyspnea, arrhythmias).
- Monitor intake–output, and note any change in renal function. Report immediately.
- Observe number, consistency, and character of stools. Fecal examinations should be repeated for up to 3 months following therapy to ensure elimination of parasites.

1. Handle solution carefully and avoid contact with eyes and mucous membranes because solution is very irritating
2. Administer by deep IM or SC injection. Inadvertent IV injection can cause severe toxic effects.

PATIENT EDUCATION
1. Instruct patient to avoid strenuous activity for several weeks after termination of therapy.

Iodoquinol (Diiodohydroxyquin)

Moebiquin, Yodoxin
(CAN) Diodoquin

An iodinated hydroxyquinoline, iodoquinol is effective in intestinal amebiasis, especially in asymptomatic carriers. It is relatively nontoxic and inexpensive and has been used for mass treatment.

MECHANISMS
Not established; exerts a direct amebicidal action against both motile and cystic forms of trophozoites; action is restricted to the intestinal tract owing to poor oral absorption

USES
Treatment of asymptomatic or mild to moderate acute or chronic intestinal amebiasis
Treatment of giardiasis (investigational use)

DOSAGE
Adults: 650 mg orally three times a day for 20 days
Children: 40 mg/kg/day in three divided doses for 20 days (maximum 2 g/day)

FATE
Largely unabsorbed from the GI tract; eliminated largely in the feces

COMMON SIDE EFFECTS
Gastric distress (diarrhea, nausea, abdominal discomfort)

SIGNIFICANT ADVERSE REACTIONS
(Rare at usual doses) Vomiting, abdominal cramping, pruritus ani, urticaria, skin eruptions, headache, vertigo, fever, chills, thyroid enlargement. Optic neuritis, optic atrophy, and peripheral neuropathy have occurred with long-term therapy

CONTRAINDICATIONS
Hypersensitivity to iodides, hepatic damage. *Cautious use* in patients with thyroid disorders and in pregnant or lactating women

NURSING CONSIDERATIONS
1. Determine whether patient is allergic to iodide before administering initial dose.
2. Question prescription of iodoquinol for prophylaxis or treatment of nonspecific or "travelers'" diarrhea. It is *not* indicated for these conditions, although it has been used for them.
3. Interpret results of thyroid function tests cautiously because drug can interfere with some of them by increasing protein-bound serum iodine levels.

PATIENT EDUCATION
1. Instruct patient to be alert for development of ocular or neurologic disturbances, especially during prolonged high-dosage therapy, and to inform drug prescriber if they occur because the drug should be discontinued. Long-term therapy should be avoided.
2. Inform patient that periodic ophthalmologic examinations are advisable during therapy, especially in young children.
3. Teach patient how to recognize signs of hypersensitivity reactions (pruritus, urticaria, chills, fever). Instruct patient to notify drug prescriber if they occur.

Metronidazole

Femazole, Flagyl, Metizole, Metro I.V., Metryl, Protostat, Satric
(CAN) Apo-Metronidazole, Neo-Tric, Novonidazol, PMS Metronidazole

Metronidazole exerts a direct amebicidal and trichomonacidal action against *Entamoeba histolytica* and *Trichomonas vaginalis,* respectively. It is considered the drug of choice for oral treatment of trichomoniasis in both females and males. In addition, it is employed in treating acute intestinal amebiasis, both symptomatic and asymptomatic as well as amebic liver abscess. The drug has been reported to be carcinogenic in mice and rats, and *unnecessary* use should be avoided. However, metronidazole remains a valuable drug for the therapy of both amebiasis and trichomoniasis.

In addition to its use as both an amebicide and trichomonacide, metronidazole is also available both orally and IV for the treatment of serious infections caused by susceptible anaerobic bacteria. Parenteral metronidazole has demonstrated clinical activity against the following organisms: anaerobic gram-negative bacilli, including *Bacteroides* and *Fusobacterium* species; anaerobic gram-positive bacilli, including *Clostridium* species; and anaerobic gram-positive cocci, including *Peptococcus* and *Peptostreptococcus* species. Necessary surgical procedures should always be performed in conjunction with drug treatment, and in mixed aerobic–anaerobic infections, appropriate antibiotics should be included in the drug regimen. The principal hazard connected with parenteral metronidazole therapy is the possibility of convulsive seizures and development of peripheral neuropathy. The benefit: risk ratio must be critically evaluated in patients who show evidence of abnormal neurologic signs.

MECHANISM
Not entirely established; appears to disrupt the structure of DNA in susceptible organisms, causing strand breakage and loss of helical structure; destroys most organisms within 24 to 48 hours

USES
Treatment of acute intestinal amebiasis (amebic dysentery) and amebic liver abscess

Treatment of symptomatic and asymptomatic trichomoniasis in both sexes (oral only)

Treatment of serious infections caused by susceptible anaerobic bacteria, especially *Bacteroides* (including strains resistant to clindamycin and chloramphenicol), *Clostridium* (including pseudomembranous colitis resulting from *Clostridium difficile* overgrowth), *Eubacterium, Peptococcus,* and *Peptostreptococcus* species (IV)

Preoperative, intraoperative, or postoperative prophylaxis of infection in patients undergoing surgery classified as potentially contaminated, such as colorectal, abdominal, or gynecologic surgery

Investigational uses include (1) hepatic encephalopathy, (2) treatment of giardiasis or *Gardnerella vaginalis* infections, (3) Crohn's disease, and (4) as a radiosensitizer to render tumors more susceptible to radiation

DOSAGE
Amebiasis
Adults: 500 mg to 750 mg three times a day orally for 5 to 10 days
Children: 35 mg/kg to 50 mg/kg/day orally in three divided doses for 10 days
Trichomoniasis
250 mg three times a day orally for 7 days *for males and females; alternatively,* 2 g in a single dose or two divided doses; allow 4 to 6 weeks between courses of therapy when a repeat treatment is necessary
Anaerobic Infections
Initially 15 mg/kg infused over 1 hour; maintenance doses, 7.5 mg/kg infused over 1 hour every 6 hours for 7 to 10 days; maximum dose, 4 g/24-hour period; may change to oral therapy (7.5 mg/kg every 6 h) as condition warrants
Prophylaxis of Postoperative Infection
15 mg/kg infused over 30 to 60 minutes and completed at least 1 hour before surgery, followed by 7.5 mg/kg infused over 30 to 60 minutes at 6 and 12 hours after the initial dose

FATE
Well absorbed from GI tract; peak serum levels occur in 1 hour to 2 hours; widely distributed in the body and diffuses well into all tissues; slightly (20%) bound to plasma proteins; plasma half-life is approximately 8 hours; excreted largely in the urine, both as unchanged drug (20%) and 2-hydroxymethyl metabolite; both parent compound and metabolite have antibacterial activity

COMMON SIDE EFFECTS
(Especially orally) Nausea, metallic taste, anorexia, epigastric distress

SIGNIFICANT ADVERSE REACTIONS

> **WARNING**
> Prolonged oral administration of metronidazole in rodents has been associated with an increased incidence of neoplastic tumors, especially hepatic and mammary. Unnecessary use of the drug for extended periods in humans should be avoided

Oral
GI: vomiting, diarrhea, abdominal cramping, furry tongue, glossitis, stomatitis, candidal overgrowth
CNS: dizziness, vertigo, incoordination, ataxia, paresthesia, numbness, confusion, depression, irritability, insomnia
Allergic/hypersensitivity: pruritus, flushing, urticaria, fever
Urinary: dysuria, cystitis, polyuria, incontinence, darkened urine
Other: leukopenia, nasal congestion, xerostomia, dyspareunia, decreased libido, proctitis, pyuria, flattened T wave, joint pain
IV
See Oral; in addition, convulsions, seizures, peripheral neuropathy, thrombophlebitis with IV infusion

CONTRAINDICATIONS
Blood dyscrasias, organic CNS disease, first trimester of pregnancy (unless absolutely necessary, e.g., *severe,* life-threatening infections). *Cautious use* in persons with liver or kidney disease, persistent fungal infections; in alcoholics (see Interactions), and in pregnant or nursing women

INTERACTIONS
Alcohol ingestion may elicit a disulfiram-like reaction (abdominal cramps, vomiting, severe headache, hypotension); see Chapter 78
Metronidazole may potentiate the effects of oral anticoagulants
The effectiveness of metronidazole may be reduced if given concurrently with phenobarbital or phenytoin, drugs that may increase its rate of metabolism
Cimetidine may reduce the metabolism of metronidazole

NURSING CONSIDERATIONS

Nursing Alerts
- Observe patient for symptoms of CNS toxicity (e.g., mood changes, incoordination, ataxia). Drug should be discontinued if these occur.
- Observe patient carefully for signs of peripheral neurologic dysfunction, especially with IV administration. Persistent peripheral neuropathy has occurred in some patients on prolonged therapy. Benefit:risk ratio of continued therapy must be critically evaluated.

1. Monitor results of total and differential leukocyte counts, which should be performed before and periodically during therapy because drug can elicit leukopenia.
2. Closely follow package instructions for preparing IV infusion solution. Order of mixing is important. Do *not* refrigerate neutralized solution because precipitate may form. Use within 24 hours.

PATIENT EDUCATION
1. Instruct patient to take oral drug with food to minimize GI upset.
2. Inform patient that drug may cause an unpleasant metallic taste.
3. Inform patient that drug may harmlessly darken urine.
4. Stress the importance of adhering to prescribed dosage (see *Warning* under Significant Adverse Reactions) and of completing the full course of therapy.
5. Inform patient that ingestion of alcohol in any form (e.g., cough preparations, mouthwashes) can result in a disulfiram-like reaction (vomiting, diarrhea, flushing, hypotension, abdominal pain).
6. Teach patient how to recognize signs of secondary fungal (candidal) overgrowth, which may result from drug use. If glossitis, stomatitis, vaginitis, vaginal discharge, diarrhea, or furry tongue occurs, appropriate antifungal medicine is required.

7. Caution woman treated for trichomoniasis that concurrent treatment of the male sexual partner is usually necessary to prevent reinfection.

Paromomycin
Humatin

An aminoglycoside-like drug, paromomycin exhibits an antibacterial action resembling that of neomycin. In addition, it exerts an amebicidal action in the intestinal tract but is not appreciably absorbed orally and is therefore ineffective in extraintestinal amebiasis.

MECHANISM
Direct amebicidal action in vivo and in vitro; may also reduce the population of intestinal microbes essential for proliferation of protozoa

USES
Treatment of acute and chronic intestinal amebiasis, usually as an alternative drug to other more potent and specific amebicides
Adjunctive therapy in management of hepatic coma

DOSAGE
Amebiasis
25 mg/kg to 35 mg/kg/day in three divided doses for 5 to 10 days
Hepatic Coma
4 g/day in divided doses for 5 to 6 days

FATE
Not significantly absorbed orally; excreted largely in the feces; systemically absorbed drug is excreted very slowly via the kidneys

COMMON SIDE EFFECTS
Nausea, anorexia, GI upset, diarrhea

SIGNIFICANT ADVERSE REACTIONS
Abdominal cramps, pruritus ani, headache, vertigo, skin rash, malabsorption state, and overgrowth of nonsusceptible organisms

CONTRAINDICATIONS
Intestinal obstruction, ulcerative bowel lesions. *Cautious use* in patients with preexisting hearing loss, vestibular damage, or renal dysfunction

NURSING CONSIDERATION
1. Note that paromomycin is an aminoglycoside derivative. Although it has the potential to elicit serious untoward reactions (nephrotoxicity, ototoxicity) and to interact with a number of other drugs (see Chap. 62 for complete discussion of aminoglycosides), the incidence of such reactions is quite low because paromomycin is poorly absorbed.

PATIENT EDUCATION
1. Instruct patient to take drug with meals to minimize GI upset.
2. Inform patient that stools are usually examined weekly during and for at least 6 weeks following termination of therapy.
3. Teach patient how to recognize signs of secondary fungal (candidal) overgrowth, which may result from drug use. If glossitis, stomatitis, vaginitis, vaginal discharge, diarrhea, or furry tongue occurs, appropriate antifungal medicine should be instituted.

Table 69-1
Amebicides Available by Request from the Centers for Disease Control[a]

Drug	Preparations	Usual Dosage Range	Remarks
Dehydroemetine Mebadin	Injection: 30 mg/mL	Adults and children: 1 mg/kg–1.5 mg/kg/day IM *or* SC for up to 5 days (maximum 100 mg/day)	Clinical indications are the same as for emetine, but the incidence and severity of cardiovascular complications may be somewhat less; usually given in combination with diloxanide and a tetracycline, followed by chloroquine if hepatic amebiasis is present; daily dose may be divided into 2 parts; use very *cautiously* in patients with cardiac disease or neuromuscular disorders
Diloxanide furoate Furamide	Tablets: 500 mg	Adults: 500 mg 3 times a day for 10 days Children: 20 mg/kg/day in 3 divided doses for 10 days; repeat in several weeks if necessary	Relatively nontoxic intestinal amebicide regarded by many as the drug of choice for asymptomatic and mild symptomatic intestinal amebiasis; ineffective alone against extraintestinal parasites; may be combined with metronidazole in moderate to severe intestinal disease; mild GI distress and flatulence have been reported; GI absorption is appreciable, and much of an oral dose is excreted in the urine within 48 h, largely as metabolites

[a] Parasitic Disease Drug Service, Centers for Disease Control, Atlanta, Georgia 30333.

Selected Bibliography

Bergan T, Thorsteinsson SB: Pharmacokinetics of metronidazole and its metabolites in reduced renal function. Chemotherapeutics 32:305, 1986

Finegold SM: Metronidazole. Ann Intern Med 93:585, 1980

Goldman P: Metronidazole. N Engl J Med 303:1212, 1980

Gupte S: Phenobarbital and metabolism of metronidazole. N Engl J Med 308:529, 1983

Harries J: Amebiasis: A review. J R Soc Med 75:190, 1982

Knight R: The chemotherapy of amebiasis. J Antimicrobial Chemotherap 6:577, 1980

Molavi A, Le Frock JL, Prince RA: Metronidazole. Med Clin North Am 66:121, 1982

Neal RA: Experimental amebiasis and the development of antiamebic compounds. Parasitology 86:175, 1983

Oldenburg B, Speck WT: Metronidazole. Pediatr Clin North Am 30:71, 1983

Ralph ED: Clinical pharmacokinetics of metronidazole. Clin Pharmacokinet 8:43, 1983

Ravdin JI, Guerrant RL: Current problems in diagnosis and treatment of amebic infections. In Remington JS and Swartz MN (eds): Current Clinical Topics in Infectious Diseases. New York, McGraw-Hill, 1986

Salvio K, Apuzzio JJ: New antibiotics in the treatment of pelvic infections. JOGN Nursing 13:308, 1984

Warren KS, Mahmoud AAF (eds): Tropical and Geographic Medicine. New York, McGraw-Hill, 1984

SUMMARY. AMEBICIDES

Drug	Preparations	Usual Dosage Range
Carbarsone Carbarsone	Capsules: 250 mg	Adults: 250 mg 2 or 3 times a day for 10 days; may repeat in 2 wk Children: 75 mg/kg over 10 days in 3 daily divided doses
Chloroquine Aralen	Tablets (phosphate): 250 mg, 500 mg Injection (hydrochloride): 50 mg/mL	Oral: 1 g/day for 2 days, then 500 mg/day for at least 2 to 3 wk IM: 200 mg–250 mg/day for 10 to 12 days
Emetine Emetine	Injection: 65 mg/mL	65 mg/day in a single dose *or* divided doses, SC or IM, for 3 to 5 days in amebic dysentery *or* for 10 days in amebic hepatitis
Iodoquinol (Dihydroxyiodoquin) Moebiquin, Yodoxin	Tablets: 210 mg, 650 mg	Adults: 650 mg 3 times a day for 20 days Children: 40 mg/kg/day in 3 divided doses for 20 days (maximum 2 g/day)
Metronidazole Femazole, Flagyl, Metro I.V., Metizole, Metryl, Protostat, Satric	Tablets: 250 mg, 500 mg Powder for injection: 500 mg/vial Injection: 5 mg/mL	*Amebiasis* Adults: 500 mg–750 mg 3 times a day orally for 5 to 10 days Children: 35 mg–50 mg/kg/day orally in 3 divided doses for 10 days *Trichomoniasis* 250 mg 3 times a day orally for 7 days *or* 2 g in a single dose or 2 divided doses *Anaerobic infections* Initially: 15 mg/kg infused over 1 h Maintenance: 7.5 mg/kg infused over 1 h every 6 h for 7 to 10 days (maximum 4 g in 24 h) *Perioperative prophylaxis* 15 mg/kg given over 30 to 60 min IV at least 1 h before surgery, followed by 7.5 mg/kg at 6 and 12 h after surgery
Paromomycin Humatin	Capsules: 250 mg	25 mg–35 mg/kg/day in 3 divided doses for 5 to 10 days *Hepatic coma* 4 g/day in divided doses for 5 to 6 days

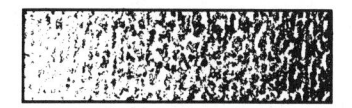

70 ANTIFUNGAL AGENTS

Fungal, or mycotic, infections are responsible for a number of pathologic conditions in humans that, with few exceptions, remain difficult to treat. Fungal diseases are conventionally categorized as either topical (cutaneous, superficial) or deep (systemic) infections. Although this classification is convenient, it should be recognized that organisms responsible for local infections of the skin, nails, vagina, or GI tract (such as *Candida*) can also invade deeper body organs, resulting in systemic involvement and serious complications. Because there are only a few effective systemic antifungal drugs, most of which are relatively toxic in the doses needed to eliminate deep mycotic infections, successful treatment of systemic fungal diseases is one of the most difficult tasks in chemotherapy.

Reflecting the classification of fungal diseases into topical or deep infections, antifungal drugs can be categorized in much the same way, although it should be noted that some drugs are used in treating *both* superficial and systemic infections. A useful classification of antifungal agents is as follows:

Drugs for treating systemic infections only
   flucytosine
Drugs for treating both systemic and topical infections
   amphotericin B
   ketoconazole
   miconazole
   nystatin
Drugs for treating topical infections only
   Oral administration only
   griseofulvin
   Cutaneous administration only
   ciclopirox   oxiconazole
   econazole   sulconazole
   haloprogin   tolnaftate
   iodochlorhydroxyquin   triacetin
   naftifine   undecylenic acid
   Vaginal administration only
   butoconazole
   terconazole
   Cutaneous and vaginal administration
   clotrimazole
Drugs for treating ophthalmic infections only
   natamycin

The organisms responsible for the common fungal infections, together with the preferred drugs for treating each disease, are listed in Table 56-1, Chapter 56. Most systemic fungal infections respond best to amphotericin B. Flucytosine is indicated for serious candidal or cryptococcal infections and is synergistic with amphotericin B against these organisms. Miconazole and ketaconazole are viewed as rather broad-spectrum antifungal agents, but some questions exist as to their clinical efficacy in many fungal diseases. In addition, relapses have frequently occurred with use of these agents. Oral nystatin is indicated for intestinal candidiasis and for local fungal infections of the mouth and throat. Topical or vaginal monilial infections due to *Candida* species can be effectively controlled by several antifungal drugs, such as butoconazole, terconazole, clotrimazole, miconazole, and nystatin. Cutaneous dermatophytal infections (e.g., tinea) of the skin, hair, or nails (including ringworm, athlete's foot, jock itch) can be controlled either by oral griseofulvin (severe ringworm) or one of the topically effective antifungal drugs such as ciclopirox, econazole, haloprogin, tolnaftate, triacetin, or undecylenic acid. Natamycin is an antifungal agent used locally in the eye for treatment of fungal conjunctivitis, blepharitis, and keratitis.

The systemic antifungal agents are reviewed individually in detail in this chapter. The topically effective drugs are then listed in Table 70-1, along with their indications, dosage ranges, and specific information relating to each drug.

SYSTEMIC ANTIFUNGAL AGENTS

Amphotericin B
   Fungizone

An antibiotic produced by a strain of *Streptomyces*, amphotericin is a first-line drug for many severe progressive and potentially fatal systemic fungal infections, but because of its serious toxicity, it should not be used to treat trivial or clinically insignificant fungal diseases. It is also used topically to treat cutaneous or mucosal candidal (monilial) infections.

MECHANISM
Fungistatic or fungicidal depending on organism and concentration of drug; binds to sterols (e.g., ergosterol) in fungal cell membrane, thus increasing cell permeability and allowing leakage of cellular constituents; no effect on bacteria, viruses, or rickettsiae; potentiates the effects of flucytosine and other antibiotics by allowing penetration of these drugs into the fungal cell

USES
Treatment of serious and potentially fatal systemic fungal infections, such as aspergillosis, blastomycosis, coccidioidomycosis, cryptococcosis, disseminated candidiasis (moniliasis), histoplasmosis, mucormycosis, and sporotrichosis (see Table 56-1)
Alternative treatment of American mucocutaneous leishmaniasis (IV only)
Treatment of cutaneous and mucocutaneous candidal (monilial) infections (topically only)

DOSAGE
IV infusion
Initially 0.25 mg/kg/day infused over 6 hours; may increase gradually to 1 mg/kg/day or 1.5 mg/kg every other day as tolerance permits; total treatment time is usually several months, although some serious infections can require 9 to 12 months of therapy; maximum daily dose is 1.5 mg/kg; total dosage can range from 1.5 g for blastomycosis up to 4 g for life-threatening infections such as rhinocerebral phycomycosis
Intrathecal/intraventricular
0.1 mg initially, increased gradually up to 0.5 mg every 48 to 72 hours (investigational use only)
Topical
Apply liberally to lesions 2 to 4 times a day for 1 to 4 weeks depending on response

FATE
Poorly absorbed from GI tract and not given orally; following IV infusion, drug is highly (90%–95%) bound to plasma proteins and has a plasma half-life of 24 hours; diffuses well into inflamed pleural and peritoneal cavities and joints but poorly into most other body tissues; slowly excreted by the kidneys (elimination half-life is 15 days), a small fraction in a biologically active form; drug can be detected in the urine for at least 7 weeks after termination of therapy

COMMON SIDE EFFECTS
IV: fever, chills, nausea, vomiting, diarrhea, headache, dyspepsia, impaired renal function (hypokalemia, azotemia, renal tubular acidosis, nephrocalcinosis), anorexia, weight loss, malaise, muscle and joint pain, abdominal cramping, pain at injection site, phlebitis, normochromic–normocytic anemia

SIGNIFICANT ADVERSE REACTIONS
IV: maculopapular rash, pruritus, tinnitus, hearing loss, blurred vision, vertigo, flushing, peripheral neuropathy, blood pressure alterations, arrhythmias, cardiac arrest, blood dyscrasias, coagulation defects, anuria, oliguria, hemorrhagic gastroenteritis, convulsions, anaphylactic reaction, acute liver failure
Topical: drying of the skin, irritation, pruritus, erythema, burning, contact dermatitis, skin discoloration

CONTRAINDICATIONS
No absolute contraindications if the situation being treated is potentially life-threatening. *Cautious use* in pregnant women and in patients with renal impairment, blood dyscrasias, neurologic disorders, or peptic ulcer

INTERACTIONS
Hypokalemia induced by amphotericin B may be increased by diuretics or corticosteroids and poses a danger in patients receiving digitalis drugs
Amphotericin B can enhance the effect of peripherally acting muscle relaxants, for example, curare, gallamine, succinylcholine
Concomitant use of corticosteroids, antibiotics, or antineoplastics with amphotericin B can increase the incidence of superinfections and blood dyscrasias
Aminoglycosides and other nephrotoxic or ototoxic drugs can have additive toxic effects with amphotericin B
Flucytosine, minocycline, and rifampin can potentiate the antifungal activity of amphotericin B

NURSING CONSIDERATIONS

Nursing Alerts
- Administer IV only to hospitalized patients with a confirmed diagnosis of progressive, potentially fatal fungal disease. Ensure that patient is closely supervised during administration.
- Monitor results of the following laboratory studies, which should be performed at least weekly during therapy: liver function studies, BUN, serum creatinine and potassium, and hemogram. Drug should be discontinued if liver function is abnormal, if BUN exceeds 40 mg/dL, or if serum creatinine exceeds 3 mg/dL.
- Monitor intake–output and observe for oliguria, hematuria, or cloudy urine. Notify drug prescriber of any change in renal function because nephrotoxicity develops after a few months in most patients. The azotemia that develops during therapy is usually reversible, but if total dose exceeds 4 g, *persistent* renal damage often ensues.
- Assess patient's auditory and vestibular function frequently, and instruct patient to report any changes immediately because drug is ototoxic.
- Monitor patient for symptoms of hypokalemia (muscle weakness or cramping, drowsiness, paresthesias). If they occur, potassium supplementation should be provided.
- Infuse IV slowly and observe infusion site for signs of inflammation. Extravasation may lead to thromboses and thrombophlebitis. Simultaneous infusion of heparin may decrease the incidence of thrombophlebitis.

1. Be prepared to administer aspirin, antihistamines, antiemetics, or small doses of corticosteroids to lessen the severity of adverse reactions (e.g., fever, headache, vomiting).
2. Add 10 mL sterile water for injection to powder, shake, then dilute further (1:50) with 5% dextrose injection of pH above 4.2. Do *not* reconstitute with saline solution because precipitate may form. Powder contains no preservative or bacteriostatic agent.
3. Store vials in refrigerator, protect against exposure to light, and use IV solutions immediately after preparing.
4. If an in-line membrane is used during IV infusion, ensure that the mean pore diameter is greater than 1 μm to allow passage of the colloidal dispersion of the drug.
5. Interpret results of the following laboratory tests cautiously because amphotericin can interfere with them: SGOT, SGPT, BUN, serum creatinine, hematocrit, hemoglobin, and platelet count.
6. Note that amphotericin B is available in combination with tetracycline (Mysteclin-F) to prevent fungal overgrowth that can occur with use of oral tetracycline.

PATIENT EDUCATION
1. Instruct patient to apply topical preparation liberally and to rub gently but well into lesions.
2. Inform patient that some skin drying and discoloration may occur with use of cream preparation, but generally not with the lotion or ointment. Lotion may stain nail lesions, however.
3. Inform patient that topical preparation can stain clothes or other fabrics, but that the stain can be removed easily by washing with soap and water or by using a standard cleaning fluid.
4. Teach patient how to recognize signs of hypersensitivity reaction to topical preparation (rash, pruritus, erythema) and report to prescriber.

Flucytosine
Ancobon
(CAN) Ancotil

A synthetic pyrimidine, structurally related to the antineoplastic drug fluorouracil, flucytosine is an orally effective systemic antifungal drug that is considered a secondary agent in treating deep-seated mycotic infections due to *Candida* and *Cryptococcus* species. It is much less toxic than amphotericin B but is less effective as well, and resistance frequently develops rapidly. Thus it is used mainly in combination with amphotericin B for treating cryptococcal infections such as meningitis.

MECHANISM
Probably converted to 5-fluorouracil in fungal cells (but not normal mammalian cells); acts as a competitive inhibitor of nucleic acid synthesis; host cells apparently lack the enzyme that converts drug to active metabolite and are thus unaffected

USES
Treatment of serious systemic candidal infections (endocarditis, septicemia, urinary) or cryptococcal infections (meningitis, septicemia, pulmonary or urinary)—frequently given in combination with amphotericin B, with which it has a synergistic effect against *Candida* and *Cryptococcus*

DOSAGE
50 mg/kg to 150 mg/kg/day orally in divided doses every 6 hours

FATE
Well absorbed orally; peak plasma concentrations occur within 1 to 2 hours; minimally bound to plasma proteins; widely distributed in the body; drug levels in cerebrospinal fluid reach 50% to 100% of those in the serum; not significantly metabolized but excreted largely unchanged (90%) in the urine; serum half-life is 3 to 6 hours

COMMON SIDE EFFECTS
Nausea, diarrhea, skin rash, vomiting

SIGNIFICANT ADVERSE REACTIONS
Anemia, leukopenia, thrombocytopenia, pancytopenia, hepatomegaly, enterocolitis, elevation of SGOT, SGPT, BUN, and serum creatinine; less frequently, headache, vertigo, drowsiness, confusion, and hallucinations

CONTRAINDICATIONS
No absolute contraindications. *Cautious use* in patients with impaired renal function, bone marrow depression, hematologic disorders; during pregnancy or lactation; and in persons receiving radiation therapy or cancer chemotherapy

INTERACTIONS
Flucytosine can potentiate the antifungal effects and toxicity of amphotericin B

Concurrent use with other bone marrow–depressing drugs (e.g., antineoplastics, pyrazolones) may increase the toxic effects of both drugs

NURSING CONSIDERATIONS

Nursing Alerts
- Ensure that the renal, hepatic, and hematologic status of patient has been determined before therapy is initiated. These parameters should also be assessed at frequent intervals during therapy. Liver enzyme levels should be ascertained frequently during therapy.
- Monitor intake–output. Serum drug levels should be assayed frequently to ensure normal excretion.

1. Administer capsules a few at a time over a 15-minute period to minimize the incidence of nausea and vomiting.
2. Monitor results of culture and sensitivity tests, which should be performed periodically during therapy, because drug resistance may develop during prolonged therapy.

Griseofulvin
Microsize—Fulvicin U/F, Grifulvin V, Grisactin
Ultramicrosize—Fulvicin P/G, Grisactin Ultra, Gris-Peg
(CAN) Grisovin-FP

An orally administered fungistatic antibiotic that is effective only against dermatophyte infections of the skin, hair, and nails, griseofulvin is available as either a microsize or ultramicrosize particle formulation. Ultramicrosize griseofulvin exhibits approximately 1.5 times the biologic activity of microsize griseofulvin largely because of improved GI absorption; thus a 330-mg dose of ultramicrosize yields antifungal activity comparable to a 500-mg dose of the microsize formulation. However, there is no evidence that the ultramicrosize formulation is clinically superior with regard to efficacy or safety.

MECHANISM
Localizes in keratin precursor cells in skin, nails, and hair and disrupts the mitotic spindle, thus arresting cell division; new keratin that is subsequently formed strongly binds griseofulvin and becomes resistant to fungal invasion; no effect on bacteria, yeasts, or fungi other than dermatophytal organisms

USES
Treatment of fungal infections of the skin, hair, or nails caused by the following dermatophytes: *Epidermophyton, Microsporum,* or *Trichophyton*

> **NOTE**
> *Not* effective in systemic mycotic infections, candidiasis, tinea versicolor, or bacterial infections—should not be used in trivial infections that respond to topical agents alone

DOSAGE
Adults: 500 mg to 1 g microsize *or* 330 mg to 750 mg ultramicrosize daily in a single dose or divided doses
Children: 11 mg/kg microsize daily *or* 7 mg/kg ultramicrosize daily in a single dose *or* divided doses

FATE
Oral absorption is somewhat variable, the ultramicrosize preparation being absorbed more efficiently than the microsize formulation. Peak plasma levels occur in about 4 hours, and drug is detectable in the skin within 4 to 8 hours. Griseofulvin exhibits a greater affinity for diseased skin than normal skin. Its plasma half-life is approximately 24 hours; it is metabolized in the liver and slowly excreted in the urine, mainly as metabolites.

COMMON SIDE EFFECTS
Skin rash, urticaria

SIGNIFICANT ADVERSE REACTIONS
GI: nausea, vomiting, diarrhea, epigastric distress, flatulence, stomatitis
Neurologic: paresthesias, fatigue, headache, dizziness, insomnia, confusion, peripheral neuritis, blurred vision, impaired motor skills, syncope
Hematologic: leukopenia, neutropenia, granulocytopenia
Allergic: angioedema, serum sickness, photosensitivity, erythema multiforme, lupuslike syndrome
Other: proteinuria, estrogenlike effects in children

CONTRAINDICATIONS

Porphyria, severe liver disease, systemic lupus erythematosus, prophylaxis of *non*established fungal infections. *Cautious use* in patients with renal dysfunction, penicillin allergy; in alcoholics (see Interactions); and in pregnant women

INTERACTIONS

Griseofulvin can reduce the activity of oral anticoagulants

Activity of griseofulvin may be diminished by barbiturates, glutethimide, diphenhydramine, orphenadrine, and phenylbutazone through enzyme induction

The effects of alcohol may be potentiated by griseofulvin, producing tachycardia and flushing

NURSING CONSIDERATION

Nursing Alert

- Monitor results of hematologic studies, which should be performed at least weekly during therapy. Renal and hepatic function should be monitored periodically during prolonged treatment. Griseofulvin has produced hepatocellular necrosis and liver tumors in mice, impaired spermatogenesis in rats, and embryotoxic and teratogenic effects in rats and dogs. Although these effects have not been demonstrated in humans, caution is required when using drug for extended periods, and it should not be used for minor or trivial fungal infections, nor for infections due to organisms other than susceptible dermatophytes.

PATIENT EDUCATION

1. Suggest taking drug with meals to reduce GI irritation and to improve absorption (a high fat diet increases absorption).
2. Stress the necessity of continuing treatment until infecting organism is completely eradicated, as indicated by clinical and laboratory examinations. Beneficial effects may not be noticeable for several weeks to months. Average duration of treatment is 4 to 6 weeks for scalp ringworm and at least 4 to 6 months for fingernail and toenail fungal infections.
3. Instruct patient to report the development of fever, sore throat, mucosal irritation, or extreme malaise because these might indicate a developing blood dyscrasia.
4. Warn patient that flushing and tachycardia can occur with ingestion of alcohol.
5. Advise patient to avoid exposure to intense sunlight because photosensitivity can occur.
6. Teach patient interventions that minimize incidence of reinfection, and instruct patient to keep infected areas dry because moisture enhances fungal growth.
7. Teach patient how to recognize and report overgrowth of nonsusceptible fungi (diarrhea, perianal itching, stomatitis, "black tongue").
8. If patient is allergic to penicillin, warn her or him to watch for early signs of a hypersensitivity reaction because cross-sensitivity to penicillins can occur.

Ketoconazole

Nizoral

Ketoconazole is used orally for treating a variety of oral and systemic fungal infections. It is less toxic than amphotericin B but somewhat less effective as well. Gastrointestinal complaints are common, and serious hepatotoxicity has been reported. A topical cream is also available (see Table 70-1).

MECHANISM

Not completely established; impairs the synthesis of ergosterol, which is a vital component of fungal cell membranes, resulting in increased permeability and subsequent leakage of cellular components

USES

Oral

Treatment of the following fungal infections: candidiasis, oral thrush, chronic mucocutaneous candidiasis, candiduria, histoplasmosis, blastomycosis, coccidioidomycosis, paracoccidioidomycosis, and chromomycosis

Treatment of severe, resistant, cutaneous dermatophytal infections not responding to topical therapy or oral griseofulvin

Investigational uses include treatment of onychomycosis (due to *Trichophyton* or *Candida* species), pityriasis versicolor (tinea versicolor), recurrent vaginal candidiasis, and advanced prostatic carcinoma

Topical

(See also Table 70-1)

Treatment of tinea corporis, tinea cruris and tinea versicolor

DOSAGE

Oral

Adults: 200 mg once daily (400 mg once daily in very serious infections)

Children (over 2 years): 3.3 to 6.6 mg/kg/day as a single daily dose

Minimum treatment is 1 to 2 weeks for candidiasis, 4 weeks for recalcitrant dermatophytal infections, and 6 months for other systemic mycotic infections.

Topical

See Table 70-1

FATE

Well absorbed orally; peak serum levels occur in 1 to 2 hours; tablet dissolution requires an acidic environment; highly (95%–99%) protein-bound; cerebrospinal fluid penetration is negligible; undergoes extensive hepatic metabolism; excreted largely (80%–90%) in the bile and feces (via enterohepatic circulation) with about 10% to 15% of drug excreted in the urine

COMMON SIDE EFFECTS

Nausea, vomiting, GI upset, pruritus; in addition, elevated serum transaminase occurs in 5% to 10% of patients

SIGNIFICANT ADVERSE REACTIONS

Abdominal pain, diarrhea, dizziness, lethargy, headache, fever, chills, photophobia, impotence, gynecomastia, thrombocytopenia, hepatic dysfunction, and oligospermia

CONTRAINDICATIONS

Treatment of fungal meningitis. *Cautious use* in persons with liver dysfunction and in pregnant or nursing women

INTERACTIONS

GI absorption of ketoconazole may be impaired by antacids, histamine-2 antagonists, anticholinergics, and other drugs that reduce stomach acidity

Ketoconazole can enhance the anticoagulant effect of coumarins and may elevate the plasma level of cyclosporine

Rifampin can reduce blood levels of ketaconazole if given concurrently

Use of ketoconazole and phenytoin may alter the metabolism of one or both drugs

NURSING CONSIDERATIONS

Nursing Alert
- Monitor results of liver function tests, which should be performed before therapy is initiated and at intervals of several weeks during treatment. *Transient* elevations in liver enzymes occur frequently and do not require discontinuation of therapy. Persistent elevations or presence of clinical signs of hepatic injury, however, require immediate termination of treatment because liver disorders, although rare, are potentially fatal.

1. Note that ketoconazole can decrease synthesis of cortisol and testosterone, especially with higher doses. The clinical significance of these effects remains to be determined.

PATIENT EDUCATION

1. Instruct patient not to take any other drugs, including OTC preparations, unless prescribed. If drugs or substances that reduce gastric acidity are taken within 2 hours of ketoconazole, GI absorption may be impaired (see Interactions).
2. Emphasize the importance of continuing treatment until *all* clinical and laboratory tests indicate that the active fungal infection has abated. In general, candidiasis requires a minimum of 2 weeks of therapy, whereas systemic mycotic infections may require 6 months or more of therapy.

Miconazole

Monistat I.V.

A broad-spectrum antifungal agent, miconazole is used intravenously for treatment of severe systemic fungal infections as well as topically and vaginally for control of cutaneous and mucocutaneous candidal and dermatophytal infections. The discussion that follows focuses on the systemic use of miconazole; its topical application is considered in Table 70-1.

MECHANISM
Alters the permeability of the fungal cell membrane, resulting in loss of cell constituents and ultimately cellular death

USES
Alternative treatment of coccidioidomycosis, paracoccidioidomycosis, cryptococcosis, petriellidiosis, and chronic mucocutaneous candidiasis

Topical treatment of cutaneous and mucocutaneous candidal and dermatophytal infections (see Table 70-1)

DOSAGE
Intravenous
Adults: 200 mg to 3600 mg/day depending on disease and severity, divided over three infusions of 30 to 60 minutes each; dilute standard injection (10 mg/mL) in 200 mL fluid before infusing
Coccidioidomycosis: 1800 mg to 3600 mg/day
Cryptococcosis: 1200 mg to 2400 mg/day
Petriellidiosis: 600 mg to 3000 mg/day
Candidiasis: 600 mg to 1800 mg/day
Paracoccidioidomycosis: 200 mg to 1200 mg/day

Children: 20 mg to 40 mg/kg/day in divided infusions; maximum is 15 mg/kg/infusion

NOTE
Treatment is continued until clinical and laboratory tests no longer indicate the presence of an active fungal infection (usually a minimum of 3–4 weeks), because inadequate treatment can result in recurrence of the infection

Intrathecal
20 mg undiluted solution every 3 days to 7 days as adjunct to IV infusion in fungal meningitis

Bladder Instillation
200 mg diluted solution (10 mg/200 mL)

FATE
Highly bound to plasma protein; penetration into cerebrospinal fluid is poor; rapidly metabolized in the liver and excreted both in the urine and feces, mainly as inactive metabolites; elimination half-life is 20 to 25 hours

COMMON SIDE EFFECTS
(IV use only) Phlebitis, pruritus, nausea, febrile reactions, rash, vomiting

SIGNIFICANT ADVERSE REACTIONS
(IV use only) Diarrhea, drowsiness, flushing, anorexia, hyponatremia, decreased hematocrit, thrombocytopenia, hyperlipemia (due to the castor oil vehicle), and arrhythmias (with too-rapid IV administration)

CONTRAINDICATIONS
No absolute contraindications. *Cautious use* in persons with anemia, hyperlipemia; in pregnant women or nursing mothers; and in young children.

INTERACTIONS
The effects of oral anticoagulants may be enhanced by IV miconazole

Miconazole and amphotericin B are mutually antagonistic and the antifungal activity of the combination is less than that of either drug used alone

Miconazole may potentiate the action of the oral hypoglycemic drugs

The metabolism of phenytoin may be reduced by concurrent use of miconazole

NURSING CONSIDERATIONS

Nursing Alerts
- Initiate administration only in hospitalized patients, and monitor patient closely during therapy. An initial dose of 200 mg should be given to assess patient's reaction.
- Administer IV infusion slowly (over a 30–60-min period) to minimize the danger of tachycardia and arrythmias.
- Monitor results of hemoglobin, hematocrit, electrolyte, and lipid determinations, which should be performed at the beginning of therapy and regularly thereafter.

1. Dilute injection in 200 mL of sodium chloride or 5% dextrose solution.
2. Observe infusion site for signs of phlebitis.
3. If nausea and vomiting become problematic, collaborate with drug prescriber to implement effective interventions (e.g., slowing infusion rate, reducing dose, avoiding mealtime drug administration, administering prophylactic antiemetic medication).

Nystatin, Oral

Mycostatin, Nilstat

(CAN) Nadostine

Nystatin is a fungicidal antibiotic obtained from a species of *Streptomyces*. It is used principally in the treatment of candidal infections of the skin, mucous membranes, and intestinal tract. Following oral administration, it is poorly absorbed and thus is effective only against candidal infections of the oral cavity and intestinal tract. The drug is available as an oral tablet (which is swallowed whole) for the treatment of intestinal candidiasis and also as an oral suspension (which is retained in the mouth as long as possible before swallowing) for the treatment of candidiasis of the oral cavity. Those indications are discussed here, while the topical use of nystatin is considered in Table 70-1.

MECHANISM

Binds to sterols in the membrane of fungal cells, altering its permeability; the resultant leakage of intracellular components leads to cellular death

USES

Treatment of intestinal candidiasis (oral tablet)

Treatment of candidiasis of the oral cavity (oral suspension)

Treatment of cutaneous and mucocutaneous candidal infections (for topical and vaginal application, see Table 70-1)

DOSAGE

Intestinal Candidiasis

500,000 U to 1 million U (1 or 2 tablets) three times a day; continue for at least 48 hours after clinical cure

Oral Candidiasis

Adults and children: 400,000 U to 600,000 U (4 mL–6 mL oral suspension) four times a day (one half dose in each side of mouth—retain for as long as possible before swallowing); continue for at least 48 hours after symptoms have disappeared

> **NOTE**
> The oral retention of the drug may be improved by the use of nystatin "popsicles," which are formulated to contain 250,000 U. Alternatively, nystatin vaginal tablets may be given orally and dissolved in the mouth.

Infants: 200,000 U four times a day, as above

FATE

No detectable systemic blood levels following oral administration; excreted largely unchanged in the stool

SIGNIFICANT ADVERSE REACTIONS

Nausea, vomiting, GI distress, and diarrhea with large oral doses

PATIENT EDUCATION

1. Urge patient to complete the entire prescribed course of therapy to minimize the danger of reinfection or relapse.
2. Instruct patient using the oral suspension to place one half of the dose in each side of the mouth, retain there as long as possible (at least several minutes), then swallow.

OPHTHALMIC ANTIFUNGAL AGENT

Natamycin

Natacyn

An antibiotic obtained from a species of *Streptomyces*, natamycin is fungicidal against a variety of organisms. It is not absorbed orally and is used only in the eye for treatment of localized fungal infections.

MECHANISM

Binds to sterols in fungal cell membrane, altering the cell permeability, thus allowing escape of essential cell constituents; not effective against bacteria

USES

Treatment of fungal blepharitis, conjunctivitis, and keratitis due to susceptible organisms (drug of choice for *Fusarium solani* keratitis)

DOSAGE

One drop in affected eye every 1 to 2 hours for 3 to 4 days, then reduce to one drop six to eight times a day for 14 to 21 days depending on the severity of the infection

FATE

No appreciable systemic absorption following topical administration

SIGNIFICANT ADVERSE REACTIONS

Conjunctival hyperemia or chemosis, blurred vision, and photosensitivity

PATIENT EDUCATION

1. Explain proper dosing procedure and importance of completing entire course of therapy to prevent recurrence.
2. Inform patient that bottle must be shaken well before use and dropper should not be contaminated by touching eyes, fingers, or other surfaces.
3. Instruct patient to wait at least 5 minutes before using any other drops in eyes.
4. Instruct patient to notify drug prescriber if irritation occurs or condition appears to deteriorate.
5. Inform patient that condition should be reevaluated if clinical improvement is not evident within 7 to 10 days. Additional laboratory tests are usually required to determine if other organisms are present.

TOPICAL/VAGINAL ANTIFUNGAL AGENTS

Amphotericin B	Miconazole
Butoconazole	Naftifine
Ciclopirox	Nystatin
Clotrimazole	Oxiconazole
Econazole	Terconazole

Haloprogin
Iodochlorhydroxyquin
Ketoconazole
Tolnaftate
Triacetin
Undecylenic acid

A number of drugs possessing antifungal activity are employed topically or intravaginally for the treatment of cutaneous infections, for example, ringworm, athlete's foot, "jock itch," or mucocutaneous infections, such as vulvovaginal moniliasis. They are listed alphabetically in Table 70-1 along with dosage and other relevant information. Griseofulvin, an orally administered drug discussed earlier in the chapter, is also employed for treating ringworm (*Tinea*) infections of the skin, hair, or nails. Ketoconazole may also be administered orally for treating recurrent, resistant vaginal candidal infections.

Table 70-1
Topical/Vaginal Antifungal Agents

Drug	Preparations	Usual Dosage Range	Nursing Implications
Amphotericin B, topical Fungizone	Cream: 3% Ointment: 3% Lotion: 3%	Apply liberally 2–4 times a day; duration of therapy ranges from 1–2 wk for simple infections (e.g., candidiasis) to several months for onychomycoses	Used for treating cutaneous and mucocutaneous candidal infections; similar to nystatin in activity; cream may have a drying effect and discolor the skin; lotion and ointment may stain nail lesions; redness, itching, and burning have occurred with all preparations; discoloration of clothing or fabrics is removable by washing in soap and water or cleaning fluid; also used parenterally; see separate discussion
Butoconazole Femstat	Vaginal cream: 2%	1 applicator full into vagina at bedtime for 3 days; may give for 6 days if necessary	Used for vulvovaginal candidiasis; a 3-day course of therapy is usually sufficient except in pregnant women, who should receive the drug for 6 days; avoid during the first trimester of pregnancy; vulvar and vaginal itching and burning can occur
Ciclopirox Loprox	Cream: 1% Lotion: 1%	Apply twice a day	Broad-spectrum antifungal used for tinea pedis, tinea cruris, tinea corporis, candidiasis, and tinea versicolor due to *Malassezia furfur*; penetrates hair, hair follicles, sebaceous glands, and dermis; do *not* use occlusive dressings; if no clinical improvement occurs within 4 wk, reevaluate therapy; very low incidence of irritation, sensitization, or phototoxicity; safety and efficacy in children less than 10 yr of age have not been established
Clotrimazole Gyne-Lotrimin, Lotrimin, Mycelex (CAN) Canestan, Myclo	Cream: 1% Solution: 1% Lotion: 1% Troches: 10 mg Vaginal tablets: 100 mg, 500 mg Vaginal cream: 1%	*Topical:* massage into infected area twice a day *Vaginal:* 1 100-mg tablet inserted at bedtime for 7 days *or* 1 applicator full of vaginal cream inserted at bedtime for 7–14 days; *alternatively,* 1 500-mg tablet used *once only* *Oral:* 1 troche dissolved in mouth 5 times a day for 14 days	Broad-spectrum antifungal used topically for dermatophytal infections, candidiasis, and tinea versicolor and vaginally for vulvovaginal candidiasis; topical application may cause burning, stinging, peeling, itching, urticaria, and edema; clinical improvement usually occurs within 7 days; discontinue if severe irritation or hypersensitivity reactions occur; vaginal application has resulted in mild burning, rash,

Continued

Table 70-1
Topical/Vaginal Antifungal Agents (continued)

Drug	Preparations	Usual Dosage Range	Nursing Implications
			urinary frequency, and lower abdominal cramping; use of a sanitary pad will prevent staining of clothing; in case of treatment failure, presence of other pathogens (e.g., *Trichomonas, Hemophilus vaginalis*) should be suspected; stress importance of taking full course of therapy; oral use results in prolonged salivary levels of drug; nausea, vomiting, and abnormal liver function test (e.g., elevated SGOT) occur in approximately 15% of patients using troches
Econazole Spectazole (CAN) Ecostatin	Cream: 1%	Apply once or twice a day	Broad-spectrum antifungal with good activity against dermatophytes, yeasts, and some gram-positive bacteria; following topical application, inhibitory concentrations of drug have been found as deep as the middle region of the dermis; low incidence of burning, itching, and erythema; apply after cleansing affected area; treat candidal infections, tinea cruris, and tinea corporis for 2 wk, and tinea pedis for 4 wk
Haloprogin Halotex	Cream: 1% Solution: 1%	Apply liberally 2 times a day for 2–4 wk	Indicated for superficial fungal infections of the skin and for tinea versicolor; side effects include irritation, burning, vesicle formation, and pruritis—may worsen preexisting lesions; avoid contact with eyes; if no improvement is noted within 4 wk, patient's condition should be reevaluated
Iodochlorhydroxyquin-clioquinol Torofor, Vioform	Cream: 3% Ointment: 3%	Apply 2–3 times a day for a maximum of 1 wk	Antibacterial and antifungal agent used in treatment of cutaneous fungal infections and inflammatory skin conditions (e.g., eczema); do *not* use in the presence of superficial viral conditions, tuberculosis, vaccinia, or varicella; infrequently elicits skin irritation but can stain skin, hair, or fabrics; may be absorbed systemically if used on widespread areas, and can interfere with thyroid function tests because drug contains iodine; available in combination with hydrocortisone (Vioform-HC) as prescription only, but can be sold over the counter when used alone

Continued

Table 70-1
Topical/Vaginal Antifungal Agents (continued)

Drug	Preparations	Usual Dosage Range	Nursing Implications
Ketoconazole Nizoral	Cream: 2%	Apply once or twice daily for at least 2 wk	Broad-spectrum antifungal used topically for treatment of tinea corporis and tinea cruris as well as tinea versicolor due to *Malassezia furfur*; resistance has not been reported; pruritis, stinging, and dermal irritation have occurred; *cautious use* in pregnant women; also used orally—see separate discussion
Miconazole Micatin, Monistat-Derm, Monistat-3, Monistat 7	Cream: 2% Lotion: 2% Powder: 2% Spray: 2% Vaginal cream: 2% Vaginal suppositories: 100 mg, 200 mg	*Topical:* apply twice a day for 2–4 wk *Vaginal:* 1 applicator full or 1 suppository (100 mg) vaginally at bedtime for 7 days *or* 1 suppository (200 mg) once daily for 3 days	Indicated for cutaneous dermatophytal and candidal infections, tinea versicolor, and vulvovaginal candidiasis; rarely causes burning or irritation topically; avoid eyes; use lotion rather than cream between the toes or fingers to avoid maceration effects; clinical improvement should occur in 1–2 wk; diagnosis should be reevaluated after 4 wk if good response is not evident; pathogens other than *Candida* should be ruled out before using drug for vaginitis, because it is effective only against candidal vulvovaginitis; 100-mg suppository (Monistat 7) is given for 7 days while 200-mg suppository (Monistat-3) is used only for 3 days; advise patient to insert high into vagina, to use sanitary napkin to prevent staining, to complete full course of therapy, and to avoid sexual intercourse during treatment to prevent reinfection; burning, itching, and irritation can occur—notify physician; use *cautiously* during pregnancy, especially the first trimester; perform urine and blood glucose studies in patients who do not respond to treatment, because persistent candidal vulvovaginitis may be related to unrecognized diabetes mellitus; also used IV for severe systemic fungal infections; see separate discussion
Naftifine Naftin	Cream: 1%	Apply twice a day for at least 2 wk	Broad-spectrum agent used for treating tinea corporis and tinea cruris; some systemic absorption occurs and drug and metabolites can appear in the urine and feces; burning, stinging, erythema, itching, dryness of skin are noted with topical use; avoid contact with eyes, nose or mouth; do *not* use occlusive dressings

Continued

Table 70-1
Topical/Vaginal Antifungal Agents (continued)

Drug	Preparations	Usual Dosage Range	Nursing Implications
Nystatin Mycostatin, Mykinac, Nilstat, Nystex, O-V Statin (CAN) Nyaderm	Cream: 100,000 U/g Ointment: 100,000 U/g Powder: 100,000 U/g Vaginal tablets: 100,000 U Troches: 200,000 U	*Topical:* apply 2–3 times a day for at least 1 wk after clinical cure *Vaginal:* 1 tablet inserted vaginally daily for 14 days *Oral:* 1–2 troches dissolved in mouth 4–5 times a day for up to 14 days	Used in treating cutaneous and vaginal infections due to *Candida* species; troches and oral suspension (see nystatin, oral) are used to treat oral candidiasis; no detectable blood levels are noted following topical application; irritation is rare and drug does not stain skin or mucous membranes; avoid contact with eyes; powder may be dusted into shoes and socks as well as onto feet; symptomatic relief of cutaneous infections usually occurs within 72 h; vaginal application should be continued for entire 14 days, even though clinical symptoms disappear within a few days; lack of response suggests presence of other pathogens besides *Candida*; no adverse effects or complications have been reported when drug is used during pregnancy; also available in oral tablets for treatment of intestinal candidiasis—see separate discussion
Oxiconazole Oxistat	Cream: 1%	Apply once daily for 2–4 wk	Broad-spectrum topical antifungal used to treat tinea pedis, tinea cruris, and tinea corporis; low incidence of itching, burning, and erythema with topical use; avoid eyes; systemic absorption is low
Sulconazole Exelderm	Topical solution: 1%	Massage small amount of solution into affected area once or twice daily	Broad-spectrum antifungal used for treating tinea cruris, tinea corporis and tinea versicolor; efficacy in tinea pedis (athlete's foot) has *not* been demonstrated; itching, burning or stinging on application is rare; avoid contact with eyes; improvement usually occurs within 1 week; continue treatment for 3–4 wk
Terconazole Terazol 7	Vaginal cream: 0.4%	1 applicator full at bedtime daily for 7 days	Effective in treating vulvovaginitis due to *Candida only*; systemic absorption can be as high as 15%; *cautious use* in pregnant and nursing women; headache is very common (25%); therapeutic effect is not altered by menstruation
Tolnaftate Aftate, Tinactin, and other manufacturers (CAN) Pitrex	Cream: 1% Gel: 1% Solution: 1% Liquid aerosol: 1% Powder: 1% Powder aerosol: 1%	Apply small amount 2–3 times a day for 2–6 wk as necessary	Effective in treating cutaneous dermatophytal infections, e.g., athlete's foot, jock itch, or ringworm; inactive systemically, virtually nontoxic, nonirritating, and

Continued

Table 70-1
Topical/Vaginal Antifungal Agents (continued)

Drug	Preparations	Usual Dosage Range	Nursing Implications
			nonsensitizing; serious or chronic fungal infections may require concomitant use of griseofulvin; powder is used only as adjunctive therapy; liquids or solutions are preferred in hairy areas; not effective against *Candida,* therefore if patient does not improve within several weeks, additional antifungal therapy is indicated; discontinue treatment if irritation occurs or condition worsens; available without prescription
Triacetin Enzactin, Fungacetin, Fungoid	Cream: 25% Ointment: 25% Liquid (Fungoid): with cetylpyridinium and chloroxylenol	Apply twice a day; continue for at least 1 wk after symptoms have subsided	Indicated for milder superficial fungal infections (e.g., athlete's foot); cleanse affected area with alcohol or soap and water before application; cover treated areas; avoid eyes; use *cautiously* in patients with impaired circulation; may stain certain fabrics; available without prescription, except Fungoid, which contains additional antiseptics
Undecylenic acid and salts Caldesene, Cruex, Desenex, Quinsana, Ting, and other manufacturers	Ointment: 5% undecylenic acid and 20% zinc undecylenate Cream: 20% total undecylenate Liquid: 10% undecylenic acid and 47% isopropyl alcohol Powder and aerosol powder: 10% calcium undecylenate *or* 2% undecylenic acid plus 20% zinc undecylenate Soap: 2% undecylenic acid Foam: 10% undecylenic acid and 35% isopropyl alcohol	Apply as needed several times a day	Fungistatic and weak antibacterial activity; mainly used for athlete's foot, jock itch, or ringworm *exclusive* of nails and hairy areas; also employed for relief or prevention of diaper rash, prickly heat, groin irritation, and other minor skin irritations; do *not* use if skin is broken or severely abraded; area should be cleansed well before application; use with *caution* in patients with impaired circulation; powder is recommended only as adjunctive therapy—ointments, creams, and liquids are used as primary therapy in most body areas

Selected Bibliography

Bennett JE: Antifungal Agents. In Mandell GL, Douglas RG, Bennett JE (eds): Principles and Practice of Infectious Diseases, 2nd ed, p 263. New York, John Wiley & Sons, 1985

Cantanzaro A et al: Ketoconazole for treatment of disseminated coccidioidomycosis. Ann Intern Med 96:436, 1982

Craven PC, Graybill JR: Combination of oral flucytosine and ketoconazole as therapy for experimental cryptococcal meningitis. J Infect Dis 149:584, 1984

Drouhet E, DuPont B: Laboratory and clinical assessment of ketoconazole in deep-seated mycoses. Am J Med 74:30, 1983

Drugs for the treatment of systemic fungal infections. Med Lett Drugs Ther 26:36, 1984

Drutz DJ: Amphotericin B in the treatment of coccidioidomycosis. Drugs 26:337, 1983

Drutz DJ: Newer antifungal agents and their use, including an update on amphotericin B and flucytosine. In Remington JS, Swartz MN (eds): Current Clinical Topics in Infectious Diseases, vol 3, p 97. New York, McGraw-Hill, 1982

Gever LN: Giving amphotericin B for systemic fungal infections. Nursing 84 14(7):8, July 1984

Hume AL, Kerkering TM: Ketoconazole. Drug Intell Clin Pharm 17:169, 1983

Janssen PA, Symoens JE: Hepatic reactions during ketoconazole treatment. Am J Med 74:80, 1983

Koldin MH, Medoff G: Antifungal chemotherapy. Pediatr Clin North Am 30:49, 1983

Medoff G, Brajtburg J, Kobayashi GS, Bolard J: Antifungal agents useful in the therapy of systemic fungal infection. Annu Rev Pharmacol Toxicol 23:303, 1983

Meunier-Carpentier F: Treatment of mycoses in cancer patients. Am J Med 74:74, 1983

New topical antifungal drugs. Med Lett Drugs Ther 25:98, 1983

Norris SM: Amphotericin B—how safe and effective? Infect Control 6:243, 1985

Odds FC: Interactions among amphotericin B, 5-fluorocytosine, ketoconazole and miconazole against pathogenic fungi in vitro. Antimicrob Agents Chemother 22:763, 1982

Owens NJ et al: Prophylaxis of oral candidiasis with clotrimazole troches. Arch Intern Med 144:290, 1984

Shechtman LB et al: Clotrimazole treatment of oral candidiasis in patients with neoplastic disease. Am J Med 76:1, 1984

Smego RA: Combined Therapy with amphotericin B and flucytosine for *Candida* meningitis. Rev Infect Dis 6:791, 1984

Stevens DA: Miconazole in the treatment of coccidioidomycosis. Drugs 26:347, 1983

Sud IJ, Feingold DS: Effect of ketoconazole on the fungicidal action of amphotericin B in *Candida albicans*. Antimicrob Agents Chemotherap 23:185, 1983

Van Cutsem J: The antifungal activity of ketoconazole. Am J Med 74:9, 1983

Waldorf AR, Polak A: Mechanisms of action of 5-fluorocytosine. Antimicrob Agents Chemother 23:79, 1983

Ward MD: Amphotericin B. Crit Care Nurs 4(6):7, Nov/Dec 1984

SUMMARY. ANTIFUNGAL AGENTS

Drug	Preparations	Usual Dosage Range
Systemic		
Amphotericin B Fungizone	Powder for injection: 50 mg/vial See also Table 70-1	*IV infusion:* initially 0.25 mg/kg/day infused over 6 h; increase gradually to 1 mg/kg/day *or* 1.5 mg/kg every other day (maximum daily dose 1.5 mg/kg) *Intrathecal/intraventricular:* 0.1 mg initially, increased gradually up to 0.5 mg every 48–72 h *Topical:* apply liberally 2–4 times a day for 1–4 wk
Flucytosine Ancobon	Capsules: 250 mg, 500 mg	50 mg–150 mg/kg/day in divided doses at 6-h intervals
Griseofulvin Fulvicin, Grifulvin, Grisactin, Gris-PEG	*Microsize* Tablets: 250 mg, 500 mg Capsules: 125 mg, 250 mg Suspension: 125 mg/5 mL *Ultramicrosize* Tablets: 125 mg, 165 mg, 250 mg, 330 mg (ultramicrosize tablets have 1.5 times the activity of microsize tablets)	Adults: 500 mg–1 g microsize or equivalent daily in a single dose or divided doses Children: 11 mg/kg/day microsize or equivalent, daily in a single dose or divided doses
Ketoconazole Nizoral	Tablets: 200 mg	Adults: 200 mg–400 mg once a day Children over 2 yr: 3.3 mg–6.6 mg/kg/day as a single daily dose
Miconazole IV Monistat IV	Injection: 10 mg/mL See also Table 70-1	Adults: 200 mg–3600 mg/day (depending on disease) by 3 equally divided IV infusions Children: 20 mg/kg–40 mg/kg/day in divided IV infusions (maximum 15 mg/kg/infusion) *Intrathecal:* 20 mg undiluted injection every 3–7 days *Bladder instillation:* 200 mg diluted solution (10 mg/200 mL)
Nystatin, Oral Mycostatin, Nilstat	Tablets: 500,000 U Oral suspension: 100,000 U/mL See also Table 70-1	*Intestinal candidiasis:* 500,000 U to 1 million U (1–2 tablets) 3 times a day *Oral candidiasis:* 400,000 U to 600,000 U (4 mL–6 mL suspension) 4 times a day; half dose in each side of the mouth Infants: 200,000 U 4 times a day
Topical/Vaginal	See Table 70-1	
Ophthalmic		
Natamycin Natacyn	Ophthalmic suspension: 5%	1 drop every 1–2 h for 3–4 days, then 1 drop 6–8 times a day for 14–21 days

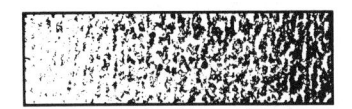

ANTIVIRAL AGENTS

Although viruses are responsible for a large number of diseases, the number of effective antiviral drugs currently available is rather small. The principal obstacle to effective antiviral treatment is the fact that virus particles replicate within host (i.e., human) cells by means of the enzyme systems of the invaded cell. Thus, drugs interfering with intracellular viral replication are likely to damage the host cell as well and are often quite toxic if given systemically. In addition, most viral diseases are of short duration and are often clinically asymptomatic until the infectious process within the host cells is well advanced, by which time the body's own defense mechanisms have already come into play. Thus, to be maximally effective, drugs that block viral replication should be administered *before* the onset of the disease. Such is the case with use of amantadine as a prophylactic agent against influenza A virus. On the other hand, some viral infections, such as herpesvirus, continue to manifest viral replication even after symptoms have appeared. In these diseases, inhibition of *further* viral replication may speed healing and thus serves as the basis for use of drugs such as acyclovir, idoxuridine, and vidarabine in herpetic infections.

Viral diseases are best managed prophylactically, either by active (attenuated or killed virus vaccines) or in some cases passive (viral antibodies) immunization. Once the disease has appeared, however, immunization is of no value, and most common viral infections (such as colds or "flu") are usually best treated symptomatically. Specific antiviral drugs have a limited therapeutic application, largely for the reasons already outlined. Only a handful of viral infections have been shown to be responsive to the available antiviral agents.

Of course, much attention has been focused recently on the AIDS virus. Although no cure for this dread disease has been attained, at least one anti-AIDS drug has become available. While far from an ideal drug in terms of side effects and cost, zidovudine has at least afforded a degree of palliation and appears to slow the progress of the disease. Many other drugs are currently being investigated for the treatment of AIDS and AIDS-related diseases, and some of these are mentioned following the discussion of zidovudine at the end of the chapter.

Acyclovir

Zovirax

Acyclovir is a nucleoside of guanine with in vitro antiviral activity against herpes simplex types 1 and 2, varicella–zoster, Epstein–Barr, and cytomegalovirus. Normal cellular thymidine kinase enzyme does not utilize acyclovir; hence, the drug *selectively* inhibits viral cell replication with minimal toxicity for normal uninfected cells and is thus well tolerated by most patients. Acyclovir is available for oral, topical, or intravenous administration. Oral acyclovir can reduce the frequency and severity of recurrences in up to 95% of patients. Topical application of the drug can also shorten healing time and reduce pain when applied to primary lesions but generally has no significant beneficial effect on *recurrent* genital lesions. Intravenous infusion is used in severe infections or in immunocompromised patients.

MECHANISM

Converted by herpes simplex virus-coded thymidine kinase into acyclovir monophosphate, which is further transformed into the diphosphate and triphosphate, the latter representing the active form of the drug; acyclovir triphosphate interferes with herpes simplex virus DNA polymerase, thus blocking viral replication, and can also be incorporated into growing chains of DNA by viral DNA polymerase, thereby terminating further growth of the DNA chain

USES
Topical

Management of initial episodes of herpes genitalis and limited, non-life-threatening mucocutaneous herpes simplex infections in immunocompromised patients

Intravenous infusion

Treatment of initial and recurrent mucosal and cutaneous herpes simplex (HSV-1 and HSV-2) infections in immunocompromised patients

Treatment of *severe* initial episodes of herpes genitalis in patients who are *not* immunocompromised

Oral

Treatment of initial episodes of genital herpes (HSV-2)

Management of recurrent episodes of genital herpes

DOSAGE
Ointment

Apply sufficient quantity to cover all lesions every 3 hours six times a day for 7 days

Intravenous infusion

Adults and children over 12 years: 5 mg/kg infused at a constant rate over 1 hour every 8 hours for 5 to 7 days

Children under 12 years: 250 mg/M^2 infused at a constant rate over 1 hour every 8 hours for 5 to 7 days

Oral

Initial infections: 200 mg every 4 hours while awake for a total of five capsules a day for 10 days

Recurrent infections: 200 mg three to five times a day for up to 6 months

FATE

Oral acyclovir is slowly and incompletely absorbed, and absorption is unaffected by food; peak plasma levels occur in 1.5 to 2 hours; widely distributed into most body tissues; concentrations in cerebrospinal fluid are approximately one half those in plasma; protein binding is low (10%–30%); plasma half-life is 2 to 3 hours in patients with normal kidney function; excreted primarily unchanged by the kidneys (60%–90%), with approximately 15% of dose excreted as a metabolite

Systemic absorption after topical application is minimal.

COMMON SIDE EFFECTS

IV: inflammation at injection site following extravasation, elevated serum creatinine, rash, urticaria

Topical: burning or stinging at application site, pruritus

Oral: nausea, vomiting, diarrhea, headache

SIGNIFICANT ADVERSE REACTIONS

IV: sweating, hypotension, headache, nausea, hematuria, thrombocytosis, nervousness, and renal damage; *rarely,* encephalopathic changes (e.g., lethargy, confusion, tremors, agitation, seizures, hallucinations, and coma)

Topical: rash, vulvitis

Oral: dizziness, vertigo, fatigue, insomnia, irritability, depression, skin rash, acne, accelerated hair loss, anorexia, arthralgia, fever, sore throat, palpitations, muscle cramping, lymphadenopathy, edema, menstrual abnormalities, and superficial thrombophlebitis

CONTRAINDICATIONS

No absolute contraindications. *Cautious use* in patients with renal, hepatic, neurologic or electrolyte abnormalities; hypoxia; dehydration; and in pregnant or nursing women

INTERACTIONS

Probenecid increases the half-life of acyclovir and reduces the rate of urinary elimination.

NURSING CONSIDERATIONS

Nursing Alerts

- Administer IV infusion *slowly* because bolus injection can cause precipitation of acyclovir crystals in renal tubules. Adequate hydration should be ensured during infusion (urine flow should be sufficient to minimize danger of precipitation).
- Be alert for development of encephalopathic changes (see Significant Adverse Reactions).
- Observe infusion site for signs of phlebitis or inflammation.
- Monitor results of complete blood counts with differentials, which should be performed prior to initiating therapy and at midtreatment each time the drug is used to detect development of blood dyscrasias.

1. Dissolve powder in 10 mL sterile water for injection, which yields a concentration of 50 mg/mL. Remove desired dose and add it to appropriate infusion solution. Infusion concentrations of 7 mg/mL or less are recommended because higher concentrations are more likely to cause inflammation and phlebitis upon extravasation.
2. Use prepared solution (50 mg/mL) within 12 hours. Once diluted, each dose should be used within 24 hours.
3. Refer to enclosed package information for dosage modification based on creatinine clearance in patient with renal impairment.
4. Use a finger cot or rubber glove when applying ointment.

PATIENT EDUCATION

1. Caution patient to adhere to prescribed dosage, frequency of administration, and length of treatment.
2. Explain to patient, as supportively as possible, that there is no evidence that episodic treatment with any acyclovir drug forms (IV, oral, or topical) eliminates either contagiousness, which is present when the virus is shedding, or recurrence.
3. Explain to patient that ointment should be applied only cutaneously (it should not be used in the eyes).
4. Warn patient to use caution in driving or engaging in other hazardous activities until drug effects are known because transient dizziness may occur.
5. Teach patient how to recognize early signs of possible blood dyscrasia (fever, sore throat, bleeding, or fatigue) and stress importance of reporting these to prescriber.
6. Urge patient to seek treatment for recurrence promptly. The sooner acyclovir therapy is initiated, the more effective it is.

Amantadine
Symmetrel

An orally effective drug that exhibits antiviral activity against influenza A viruses as well as an antiparkinsonian action, amantadine is used for the *prevention* of Asian (A) type viral infections in high-risk patients and as adjunctive therapy in Parkinson's disease and in drug-induced extrapyramidal reactions. In addition, the drug may also be effective in shortening the duration of viral symptoms (fever, chills) if taken early in the course of infection. The antiviral activity of amantadine appears to be specific for A virus strains, and there is no evidence that the drug is effective for either prophylaxis or treatment of other viral diseases. The antiparkinsonian actions of the drug are discussed in detail in Chapter 26, and only its antiviral activity is considered here.

MECHANISM

Inhibits viral replication at an early stage, probably by preventing the uncoating of viral nucleic acid and blocking the release of nucleic acids into host cells; increases release of dopamine from nerve endings in the CNS (see Chap. 26)

USES

Prevention and symptomatic management of Asian (A) influenza infections, especially in high-risk patients (e.g., those with heart disease, pulmonary disease, or immunodeficiency states) or in cases in which contact with the virus is likely, for example, in hospital wards or infected households

Symptomatic treatment of parkinsonian or drug-induced extrapyramidal reactions, usually in combination with levodopa (see Chap. 26)

DOSAGE
Influenza

Adults and children 12 and over: 200 mg/day, in a single dose or two divided doses

Children 1 through 8 years: 4.4 mg/kg to 8.8 mg/kg/day (maximum 150 mg/day) in two or three equally divided doses

Children 9 through 12 years: 100 mg twice a day

Parkinson's Disease

100 mg twice a day; may increase to 400 mg/day if necessary

FATE

Readily absorbed orally; peak serum levels occur in 2 to 4 hours but 48 hours is required for drug to reach maximal tissue concentrations; excreted largely unchanged in the urine, 50% of a dose within 20 to 24 hours

COMMON SIDE EFFECTS

Dizziness, lightheadedness, anxiety, irritability, confusion, mild depression, orthostatic hypotension, urinary hesitancy, and constipation

SIGNIFICANT ADVERSE REACTIONS

Cardiovascular: congestive heart failure

Neurologic: fatigue, weakness, headache, nervousness, insomnia, tremors, convulsions, slurred speech, blurred vision, oculogyric crisis. Hallucinations and psychotic reactions have occurred, especially in older persons

GI: nausea, vomiting, anorexia, dry mouth

Others: leukopenia, neutropenia, livedo reticularis (skin mottling), skin rash, eczematoid dermatitis, peripheral edema

CONTRAINDICATIONS
Pregnancy. *Cautious use* in patients with epilepsy or a history of convulsive disorders, congestive heart failure, peripheral edema, renal impairment, orthostatic hypotension, liver disease, history of skin rash or other allergic dermatoses; in psychotic patients; and in elderly or debilitated patients

INTERACTIONS
Amantadine may exhibit additive atropine-like effects with anticholinergic drugs, tricyclic antidepressants, or antihistamines

Excessive CNS stimulation may occur with combined use of amantadine and other CNS stimulants (e.g., amphetamines, methylphenidate)

Decreased urinary excretion of amantadine has occurred when hydrochlorothiazide plus triamterene was administered concurrently

NURSING CONSIDERATION
See also Chapter 26.

1. Note that amantadine does *not* suppress antibody response and can therefore be used in conjunction with influenza A virus vaccine until antibody response develops. It is administered for 2 to 3 weeks after the vaccine has been given. When given alone for prophylaxis, it should be continued for the duration of the epidemic, usually 6 to 8 weeks.

PATIENT EDUCATION
See also Chapter 26.

1. Instruct patient to avoid taking drug too close to bedtime because insomnia may occur.
2. Warn patient not to engage in hazardous activities because dizziness, confusion, and blurred vision can occur, especially early in therapy.
3. Instruct patient to change position slowly to minimize the danger of orthostatic hypotension (see **Plan of Nursing Care 8** in Chap. 31).
4. Inform patient that livedo reticularis (mottling of skin, usually of lower extremities) may occur but that it will subside when drug is discontinued or dosage is reduced.

Ganciclovir
Cytovene

Ganciclovir is a synthetic nucleoside analog of 2-deoxyguanosine that is active against several types of viruses, including cytomegalovirus (CMV), herpes types 1 and 2, varicella-zoster and Epstein-Barr. It is indicated *only* for treatment of CMV retinitis in immunocompromised patients, but it is being evaluated for use in other CMV infections.

MECHANISM
Converted to the triphosphate by cellular kinases on entry into host cells; ganciclovir triphosphate inhibits viral DNA synthesis by competitive inhibition of viral DNA polymerases and by direct incorporation into viral DNA, resulting in termination of viral DNA elongation

USES
Treatment of cytomegalovirus retinitis in immunocompromised patients, including individuals with AIDS

Investigational uses include treatment of other CMV infections such as pneumonitis or colitis and treatment of CMV infections in noncompromised patients

DOSAGE
Initially, 5 mg/kg by IV infusion over 1 hour every 12 hours for 14 to 21 days. For maintenance, 5 mg/kg may be given by IV infusion once daily. Dosage is reduced in the presence of renal impairment according to creatinine clearance

FATE
Following IV infusion, plasma half-life is 2 to 4 hours; the major route of elimination is glomerular filtration and renal excretion, with more than 90% of the dose appearing as unmetabolized drug in the urine

COMMON SIDE EFFECTS
Granulocytopenia, thrombocytopenia

> **NOTE**
> The above two adverse effects occur in 20% to 40% of immunocompromised patients who receive ganciclovir. Granulocytopenia usually occurs within the first 2 weeks of therapy but may occur anytime. Withdrawal of ganciclovir usually results in recovery of cell counts within 3 to 7 days

SIGNIFICANT ADVERSE REACTIONS
CNS: ataxia, confusion, bizarre dreams, dizziness, headache, somnolence, tremor, psychosis, coma
GI: nausea, diarrhea, anorexia, vomiting, abdominal pain
Cardiovascular: hypertension, arrhythmia
Dermatologic: pruritus, urticaria, alopecia
Genitourinary: increased BUN and serum creatinine, hematuria
Other: fever, rash, anemia, chills, edema, malaise, dyspnea, decreased blood glucose, abnormal liver function values, anemia, pain and inflammation at injection site

CONTRAINDICATIONS
No absolute contraindications. *Cautious use* in patients with preexisting cytopenias, reduced renal function, liver impairment, in elderly persons, in pregnant or nursing women, and in children

INTERACTIONS
Other cytotoxic drugs, such as dapsone, flucytosine, vincristine, vinblastine, amphotericin B, adriamycin and pentamidine may have additive effects with ganciclovir

Probenecid may reduce the renal clearance of ganciclovir

Concurrent use of ganciclovir and imipenem–cilastatin has resulted in generalized seizures

Concurrent use of ganciclovir and zidovudine may result in severe granulocytopenia

NURSING CONSIDERATIONS

Nursing Alerts
- Because of the frequency of granulocytopenia and thrombocytopenia, perform neutrophil and platelet counts every 2 days during twice daily dosing and weekly thereafter. Severe neutropenia (500 cells/mm^3) or thrombocytopenia (25000 platelets/mm^3) necessitates dose interruption until marrow recovery is evident.

- Monitor serum creatinine or creatinine clearance every 2 weeks. Dosage is reduced accordingly if creatinine clearance falls below 80 ml/1.73 m²/min.
- Do not exceed recommended dosage, because doses above 6 mg/kg or rates of infusion faster than 1 hour usually result in increased toxicity.
- Do not administer ganciclovir IM or SC, because severe tissue irritation can occur because of the high pH (11) of the solution.

1. Note than ganciclovir was carcinogenic and teratogenic, and caused impaired spermatogenesis in animals, although human studies are lacking. Use during pregnancy and in women of childbearing potential with caution.
2. Ensure adequate hydration during administration of ganciclovir because drug is eliminated largely unchanged in the kidneys.
3. Use care to avoid extravasation during infusion, because drug solution is quite irritating; use veins with adequate blood flow to facilitate rapid dilution and distribution of drug.

PATIENT EDUCATION

1. Urge patients to have regular ophthalmologic examinations because retinitis is not cured by ganciclovir and condition ultimately deteriorates.
2. Impress patients with the necessity of using contraceptive measures during treatment, because drug may cause birth defects.

Idoxuridine

Herplex, Stoxil

Idoxuridine (IDU) is a structural analog of thymidine, an essential intermediate in DNA synthesis. Because it is rapidly inactivated by enzymes, IDU is used only locally in the eye for the treatment of herpes simplex keratitis, a viral disease that affects the cornea.

MECHANISM

Incorporated into viral DNA, producing a faulty molecule incapable of reproduction, thus blocking herpes viral cell replication

USE

Treatment of herpes simplex (herpetic) keratitis

NOTE
Idoxuridine will control the infection but has no effect on accumulated scarring or progressive loss of vision

DOSAGE

Ophthalmic solution: one drop in infected eye every hour during the day and every 2 hours at night; reduce to every 2 hours during the day and every 4 hours at night when improvement is noted; continue for 5 to 7 days after healing is complete

Ophthalmic ointment: instill into lower conjunctival sac five times a day, every 4 hours; continue for 5 to 7 days after healing is complete

Antibiotics or corticosteroids may be used concurrently with idoxuridine as the condition warrants.

FATE

Short acting and quickly inactivated by nucleotidases

COMMON SIDE EFFECTS

Periorbital burning, irritation, lacrimation

SIGNIFICANT ADVERSE REACTIONS

Pain, inflammation, pruritus, and edema of eyes and eyelids; photophobia; local allergic reactions; corneal clouding, vascularization or stippling; prolonged use can result in follicular conjunctivitis, blepharitis, conjunctival hyperemia, and corneal epithelial staining

INTERACTIONS

Concurrent use of a boric acid solution may increase the severity of local irritation

NURSING CONSIDERATION

1. Note that improvement of keratitic lesions may be enhanced by concomitant use of topical corticosteroids. Steroid should be withdrawn several days before discontinuing idoxuridine. Corticosteroids should *not* be used without idoxuridine.

PATIENT EDUCATION

1. Teach patient how to administer eye drops or ointment (see Chap. 1).
2. Instruct patient to store ophthalmic solution in refrigerator, except for Herplex Liquifilm, which requires no refrigeration.
3. Stress the importance of continuing therapy for at least 5 to 7 days after healing is complete to prevent recurrence of infection, which is common with short courses of therapy.
4. Instruct patient to notify drug prescriber if improvement is not noted within 7 or 8 days, in epithelial infections, or if pain, itching, or swelling occurs, because drug should be discontinued.

Ribavirin

Virazole

Ribavirin has demonstrated antiviral activity against respiratory syncytial virus (RSV), influenza A and B viruses, and herpes simplex virus. When administered as an aerosol, ribavirin retards replication of RSV in infants and reduces the severity and duration of the illness. Aerosol ribavirin has also been shown to be effective against influenza A and B, and oral ribavirin (an investigational dosage form) has been reported to be active in other viral diseases such as acute and chronic hepatitis, herpes genitalis, measles, and Lassa fever.

MECHANISM

Not completely established; appears to interfere with guanidine monophosphate formation and subsequent nucleic acid synthesis in viral particles

USES

Treatment of selected hospitalized infants and young children with severe lower respiratory tract infections due to respiratory syncytial virus

Investigational uses include aerosol treatment of influenza A and B virus infection and oral therapy of hepatitis virus, measles, and Lassa fever

DOSAGE

Solution containing 20 mg/mL is aerosolized and delivered to an infant oxygen hood using the Viratek Small Particle Aerosol Generator.

Treatment is carried out for 12 to 18 hours a day for 3 to 7 days.

A face mask or oxygen tent may be used if an oxygen hood is unavailable

NOTE

Do not use in infants requiring assisted ventilation because drug particles can precipitate in respiratory equipment

FATE

Administration by aerosolization results in significant systemic absorption; plasma half-life is 8 hours to 10 hours; ribavirin and its metabolites accumulate in red blood cells, with a half-life of approximately 40 days

SIGNIFICANT ADVERSE REACTIONS

Rash, hypotension, conjunctivitis, reticulocytosis, worsening of respiratory status, bacterial pneumonia, pneumothorax, apnea, cardiac arrest (rare)

CONTRAINDICATIONS

Pregnancy (drug is potentially teratogenic). *Cautious use* in persons with chronic obstructive lung disease, persons taking digitalis drugs (see Interaction) and in nursing mothers

INTERACTIONS

Use of ribavirin can increase the likelihood of digitalis toxicity

NURSING CONSIDERATIONS

Nursing Alerts

- Administer by aerosol only, use only a Viratek small particle aerosol generator (SPAG) Model-2 (operator's manual contains operating instructions), and avoid concomitant administration of other aerosol preparations.
- Closely monitor patient's respiratory status. Assess rate and character of respirations, and auscultate lungs for abnormal breath sounds prior to initiation of therapy and frequently thereafter. Observe patient for signs of dyspnea; apnea; rapid, shallow respirations; intercostal and substernal retraction; nasal flaring; limited lung excursion; cyanosis; and evidence of pneumothorax.
- Monitor cardiac rhythm continuously to detect cardiac arrythmias.
- Check blood pressure frequently to detect hypotension.
- Monitor intake–output and assess fluid status frequently.
- Monitor results of complete blood counts with differentials, which should be performed frequently during therapy, especially if treatment is prolonged, because drug may cause a precipitous drop in hemoglobin, hematocrit, and red blood cells.
- Observe patient simultaneously receiving mechanical ventilation for signs of worsening pulmonary function. Obstruction may cause inadequate ventilation and gas exchange if ribavirin precipitates or fluid accumulates in tubing. Check equipment, including endotracheal tube, every 2 hours.

1. Prepare aerosol solution with either sterile water for injection or sterile water for inhalation without preservatives or any other additive. Package insert contains preparation instructions.
2. Inspect solution before using. Discard if discolored or cloudy.

Trifluridine

Viroptic

A halogenated pyrimidine, trifluridine exhibits in vivo antiviral activity against herpes simplex virus types 1 and 2 and vaccinia virus. The drug is also active in vitro against some strains of adenovirus. Its clinical application is presently restricted to ophthalmic infections due to sensitive organisms, and the drug is often effective in patients unresponsive to idoxuridine and vidarabine.

MECHANISM

Not established; interferes with DNA synthesis in cultured mammalian cells

USES

Treatment of primary keratoconjunctivitis and recurrent epithelial keratitis due to herpes simplex viruses 1 and 2
Treatment of epithelial keratitis in patients intolerant of or unresponsive to idoxuridine or vidarabine
Treatment of ophthalmic infections due to vaccinia virus or adenovirus (clinical efficacy not definitely established)
Prophylaxis of herpes simplex virus keratoconjunctivitis and epithelial keratitis (efficacy not definitely established)

DOSAGE

One drop onto cornea every 2 hours *while awake* (maximum 9 drops/day) until corneal ulcer has completely reepithelialized, then one drop every 4 hours (maximum 5 drops/day) for an additional 7 days

FATE

Intraocular penetration following topical application is good; systemic absorption is negligible; half-life is approximately 15 minutes

COMMON SIDE EFFECTS

Mild, transient burning or stinging

SIGNIFICANT ADVERSE REACTIONS

Palpebral edema, superficial punctate keratopathy, epithelial keratopathy, stromal edema, irritation, hypersensitivity reactions, hyperemia, and increased intraocular pressure

CONTRAINDICATIONS

No absolute contraindications. *Cautious use* in patients with glaucoma and in pregnancy or lactation

NURSING CONSIDERATION

Nursing Alert

- Administer only after diagnosis of herpetic keratitis has been established because drug is ineffective against bacterial, fungal, or chlamydial infections. Recommended dosage should not be exceeded. Alternative forms of therapy should be considered if clinical improvement does not occur within 7 days or if *complete* reepithelialization is not evident within 14 days. To avoid ocular toxicity, drug should not be used longer than 21 days under any circumstances.

PATIENT EDUCATION

1. Teach patient how to administer eye drops (see Chap. 1).
2. Inform patient that a transient stinging sensation may occur upon instillation.
3. Instruct patient to store drug under refrigeration because elevated temperatures accelerate its degradation.

Vidarabine

Vira-A

Vidarabine is a pyrimidine derivative that possesses antiviral activity against herpes simplex virus types 1 and 2. It may be used systemically in the treatment of herpes simplex virus encephalitis, or ophthalmically for keratoconjunctivitis and epithelial keratitis. Prompt diagnosis of herpes encephalitis, a frequent complication of cancer immunosuppressive therapy, and treatment by vidarabine can reduce mortality from 70% to approximately 25%. However, patients already in a comatose state at the time therapy is initiated do not appear to benefit from the drug. When applied locally in the eye, vidarabine is often effective in patients resistant to or intolerant of idoxuridine.

MECHANISM

Converted into nucleotides, which can inhibit viral DNA synthesis, presumably by interfering with viral DNA polymerase; mammalian cell DNA synthesis is also inhibited, but to a lesser extent; metabolized to hypoxanthine arabinoside, which may act synergistically with the parent compound against DNA viruses

USES

Treatment of herpes simplex virus encephalitis (IV only)
Treatment of superficial and recurrent epithelial keratitis and acute keratoconjunctivitis due to herpes simplex virus types 1 and 2 (ophthalmic only)

DOSAGE

IV: 15 mg/kg/day for 10 days, infused slowly over a 12- to 24-hour period
Ophthalmic: one half inch of ophthalmic ointment into lower conjunctival sac five times a day at 3-hour intervals until reepithelialization has occurred, then twice a day for an additional 7 days

FATE

IV infusion: rapidly deaminated to hypoxanthine arabinoside, the principal metabolite, which is quickly distributed in the body but possesses only one-tenth the in vitro antiviral activity of vidarabine; half-life of vidarabine is 1 hour, and hypoxanthine arabinoside is 3.5 hours; excreted primarily by the kidneys
Ophthalmic application: if cornea is normal, only trace amounts of drug or metabolite are detectable in the aqueous humor; systemic absorption following ocular administration is negligible

COMMON SIDE EFFECTS

Temporary visual haze with ophthalmic application

SIGNIFICANT ADVERSE REACTIONS

IV: anorexia, nausea, vomiting, diarrhea; tremor, dizziness, ataxia, confusion, hallucinations, psychosis; decreased hemoglobin and hematocrit values, hematemesis, reduced white blood cell count and platelet count; weight loss, malaise; rash, pruritus, pain at injection site, and elevated total bilirubin and SGOT
Ophthalmic: irritation, ocular pain, photophobia, lacrimation, burning, superficial punctate keratitis, punctal occlusion, foreign body sensation, hypersensitivity reactions

CONTRAINDICATIONS

No absolute contraindications. *Cautious use* of IV infusion during pregnancy and lactation, and in patients with impaired renal or liver function or in CNS infections other than herpes encephalitis

INTERACTIONS

Concurrent use of allopurinol may interfere with vidarabine metabolism

NURSING CONSIDERATIONS

Nursing Alerts

- Administer only after diagnosis of herpes simplex virus has been established because drug is ineffective against infections due to other viral species or bacterial and fungal infections. Drug should not be used to treat trivial infections, and recommended dosage and duration of therapy should not be exceeded because vidarabine has exhibited mutagenic and carcinogenic potential in laboratory animals, although the significance of this for humans is not yet known.
- Avoid rapid or bolus IV injections, and do not administer SC or IM because drug is poorly soluble and erratically absorbed.
- Monitor results of hematologic tests (e.g., hemoglobin, hematocrit, white blood cells, platelets), which should be performed periodically during systemic therapy because vidarabine can alter them.

1. Prepare infusion just prior to administration. To prepare, shake vial well, then withdraw and transfer desired dose (solution contains 200 mg/mL) into prewarmed (35°C–40°C) fluid (any IV solution is suitable *except* biologic or colloidal fluids such as protein solutions or blood products). Thoroughly agitate until completely clear, then run through an in-line filter (0.45 μm or smaller) to ensure that undissolved particles are removed. Do not refrigerate. Use within 48 hours.

PATIENT EDUCATION

1. Teach patient how to administer ophthalmic ointment.
2. Inform patient using ophthalmic preparation that photophobia or a temporary clouding of vision may occur. Advise caution in operating machinery or performing other hazardous tasks.
3. Stress importance of adhering to prescribed ophthalmic dosage and frequency of administration. Drug prescriber should be notified if improvement is not observed

within 7 days or if condition worsens during therapy. If complete reepithelialization has not occurred within 21 days, alternative treatment may be prescribed.

Zidovudine

Retrovir

Zidovudine, formerly known as azidothymidine (AZT), is the first available anti-AIDS drug. It appears to slow the replication of the human immunodeficiency virus (HIV), the causative agent of AIDS, thus allowing for some immunologic reconstruction in persons afflicted with the virus. To date, however, *no* cures have been reported in HIV-infected patients and the drug must be viewed as merely palliative.

MECHANISM

Thymidine analog converted by thymidine kinase into the triphosphate derivative, which is the active form; inhibits monophosphate and ultimately into the replication of the human immunodeficiency virus (HIV) by blocking viral RNA-dependent DNA polymerase (reverse transcriptase); drug is incorporated into growing chains of DNA by viral reverse transcriptase and thus terminates the incorporation of the DNA chain. Treatment with zidovudine does *not* reduce the risk of transmission of the virus through sexual contact or blood contamination

USES

Management of patients with symptomatic HIV infection (i.e., AIDS or AIDS-related complex—ARC) who have a history of cytologically confirmed *Pneumocystis carinii* pneumonia *or* an absolute CD4 (T$_4$ helper/inducer) lymphocyte count of less than 200/mm^2

DOSAGE

200 mg every 4 hours *around the clock*. If anemia or granulocytopenia occur (see Significant Adverse Reactions), dosage reduction or temporary interruption may be necessary.

FATE

Oral absorption is rapid and peak plasma levels occur within 1 hour; plasma protein binding is 35% to 40%; drug is quickly metabolized in the liver; plasma half-life is about 1 hour; metabolites and some unchanged drug are eliminated in the urine

COMMON SIDE EFFECTS

See *Warning* below

Also: headache, nausea, GI pain, skin rash, fever, myalgia, insomnia, asthenia

SIGNIFICANT ADVERSE REACTIONS

WARNING

The most frequent adverse effects occurring with zidovudine are anemia and granulocytopenia. The frequency of occurrence is directly related to dosage and duration of therapy and inversely related to T$_4$ lymphocyte number, hemoglobin, and granulocyte count at the outset of therapy. Anemia usually occurs within 4 to 6 weeks of therapy and frequently requires blood transfusion. Myelosuppression is generally reversible but often recurs even with dosage reduction, which may necessitate repeated transfusions.

GI: anorexia, diarrhea, vomiting, dysphagia, flatulence, mouth ulcers, bleeding gums, edema of the tongue, rectal bleeding

CNS: dizziness, paresthesias, somnolence, anxiety, confusion, nervousness, syncope, depression

Respiratory: dyspnea, cough, nosebleed, sinusitis, pharyngitis, hoarseness, rhinitis

Urinary: dysuria, polyuria, urinary frequency

Dermatologic/hypersensitivity: pruritus, urticaria, acne

Other: vasodilation, arthralgia, muscle spasm, tremor, photophobia, hearing loss, amblyopia, chills, body odor, hyperalgesia, lymphadenopathy, altered taste

CONTRAINDICATIONS

No absolute contraindications. *Cautious use* in the presence of liver or kidney disease, compromised bone marrow function, and in pregnant or nursing women

INTERACTIONS

Use of drugs that are nephrotoxic or cytotoxic (e.g., amphotericin B, flucytosine, dapsone, pentamidine, vincristine, vinblastine) may increase the risk of toxicity during zidovudine administration

Drugs that are likely to produce hematologic toxicity (chloramphenicol, carbamazepine, adriamycin, interferon) will increase the likelihood of such effects with zidovudine

Drugs that can inhibit the metabolism (glucuronidation) of zidovudine (such as probenecid, indomethacin, aspirin, acetaminophen) by competitive antagonism may potentiate the toxic effects of the drug

NURSING CONSIDERATIONS

Nursing Alerts

- Monitor results of complete blood counts with differentials, which should be performed prior to initiation of therapy and at least every 2 weeks thereafter because hematologic toxicity is common (see *Warning* under Significant Adverse Reactions).
- Assess patient for evidence of opportunistic infection. Zidovudine does not reduce patient's predisposition to infection. It may, in fact, increase it by suppressing bone marrow.

PATIENT EDUCATION

1. Ensure that patient understands dosage regimen: Drug is to be taken every 4 hours around the clock.
2. Warn patient not to take any other drugs, including OTC preparations, unless specifically ordered (see Interactions).
3. Explain the importance of maintaining close medical supervision. The patient should be evaluated at least weekly during early stages of therapy.
4. Supportively explain to patient that drug does not reduce risk of transmitting HIV.
5. Advise patient to notify drug prescriber if condition worsens or any unusual symptoms develop.

Zidovudine is the forerunner for what is hoped to be a spate of new drugs that will provide improved quality and length of life to AIDS victims and perhaps ultimately a cure for this dread disease. As many as 50 antiviral and immunomodulating drugs are currently undergoing clinical trials for the treatment of AIDS, ARC, and AIDS-associated diseases, such as pneumocystis pneumonia and Kaposi's sarcoma. Among these investigational drugs are ampligen, eflornithine, alpha- and beta-interferons, interleukin-2, ribavirin (see earlier discussion), thymopentin, and thymostimuline.

Selected Bibliography

Bennett JA: What we know about AIDS. Am J Nurs 86:1016, 1986

Corey L, Holmes KK: Genital herpes simplex virus infections, Current concepts in diagnosis, therapy and prevention. Ann Intern Med 98:973, 1983

deMiranda P, Blum MR: Pharmacokinetics of acyclovir after intravenous and oral administration. J Antimicrob Chemother 12(Suppl B):29, 1983

Douglas RG: Antiviral drugs. Med Clin North Am 67:1163, 1983

Elion CB: Mechanism of action and selectivity of acyclovir. Am J Med 73:7, 1982

Fischl MA et al: The efficacy of azidothymidine (AZT) in the treatment of patients with AIDS and AIDS-related complex. A double blind, placebo-controlled trial. N Engl J Med 317:185, 1987

Halpern JS: Acyclovir: A respite, not a cure for primary genital herpes. J Emer Nursing 10:268, 1984

Hayden FG, Douglas RG: Antiviral agents. In Mandell GL, Douglas RG, Bennett JE (eds): Principles and Practice of Infectious Diseases, 2nd ed, p 270. New York, John Wiley & Sons, 1985

Hirsch MS, Schooley RT: Treatment of herpes virus infections. N Engl J Med 309:963, 1983

Keay S, Bissett J, Merigan TC: Ganciclovir treatment of cytomegalovirus infections in iatrogenically immunocompromised patients. J Infect Dis 156:1016, 1987

Keeney RE, Kirk LE, Bridgen D: Acyclovir tolerance in humans. Am J Med 75(Suppl):176, 1983

Laskin OL: Acyclovir. Ration Drug Ther 18(5):1, 1984

Laskin OL et al: Use of ganciclovir to treat serious cytomegalovirus infections in patients with AIDS. J Infect Dis 155:323, 1987

Oral acyclovir for genital herpes simplex infections. Med Lett Drugs Ther 27:41, 1985

Sasso CS: Acyclovir for herpes infections. MCN 8:433, 1983

Schinazi RF, Prusoff WH: Antiviral agents. Pediatr Clin North Am 30:77, 1983

Scott TM, Parish LC, Witkowski JA: Herpes simplex virus infections. II, Diagnosis and treatment. Drug Ther 15:135, 1985

Stuart-Harris CH, Oxford JS (eds): Problems of Antiviral Therapy: The Fifth Beecham Colloquium, p 71. London, Academic Press, 1983

Wade JC, Newton B, Flournoy N, Meyers JD: Oral acyclovir for prevention of herpes simplex virus reactivation after marrow transplantation. Ann Intern Med 100:823, 1984

Whitley RJ et al: Viderabine versus acyclovir therapy in herpes simplex encephalitis. N Engl J Med 314:144, 1986

SUMMARY. ANTIVIRAL AGENTS

Drug	Preparations	Usual Dosage Range
Acyclovir Zovirax	Powder for injection: 500 mg/vial Topical ointment: 5% Capsules: 200 mg	*IV infusion* Adults: 5 mg/kg infused over 1 h every 8 h for 5 to 7 days Children under 12 yr: 250 mg/M² infused over 1 h every 8 h for 7 days *Topical* Apply sufficient quantity to cover all lesions every 3 h 6 times a day for 7 days *Oral* 200 mg every 4 h (5 times a day) for 10 days
Amantadine Symmetrel	Capsules: 100 mg Syrup: 50 mg/5 mL	Adults and children 12 and over: 200 mg/day, either as a single dose or 2 equally divided doses Children 1 through 8 yr: 4.4 mg/kg–8.8 mg/kg/day in 2 to 3 divided doses (maximum 150 mg/day) Children 9 through 11 yr: 100 mg twice a day
Ganciclovir Cytovene	Powder for injection: 500 mg/vial	Initially, 5 mg/kg IV (over 1 h) every 12 h for 14 to 21 days Maintenance: 5 mg/kg IV (over 1 h) once daily
Idoxuridine Herplex, Stoxil	Ophthalmic solution: 0.1% Ophthalmic ointment: 0.5%	*Solution* 1 drop every hour during the day and every 2 h at night; reduce to every 2 h during the day and every 4 h at night when improvement is noted *Ointment* Instill into lower conjunctival sac 5 times a day, every 4 h

Continued

SUMMARY. ANTIVIRAL AGENTS (continued)

Drug	Preparations	Usual Dosage Range
Ribavirin Virazole	Powder for reconstitution as aerosol: 20 mg/mL	Use in an oxygen hood for 12 to 18 h a day for 3 to 7 days
Trifluridine Viroptic	Ophthalmic solution: 1%	1 drop every 2 h while awake until corneal ulcer has healed, then 1 drop every 4 h for an additional 7 days
Vidarabine Vira-A	Injection: 200 mg/mL Ophthalmic ointment: 3%	*IV* 15 mg/kg/day for 10 days, infused over 12 to 24 h *Ophthalmic* ½ inch of ointment into lower conjunctival sac 5 times a day at 3-h intervals until reepithelialization occurs, then twice a day for an additional 7 days
Zidovudine Retrovir	Capsules: 100 mg	200 mg every 4 h around the clock

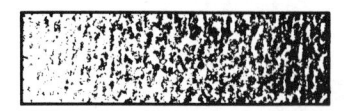

72 ANTINEOPLASTIC AGENTS

Cancer, a disease that occurs in all human and animal populations, affects tissues composed of dividing cells. The exact etiology of most cancers is still unknown, but infections as well as environmental factors (chemicals, fiber particles, radiation) and genetic factors are all capable of inducing a normal cell to become neoplastic—that is, to multiply abnormally.

Cancer may be characterized by the following:

- Cells grow excessively because normal growth-controlling mechanisms are impaired.
- Cells and tissues are undifferentiated.
- Cells exhibit invasiveness and have the ability to metastasize (i.e., establish themselves at sites distant from their original location).
- Cells have acquired heredity (i.e., properties of the original cancerous cells).
- Cells demonstrate increased synthesis of macromolecules from nucleosides and amino acids.

Treatment of cancer many involve surgery, radiation, immunotherapy, or chemotherapy. Until recently, chemotherapy with antineoplastic drugs was used mainly to supplement surgery or radiation therapy in an attempt to eradicate any remaining metastatic tumor cell foci. At present, however, chemotherapy is an accepted and vital part of most cancer regimens. Some neoplastic diseases are, in fact, treated primarily with chemotherapy. In many patients undergoing cancer chemotherapy, a significantly prolonged survival time and, in some cases, complete remission have been achieved (see Table 72-1).

The antineoplastic agents may be classified in a variety of ways. The broadest classification and the one used for this discussion is based on mechanism of action and source of the drug. Thus, the antineoplastic drugs include the following:

- Alkylating agents
- Antimetabolites
- Natural products
- Hormones
- Miscellaneous agents

Antineoplastic agents may also be classified on the basis of their differential effects on normal and malignant cell metabolism. To understand this classification it is important to review the phases of cell division:

G_1—*post*mitotic phase; a number of enzymes are synthesized during this phase

S—period of DNA synthesis for chromosomes

G_2—*pre*mitotic phase; specialized protein and RNA synthesis and formation of mitotic spindle

M—mitosis

G_0—temporarily nondividing cells, cell differentiation, or cell death

Some antineoplastic agents inhibit cells during a specific phase of the mitotic cycle and are referred to as *cell-cycle specific* (CCS). The therapeutic response to cell-cycle specific agents is usually schedule dependent; that is, therapeutic blood levels must be maintained for a sufficient period to allow large numbers of cells to enter the S phase so that the greatest possible number of cells will be killed. Other antineoplastic agents are cytotoxic during any phase of the cell cycle and are referred to as *cell-cycle nonspecific* (CCNS). Cell-cycle nonspecific agents are dose-dependent and are usually more effective if given in large intermittent doses. Cell-cycle specific and cell-cycle nonspecific agents are listed in Table 72-2.

To understand the complex pharmacology of the antineoplastic agents more fully, it is necessary to review the general principles of cancer chemotherapy.

- The goal of cancer therapy is to destroy or remove all neoplastic cells with minimal effect upon normal host cells.
- The maximum chance for cure exists when the tumor cell burden is at a minimum and tumors have a high growth fraction (i.e., a high proportion of tumor cells are actively dividing).
- A given dose of antineoplastic agent kills a constant *percentage* of cells, not a constant *number.*
- Cell-cycle specific agents are more effective than cell-cycle nonspecific agents in tumors with a large, bulky mass.
- Before a change to another agent, treatment with an antineoplastic agent should continue until either the desired response is obtained or toxicity occurs.
- Toxicity is often the limiting factor in the usefulness of an antineoplastic agent, and the risk of toxicity is increased if the patient has received prior chemotherapy or radiation treatment. Because the disease is so often fatal, however, the risk of serious toxicity is relatively acceptable in most instances.
- Malignant cells may exhibit resistance to some antineoplastic agents, thus limiting their usefulness. Resistance may be natural or acquired, that is, either the tumor is resistant from the start of therapy (natural), or resistance occurs after therapy has begun and results from drug-induced adaptation or mutation of malignant cells (acquired).
- Drug scheduling is important. High-dose intermittent therapy is usually more effective, less toxic, and less immunosuppressive than low-dose, continuous therapy. Toxicity may be reduced and cell resistance delayed by administering combinations of drugs in cycles or sequence (see discussion of combination chemotherapy at the end of the chapter).
- Factors such as the age, sex, and physical condition of the patient, prior treatment, and altered renal or hepatic function can influence the outcome of chemotherapy.
- When dosage of antineoplastic agents is based on weight, children tolerate relatively larger doses of drugs than do older patients. Dosage may be more accurately calculated in adults and children using body surface area; mg/kg doses may be conveniently converted to mg/m² doses by multiplying by 40.

Although a variety of drugs are employed in cancer chemotherapy, a number of nursing alerts and nursing considerations are common to all antineoplastic drugs; these are outlined below. Specific alerts and considerations pertaining to individual drugs are given with the respective discussions of each group.

GENERAL NURSING CONSIDERATIONS: ANTINEOPLASTIC AGENTS

Nursing Alerts
- Avoid skin or eye contact and inhalation of vapors or powders when handling cytotoxic drugs. Protective gloves should be worn, particularly when working with

Table 72-1
Neoplastic Diseases Showing a Good Response to Chemotherapy

Disease	Antineoplastic Agents[a]
Acute lymphocytic leukemia (pediatric)	*Induction:* vincristine + prednisone ± asparaginase or doxorubicin *Maintenance:* methotrexate + 6-mercaptopurine
Acute myelogenous leukemia (adult)	Doxorubicin or daunorubicin + cytarabine *or* mitoxantrone + cytarabine ± daunorubicin
Breast cancer	Estrogens, progestins, and tamoxifen Cyclophosphamide + methotrexate + fluorouracil ± prednisone *or* cycloposphamide + doxorubicin ± fluorouracil
Burkitt's lymphoma	Cyclophosphamide *or* cyclophosphamide + methotrexate + vincristine
Choriocarcinoma	Methotrexate ± dactinomycin
Diffuse histiocytic lymphoma	CHOP (cyclophosphamide, doxorubicin, vincristine, prednisone) *or* BACOP (bleomycin, doxorubicin, cyclophosphamide, vincristine, prednisone) *or* COMA (cyclophosphamide, vincristine, methotrexate, cytarabine) *or* COPP (cyclophosphamide, vincristine, procarbazine, prednisone) *or* MACOP-B (methotrexate, bleomycin, doxorubicin, cyclophosphamide, vincristine, prednisone) *or* ProMACE-MOPP (prednisone, methotrexate, doxorubicin, cyclophosphamide, etoposide–mechlorethamine, vincristine, procarbazine, prednisone) *or* COP-BLAM (cyclophosphamide, vincristine, prednisone, bleomycin, doxorubicin, procarbazine)
Ewing's sarcoma	Cyclophosphamide + doxorubicin + vincristine
Hairy cell leukemia	Interferon
Hodgkin's disease	MOPP (mechlorethamine, vincristine, procarbazine, prednisone) *or* ABVD (doxorubicin, bleomycin, vinblastine, dacarbazine) *or* CVPP (chlorambucil, vinblastine, procarbazine, prednisone) ± carmustine
Lung cancer (small cell)	CAV (cyclophosphamide, doxorubicin, vincristine) *or* etoposide + cisplatin *or* CEP (cyclophosphamide, etoposide, cisplatin)
Retinoblastoma	Cyclophosphamide
Rhabdomyosarcoma	VAC (vincristine, dactinomycin, cyclophosphamide) ± doxorubicin
Testicular cancer	Vinblastine + bleomycin + cisplatin *or* cisplatin + etoposide + bleomycin
Wilms' tumor	Dactinomycin + vincristine ± doxorubicin ± cyclophosphamide

[a] (±) indicates a possibly beneficial addition.

---

solutions, because many of these drugs are potent vesicants and all are potential carcinogens. Guidelines for handling cytotoxic drugs have been published by several national agencies.
- Monitor results of blood, liver, and renal studies, which should be performed prior to initiation of therapy and periodically during therapy, to assess the effectiveness and toxicity of therapy. The frequency at which studies are done varies with the agent or agents used and the patient's clinical status.
- Frequently assess patient for signs of developing myelosuppression (unusual bleeding or bruising, fever, sore throat, mucosal ulceration, weakness).
- Check patient's temperature frequently, especially if the granulocyte count is very low, because susceptibility to infection is increased by these drugs. If potential for rectal irritation exists, avoid taking the temperature rectally, because thermometer may irritate rectal mucosa.
- Inspect patient's mouth frequently, particularly for evidence of stomatitis or infection.
- If bone marrow depression becomes severe, place patient in protective isolation and monitor carefully for signs of infection.
- Assess patient's hepatic status frequently for signs of developing dysfunction (jaundice, yellowing of eyes, hepatomegaly, anorexia, right hypochondriac tenderness, clay-colored stools, dark urine).
- Assess patient's pulmonary status frequently for signs of possible pulmonary fibrosis (fever, cough, shortness of breath).
- Be alert for indications of CNS toxicity (dizziness, headache, convulsions, confusion, fatigue, slurred speech, paresthesias).
- Assess patient frequently for loss of taste or tingling in face, fingers, or toes, symptoms of possible peripheral neuropathy.

Table 72-2
Cell-Cycle Specific and Cell-Cycle Nonspecific Agents

Cell-Cycle Specific	Cell-Cycle Non-specific
Antimetabolites	*Alkylating agents*
Cytarabine	Busulfan
Mercaptopurine	Carboplatin
Methotrexate	Carmustine
Thioguanine	Chlorambucil
	Cisplatin
	Cyclophosphamide
	Dacarbazine
	Ifosfamide
	Lomustine
	Mechlorethamine
	Melphalan
	Pipobroman
	Streptozocin
	Triethylenethiophosphoramide
Natural products	*Natural products*
Bleomycin	Dactinomycin
Etoposide	Daunorubicin
Vinblastine	Doxorubicin
Vincristine	Mitoxantrone
	Antimetabolites
	Floxuridine
	Fluorouracil
Miscellaneous	*Miscellaneous*
Hydroxyurea	Procarbazine

- Monitor patient for indications of hyperuricemia (swelling of feet or lower legs, joint pain, stomach pain), which can lead to uric acid nephropathy.
- Observe patient for rash or dermatitis, which may signal drug hypersensitivity.
- If cytotoxic drugs are given IV, assess administration site frequently for earliest signs of extravasation. Certain agents cause thrombophlebitis and severe tissue necrosis; among these are carmustine, dacarbazine, dactinomycin, daunorubicin, doxorubicin, etoposide, mechlorethamine, mithramycin, mitomycin, streptozocin, vinblastine, and vincristine. The following guidelines are recommended to reduce the risk of extravasation and to treat it:

To reduce the risk of extravasation:
—Choose a vein that travels a straight course long enough to accept the length of the needle. Veins of the dorsum of the hand, ventral surface of the forearm, or antecubital fossa are preferred.
—Avoid bruised, sclerosed, or inflamed veins and veins that travel through hematomas or ecchymotic areas.
—Avoid using an arm where axillary node dissection has been performed or an arm affected by the superior vena cava syndrome.
—Alternate sites of drug administration.
—When possible, use 21-, 23- or 25-gauge butterfly needle because it can be secured easily and causes minimal irritation. The small needle is easy to position, and the presence of blood return can be noted in the tubing.
—When securing a butterfly catheter or tubing, allow for visualization of the injection site, the proximal portion of the butterfly tubing, and the surrounding area, including most of the arm.
—Always check needle position and flow by administering 5 ml to 10 ml of normal saline before injecting cytotoxic agent.
—Administer drug by slow, steady IV push or by IV infusion through injection port of tubing.
—Flush tubing and vein with 5 ml to 10 ml of normal saline after administration of drug.
—Instruct patient to immediately report any discomfort or other unusual sensation.
—If there is any doubt about patency of vein (e.g., redness, swelling), stop injection immediately and administer drug via another site.

To treat extravasation:
—Stop infusion. Leave needle in place.
—Aspirate as much of drug as possible.
—Administer specific antidote, if available.
—Through the *same* needle, administer 100 mg to 200 mg of hydrocortisone *or* 4 mg dexamethasone.
—Inject 1% to 2% lidocaine into area to reduce pain (optional).
—Apply ice packs for 24 to 36 hours.
—Apply warm, moist compresses after the first 24 to 36 hours. Check site frequently.
—Elevate injection site above the level of the heart.
—Tissue necrosis may be treated by surgically excising the ulcer and covering the wound with a xenograft (usually pigskin) for 48 to 72 hours. The xenograft is then replaced by a split-thickness skin graft, and the extremity is immobilized for 5 to 7 days.

1. Provide appropriate emotional support. Involve other health team members, patient, and patient's significant others in nursing care plans to ensure consistency and continuity of care.
2. Ensure that patient has opportunities to privately discuss self-concept, body image, and sexuality. Many anticancer drugs cause both subjective and objective changes that elicit widespread alterations in feelings about self.
3. Obtain patient's *lean* body weight. Medication dosages should be calculated on this basis, particularly if patient is obese or has edema or ascites. Dosages should, however, be adjusted, wherever possible, to account for clinical response and development of adverse reactions.
4. If platelet count is low, implement nursing interventions to prevent or minimize bleeding. Avoid giving injections.
5. Collaborate with dietician, physician, patient, and family to plan measures to help maintain or attain optimal nutritional status. In addition to the usual reasons for concern with nutritional status, therapy is most successful when the patient is well nourished.
6. Implement nursing interventions to prevent or minimize nausea and vomiting. With certain antineoplastics, it is often necessary to give an effective dose of an appropriate antiemetic drug 30 to 60 minutes before the antineoplastic agent is administered. Bland food or antacids given prior to administration of an oral agent may reduce nausea and vomiting caused by local irritation, but the presence of food in the stomach may impair absorption of some agents.
7. Monitor intake and output, and collaborate with patient to develop plan to maintain fluid intake at 2 L to 3 L/day to ensure that urine output is adequate for drug excretion,

to prevent dehydration related to excessive vomiting, and to minimize risks of hyeruricemia and uric acid nephropathy.
8. Inform physician if patient vomits after receiving an oral antineoplastic agent. If the medication was not absorbed, a dosage adjustment may be required.
9. Use appropriate interventions for mouth care. Anorexia, nausea and vomiting, xerostomia, increased risk of dental caries, bleeding tendencies, heightened susceptibility to infection, and numerous other potential problems need to be considered. Soft-bristled toothbrushes, special mouth rinses, avoidance of certain foods (tart, spicy, hot, rough-textured), and use, when prescribed, of antifungal agents formulated for intraoral use to treat fungal overgrowth of the mouth may all be helpful, depending on the patient's condition.
10. If medication is given by IV push and if widely metastatic tumors (i.e., leukemia) are *not* being treated, be prepared to assist with one of the following procedures to minimize hair loss: (1) apply scalp tourniquet before drug administration and retain for at least 5 minutes afterwards; (2) apply ice compress to scalp 15 minutes before and for 30 minutes after drug administration.
11. Be prepared to administer antihistamines, steroids, epinephrine, and oxygen to treat hypersensitivity reaction.

PATIENT EDUCATION: ANTINEOPLASTIC AGENTS

1. Instruct patient to notify prescriber if a dose of medication is missed. The next dose should not be doubled; instead, the regular dosing schedule should be resumed.
2. Explain that drug effects may not become manifest for several weeks.
3. Stress the importance of adhering to prescribed regimen and avoiding all nonprescribed drugs, including OTC medications. See **Plans of Nursing Care** 1, **Knowledge Deficit,** and 2, **Noncompliance.**
4. Discuss the importance of observing for development of side effects and informing appropriate care provider if they occur.
5. Reassure patient that dosage adjustment can often reduce incidence and severity of untoward reactions.
6. Inform patient that alopecia may occur, but that it is transient. Encourage use of wigs, scarves, and hats until normal regrowth occurs, usually 4 to 8 weeks after therapy ends. Transient regrowth may occur during therapy, but hair is often of a different texture, and color will be lost as therapy continues.
7. Counsel male or female patient regarding the possibility of birth defects or sterility, which can occur after therapy is terminated as well as during therapy.

ALKYLATING AGENTS

Busulfan	Lomustine
Carboplatin	Mechlorethamine
Carmustine	Melphalan
Chlorambucil	Pipobroman
Cisplatin	Streptozocin
Cyclophosphamide	Thiethylenethiophosphor-
Dacarbazine	amide
Ifosfamide	Uracil mustard

The alkylating agents were developed during the 1940s as a result of research on chemical warfare agents, notably the mustard gases. Of these compounds, the nitrogen mustards were found to have a marked cytotoxic action on lymphoid tissue, and clinical research was then initiated that led to development of chemically related derivatives.

The alkylating agents used in chemotherapy may be divided into six different chemical groups as follows:

Nitrogen mustards: chlorambucil, cyclophosphamide, ifosfamide, mechlorethamine, melphalan, uracil mustard
Ethylenimines: thiotepa
Alkyl sulfonates: busulfan
Triazenes: dacarbazine
Nitrosoureas: carmustine, lomustine, streptozocin
Miscellaneous alkylator-like agents: carboplatin, cisplatin, pipobroman

The alkylating agents are discussed as a group, then individual drugs are listed in Table 72-3.

MECHANISM

Alkylating agents are polyfunctional compounds that produce highly reactive carbonium ions that form covalent linkages with nucleophilic centers such as amino, carboxyl, hydroxyl, imidazole, phosphate, and sulfhydryl groups. The most important site of alkylation is the number 7 nitrogen in the purine base guanine. This may cause cross-linking of DNA strands and miscoding of the genetic message, resulting in abnormal base pairing. Destruction of the guanine ring and DNA chain breakage ensues, inhibiting DNA replication, transcription of RNA, and normal nucleic acid function. Cross-linking of DNA strands thus appears to be the major cytotoxic effect of the alkylating agents

USES
See Table 72-3

DOSAGE
See Table 72-3

FATE
The oral agents busulfan, chlorambucil, cyclophosphamide, lomustine, melphalan, pipobroman, and uracil mustard generally exhibit rapid absorption, but melphalan and uracil mustard may be incompletely absorbed. All alkylating agents are widely distributed throughout the body and exhibit some protein binding. Carmustine and lomustine are rapidly transported across the blood–brain barrier. Most agents are metabolized in the liver to inactivate metabolites; however, cyclophosphamide and ifosfamide must be metabolized in order to become active. All alkylating agents are eliminated by way of the kidney as both inactive metabolites and unchanged drug

COMMON SIDE EFFECTS
Myelosuppression (leukopenia, thrombocytopenia, anemia), nausea, vomiting, and anorexia

Cisplatin: nephrotoxicity and hyperuricemia
Cyclophosphamide: gonadal suppression
Streptozocin: nephrotoxicity

SIGNIFICANT ADVERSE REACTIONS
(Not all reactions observed with all drugs)

GI: diarrhea, abdominal cramping, stomatitis, glossitis, colitis
Renal: hyperuricemia, uric acid nephropathy, hemorrhagic cystitis (especially ifosfamide)

Hypersensitivity: dermatitis, maculopapular skin eruption, urticaria, fever, alopecia, pruritis, facial edema, anaphylactic-like reaction, erythema multiforme

Neurologic: headache, confusion, tinnitus, weakness, ataxia, peripheral neuropathies, dizziness, paralysis, depression, hyperactivity, convulsions

Respiratory: pulmonary fibrosis, dyspnea, wheezing

Cardiovascular: tachycardia, hypotension, flushing, sweating

Other: hepatic dysfunction, jaundice, hepatitis, gynecomastia, impotence, myxedema, myalgia, metallic taste, melanoderma, hyperpigmentation, pain at IV injection site or along vein

> *NOTE*
> All alkylating agents have been shown to be teratogenic, carcinogenic (owing to a direct cellular action or immunosuppression), and to cause testicular and ovarian suppression

CONTRAINDICATIONS

Leukopenia, thrombocytopenia or anemia caused by previous chemotherapy or radiation therapy, hepatoxicity, renal toxicity, and known hypersensitivity

INTERACTIONS

The toxicity of *chlorambucil* and *cyclophosphamide* may be increased when used concurrently with barbiturates, chloral hydrate, or phenytoin owing to induction of liver microsomal enzymes.

Cisplatin used concurrently with aminoglycosides may increase nephrotoxicity and ototoxicity.

Allopurinol and chloramphenicol may increase the toxicity of *cyclophosphamide*.

Corticosteroids may decrease the activity of *cyclophosphamide* by inhibiting microsomal enzymes.

Cyclophosphamide and *thiotepa* may decrease serum pseudocholinesterase and thereby enhance the effect of succinylcholine.

Cyclophosphamide used concurrently with daunorubicin or doxorubicin may increase cardiotoxicity.

Dacarbazine may potentiate the activity of allopurinol by inhibiting xanthine oxidase.

The metabolism of *dacarbazine* may be enhanced by phenobarbital and phenytoin owing to induction of liver microsomal enzymes.

Most *alkylating agents* may antagonize the effects of antigout medications by increasing serum uric acid levels; dosage adjustments of the antigout medications may be necessary.

Alkylating agents cause immunosuppression, which may result in a generalized vaccinia following immunization with smallpox vaccine.

Corticosteroids used concurrently with *streptozocin* may increase the hyperglycemic effect of *streptozocin*.

Streptozocin should not be used concurrently with nephrotoxic medications such as aminoglycoside antibiotics, cephalothin, cisplatin, or polymyxins.

Phenytoin may protect pancreatic beta cells from the cytotoxic effects of *streptozocin*, thus reducing its therapeutic effect in patients with islet cell tumors.

Myelosuppression caused by *carmustine* may be enhanced by cimetidine.

Carmustine and *cyclophosphamide* may decrease the effects of digoxin by decreasing its GI absorption.

Carmustine and *cisplatin* may decrease the effects of phenytoin.

Cisplatin used concurrently with loop diuretics (bumetanide, ethacrynic acid, furosemide) may increase the ototoxicity of both drugs.

Cyclophosphamide may increase the effects of succinylcholine, resulting in periods of prolonged respiratory depression.

Carboplatin may potentiate the renal effects of other nephrotoxic drugs.

Note: Ifosfamide is a new antineoplastic agent with no reported drug interactions at this time. However, owing to its structural similarity to cyclophosphamide, similar drug interactions to those seen with cyclophosphamide may occur when using ifosfamide.

NURSING CONSIDERATIONS

See general discussion of nursing considerations for all antineoplastic drugs. In addition:

Nursing Alerts
- When administering carboplatin, cisplatin, or mechlorethamine, monitor patient for tachycardia, hypotension, or shortness of breath because anaphylactoid reactions, which necessitate supportive measures, can occur.
- Check patient receiving cyclophosphamide or ifosfamide for hematuria or dysuria. Withhold drug and notify physician at first sign of hemorrhagic cystitis.
- If patient is receiving cisplatin or mechlorethamine, assess auditory function frequently. Tinnitus or impaired hearing may signal ototoxicity. Periodic audiometric testing is recommended.
- Closely monitor patient receiving first dose of streptozocin for signs of hypoglycemia due to sudden release of insulin. Have IV dextrose available.

1. If cyclophosphamide or ifosfamide is prescribed, work with patient in planning to maintain adequate hydration to reduce risk of hemorrhagic cystitis. Give drug early in morning to prevent accumulation in bladder during night.

ANTIMETABOLITES

Cytarabine	Mercaptopurine
Floxuridine	Methotrexate
Fluorouracil	Thioguanine

The *antimetabolites* are structural analogs of normally occurring metabolites that interfere with the synthesis of nucleic acids by competing with purines or pyrimidines in metabolic pathways. The antimetabolites themselves may also be incorporated into nucleic acids, resulting in a cell product that fails to function. Antimetabolites act during the S phase of the cell cycle (see introduction). They can be divided into three groups: folic acid antagonists (methotrexate), purine antagonists (mercaptopurine, thioguanine), and pyrimidine antagonists (floxuridine, fluorouracil, cytarabine). They are considered here as a group, then listed individually in Table 72-4.

(Text continued on page 718)

Table 72-3
Alkylating Agents

Drug	Preparations	Usual Dosage Range	Uses	Nursing Implications
Busulfan Myleran	Tablets: 2 mg	**Adults** Initially: 4 mg–12 mg/day Maintenance: 2 mg once or twice a week to 1 mg–4 mg/day **Children** Induction: 0.06 mg/kg–0.12 mg/kg/day *or* 1.8 mg–4.6 mg/m²/day	Chronic myelogenous leukemia (DOC) Polycythemia vera	May increase uric acid levels in blood and urine; pulmonary fibrosis usually occurs with long-term therapy—onset after 8 mo–10 yr (average 4 yr); treatment is usually unsatisfactory and death usually occurs within 6 mo of diagnosis
Carmustine BiCNU, BCNU	Injection: 100 mg/vial	75 mg–100 mg/m² by IV infusion over 1–2 h for 2 consecutive days *or* 200 mg/m² in a single dose no more frequently than every 6–8 wk A suggested guide for subsequent dosage adjustment is the following: *Nadir after Prior Dose* Leukocytes / Platelets / % of Prior Dose to be Given Above 4000 / Above 100,000 / 100% 3000–3999 / 75,000–99,999 / 100% 2000–2999 / 25,000–74,999 / 70% Below 2000 / Below 25,000 / 50%	Brain tumors (DOC) Multiple myeloma (in combination with prednisone) Hodgkin's disease (in combination with other approved drugs in patients who experience relapse while on primary therapy or fail to respond to the primary therapy) Non-Hodgkin's lymphomas (in combination with other drugs; see above) May also be useful in Burkitt's tumor, Ewing's sarcoma, malignant melanoma (in combination with vincristine), in hepatic carcinoma when given by intraarterial injection, and in mycosis fungoides	Unopened vials of dry powder must be stored under refrigeration—oily film on bottom of the vial is sign of decomposition, and vial should be discarded; preparation of solution: dissolve contents of vial with 3 mL absolute alcohol diluent and then add 27 mL of sterile water for injection—resulting solution contains 3.3 mg/mL; further dilution in 500 mL of 0.5% dextrose or 0.9% sodium chloride results in a solution stable for 48 h when refrigerated and protected from light; contact with skin may cause transient hyperpigmentation; may increase bilirubin, alkaline phosphatase, SGOT, and BUN levels; a 0.1%–0.4% solution in 95% alcohol applied topically 1–2 times/day for 2 wk has been used to treat mycosis fungoides; pulmonary fibrosis and pneumonitis occur, primarily with high cumulative dose (1200–1400 mg/m²) or long-term therapy (5 mo) but may also occur with short-term, low-dose therapy
Carboplatin Paraplatin	Injection: 50 mg/vial, 150 mg/vial, 450 mg/vial	360 mg/m² by infusion over 15 min–1 h; repeat every 4 wk A suggested guide for subsequent dosage adjustment is the following: *Nadir after Prior Dose* Neutrophils / Platelets / % of Prior Dose to be Given Above 2000 / Above 100,000 / 125% 500–2000 / 50,000–100,000 / 100% Below 500 / Below 50,000 / 75% *Renal Impairment* Creatinine Clearance / Dose 41–59 mL/min / 250 mg/m² 16–40 mL/min / 200 mg/m²	Palliative treatment of ovarian carcinoma May also be useful in small cell and non-small cell lung carcinoma and head and neck tumors	To prepare solution, dissolve contents of vials in sterile water for injection, 5% dextrose, or 0.9% sodium chloride; solutions are stable for 8 h at room temperature; do *not* use needles, IV sets, or other equipment containing aluminum, as drug may form a precipitate with loss of potency; drug may be used in patients previously treated with cisplatin; no pre- or posttreatment hydration or forced diuresis is required; *reduce dosage* in patients with impaired kidney function
Chlorambucil Leukeran	Tablets: 2 mg	**Adults** Initially: 0.1 mg/kg–0.2 mg/kg/day for 3–6 wk (4 mg–12 mg/day for the average patient) Maintenance: 2 mg–6 mg/day, *not* to exceed 0.1 mg/kg/day; may be as low as 0.03 mg/kg/day	Chronic lymphocytic leukemia (DOC) Malignant lymphomas Hodgkin's disease Choriocarcinoma Ovarian carcinoma Breast carcinoma Macroglobulinemia Nephrotic syndrome	Give dose 1 h before breakfast or 2 h after evening meal; may increase serum and urine uric acid levels

DOC, drug of choice.

Continued

Table 72-3
Alkylating Agents (continued)

Drug	Preparations	Usual Dosage Range	Uses	Nursing Implications
Chlorambucil (cont'd)		Macroglobulinemia: 2 mg–10 mg/day *or* 8 mg/m²/day for 10 days; repeat every 6–8 wk Nephrotic syndrome: 0.1 mg/kg–0.2 mg/kg/day for 8–12 wk Uveitis: 0.1 mg/kg/day *Children* 0.1 mg/kg–0.2 mg/kg/day or 4.5 mg/m²/day	Uveitis, intractable, idiopathic	
Cisplatin Platinol, Platinol-AQ	Powder for injection: 10 mg/vial, 50 mg/vial Injection solution: 1 mg/mL in 50 mL, and 100 mL vials	*As a single agent* 100 mg/m² IV once every 4 wk *Testicular tumors* 20 mg/m² IV for 5 days every 3 wk for 3 courses *in combination with* Bleomycin: 30 U IV on day 2 of each week for 12 doses and Vinblastine: 0.15 mg/kg–0.2 mg/kg IV on days 1 and 2 of each week every 3 wk for 4 courses Maintenance for patients who respond: vinblastine 0.2 mg/kg IV every 4 wk for 2 yr *Ovarian tumors* 50 mg/m² IV once every 3 wk on day 1 *in combination with* Doxorubicin: 50 mg/m² IV once every 3 wk on day 1 A repeat dose should *not* be given until serum creatinine is below 1.5 mg/dL or BUN is below 25 mg/dL platelets are over 100,000/mm³, and WBCs are over 4000/mm³ *Advanced bladder carcinoma* 50 mg to 70 mg/m² IV once every 3–4 wk; patients receiving prior radiation or chemotherapy should start at 50 mg/m² IV once every 4 wk *Non-small cell lung carcinoma* 75 mg–120 mg/m² IV once every 3–6 wk *Neuroblastoma and osteosarcoma in children* 90 mg/m² IV once every 3 wk *or* 30 mg/m² IV once weekly	Metastatic testicular tumors (DOC) Metastatic ovarian tumors (DOC) Lymphoma Squamous cell carcinoma of head and neck Advanced bladder carcinoma (DOC) Cervical cancer (DOC) Prostatic carcinoma Non-small cell lung carcinoma Neuroblastoma Osteosarcoma	Preparation of solution: dissolve contents of vial in 10 mL sterile water for injection; solution is stable for 20 h at room temperature—do *not* refrigerate; hydrate patient with 1–2 L fluid infused over 8–12 h before treatment; dilute drug in 1–2 L 5% dextrose in 0.3% or 0.45% saline containing 37.5 g mannitol, and infuse over 6–8 h; maintain urinary output of 100 mL/h for 24 h after therapy to reduce danger of nephrotoxicity; do *not* use needles, IV sets, or equipment containing aluminum to administer cisplatin—a black precipitate of platinum will form; may increase BUN, serum creatinine, SGOT, and serum uric acid levels; may decrease creatinine clearance and serum calcium, magnesium, and potassium levels; high-frequency hearing loss may occur in one or both ears, more commonly in children

DOC, drug of choice.

Table 72-3
Alkylating Agents (continued)

Drug	Preparations	Usual Dosage Range	Uses	Nursing Implications
		Renal Impairment Creatinine Clearance — Dosage 10 mL–50 mL/min — 75% usual dose <10 mL/min — 50% usual dose		

Cyclophosphamide
Cytoxan, Neosar
	Tablets: 25 mg, 50 mg
	Powder for injection (regular or lyophilized: 100 mg/vial, 200 mg/vial, 500 mg/vial, 1 g/vial, 2 g/vial
		Oral
		Adult: 1 mg/kg–5 mg/kg/day
		Children: induction: 2 mg/kg–8 mg/kg or 60 mg–250 mg/m² for 6 or more days
		Maintenance: 2 mg/kg–5 mg/kg or 50 mg–150 mg/m² twice a week
		IV
		Adult: induction—40 mg/kg–50 mg/kg in divided doses over 2–5 days. Maintenance: 10 mg/kg–15 mg/kg every 7–10 days or 3 mg/kg–5 mg/kg twice a week or 1.5 mg/kg–3 mg/kg daily
		Children: induction—2 mg/kg–8 mg/kg or 60 mg–250 mg/m² in divided doses for 6 or more days: Maintenance: 10 mg/kg–15 mg/kg every 7–10 days or 30 mg/kg every 3–4 wk
		Reduce induction dose by 1/3–1/2 in patients with bone marrow depression
		Hepatic impairment: bilirubin 3.1 mg/dL to 5.0 mg/dL or SGOT > 180, reduce dose by 25%; bilirubin > 5.0 mg/dL omit dose
		Renal impairment: GFR < 10 mL/min, decrease dose by 50%
		Immunosuppressant nephrotic syndrome: 2 mg/kg–2.5 mg/kg/day
		Rheumatoid arthritis: 1.5 mg/kg–3 mg/kg/day
			Hodgkin's disease
			Non-Hodgkin's lymphomas (DOC)
			Follicular lymphomas
			Lymphocytic lymphosarcoma
			Reticulum cell sarcoma
			Lymphoblastic lymphosarcoma
			Burkitt's lymphoma (DOC)
			Multiple myeloma (DOC)
			Leukemias:
			  Chronic lymphocytic leukemia
			  Chronic granulocytic leukemia
			  Acute myelogenous and monocytic leukemia
			  Acute lymphoblastic leukemia
			Mycosis fungoides
			Neuroblastoma (DOC)
			Adenocarcinoma of ovary (DOC)
			Retinoblastoma (DOC)
			Carcinoma of breast or lung (DOC)
			Ewing's sarcoma (DOC)
			Other uses:
			  Prevent transplant rejection
			  Rheumatoid arthritis
			  Nephrotic syndrome
			  Systemic lupus erythematosus
				To prepare solution: Reconstitute with sterile water for injection or bacteriostatic water for injection (paraben preserved only); use 5 mL for the 100-mg vial, 10 mL for the 200-mg vial, 25 mL for the 500-mg vial, 50 mL for the 1-g vial, and 100 mL for the 2-g vial; lyophilized powder dissolves much more quickly than regular powder; solution is stable for 24 h at room temperature or 6 days refrigerated; may be given IM, IV push, intraperitoneally, intrapleurally, or by IV infusion in 5% dextrose, 5% dextrose in 0.9% saline; may suppress positive reactions to skin tests; may increase uric acid levels of urine and serum; may produce false-positive Pap test; secondary malignancies have been observed, most frequently of the urinary bladder; may cause syndrome of inappropriate antidiuretic hormone secretion (SIADH); manifested as tiredness, weakness, confusion, agitation; an oral solution may be prepared by dissolving the powder for injection in aromatic elixir to a concentration of 1 mg–5 mg/mL—refrigerate and use within 14 days; tablets contain tartrazine

Dacarbazine
DTIC-Dome
	Injection: 100-mg vial, 200-mg vial, 500-mg vial	IV: 2 mg/kg–4.5 mg/kg/day for 10 days, repeated every 28 days or 250 mg/m²/day for 5 days, repeated every 21 days	Metastatic malignant melanoma (DOC)
			Hodgkin's disease
			Investigational uses include:
			  Soft tissue sarcomas
			  Neuroblastoma
				To prepare solution: Add 9.9 mL sterile water for injection to 100 mg vial or 19.7 mL sterile water for injection to 200-mg vial giving a concentration of 10 mg/mL; solution, colorless or clear yellow in color, is stable 8 h at room temperature or 72 h refrigerated, and protected from light—a change in color to pink indicates decomposition; may be given by IV push over 1 min or by IV infusion over 30 min, diluted in 250 mL 5% dextrose in water or 0.9% sodium chloride; severe pain along injected vein can occur—dilute drug, infuse slowly, and avoid extravasation; may increase alkaline phosphatase, BUN, SGOT, SGPT

DOC, drug of choice.

Continued

Table 72-3
Alkylating Agents (continued)

Drug	Preparations	Usual Dosage Range	Uses	Nursing Implications
Ifosfamide Ifex	Injection: 1 g/vial	IV: 1.2 g/m²/day for 5 days; repeat every 21 days *or* when leukocytes are more than 4000 and platelets are more than 100,000	Germ cell testicular cancer *Other uses:* Lung, breast, ovarian, pancreatic, and gastric cancer; acute leukemias (except AML) and malignant lymphoma	To prepare solution: Use 20 mL of sterile water for injection *or* bacteriostatic water for injection; solutions are stable for 1 wk at room temperature or up to 3 wk when refrigerated; solutions may be further diluted in 5% dextrose, 0.9% saline, lactated Ringer's solution or sterile water for injection and are stable up to 6 wk when refrigerated; to prevent bladder toxicity (gross hematuria, hemorrhagic cystitis), patient should be hydrated with 2 L of oral or IV fluid daily; incidence of hemorrhagic cystitis may be reduced by IV administration of mesna (Mesnex) in a dosage equal to 20% of the ifosfamide dose, given with ifosfamide and again at 4 and 8 h after ifosfamide
Lomustine CCNU, CeeNU	Capsules: 10 mg, 40 mg, 100 mg	*Oral* Adults and children: 100 mg–130 mg/m² as a single dose, repeated every 6 wk A suggested guide for subsequent dosage adjustment is the following: *Nadir after Prior Dose* Leukocytes / Platelets / % of Prior Dose to be Given Above 4000 / Above 100,000 / 100% 3000–3999 / 75,000–99,999 / 75%–100% 2000–2999 / 25,000–74,999 / 50%–75% Below 2000 / Below 25,000 / 0–50%	Brain tumors (DOC) Hodgkin's disease Investigation uses include: Lung and breast carcinoma Malignant melanoma Multiple myeloma Gastrointestinal carcinoma Renal cell carcinoma	May cause transient elevation of liver function tests; available as a dose pack containing two 10-mg capsules, two 40-mg capsules, and two 100-mg capsules
Mechlorethamine Mustargen, Nitrogen Mustard	Injection: 10 mg/vial	IV: 0.4 mg/kg as a single dose *or* in divided doses of 0.1 mg/kg–0.2 mg/kg/day; repeat every 3–6 wk Intracavitary: 0.4 mg/kg diluted in 50 mL to 100 mL 0.9% saline; 0.2 mg/kg may be used intrapericardially Ointment and solution: apply once daily (up to 4 times/day in severe cases) to entire skin surface for 6–12 mo until response has occurred, then every 2–7 days for up to 3 yr	Hodgkin's disease (DOC) Lymphosarcoma Chronic myelocytic and lymphocytic leukemia Bronchogenic carcinoma Polycythemia vera Mycosis fungoides (DOC) Intracavitary injection to control malignant effusions	Do *not* use drug if vial contains water droplets before reconstitution. To prepare solution: Reconstitute with 10 mL sterile water for injection or 0.9% sodium chloride injection; use immediately; discard unused portion after neutralizing with aqueous solution containing equal parts of 5% sodium bicarbonate and 5% sodium thiosulfate; any equipment used for administration (gloves, tubing, glassware) should be neutralized for 45 min in this solution; avoid inhalation of powder or vapors; avoid contact with skin or mucous membranes—if contact occurs, wash 15 min with water, followed by 2% sodium thiosulfate solution; administer IV dose by injection into tubing of running IV; change position of patient every 5–10 min for 1 h after intracavitary injection. A topical solution may be prepared by dissolving 10 mg in 20 mL–60 mL of water or sodium chloride and made fresh daily; an ointment may be prepared (0.01%–0.04%) by dissolving drug in absolute alcohol and mixing into an anhydrous ointment base; use protective gloves to apply topical preparations; use minimal application to perineum, axillary, inguinal, inframammary areas and inside bends of elbows and backs of knees

DOC, drug of choice.

Continued

Table 72-3
Alkylating Agents (continued)

Drug	Preparations	Usual Dosage Range	Uses	Nursing Implications
Melphalan Alkeran, PAM, L-PAM, Phenylalanine Mustard, L-Sarcolysin	Tablets: 2 mg	0.15 mg/kg/day for 7 days followed by a rest period of 2–6 wk, then 0.05 mg/kg/day maintenance *or* 0.1 mg/kg–0.15 mg/kg/day for 2–3 wk *or* 0.25 mg/kg/day for 4 days followed by a rest period of 2–4 wk, then 2 mg–4 mg/day maintenance *or* 0.2 mg/kg/day for 5 days followed by a rest period of 4–5 wk (for ovarian carcinoma) *or* 7 mg/m^2/day for 5 days every 5–6 wk	Multiple myeloma (DOC) Malignant melanoma Breast, lung, and ovarian carcinoma Testicular seminoma Reticulum cell and osteogenic sarcoma Polycythemia vera Amyloidosis	May increase uric acid levels in blood and urine; acute, nonlymphatic leukemia has developed in some patients with multiple myeloma treated with melphalan; benefit/risk ratio must be determined on an individual basis
Pipobroman Vercyte	Tablets: 10 mg, 25 mg	Polycythemia vera: 1 mg/kg/day for 30 days, then increase to 1.5 mg/kg–3 mg/kg/day if no response. Maintenance—0.1 mg/kg–0.2 mg/kg/day when hematocrit has been reduced to 50%–55% Chronic myelocytic leukemia: 1.5 mg/kg–2.5 mg/kg/day until leukocyte count approaches 10,000, then maintenance dose of 7 mg–175 mg/day as required	Polycythemia vera Chronic myelocytic leukemia (resistant to other therapy)	May increase uric acid levels in blood and urine; may increase serum potassium. *Not* recommended for children under 15 yr
Streptozocin Zanosar	Injection: 1 g/vial	IV: 500 mg/m^2/day for 5 consecutive days every 4–6 wk *or* 1 g/m^2 once a week for 2 wk; thereafter, dosage may be increased to a maximum of 1.5 g/m^2 weekly for 2–4 wk; may be given by rapid IV injection, short infusion (10–15 min), long infusion (6 hr) or continuous 5-day infusion Renal impairment: 50% to 75% of usual dose based on creatinine clearance	Metastatic islet cell carcinoma of the pancreas (DOC) Advanced Hodgkin's disease Investigational use: malignant carcinoid tumors, palliative treatment of metastatic colorectal cancer	Dry powder must be stored under refrigeration and protected from light; preparation of solution: reconstitute with 9.5 mL of 5% dextrose in water or 0.9% sodium chloride; solution is stable for 12 h at room temperature; solution is preservative-free and should *not* be used for more than one dose; a change in color from pale gold to brown indicates decomposition; adequate patient hydration may reduce renal toxicity; hypophosphatemia may be first sign of renal toxicity
Triethylene-thiophosphor-amide Thiotepa	Injection: 15 mg/vial	IV: 0.3 mg/kg–0.4 mg/kg at 1–2-wk intervals, *or* 0.5 mg/kg every 1–4 wk, *or* 0.2 mg/kg/day for 5 days repeated every 2–4 wk; may be given by IV push Local, intratumor: 0.6 mg/kg–0.8 mg/kg; maintenance dose 0.07 mg/kg–0.8 mg/kg every 1–4 wk Intracavitary: 0.6 mg/kg–0.8 mg/kg diluted in 10 mL–20 mL 0.9% saline	Superficial papillary carcinoma of the urinary bladder (DOC) Adenocarcinoma of the breast and ovary Intracavitary injection to control malignant effusions Lymphomas Investigational uses: Malignant meningeal neoplasms	Dry powder must be stored under refrigeration. To prepare solution: Reconstitute with 1.5 mL sterile water for injection; solution should be clear to slightly opaque—if *grossly* opaque, discard; solution is stable 5 days under refrigeration; compatible with procaine 2% and epinephrine HCl 1:1000 for local injection; dehydrate patients 8–12 h before bladder instillation; may increase uric acid levels in blood and urine; has been used IM, although not approved by the FDA

DOC, drug of choice.

Continued

Table 72-3
Alkylating Agents (continued)

Drug	Preparations	Usual Dosage Range	Uses	Nursing Implications
Triethylene-thiophos-phoramide (cont'd)		Bladder instillation: 30 mg–60 mg at weekly intervals diluted in 30 mL–60 mL sterile water for injection; patient should retain for 2 h with frequent repositioning; repeat once weekly for 4 wk; volume may be reduced to 30 mL if discomfort occurs Intrathecal (investigational): 1 mg/m²–10 mg/m² 1 or 2 times/wk (1 mg/mL)		
Uracil Mustard	Capsules: 1 mg	Initially 1 mg–2 mg/day until improvement or bone marrow depression occurs; then 1 mg/day for 3 out of 4 wk maintenance *or* Initially 3 mg–5 mg/day for 7 days not to exceed 0.5 mg/kg during this period, then 1 mg/day for 3 out of 4 wk maintenance	Chronic lymphocytic leukemia Non-Hodgkin's lymphomas Chronic myelocytic leukemia Polycythemia vera (early stage) Mycosis fungoides	May increase uric acid levels in blood and urine; total dosage of 1 mg/kg greatly increases the risk of irreversible bone marrow depression; capsules contain tartrazine

DOC, drug of choice.

MECHANISM

Folic acid antagonists bind to the enzyme dihydrofolate reductase, thereby preventing reduction of folic acid to tetrahydrofolic acid. This limits the availability of one-carbon fragments necessary for purine and thymidine synthesis, thereby blocking DNA synthesis and cell replication.

Purine antagonists are analogs of the natural purines hypoxanthine, guanine, and adenine. These agents must be metabolized to active nucleotides which then can interfere with the synthesis of natural purines, thus preventing normal nucleic acid synthesis.

The *pyrimidine antagonists* floxuridine and fluorouracil compete for the enzyme thymylate synthetase, preventing synthesis of thymidine, an essential substrate of DNA, and thereby blocking DNA synthesis. Cytarabine is metabolized by deoxycytidine kinase to the nucleotide triphosphate (ARA–CTP), which is an inhibitor of DNA polymerase, an enzyme necessary for the conversion of RNA into DNA

USES
See Table 72-4

DOSAGE
See Table 72-4

FATE
The oral agents mercaptopurine and methotrexate are well absorbed from the GI tract, whereas thioguanine is poorly absorbed. Cytarabine and methotraxate are widely distributed and cross the blood–brain barrier. Mercaptopurine and methotrexate are moderately protein-bound. All agents are largely metabolized in the liver (except methotrexate) and are excreted by the kidneys as inactive metabolites and unchanged drug. Floxuridine and fluorouracil are also partially eliminated by the lungs as carbon dioxide

COMMON SIDE EFFECTS
Myelosuppression (leukopenia, thrombocytopenia, anemia); nausea, vomiting, diarrhea, stomatitis, glossitis, hepatotoxicity (thioguanine and methotrexate), gastritis (fluorouracil and methotrexate); hyperuricemia, renal toxicity; interstitial pneumonitis; CNS disturbances (methotrexate)

SIGNIFICANT ADVERSE REACTIONS
(Not all reactions observed with all drugs)

Dermatologic: skin rash, freckling, dermatitis, hyperpigmentation, alopecia
CNS: ataxia, vertigo, anorexia
Ocular: blurred vision, photophobia, lacrimation
Renal/hepatic: hyperuricemia, uric acid nephropathy, hepatic dysfunction, cholestasis
Cardiovascular: myocardial ischemia, angina
Hypersensitivity: fever, anaphylaxis, arthralgia
Other: GI ulceration, osteoporosis, pneumonia, thrombophlebitis, cellulitis, Guillain–Barré syndrome

NOTE
Antimetabolite agents have been shown to be carcinogenic in animal studies and thus may present an oncogenic risk in humans. The antimetabolites are potential mutagens and teratogens and also cause ovarian and testicular suppression

CONTRAINDICATIONS

Leukopenia, thrombocytopenia or anemia caused by previous chemotherapy or radiation therapy; hepatoxicity; and renal toxicity

In addition, do not use mercaptopurine or thioguanine in a patient who has demonstrated prior resistance to either of the two agents because there is usually complete cross-resistance.

INTERACTIONS

Cytarabine and *methotrexate* used concurrently can have either a synergistic or antagonistic effect.

Fluorouracil is incompatible with cytarabine, diazepam, doxorubicin, and methotrexate; complete flushing of IV line between injections is recommended.

The absorption of *fluorouracil* when given orally is decreased by the presence of food.

Concomitant administration of *mercaptopurine* and allopurinol increases both the antineoplastic and toxic effects of mercaptopurine; reduce the dose of mercaptopurine to one third to one fourth the usual dose.

Alcohol may enhance the possibility of *methotrexate*-induced hepatotoxicity.

Chloramphenicol, phenylbutazone, phenytoin, para-aminobenzoic acid, salicylates, sulfonamides, and tetracyclines can displace *methotrexate* from binding sites and cause increased toxicity.

Probenecid, salicylates, and nonsteroidal antiinflammatory agents can block the tubular secretion of *methotrexate* and thus increase its toxicity.

Pyrimethamine used concurrently with *methotrexate* can cause increased toxicity because of similar folic acid antagonist actions.

Concurrent use of high-dose methotrexate and procarbazine may increase the nephrotoxicity of methotrexate

Methotrexate may enhance the hypoprothrombinemic effect of oral anticoagulants such as warfarin.

Concurrent use of *methotrexate* and asparaginase may block the antineoplastic action of methotrexate by inhibiting cell synthesis; administer asparaginase 9 days to 10 days before or within 24 hours after administering methotrexate; the toxic effect of methotrexate may also be reduced.

Vitamin preparations containing folic acid may decrease the effect of *methotrexate*.

Most *antimetabolite agents* may antagonize the effects of antigout medications by increasing serum uric acid levels; dosage adjustments of the antigout medications may be necessary.

Antimetabolite agents cause immunosuppression, which may result in a generalized vaccinia following immunization with smallpox vaccine.

Concurrent use of *fluorouracil* and allopurinol may reduce the hematologic toxicity of fluorouracil.

Mercaptopurine may increase or decrease the anticoagulant effect of warfarin.

Cytarabine and *methotrexate* may decrease the effects of digoxin by impairing its GI absorption.

Absorption from digoxin capsules (Lanoxicaps) may *not* be decreased.

The toxicity of *fluorouracil* and *methotrexate* may be increased when used concurrently with thiazide diuretics.

Mercaptopurine may reverse the effects of nondepolarizing muscle relaxants, such as pancuronium and atracurium.

Mercaptopurine and *methotrexate* may decrease the effects of phenytoin.

The toxic effects of *methotrexate* may be enhanced when used concurrently with etretinate to treat psoriasis.

NURSING CONSIDERATIONS

See general discussion of nursing considerations for all antineoplastic drugs. In addition:

Nursing Alert
- When administering cytarabine or methotrexate, monitor patient for tachycardia, hypotension, and shortness of breath because anaphylactoid reactions, which require supportive measures, can occur

1. When administering fluorouracil, mercaptopurine, or thioguanine, do *not* confuse the notations 5-FU, 6-MP, or 6-thioguanine, which is how these drugs are often written, with the numbers of vials or tablets to be administered. In these instances, these numbers are part of the drug names.
2. To administer floxuridine, which is given intraarterially, use an IV infusion pump.

NATURAL PRODUCTS

Asparaginase	Mitomycin
Bleomycin	Mitoxantrone
Dactinomycin	Plicamycin
Daunorubicin	Vinblastine
Doxorubicin	Vincristine
Etoposide	

The natural products commercially available for use as chemotherapeutic agents include an enzyme, antibiotics, and plant derivatives. Asparaginase, an enzyme isolated from *Escherichia coli*, is used to treat acute lymphocytic leukemia. Bleomycin, dactinomycin, daunorubicin, doxorubicin, mithramycin, and mitomycin are antineoplastic antibiotics produced from fermentation processes of several different strains of the *Streptomyces* fungus and are used to treat a wide range of malignant diseases. Mitoxantrone is a synthetic anthracenedione that is structurally related to the anthracyclines such as daunorubicin and doxorubicin. Vinblastine and vincristine are plant alkaloids isolated from periwinkle (*Vinca rosea*); both agents have a broad spectrum of antitumor activity. Etoposide is a semisynthetic podophyllotoxin derived from the root of the May apple or mandrake plant (*Podophyllum*) and is used to treat testicular and lung carcinomas (see Table 72-5).

MECHANISM

Asparaginase: Because they lack the enzyme asparagine synthetase, some tumor cells are unable to synthesize asparagine, an amino acid necessary for the synthesis of DNA and essential cellular proteins. Such cells must rely on an exogenous source of asparagine from the bloodstream. The administration of asparaginase hydrolyzes serum asparagine to aspartic acid, which the tumor cells cannot use. Normal cells are able to synthesize asparagine and are therefore much less affected by the agent.

Antibiotics: The antibiotics work by inhibiting synthesis of DNA or RNA. Bleomycin causes rupture of DNA strands,

(*Text continued on page 722*)

Table 72-4
Antimetabolites

Drug	Preparations	Usual Dosage Range	Uses	Nursing Implications
Cytarabine Cytosine Arabinoside, ARA-C, Cytosar-U	Injection: 100-mg vial, 500-mg vial, 1-g vial, 2-g vial	*Induction—IV infusion:* 100 mg–200 mg/m^2/day or 3 mg/kg/day as a continuous IV infusion over 24 h (or in divided doses by rapid IV injection) for 5–10 days and repeated approximately every 2 wk *Maintenance—IM, SC:* 1 mg/kg–1.5 mg/kg once or twice a week at 1–4 wk intervals or 70 mg–200 mg/m^2/day by rapid IV injection in divided doses or continuous IV infusion for 2–5 days repeated every 30 days *Investigational use for refractory acute myelogenous leukemia:* 2 gm–3 gm/m^2 IV infusion over 1–2 h every 12 h for 4–12 doses Combination therapy: See Table 72-8 *Stop therapy* if leukocyte count falls below 1000 or platelet count below 50,000; resume usually after 5–7 drug-free days and when above levels are reached *Intrathecal injection (investigational):* 5 mg–75 mg/m^2 or 30 mg–100 mg every 3–7 days or once daily for 4–5 days	Acute myelogenous leukemia (DOC) Also useful for: Acute lymphocytic leukemia Chronic myelogenous leukemia Meningeal leukemia Non-Hodgkin's lymphomas	To prepare solution: Reconstitute vials with bacteriostatic water for injection (0.9% benzyl alcohol) 5 mL/100-mg vial; 10 mL/500-mg vial; 10 mL/1-g vial, 20 mL/2-g vial; use 5 mL to 10 mL Elliott's B solution, Lactated Ringer's solution or patient's own cerebrospinal fluid to reconstitute for intrathecal injection; solution may be stored at room temperature for 48 h; discard any hazy or cloudy solution; infusion solutions may be prepared in 0.9% sodium chloride or dextrose 5%; solutions are stable at room temperature for 7 days; reconstitute with smaller volumes (1 mL–2 mL) for SC injection; may increase SGOT levels and uric acid levels in blood and urine; usual pediatric dose is equivalent to the adult dose; less nausea, vomiting, diarrhea if given IV infusion rather than IV injection, but danger of hematologic toxicity is increased
Floxuridine FUDR	Injection: 500 mg/vial	Intra-arterial infusion *only:* 0.1 mg/kg–0.6 mg/kg/day by continuous infusion; 0.4 mg/kg–0.6 mg/kg/day for hepatic artery infusion; continue therapy until toxicity occurs, usually 14–21 days, with 2 wk rest between courses	Palliative management of GI adenocarcinoma metastatic to liver, pancreas, or biliary tract Head and neck tumors Also, bladder, breast, cervical, ovarian and prostatic carcinoma	Reconstitute with 5 mL sterile water for injection; solution stable for 14 days under refrigeration; further dilution in 0.9% sodium chloride or 5% dextrose is necessary for infusion; dilution is stable for 24 h; may increase serum alkaline phosphatase, LDH, SGOT, SGPT, and bilirubin levels
Fluorouracil 5-Fluorouracil, 5-FU, Adrucil	Injection: 500 mg/10 mL, 5000 mg/100 mL	*Initially:* 12 mg/kg IV injection over 1–2 min once daily for 4 days; maximum daily dose 800 mg; if no toxicity, give 6 mg/kg on days 6, 8, 10, and 12 (For *poor-risk patients,* reduce dose 50%) *Maintenance:* repeat above schedule every 30 days after last day of previous treatment or 10 mg/kg–15 mg/kg IV once a week, not to exceed 1 g/wk; dosage based on actual body weight unless patient is obese or has fluid retention	Palliative management of carcinoma of colon, rectum, stomach, and pancreas (DOC) Treatment of breast, ovarian, cervical, and liver carcinomas	Solution may discolor slightly during storage but may still be used safely; crystal precipitate may be redissolved by heating to 60°C—allow to cool to body temperature before using; infusions may be prepared using 0.9% sodium chloride or 5% dextrose; solutions are stable for 24 h; incompatible with cytarabine and methotrexate; may increase 5-hydroxyindole acetic acid (5-HIAA) in urine; may decrease plasma albumin; FDA has *not* approved the drug for oral use; oral doses are associated with a very brief clinical response

Continued

Table 72-4
Antimetabolites (continued)

Drug	Preparations	Usual Dosage Range	Uses	Nursing Implications
		Oral: 15 mg/kg–20 mg/kg/day for 5–8 days; dilute in water or bicarbonate buffer solution rather than juice		
Mercaptopurine 6-Mercaptopurine, 6-MP, Purinethol	Tablets: 50 mg	*Adults* Initially 2.5 mg/kg or 80 mg to 100 mg/m^2 daily in single or divided doses; if no response and no toxicity after 4 wk increase to 5 mg/kg/day *Maintenance:* 1.5 mg–2.5 mg/kg or 50 mg–100 mg/m^2 daily *Children* 2.5 mg/kg or 75 mg/m^2 daily (Calculate all doses to nearest 25 mg) *Inflammatory bowel disease* 1.5 mg/kg/day; gradually increase to 2.5 mg/kg/day as necessary	Acute lymphocytic (DOC) and myelogenous leukemia Chronic myelogenous leukemia Other uses: Non-Hodgkin's lymphoma Polycythemia vera Inflammatory bowel disease Psoriatic arthritis	Decrease dose of mercaptopurine to $^1/_3$–$^1/_4$ usual dose if given concurrently with allopurinol; may increase uric acid levels in blood and urine; rarely used as a single agent for maintenance of remissions in acute leukemia; may falsely increase serum glucose and uric acid levels when the SMA (sequential multiple analyzer) is used
Methotrexate Amethopterin, Folex, MTX, Mexate, Mexate-AQ, Folex-PFS, Abitrexate, Methotrexate-LPF, Rheumatrex DosePak	Tablets: 2.5 mg Injection: 2.5 mg/mL, 25 mg/mL Powder for injection: 20 mg/vial, 50 mg/vial, 100 mg/vial, 250 mg/vial, 1 g/vial	*Choriocarcinoma:* 15 mg–30 mg/day orally or IM for 5 days; repeat for 3–5 courses with 1–2 wk rest between courses *Leukemia:* induction—3.3 mg/m^2 IM, IV or orally daily for 4–6 wk combined with prednisone 60 mg/m^2 daily; maintenance—30 mg/m^2 orally or IM twice a week or 2.5 mg/kg IV every 14 days Children: 20 mg–30 mg/m^2 orally or IM once a week *Meningeal leukemia:* 10 mg–15 mg/m^2 intrathecally very 2–5 days; maximum 15 mg; maximum pediatric dose, 12 mg *Burkitt's lymphoma* Stage I & II: 10 mg–25 mg orally daily for 4–8 days then rest 1 wk Stage III: Up to 1 g/m^2/day combined with cyclophosphamide and vincristine *Mycosis fungoides* Oral: 2.5–10 mg/day for weeks or months as needed IM: 50 mg once a week or 25 mg twice a week *Psoriasis* Oral: Three schedules may be used:	Trophoblastic tumors such as gestational choriocarcinoma, chorioadenoma destruens, or hydatidiform mole (DOC) Acute lymphocytic leukemia (DOC), prophylaxis of meningeal leukemia (DOC), breast, lung, and epidermoid cancers of head and neck, Burkitt's lymphoma (DOC), lymphosarcoma, mycosis fungoides, severe psoriasis, rheumatoid arthritis, osteosarcoma	Monitor urinary chorionic gonadotropin to determine effectiveness of therapy in choriocarcinoma; level should return to less than 50 IU/24 h after 3–4 courses of therapy; use preservative-free solution in treating meningeal leukemia; reconstitute with Elliott's B solution, 0.9% sodium chloride, lactated Ringer's solution, or patient's own cerebrospinal fluid; powders may be reconstituted with sterile water for injection, 0.9% sodium chloride injection, of 5% dextrose in water; solution is stable for 7 days at room temperature but should be used within 24 h because it is not preserved; for high-dose methotrexate therapy use prevervative-free solution and dilute in 0.9% sodium chloride or 5% dextrose in water; patient should be well hydrated and urine alkalinized with sodium bicarbonate (3 g every 3 h for 12 h before therapy) to prevent renal toxicity; may increase uric acid levels in blood and urine; CNS toxicity is commonly associated with intrathecal injection; methotrexate is excreted in breast milk; calcium leucovorin is used to "rescue" from high methotrexate doses (see Usual Dosage Range)—dose of calcium leucovorin should be equal to or higher than dose of methotrexate

Continued

Table 72-4
Antimetabolites (continued)

Drug	Preparations	Usual Dosage Range	Uses	Nursing Implications
Methotrexate (cont'd)		10 mg to 25 mg once a week to a maximum of 50 mg/wk *or* 2.5 mg every 12 h for 3 doses or every 8 h for 4 doses once a week, to a maximum of 30 mg/wk *or* 2.5 mg/day for 5 days, skip 2 days, and repeat; maximum 6.25 mg/day (this schedule may cause increased liver toxicity) IM, IV: 10 mg–25 mg once a week to a maximum of 50 mg/wk *High-dose methotrexate* IV infusion: 100 mg/m^2–15 g/m^2 over 4–24 h every 1–3 wk; follow with calcium leucovorin rescue (see below) *Calcium leucovorin "rescue"* Oral, IV, IM: 10 mg–15 mg/m^2 every 6 h starting 1–24 h after methotrexate and continue for 24–72 h; (dosage and schedule vary according to protocol and methotrexate dose) *Rheumatoid arthritis:* 2.5 mg orally every 12 h for 3 doses, *or* 7.5 mg orally as a single dose once a week; may increase to a maximum of 20 mg/wk Alternatively, 7.5–15 mg IM once a week		
Thioguanine TG, 6-Thio-guanine	Tablets: 40 mg	*Induction* Adults and children: 2 mg/kg/day, *or* 75–200 mg/m^2/day in 1–2 divided doses; may increase to 3 mg/kg/day *Maintenance* Adults and children: 2 mg/kg–3 mg/kg/day *or* 75 mg–400 mg/m^2/day Calculate all doses to nearest 20 mg	Acute lymphocytic and myelogenous leukemia (DOC) Chronic myelogenous leukemia	May increase uric acid levels of blood and urine

thereby inhibiting DNA synthesis. Dactinomycin and plicamycin anchor to DNA and inhibit DNA-dependent RNA synthesis. Daunorubicin and doxorubicin bind to adjoining nucleotide pairs of DNA and inhibit DNA and DNA-dependent RNA synthesis. Mitoxantrone inhibits DNA synthesis and possesses cytocidal action on both proliferating and nonproliferating cells. Mitomycin acts like an alkylating agent causing cross-linking between DNA strands, thus inhibiting duplication.

Plant derivatives: Vinblastine and vincristine inhibit mitosis during metaphase by binding to or crystallizing microtubular proteins, thus preventing their proper polymerization. At high concentrations, these agents also inhibit DNA-dependent synthesis. Etoposide inhibits mitosis at high concentrations (>10 µg/mL) by causing lysis of cells entering mitosis, and at low concentrations (0.3 µg-10 µg/mL) by inhibiting cells from entering prophase; the net effect is inhibition of DNA synthesis

USES
See Table 72-5

DOSAGE
See Table 72-5

FATE
All of the natural products are administered parenterally and for the most part are widely distributed to most body tissues and organs, primarily the liver, kidneys, heart, and lungs. Asparaginase is not extensively distributed and its metabolic fate is not well known. Plicamycin is the only natural product that crosses the blood–brain barrier. The agents are metabolized in the liver to some degree and are excreted in the urine or feces (via the bile) as inactive metabolites or unchanged drug

COMMON SIDE EFFECTS
Myelosuppression (leukopenia, thrombocytopenia, anemia; less commonly, agranulocytosis and pancytopenia), nausea, vomiting, alopecia, and anorexia

Daunorubicin and doxorubicin: congestive heart failure
Asparaginase: hypersensitivity reactions, pancreatitis, hepatotoxicity, hypofibrinogenemia
Bleomycin: pneumonitis, hyperpigmentation, erythema, cutaneous edema and tenderness, hyperthermia
Dactinomycin: GI ulceration
Dactinomycin and doxorubicin: stomatitis, esophagitis
Plicamycin: hemorrhagic diathesis
Vincristine: neurotoxicity, hyperuricemia, paralytic ileus, constipation

SIGNIFICANT ADVERSE REACTIONS
(Not all reactions observed with all drugs)

GI: diarrhea, cheilitis, pharyngitis, esophagitis, hemorrhagic colitis, rectal bleeding
Hypersensitivity: skin rash, fever, chills, urticaria, angioedema, pruritus, anaphylactic reaction
Neurologic: agitation, drowsiness, headache, hypothermia, lethargy, malaise, irritability, confusion, syncope, paresthesias, peripheral neuritis, convulsions, motor incoordination
Ocular: blurred vision, conjunctivitis, lacrimation
Dermatologic: acne, hyperpigmentation, hyperkeratosis, thickening of nail beds, photosensitivity
Renal/hepatic: cystitis, polyuria, dysuria, uric acid nephropathy, electrolyte abnormalities, hepatotoxicity
Other: hyperglycemia, ototoxicity, Raynaud's phenomenon, pain at tumor or injection site, phlebitis, tissue necrosis upon extravasation, pulmonary fibrosis

> **NOTE**
> Natural products have been shown to be carcinogenic in animal studies and may present oncogenic risk. These agents are also potential mutagens and teratogens and can cause ovarian and testicular suppression

CONTRAINDICATIONS
Leukopenia, thrombocytopenia, or anemia caused by previous chemotherapy or radiation therapy; hepatotoxicity; renal toxicity; and known hypersensitivity

The use of *daunorubicin and doxorubicin* in patients with preesixting cardiac disease may increase the risk of cardiotoxicity (toxicity may occur at cumulative doses higher than 550 mg/m^2). Daunorubicin and doxorubicin are contraindicated in patients who have received previous treatment with complete cumulative doses of one of the agents. *Asparaginase* should not be used in patients with a history of pancreatitis

INTERACTIONS
Most *natural products* may antagonize the effects of antigout medications by increasing serum uric acid levels; dosage adjustment of the antigout medications may be necessary.

Concurrent use of *asparaginase* and methotrexate may block the antineoplastic action of methotrexate by inhibiting cell synthesis; administer asparaginase 9 to 10 days before or within 24 hours after administering methotrexate; the toxic effect of methotrexate may also be reduced by this regimen.

The concurrent administration of *asparaginase, vincristine,* and prednisone may enhance the hyperglycemic effect, neurotoxicity, and myelosuppression of asparaginase; toxicity does not appear to be enhanced when asparaginase is administered *after* vincristine and prednisone.

Because *asparaginase* causes hyperglycemia, dosage adjustment of hypoglycemic medications may be necessary during asparaginase therapy.

Raynaud's phenomenon has occurred in patients with testicular carcinoma being treated with a combination of *bleomycin* and *vinblastine*; whether the cause is the disease, the chemotherapeutic agents, or a combination of these factors is not known.

Dactinomycin may decrease the effect of vitamin K, requiring an increase in the dose of vitamin K and close observation of the patient.

Daunorubicin is incompatible with heparin sodium and dexamethasone phosphate when mixed together.

Concurrent use of cyclophosphamide, *dactinomycin,* or *mitomycin* with *doxorubicin* may result in increased cardiotoxicity; the total dose of doxorubicin should not exceed 400 mg/m^2.

Doxorubicin is incompatible in solution with aminophylline, cephalothin, dexamethasone, fluorouracil, hydrocortisone, and sodium heparin.

Concurrent use of cyclophosphamide with *daunorubicin* may increase cardiac toxicity; the total dose of daunorubicin should not exceed 450 mg/m^2.

Administration of *doxorubicin* to a patient who has received *daunorubicin* or vice versa, increases the risk of cardiotoxicity; neither agent should be used in a patient who has previously received complete cumulative doses of the other agent.

Concurrent use of *vincristine* with *doxorubicin* and prednisone can increase myelosuppression; avoid this combination.

Patients receiving *natural product antineoplastic agents* may develop a viral disease following immunization with a live virus vaccine for that disease.

Asparaginase may interfere with the interpretation of thyroid function tests by causing a rapid decrease of serum thyroxine–binding globulin within 2 days of administration of the drug; concentrations return to pretreatment levels within 4 weeks following the last dose of asparaginase.

Concurrent use of *dactinomycin* and radiation therapy may potentiate the effects of both and increase the toxicities of both; lower doses of both are suggested.

Concurrent use of *doxorubicin* with streptozocin may prolong the half-life of doxorubicin; therefore a reduction in dosage of doxorubicin is recommended.

The elimination of *etoposide* may be impaired in patients who have been previously treated with cisplatin.

Plicamycin can cause hypoprothrombinemia and inhibit platelet aggregation and therefore increase the risk of hemorrhage in patients receiving warfarin, heparin, thrombolytic agents, aspirin, dextran, dipyridamole, or valproic acid.

Concurrent use of *vincristine* with other neurotoxic drugs and spinal cord radiation therapy may produce increased neurotoxicity.

Bleomycin, doxorubicin, and *vincristine* may decrease the GI absorption of digoxin.

The concurrent administration of *bleomycin, vinblastine,* or *vincristine* with phenytoin may decrease the plasma levels of phenytoin.

Barbiturates can enhance the plasma clearance of *doxorubicin.*

Concomitant use of *etoposide* and warfarin may increase the effects of warfarin.

Adminstration of *vinblastine* or *vincristine* may cause pulmonary distress in patients who are receiving or have received *mitomycin.*

NURSING CONSIDERATIONS

See general discussion of nursing considerations for all antineoplastic drugs. In addition:

Nursing Alerts

- In patients treated with *asparaginase:*
  —Observe for laryngeal constriction, hypotension, diaphoresis, facial edema, respiratory distress, fever, aches, chills, and loss of consciousness because hypersensitivity or acute anaphylactic reactions frequently occur. Because incidence increases with repeated doses, intradermal skin test should be repeated when more than 1 week passes between administration.
  —Assess frequently for severe stomach pain with nausea and vomiting, possible indications of pancreatitis. Monitor results of serum amylase determinations, which should be performed often.
  —Observe for polyuria and polydipsia, potential signs of hyperglycemia. Monitor serum glucose determinations and check urine for glucose.
- Monitor respiratory status of patient receiving *bleomycin* or *mitomycin.* Cough or shortness of breath may indicate pulmonary toxicity.
- If patient is receiving *bleomycin,* assess frequently for wheezing, hypotension, and mental confusion during first 12 to 24 hours after administration of first two doses because incidence of idiosyncratic anaphylactoid reaction is 1%. Risk of reaction may be reduced by giving diphenhydramine before administering bleomycin.
- If patient is receiving *daunorubicin* or *doxorubicin,* assess cardiac status frequently. Dyspnea, tachycardia, hepatomegaly, and swelling of feet and lower legs may indicate cardiotoxicity.
- If patient is receiving *plicamycin,* check laboratory findings for platelet count, bleeding time, and prothrombin time, which should be tested frequently during therapy, and monitor patient for episodes of epistaxis of hematemesis, signs of impending hemorrhagic syndrome.
- During therapy with *plicamycin,* monitor patient for tetany or muscle cramps, possible indications of hypocalcemia. Monitor results of serum calcium, phosphorus, and potassium determinations, which should be obtained before, and at regular intervals during, therapy.
- If patient is receiving *vincristine* or *vinblastine,* assess neurologic status often. Signs and symptoms of neurotoxicity (peripheral neuropathy) include loss of deep tendon reflexes, numbness, weakness, myalgias, motor difficulties, and visual disturbances.
- During therapy with *vincristine,* implement nursing interventions to prevent constipation and monitor bowel function because severe constipation may occur. Bulk-forming laxatives and/or stool softeners are often prescribed.
- When *etoposide* is administered, be alert for development of anaphylactic-like reactions (e.g., chills, fever, tachycardia, bronchospasm, dyspnea, hypotension). Incidence is 1% to 2%.

1. Inject no more than 2 mL of *asparaginase* IM at one site.
2. Inject *daunorubicin* and *doxorubicin* slowly. Facial flushing and erythematous streaking along the vein indicate that injection is too rapid.
3. Ensure that chest radiograph, ECG, and echocardiogram are obtained prior to, and every month during, therapy with daunorubicin or *doxorubicin.*
4. Ensure that pulmonary function studies have been completed before *bleomycin* therapy is initiated. Chest radiographs should be repeated every 2 weeks. Carbon dioxide diffusion capacity should be monitored monthly. Therapy should be discontinued if capacity falls below 30% to 35% of pretreatment value.

PATIENT EDUCATION

See general discussion of Patient Education for all antineoplastic drugs. In addition:

1. Inform patient receiving *daunorubicin* or *doxorubicin* that urine will be red for 24 to 48 hours after drug administration.
2. Explain to patient receiving mitomycin that purple bands in the nail beds may appear with repeated doses.

HORMONAL, ANTIHORMONAL, AND GONADOTROPIN RELEASING—HORMONE ANALOG AGENTS

Hormonal agents have been used to successfully treat a variety of different types of neoplasms. Tumors that are sensitive to hormones may respond to the administration of natural or synthetic hormonal agents that delay tumor growth. Hormonal agents are not curative, however, because most lack a cytoxic action. Still, they may provide the patient with prolonged palliation without major toxicities.

The principal hormones used as antineoplastic drugs are the sex hormones (androgens, estrogens, progestins) and the corticosteroids. Androgens, derivatives of testosterone, are used for the palliative treatment of advanced or disseminated breast cancer in *post*menopausal women when hormonal therapy is indicated. The androgens discussed in this section include the 17-alkylated compounds (dromostanolone, fluoxymesterone, testolactone) and testosterone propionate.

Estrogens are used for the palliative treatment of *post*-menopausal breast cancer, advanced prostatic cancer, and male

(*Text continued on page 730*)

Table 72-5
Natural Products

Drug	Preparations	Usual Dosage Range	Uses	Nursing Implications
Asparaginase Elspar, L-Asparaginase	Injection: 10,000 IU/vial	**Children** *Regimen 1* Asparaginase: 1000 IU/kg/day IV for 10 days starting day 22 Vincristine: 2 mg/m² IV once a week on days 1, 8, 15; maximum single dose is 2 mg Prednisone: 40 mg/m²/day in 3 divided doses for 15 days, then 20 mg/m² for 2 days, 10 mg/m² for 2 days, 5 mg/m² for 2 days, and 2.5/m² for 2 days *Regimen 2* Asparaginase: 6000 IU/m² IM every 3 days for 9 doses starting day 4 Vincristine: 1.5 mg/m² IV for 4 doses on days 1, 8, 15, 22 Prednisone: 40 mg/m²/day in 3 divided doses for 28 days, then taper over 14 days Sole induction agent: 200 IU/kg IV daily for 28 days **Adults** Induction: 10,000 IU/m² every 1–2 wk Intra-arterial: 20,000 IU/day for 7–10 days	Acute lymphocytic leukemia in children *Other uses* Acute myelocytic leukemia, chronic lymphocytic leukemia, Hodgkin's disease, lymphosarcoma, reticulum cell sarcoma, melanosarcoma, hypoglycemia due to islet cell tumors	Adult usage is primarily investigational; may be administered via the hepatic artery for insulin-secreting pancreatic islet cell tumors; store intact vial under refrigeration; for IV use, reconstitute with 5 mL 0.9% sodium chloride for injection and inject over at least 30 min into running IV of 0.9% sodium chloride *or* 5% dextrose; for IM use reconstitute with 2 mL 0.9% sodium chloride; do *not* inject more than 2 mL into one site; avoid vigorous shaking during reconstitution; solution is stable for 8 h at room temperature—discard solution if cloudy; *not* recommended as the sole induction agent unless combined chemotherapy is inappropriate owing to toxicity or other factors; intradermal skin test is recommended prior to initiation of therapy and when more than 7 days have elapsed between doses (up to 35% of patients exhibit hypersensitivity reactions); give 0.1 mL (2 IU) of test solution and observe for at least 1 h for erythema or wheal; to prepare skin test solution reconstitute vial with 5 ml 0.9% sodium chloride; withdraw 0.1 mL (200 IU) and inject into 9.9 mL 0.9% sodium chloride for injection giving test solution of 20 IU/mL; densensitization should be used on any positive reactors; inject 1 IU IV and double the dose every 10 min, provided there is no reaction, until total accumulated dose is equal to the dose for that day; may increase SGOT, SGPT, alkaline phosphatase, bilirubin values; may increase blood ammonia, glucose, and uric acid levels; may increase urinary uric acid levels and decrease serum albumin and calcium; gelatinous fiberlike particles may develop in IV infusion on standing; solution may be administered through a 5-μm filter to remove particles without loss of potency; do not administer thru a 0.2 μm filter, loss of potency may result; asparaginase derived from *Erwinia carotovora* (investigational from the NCI) may be used in patients allergic to the commercial preparation
Bleomycin Blenoxane	15 U/ampule	*Squamous cell carcinoma, lymphosarcoma, reticulum cell sarcoma, testicular carcinoma:* 0.25 U–0.5 U/kg (10 U–20 U/m²) IV, IM, or SC once or twice a week to a total of 300 U–400 U IV infusion: 0.25 U/kg/day or 15 U/m²/day over 24 h for 4–5 days *Hodgkin's disease:* as above until 50% response oc-	*Squamous cell carcinoma* of head and neck (DOC), mouth, tongue, nasopharynx, oropharynx, sinus, palate, lip, buccal mucosa, gingiva, epiglottis, skin, larynx, penis, cervix, vulva *Lymphomas* Hodgkin's disease Reticulum cell sarcoma Lymphosarcoma Testicular carcinomas (DOC)	For IM or SC use, reconstitute with 1 mL–5 mL of sterile water for injection, 0.9% sodium chloride, 5% dextrose, or bacteriostatic water for injection; for IV use, reconstitute with 5 mL 0.9% sodium chloride or 5% dextrose and administer slowly over 10 min; solution is stable 14 days at room temperature and 28 days refrigerated; give test dose of 2 U for first 2 doses in lymphoma patients because of possibility of anaphylactoid reaction; pneumonitis occasionally progressing to pulmonary fibrosis occurs in 10% to 40% of pa-

Continued

Table 72-5
Natural Products (continued)

Drug	Preparations	Usual Dosage Range	Uses	Nursing Implications
Bleomycin (cont'd)		curs, then 1 U daily *or* 5 U weekly IV or IM Intra-arterial infusion for squamous cell carcinoma of head, neck, or cervix: 30 U–60 U/day over 1–24 h *Malignant effusion* Intrapleural: 15 U–120 U in 100 mL of 0.9% sodium chloride allowed to dwell for 24 h Intraperitoneal: 60 U–120 U in 100 mL of 0.9% sodium chloride allowed to dwell for 24 h *Warts:* 0.2 U–0.8 U intralesionally every 2–4 wk to a maximum of 2 U (prepare solution of 15 U/15 mL of 0.9% sodium chloride) Reduce dose in patients with impaired renal function *Serum* *Creatinine* *Dose* 1.5–2.5 ½ normal dose 2.5–4.0 ¼ normal dose 4.0–6.0 ⅕ normal dose 6.0–10.0 1/10–1/20 normal dose	Embryonal cell carcinoma Choriocarcinoma Teratocarcinoma (DOC) Malignant effusions Verruca vulgaris (warts)	tients at total doses of 200 U–400 U; if bleomycin has been used to treat malignant effusions, ½ of the administered dose should be counted toward this total; be alert for symptoms such as dry cough, dyspnea, and fine rales; fatal in 1% of patients; cutaneous allergic reactions are also common; fever and chills occur in 25% of patients 3–6 h after administration and last 4–12 h; becomes less frequent with continued use
Dactinomycin Actinomycin D, Cosmegen	Injection: 0.5 mg/vial	Adults: 0.01 mg/kg–0.015 mg/kg/day IV for 5 days every 4–6 wk, *or* 0.5 mg/m² (maximum 2 mg) IV once a week for 3 wk Children: 0.01 mg/kg–0.015 mg/kg/day IV for 5 days or a total dose of 2.5 mg/m² IV in divided doses over 7 days; may repeat every 4–6 wk *Isolation perfusion* Upper extremity: 0.035 mg/kg Lower extremity: 0.05 mg/kg Dosage should be based on body surface area in obese or edematous patients	Wilms' tumor (DOC) Rhabdomyosarcoma Carcinoma of testis and uterus Ewing's sarcoma Osteosarcoma Choriocarcinoma Investigational uses: Kaposi's sarcoma, malignant melanoma, Paget's disease, management of acute organ rejection in kidney and heart transplants	Reconstitute with 1.1 mL sterile water for injection (preservative-free); administer directly into tubing of running IV of 0.9% sodium chloride or 5% dextrose; may dilute and infuse over 10–15 min; AVOID EXTRAVASATION; NEVER administer IM or SC; solution is *theoretically* stable at room temperature for long periods but should be discarded within 24 h to prevent bacterial contamination; may increase uric acid levels of blood and urine; hyperpigmentation occurs if skin has been previously irradiated; nausea and vomiting are common during first few hours and may persist for up to 24 h
Daunorubicin Cerubidine	Injection: 20 mg/vial	**Adults** *Single agent* 30 mg–60 mg/m²/day IV on days 1–3 every 3–4 wk *or* 0.8 mg/kg–1 mg/kg/day IV for 3–6 days repeated every 3–4 wk *Combination* Daunorubicin:; 45 mg/m²/day IV on days 1–3 of first course and days 1 and 2 of subsequent courses	Acute myelogenous leukemia (DOC) Acute lymphocytic leukemia *Other uses* Neuroblastoma Ewing's sarcoma Wilm's tumor Non-Hodgkin's lymphoma Chronic myelogenous leukemia	Reconstitute with 4 mL sterile water for injection; solution is stable for 24 h at room temperature and 48 h under refrigeration; protect from exposure to sunlight; a change from red to blue-purple indicates deterioration; administer into the tubing of a rapidly flowing IV of 0.9% sodium chloride or 5% dextrose; AVOID EXTRAVASATION; NEVER administer IM or SC; may increase uric acid levels of blood and urine

Continued

Table 72-5
Natural Products (continued)

Drug	Preparations	Usual Dosage Range	Uses	Nursing Implications
		Cytarabine: 100 mg/m²/day IV infusion daily for 7 days for the first course and daily for 5 days for subsequent courses Total cumulative dose of daunorubicin should not exceed 550 mg/m² in adults, 300 mg/m² in children over 2 yr or 10 mg/kg in children under 2 yr **Children** (see also below) *Combination* Daunorubicin: 25 mg–45 mg/m² IV once a week for 4–6 wk Vincristine: 1.5 mg/m² IV once a week for 4–6 wk Prednisone: 40 mg/m² daily orally *Note:* For children under 2 yr or less than 0.5 m² body surface, dosage is based on body weight Reduce dose in patients with impaired hepatic or renal function *Serum Bilirubin* / *Serum Creatinine* / *Dose* 1.2 mg to 3 mg/dL — ¾ normal dose Above 3 mg/dL / Above 3 mg/dL — ½ normal dose		
Doxorubicin Adriamycin-RDF, Adriamycin-PFS	Injection: 2 mg/mL Powder for injection: 10-mg/vial, 20-mg/vial, 50-mg/vial, 150-mg/vial	*Adults:* 60 mg–75 mg/m²/day IV repeated every 21 days *or* 25 mg–30 mg/m²/day IV for 3 days repeated every 4 wk Alternatively, 20 mg/m² IV once weekly cause less cardiotoxicity Bladder instillation: 30 mg/30 mL of 0.9% sodium chloride instilled and retained for 30 min; repeat monthly *Children:* 30 mg/m²/day IV for 3 days repeated every 4 wk Total cumulative dose should not exceed 550 mg/m² Reduce dose in patients with impaired hepatic function *Serum Bilirubin* / *BSP Retention* / *Dose* 1.2 mg–3 mg/dL / 9%–15% — ½ normal dose Above 3 mg/dL / Above 15% — ¼ normal dose	Acute lymphocytic and myelogenous leukemia Wilm's tumor Neuroblastoma (DOC) Soft tissue and bone sarcomas (DOC) Thyroid carcinoma Hodgkin's disease Non-Hodgkin's lymphomas (DOC) Breast and ovarian carcinoma Bronchogenic carcinoma (DOC) Bladder carcinoma (DOC) Endometrial carcinoma Gastric carcinoma Retinoblastoma Pancreatic carcinoma Prostatic carcinoma Testicular carcinoma	Reconstitute powder with 0.9% sodium chloride injection according to package directions; solution is stable for 24 h at room temperature and 48 h under refrigeration; protect from exposure to sunlight; administer into the tubing of a rapidly flowing IV of 0.9% sodium chloride or 5% dextrose; local erythematous streaking along the vein or facial flushing may indicate too rapid administration; AVOID EXTRAVASATION; NEVER administer IM or SC; may increase uric acid levels of blood and urine; cardiotoxic effects can occur at cumulative doses above 550 mg/m² in most patients but may be seen at lower doses in patients who have received previous mediastinal irradiation or cyclophosphamide, dactinomycin or mitomycin therapy; in latter instances, dose should not exceed 400 mg/m²–450 mg/m²

Continued

Table 72-5
Natural Products (continued)

Drug	Preparations	Usual Dosage Range	Uses	Nursing Implications
Etoposide VePesid, VP-16-213, VP-16	Injection: 100 mg/5 mL Capsules: 50 mg	*Testicular carcinoma* IV: 50 mg–100 mg/m^2/day for 5 days repeated every 3–4 wk In combination with other agents: 100 mg/m^2/day on days 1, 3, and 5 repeated every 3–4 wk *Small cell lung carcinoma*: 35 mg/m^2/day IV for 4 days to 50 mg/m^2/day for 5 days; repeat every 3–4 wk; alternatively, 2 times IV dose orally rounded to the nearest 50 mg *Kaposi's sarcoma in AIDS patients* (investigational use): 150 mg/m^2/day for 3 days; repeat every 4 wk	Refractory testicular tumors Small cell lung carcinoma *Investigational uses* Acute myelogenous leukemia Hodgkin's disease Non-Hodgkin's lymphomas Kaposi's sarcoma	Do *not* give by rapid IV push: severe hypotension may result. IV infusion prepared in 5% dextrose or 0.9% sodium chloride injection may be given over 30–60 min; infusion concentrations of 0.2 mg/mL are stable for 96 h at room temperature, and concentrations of 0.4 mg/mL are stable for 48 h in both glass and plastic containers; capsules must be stored under refrigeration; oral form is *not* indicated for testicular tumors; dosage reductions may be indicated in patients with impaired hepatic and renal function, although precise criteria for dosage adjustment have not been established
Mitomycin Mutamycin	Injection: 5 mg/vial, 20 mg/vial, 40 mg/vial	IV: 10 mg–20 mg/m^2 as a single dose repeated every 6–8 wk *or* 2 mg/m^2/day IV for 5 days, skip 2 days, and repeat 2 mg/m^2/day for 5 days; cycle may be repeated every 6–8 wk A suggested guide for subsequent dosage adjustment is the following: | Nadir after Prior Dose Leukocytes	Platelets	% of Prior Dose to be Given
---	---	---
Above 4000	Above 100,000	100%
3000–3999	75,000–99,999	100%
2000–2999	25,000–74,999	70%
Below 2000	Below 25,000	50% | Doses greater than 20 mg/m^2 are no more effective than lower doses, but toxicity increases *Bladder instillation*: 20 mg–40 mg of a solution of 1 mg/ml in water retained for 2–3 h; repeat weekly for 8 wk	Adenocarcinoma of stomach, pancreas, colon, rectum, and breast Squamous cell carcinoma of head, neck, lungs, and cervix (DOC) Malignant melanoma Chronic myelogenous leukemia Bladder carcinoma	Reconstitute with sterile water for injection: according to package directions; solution is stable 7 days at room temperature and 14 days if refrigerated; protect from light; may be diluted for IV infusion (5% dextrose, stable for 3 h at room temperature; 0.9% sodium chloride, stable 12 h; sodium lactate, stable 24 h); AVOID EXTRAVASATION; NEVER administer IM or SC; may increase BUN and serum creatinine levels; vomiting is usually transient (3–4 h), but nausea may persist up to 72 h; if disease shows no response after 2 courses of therapy, discontinue because likelihood of response is minimal
Mitoxantrone Novantrone	Injection: 2 mg/mL, 20 mg/vial, 25 mg/vial, 30 mg/vial	Initially, 12 mg/m^2/day on days 1–3 as an IV infusion with 100 mg/m^2 of cytosine arabinoside for 7 days as a continuous 24-h infusion; a second course of therapy may be given if response is incomplete as follows: 12 mg/m^2/day of mitoxantrone on days 1 and 2 and 100 mg/m^2 of cytosine arabinoside on days 1–5	Acute nonlymphocytic leukemia Breast carcinoma Lymphoma Hepatic carcinoma	Solution must be diluted prior to IU administration with 0.9% sodium chloride or 5% dextrose injection; extravasation reactions are rare; avoid contact with skin (rinse immediately if contact occurs); do not mix in same syringe with heparin, as precipitate may form; spills may be cleaned using an aqueous solution of 5.5 parts calcium hypochlorite in 13 parts of water for each 1 part of mitoxantrone; may increase serum uric acid levels; urine may be blue-green for 24 h after administration and sclerae may be blue; cardiac toxicity may be less than that observed with daunorubicin or doxorubicin

Continued

Table 72-5
Natural Products (continued)

Drug	Preparations	Usual Dosage Range	Uses	Nursing Implications
Plicamycin Mithracin (formerly mithramycin)	Injection: 2.5 mg/vial	*Testicular carcinoma:* 0.025 mg/kg–0.03 mg/kg/day IV infusion for 8 days to 10 days *or* 0.025 mg/kg–0.05 mg/kg/day IV on alternate days for 3–8 doses; repeat every 4 wk *Hypercalcemia and hypercalciuria:* 0.015 mg/kg–0.025 mg/kg/day for 3–4 days; may repeat at 1-wk intervals *or* 0.025 mg/kg IV over 4–6 h as a single dose; if no response in 48 h, a second dose may be given; subsequent doses are given every 3–7 days depending on serum calcium level *Paget's disease:* 0.015 mg/kg/day IV for 10 days; reduce dose (by 25%–50%) in patients with impaired hepatic and renal function	Testicular carcinoma Hypercalcemia and hypercalciuria (not responsive to conventional treatment) associated with advanced neoplasms (see Chap. 41) Investigational use: Paget's disease	Store intact vial under refrigeration; alternate-day dosing may reduce toxicity; delayed toxicity may occur up to 72 h after medication has been discontinued following daily administration but *not* alternate-day administration; reconstitute with 4.9 mL sterile water for injection; stable 24 h at room temperature and 48 h refrigerated; dilute in 5% dextrose or 0.9% sodium chloride, and infuse over 4–6 h; AVOID EXTRAVASATION; may increase SGOT, SGPT, LDH, BUN, serum creatinine levels; may decrease serum calcium, phosphorus, and potassium levels; be alert for epistaxis or hematemesis, early signs of possible hemorrhagic diathesis—inform physician immediately; dosages greater than 0.03 mg/kg/day or a duration of therapy longer than 10 days increases the potential of hemorrhagic diathesis
Vinblastine Alkaban-AQ, Velsar, Velban	Injection: 10 mg vial	*Adults:* initially, 0.1 mg/kg or 3.7 mg/m^2 once every 7 days; increase in increments of 0.05 mg/kg or 1.8 mg–1.9 mg/m^2 until tumor size decreases, leukocyte count falls to 3000, or a maximum dose of 0.5 mg/kg or 18.5 mg/m^2 is reached (usual range is 0.15 mg–0.2 mg/kg or 5.5 mg–7.4 mg/m^2); maintenance dose is 1 increment smaller than final initial dose repeated every 7–14 days *or* 10 mg once or twice a month *Children:* initially, 2.5 mg/m^2 once every 7 days; increase in increments of 1.25 mg/m^2 until leukocyte count falls to 3000, tumor size decreases, or maximum dose of 7.5 mg/m^2 is reached; maintenance dose is 1 increment smaller than final initial dose repeated every 7–14 days Subsequent maintenance doses should not be given to adults *or* children until leukocyte count exceeds 4000 Reduce dose by 50% in patients with a direct serum bilirubin greater than 3 mg/dL	*Frequently responsive* Hodgkin's disease Lymphosarcoma Renal carcinoma Reticulum cell sarcoma Neuroblastoma Advanced mycosis fungoides Histiocytosis X (Letterer-Siwe disease) Testicular carcinoma (DOC) Kaposi's sarcoma *Less responsive* Choriocarcinoma Breast carcinoma Chronic myelogenous leukemia *Investigational uses* Idiopathic thrombocytopenic purpura Auto-immune hemolytic anemia	Store unopened vial under refrigeration; reconstitute with 10 mL 0.9% sodium chloride; solution is stable 30 days under refrigeration; administer by IV push or through tubing of a running IV (0.9% sodium chloride or 5% dextrose) over 1 min; AVOID EXTRAVASATION; rinse syringe and needle with venous blood before withdrawing; if extravasation occurs, damage may be minimized by local injection of hyaluronidase and by following guidelines for treatment of extravasation outlined in general nursing considerations at the beginning of the chapter; may increase uric acid levels of blood and urine; Raynaud's phenomenon is seen with combined use of vinblastine and bleomycin for testicular carcinoma; response may not be seen in some patients until 4–12 wk of therapy has been completed

Continued

Table 72-5
Natural Products (continued)

Drug	Preparations	Usual Dosage Range	Uses	Nursing Implications
Vincristine Oncovin, Vincasar PFS	Injection: 1 mg/mL, 2 mg/2 mL, 5 mg/5mL	*Adults:* 0.01 mg/kg–0.03 mg/kg *or* 0.4 mg/m^2 to 1.4 mg/m^2 IV every 7 days as a single dose *Children ≥10 kg:* 1.5 mg–2 mg/m^2 IV every 7 days as a single dose *Children < 10 kg:* 0.05 mg/kg IV once weekly Reduce dosage by 50% in patients with a direct serum bilirubin greater than 3 mg/dL Small daily doses are not recommended because severe toxicity can occur with no increased benefits	Acute lymphocytic leukemia (DOC) Hodgkin's disease (DOC) Lymphosarcoma Rhabdomyosarcoma (DOC) Neuroblastoma (DOC) Wilms' tumor (DOC) Carcinoma of lung and breast Cervical carcinoma Burkitt's lymphoma *Investigational uses* Ewing's sarcoma Multiple myeloma Idiopathic thrombocytopenic purpura Kaposi's sarcoma	Store unopened vial under refrigeration; protect from light; administer by IV push or through tubing of running IV (0.9% sodium chloride or 5% dextrose) over 1 min; for IV use *only*—intrathecal administration may be fatal; AVOID EXTRAVASATION (see vinblastine); neurotoxicity (numbness, weakness, myalgia, jaw pain, loss of deep tendon reflexes, motor difficulties, visual disturbances) can occur as soon as 2 mo after start of therapy and is usually progressive as long as treatment is continued; paralytic ileus can occur, more commonly in young children; syndrome of inappropriate antidiuretic hormone secretion has been noted, resulting in hyponatremia

breast cancer in selected patients. The estrogens reviewed in this section include the estradiol compounds whose steroidal structures closely resemble the natural hormone, estramustine, a phosphorylated combination of estradiol and mechlorethamine, and several nonsteroidal agents possessing estrogenic activity, such as chlorotrianisene and diethylstilbestrol (DES).

Progestins are steroidal compounds related to the natural hormone progesterone. Progestins have been used in the palliative treatment of carcinoma of the breast, endometrium, and renal cells. The progestational agents discussed in this section include hydroxyprogesterone caproate, medroxyprogesterone acetate, and megestrol acetate.

Corticosteroids are synthetic steroidal agents derived from the natural adrenal hormone cortisol (hydrocortisone). Corticosteroids, primarily prednisone, are used frequently in combination chemotherapy regimens for the treatment of acute and chronic lymphocytic leukemia, Hodgkin's and non-Hodgkin's lymphomas, multiple myeloma, and some breast cancers.

In addition to the hormonal drugs, five other agents are considered in this section. *Aminoglutethimide* is an antiadrenal agent used in the palliative treatment of *post*menopausal breast carcinoma and prostatic carcinoma. *Flutamide* is a nonsteroidal antiandrogen agent used in combination with leuprolide (see below) for the treatment of metastatic prostatic carcinoma. *Mitotane*, a derivative of the insecticide DDT, is used in the palliative treatment of inoperable adrenal cortical carcinoma. *Tamoxifen*, a nonsteroidal antiestrogen, is used for the palliative treatment of advanced breast cancer in pre- *and* postmenopausal women with estrogen receptor (ER)–positive tumors. *Leuprolide* is a gonadotropin releasing–hormone analog used in the palliative treatment of advanced prostatic cancer when orchiectomy or estrogen therapy is either not indicated or is unacceptable to the patient.

The general discussion of these agents presented below is followed by a listing of individual agents in Table 72-6, where specific characteristics of each drug are given.

MECHANISM
Hormonal agents

Androgens: The exact mechanism of the antitumor effect of androgens is unknown. In most cases, hormone receptors must be present in the tumor cell cytosol. Androgens bind to the receptor site, are transported into the cell nucleus, and block normal cell growth by inhibiting the transport of the natural growth hormone into the cell. In addition, androgens may inhibit estrogen synthesis, thus causing androgen-induced estrogen depletion.

Estrogens: The mechanism is thought to be essentially the same as proposed for androgens; the estrogens bind to the cell cytosol receptor, and this complex then translocates to the cell nucleus and blocks normal growth of the cell. Estrogens can also cause regression of some tumors by suppressing normal pituitary function. In males with prostatic cancer, estrogens decrease the amount of luteinizing hormone (i.e., interstitial cell–stimulating hormone) secreated by the pituitary, which in turn decreases the amount of androgen secreted by the testes. The antitumor effect of estramustine may be due to estradiol, the alkylating activity of mechlorethamine, a direct effect of estramustine, or to a combination of these effects.

Progestins: The progestins may have a direct local effect on hormonally sensitive endometrial cells and may also decrease the amount of luteinizing hormone secreted by the pituitary gland. The antineoplastic effect of progestins on carcinoma of the breast is unclear.

Corticosteroids: The corticosteroids produce their antitumor effects by binding to corticosteroid receptors present in high numbers on lymphoid tumors. This binding appears to inhibit both cellular glucose transport and phosphorylation, thereby decreasing the amount of energy available for mitosis and protein synthesis, and ultimately resulting in cell lysis.

Antihormonal agents

Aminoglutethimide: This agent blocks the conversion of cholesterol to pregnenolone by inhibiting the desmolase complex

(Text continued on page 734)

Table 72-6
Hormonal, Antihormonal, and Gonadotropin-Releasing Hormones

Drug	Preparations	Usual Dosage Range	Uses	Nursing Implications
Androgens				
Fluoxymesterone Android-F, Halotestin, Ora-Testryl	Tablets: 2 mg, 5 mg, 10 mg	10 mg to 40 mg/day in divided doses (0.05 mg/kg–1 mg/kg/day)	Advanced breast carcinoma	Indicated for women with inoperable cancer who are 1–5 yr *post*-menopausal; continue treatment 8–12 wk to determine efficacy; if disease progresses during first 6–8 wk of IV therapy, consider alternate therapy; fewer androgenic side effects than testosterone; higher incidence of biliary stasis and jaundice than other androgens. Halotestin tablets contain tartrazine
Testolactone Teslac	Tablets: 50 mg	Oral: 250 mg 4 times/day	Advanced breast carcinoma in women only	*See* Fluoxymesterone; may be used in *pre*menopausal women whose ovarian function has been terminated; devoid of androgenic activity at normal dosages
Methyltestosterone Android, Metandren, Oreton Methyl, Testred, Virilon	Tablets: 10 mg, 25 mg Buccal tablets: 5 mg, 10 mg	Oral: 50 mg–200 mg/day Buccal: 25 mg–100 mg/day	Advanced breast carcinoma	*See* Fluoxymestrone; also, androgenic side effects are more common; painful, erythematous local reactions can occur at injection site; hypercalcemia may result if patient is immobilized or if bony metastases are present; crystals may develop at low temperatures but warming and shaking will redissolve them; moisture from wet needle or syringe may cloud solution but potency is not affected
Testosterone Cypionate Andro-Cyp, Andronate, Depo-Testosterone, Depotest, Duratest, Testoject, and others	Injection: 50 mg/mL, 100 mg/mL, 200 mg/mL	IM: 200 mg–300 mg every 2–4 wk		
Testosterone Enanthate Andryl 200, Delatestryl, Everone, Testrin PA, and others	Injection: 100 mg/mL, 200 mg/mL	IM: 200 mg–400 mg every 2–4 wk		
Testosterone Propionate Testex	Injection: 25 mg/mL, 50 mg/mL, 100 mg/mL	IM: 50 mg–100 mg 3 times/wk		
Estrogens				
Chlorotrianisene Tace	Capsules: 12 mg, 25 mg, 72 mg	Oral: 12 mg–25 mg/day	Advanced prostatic carcinoma (DOC)	Also used for symptomatic treatment of menopausal symptoms and relief of postpartum breast engorgement (72-mg capsules; see Chap. 44)
Diethylstilbestrol DES	Tablets: 0.1 mg, 0.25 mg, 0.5 mg, 1 mg, 5 mg	*Breast cancer* Oral: 1 mg–5 mg 3 times day *Prostatic cancer* Oral: 1 mg–3 mg/day initially, then decrease to 1 mg/day	Advanced breast and prostatic carcinoma (DOC)	Dosage may be increased in advanced prostatic carcinoma, but incidence of thromboembolic complications increases with doses above 1 mg/day
Diethylstilbestrol Diphosphate Stilphostrol	Tablets: 50 mg Injection: 250 mg/5 mL	Oral: 50 mg–200 mg 3 times/day IV: 500 mg on day 1, 1000 mg on days 2–5, then 250 mg–500 mg 1–2 times/wk	Advanced prostatic carcinoma (DOC)	Mix drug in 300 mL 5% dextrose or normal saline solution; administer slowly for 10–15 min at 20–30 drops/min, then increase rate to run entire infusion in over 1 h

DOC, drug of choice.

Continued

Table 72-6
Hormonal, Antihormonal, and Gonadotropin-Releasing Hormones (continued)

Drug	Preparations	Usual Dosage Range	Uses	Nursing Implications
		Maintenance: 250 mg–500 mg IV once or twice a week		
Estradiol Estrace	Tablets: 1 mg, 2 mg	*Breast cancer* 10 mg 3 times/day *Prostatic cancer* 1 mg–2 mg 3 times/day	Advanced breast and prostatic carcinoma	Continue breast cancer treatment for a minimum of 3 mo to determine efficacy
Estradiol Cypionate Depo-Estradiol, Depestro, DepGynogen, Depogen, Dura-Estrin, Estra-D, Estro-Cyp, Estrofem, Estroject-LA, Estronol-LA, Hormogen-Depot	Injection: 1 mg/mL, 5 mg/mL	IM: initially 1 mg–5 mg/wk Maintenance: 2 mg–5 mg every 3–4 wk	Advanced prostatic carcinoma (DOC)	
Estradiol Valerate Delestrogen, Dioval, Duragen, Estradiol-LA, Estraval, Gynogen LA, Valergen	Injection: 10 mg/mL, 20 mg/mL, 40 mg/mL	IM: 30 mg or more every 1–2 wk	Advanced prostatic carcinoma (DOC)	
Estramustine Phosphate Sodium EMCYT	Capsules: 140 mg	14 mg/kg/day in 3–4 divided doses; maintenance therapy 10 mg/kg to 16 mg/kg/day in divided doses	Advanced prostatic carcinoma	Store in refrigerator and protect from light; continue treatment 1–3 mo to determine efficacy; may increase serum bilirubin, LDH, and SGOT concentrations
Estrogens, conjugated Premarin, Progens **Estrogens, esterified** Estratab, Menest	Tablets: 0.3 mg, 0.625 mg, 0.9 mg, 1.25 mg, 2.5 mg	*Breast cancer* 10 mg 3 times a day *Prostatic cancer* 1.25 mg–2.5 mg 3 times/day	Advanced breast and prostatic carcinoma (DOC)	Continue breast cancer treatment 8–12 wk to determine efficacy; determine effectiveness in prostatic cancer by monitoring serum phosphate levels, which should decrease.
Estrone Bestrone, Estrone-A, Estronol, Theelin Aqueous	Injection: 2 mg/mL, 5 mg/mL	IM: 2 mg–4 mg 2–3 times/wk	Advanced prostatic carcinoma (DOC)	Continue treatment for 3 mo to determine efficacy
Ethinyl Estradiol Estinyl, Feminone	Tablets: 0.02 mg, 0.05 mg, 0.5 mg	*Breast cancer* 1 mg 3 times/day *Prostatic cancer* 0.15 mg to 2 mg/day	Advanced breast and prostatic carcinoma (DOC)	
Polyestradiol Phosphate Estradurin	Injection: 40 mg	IM: 40 mg every 2–4 wk; may increase to 80 mg	Advanced prostatic carcinoma (DOC)	Continue treatment for 3 mo to determine efficacy; reconstitute with sterile diluent provided; do *not* agitate violently; store at room temperature away from light for 10 days and discard at first sign of cloudiness or precipitate

DOC, drug of choice.

Continued

Table 72-6
Hormonal, Antihormonal, and Gonadotropin-Releasing Hormones (continued)

Drug	Preparations	Usual Dosage Range	Uses	Nursing Implications
Progestins				
Hydroxyprogesterone caproate Gesterol LA, Hylutin, Hyprogest, Hyproval P.A., Hyroxon, Pro-Depo	Injection: 125 mg/mL, 250 mg/mL	IM: 1 g–7 g/wk	Advanced endometrial carcinoma (stage III or IV)(DOC)	Stop therapy when relapse occurs or after 12 wk with no obejctive response
Medroxyprogesterone Acetate Amen, Curretab, Cycrin, Provera, Depo-Provera	Tablets: 2.5 mg, 5 mg, 10 mg Injection: 100 mg/mL, 400 mg/mL	Oral, IM: 400 mg–1000 mg/wk Maintenance: 400 mg/mo or adjusted to patient's needs	Endometrial and renal carcinoma (DOC)	Recommended *only* as adjunctive and palliative therapy in advanced inoperable cases; usually well tolerated even in large doses; gluteal abscesses have occurred
Megestrol Acetate Megace	Tablets: 20 mg, 40 mg	*Breast cancer* 40 mg 4 times/day *Endometrial cancer* 40 mg–320 mg/day in 4 divided doses	Breast and endometrial carcinoma (DOC) Investigational use: anorexia due to AIDS	Continue treatment at least 2 mo to determine efficacy; relatively nontoxic in doses up to 800 mg/day
Corticosteroids				
Prednisone Deltasone, Liquid Pred, Prednisone Intensol, Orasone	Tablets: 1 mg, 2.5 mg, 5 mg, 10 mg, 20 mg, 25 mg, 50 mg Syrup: 5 mg/5 mL Solution: 5 mg/5 mL Solution concentrate: 5 mg/mL	*Acute and chronic lymphocytic leukemia* 40 mg–60 mg/m^2/day *Hodgkin's disease and non-Hodgkin's lymphomas* 40 mg–100 mg/m^2/day *Multiple myeloma* 75 mg/m^2/day *Breast cancer* 40 mg/m^2/day	Acute and chronic lymphocytic leukemia (DOC) Hodgkin's disease (DOC) Non-Hodgkin's lymphomas (DOC) Multiple myeloma (DOC) Some breast cancers	Never used alone but always as a part of combination chemotherapy regimens; side effects are minimized by alternate-day or intermittent therapy; concentrate solution is 30% alcohol and dye free
Antihormonal Agents				
Aminoglutethimide Cytadren	Tablets: 250 mg	*Antiadrenal:* 250 mg 2–3 times/day for 2 wk; maintenance—250 mg 4 times day to a maximum of 2 g/day *Breast and prostatic cancer* 250 mg 2–3 times/day for 2 wk; maintenance—250 mg 4 times/day in combination with hydrocortisone, 40 mg/day in 3 divided doses	Cushing's syndrome associated with adrenal carcinoma Investigational uses: Postmenopausal metastatic breast cancer and prostatic carcinoma	Serum acid phosphatase levels should decrease in patients with prostatic cancer if aminoglutethimide is producing a positive clinical response; replacement glucocorticoid therapy is usually required in patients with breast and prostatic cancer; replacement mineralocorticoid (fludrocortisone) may be necessary in 25%–50% of patients with Cushing's syndrome to prevent reduction of aldosterone which could lead to hyponatremia and orthostatic hypotension; monitor thyroid function during prolonged therapy
Flutamide Eulexin	Capsules: 125 mg	Oral: 250 mg 3 times/day at 8-h intervals	Metastatic prostatic carcinoma	Used in combination with gonadotropin–releasing hormone analog agents (leuprolide); to provide maximal benefit, therapy must be started simultaneously with both drugs; monitor

DOC, drug of choice.

Continued

Table 72-6
Hormonal, Antihormonal, and Gonadotropin-Releasing Hormones (continued)

Drug	Preparations	Usual Dosage Range	Uses	Nursing Implications
				liver function in patients on long-term therapy; side effects include hot flashes, loss of libido, impotence, nausea, gynecomastia
Mitotane Lysodren	Tablets: 500 mg	**Adults** Initially 8 g–10 g/day in 3 or 4 divided doses; adjust dosage to maximum tolerated dose (usually 2 g–16 g/day); maximum dose 18–19 g/day *Cushing's syndrome:* Initially, 3 g–6 g/day in 3–4 divided doses; maintenance range is 500 mg twice a week to 2 g/day **Children** 0.1 mg/kg–0.5 mg/kg/day in divided doses *or* 1 g–2 g/day in divided doses; may be gradually increased to 5 g–7 g/day	Functional and nonfunctional adrenal cortical carcinoma (DOC) *Investigational use:* Cushing's syndrome	Continue therapy 3 mo to determine efficacy; may decrease protein-bound iodine and urinary 17-hydroxycorticosteroid levels; adrenocortical insufficiency can occur; replacement therapy may be necessary; periodic neurologic assessments are recommended for patients on therapy longer than 2 yr
Tamoxifen Nolvadex	Tablets: 10 mg	10 mg–20 mg twice a day	Advanced breast carcinoma (DOC)	May increase serum calcium levels; transient "flaring" of disease may occur during initial therapy—usually subsides rapidly; ocular toxicity is associated with long-term, high-dose therapy; can induce ovulation
Gonadotropin Releasing–Hormone Analog Agent				
Leuprolide Leupron	Injection: 5 mg/mL; available as 2.8-mL or 5.6-mL kits (14- or 28-day supply) Depot injection: 7.5 mg/ml	*SC:* 1 mg/day Depot: 7.5 mg IM every 28–33 days	Advanced prostatic carcinoma (DOC) *Investigational uses* Pre- and postmenopausal breast cancer, polycystic ovarian disease, endometriosis, anovulation, amenorrhea	Patients may experience an increase in testosterone levels and worsening of signs and symptoms early in treatment; refrigerated prior to dispensing but may be stored at room temperature while in use; serum testosterone and prostatic acid phosphatase (PAP) levels should be assessed periodically to monitor therapeutic response; depot may be stored at room temperature

DOC, drug of choice.

enzyme system in adrenal mitochondria, thus blocking the biosynthesis of all steroid hormones. Additionally, aminoglutethimide blocks the conversion of androgens to estrogens in peripheral tissues by blocking the aromatase enzyme. The net result is a medical adrenalectomy due to the complete suppression of the adrenal cortex by aminoglutethimide.

Flutamide: This nonsteroidal antiandrogen exerts its antiandrogenic effect by competing with testosterone and its metabolites for the androgen binding sites on the receptor proteins in the cytoplasm of the prostate cells. Flutamide or a metabolite also interferes with the retention of the androgen-receptor complex in the nucleus, thus inhibiting prostatic-stimulated DNA synthesis.

Mitotane: This adrenal cytoxic agent causes adrenal inhibition, apparently without cellular destruction. It exerts its principal action on the mitochondria of the adrenal cortex, although the exact biochemical mechanism of action is unknown. Mitotane modifies the peripheral metabolism of steroids and directly suppresses the adrenal cortex. Mitotane also alters the extra-adrenal metabolism of cortisol, even though plasma levels of corticosteroids do not fall. The drug apparently causes increased formation of 6 beta-hydroxycortisol.

Tamoxifen: Tamoxifen is a nonsteroidal estrogen antagonist that binds to estrogen receptor sites in the cytosol of the cell. This complex is translocated to the nucleus of the cell where it acts as a false messenger and ultimately inhibits DNA synthesis. Tamoxifen is unlikely to cause a response in patients who have had a negative estrogen-receptor (ER) assay.

Gonadotropin Releasing–Hormone Analog

Leuprolide, a gonadotropin releasing–hormone (GnRH) analog, has the same action as the naturally occurring hormone. Long-term administration of leuprolide inhibits gonadotropin secretion and suppresses ovarian and testicular steroidogenesis. Leuprolide reduces the number of pituitary GnRH or testicular luteinizing hormone (LH) receptors, causing pituitary or testicular desensitization, respectively. Leuprolide may also inhibit the enzymes necessary for steroidogenesis.

In males, leuprolide decreases serum levels of LH, follicle-stimulating hormone (FSH), testosterone, and dihydrotestosterone, with serum testosterone levels reaching castration levels after 2 to 4 weeks of continuous therapy. In females, leuprolide decreases serum levels of LH, FSH, progesterone, and estrogen; it suppresses ovarian estrogen and androgen production by inhibiting pituitary gonadotropin release; serum estrogen levels in premenopausal women may be reduced to postmenopausal levels after 2 to 4 weeks of therapy

USES
See Table 72-6

DOSAGE
See Table 72-6

FATE

The fate of the androgen, estrogen, progestin, and corticosteroid agents are reviewed in Chapters 43, 44, and 46. *Aminoglutethimide* is well absorbed from the GI tract, exhibits low protein binding, is metabolized in the liver, and is about 50% renally excreted. *Flutamide* is rapidly and completely absorbed orally, highly protein bound, rapidly and extensively metabolized in the liver, and excreted mainly in the urine. The antihormonal agent *mitotane* is approximately 40% absorbed from the GI tract and is excreted by the kidneys (10%–25%) as a water-soluble metabolite, in the bile (a small amount), and largely unchanged in the feces (60%). Mitotane is stored primarily in fatty tissues throughout the body, and blood levels are detectable up to 10 weeks after the medication has been discontinued. *Tamoxifen* is well absorbed orally, metabolized in the liver, and excreted primarily in the feces. *Leuprolide* is rapidly absorbed following subcutaneous administration. Its distribution, metabolism, and excretion have not been conclusively determined

COMMON SIDE EFFECTS

See Chapters 43, 44, and 46 for common side effects of corticosteroids, estrogens and progestins, and androgens, respectively.

Mitotane: anorexia, nausea, vomiting, diarrhea, skin rash, skin darkening; CNS toxicity (drowsiness, dizziness, depression)
Tamoxifen: nausea, vomiting, hot flashes
Aminoglutethimide: anorexia, nausea, vomiting; measles-like rash, itching (starting 10–15 days after initiation of therapy and lasting for 5–7 days), skin darkening; drowsiness, dizziness, lethargy, uncontrolled eye movements, headache, depression
Flutamide: hot flashes, loss of libido, gynecomastia, impotence; diarrhea, nausea, vomiting
Leuprolide: hot flashes, gynecomastia, impotence; rash, itching; dizziness, headache, blurred vision, paresthesias; GI distress

SIGNIFICANT ADVERSE REACTIONS

See Chapters 43, 44, and 46 for significant adverse reactions of corticosteroids, estrogens and progestins, and androgens, respectively.

Mitotane: visual disturbances, hypersensitivity reactions (dyspnea, wheezing), generalized aching, hyperpyrexia, muscle twitching, hematuria, proteinuria, hemorrhagic cystitis
Tamoxifen: leukopenia, thrombocytopenia, hypercalcemia, increased bone pain, vaginal bleeding, menstrual irregularities, lactation, alopecia, photosensitivity, dizziness, headache, depression, anorexia, retinopathy, corneal changes, decreased visual acuity
Aminoglutethimide: myelosuppression (rare), hypotension, hypothyroidism (rare), hypersensitivity reactions (fever, skin rash, cholestatic jaundice, increased SGOT; rare)
Flutamide: elevated liver enzymes, hepatitis, edema, hypertension, myelosuppression (rare)
Leuprolide: congestive heart failure, thrombophlebitis, peripheral edema, myalgia, increased bone or tumor pain at start of therapy, myocardial infarction (rare), pulmonary embolism (rare)

CONTRAINDICATIONS

(Especially as they apply to the use of these agents as antineoplastic drugs)

Androgens are contraindicated in carcinoma of the male breast, known or suspected prostatic cancer, and *pre*menopausal women
Estrogens are contraindicated in men or women with known or suspected cancer of the breast, except in appropriately selected patients being treated for metastatic disease
Estrogen usage is contraindicated in known or suspected estrogen-dependent neoplasia
Estrogen and *progestin* usage is contraindicated in active thrombophlebitis or thromboembolic disorders and in markedly impaired liver function
The progestins *hydroxyprogesterone* and *medroxyprogesterone* are contraindicated in known or suspected breast carcinoma, known or suspected genital malignancy, and undiagnosed vaginal bleeding
Aminoglutethimide is contraindicated in patients allergic to glutethimide (Doriden)

(See Chaps. 43, 44, and 46 for additional information on contraindications of hormonal agents.)

INTERACTIONS

The androgens, particularly *fluoxymesterone* and *methyltestosterone*, may increase sensitivity to anticoagulants; the dosage of the anticoagulant may have to be decreased.
Androgens may enhance the effect of hypoglycemic agents.
Estrogens may reduce the effect of oral anticoagulants by increasing certain clotting factors in the blood.
The anticonvulsants carbamazepine, phenobarbital, phenytoin, and primidone may reduce the effect of *estrogens* owing to increased estrogen metabolism caused by the induction of liver enzymes.
Concurrent use of rifampin and *estrogens* may result in decreased estrogenic activity due to enzyme induction.
Large doses of *estrogens* may enhance the side effects of tricyclic antidepressants and diminish their antidepressant effect.

Antiinfective and Chemotherapeutic Agents

Corticosteroids, when used concurrently with amphotericin B, may cause increased potassium depletion leading to hypokalemia.

Corticosteroids may increase *or* decrease the response to oral anticoagulants.

Corticosteroids cause hyperglycemia and thus may increase requirements for insulin or oral hypoglycemic agents.

Ephedrine, phenobarbital, phenytoin, and rifampin enhance the metabolism of *corticosteroids* through enzyme induction, thus decreasing corticosteroid activity.

Patients taking potassium-depleting diuretics and *corticosteroids* concomitantly may develop hypokalemia.

Corticosteroids may decrease blood salicylate levels by increasing the glomerular filtration rate and by decreasing renal tubular reabsorption of water.

Mitotane alters *corticosteroid* metabolism, and higher doses of corticosteroids may be needed to treat adrenal insufficiency.

Mitotane and CNS depressants used concurrently may cause additive CNS depression.

Milk, milk products, and calcium rich foods or drugs should not be taken with *estramustine phosphate sodium* since an insoluble, nonabsorbable calcium salt may be formed.

Concurrent administration of spironolactone and *mitotane* may antagonize the effects of mitotane.

Concurrent administration of *aminoglutethimide* and theophylline or digitoxin may decrease the effects of the latter two drugs.

Aminoglutethimide may reduce the anticoagulant effect of warfarin, whereas *tamoxifen* may increase warfarin's action.

The effects of dexamethasone and medroxyprogesterone may be decreased by *aminoglutethimide,* even for several days after discontinuation of aminoglutethimide.

NURSING CONSIDERATIONS

See individual Nursing Considerations for androgens, estrogens, progestins, and corticosteroids. In addition:

Nursing Alerts

- Monitor patient with metastatic breast cancer being treated with an *androgen, estrogen, progestin,* or *tamoxifen* for signs of hypercalcemia (polyuria, polydipsia, weakness, constipation, mental sluggishness or disorientation). Check results of serum calcium determinations, which should be obtained periodically.
- Consider the possibility of intermittent porphyria if patient experiences moderate to severe abdominal pain during therapy with an *androgen, estrogen,* or *progestin.*
- Frequently assess neurologic status of patient receiving *testolactone.* Numbness or tingling of fingers, toes, or face may indicate peripheral neuropathy.
- If patient receiving *aminoglutethimide* or *mitotane* experiences unusual stress, shock, or severe trauma, be prepared to discontinue drug and administer steroids because normal adrenal response is suppressed.

1. Provide opportunity (i.e., time, privacy) for patient to discuss feelings about potential or actual changes in body image and sexuality.
2. To reduce susceptibility to hypercalcemia, implement interventions to increase patient mobility, as needed.
3. Monitor patient receiving aminoglutethimide for signs of hypotension related to reduced aldosterone production.

PATIENT EDUCATION

See Patient Education for androgens, estrogens, progestins, or corticosteroids. In addition:

1. Warn patient receiving mitotane or aminoglutethimide to exercise caution in performing hazardous tasks because drowsiness, dizziness, or weakness may occur, especially during early therapy.
2. Teach patient receiving aminoglutethimide precautions to prevent postural hypotension (see **Plan of Nursing Care 8** in Chapter 31).
3. Review patient-information package insert with patient before therapy with an *estrogen, leuprolide,* or a *progestin* is initiated to ensure that patient understands information.
4. Warn patient treated with *leuprolide* or *tamoxifen* that a transient flare of disease, with increased symptoms and bone pain, often occurs. Hot flashes may also occur with leuprolide.
5. Recommend use of contraceptive measures if patient is receiving an *estrogen, progestin, tamoxifen,* or *mitotane.*
6. Inform male receiving an estrogen that the gynecomastia that can occur may be prevented by pretreatment low-dose breast irradiation.
7. Explain that *leuprolide* therapy may impair fertility and decrease libido.

MISCELLANEOUS ANTINEOPLASTIC AGENTS

Hydroxyurea Procarbazine
Interferon

The agents discussed in this section (hydroxyurea; interferon alfa-2a, recombinant; interferon alfa-2b, recombinant; and procarbazine) are classified as miscellaneous agents because their mechanism(s) of action or source does not correspond with the other classes of antineoplastic agents.

The interferons are synthetic protein chains consisting of 165 amino acids produced by recombinant DNA technology using genetically engineered *Escherichia coli.* Interferon alfa-2a, recombinant, has lysine at position 23 whereas interferon alfa-2b, recombinant, has an arginine group at position 23 (see Table 72-7).

MECHANISM

Hydroxyurea: The exact mechanism of action is not completely established. Hydroxyurea causes an immediate inhibition of DNA synthesis without interfering with the synthesis of RNA or protein. It is a cell-cycle specific agent for the S phase of cell division.

Interferon: The exact mechanism of action of the interferons is unknown; however, it is known that interferons have antiviral, antiproliferative, and immunomodulatory activities, and any or all of these activities are important to the antitumor action of the interferons.

The interferons bind to specific membrane receptors on the surface of the cell and initiate a complex sequence of intracellular events that includes the induction of several enzymes (synthetases, protein kinases, and endonucleases). This process, in part, is responsible for the cellular responses to interferon: inhibition of virus replication in virus-infected cells, suppression of cell proliferation, and enhancement of the phagocytic activity of macrophages and augmentation of the specific cytotoxicity of lymphocytes for target cells.

Procarbazine: The exact mechanism of action is not completely established. Procarbazine may inhibit DNA, RNA, and protein synthesis; however, no cross-resistance with other alkylating agents has been demonstrated. It is cell-cycle specific for the S phase of cell division

USES
See Table 72-7

DOSAGE
See Table 72-7

FATE
Hydroxyurea is readily absorbed from the GI tract and readily crosses the blood–brain barrier. It is metabolized in the liver and excreted by the kidneys as urea and hydroxyurea and by the lungs as carbon dioxide.

Interferon is readily absorbed from IM or SC injection sites and is distributed principally to the blood and kidneys. It is metabolized in the kidneys, and the products of renal catabolism are almost completely reabsorbed with negligible renal excretion

Procarbazine is rapidly and completely absorbed from the GI tract and readily crosses the blood–brain barrier. It is metabolized by the liver to active metabolites and excreted by the kidneys and lungs

COMMON SIDE EFFECTS
Hydroxyurea: myelosuppression (leukopenia), drowsiness
Interferon: leukopenia and thrombocytopenia (occur frequently but are generally mild); flu-like syndrome—anorexia, nausea, vomiting, diarrhea; altered taste sensation, dizziness, tiredness
Procarbazine: myelosuppression (leukopenia, thrombocytopenia, anemia); nausea, vomiting, diarrhea; fever, chills, sweating, myalgia, arthralgia

SIGNIFICANT ADVERSE REACTIONS
Hydroxyurea: GI disturbances, stomatitis, neurotoxicity (headache, dizziness, disorientation, hallucinations, convulsion), hyperuricemia, dysuria, uric acid nephropathy, maculopapular rash, facial edema, alopecia
Interferon: cardiotoxicity (edema, hypotension, angina, arrhythmias, tachycardia, congestive heart failure, myocardial infarction [high doses]); neurotoxicity (paresthesias, numbness, depression, nervousness, sleep disturbances, seizures, hallucinations); hyperuricemia; proteinuria; elevated serum creatinine and BUN; alopecia with long-term therapy
Procarbazine: neurotoxicity (paresthesias, decreased tendon reflexes, peripheral neuropathies, depression, insomnia, nightmares, tremors, ataxia, convulsions); dermatological toxicity (pruritus, dermatitis, alopecia, photosensitivity, hyperpigmentation); ophthalmic toxicity (diplopia, nystagmus, photophobia, papilledema, retinal hemorrhage); pneumonitis, hepatotoxicity, dysuria, orthostatic hypotension, tachycardia, hypertensive crisis, impaired hearing

CONTRAINDICATIONS
Hydroxyurea and *procarbazine* therapy should not be initiated in any patient with marked bone marrow depression. Patients hypersensitive to any alfa interferon may also be intolerant of *recombinant interferon alfa-2a* or *alfa-2b*. Also patients hypersensitive to mouse immunoglobulin may also be hypersensitive to *interferon alfa-2a, recombinant*

INTERACTIONS
Hydroxyurea may antagonize the effects of antigout medications by increasing serum uric acid; dosage adjustment of the antigout medications may be necessary.
Procarbazine and ethanol ingestion may cause a disulfiram-like reaction and have an additive CNS-depressant effect.
Concurrent use of *procarbazine* with tricyclic antidepressants, monoamine oxidase (MAO) inhibitors, or phenothiazines, may cause a severe hypertensive crisis.
Thiazide diuretics administered concurrently with *procarbazine* may cause enhanced hypotension.
CNS depressants such as narcotic analgesics and barbiturates used concurrently with *procarbazine* may cause enhanced CNS depression and hypotension in some patients but may cause excitation, rigidity, sweating, hyperpyrexia, and hypertension in others.
Procarbazine may enhance the effects of insulin and oral hypoglycemic medications; dosage adjustment of hypoglycemic agents may be necessary.
Guanethidine, levodopa, methyldopa, or reserpine used concurrently with *procarbazine* may result in hypertension and excitation.
Sympathomimetics such as amphetamines, epinephrine, ephedrine, isoproterenol, methylphenidate, and phenylpropanolamine used concurrently with *procarbazine* may cause hyperpyrexia and a severe hypertensive crisis.
Ingestion of foods with a high tyramine content (see Nursing Alerts) may cause a severe hypertensive crisis in a patient on *procarbazine* therapy.
Concurrent use of any of the miscellaneous agents with live virus vaccines may potentiate the replication of the vaccine virus, increase the side effects and adverse reactions of the vaccine virus, or decrease the patient's antibody response to the vaccine because the patient's normal defense mechanisms are suppressed.
Concurrent use of *procarbazine* with dextromethorphan (a cough suppressant found in many nonprescription cough preparations) may cause excitation and hyperpyrexia.
Interferon may increase the effects of theophylline and aminophylline by decreasing their clearance.
The gastrointestinal absorption of digoxin may be impaired by concurrent administration of *procarbazine.*
Concurrent administration of *procarbazine* and high-dose methotrexate may increase the nephrotoxicity of methotrexate.

NURSING CONSIDERATIONS
See general discussion of Nursing Considerations for all antineoplastic agents. In addition:

Nursing Alerts
- During therapy with hydroxyurea, carefully monitor intake and output as well as results of BUN and serum creatinine determinations because renal function may be

temporarily impaired. If patient with renal impairment receives hydroxyurea, auditory and visual hallucinations or increased hematologic toxicity may develop.
- The following points pertain to a patient receiving *procarbazine:*
  — Before initiating therapy, be sure that the patient has not taken another MAO inhibitor within the previous 14 days or tricyclic antidepressants within the previous 10 days.
  — Check ingredients of all medications before administering. Sympathomimetic agents, which can precipitate potentially lethal hypertensive crises, are present in many prescription and OTC preparations, such as cough, cold, asthma, hay fever, and allergy formulations, appetite depressants, and antiemetics.
  — Institute preventive measures and monitoring procedures appropriate for MAO inhibitors (see MAO inhibitors).
- The following points pertain to a patient receiving *interferon.*
  — Ensure that baseline laboratory determinations of complete blood count, peripheral and bone marrow hairy cells, and liver and renal function are obtained before initiating administration. Monitor results of tests obtained during therapy, usually every month, to assess response to drug.
  — Monitor intake and output, and work with patient to develop plan to maximize fluid intake. Patient should be well hydrated, especially during initial stages of therapy, to prevent hypotension from fluid depletion.
  — Monitor blood pressure and vital signs because cardiotoxicity may occur, particularly if patient has a history of heart disease or cancer is in advanced stage.
  — Carefully evaluate for evidence of neuropsychiatric changes such as depression, sleep disturbances, or hallucinations, because neurotoxicity may occur.

1. When possible, administer *alfa-2a interferon* in the morning to maximize accuracy of assessment for toxicity. A consistent time of administration is also important.
2. When possible, administer *alfa-2b interferon* at night to minimize impact of side effects.
3. If patient is receiving interferon, take measures to prevent falls because neurotoxicity, which may be manifested by gait alterations, can occur.

PATIENT EDUCATION

See general discussion of Patient Education for all antineoplastic agents. In addition:

1. The following points pertain to a patient receiving; *procarbazine:*
   — Teach precautions appropriate for MAO inhibitors (see discussion of MAO inhibitors).
   — Warn patient to exercise caution while performing potentially hazardous tasks because drowsiness, dizziness, or blurred vision may occur.
   — Warn fertile woman to use effective contraceptive measures.
2. Inform patient that flulike symptoms may occur during initiation of *procarbazine* therapy and usually occur 2 to 6 hours after a dose of *interferon.* Reassure patient that symptoms tend to abate with continued therapy. Premedication with acetaminophen may help control this response to interferon.
3. If patient receiving *hydroxyurea* has had previous radiation therapy, inform patient that postirradiation erythema may be exacerbated.

COMBINATION CHEMOTHERAPY

Combination chemotherapy is currently in wide use in many neoplastic diseases to produce higher response rates and longer periods of remission than can be obtained with single-agent therapy. Combinations of agents are also used to delay the emergence of resistance in the tumor cells and to obtain a synergistic therapeutic effect with minimal toxicity.

The general principles used for the selection of agents to be used for a combination chemotherapeutic regimen are as follows:

Table 72-7
Miscellaneous Antineoplastic Agents

Drug	Preparations	Usual Dosage Range	Uses	Nursing Implications
Hydroxurea Hydrea	Capsules: 500 mg	*Solid tumors* Intermittent therapy: 80 mg/kg as a single dose every third day Continuous therapy: 20 mg/kg–30 mg/kg daily as a single dose *Carcinoma of head and neck* 80 mg/kg as a single dose every third day; used concomitantly with radiation	Acute and chronic myelocytic leukemia Malignant melanoma Ovarian carcinoma Squamous cell carcinoma of head and neck (excluding the lip) *Investigational uses* Advanced prostatic carcinoma Lung carcinoma Psoriasis Hypereosinophilia syndrome	Discontinue therapy if leukocytes are less than 2500 and platelets are less than 100,000; drowsiness occurs with large doses; hydroxyurea should be started at least 7 days before radiation therapy and continued during and after radiation therapy; contents of capsules may be emptied into a glass of water and taken immediately if patient is unable to swallow capsules (some inert material may not dissolve and may float on the surface); may increase serum uric acid, BUN, and creatinine levels; dysuria may occur but is usually temporary; intermittent therapy causes less

Continued

Table 72-7
Miscellaneous Antineoplastic Agents (continued)

Drug	Preparations	Usual Dosage Range	Uses	Nursing Implications
		Myelocytic leukemia 20 mg/kg–30 mg/kg daily as a single dose *Malignant melanoma* 60 mg/kg–80 mg/kg as a single dose every third day either alone or in combination with radiation *or* 20 mg/kg–30 mg/kg daily as a single dose		toxicity; continue therapy 6 wk to determine efficacy
Interferon Alfa-2a, Recombinant Roferon-A	Injection solution: 3 million IU/mL, 18 million IU/3 mL Lyophilized powder: 3 million IU/vial, 18 million IU/vial	*Hairy cell leukemia* IM, SC Induction: 3 million IU/day for 16–24 wk Maintenance: 3 million IU 3 times/wk; reduce dose by 50% if severe adverse effects occur *Kaposi's sarcoma* Induction: 36 million IU daily IM or SC for 10–12 wk Maintenance: 3 million IU 3 times/wk; reduce dose by 50% if severe adverse effects occur Some dosage regimens for investigational uses *Chronic myelogenous leukemia* IM: 5 million IU/m^2/day *Non-Hodgkin's lymphomas* IM: 50 million IU/m^2 3 times/wk; reduce a dose as needed if side effects occur *Renal cell carcinoma* IM: 20 million IU/m^2/day *or* 5 times a week *or* 3 times/wk *Malignant melanoma* IM: 12 million IU–50 million IU/m^2 3 times/wk *Mycosis fungoides* IM: 50 million IU/m^2 3 times/wk *Multiple myeloma* IM: 2 million IU–100 million IU/m^2/day	Hairy cell leukemia and Kaposi's sarcoma (in patients 18 yr and older) *Investigational uses* Renal carcinoma Bladder carcinoma (instillation) Non-Hodgkin's lymphomas Malignant melanoma Mycosis fungoides Condylomata accuminata (genital warts) (by intralesional injection) Chronic myelogenous leukemia Multiple myeloma Cervical and ovarian cancer Osteosarcoma Cutaneous T-cell lymphoma Chronic non-A, non-B hepatitis Cytomegaloviruses Cutaneous warts Herpes keratoconjunctivitis Herpes simplex Papillomaviruses Rhinoviruses *Vaccinia* virus *Varicella zoster* Viral hepatitis B	Interferon alfa-2a and 2b are *not* interchangeable; store solution in refrigerator; do *not* shake or freeze; patients should be well hydrated during initiation of therapy to prevent hypotension due to fluid depletion; patients should be treated for 6 mo to determine efficacy of therapy; maintenance therapy may be continued for up to 20 mo; neutralizing antibodies to alfa-2a have been detected in 27% of patients but *no* clinical significance has been determined; patients with platelet counts less than 50,000/mm^3 should receive SC injection *not* IM injection; premedicate patient with acetaminophen to minimize flulike syndrome and administer at night to minimize persistent fatigue; lyophilized powder is stable for 30 days when refrigerated after reconstitution
Interferon Alfa-2b, Recombinant Intron-A	Lyophilized powder for injection: 3 million IU/vial, 5 million IU/vial, 10 million IU/vial, 25 million IU/vial, 50 million IU/vial	*Hairy cell leukemia:* 2 million IU/m^2 IM or SC 3 times/wk; may require 6 mo or longer therapy; reduce dose by 50% if severe adverse effects occur *Condylomata accuminata:* 1 million IU/lesion 3 times/wk for 3 wk (maximum response usually occurs within 4–8 wk—if response is inadequate after 12 wk, a second course may be initiated	Hairy cell leukemia and Kaposi's sarcoma (in patients 18 years of age or older) Condylomata accuminata *Investigational uses* See Interferon alfa-2A	*See* interferon alfa-2A, recombinant Use only the 10-million IU vial reconstituted with 1 mL or diluent for intralesional injection; use of other strengths results in a hypertonic solution; after reconstitution with bacteriostatic water for injection the clear, colorless to light yellow solution is stable for 30 days when refrigerated; prothrombin time (PT) and partial thromboplastin time (PTT) may be increased

Continued

Table 72-7
Miscellaneous Antineoplastic Agents (continued)

Drug	Preparations	Usual Dosage Range	Uses	Nursing Implications
Interferon Alfa-2b, Recombinant (cont'd)		*Kaposi's sarcoma:* 30 million IU/m² IM or SC 3 times/wk; reduce dose by 50% if severe adverse effects occur *Preparation of Solution* Vial Strength / Amount of Diluent / Final Concentration 3 million IU / 1 mL / 3 million IU/mL 5 million IU / 1 mL / 5 million IU/mL 10 million IU / 2 mL / 5 million IU/mL 25 million IU / 5 mL / 5 million IU/mL 50 million IU / 1 mL / 50 million IU/mL		
Procarbazine Matulane	Capsules: 50 mg	**Adults** *Initially* 2 mg/kg–4 mg/kg/day (to the nearest 50 mg) in single or divided doses the first week; then 4 mg/kg–6 mg/kg/day until leukocytes fall below 4000, platelets below 100,000 or a maximum clinical response is obtained *Following recovery from hematologic toxicity:* 1 mg–2 mg/kg/day; maintenance—1 mg/kg–2 mg/kg/day **Children** *Initially* 50 mg/m² daily for 1 wk; then 100 mg/m² daily (to the nearest 50 mg) until hematologic toxicity occurs or maximum response occurs, then 50 mg/m² daily after recovery; maintenance—50 mg/m² daily	Hodgkin's disease (DOC) Non-Hodgkin's lymphomas (DOC) *Investigational uses* Lung carcinoma Malignant melanoma Brain tumors Multiple myeloma Polycythemia vera Mycosis fungoides	Tolerance to GI side effects usually develops within several days; fever, chills, and sweating are most common during early stages of therapy; use in children is limited; undue toxicity such as tremors, coma, and convulsions have occurred; dosage must be individually adjusted

DOC, drug of choice.

I. Each agent used in the regimen must be *clinically active* in the specific disease.
II. To obtain synergism, each agent must have a *different mechanism* of action. Agents are used to block different sites in biochemical pathways or to inhibit critical cell functions. Three different types of blockade have been described:
   A. *Sequential blockade:* the inhibition of two different steps of the same biochemical pathway
   B. *Concurrent blockade:* the blockade of parallel metabolic pathways leading to a common end product
   C. *Complementary inhibition:* inhibition at different sites in the synthesis of large polymeric molecules
III. The agents used must have *different toxicities* or *different timing* of a similar toxicity. This reduces cumulative toxicity to a single organ system and allows for individual agents to be used in full clinical doses.
IV. Agents are *scheduled* with respect to tumor cell kinetics to potentiate the effect of each agent in the regimen. Both cell-cycle specific and cell-cycle nonspecific agents are used in regimens to simultaneously kill both dividing and nondividing cell fractions in the tumor. Careful intermittent scheduling has also proved to be less immunosuppressive and less toxic than continuous daily therapy.
V. Each agent should be administered at the maximum dose tolerated by the patient, and such dose should be close to or beyond the *minimum effective dosage* of each agent as a single agent.

Table 72-8 lists a number of currently used combination chemotherapeutic regimens according to their commonly known acronym. Individual drug components of the combination are given along with the recommended dosage and indications.

(*Text continued on page 753*)

Table 72-8
Combination Chemotherapeutic Regimens

Acronym	Drug	Dosage	Indications
ABVD	A—doxorubicin B—bleomycin V—vinblastine D—dacarbazine	25 mg/m² IV days 1 and 14 10 U/m² IV days 1 and 14 6 mg/m² IV days 1 and 14 375 mg/m² IV days 1 and 14 Repeat every 28 days for 6–8 cycles	Hodgkin's disease
AC-BCG	A—doxorubicin C—cyclophosphamide BCG—bacille Calmette Guérin	40 mg/m² IV days 1 and 14 200 mg/m² IV days 3–6 1 vial by scarification on days 8 and 15 Repeat every 3–4 wk	Ovarian carcinoma
A Ce (AC)	A—doxorubicin Ce—cyclophosphamide	40 mg/m² IV day 1 200 mg/m² PO days 3–6 Repeat every 21–28 days	Breast carcinoma
ACE	A—doxorubicin C—cyclophosphamide E—etoposide	45 mg/m² IV day 1 1 g/m² IV day 1 50 mg/m²/day IV days 1–5 Repeat every 21 days	Small cell lung carcinoma
ACMF	A—doxorubicin C—cyclophosphamide M—methotrexate F—fluorouracil	40 mg/m² IV day 1 1 g/m² IV day 1 30 mg to 40 mg/m² IV days 21, 28 and 35 400 mg to 600 mg/m² IV days 21, 28, and 35 Repeat every 42 days	Breast carcinoma
A-COPP	A—doxorubicin C—cyclophosphamide O—vincristine P—procarbazine P—prednisone	60 mg/m² IV day 1 300 mg/m² IV days 14 and 20 1.5 mg/m² IV days 14 and 20 (maximum 2 mg) 100 mg/m² PO days 14–28 40 mg/m² PO days 1–27 (first and fourth cycles) days 14–27 (second, third, fifth, and sixth cycles) Repeat every 42 days for 6 cycles	Hodgkin's disease
ACV	A—doxorubicin C—cyclophosphamide V—vincristine	75 mg/m² IV days 1 and 43 40 mg/kg IV day 21 0.04 mg/kg IV day 22	Ewing's sarcoma
AD	A—doxorubisin D—dacarbazine	60 mg/m² IV day 1 (adequate marrow) 45 mg/m² IV day 1 (inadequate marrow) 250 mg/m² IV days 1–5 (adequate marrow) 200 mg/m² IV days 1–5 (inadequate marrow)	Soft tissue and bony sarcomas
ADIC	A—doxorubicin DIC—dacarbazine	50 mg/m² IV day 1 250 mg/m² IV days 1–5 Repeat every 3–4 wk	Advanced sarcomas
Ad-OAP (AOAP)	Ad—doxorubicin O—vincristine A—cytarabine P—prednisone	40 mg/m² IV day 1 2 mg IV day 1 70 mg/m² continuous infusion days 1–7 or 100 mg/m² continuous infusion days 5–9 100 mg/day on days 1–5 Repeat after 2 wk	Acute myelocytic leukemia
Adria + BCNU	Adria—doxorubicin BCNU—carmustine	30 mg/m² IV day 1 30 mg/m² IV day 1 Repeat every 21 days–28 days	Multiple myeloma
AMV	A—doxorubicin M—mitomycin V—vinblastine	30 mg/m² IV every 4 wk 10 mg/m² IV every 8 wk 6 mg/m² IV every 4 wk	Breast carcinoma
AP	A—doxorubibin P—cisplatin	50 mg/m² IV every 21 days 50 mg/m² IV every 21 days	Ovarian carcinoma
Ara-C + ADR	Ara-C—cytarabine ADR—doxorubicin	100 mg/m² continuous IV infusion for 7–10 days 30 mg/m² IV days 1–3	Acute myelocytic leukemia

Continued

Table 72-8
Combination Chemotherapeutic Regimens (continued)

Acronym	Drug	Dosage	Indications
Ara-C + DNR + PRED + MP	Ara-C—cytarabine DNR—daunorubicin PRED—prednisone MP—mercaptopurine	80 mg/m^2 IV days 1–3 25 mg/m^2 IV day 1 40 mg/m^2 PO daily 100 mg/m^2 PO daily Repeat weekly until remission, then monthly for maintenance	Acute myelocytic leukemia (in children)
Ara-C + 6-TG	Ara-C—cytarabine 6-TG—thioguanine	100 mg/m^2 IV every 12 h for 10 days 100 mg/m^2 PO every 12 h for 10 days Repeat every 30 days until remission, then repeat monthly for 5 days for maintenance	Acute myelocytic leukemia
AV	A—doxorubicin V—vincristine	60 mg–75 mg/m^2 day 1 1.4 mg/m^2 days 1 and 8 Repeat every 3 wk	Breast carcinoma
BACON	B—bleomycin A—doxorubicin C—lomustine O—vincristine N—mechlorethamine	30 U IV (6 h after vincristine) 40 mg/m^2 IV day 1; repeat every 4 wk 65 mg/m^2 PO day 1; repeat every 4–8 wk 0.75 mg–1 mg IV day 2; repeat every week for 6 wk 8 mg/m^2 IV day 1 (30 min after lomustine); repeat every 4 wk	Squamous cell carcinoma of lung
BACOP	B—bleomycin A—doxorubicin C—cyclophosphamide O—vincristine P—prednisone	5 U/m^2 IV days 15 and 22 25 mg/m^2 IV days 1 and 8 650 mg/m^2 IV days 1 and 8 1.4 mg/m^2 IV day 1 and 8 60 mg/m^2 PO days 15–28 Repeat every 28 days for 6 cycles	Non-Hodgkin's lymphomas
BCAP	B—carmustine C—cyclophosphamide A—doxorubicin P—prednisone	50 mg/m^2 IV day 1 200 mg/m^2 IV day 1 20 mg/m^2 IV day 2 60 mg/m^2 PO days 1–5 Repeat every 4 wk	Multiple myeloma
B-CAVe	B—bleomycin C—lomustine A—doxorubicin Ve—vinblastine	5 U/m^2 IV days 1, 28, 35 100 mg/m^2 PO day 1 60 mg/m^2 IV day 1 5 mg/m^2 IV day 1 Repeat every 6 weeks for 9 cycles	Hodgkin's disease
BCMF	B—bleomycin C—cyclophosphamide M—methotrexate F—fluorouracil	7.5 U/m^2 continuous infusion days 1–3 300 mg/m^2 IV day 5 30 mg/m^2 IV day 5 300 mg/m^2 IV day 5 Repeat every 3 wk	Squamous cell carcinoma of head and neck
BCNU + 5-FU	BCNU—carmustine 5-FU—fluorouracil	40 mg/m^2 IV days 1–5 10 mg/kg IV days 1–5 Repeat every 6 wk	Gastric carcinoma
BCOP	B—carmustine C—cyclophosphamide O—vincristine P—prednisone	100 mg/m^2 IV day 1 600 mg/m^2 IV day 1 1 mg/m^2 IV days 1 and 14 40 mg/m^2 PO days 1–7 Repeat every 28 days	Non-Hodgkin's lymphomas
BCVPP	B—carmustine C—cyclophosphamide V—vinblastine P—procarbazine P—prednisone	100 mg/m^2 IV day 1 600 mg/m^2 IV day 1 5 mg/m^2 IV day 1 100 mg/m^2 PO days 1–10 60 mg/m^2 PO days 1–10 Repeat every 28 days for 6 cycles	Hodgkin's disease
B-DOPA	B—bleomycin D—dacarbazine O—vincristine P—prednisone A—doxorubicin	4 U mg/m^2 IV days 2 and 5 150 mg/m^2 IV days 1–5 1.5 mg/m^2 PO days 1 and 5 40 mg/m^2 PO days 1–6 60 mg/m^2 IV day 1 Repeat every 21 days	Hodgkin's disease
BEP	B—bleomycin E—etoposide	30 U IV weekly 100 mg/m^2/day IV days 1–5	Testicular carcinoma

Continued

Table 72-8
Combination Chemotherapeutic Regimens (continued)

Acronym	Drug	Dosage	Indications
	P—cisplatin	20 mg/m^2/day IV days 1–5 Repeat every 3 wk for 4 cycles Reduce dose of etoposide by 20% if patient received prior radiotherapy	
BHD	B—carmustine	100 mg or 150 mg/m^2 IV day 1; repeat every 6 wk	Malignant melanoma
	H—hydroxyurea	1480 mg/m^2/day PO days 1–5; repeat every 3 wk	
	D—dacarbazine	100 mg or 150 mg/m^2/day IV days 1–5; repeat every 3 wk	
BLEO-MTX	BLEO—bleomycin	15 U IV every 4 days–14 days	Head and neck carcinoma
	MTX—methotrexate	15 mg/m^2 IV every 4–14 days	
B-MOPP	B—bleomycin	2 U/m^2 IV days 1 and 8	Hodgkin's disease
	M—mechlorethamine	6 mg/m^2 IV days 1 and 8	
	O—vincristine	1.4 mg/m^2 IV days 1 and 8	
	P—procarbazine	100 mg/m^2 PO days 1–4	
	P—prednisone	50 mg/m^2 PO days 1–14 cycles 1 and 4 only Repeat every 28 days	
BM	B—bleomycin	5 U/day IV days 1–7	Carcinoma of cervix
	M—mitomycin	10 mg IV day 8 Repeat every 2 wk	
BOPP	B—carmustine	80 mg/m^2 IV day 1	Hodgkin's disease
	O—vincristine	1.4 mg/m^2 IV days 1 and 8	
	P—procarbazine	50 mg PO day 1; 100 mg PO day 2; 100 mg/m^2/day PO days 3–14	
	P—prednisone	40 mg/m^2 PO days 1–14 Repeat every 28 days for 6 cycles	
BVD	B—carmustine	65 mg/m^2 IV days 1–3	Malignant melanoma
	V—vincristine	1 mg–1.5 mg IV weekly	
	D—dacarbazine	250 mg/m^2 IV days 1–3 Repeat every 6 wk	
CAF	C—cyclophosphamide	100 mg/m^2 PO days 1–14	Breast carcinoma
	A—doxorubicin	30 mg/m^2 IV days 1 and 8	
	F—fluorouracil	500 mg/m^2 IV days 1 and 8 Repeat every 4 wk until total dose of 450 mg/m^2 doxorubicin is administered; then discontinue doxorubicin and replace with methotrexate 40 mg/m^2 IV and increase fluorouracil to 600 mg/m^2 IV	
CAM	C—cyclophosphamide	600 mg/m^2 IV day 1	Prostatic carcinoma (advanced)
	A—doxorubicin	40 mg/m^2 IV day 1	
	M—methotrexate	15 mg/m^2 PO days 9, 13, 16, 20 Repeat every 21 days	
CAMP	C—cyclophosphamide	300 mg/m^2 IV days 1 and 8	Lung carcinoma (non–oat cell)
	A—doxorubicin	20 mg/m^2 IV days 1 and 8	
	M—methotrexate	15 mg/m^2 IV days 1 and 8	
	P—procarbazine	100 mg/m^2 PO days 1–10 Repeat every 28 days	
CAP	C—cyclophosphamide	400 mg/m^2 IV day 1	Adenocarcinoma of lung
	A—doxorubicin	40 mg/m^2 IV day 1	
	P—cisplatin	60 mg/m^2 IV day 1 Repeat every 4 wk for 10 cycles	
CAP	C—cyclophosphamide	650 mg/m^2 IV day 1	Bladder carcinoma
	A—doxorubicin	50 mg/m^2 IV day 1	
	P—cisplatin	100 mg/m^2 IV day 1 or 2 Repeat every 3–4 wk	
CAV	C—cyclophosphamide	500 mg/m^2 IV day 1	Non-small cell lung carcinoma
	A—doxorubicin	50 mg/m^2 IV day 1	
	V—vincristine	1.4 mg/m^2 IV day 1 (not to exeed 2 mg) Repeat every 28 days	
	or		
	C—cyclophosphamide	750 mg/m^2 IV day 1	Small-cell lung carcinoma
	A—doxorubicin	50 mg/m^2 IV day 1	
	V—vincristine	2 mg IV day 1 Repeat every 21 days	

Continued

Table 72-8
Combination Chemotherapeutic Regimens (continued)

Acronym	Drug	Dosage	Indications
CAVe	C—lomustine A—doxorubicin Ve—vinblastine	100 mg/m² PO day 1 60 mg/m² IV day 1 5 mg/m² IV day 1 Repeat every 6 wk for 9 cycles	Hodgkin's disease
CCV	C—cyclophosphamide C—lomustine V—vincristine	700 mg/m² IV days 1 and 22 70 mg/m² PO day 1 2 mg IV days 1 and 22 Repeat ever 6 wk	Oat-cell carcinoma of lung
CCV-AV	C—lomustine C—cyclophosphamide V—vincristine AV—doxorubicin	100 mg/m² PO day 1 1 g/m² IV days 1 and 22 2 mg IV days 1, 22, 42, 63 75 mg/m² IV days 42 and 63 Repeat every 12 wk	Oat-cell carcinoma of lung
CD	C—cisplatin D—doxorubicin or C—cytarabine D—daunorubicin	50 mg–60 mg/m² IV day 1 50 mg–60 mg/m² IV day 1 Repeat every 21–28 days 100 mg/m² IV infusion over 24 h daily for 7 days 45 mg/m² IV days 1–3	Prostatic carcinoma (advanced) Acute myelocytic leukemia
CDC	C—carboplatin D—doxorubicin C—cyclophosphamide	300 mg/m² IV day 1 40 mg/m² IV day 1 500 mg/m² IV day 1 Repeat every 28 days	Ovarian carcinoma
CDV	C—cyclophosphamide D—dacarbazine V—vincristine	750 mg/m² IV day 1 250 mg/m² IV days 1–5 1–5 mg/m² IV day 1 Repeat every 22 days	Neuroblastoma
CEV	C—cyclophosphamide E—etoposide V—vincristine	1000 mg/m² IV day 1 50 mg/m² IV day 1, then 100 mg/m²/day PO on days 2–5 1.4 mg/m² IV day 1 Repeat every 3 wk	Small-cell lung carcinoma
CFB	C—cisplatin F—fluorouracil B—bleomycin	100 mg/m²/day continuous IV infusion day 1 1000 mg/m²/day continuous IV infusion days 1–4 30 U/m² continuous IV infusion day 1, then 7.5 U/day continuous IV infusion days 2–4	Head and neck carcinoma
CFD	C—cyclophosphamide F—fluorouracil D—doxorubicin	500 mg/m² IV day 1 500 mg/m² IV day 1 50 mg/m² IV day 1 Repeat every 21 days	Prostatic carcinoma (advanced)
CHL + PRED	CHL—chlorambucil PRED—prednisone	0.4 mg/kg PO 1 day every other week, increase by 0.1 mg/kg every 2 wk until toxicity or control 100 mg PO days 1 and 2 every other week	Chronic lymphocytic leukemia
CHOP	C—cyclophosphamide H—doxorubicin O—vincristine P—prednisone	750 mg/m² IV day 1 50 mg/m² IV day 1 1.4 mg/m² IV day 1 (maximum 2 mg) 60 mg/day PO days 1–5 Repeat every 21–28 days for 6 cycles	Non-Hodgkin's lymphoma
CHOP-BCG	CHOP—(as above) plus BCG—bacille Calmette Guérin	1 vial by scarification days 7 and 14	Non-Hodgkin's lymphoma
CHOP-Bleo	C—cyclophosphamide H—doxorubicin O—vincristine P—prednisone Bleo—bleomycin	750 mg/m² IV day 1 50 mg/m² IV day 1 1.4 mg/m² IV day 1 (maximum 2 mg) 100 mg/m²/day days 1–5 4 U IV days 1 and 8 or 15 U IV days 1 and 5 Repeat every 21–28 days	Non-Hodgkin's lymphoma
CHOR	C—cyclophosphamide H—doxorubicin	750 mg/m² IV days 1 and 22 50 mg/m² IV days 1 and 22	Lung carcinoma

Continued

Table 72-8
Combination Chemotherapeutic Regimens (continued)

Acronym	Drug	Dosage	Indications
	O—vincristine	1 mg IV days 1, 8, 15, 22	
	R—radiation	3000 rad total dose in daily fractions over 2 wk starting day 36	
CISCA	CIS—cisplatin	100 mg/m^2 IV infusion over 2 h day 2	Urinary carcinoma
	C—cyclophosphamide	650 mg/m^2 IV day 1 Increase to 1000 mg/m^2 when doxorubicin is discontinued	
	A—doxorubicin	50 mg/m^2 IV day 1; discontinue at 450 mg/m^2 total dose; repeat every 21 days	
CISCA$_{II}$VB$_{IV}$	CIS—cisplatin	100 mg–120 mg/m^2 IV day 3	Testicular carcinoma
	C—cyclophosphamide	500 mg/m^2 IV days 1 and 2	
	A—doxorubicin	40–45 mg/m^2 IV days 1 and 2 *alternating with*	
	V—vinblastine	3 mg/m^2/day IV as a continuous infusion for 5 days	
	B—bleomycin	30 U/day IV as a continuous infusion for 5 days	
CMC-High dose	C—cyclophosphamide	1000 mg/m^2 IV days 1 and 29	Lung carcinoma
	M—methotrexate	15 mg/m^2 IV twice wk for 6 wk	
	C—lomustine	100 mg/m^2 PO day 1	
CMC-V	C—cyclophosphamide	700 mg/m^2 IV day 1	Small-cell carcinoma of the lung
	M—methotrexate	20 mg/m^2 PO days 18 and 21	
	C—lomustine	70 mg/m^2 PO day 1; repeat every 28 days	
	V—vincristine	2 mg IV days 1, 8, 15, 22; then 1.3 mg/m^2 IV every 4 wk	
CMF	C—cyclophosphamide	100 mg/m^2 PO days 1–14	Breast carcinoma
	M—methotrexate	40 mg–60 mg/m^2 IV days 1 and 8	
	F—fluorouracil	600 mg/m^2 IV days 1 and 8 Repeat every 28 days; above age 60, reduce methotrexate dose to 30 mg/m^2 and fluorouracil dose to 400 mg/m^2	
CMFP	C—cyclophosphamide	100 mg/m^2 PO days 1–14	Breast carcinoma
	M—methotrexate	60 mg/m^2 IV days 1 and 8	
	F—fluorouracil	700 mg/m^2 IV days 1 and 8	
	P—prednisone	40 mg/m^2 PO days 1–14 Repeat every 28 days	
CMFT	C—cyclophosphamide	100 mg/m^2/day PO days 1–14	Breast carcinoma
	M—methotrexate	40 mg/m^2 IV day 1 and 8	
	F—fluorouracil	400 mg/m^2/day IV days 1 and 8	
	T—tamoxifen	10 mg PO 2 times/day ongoing Repeat every 4 wk	
CMFVP (Cooper's regimen)	C—cyclophosphamide	2 mg/kg PO daily	Breast carcinoma
	M—methotrexate	0.75 mg/kg IV weekly for 8 wk; then every other week	
	F—fluorouracil	12 mg/kg IV weekly for 8 wk, then every other week	
	V—vincristine	0.035 mg/kg IV weekly (maximum 2 mg)	
	P—prednisone	0.75 mg/kg PO days 1–10 then taper	
COMA or COMLA	C—cyclophosphamide	1.5 g/m^2 IV	Non-Hodgkin's lymphoma
	O—vincristine	1.4 mg/m^2 IV days 1, 8, 15	
	M—methotrexate	120 mg/m^2 PO	
	L—leucovorin	Give leucovorin 25 mg PO every 6 h 4 doses starting 6 h after methotrexate	
	A—cytarabine	300 mg/m^2 IV bolus 16 h after methotrexate Repeat every 7–14 days for 8 cycles through days 22–71	
COAP	C—cyclophosphamide	100 mg/m^2 IV days 1–5	Acute myelocytic leukemia
	O—vincristine	1 mg IV days 1, 8, 15, 22	
	A—cytarabine	200 mg/m^2 IV days 1–5 or 100 mg/m^2 IV days 1–10	
	P—prednisone	100 mg/day PO days 1–5 Repeat after 2-wk interval	

Continued

Table 72-8
Combination Chemotherapeutic Regimens (continued)

Acronym	Drug	Dosage	Indications
COP	C—cyclophosphamide O—vincristine P—prednisone	1000 mg/m^2 IV day 1 1.4 mg/m^2 IV day 1 (maximum 2 mg) 60 mg/m^2 PO days 1–5 Repeat every 21 days for 6 cycles	Non-Hodgkin's lymphoma
COP-BLAM	C—cyclophosphamide O—vincristine P—prednisone BL—bleomycin A—doxorubicin M—procarbazine	400 mg/m^2 day 1 1 mg/m^2 IV day 1 40 mg/m^2 PO days 1–10 15 U IV day 14 40 mg/m^2 IV day 1 100 mg/m^2 PO days 1–10 Repeat every 21 days	Histiocytic lymphoma
COPP or C-MOPP	C—cyclophosphamide O—vincristine P—procarbazine P—prednisone	650 mg/m^2 IV days 1 and 8 1.4 mg/m^2 IV days 1 and 8 (maximum 2 mg) 100 mg/m^2 PO days 1–14 40 mg/m^2 PO days 1–14 Repeat every 28 days for 6 cycles	Non-Hodgkin's lymphoma
CP	C—carmustine P—prednisone	150 mg/m^2 IV day 4 60 mg/m^2 PO days 1–4 Repeat every 42 days	Multiple myeloma
Hi-CP	C—cyclophosphamide P—prednisone	1000 mg/m^2 IV day 1 60 mg/m^2 days 1–4 Repeat every 42 days	Multiple myeloma
CT	C—cytarabine T—thioguanine	1 mg–3 mg/kg IV daily for 8–32 days 2 mg–2.5 mg/kg PO daily for 8–32 days Thioguanine usualy given in morning and cytarabine 8–10 h later	Acute myelocytic leukemia
CV	C—cyclophosphamide V—vincristine	10 mg/kg IV every other week 0.05 mg/kg IV on the alternate weeks Continue treatment 12 wk or longer	Neuroblastoma
CVB	C—cisplatin V—vinblastine B—bleomycin	20 mg/m^2 IV days 1–5; repeat every 3 wk for 3 cycles 0.2 mg/kg IV days 1 and 2; repeat every 3 wk for 12 wk; then 0.3 mg/kg IV every 4 wk for 2 yr 30 U IV weekly for 12 wk	Testicular carcinoma
CVB	C—lomustine V—vinblastine B—bleomycin	100 mg/m^2 PO day 1 6 mg/m^2 IV days 1 and 8 15 U/m^2 IV days 1 and 8 Repeat every 28 days	Hodgkin's disease
CVI	C—carboplatin V—etoposide I—ifosfamide	300 mg/m^2 IV day 1 60–100 mg/m^2 IV day 1 1.5 g/m^2 IV days 1, 3 and 5 Repeat cycle every 28 days	Non-small cell lung carcinoma
CVP	C—cyclophosphamide V—vincristine P—prednisone	400 mg/m^2 PO days 2–6 1.4 mg/m^2 IV day 1 (maximum 2 mg) 40 mg/m^2 PO days 1–14 Repeat every 28 days for 6 cycles	Non-Hodgkin's lymphoma
CVPP	C—cyclophosphamide V—vinblastine P—procarbazine P—prednisone	300 mg/m^2 IV days 1 and 8 10 mg/m^2 IV days 1, 8, 15 100 mg/m^2 PO days 1–15 40 mg/m^2 PO days 1–15 (cycles 1 and 4 only) Repeat every 28 days	Hodgkin's disease
CVPP/CCNU	C—cyclophosphamide V—vinblastine P—procarbazine P—prednisone CCNU—lomustine	600 mg/m^2 IV day 1 6 mg/m^2 IV day 1 100 mg/m^2 PO days 1–14 40 mg/m^2 days 1–14 75 mg/m^2 day 1 (alternate cycles) Repeat every 28 days	Hodgkin's disease
CY-VA-DIC	CY—cyclophosphamide V—vincristine	500 mg/m^2 IV day 1 1.4 mg/m^2 IV days 1 and 5 (maximum 2 mg)	Soft tissue sarcomas

Continued

Table 72-8
Combination Chemotherapeutic Regimens (continued)

Acronym	Drug	Dosage	Indications
	A—doxorubicin	50 mg/m² IV day 1	
	DIC—dacarbazine	250 mg/m² IV days 1–5 Repeat every 21 days	
DA	D—daunorubicin	45 mg/m² IV days 1–3	Acute myelocytic leukemia
	A—cytarabine	100 mg/m² IV days 1–10 Repeat as needed	
DAT	D—daunorubicin	60 mg/m² IV days 5–7	Acute myelocytic leukemia
	A—cytarabine (Ara-C)	100 mg/m² IV over 30 min twice a day for 7 days	
	T—thioguanine	100 mg/m² PO every 12 h for 7 days Repeat every 30 days with 5 days' therapy of cytarabine and thioguanine alternating with a single dose of daunorubicin	
DC	D—doxorubicin	60 mg/m² IV day 1 at 6 A.M.	Ovarian carcinoma
	C—cisplatin	60 mg/m² IV day 1 at 6 P.M.	
DMC	D—doxorubicin	2.5 mg/kg/day IV days 1–3	Osteogenic sarcoma
	M—methotrexate	200 mg–750 mg/kg/24 h IV infusion day 14	
	C—citrovorum factor (calcium leucovorin)	9 mg PO every 6 h for 12 doses starting 12 h after methotrexate infusion Repeat every 28 days	
DOAP	D—daunorubicin	60 mg/m² IV day 1	Acute myelocytic leukemia
	O—vincristine	1 mg IV days 1, 8, 15, 22	
	A—cytarabine	200 mg/m² IV days 1–5 or 100 mg/m² IV days 1–10	
	P—prednisone	100 mg/day PO days 1–5 Repeat after 2-wk interval	
FAC	F—fluorouracil	500 mg/m² IV days 1 and 8	Breast carcinoma
	A—doxorubicin	50 mg/m² IV day 1	
	C—cyclophosphamide	500 mg/m² IV day 1 Repeat every 3 wk	
FAM	F—fluorouracil	600 mg/m² IV days 1, 2, 28, 36	Lung or gastric carcinoma
	A—doxorubicin	30 mg/m² IV days 1 and 28	
	M—mitomycin or	10 mg/m² IV day 1 Repeat eveyr 8 wk	
	F—fluorouracil	600 mg/m² IV wk 1, 2, 5, 6, 9	Pancreatic carcinoma
	A—doxorubicin	30 mg/m² IV wk 1, 5, 9	
	M—mitomycin	10 mg/m² IV wk 1 and 9	
FAP	F—fluorouracil	500 mg/m² IV day 1	Bladder carcinoma
	A—doxorubicin	50 mg/m² IV day 1	
	P—cisplatin	100 mg/m² IV day 1; reduce to 50 mg–75 mg/m² after 3 doses Repeat every 4 wk	
FCP	F—fluorouracil	8 mg/kg/day IV for 5 days	Breast carcinoma
	C—cyclophosphamide	4 mg/kg/day for 5 days	
	P—prednisone	30 mg/day PO tapered to 10 mg/day	
	(±)vincristine	1.4 mg/m² IV days 1 and 5	
FIVB (FDVB)	F—fluorouracil	10 mg/kg IV days 1–5	Colorectal carcinoma
	I—dacarbazine	3 mg/kg IV days 1 and 2	
	V—vincristine	0.025 mg/kg IV day 1	
	B—carmustine	1.5 mg/kg IV day 1 Repeat every 4 wk–6 wk	
FL	F—flutamide	250 mg PO 3 times/day	Prostatic carcinoma
	L—leuprolide	1 mg sc daily or 7.5 mg depot injection IM every 28 days	
FOMi	F—fluorouracil	300 mg/m² IV days 1–4	Lung carcinoma (non–small cell)
	O—vincristine	2 mg IV day 1	
	Mi—mitomycin	10 mg/m² IV day 1 Repeat every 3 wk for 3 cycles then every 6 wk	
HOP	H—doxorubicin	80 mg/m² IV day 1	Non-Hodgkin's lymphoma
	O—vincristine	1.4 mg/m² IV day 1 (maximum 2 mg)	
	P—prednisone	100 mg/m² PO days 1–5 Repeat every 3 wk	

Continued

Table 72-8
Combination Chemotherapeutic Regimens (continued)

Acronym	Drug	Dosage	Indications
ID	I—Ifosfamide	5 g/m^2 IV over 24 h day 1 along with mesna 1 g/m^2 IV bolus prior to ifosfamide, then 4 g/m^2 IV continuous over 32h	Soft tissue sarcoma
	D—Doxorubicin	40 mg/m^2 IV day 1 Repeat cycle every 21 days	
IMF	I—Ifosfamide	1.5 g/m^2 IV days 1 and 8 along with mesna IV at 20% of ifosfamide dose given before ifosfamide and again at 4 h and 8 h after ifosfamide	Breast carcinoma
	M—Methotrexate	40 mg/m^2 IV days 1 and 8	
	F—Fluorouracil	600 mg/m^2 IV days 1 and 8 Repeat cycle every 28 days	
M-2 Protocol	vincristine	0.03 mg/kg IV day 1 (maximum 2 mg)	Multiple myeloma
	carmustine	0.5 mg/kb IV day 1	
	cyclophosphamide	10 mg/kg IV day 1	
	melphalan	0.25 mg/kg PO days 1–14	
	prednisone	1 mg/kg PO days 1–7, then taper to day 21 Repeat every 35 days	
MA	M—mitomycin	10 mg/m^2 IV day 1	Breast carcinoma
	A—doxorubicin	50 mg/m^2 IV days 1 and 22 Repeat every 6 wk	Adenocarcinoma of lung
MAC	M—methotrexate	15 mg IM days 1–5	Choriocarcinoma
	A—dactinomycin	8 µg–10 µg/kg IV days 1–5	
	C—chlorambucil	8 mg–10 mg PO days 1–5 Repeat every 10–14 days	
MACC	M—methotrexate	40 mg/m^2 IV day 1	Lung carcinoma (non–oat cell)
	A—doxorubicin	40 mg/m^2 IV day 1	
	C—cyclophosphamide	400 mg/m^2 IV day 1	
	C—lomustine	30 mg/m^2 PO day 1 Repeat every 21 days	
MACM	M—mitomycin	8 mg/m^2 IV day 1	Squamous cell carcinoma of lung
	A—doxorubicin	60 mg/m^2 IV day 1	
	C—lomustine	60 mg/m^2 PO day 1	
	M—methotrexate	40 mg/m^2 IV day 1 Repeat every 4 wk	
MACOP-B	M—methotrexate	400 mg/m^2 IV wk 2, 6, 10 given as 100 mg/m^2 IV bolus and 300 mg/m^2 IV infusion over 4 h followed in 24 h by leucovorin calcium 15 mg PO every 6 h for 6 doses	Non-Hodgkin's lymphoma
	A—doxorubicin	50 mg/m^2 IV weeks 1, 3, 5, 7, 9, 11	
	C—cyclophosphamide	350 mg/m^2 IV weeks 1, 3, 5, 7, 9, 11	
	O—vincristine	1.4 mg/m^2 IV wks 2, 4, 6, 8, 10, 12	
	P—prednisone	75 mg/day PO daily; dose tapered over the last 15 days	
	B—bleomycin	10 U/m^2 IV weeks 4, 8, 12	
	Co-trimoxazole	Two tablets twice a day throughout 12-week course of therapy	
MAID	M—mesna	2500 mg/m^2/day continuous IV infusion on days 1–4	Advanced sarcomas
	A—doxorubicin	20 mg/m^2/day continuous IV infusion days 1–3	
	I—ifosfamide	2500 mg/m^2/day continuous IV infusion days 1–3	
	D—dacarbazine	300 mg/m^2/day continuous IV infusion days 1–3	
MAP	M—melphalan	6 mg/m^2 PO days 1–4	Multiple myeloma
	A—doxorubicin	25 mg/m^2 IV day 1	
	P—prednisone	60 mg/m^2 PO days 1–4 Repeat every 4 wk	
M-BACOD	M—methotrexate	3 g/m^2 IV day 14 followed by leucovorin calcium 10 mg/m^2 IV in 24 h and 10 mg/m^2 PO every 6 h for 72 h	Non-Hodgkin's lymphoma

Continued

Table 72-8
Combination Chemotherapeutic Regimens (continued)

Acronym	Drug	Dosage	Indications
	B—bleomycin	4 U/m^2 IV day 1	
	A—doxorubicin	45 mg/m^2 IV day 1	
	C—cyclophosphamide	600 mg/m^2 IV day 1	
	O—vincristine	1 mg/m^2 IV day 1	
	D—dexamethasone	6 mg/m^2 PO days 1–5	
		Repeat every 21 days	
MBD	M—methotrexate	40 mg/m^2 IM days 1 and 15	Head and neck carcinoma
	B—bleomycin	10 U IM weekly	
	D—cisplatin (*cis*-diamminedichloroplatinum)	50 mg/m^2 IV day 4 Repeat every 21 days	
MC	M—mitoxantrone	12 mg/m^2/day IV days 1 and 2	Acute myelocytic leukemia
	C—cytorabine	100 mg/m^2/day IV days 1–5 by continuous infusion	
		Repeat cycle in 4 wk	
MCBP	M—melphalan	4 mg/m^2 PO days 1–4	Multiple myeloma
	C—cyclophosphamide	300 mg/m^2 IV day 1	
	B—carmustine	30 mg/m^2 IV day 1	
	P—prednisone	60 mg/m^2 PO days 1–4	
		Repeat every 4 wk	
MCC	M—methotrexate	10 mg/m^2 PO twice a week	Non-small cell lung carcinoma
	C—cyclophosphamide	500 mg/m^2 IV every 21 days	
	C—lomustine (CCNU)	50 mg/m^2 PO every 42 days	
MCP	M—melphalan	6 mg/m^2 PO days 1–4	Multiple myeloma
	C—cyclophosphamide	500 mg/m^2 PO day 1	
	P—prednisone	60 mg/m^2 PO days 1–4	
		Repeat every 4 wk	
MF	M—mitomycin	15 mg–20 mg/m^2 IV day 1; repeat every 8 wk; reduce dose 50% after second dose	Colorectal carcinoma
	F—fluorouracil	1 g/m^2 continuous IV infusion over 24 h days 1–4	
		Repeat every 4 wk	
M-F	M—methotrexate	125 mg–250 mg/m^2 IV	Head and neck carcinoma
	F—fluorouracil	600 mg/m^2 IV 1 h later	
	Leucovorin rescue	10 mg/m^2 IV or PO at 24 h then 10 mg/m^2 PO every 6 h for 5 doses	
		Repeat every 7 days	
MOB	M—mitomycin	20 mg/m^2 IV day 1	Squamous cell carcinoma of cervix
	O—vincristine	0.5 mg/m^2 IV twice a week for 12 wk	
	B—bleomycin	6 U/m^2 IM or IV 6 h after vincristine twice a week for 12 wk	
		Repeat every 6 wk	
MOPP	M—mechlorethamin	6 mg/m^2 IV days 1 and 8	Hodgkin's disease
	O—vincristine	1.4 mg/m^2 IV days 1 and 8 (maximum 2 mg)	
	P—procarbazine	100 mg/m^2 PO days 1–14	
	P—prednisone	40 mg/m^2 PO days 1–14	
		Repeat every 28 days for 6 to 8 cycles	
MOPP-LO BLEO	M—mechlorethamine	6 mg/m^2 IV days 1 and 8	Hodgkin's disease
	O—vincristine	1.5 mg/m^2 IV days 1 and 8 (maximum 2 mg)	
	P—procarbazine	100 mg/m^2 PO days 2–7, 9–12	
	P—prednisone	40 mg/m^2 PO days 2–7, 9–12	
	BLEO—bleomycin	2 U/m^2 IV days 1 and 8	
		Repeat every 28 days for 6 cycles	
MP	M—melphalan	0.25 mg/kg PO days 1–4	Multiple myeloma
	P—prednisone	2 mg/kg PO days 1–4	
		Repeat every 6 wk	
MPL + PRED (MP)	MPL—melphalan	8 mg/m^2 PO days 1–14	Multiple myeloma
	PRED—prednisone	75 mg/m^2 PO days 1–7	
		Repeat every 28 days for 6 cycles	
MTX + MP	MTX—methotrexate	20 mg/m^2 IV weekly	Acute lymphocytic leukemia
	MP—mercaptopurine	50 mg/m^2/day PO	
		Continue until relapse or remission for 3 yr	

Continued

Table 72-8
Combination Chemotherapeutic Regimens (continued)

Acronym	Drug	Dosage	Indications
MTX + MP + CTX	MTX—methotrexate MP—mercaptopurine CTX—cyclophosphamide	20 mg/m^2 IV weekly 50 mg/m^2/day PO 200 mg/m^2 IV weekly Continue until relapse or remission for 3 yr	Acute lymphocytic leukemia
MV	M—mitomycin V—vinblastine	20 mg/m^2 IV day 1 0.15 mg/kg IV days 1 and 22 Repeat every 6–8 wk	Breast carcinoma
M-VAC	M—methotrexate V—vinblastine A—doxorubicin C—cisplatin	30 mg/m^2 IV days 1, 15, 22 3 mg/m^2 IV day 2, 15, 22 30 mg/m^2 IV day 2 70 mg/m^2 IV day 2 Repeat every 28–35 days	Genitourinary carcinoma
MVPP	M—mechlorethamine V—vinblastine P—procarbazine P—prednisone	6 mg/m^2 IV days 1–8 6 mg/m^2 IV days 1 and 8 100 mg/m^2 PO days 1–14 40 mg/day PO days 1–14 Rest 28 days and repeat for 6 or more cycles	Hodgkin's disease
MVVPP	M—mechlorethamine V—vincristine V—vinblastine P—procarbazine P—prednisone	0.4 mg/kg IV day 1 1.4 mg/m^2 IV days 1, 8, 15 6 mg/m^2 IV days 22, 29, 36 100 mg/m^2 PO days 22–43 40 mg/m^2 PO days 1–22 (taper over 14 days) Repeat every 57 days	Hodgkin's disease
OAP	O—vincristine A—cytarabine P—prednisone	1 mg IV days 1, 8, 15, 22 200 mg/m^2 IV days 1–5 or 100 mg/m^2 IV days 1–10 100 mg PO days 1–5 Repeat after 2-wk interval	Acute myelocytic leukemia
PA	P—cisplatin A—doxorubicin	50 mg–60 mg/m^2 IV 50 mg–60 mg/m^2 IV Repeat every 3–4 wk	Adenocarcinoma of prostate
PAC-5	P—cisplatin A—doxorubicin C—cyclophosphamide	20 mg/m^2 IV days 1–5 (total dose 300 mg/m^2) 50 mg/m^2 IV day 1 (total dose 450 mg/m^2) 750 mg/m^2 IV day 1 (increase dose 20% after stopping cisplatin and doxorubicin) Repeat every 3 wk	Ovarian carcinoma
PCV	P—procarbazine C—lomustine V—vincristine	60 mg/m^2 PO days 8–21 110 mg/m^2 PO day 1 1.4 mg/m^2 IV days 8 and 29 Repeat every 6–8 wk	Primary malignant brain tumors
PEB	P—cisplatin E—etoposide B—bleomycin	20 mg/m^2 IV days 1–5 100 mg/m^2 IV days 1–5 30 U/day IV on day 2, then weekly for 12 consecutive wk	Testicular carcinoma
POCC	P—procarbazine O—vincristine C—cyclophosphamide C—lomustine	100 mg/m^2 PO days 1–14 2 mg IV days 1 and 8 600 mg/m^2 IV days 1 and 8 60 mg/m^2 PO day 1 Repeat every 28 days	Lung carcinoma
POMP (low dose)	P—prednisone O—vincristine M—methotrexate P—mercaptopurine	150 mg/day PO days 1–5 2 mg/day IV day 1 5 mg/m^2/day IV days 1–5 500 mg/m^2 IV days 1–5 Repeat every 2–3 wk as tolerated	Acute myelocytic leukemia
Pro-MACE-MOPP	Pro—prednisone M—methotrexate A—doxorubicin C—cyclophosphamide	60 mg/m^2 PO days 1–14 1500 mg/m^2 IV day 14 followed in 24 h by *leucovorin calcium* 50 mg/m^2 PO every 6 h for 5 doses 25 mg/m^2 IV days 1 and 8 650 mg/m^2 IV days 1 and 8	Non-Hodgkin's lymphomas

Continued

Table 72-8
Combination Chemotherapeutic Regimens (continued)

Acronym	Drug	Dosage	Indications
	E—etoposide	120 mg/m² IV days 1 and 8 Repeat every 28 days	
	MOPP	Standard MOPP therapy after remission and repeated every 28 days	
PVB	P—cisplatin	20 mg/m²/day IV days 1–5 every 3 wk for 4 doses	Testicular carcinoma
	V—vinblastine	0.2 mg–0.4 mg/kg IV day 1 every 3 wk for 4 doses	
	B—bleomycin	30 U IV day 2 and then weekly for 12 consecutive wk	
SCAB	S—streptozocin	500 mg/m² IV days 1 and 15	Hodgkin's disease
	C—lomustine	100 mg/m² PO day 1	
	A—doxorubicin	45 mg/m² IV day 1	
	B—bleomycin	15 U/m²mg/m²s 1 and 8 Repeat every 28 days	
SMF (or FMS)	S—streptozocin	1000 mg/m² IV days 1, 8, 29, 35	Pancreatic carcinoma
	M—mitomycin	10 mg/m² IV day 1	
	F—fluorouracil	600 mg/m² IV days 1, 8, 29, 35 Repeat every 8 wk	
T-2 protocol	*Cycle No. 1* Month 1		Ewing's sarcoma
	dactinomycin	0.45 mg/m² IV days 1–5	
	doxorubicin	20 mg/m² IV days 20–22	
	radiation	Days 1–21, then rest 2 wk	
	Month 2		
	doxorubicin	20 mg/m² IV days 8–10	
	vincristine	1.5 mg–2 mg/m² IV day 24 (maximum 2 mg)	
	cyclophosphamide	1200 mg/m² IV day 24	
	radiation	Days 8–28	
	Month 3		
	vincristine	1.5 mg–2 mg/m² IV days 3, 9, 15 (maximum 2 mg)	
	cyclophosphamide	1200 mg/m² IV day 1	
	Cycle No. 2 Repeat Cycle No. 1 without radiation. *Cycle No. 3* Month 1		
	dactinomycin	0.45 mg/m² IV days 1–5	
	doxorubicin	20 mg/m² IV days 20–22	
	Month 2		
	vincristine	1.5 mg–2 mg/m² IV days 8, 15, 22, 28 (maximum 2 mg)	
	cyclophosphamide	1200 mg/m² IV days 8 and 22	

	Month 3
	  No drugs given for 28 days
	Cycle No. 4
	  Repeat Cycle No. 3.		

TODD	T—thioguanine	2 mg/kg PO days 1–5	Acute lymphocytic leukemia
	O—vincristine	2 mg/m² IV day 1	
	D—pyrimethamine	1.5 mg/kg PO days 1–5	
	D—dexamethasone	2 mg/m² PO 3 times/day on days 1–5 Repeat every 11 days with 6-day rest period	
TRAMPCO(L)	T—thioguanine	100 mg/m² PO days 1–3 Increase to 4–5 days after first course	Acute leukemia
	R—daunorubicin	40 mg/m² IV day 1	
	A—cytarabine	100 mg/m² IV days 1–3 Increase to 4–5 days after first course	
	M—methotrexate	7.5 mg/m² IV or IM days 1–3 Increase to 4–5 days after first course	
	P—prednisolone	200 mg PO days 1–3 Increase to 4–5 days after first course	
	C—cyclophosphamide	100 mg/m² IV days 1–3 Increase to 4–5 days after first course	

Continued

Table 72-8
Combination Chemotherapeutic Regimens (continued)

Acronym	Drug	Dosage	Indications
TRAMPCO(L) (cont'd)	O—vincristine	2 mg IV day 1	
	L—L-asparaginase	8000 U/m² IV days 1–28 in first 2 courses Repeat every 2–4 wk with wider spacing in patients with good response	
TRAP	T—thioguanine	100 mg/m²/day PO days 1–5	Acute myelocytic leukemia
	R—daunorubicin (rubidomycin)	40 mg/m²/day IV day 1	
	A—cytarabine	100 mg/m²/day IV or IM days 1–5	
	P—prednisone	30 mg/m²/day PO days 1–5	
VAC	V—vincristine	1.5 mg/m² IV every week for 10–12 wk	Ovarian carcinoma
	A—dactinomycin	0.5 mg/day IV days 1–5; repeat every 4 wk	
	C—cyclophosphamide	5 mg–7 mg/kg/day IV days 1–5; repeat every 4 wk	
VAC	V—vincristine	1 mg IV day 1	Lung carcinoma
	A—doxorubicin	50 mg/m² IV day 1	
	C—cyclophosphamide	750 mg/m² IV day 1	
VAC Pulse	V—vincristine	2 mg/m² IV weekly for wk 1–12 (maximum 2 mg)	Sarcoma
	A—dactinomycin	0.015 mg/kg IV days 1–5 of wk 1 and 13, then every 3 mo for 5 or 6 courses (maximum 0.5 mg a day)	
	C—cyclophosphamide	10 mg/kg IV or PO for 7 days Repeat every 6 wk for 2 yr	
VAC Standard	V—vincristine	2 mg/m² IV weekly for wk 1–12 (maximum 2 mg)	Sarcoma
	A—dactinomycin	0.015 mg/kg IV days 1–5; repeat every 3 mo for 5 or 6 courses (maximum 0.5 mg a day)	
	C—cyclophosphamide	2.5 mg/kg PO daily for 2 yr	
VAD	V—vincristine	0.4 mg/day IV continuous infusion days 1–4	Multiple myeloma
	A—doxorubicin	9 mg/m²/day continuous IV infusion days 1–4	
	D—dexamethasone	40 mg PO daily, days 1–4	
VAP	V—vincristine	2 mg/m² IV weekly for 6 wk	Acute lymphocytic leukemia
	A—doxorubicin	25 mg/m² IV weekly for 6 wk	
	P—prednisone	60 mg/m² PO days 1–28	
VBAP	V—vincristine	1 mg IV day 1	Multiple myeloma
	B—carmustine	30 mg/m² IV day 2	
	A—doxorubicin	30 mg/m² IV day 2	
	P—prednisone	60 mg/m² PO days 2–5 Repeat every 3 wk	
VBD	V—vinblastine	6 mg/m² IV days 1 and 2	Melanoma
	B—bleomycin	15 U/m² IV days 1–5 by 24-h infusion	
	D—cisplatin	50 mg/m² IV day 5 Repeat every 28 days	
VBP	V—vinblastine	0.2 mg/kg IV days 1 and 2; repeat every 3 wk for 5 courses	Testicular carcinoma
	B—bleomycin	30 U/week IV 6 h after vinblastine on the second day of each week for 12 wk until total dose of 360 U	
	P—cisplatin	20 mg/m² IV days 1–5, 6 h after vinblastine Repeat every 3 wk for 3 courses	
VC	V—etoposide	100–200 mg/m² IV days 1–3	Small cell lung carcinoma
	C—carboplatin	50–125 mg/m² IV days 1–3 Repeat cycle every 28 days	
VCAP	V—vincristine	1 mg IV day 1	Multiple myeloma
	C—cyclophosphamide	100 mg/m² PO days 1–4	
	A—doxorubicin	25 mg/m² IV day 2	
	P—prednisone	60 mg/m² PO days 1–4 Repeat every 4 wk	

Continued

Table 72-8
Combination Chemotherapeutic Regimens (continued)

Acronym	Drug	Dosage	Indications
VCR-MTX-CF or VMC	VCR—vincristine	2 mg/m^2 IV for one dose (maximum 2 mg)	Osteogenic sarcoma
	MTX—methotrexate	3000 mg–7500 mg/m^2 IV 6-h infusion starting 30 min after vincristine	
	CF—citrovorum factor (calcium leucovorin)	15 mg IV every 3 h for 8 doses, then 15 mg PO every 3 h for 8 doses	
VM	V—vinblastine	5 mg/m^2 IV	Adenocarcinoma of lung
	M—mitomycin	6 mg/m^2 IV Repeat every 2 wk	
VMCP	V—vincristine	1 mg IV day 1	Multiple myeloma
	M—melphalan	5 mg/m^2 PO days 1–4	
	C—cyclophosphamide	100 mg/m^2 PO days 1–4	
	P—prednisone	60 mg/m^2 PO days 1–4 Repeat every 3 wk	
VP	V—vincristine	2 mg/m^2 IV every week for 4–6 wk (maximum 2 mg)	Acute lymphocytic leukemia
	P—prednisone	60 mg/m^2 PO daily for 4 wk, then taper weeks 5–7	
VP-L-Asparaginase (VPAsp)	V—vincristine	2 mg/m^2 IV every week for 4–6 wk (maximum 2 mg)	Acute lymphocytic leukemia
	P—prednisone	60 mg/m^2 PO daily for 4 wk–6 wk, then taper	
	Asp—L-asparaginase	10,000 U/m^2 IV days 1–14	
VP plus Daunorubicin	V—vincristine	1.5 mg/m^2 IV weekly for 4–6 wk	Acute lymphocytic leukemia
	P—prednisone	40 mg/m^2 PO daily for 4–6 wk	
	daunorubicin	25 mg/m^2 IV weekly for 4–6 wk	

Selected Bibliography

Aronin PA, Mahaley MS, Rudnick S et al: Prediction of BCNU pulmonary toxicity in patients with malignant gliomas: An assessment of risk factors. N Engl J Med 303(4):183, 1980

Barnett M, Waxman J, Richards M et al: Central nervous system toxicity of high dose cytosine arabinoside. Semin Oncol 12(2):133, 1985

Baxley K, Erdman L, Henry E, Roof B: Alopecia: Effect on cancer patient's body image. Cancer Nurs 7:499, 1984

Becker T: Cancer Chemotherapy: A Manual for Nurses. Boston, Little Brown, 1981

Brager B, Yasko J: Care of the Client Receiving Chemotherapy. Reston, Reston Publishing, 1984

Brandt B: A nursing protocol for the client with neutropenia. Oncol Nurs Forum 11(2):24, 1984

Calabresi P, Schein PS, Rosenberg SA (eds): Medical Oncology. New York, MacMillan, 1985

Cancer chemotherapy. Med Lett Drug Ther 29:29, 1987

Cline B: Prevention of chemotherapy-induced alopecia: A review of the literature. Cancer Nurs 7(3):221, 1984

Conrad K: Cerebellar toxicities associated with cytosine arabinoside: A nursing perspective. Oncol Nurs Forum 13(5):57, 1986

Cooley M, Cobb S: Sexual and reproductive issues for women with Hodgkins disease: I. Overview of issues. Cancer Nurs 9(4):188, 1986

Dellefield ME: Caring for the elderly patient with cancer. Oncol Nurs Forum 13(3):19, 1986

DeVita VT, Helman S, Rosenberg SA (eds): Cancer: Principles and Practice of Oncology, 2nd ed. Philadelphia, JB Lippincott, 1985

Engelking C, Steele N: A model for pretreatment nursing assessment of patients receiving cancer chemotherapy. Cancer Nurs 7(3):203, 1984

Furr BJ, Jordan VC: Pharmacology and clinical uses of tamoxifen. Pharmacol Ther 25:127, 1984

Glazer RI (ed): Developments in Cancer Chemotherapy. Boca Raton, CRC Press, 1984

Goodman M: Cisplatin: Outpatient and office hydration regimens. Semin Oncol Nurs 3(Suppl 1):36, 1987

Goodman M: Management of nausea and vomiting induced by outpatient cisplatin therapy. Semin Oncol Nurs 3(Suppl 1):23, 1987

Griffiths MJ, Murray KH, Russo DC: Oncology Nursing: Pathophysiology Assessment and Intervention. New York, MacMillan, 1985

Hacker MP, Douple EB, Krakoff IH (eds): Platinum co-ordination complexes in cancer chemotherapy. Boston, Martinus Nijhoff, 1984

Holden S, Felde G: Nursing care of patients experiencing cisplatin-related peripheral neuropathy. Oncol Nurs Forum 14(1):13, 1987

Hughes CB: Giving cancer drugs IV: Some guidelines. Am J Nurs 86(1):34, Jan 1986

Hunter R: Hodgkin's disease: A critical review. Cancer Chemother Update 1(2): Sept/Oct 1983

Ignoffo RJ: Oncology. In Kotcher BS, Young LY, Koda-Kimble MA (eds): Applied Therapeutics—The Clinical Use of Drugs, p 899. Spokane, Applied Therapeutics, Inc, 1983

Kaempfer S, Wiley F, Hoffman D, Rhodes E: Fertility considerations and procreative alternatives in cancer care. Semin Oncol Nurs 1(1):25, 1985

Knobf MK, Fischer DS, Welch-McCaffrey D: Cancer Chemotherapy: Treatment and Care. Boston, GK Hall Medical Publishers, 1984

Lauer P: Learning needs of cancer patients: A comparison of nurse and patient's perceptions. Nurs Res 31(1):11, 1982

Lydon J: Nephrotoxicity of cancer treatment. Oncol Nurs Forum 13(2):68, 1986

Miller S, Dodd M, Goodman M, et al: Cancer Chemotherapy: Guidelines and Recommendations for Nursing Education and Practice. Oncology Nursing Society, 1984

Miller S: Considerations in the outpatient and office administration of cisplatin. Semin Oncol Nurs 3(1, Suppl 1):3, 1987

Muggia EM, Nishoff M (eds): Cancer Chemotherapy, Vol. II. Boston, Martinus Nijhoff, 1985

O'Dwyer PJ, Leyland-Jones B, Alonso MT et al: Etoposide (VP-16-213): Current status of an active anticancer drug. N Engl J Med 312:692, 1985

Riggs CE: Combination Chemotherapy. In Moossa AR, Robsen MC, Schimpf SC (eds): Comprehensive Testbook of Oncology. Baltimore, Williams & Wilkins, 1986

Rubin P: Clinical Oncology, 6th ed. New York, American Cancer Society, 1983

Solimando DA: Myelosuppressive effects of antineoplastic agents. Highlights on Antineoplastic Drugs 4(2):1, May/June 1986

Welch-McCaffrey D: Evolving patient education needs in cancer. Oncol Nurs Forum 12(5):62, 1985

Welch-McCaffrey D (ed): Nursing Considerations in Geriatric Oncology. Columbus, OH Adria Laboratories, 1986

Wickham P: Pulmonary toxicity secondary to cancer treatment. Oncol Nurs Forum 13(5):69, 1986

Wojciechowski NJ, Carter CA, Skoutakis VA et al: Leuprolide: A gonadotropin-releasing hormone analog for the palliative treatment of prostatic cancer. Drug Intell Clin Pharm 20:746, 1986

Wolfe CA, Linkewich JA: Preparation of guidelines for the avoidance and treatment of extravasation due to antineoplastic drugs. Hosp Pharm 22:125, 1987

Yarbo C, Perry M: The effect of cancer therapy on gonadal function. Semin Oncol Nurs 1(1):3, 1985

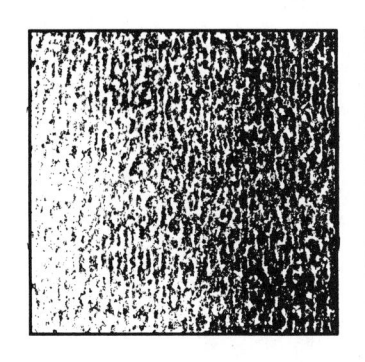

IX Nutrients, Fluids, and Electrolytes

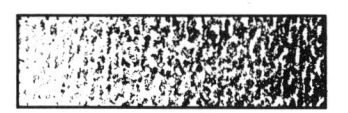

73 WATER-SOLUBLE VITAMINS: VITAMINS B AND C

Vitamins are commonly classified as either water soluble (B complex, C) or fat soluble (A, D, E, K). The water-soluble vitamins are reviewed in this chapter and the fat-soluble vitamins are discussed in Chapter 74.

VITAMINS: GENERAL CONSIDERATIONS

Vitamins are organic substances required by the body for synthesis of essential cofactors that catalyze metabolic reactions. The body does not have the capacity to provide enough of all the essential vitamins, hence dietary sources are necessary. Since the average diet is usually more than adequate in supplying most required vitamins, there is rarely a need for additional vitamins in the majority of persons, and indiscriminate use of single- or multiple-vitamin preparations should be discouraged.

There are, however, certain situations in which vitamin supplementation can be justified. Vitamin deficiency states can result from inadequate nutritional intake, impaired absorption; increased requirements, malnutrition (e.g., from starvation, anorexia, extreme diets, food faddism), pathologic conditions (GI disorders, hyperthyroidism, intestinal surgery, carcinomas), alcoholism, prolonged stress, dialysis, and a variety of other conditions. Provided that a definite vitamin deficiency can be demonstrated on the basis of clinical symptoms, *selective* replacement of those vitamins that are lacking is indicated. Use of multivitamin formulations for replacement therapy, however, is usually unnecessary and can become a significant expense as well. A much more reasonable approach is to supply the deficient vitamins in the amounts required to eliminate the symptoms of the vitamin deficiency state. For example, thiamine is indicated for beriberi, niacin for pellagra, ascorbic acid for scurvy, and cyanocobalamin for pernicious anemia. It is important, however, to regard vitamins as *drugs;* as such, they should be used only where there is valid indication. Injudicious or excessive intake of vitamins is at best wasteful and can lead to untoward reactions, especially in the case of the fat-soluble vitamins (A, D, E, K). Moreover, continued self-medication with vitamin preparations may delay recognition or mask the symptoms of a more serious underlying disease. Vitamin supplementation should be undertaken only after consultation with a health care professional, and the type and amount of individual vitamins prescribed should be based upon thorough clinical assessment of the patient's diet, health status, and presenting symptoms.

The Food and Nutrition Board of the National Academy of Sciences periodically provides guidelines for recommended intake of individual nutrients, including vitamins. The recommended dietary allowances (RDAs) are *not* requirements but are suggested daily intakes of vitamins and other nutrients that, based on current scientific data, are believed to be adequate for the nutritional needs of most healthy persons under normal environmental conditions. RDAs will vary with sex and age, and additional allowances are made for special circumstances, such as during pregnancy and lactation. As noted, RDA values apply to *healthy* persons and are not intended to cover nutritional requirements in disease or other abnormal situations. RDAs are subject to periodic revision, and values do change as population subgroups with unique nutritional requirements emerge.

The U.S. Food and Drug Administration (FDA) regulates the labeling of vitamin and mineral products sold as foods or drugs and has designated an "official" U.S. RDA for each substance, which serves as the legal standard for nutritional labeling of those products controlled by the administration. In general, U.S. RDAs represent the highest male or female RDA for each nutrient. Previously, these U.S. RDAs were labeled "minimum daily requirements" (MDRs), but this term has become obsolete.

The current RDAs for the B complex and C vitamins are listed in Table 73-1 and those for the fat-soluble vitamins (A, D, E, K) are listed in Table 74-1 in Chapter 74.

There is no convincing evidence that use of excessive amounts (i.e., megadoses) of certain vitamins can cure or prevent nonnutritional diseases. Despite the many, usually anecdotal, claims made by proponents of megadose vitamin therapy for beneficial effects in diseases ranging from alopecia to warts, use of quantities of vitamins beyond those needed for normal body functioning is at the very least wasteful and can be potentially quite hazardous.

WATER-SOLUBLE VITAMINS

Certain vitamins are readily soluble in water and are found together in many of the same foods. They are therefore usually grouped together as the water-soluble vitamins. They include the B complex group and ascorbic acid (vitamin C). These substances are readily excreted in the urine and thus are potentially much less toxic following large doses than are the fat-soluble vitamins, which are metabolized slowly and can be stored in significant amounts in the body. Table 73-1 lists the water-soluble vitamins together with their RDAs, dietary sources, and other pertinent information.

B Complex Vitamins

The vitamin B complex group is composed of a number of compounds that differ in structure and biological activity but are obtained from many of the same sources, most notably liver and yeast. Two B complex vitamins, cyanocobalamin (vitamin B_{12}) and folic acid (vitamin B_9) have been reviewed in Chapter 34, because they are primarily indicated in the treatment of pernicious anemia; cyanocobalamin is discussed here only as a nutritional supplement. The remaining B complex vitamins are examined individually in this chapter.

Vitamin B_1 (Thiamine)

Betalin S, Biamine

(CAN) Betaxin, Bewon

Thiamine, or vitamin B_1, is an organic molecule that combines with ATP to form thiamine pyrophosphate, a coenzyme essential for carbohydrate metabolism. Thiamine requirements are closely linked to caloric intake, and clinical manifestations of thiamine deficiency can range from mild (anorexia, weakness, paresthesias, hypothermia, hypotension) to moderate (polyneuritis, sensory and motor defects, cardiovascular disease) to

Table 73-1
Water-Soluble Vitamins

Vitamin	Major Dietary Sources	RDA Infants	RDA Children	RDA Adults	Principal Symptoms of Deficiency States
B Complex					
Thiamine (B$_1$)	Liver; whole grain, enriched bread and cereals; pork	0.3 mg–0.5 mg	0.7 mg–1.2 mg	1.0 mg–1.4 mg	Anorexia, constipation, beriberi (cardiac complications, peripheral neuritis)
Riboflavin (B$_2$)	Organ meats, milk, eggs, green vegetables, enriched bread and flour	0.4 mg–0.6 mg	0.8 mg–1.4 mg	1.2 mg–1.7 mg	Stomatitis, glossitis, ocular itching or burning, photophobia, facial dermatitis, cheilosis, corneal vascularization
Nicotinic acid (Niacin, B$_3$)	Liver, fish, poultry, red meat, enriched bread and cereals	6 mg–8 mg	9 mg–16 mg	13 mg–18 mg	Pellagra (nervousness, insomnia, dermatitis, diarrhea, confusion, delusions)
Pantothenic acid (B$_5$)	Organ meats, egg yolks, beef, peanuts, whole grains, cauliflower	[a]	[a]	[a]	Weakness, fatigue, mood changes, dizziness, "burning-foot" syndrome
Pyridoxine (B$_6$)	Red meat, liver, yeast, whole grains, soybeans, green vegetables	0.3 mg–0.6 mg	0.9 mg–1.6 mg	1.8 mg–2.2 mg	Anemia, CNS lesions, epileptic convulsions in children
Cyanocobalamin (B$_{12}$)	Red meat, milk, egg yolk, oysters, clams	0.5 μg–1.5 μg	2 μg–3 μg	3 μg	Pernicious anemia, glossitis, paresthesias, muscle incoordination, confusion
Vitamin C (Ascorbic acid)	Citrus fruits, tomatoes, green vegetables, potatoes, strawberries, green peppers	35 mg	45 mg	50 mg–60 mg	Scurvy (petechiae, bleeding gums, bruising, impaired wound healing, loosened teeth)

[a] RDA is not established

---

severe (Wernicke's encephalopathy, Korsakoff's psychosis). Beriberi, a thiamine deficiency characterized by GI disturbances, peripheral neurologic complications ("dry beriberi"), and cardiovascular disease ("wet beriberi"), is frequently observed in far eastern countries where the diet consists largely of polished rice, which is very low in thiamine. In contrast, in the United States, alcoholism is the most common cause of thiamine deficiency.

MECHANISM
Interacts with ATP to form thiamine pyrophosphate, a coenzyme that functions in the decarboxylation of alpha-keto and pyruvic acids and in the utilization of pentose by the hexose–monophosphate shunt

USES
Prevention and treatment of thiamine deficiency states (see Table 73-1)

DOSAGE
Oral: 5 mg to 30 mg/day

IM (Beriberi): 10 mg to 20 mg three times a day for 2 weeks, supplemented with a daily oral multivitamin containing 5 mg to 10 mg thiamine

IV (Beriberi with myocardial failure; Wernicke–Korsakoff syndrome): up to 30 mg three times a day

> NOTE
> When thiamine is to be administered IV, perform an intradermal sensitivity test before injection, because deaths have resulted from thiamine hypersensitivity following IV use

FATE
Oral absorption is limited to 8 mg to 15 mg/day. As intake exceeds the minimal requirement (1 mg–2 mg), tissue stores

become saturated, and the excess appears in the urine, either as unchanged thiamine or as a pyrimidine metabolite

SIGNIFICANT ADVERSE REACTIONS

(Usually with large doses) Feeling of warmth, pruritus, urticaria, sweating, nausea, restlessness, weakness, cyanosis, dyspnea, tightness of the throat, angioedema, pulmonary edema, and GI hemorrhage

INTERACTIONS

Thiamine can enhance the response to peripherally acting muscle relaxants

Thiamine is unstable in alkaline solutions, for example, with carbonates, citrates, or barbiturates

NURSING CONSIDERATIONS

1. Be prepared to administer thiamine to thiamine-deficient patient before a glucose load is delivered to avert the sudden worsening of symptoms of Wernicke's encephalopathy (e.g., ataxia, diplopia, tremor, agitation) that may occur following IV glucose administration.
2. Expect appropriate supplementary therapy to be instituted because multiple vitamin and nutrient deficiencies usually accompany thiamine deficiency.
3. Do *not* use thiamine in combination with alkaline solutions (e.g., citrates, carbonates, bicarbonates, barbiturates) because it is unstable in alkaline or neutral solutions.
4. Note that clinically significant thiamine depletion can occur within 3 weeks in the total absence of dietary thiamine.

Vitamin B₂ (Riboflavin)

Riboflavin, or vitamin B$_2$, derives its name from the presence of the sugar ribose as a component of the molecule and from the fact that the remainder of the structure is a yellow-pigmented compound termed a *flavin*. Riboflavin functions as a coenzyme that plays an essential role in the metabolism of a variety of cellular respiratory proteins.

MECHANISM

Converted to one of two riboflavin-containing biologically active coenzymes, flavin mononucleotide (FMN) and flavin adenine dinucleotide (FAD), which play a vital metabolic role in the action of tissue respiratory flavoproteins

USES

Prevention and treatment of riboflavin deficiency (ariboflavinosis)—see Table 73-1

DOSAGE

Oral: 5 mg to 10 mg/day

FATE

Well absorbed orally; widely distributed in the body but very little is stored; in small amounts, approximately 10% is excreted in the urine; larger doses are eliminated in increasing proportion in the urine; drug is present in the feces but probably represents vitamin synthesized by intestinal microorganisms

INTERACTIONS

Riboflavin may inhibit the activity of tetracyclines when mixed together in solution

Riboflavin can reduce chloramphenicol-induced bone marrow depression and optic neuritis

NURSING CONSIDERATION

1. Expect appropriate supplementary therapy to be instituted because multiple vitamin and nutrient deficiencies usually accompany riboflavin deficiency.

PATIENT EDUCATION

1. Reassure patient that symptoms of riboflavin deficiency (sore throat, stomatitis, glossitis, corneal vascularization, cheilosis, seborrheic dermatitis, blepharospasm, photophobia) usually disappear shortly after beginning replacement therapy.
2. Inform patient that riboflavin will impart a harmless yellowish color to urine. The color may, however, interfere with urinary catecholamine determinations.

Vitamin B₃ (Nicotinic Acid, Niacin)

Niac, Niacels, Nico-400, Nicobid, Nicolar, Nicotinex, Span-Niacin

(CAN) Novoniacin, Tri-B3

Nicotinic acid or niacin (vitamin B$_3$) is a B complex vitamin that serves as a constituent of two important coenzymes, NAD (coenzyme I) and NADP (coenzyme II). These coenzymes function in several oxidation–reduction reactions required for cellular and tissue respiration. Niacin is an essential dietary constituent, the lack of which results in pellagra, a condition that primarily affects the skin, GI tract, and CNS, and is often characterized by the three "D's," that is, dermatitis, diarrhea, and dementia. In addition to its value in treating pellagra and other nicotinic acid deficiency states, niacin is also employed in large doses as adjunctive therapy in several forms of hyperlipidemia and hypercholesterolemia. These latter indications are reviewed in Chapter 33. Finally, its vasodilatory action has led to its use as a circulatory aid in peripheral vascular diseases, but there is no conclusive evidence that the drug has a clinically beneficial effect in patients with circulatory impairment.

Large doses of nicotinic acid have been employed in treating schizophrenia as part of what has been termed *orthomolecular psychiatry*. There is no convincing evidence that such treatment is effective, and use of high doses of nicotinic acid may be associated with significant toxicity, including liver damage, arrhythmias, peptic ulceration, sensory neuropathy, hyperglycemia, dermatoses, and GI distress.

MECHANISM

Niacin is converted to either NAD or NADP, enzymes vital to cellular metabolism. Large doses exert a hypolipemic effect, presumably by reducing triglyceride synthesis and blocking the release of very low-density lipoproteins (VLDLs) from the liver; may also increase cholesterol oxidation and inhibit mobilization of free fatty acids; exerts a direct, although relatively weak relaxing effect on peripheral vascular smooth muscle

USES

Prevention and treatment of pellagra and other niacin deficiency states

Adjunctive therapy of hypercholesterolemia and hyperbetalipoproteinemia (Types IIb, III, IV, and V); see Chapter 33

Symptomatic treatment of peripheral vascular disorders (conclusive evidence of beneficial effect is lacking)

DOSAGE

Oral

Niacin deficiency: 10 mg to 20 mg/day

Pellagra: up to 500 mg/day, depending on severity of symptoms

Hyperlipidemias: 1 g to 2 g three times a day (maximum 6 g/day)
IV (vitamin deficiencies only)
Dosage and duration of therapy dependent on patient response

FATE
Readily absorbed orally and widely distributed; peak serum concentrations occur in 45 minutes; approximately one third of a normal oral dose is excreted unchanged in the urine; with very large doses, the principal urinary excretory product is the unchanged drug

COMMON SIDE EFFECTS
Cutaneous flushing and sensation of warmth, especially in the face or neck area; GI distress

SIGNIFICANT ADVERSE REACTIONS
(Especially with large doses) Headache, tingling, skin rash, pruritus, increased sebaceous gland activity, dryness of the skin, jaundice, allergic reactions, keratosis nigricans, activation of peptic ulcer, abdominal pain, vomiting, diarrhea, hypotension (orthostatic), dizziness, hyperuricemia, toxic amblyopia, and decreased glucose tolerance

CONTRAINDICATIONS
Active peptic ulcer, severe hepatic dysfunction, severe hypotension, hemorrhaging or arterial bleeding. *Cautious use* in patients with glaucoma, jaundice, liver disease, peptic ulcer, gallbladder disease, diabetes, gout, or angina; in children, and in pregnant or nursing women

INTERACTIONS
Niacin may have additive blood pressure–lowering effects with antihypertensive drugs
Niacin can reduce the effectiveness of oral hypoglycemic agents by elevating blood glucose levels
Niacin may reduce the uricosuric action of sulfinpyrazone or probenecid

NURSING CONSIDERATIONS
1. Expect therapy to begin with small doses to minimize untoward reactions. Dosage should be increased gradually to optimal level. Initial therapeutic response usually occurs within 24 to 48 hours.
2. Administer parenteral therapy, which is indicated only for severe niacin deficiency (not for hyperlipidemia), by slow IV injection, if possible.

PATIENT EDUCATION
1. Instruct patient to take drug during meals to minimize GI upset and to swallow with cold water. Hot beverages should be avoided because they may intensify vasodilation.
2. Inform patient that tingling, itching, headache, or a sensation of warmth, especially in the area of the head, neck, and ears, can occur shortly after administration, but that these effects usually subside with continued therapy. For vitamin replacement therapy, niacinamide may be used instead of niacin if flushing is severe or bothersome (see nicotinamide).
3. Warn patient not to engage in hazardous activities because dizziness or weakness can occur, especially during early therapy.
4. Advise patient to avoid prolonged exposure to bright sunlight.

Nicotinamide
Niacinamide

An amide of nicotinic acid, nicotinamide provides a source of niacin that can be utilized by the body but is devoid of hypolipidemic and vasodilatory effects. Thus, it is indicated only for treatment of niacin deficiency states, in which it is preferred by many patients who find the flushing and paresthesias resulting from niacin itself unpleasant. Nicotinamide is available for oral or parenteral administration, and dosage is highly individual and based on symptoms and response. The usual dosage range is 50 mg three to ten times a day. Other than a reduced incidence of circulatory side effects, the pharmacology of nicotinamide is essentially similar to that of nicotinic acid.

Vitamin B$_5$ (Calcium Pantothenate)

Pantothenic acid is often referred to as vitamin B$_5$. Because pantothenic acid is found abundantly in the normal diet, deficiency states are quite rare. Although it is a necessary nutrient, the daily requirement is not known and no RDAs are available. Pantothenic acid in the form of its calcium salt is commonly found in multivitamin preparations, but its presence is probably unnecessary.

MECHANISM
Incorporated in coenzyme A, which functions as a cofactor for a variety of essential metabolic activities such as oxidative metabolism of carbohydrates, gluconeogenesis, synthesis and degradation of fatty acids, and synthesis of sterols and steroid hormones

USES
Treatment of pantothenic acid deficiency, although this condition has *not* been recognized in humans with an ordinary diet

DOSAGE
5 mg to 10 mg/day. Up to 10 g/day has been employed

FATE
Readily absorbed orally; widely distributed in the body; not metabolized to any extent but excreted largely unchanged in the urine

NURSING CONSIDERATIONS
1. Note that no spontaneously occurring pantothenic acid deficiency state has been reported in humans.

Vitamin B$_6$ (Pyridoxine)
Beesix, Hexa-Betalin, Nestrex, Pyroxine

Naturally occurring substances that exhibit vitamin B$_6$ activity include pyridoxine in plants and pyridoxal and pyridoxamine in animals. All three compounds possess similar biologic activity and thus should be regarded as different forms of vitamin B$_6$, although pyridoxine is the most commonly used term. Pyridoxine functions as a coenzyme at different stages in the metabolism of carbohydrates, fats, and proteins. The need for pyridoxine increases with the amount of protein in the diet, and RDAs are listed in Table 73-1.

MECHANISM
All three forms of vitamin B$_6$ are converted in vivo to pyridoxal phosphate or pyridoxamine phosphate, the physiologically active forms that serve as coenzymes for a number of essential metabolic reactions. Such reactions include decarboxylation,

transamination, and transulfuration of amino acids, conversion of tryptophan to serotonin or niacin, and glycogenolysis.

USES

Treatment of pyridoxine deficiency, as seen, for example, with inadequate dietary intake, inborn errors of metabolism (e.g., pyridoxine-dependent convulsions, pyridoxine-responsive anemia) or drug-induced depletion (e.g., from isoniazid, alcohol, oral contraceptives)

Control of nausea and vomiting in pregnancy or that resulting from radiation (effectiveness *not* conclusively demonstrated)

Investigational uses include reversal of the neurologic symptoms of hydrazine poisoning, symptomatic treatment of the premenstrual syndrome, and treatment of oxalate kidney stones

DOSAGE

Dietary deficiency: 10 mg to 20 mg/day orally for 3 weeks, followed by an oral multivitamin containing 2 mg to 5 mg pyridoxine (see Nursing Considerations)

Pyridoxine dependency syndrome: up to 600 mg/day initially, reduced to 25 to 50 mg/day for life

Isoniazid-induced deficiency: 50–300 mg daily

Isoniazid overdosage (10 g or more): give an equal amount of pyridoxine (4 g IV injection, followed by 1 g IM every 30 min)

FATE

Well absorbed orally; converted to pyridoxal phosphate; and pyridoxamine phosphate; half-life is 15 days to 20 days; metabolized in the liver to 4-pyridoxic acid, which is excreted in the urine

SIGNIFICANT ADVERSE REACTIONS

(Usually only with large doses) Paresthesias, somnolence, flushing, reduced serum folic acid levels, and pain at injection site

CONTRAINDICATIONS

No absolute contraindications. *Cautious use* in nursing mothers (may inhibit lactation)

INTERACTIONS

Pyridoxine can reduce the effectiveness of levodopa by accelerating its peripheral metabolism

Pyridoxine requirement may be increased in patients taking isoniazid, cycloserine, oral contraceptives, hydralazine, or penicillamine

Chloramphenicol-induced optic neuritis can be prevented by pyridoxine

Concomitant administration of pyridoxine may decrease serum levels of phenobarbital and phenytoin

NURSING CONSIDERATIONS

Nursing Alert
- Advocate pyridoxine supplementation for alcoholic patient to prevent neurologic complications because a substantial number of alcoholics have a significant deficiency. Pyridoxine deficiency is also common in patients taking isoniazid, and it may occur with use of oral contraceptives and certain other drugs (see Interactions).

1. Expect symptoms to be controlled with a multivitamin preparation once pyridoxine levels are restored because selective pyridoxine dietary deficiency is rare.

Vitamin B₁₂ (Cyanocobalamin)

Cyanocobalamin, or vitamin B$_{12}$, is essential for normal growth and development, cell reproduction, hematopoiesis, and nucleoprotein and myelin synthesis. Insufficient GI absorption of cyanocobalamin, due primarily to decreased availability of intrinsic factor, leads to pernicious anemia and is treated with large oral or parenteral doses (see Chap. 34). Oral preparations containing less than 500 μg cyanocobalamin are *not* indicated for pernicious anemia but are employed solely as a nutritional supplement, especially in persons on strict vegetarian diets. The recommended dosage range is 25 μg to 250 μg/day, although it should be remembered that the RDA for cyanocobalamin is only 3 μg in adults.

Vitamin C

Ascorbic Acid
various manufacturers
Calcium Ascorbate
Sodium Ascorbate
Cenolate, Cevita

Vitamin C, or ascorbic acid, is an essential dietary substance that plays a major role in many metabolic reactions as well as the formation and maintenance of collagen and intracellular ground substance. The name *ascorbic acid* is a condensation of the term *antiscorbutic vitamin*. It is derived from the compound's ability to prevent scurvy, the principal ascorbic acid deficiency state. In normal therapeutic doses, ascorbic acid elicits few demonstrable pharmacologic effects except in the scorbutic person (i.e., the patient with symptoms of scurvy). This disease is occasionally observed in elderly or debilitated persons, drug addicts, alcoholics, and others with poor diets. It is characterized by degenerative changes in connective tissue, bones, and capillaries. The symptoms of ascorbic acid deficiency (swollen and bleeding gums, petechiae, easy bruising, delayed wound healing, loosened teeth, joint pain, and bloody stools) are usually readily relieved by 200 mg to 400 mg ascorbic acid daily for several days; they can be prevented from recurring by small (50 mg–100 mg) daily supplemental doses of the vitamin. Although very large amounts (megadoses) of ascorbic acid have been advocated for a wide variety of disease states, ranging from prophylaxis of the common cold to treatment of carcinomas, *conclusive evidence* for the vitamin's effectiveness in megadose quantities for any of the proposed indications is lacking.

MECHANISM

Participates in a number of essential biologic functions, for example, formation of collagen and intracellular ground substance, cellular respiration, microsomal drug metabolism, steroid synthesis, tyrosine metabolism, and conversion of folic acid to folinic acid; important for the maintenance of tooth and bone matrix and capillary integrity, and may aid wound healing; reduces pH of the urine

USES

Prevention and treatment of scurvy and other ascorbic acid deficiency states

Adjunctive therapy in extensive or deep burns, delayed wound healing, chronic or severe illnesses, and a variety of other disease states and stressful situations (effectiveness has not been conclusively demonstrated)

Acidification of the urine, usually in conjunction with a urinary anti-infective

DOSAGE

Oral

Treatment of deficiency states: 300 mg to 1000 mg/day as needed

Prophylaxis: 75 mg to 150 mg/day

Wound healing: 300 mg to 500 mg/day for 7 to 10 days; much larger amounts have been used

Burns: 1 g to 2 g/day

IM, SC, IV

Up to 2 g/day may be given as needed for severe deficiency states; maintenance dose is 100 mg to 250 mg once or twice a day

FATE

Readily absorbed orally or parenterally and widely distributed; partly metabolized and excreted in the urine both as metabolites and unchanged drug; renal threshold is 1.5 mg/dL plasma, and the amount excreted markedly increases with large doses

SIGNIFICANT ADVERSE REACTIONS

(Usually with large doses) Diarrhea, precipitation of oxalate or urate renal stones, soreness at IM or SC injection sites, and dizziness or faintness with too rapid IV injection

CONTRAINDICATIONS

Use of sodium ascorbate injection in patients on sodium-restricted diets. *Cautious use* in patients with glucose-6-phosphate dehydrogenase deficiency, hyperuricemia, or renal impairment, and in pregnant women

INTERACTIONS

Large doses of ascorbic acid lower urinary pH and thus may reduce excretion of acidic drugs (e.g., salicylates, barbiturates) and increase excretion of basic drugs (e.g., quinidine, atropine, amphetamines, tricyclic antidepressants, phenothiazines)

Ascorbic acid increases the possibility of crystalluria with the sulfonamides

Large doses of ascorbic acid may shorten the prothrombin time in patients receiving oral anticoagulants

Ascorbic acid can interfere with the effectiveness of disulfiram when it is used in the alcoholic patient (see Chap. 78).

Ascorbic acid in large doses may enhance the absorption of oral iron

Mineral oil can retard absorption of ascorbic acid

Ascorbic acid is chemically incompatible with penicillin G potassium and should not be mixed in the same syringe

Intermittent administration of ascorbic acid may increase the risk of oral contraceptive failure

Smoking may slightly reduce ascorbic acid serum levels; conversely, ascorbic acid can enhance excretion of nicotine, perhaps resulting in an increased desire to smoke

NURSING CONSIDERATIONS

1. Inject slowly IV to avoid dizziness and possible fainting.
2. Interpret results of urine glucose, serum uric acid, and urinary steroid determinations cautiously because large doses may result in false readings.

Selected Bibliography

Cerrato PL: When to worry about vitamin overdose? RN 48(10):69, Oct, 1985

Food and Nutrition Board, National Research Council: Recommended Dietary Allowances, 9th ed. Washington, DC, National Academy of Sciences, 1980

Halpern JS: Megavitamins: Therapeutic or a threat to health? J Educ Nurs 9:346, 1983

Luke B: Megavitamins and pregnancy: A dangerous combination. Matern Child Nurs 10:18, 1985

Miller DR, Hayes KC: Vitamin excess and toxicity In Nutritional Toxicology, vol 1, p 18. New York, Academic Press, 1982

Toxic Effects of Vitamin Overdosage. Med Lett Drugs Ther 26:73, 1984

SUMMARY. WATER-SOLUBLE VITAMINS

Drug	Preparations	Usual Dosage Range
B Complex Vitamins		
Thiamine *Betalin S, Biamine*	Tablets: 5 mg, 10 mg, 25 mg, 50 mg, 100 mg, 250 mg, 500 mg Injection: 100 mg/mL, 200 mg/mL	*Oral:* 5 mg–30 mg/day *IM:* 10 mg–20 mg 3 times a day for 2 wk, supplemented with 5 mg–10 mg orally/day *IV:* up to 30 mg 3 times/day
B₂ (Riboflavin)	Tablets: 5 mg, 10 mg, 25 mg, 50 mg, 100 mg, 250 mg	*Oral:* 5 mg–10 mg/day
B₃ (Niacin, Nicotinic Acid)	Tablets: 25 mg, 50 mg, 100 mg, 250 mg, 500 mg Tablets (timed-release): 150 mg, 250 mg, 500 mg, 750 mg Capsules (timed-release): 125 mg, 250 mg, 300 mg, 400 mg, 500 mg Elixir: 50 mg/5 mL Injection: 50 mg/mL, 100 mg/mL	Oral Niacin deficiency: 10 mg–20 mg/day Pellagra: up to 500 mg/day Hyperlipidemia: 1 g–2 g 3 times/day (maximum 6 g/day) IV Dose and duration are variable

Continued

SUMMARY. WATER-SOLUBLE VITAMINS (continued)

Drug	Preparations	Usual Dosage Range
Nicotinamide (Niacinamide)	Tablets: 50 mg, 100 mg, 500 mg Tablets (timed-release): 1000 mg Injection: 100 mg/mL	*Oral or parenteral:* 50 mg 3–10 times/day depending on severity of deficiency and clinical response
B₅ (Calcium Pantothenate)	Tablets: 25 mg, 30 mg, 100 mg, 200 mg, 218 mg, 250 mg, 500 mg, 545 mg	*Oral* 5 mg–10 mg/day; up to 10 g/day has been used
B₆ (Pyridoxine) Beesix, Hexa-Betalin, Nestrex, Pyroxine	Tablets: 10 mg, 25 mg, 50 mg, 100 mg, 200 mg, 250 mg, 500 mg Injection: 100 mg/mL	*Dietary deficiency:* 10 mg–20 mg/day for 3 wk then 2 mg to 5 mg/day *Pyridoxine dependency syndrome:* up to 600 mg/day initially, then 25–50 mg/day *Isoniazid-induced deficiency:* 50 mg–300 mg a day *Isoniazid overdosage:* 4 g IV, then 1 g IM every 30 min until an equal amount of pyridoxine is given
B₁₂ (Cyanocobalamin)	Tablets: 25 μg, 50 μg, 100 μg, 250 μg, see also Chap. 34	25 μg–250 μg/day
Vitamin C **Ascorbic Acid** **Calcium Ascorbate** **Sodium Ascorbate** Cenolate, Cevita	Tablets: 50 mg, 100 mg, 250 mg, 500 mg, 1000 mg Chewable tablets: 100 mg, 250 mg, 500 mg Tablets (sustained-release): 500 mg, 1500 mg Capsules (timed-release): 500 mg Syrup: 500 mg/5 mL Solution: 100 mg/mL Drops: 35 mg/0.6 mL Injection (ascorbic acid): 100 mg/mL, 250 mg/mL, 500 mg/mL Injection (sodium ascorbate): 222 mg/mL, 500 mg/mL	*Oral* Deficiency states: 300 mg–1000 mg/day as required *Prophylaxis:* 75 mg–150 mg/day *Wound healing:* 300 mg–500 mg/day for 7–10 days *IM, SC IV:* up to 2 g/day; maintenance dose is 100 mg–250 mg once or twice a day

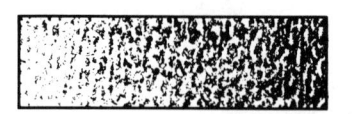

FAT-SOLUBLE VITAMINS: VITAMINS A, D, E, AND K

Unlike the B complex and C vitamins discussed in Chapter 73, vitamins A, D, E, and K are poorly soluble in water but dissolve readily in fats. This property is responsible for certain characteristics that distinguish the fat-soluble vitamins from their water-soluble counterparts. Whereas the B and C vitamins are readily absorbed orally, the fat-soluble vitamins require the presence of sufficient amounts of bile salts in the GI tract for adequate absorption. However, their absorption may be impaired by the presence of mineral oil or other fatty vehicles that can sequester the vitamins in the lumen of the intestine. Compared to the water-soluble vitamins, vitamins A, D, E, and K are stored in much larger amounts in body tissues such as adipose tissue, liver, and muscles. From these storage depots, small amounts are released over extended periods to meet nutritional needs; hence symptoms of a fat-soluble vitamin deficiency usually develop only after long periods of inadequate intake, that is, not until body stores are depleted. Loss of fat-soluble vitamins in the urine is minimal, and excretion proceeds at a slow rate. The inefficient excretion of most fat-soluble vitamins can result in accumulation to toxic levels if excessive quantities of the vitamins are ingested to supplement the diet, and such a practice should be discouraged.

Characteristics of the fat-soluble vitamins are listed in Table 74-1, along with their recommended dietary allowances where available. The four vitamins making up the fat-soluble group are reviewed below.

In addition, two vitamin D metabolites, calcifediol and calcitriol, as well as a synthetic sterol, dihydrotachysterol, which is structurally and functionally related to ergocalciferol, are considered in this chapter. Finally, two vitamin A analogs (tretinoin, isotretinoin) used in severe acne, and a third analog (etretinate) useful in recalcitrant psoriasis are also reviewed in this chapter.

VITAMIN A

Aquasol A, Del-Vi-A

The term *vitamin A* is commonly used to refer to a group of several biologically active compounds. Vitamin A_1 (retinol) is the principal naturally occurring substance and is formed from precursors termed *carotenes,* the most important of which is beta-carotene (provitamin A). The average adult receives about one half of the daily dietary intake of vitamin A as preformed retinol and the remainder as carotene precursors. Vitamin A_2 (3-dehydroretinol) occurs mixed with retinol in many dietary sources. Most currently used preparations are synthetic retinol esters, which have largely replaced the natural vitamin A products previously extracted from fish liver oils, inasmuch as they are generally better absorbed and provide more consistent blood levels of the vitamin.

The potency of vitamin A preparations is expressed as international units (IU), one IU being equal to 0.3 μg retinol or 0.6 μg beta-carotene. Vitamin A is required for growth of bones and teeth, integrity of epithelial tissue, normal functioning of the retina (especially visual adaptation to darkness), reproduction, and embryonic development. In addition, vitamin A deficiency can lower resistance to infection and reduce adrenal cortical steroid production. Deficiencies are rarely observed when reasonable dietary practices are followed, and liver stores of vitamin A are usually sufficient to satisfy requirements of the vitamin for up to 2 years.

MECHANISM
Complex and incompletely understood; among the actions ascribed to vitamin A are increased synthesis of RNA, proteins, steroids, mucopolysaccharides, and cholesterol; prevents growth retardation and preserves the integrity of epithelial cells; also necessary for formation of rhodopsin, a photosensitive pigment important for vision in dim light; may enhance healing of wounds

USES
Treatment of vitamin A deficiency states (e.g., biliary or pancreatic disease, colitis, hepatic cirrhosis, celiac disease, regional enteritis)
Prophylaxis of vitamin A deficiency during periods of increased requirements, for example, infancy, pregnancy, lactation, severe illness

DOSAGE
Adults
Oral: 100,000 IU to 500,000 IU/day for 3 days, then 50,000 IU/day for 2 weeks, then 10,000 IU to 20,000 IU/day for 2 months
IM: 100,000 IU/day for 3 days, then 50,000 IU/day for 2 weeks
Children
Oral: 10,000 IU to 15,000 IU/day as a dietary supplement
IM (1 yr–8 yr): 17,500 IU to 35,000 IU/day for 10 days
Infants
IM: 7500 IU to 15,000 IU/day for 10 days

FATE
GI absorption of vitamin A preparations is good in the presence of bile acids, pancreatic lipase, and dietary fat; aqueous dispersions of the synthetic vitamin are more rapidly absorbed than oil solutions; peak plasma concentrations occur in about 3 to 4 hours; most of a dose is stored in the liver, with smaller amounts stored in many other body tissues; vitamin E increases tissue storage of vitamin A; plasma levels increase substantially when hepatic storage sites are saturated; slowly released from liver; serum concentrations can be maintained for months by hepatic stores; transported in the plasma as retinol bound to retinol-binding protein; excretion probably occurs primarily in the bile as a glucuronide, with small amounts appearing in the urine

SIGNIFICANT ADVERSE REACTIONS
(Due to overdosage: hypervitaminosis A syndrome)

CNS: fatigue, irritability, malaise, lethargy, night sweats, vertigo, headache, increased intracranial pressure (may be manifested as papilledema)
Dermatologic: drying and fissuring of skin and lips, alopecia, gingivitis, pruritus, desquamation, increased pigmentation, tender swellings on the extremities
Musculoskeletal: retarded growth, arthralgia, premature closure of the epiphyses, bone pain
GI: abdominal pain, vomiting, anorexia
Other: liver and spleen enlargement, jaundice, leukopenia, hypomenorrhea, polydipsia, polyuria, hypercalcemia

Table 74-1
Fat-Soluble Vitamins

Vitamin	Major Dietary Source	Infants (RDA)	Children (RDA)	Adults (RDA)	Principal Symptoms of Deficiency States
Vitamin A	Fish liver oils, eggs, milk, butter, green and yellow vegetables, tomatoes, squash	2000 IU–2100 IU	2500 IU–3500 IU	4000 IU–5000 IU	Night blindness, xerophthalmia, keratinization of epithelial tissues, increased susceptibility to infection, retarded growth and development
Vitamin D	Fish liver oils, egg yolk, milk, butter, margarine, salmon, sardines	400 IU	400 IU	200 IU–400 IU	Rickets, osteomalacia
Vitamin E	Wheat germ, vegetable oils, green leafy vegetables, nuts, cereals, eggs, dairy products, meats	4 IU–6 IU	7 IU–10 IU	12 IU–15 IU	Not established in humans; *possibly* hemolytic anemia, muscular lesions and necrosis, creatinuria
Vitamin K	Green leafy vegetables, liver, cheese, egg yolks, tomatoes, meats, cereals	[a]	[a]	[a]	Hypoprothrombinemia, hemorrhage

[a] RDAs are not established.

CONTRAINDICATIONS
Oral administration in patients with malabsorption syndrome, hypervitaminosis A; administration by the IV route. *Cautious use* in the presence of impaired renal or hepatic function and in pregnant women

INTERACTIONS
Mineral oil, cholestyramine resin, and colestipol may impair absorption of vitamin A

Increased plasma vitamin A levels have occurred in women taking oral contraceptives

NURSING CONSIDERATIONS
1. Administer IM *only* when oral administration is not feasible, as, for example, when vomiting, unconsciousness, steatorrhea, or other malabsorption states are present.
2. Question administration of large doses over prolonged periods because tissue accumulation can occur. Blood levels do not necessarily reflect total body concentration because liver storage is usually extensive.
3. Note that preparations containing up to 25,000 IU are available without prescription. Stronger preparations require a prescription.

PATIENT EDUCATION
1. Warn fertile woman that use of vitamin A in excess of the RDA (i.e., 6000 IU) during pregnancy can cause fetal abnormalities.
2. Instruct patient to avoid using mineral oil while taking vitamin A (see Interactions).
3. Instruct patient to discontinue drug and notify prescriber if signs of hypervitaminosis A appear (see Significant Adverse Reactions). Symptoms subside quickly, but some, such as tender swellings in the extremities, may remain for months.

VITAMIN A ANALOGS

Etretinate
Tegison

Etretinate is related to vitamin A and is used in certain severe forms of psoriasis that have not responded to other modes of treatment. The drug is potentially toxic and is associated with a risk of fetal abnormalities. Patients using the drug must be closely supervised.

MECHANISM
Decreases erythema and thickness of psoriatic lesions and promotes normalization of epidermal differentiation; may also decrease inflammation of the epidermis and dermis; can produce a wide range of adverse effects, and its use is restricted to patients unresponsive to or intolerant of conventional modes of antipsoriatic therapy

USES
Treatment of *severe, recalcitrant* psoriasis in patients unresponsive to systemic corticosteroids, methotrexate, psoralens plus UV light, or topical tar plus UV light

DOSAGE
Initially: 0.75 mg to 1.0 mg/kg/day orally in divided doses
Maintenance dose: 0.5 mg to 0.75 mg/kg/day after 8 to 16 weeks of therapy

FATE
Oral absorption is good and may be increased by a high-lipid diet; drug undergoes significant first-pass hepatic metabolism and is more than 99% protein bound; has an extremely long half-life, and elimination is very slow. Prolonged dosing has been associated with the maintenance of detectable serum levels up to 3 years after therapy was discontinued. Excretion is by way of both the urine and bile

COMMON SIDE EFFECTS

Dry nose, sore mouth, chapped lips, thirst, nosebleed, dry skin, hair loss, itching, bone or joint pain, bruising, fatigue, muscle cramping, headache, fever, eye irritation, visual disturbances, nausea, anorexia

Also, increased triglycerides, SGOT, SGPT, alkaline phosphatase and cholesterol can occur, as well as changes in serum potassium, calcium, and phosphorus

SIGNIFICANT ADVERSE REACTIONS

> **WARNING**
> Etretinate must not be used by women who are pregnant during therapy, and contraception should be practiced for some time following discontinuation of therapy (at least 2 years, owing to the drug's extremely slow elimination). Fetal abnormalities have been reported (see also under isotretinoin)

CNS: dizziness, lethargy, pain, anxiety, depression, emotional lability, flulike symptoms, abnormal thinking, pseudotumor cerebri (benign intracranial hypertension)
Sensory: earache, otitis externa, lacrimation, hearing changes, photophobia, decreased night vision, scotoma
GI: constipation, diarrhea, weight loss, oral ulcers, altered taste, tooth cavities
Cardiovascular: chest pain, postural hypotension, phlebitis, syncope, arrhythmias
Dermatologic: bullous eruption, urticaria, pyogenic granuloma, onycholysis, hirsutism, impaired wound healing, herpes simplex infections, skin odor, fissures, skin atrophy, gingival bleeding, decreased mucus secretion, rhinorrhea
Musculoskeletal: myalgia, gout, hyperostosis (see under Contraindications), hyperkinesia
Other: coughing, dysphonia, pharyngitis, proteinuria, glycosuria, urinary casts, hemoglobinuria, kidney stones, abnormal menses, atrophic vaginitis dysuria, polyuria or urinary retention, hepatotoxicity (see under Contraindications)

CONTRAINDICATIONS

Use in women who are pregnant or who may become pregnant during or for up to 2 years after therapy. *Cautious use* in patients with liver dysfunction, hypertension, visual disturbances, and elevated serum lipids

INTERACTIONS

The oral absorption of etretinate may be increased by the presence of milk

NURSING CONSIDERATIONS

Nursing Alerts

- Monitor results of liver function tests, which should be performed prior to initiation of therapy, every few weeks for several months after treatment is started, then every few months until therapy is discontinued because hepatotoxicity may occur.
- Monitor results of blood lipid determinations, which should be performed prior to initiation of therapy, then every few weeks until lipid response is ascertained because serum lipids may rise, predisposing patient to cardiovascular risks.

PATIENT EDUCATION

With fertile woman (and sexual partner, as appropriate):
1. Ensure that patient is fully aware of drug's teratogenic potential (see *Warning* under Significant Adverse Reactions).
2. Verify that patient clearly understands the importance of effective contraception.
3. Explain that contraception needs to be employed at least 1 month prior to the start of treatment, during treatment, and for as long as 2 years after cessation of treatment. As appropriate, help patient determine preferred form of contraception or refer her and her partner to available resources.
4. Explain that a pregnancy test will be performed several weeks before therapy is initiated and that the drug will be started shortly after the onset of the next normal menstrual period.

With any patient:
1. Discuss the need to control dietary fat intake because drug may cause elevation of serum lipids. Refer patient to dietitian for additional counseling as needed.
2. Instruct patient to avoid vitamin A supplements because of possible additive toxicity.
3. Inform patient that psoriasis may temporarily worsen during early treatment.
4. Instruct patient to notify drug prescriber immediately if pain or limitation of motion is experienced in ankles, pelvis, or knees. Periodic x-rays may be recommended to detect early hyperostosis (abnormal growth of bone tissue). Evidence of emerging calcification of tendons or ligaments requires drug discontinuation.
5. Teach patient how to recognize possible early indications of hepatitis (yellow skin and sclerae, light-colored stools, dark urine, flulike symptoms) and stress importance of notifying prescriber. If hepatitis is diagnosed, drug will be discontinued.
6. Instruct patient to notify drug prescriber of any visual difficulties, which call for an ophthalmologic examination and, usually, drug discontinuation.
7. Teach patient how to recognize possible early symptoms of pseudotumor cerebri (headache, nausea, vomiting, blurred vision) and to report them. If papilledema is present, drug will be discontinued and patient will be referred for neurologic evaluation.
8. Warn patient who wears contact lenses that dry eyes may cause lens discomfort. Eye lubricants such as artificial tears may help.
9. Caution patient to avoid excessive exposure to sun because photophobia and photosensitivity may occur. Use of sunglasses and sun screen is recommended.
10. Teach patient interventions to relieve xerostomia (see **Plan of Nursing Care 4** in Chapter 14). Frequent dental care is recommended to monitor for development of caries. Drug may be discontinued if periodontal disease or candidal infection occurs.
11. Caution patient not to donate blood until several years after therapy has terminated to prevent transmission of teratogen to a pregnant woman.

Isotretinoin

Accutane

Isotretinoin is an isomer of retinoic acid, a metabolite of retinol. It is used orally for treatment of *severe* acne and other cutaneous disorders of keratinization, such as ichthyosis, pityriasis, and other hyperkeratotic skin conditions. Because of its potential for eliciting serious untoward reactions, isotretinoin should be used with utmost caution and only under close supervision.

MECHANISM
Not completely established; reduces sebum secretion and inhibits sebaceous gland differentiation; keratinization is also inhibited; elevates plasma triglycerides and cholesterol

USES
Treatment of severe, recalcitrant cystic acne in patients unresponsive to conventional therapy, including antibiotics (e.g., tetracyclines)

Treatment of disorders of excessive keratinization (e.g., ichthyosis, pityriasis, hyperkeratosis plantaris, rubra pilaris)

Treatment of cutaneous T-cell lymphoma (mycosis fungoides)

DOSAGE
Usually, 1 mg/kg to 2 mg/kg/day in two divided doses for 15 weeks to 20 weeks; a second course of therapy may be initiated after a 2-month drug-free interval. Doses of 0.05 mg/kg to 0.5 mg/kg/day have been effective in some patients, but relapses are more common

FATE
Oral bioavailability of the capsule dosage form is approximately 25%; peak plasma levels occur in about 3 hours; the drug is almost completely protein-bound; elimination half-life averages 10 hours (range 7–35 h); excreted in the urine and feces in approximately equal amounts

COMMON SIDE EFFECTS
Cheilitis, eye irritation, conjunctivitis; dry skin, skin fragility, pruritus; nosebleed, dryness of the nose and mouth; nausea, vomiting, abdominal pain; lethargy; white cells in urine; triglyceride elevation, elevated sedimentation rate

SIGNIFICANT ADVERSE REACTIONS

> **WARNING**
> Isotretinoin should not be used in women who are pregnant or who intend to become pregnant, because numerous fetal abnormalities and spontaneous abortions have occurred. An effective means of contraception must be employed during therapy and for at least 1 month before *and* after therapy

Dermatologic: facial skin desquamation, nail brittleness, rash, alopecia, photosensitivity, skin infections, erythema nodosum, pigmentary changes, urticaria

GI: anorexia, regional ileitis, mild GI bleeding, inflammatory bowel disease, weight loss

CNS: insomnia, fatigue, paresthesias, headache, dizziness, visual disturbances, papilledema, corneal opacities

Musculoskeletal: arthralgia, joint and muscle pain and stiffness

Urinary: proteinuria, hematuria

Other: bruising, edema, respiratory infections, abnormal menses, herpes simplex infections, increased SGOT, SGPT, alkaline phosphatase and fasting serum glucose, elevated platelet counts, hyperuricemia, elevated cholesterol, decreased high-density lipoproteins

CONTRAINDICATIONS
Pregnancy (drug causes fetal abnormalities), patients sensitive to parabens (preservatives in the formulation). *Cautious use* in obese, diabetic, or alcoholic patients, as triglyceride levels may be excessively high

INTERACTIONS
Vitamin A supplements together with isotretinoin may result in increased toxicity

Tetracyclines and isotretinoin can lead to pseudotumor cerebri or papilledema

Concomitant ingestion of alcohol may further increase serum triglyceride levels

NURSING CONSIDERATIONS

Nursing Alert
- Monitor results of serum lipid determinations, which should be performed prior to initiation of therapy and at weekly or biweekly intervals during therapy. Increased triglyceride and cholesterol levels and decreased high-density lipoprotein levels occur in up to 25% of patients, but they revert to pretreatment levels when therapy is terminated.

1. Provide emotional support, as appropriate, during drug treatment of severe acne.

PATIENT EDUCATION
With fertile woman, see *Warning* under Significant Adverse Reactions and see also applicable portions of Patient Education for etretinate.

1. Explain that periodic ophthalmic examinations should be performed during treatment and that any changes in visual function should be reported to drug prescriber.
2. Inform patient that acne may temporarily worsen during initial stages of therapy.
3. Instruct patient to avoid prolonged exposure to sun because photosensitivity reactions can occur.
4. Discuss the importance of reducing caloric intake, dietary fat, and alcohol consumption to minimize elevations in serum triglyceride levels.
5. Inform patient that musculoskeletal disorders may occur (incidence is 15%–20%) but that symptoms are usually mild, seldom require discontinuation of therapy, and disappear upon cessation of drug.
6. If a second course of therapy is required, inform patient that it will probably not begin until at least 8 weeks after termination of the first course. Clinical improvement may, however, continue during drug-free periods.

Tretinoin
Retin-A
(CAN) Stie VAA, Vitamin A Acid

Tretinoin (retinoic acid) is available for topical application in the treatment of acne vulgaris. Its effectiveness approaches that of steroid–antibiotic combinations and generally surpasses that of most other currently available topical acne preparations. Its use is frequently associated with erythema and desquamation, however, and some patients do not tolerate the drug. Tretinoin is available as a gel, cream, or liquid.

In addition to its usefulness in treating acne, topical tretinoin has been advocated as a "wrinkle remover" for photoaged skin. Although much publicity has surrounded this potential applica-

MECHANISM
Promotes epidermal cell turnover and facilitates desquamation; suppresses keratin synthesis and prevents formation of comedones

USES
Treatment of acne vulgaris, especially grades I, II, and III; not effective against acne conglobata (i.e., deep cystic nodules and extensive pustules)
Treatment of several forms of skin cancer (investigational use)
Treatment of premature skin aging and wrinkling (investigational use)

DOSAGE
Apply once a day for at least 4 to 6 weeks, at bedtime, and cover entire area lightly; reduce frequency of application as lesions respond

COMMON SIDE EFFECTS
Stinging, feeling of warmth, dryness, peeling, erythema

SIGNIFICANT ADVERSE REACTIONS
Edema, blistering, pigmentary changes, photosensitivity, and contact dermatitis (rare)

CONTRAINDICATIONS
No absolute contraindications. *Cautious use* in persons with eczema and in pregnant or nursing women

INTERACTIONS
Increased skin peeling can occur if tretinoin is used with sulfur, resorcinol, benzoyl peroxide, or salicylic acid
Excessive skin drying can result from concomitant use of tretinoin and products containing high concentrations of alcohol, astringents, or lime

PATIENT EDUCATION
1. Caution patient to minimize exposure to sunlight or sunlamps because photosensitivity reactions can occur. Experimental animal studies have indicated a tumorigenic potential for tretinoin upon exposure to ultraviolet light, although the significance of this effect in humans is not clear.
2. Warn patient to keep drug away from eyes, mouth, and other mucous membranes because irritation can occur.
3. Inform patient that slight stinging and feelings of warmth frequently occur, and dryness and peeling of skin are to be expected.
4. Inform patient that condition may *temporarily* worsen early in therapy owing to drug action on deeper, previously invisible lesions.
5. Instruct patient to notify drug prescriber if significant erythema or irritation occurs because the frequency of application may need to be reduced or the medication may need to be temporarily discontinued.

VITAMIN D PREPARATIONS

Calciferol
Calcitriol
Cholecalciferol
Dihydrotachysterol
Ergocalciferol

The term *vitamin D* is commonly applied to two related fat-soluble substances, ergocalciferol (D_2) and cholecalciferol (D_3), which are formed from the provitamins ergosterol and 7-dehydrocholesterol, respectively, by ultraviolet (UV) irradiation. The principal source of endogenous vitamin D in humans is the synthesis of D_3 from 7-dehydrocholesterol upon exposure to the UV rays of the sun. Vitamin D_3 is then converted by hepatic microsomal enzymes to calcifediol (25-hydroxycholecalciferol), the principal transport form of vitamin D_3. Calcifediol possesses minor intrinsic vitamin D activity and is further metabolized in the kidney to calcitriol (1,25 dihydroxycholecalciferol), the most active form of vitamin D_3. Ergocalciferol and cholecalciferol, as well as calcifediol and calcitriol, are available for clinical use, as is dihydrotachysterol, a vitamin D analog that is converted by the liver to 25-hydroxydihydrotachysterol, which elevates serum calcium levels.

Vitamin D_2 is the form usually found in commercial vitamin preparations and in fortified milk, bread, and cereals. Because in humans there is no difference in activity between vitamin D_2 and D_3, *vitamin D* will be used as the collective term for all substances, natural and synthetic, having similar activity.

Dosage of the vitamin is measured in international units (IU), one IU of vitamin D activity being equal to 0.025 μg ergocalciferol.

Following a general discussion of vitamin D, the individual vitamin D preparations are listed in Table 74-2.

MECHANISM
Enhances the active absorption of calcium and phosphorus from the small intestine, facilitates their resorption from bone, and promotes their reabsorption by the renal tubules; plasma levels of calcium and phosphorus are therefore maintained at levels adequate for neuromuscular activity, mineralization of bone, and other calcium-dependent functions

USES
Prevention or treatment of vitamin D deficiency (cholecalciferol)
Treatment of refractory (vitamin D–resistant) rickets (ergocalciferol)
Treatment of familial hypophosphatemia and hypoparathyroidism (ergocalciferol, dihydrotachysterol)
Treatment of metabolic bone disease or hypocalcemia in patients on chronic renal dialysis (calcifediol, calcitriol)
Treatment of acute, chronic, or latent forms of postoperative tetany or idiopathic tetany

DOSAGE
See Table 74-2

FATE
Well absorbed from the intestine, D_3 more completely and more rapidly than D_2; bile is essential for absorption; stored

primarily in the liver, with small amounts in skin, bones, and CNS; in the plasma, vitamin D is bound to albumin and alpha globulins; plasma half-life of the various derivatives varies from 24 hours (ergocalciferol) up to 20 days (calcifediol); primary route of excretion is the bile; very small amounts are found in the urine

SIGNIFICANT ADVERSE REACTIONS

(Usually due to overdosage: hypervitaminosis D syndrome)

Renal: polyuria, nocturia, elevated BUN, hypercalciuria, azotemia, nephrocalcinosis, proteinuria, urinary casts, renal insufficiency

GI: anorexia, nausea, vomiting, constipation or diarrhea, metallic taste, dry mouth

Other: acidosis, anemia, weakness, headache, irritability, photophobia, conjunctivitis, pancreatitis, hypertension, arrhythmias, vascular and soft-tissue calcification, muscle stiffness and pain, bone demineralization, mental retardation in children, dwarfism, hyperthermia, elevated SGOT and SGPT

CONTRAINDICATIONS

Hypercalcemia, malabsorption syndrome, hypervitaminosis D, and renal osteodystrophy with hyperphosphatemia. *Cautious use* in patients with a history of renal stones and in pregnant or nursing women and young children

INTERACTIONS

Mineral oil and cholestyramine resin can impair vitamin D absorption

Phenytoin, primidone, and barbiturates may reduce the effectiveness of vitamin D by increasing its metabolic inactivation

Thiazide diuretics may potentiate vitamin D–induced hypercalcemia in hypoparathyroid patients

Vitamin D may increase the likelihood of cardiac arrhythmias with digitalis drugs

The effects of verapamil and other calcium channel blockers may be reduced by vitamin D–induced hypercalcemia

Magnesium-containing antacids used together with vitamin D may result in development of hypermagnesemia

Table 74-2
Vitamin D Preparations

Drug	Preparations	Usual Dosage Range	Nursing Implications
Calcifediol Calderol	Capsules: 20 μg, 50 μg	Initially, 300 μg–350 μg/wk, on a daily or alternate-day schedule; may increase at 4-wk intervals as needed. Usual maintenance range, 50 μg–100 μg/day	Hydroxylated metabolite of cholecalciferol; principal serum transport form of vitamin D_3; converted in the kidneys to calcitriol; increases serum calcium and decreases alkaline phosphatase and parathyroid hormone levels
Calcitriol Calcijex, Rocaltrol	Capsules: 0.25-μg, 0.5 μg. Injection: 1 μg/mL, 2 μg/mL	Initially, 0.25 μg/day; increase by 0.25-μg/day increments at 4–8-wk intervals; hemodialysis patients generally require doses of 0.5 μg–1 μg/day. *Hypoparathyroidism:* 0.5 μg–2.0 μg daily	Most active metabolite of vitamin D; potent hypercalcemic agent primarily used for treating hypocalcemia in patients undergoing renal dialysis; avoid magnesium-containing antacids because hypermagnesemia may occur, and do not give other vitamin D supplements during therapy; advise patients to note occurrence of weakness, vomiting, or muscle or bone pain, as these may indicate hypercalcemia
Cholecalciferol Delta-D	Tablets: 400 IU, 1000 IU	400 IU–1000 IU daily	Used as a dietary supplement in vitamin D deficiency states; precursor of calcifediol and calcitriol
Dihydrotachysterol DHT, Hytakerol	Tablets: 0.125 mg, 0.2 mg, 0.4 mg. Capsules: 0.125 mg. Oral solution: 0.25 mg/mL, 0.2 mg/5 mL	Initially, 0.8 mg–2.4 mg daily for several days. Maintenance doses are 0.2 mg–1 mg daily as needed to maintain normal serum calcium levels	Potent vitamin D preparation that is more effective than ergocalciferol in mobilizing calcium from bone but shorter acting; primarily used in treating tetany and symptoms of hypoparathyroidism; maximal hypercalcemic effects require 1–2 wk to develop; safety margin with drug is rather small; be alert for symptoms of hypercalcemia
Ergocalciferol Calciferol, Drisdol	Capsules: 50,000 IU. Tablets: 50,000 IU. Liquid: 8,000 IU/mL. Injection: 500,000 IU/mL	*Vitamin D–resistant rickets:* 50,000 IU–500,000 IU daily depending on severity of disease. *Hypoparathyroidism:* 50,000 IU–200,000 IU daily *plus* 4 g calcium lactate 6 times/day	IM administration is necessary in patients with GI, liver, or biliary disease associated with malabsorption of vitamin D; range between therapeutic and toxic doses is small; serum calcium concentration is maintained between 9 mg and 10 mg/dL; use with *caution* in patients with impaired kidney function or kidney stones

NURSING CONSIDERATIONS

Nursing Alerts
- Closely monitor results of serum calcium level determinations (normal range 9 mg–11 mg/dl), which should be obtained biweekly during early therapy, and assess patient for evidence of hypercalcemia or hypervitaminosis D (see Significant Adverse Reactions), because the range between therapeutic and toxic doses of vitamin D is very small. If hypercalemia occurs, drug should be discontinued and supportive measures instituted (e.g., high fluid intake, restriction of dietary calcium, laxatives).
- If overdosage is severe, be prepared to administer intravenous diuretics, corticosteroids (150 mg/day cortisone or equivalent), and sodium citrate (2.5% IV infusion).
- Monitor results of serum phosphorus, magnesium, and alkaline phosphatase and 24-hour urinary calcium and phosphorus determinations, which should be obtained periodically during treatment.

1. Ensure that patient's diet is critically evaluated before vitamin D supplementation is initiated. Supplementation is usually unnecessary for patient who eats fortified foods and is exposed to normal amounts of sunlight.
2. Be prepared to administer ergocalciferol IM in patient with gastrointestinal, biliary, or liver disease associated with vitamin D malabsorption.
3. Collaborate with drug prescriber and dietician regarding calcium intake during treatment. Drug is often given with supplemental calcium salts and/or high-calcium foods because proper amount of additional calcium enhances therapeutic response.
4. Institute appropriate interventions to enhance patient's compliance with drug regimen, dietary recommendations, and calcium supplementation (when indicated) to minimize danger of untoward reactions (see **Plans of Nursing Care 1** in Chapter 4 and **2** in Chapter 7).

PATIENT EDUCATION
1. Warn pregnant women not to exceed RDA (400 IU/day) because high doses have been associated with fetal abnormalities in animal studies.
2. Warn patient of the hazards of excessive or indiscriminate use of vitamin D, and explain that dosage levels are individually adjusted as the deficiency abates.
3. Inform patient that improvement may develop slowly (7–10 days) and that effects may persist for up to 30 days after therapy is terminated.

VITAMIN E

Aquasol E and Other Manufacturers

The term *vitamin E* is commonly used generically to describe eight naturally occurring tocopherols possessing vitamin E activity. Alpha-tocopherol comprises about 90% of the tocopherols found in animal tissues, is the most biologically active of the eight, and is available both naturally in vegetable oils and other foods as well as synthetically. Because the potencies of the different forms of vitamin E vary somewhat, dosage is standardized in international units (IUs) according to activity. The following list indicates relative potencies of *1 mg* of the various clinically available tocopherols:

d-alpha tocopherol = 1.49 IU
dl-alpha tocopherol = 1.1 IU
d-alpha tocopheryl acetate = 1.36 IU
dl-alpha tocopheryl acetate = 1.0 IU
d-alpha tocopheryl acid succinate = 1.21 IU
dl-alpha tocopheryl acid succinate = 0.89 IU

Although RDAs have been published for vitamin E, there is little conclusive evidence that it is of significant nutritional or therapeutic value. Deficiencies of vitamin E in humans are rare, inasmuch as adequate amounts are supplied in the ordinary diet. Low levels have occasionally been noted in severely malnourished infants and in patients with prolonged fat malabsorption or acanthocytosis. On the basis of occasional relief of experimentally produced deficiency symptoms in laboratory animals, vitamin E has been advocated by some for treatment of an imposing array of human ills, including sterility, habitual abortion, muscular dystrophy, cardiovascular and peripheral vascular disorders, fever blisters, and schizophrenia as well as for improvement of athletic performance. These claims have not been substantiated, and use of vitamin E supplementation, other than in clearly established deficiency states, cannot be justified.

MECHANISM
Incompletely understood; action appears to be due to its antioxidant properties; prevents oxidation of essential cellular constituents and products; may serve as a cofactor in enzyme reactions, play a role in hematopoiesis and hemoglobin formation, protect red blood cells from hemolysis, interfere with platelet aggregation, and enhance utilization of vitamin A

USES
Prevention or treatment of vitamin E deficiency states

Control of dry or chapped skin and temporary relief of minor skin disorders, for example, itching, sunburn, abrasions (topical use only)

Investigational uses include reduction of the toxic effects of oxygen therapy on lung parenchyma (bronchopulmonary dysplasia) and the retina (retrolental fibroplasia) in premature infants and adjunctive treatment of hemolytic anemia in infants

DOSAGE
Oral (deficiency states): 50 IU to 1000 IU/day have been employed, depending on severity (RDA is approximately 15 IU)
Topical: apply as needed

FATE
Readily absorbed from GI tract if fat absorption is adequate; widely distributed in the body and stored in tissues for extended periods, providing a continual source of the vitamin; placental transfer is poor; largely excreted in the feces by way of the bile, smaller amounts appearing as metabolites in the urine

SIGNIFICANT ADVERSE REACTIONS
Minimal, even at very large doses; occasionally GI distress, muscle weakness

A *hypervitaminosis E syndrome* has been described, characterized by fatigue, headache, nausea, weakness, diarrhea, flatulence, blurred vision, and dermatitis.

INTERACTIONS
Vitamin E may enhance the action of oral anticoagulants by reducing levels of vitamin K–dependent clotting factors

Vitamin E can reduce the efficacy of oral iron preparations

Vitamin E requirements may be *increased* in patients taking large doses of oral iron and *decreased* in persons receiving selenium, antioxidants, or sulfur-containing amino acids

NURSING CONSIDERATION

1. Note that there is *no* conclusive evidence that vitamin E is beneficial for any condition other than those listed under Uses

VITAMIN K

Menadiol sodium diphosphate (K_4)   Phytonadione (K_1)

The term *vitamin K* refers to two structurally similar compounds that possess the ability to promote hepatic synthesis of certain blood clotting factors. The primary source of vitamin K in humans is via absorption of phytonadione (vitamin K_1) synthesized in the gut by intestinal bacteria. In addition, vitamin K is found in many foods (see Table 74-1), although in most cases these represent a minor source of utilizable vitamin. Vitamin K_1 (phytonadione) is the only naturally occurring vitamin K used clinically; however, this lipid-soluble derivative is also prepared synthetically. The other synthetic vitamin K compound employed therapeutically is menadiol sodium diphosphate (vitamin K_4), a water-soluble analog that is approximately one half as potent as menadione (K_3), to which it is converted in vivo. Phytonadione is the preferred drug for treating hypoprothrombinemia, because it is the most potent of the derivatives and exhibits the fastest onset and longest duration of action. However, adequate absorption of phytonadione occurs only in the presence of bile salts, whereas K_4 can be adequately absorbed without bile salts.

The available vitamin K derivatives are discussed as a group, then listed individually in Table 74-3. Phytonadione has been reviewed previously in Chapter 35 as an antidote to overdosage with oral anticoagulants and is considered only briefly here.

MECHANISM

Promote hepatic synthesis of blood clotting factors II, VII, IX, and X, probably by functioning as an essential cofactor for microsomal enzyme systems that activate the precursors of these clotting factors

USES

Treatment of vitamin K deficiency due to antibacterial therapy

Treatment of hypoprothrombinemia secondary to impaired ab-

Table 74-3
Vitamin K Preparations

Drug	Preparations	Usual Dosage Range	Nursing Implications
K_1 (Phytonadione) AquaMEPHYTON, Konakion, Mephyton	Tablets: 5 mg Injection: 2 mg/mL, 10 mg/mL	*Hypoprothrombinemia and anticoagulant-induced prothrombin deficiency* 2.5 mg–25 mg initially; repeat in 6–8 h after parenteral injection *or* 12–48 h after oral administration until prothrombin time is in desired range *Hemorrhagic disease of newborn* Prophylaxis: 0.5 mg–2 mg IM *or* (less desirable) 1 mg–5 mg to the mother 12–24 h before delivery Treatment: 1 mg–2 mg SC *or* IM daily	Fat-soluble derivative that is the preferred antidote to oral anticoagulant overdose; only vitamin K preparation indicated for hemorrhagic disease of the newborn; requires bile salts for oral absorption; injection is available as an aqueous colloidal solution (AquaMEPHYTON) for IV, SC, or IM use and as an aqueous dispersion (Konakion) for IM use only; do *not* exceed 1 mg/min when injecting IV; use smaller doses as antidote for short-acting anticoagulants and larger doses for longer-acting anticoagulants; protect solutions from light
K_4 (Menadiol sodium diphosphate) Synkayvite	Tablets: 5 mg Injections: 5 mg/mL, 10 mg/mL, 37.5 mg/mL	*Oral* 5 mg–10 mg/day *Parenteral (SC, IM, IV)* Adults: 5 mg–15 mg 1–2 times a day Children: 5 mg–10 mg 1–2 times a day	Water-soluble derivative of vitamin K that is converted to menadione in vivo; approximately one half as potent as menadione; well absorbed orally and does not require presence of bile salts; used principally for hypoprothrombinemia due to obstructive jaundice, biliary fistulas, or administration of salicylates or antibiotics; single dose usually restores prothrombin time within 8–24 h; may induce hemolysis of erythrocytes in glucose-6-phosphate dehydrogenase–deficient patients; do not infuse together with other drugs; may be given with any IV fluid

sorption or synthesis of vitamin K, for example, obstructive jaundice, biliary fistulas, ulcerative colitis, sprue, celiac disease, regional enteritis, intestinal resection, cystic fibrosis, salicylate therapy

Treatment of oral anticoagulant–induced prothrombin deficiency (phytonadione *only*)

Prophylaxis and treatment of hemorrhagic disease of the newborn (phytonadione *only*)

DOSAGE
See Table 74-3

FATE
Phytonadione is absorbed from the GI tract by way of the lymph and only in the presence of bile salts. Menadiol is absorbed directly into the bloodstream even in the absence of bile. Bleeding is controlled within 6 hours to 12 hours following oral administration and within 3 hours to 6 hours following parenteral injection. It is initially concentrated in the liver, but levels decline very rapidly. There is little accumulation in other tissues, and the drug is rapidly metabolized. It is excreted both in the bile and urine.

COMMON SIDE EFFECTS
Flushing sensation with IV injection

SIGNIFICANT ADVERSE REACTIONS
Oral: GI upset, nausea, vomiting, headache

Parenteral: dizziness, tachycardia, weak pulse, chills, fever, sweating, hypotension, dyspnea, cyanosis, hypersensitivity reactions, anaphylaxis, pain and swelling at injection site, and erythematous skin reactions; in newborns, hyperbilirubinemia, kernicterus, and hemolytic anemia have occurred, especially with menadiol

CONTRAINDICATIONS
Menadiol is contraindicated in infants and in women during the last few weeks of pregnancy and during labor (see Significant Adverse Reactions). *Cautious use* in patients with liver disease

INTERACTIONS
Vitamin K antagonizes the anticoagulant action of coumarins and indandiones, but not heparin

Mineral oil or cholestyramine may impair GI absorption of K_1 but *not* K_4

Antibiotics may reduce endogenous vitamin-K activity by decreasing its synthesis by intestinal flora. Increased bleeding can result

NURSING CONSIDERATIONS
See phytonadione in Chapter 35. See also Table 74-3 for specific information on each derivative. In addition:

Nursing Alerts
- Seek clarification before administering repeated large doses if initial response is poor because excessive dosage can further depress hepatic function.
- Note that phytonadione is the only vitamin K analog indicated for treating hemorrhagic disease of the newborn, especially in premature infants, because increased bilirubinemia, severe hemolytic anemia, and kernicterus, possibly resulting in brain damage or death, can occur with use of menadiol (K_4).

Selected Bibliography
Alperin JB: Coagulopathy caused by vitamin K deficiency in critically ill hospitalized patients. J Am Med Assoc 258:1916, 1987

Bieri JG, Corash L, Hubbard VS: Medical uses of vitamin E. N Engl J Med 308:1063, 1983

Bieri JG, McKenna MC: Expressing dietary values for fat-soluble vitamins: Changes in concepts and terminology. Am J Clin Nutr 34:289, 1981

Bigby M, Stern RS: Adverse reactions to isotretinoin. J Am Acad Dermatol 18:543, 1988

Cerrato PL: When to worry about vitamin overdose. RN 48(10):69, 1985

Deluca HF, Schnoes HK: Vitamin D: Recent advances. Annu Rev Biochem 52:411, 1983

Herbert V: Toxicity of 25,000 IV vitamin A supplements in "health" food users. Am J Clin Nutr 36:185, 1982

Leo MA, Lieber CS: Hepatic vitamin A depletion in alcoholic liver injury. N Engl J Med 307:597, 1982

Luke B: Megavitamins and pregnancy: A dangerous combination. MCN 10:18, 1985

Machlin LJ (ed): Vitamin E: A Comprehensive Treatise. New York, Marcel Dekker, 1980

O'Connor ME, Livingstone DS, Hannah J, Wilkins D: Vitamin K deficiency and breast feeding. Am J Dis Child 137:601, 1983

Orfanos CE, Ehlert R, Gollnick, H: The retinoids: A review of their clinical pharmacology and therapeutic use. Drugs 34:459, 1987.

Spron MB, Roberts AB, Goodman DS (eds): The Retinoids, vols 1 and 2. New York, Academic Press, 1984

SUMMARY. FAT-SOLUBLE VITAMINS

Drug	Preparations	Usual Dosage Range
Vitamin A Aquasol A, Del-Vi-A	Capsules: 10,000 IU, 25,000 IU, 50,000 IU Drops: 5000 IU/0.1 mL Injection: 50,000 IU/mL	*Oral* Adults: 100,000 IU–500,000 IU/day for 3 days, then 50,000 IU/day for 2 wk, then 10,000 IU–20,000 IU/day for 2 mo Children: 10,000 IU–15,000 IU/day *IM* Adults: 100,000 IU/day for 3 days, then 50,000 IU/day for 2 wk Children 1–8 yr: 17,500 IU–35,000 IU/day for 10 days Infants: 7500–15,000 IU/day for 10 days
Vitamin A Analogs		
Etretinate Tegison	Capsules: 10 mg, 25 mg	0.75–1.0 mg/kg/day initially in divided doses; reduce to 0.5–0.75 mg/kg/day after 8–16 wk
Isotretinoin Accutane	Capsules: 10 mg, 20 mg, 40 mg	1–2 mg/kg/day in 2 divided doses for 15–20 wk
Tretinoin Retin-A	Cream: 0.05%, 0.1% Gel: 0.025%, 0.01% Liquid: 0.05%	Apply daily at bedtime and cover lightly; continue until lesions have responded (4–6 wk), then reduce frequency of application
Vitamin D Preparations	*See* Table 74-2	
Vitamin E	Capsules: 100 IU, 200 IU, 400 IU, 600 IU, 1000 IU Capsules: 73.5 mg, 165 mg, 294 mg, 330 mg Tablets: 200 IU, 400 IU Drops: 50 mg/mL Injection: 200 IU/mL	*Deficiency states* 50 IU–1000 IU/day depending on severity *Topical:* apply several times a day as needed
Vitamin K	*See* Table 74-3	

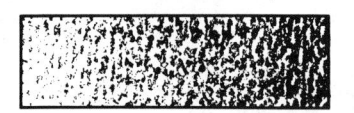

75 NUTRIENTS, MINERALS, FLUIDS, AND ELECTROLYTES

The fluid composition of the body is normally kept reasonably constant despite the many stresses placed upon it. Significant alterations in the volume and composition of the internal fluid environment can, however, result from disease, trauma, or drug therapy, as well as from a number of other external factors. Disturbances in fluid and electrolyte balance may involve changes in pH, volume, osmolarity, or concentrations of individual ions, and can seriously impair the normal metabolic activity of body organs. Thus, the chemical constituents of the body (i.e., electrolytes, minerals, amino acids, fluids, proteins, lipids) are often administered either individually or in combination to correct acute or chronic deficiency states, and such a procedure is termed *nutritional replacement therapy*.

This chapter considers those nutrients, fluids, and electrolytes, both orally and parenterally administered, that are commonly used to supply the nutritional needs of patients suffering from a deficiency of one or more of these substances. The oral nutritional supplements are reviewed first, followed by a discussion of parenteral nutrients. Not all of the substances used as nutritional supplements are considered here, inasmuch as several have been mentioned in other chapters dealing with drugs affecting specific organs with which a particular mineral or electrolyte is intimately associated. Thus, calcium is discussed with parathyroid hormone and calcitonin in Chapter 41, iron is reviewed along with other drugs used to treat anemia in Chapter 34, and iodine and iodide salts are considered in Chapter 40 with the thyroid hormones. The vitamins are discussed individually in Chapters 73 and 74.

ORAL NUTRITIONAL SUPPLEMENTS

Bioflavonoids
Calcium caseinate
l-Carnitine
Choline
Corn oil
Fluoride
Glucose polymers
Inositol
Lactase
Lecithin
l-Lysine
Magnesium
Manganese
Medium-chain triglycerides
Omega-3 polyunsaturated fatty acids
Oral electrolyte mixture
Para-aminobenzoic acid
Phosphorus
Potassium
Protein hydrolysates
Safflower oil
Sodium bicarbonate
Sodium chloride
l-Tryptophan
Zinc

The substances used orally for correcting nutritional deficiency states include minerals, electrolytes, amino acids, proteins, and lipids, as well as a few other miscellaneous drugs. Perhaps the most widely used oral electrolytes are potassium and fluoride, and these preparations are considered individually in detail below. The remaining oral nutritional supplements are listed in Table 75-1.

Potassium
Several manufacturers

Potassium is the principal intracellular cation and is essential for many vital physiologic processes, including nerve impulse transmission; skeletal, cardiac, and smooth muscle contraction; and maintenance of intracellular tonicity and renal function. Potassium depletion occurs most frequently as a result of diuretic therapy but may also be due to hyperaldosteronism, severe diarrhea, or diabetic ketoacidosis. It is usually accompanied by chloride loss as well and is therefore frequently associated with metabolic alkalosis. Symptoms of potassium depletion include muscle weakness, cramping, fatigue, disturbances in cardiac rhythm, and inability to concentrate urine. The salts of potassium available for oral use are the chloride, gluconate, acetate, citrate, and bicarbonate. When hypokalemia is associated with alkalosis, the chloride salt should be used. When acidosis is present, one of the other salts is indicated. When oral replacement therapy is not feasible (as with severe vomiting, prolonged diuresis, marked diabetic acidosis) parenteral (IV infusion) therapy is indicated (see Table 75-2).

The usual adult dietary intake of potassium ranges from 40 mEq to 150 mEq/day. Despite this variability in intake, renal regulatory mechanisms normally maintain plasma potassium levels within the narrow physiologic range.

MECHANISM
Essential ion for maintenance of excitability of nerves and muscles, as well as acid–base balance

USES
Prevention and treatment of hypokalemia, for example, resulting from diuretic therapy, prolonged vomiting or diarrhea, diabetes, hepatic cirrhosis, inadequate dietary intake, malabsorption, hyperaldosteronism, or nephropathy

DOSAGE
NOTE
The dosage of potassium (K^+) is given in milliequivalents (mEq) of the ion. Clinically available salts of potassium (with the potassium content) are as follows:

Potassium acetate 10.2 mEq K^+/g
Potassium bicarbonate 10 mEq K^+/g
Potassium chloride 13.4 mEq K^+/g
Potassium citrate 9.25 mEq K^+/g
Potassium gluconate 4.3 mEq K^+/g

Prevention of hypokalemia: 16 mEq to 24 mEq/day
Treatment of deficiency states: 40 mEq to 100 mEq/day

FATE
Oral potassium is well absorbed; renal excretion occurs primarily by secretion in the distal portion of the nephron; most of the filtered load of potassium is reabsorbed in the proximal tubule; fecal excretion is minimal and does not play a significant role in potassium hemostasis

COMMON SIDE EFFECTS
Nausea, abdominal discomfort, vomiting, diarrhea

SIGNIFICANT ADVERSE REACTIONS
GI bleeding and perforation, hyperkalemia (paresthesias, flaccid paralysis, confusion, weakness, hypotension, respiratory distress, arrhythmias, cardiac depression, heart block)

CONTRAINDICATIONS
Severe renal impairment with oliguria, anuria or azotemia; Addison's disease; acute dehydration; heat cramps; hyperkalemia in patients receiving potassium-sparing diuretics; in addition, solid dosage forms of potassium are contraindicated in patients in whom there is delayed passage of contents through the GI tract. *Cautious use* in patients with systemic acidosis, acute dehydration, chronic renal dysfunction, cardiac disease, adrenal insufficiency, or peptic ulcer

INTERACTIONS
Combinations of potassium salts with potassium-sparing diuretics can result in severe hyperkalemia

Increased serum potassium decreases both toxicity and effectiveness of digitalis drugs

Concurrent use of salt substitutes with potassium supplements can lead to hyperkalemia

Concomitant administration of anticholinergics and oral potassium products may increase the likelihood of GI erosion owing to slowed GI motility and delayed gastric emptying

Captopril can cause potassium retention, leading to hyperkalemia

NURSING CONSIDERATIONS

Nursing Alerts
- Do *not* administer potassium chloride by IV push or in concentrated amounts by any route.
- Administer only liquid dosage forms, never solid forms (i.e., tablets, capsules, powders) to patient with reduced GI passage because gastric and intestinal ulceration can occur.
- Observe patient for development of severe vomiting, GI bleeding (i.e., black stools), weakness, and abdominal pain or distention. Drug should be discontinued immediately if these occur.
- Closely monitor results of acid–base balance, serum electrolyte, and ECG determinations during treatment to avoid potassium intoxication, which can result in arrythmias and cardiac depression.

1. Monitor intake–output ratio and immediately report any significant change in renal function. Potassium intoxication with oral administration is rare in persons with normal kidney function.
2. Assist with evaluation of drug effects. *Serum* potassium concentrations are not always an accurate indication of total *intracellular* potassium levels. Treatment of potassium depletion, therefore, requires careful assessment of clinical status as well as laboratory evaluations.

PATIENT EDUCATION
1. Instruct patient to swallow coated tablets whole because chewing them will increase likelihood of GI irritation. They should be taken with a full glass of water, preferably after meals or with food.
2. Instruct patient to avoid use of salt substitutes, many of which contain potassium, and excessive use of laxatives, which can alter electrolyte balance.
3. Instruct patient to dissolve powders or effervescent tablets in 4 to 8 oz of cold water, juice, or other beverage, and to sip slowly.

Fluoride

Luride, Pediaflor, Phos-Flur, and other manufacturers
(CAN) Fluoron, Karidium

The fluoride ion, used either orally or topically, is employed as an aid in the prevention of dental caries. It is most commonly administered to young children in combination with vitamins and minerals in the form of drops or tablets. Fluoride can also be used locally as a mouthwash by persons susceptible to dental caries.

MECHANISM
Incorporated into external layers of dental enamel, making it more resistant to erosion by acid; may also facilitate osteoblastic activity of bone

USES
Aid in prevention of dental caries where community water supplies are low in fluoride

Treatment of osteoporosis; doses up to 60 mg/day, in combination with calcium, vitamin D, and/or estrogen (investigational use only)

DOSAGE
(Prevention of dental caries)
Oral: 0.25 mg to 1 mg/day, depending on age
Topical: 5 mL to 10 mL once a day as a mouth rinse after brushing; rinse for 1 minute, then expectorate

FATE
Rapidly absorbed orally; widely distributed and quickly deposited in teeth and bone; quickly excreted by the kidneys

SIGNIFICANT ADVERSE REACTIONS
Eczema, atopic dermatitis, urticaria, nausea, GI distress, headache, weakness, staining of the teeth (topical only)

Prolonged overdosage can lead to mottling of the tooth enamel. Acute ingestion of large doses of fluoride may cause excessive salivation, GI disturbances, irritability, tetany, hyperreflexia, seizures, and cardiac failure

CONTRAINDICATIONS
Intake of drinking water containing 0.7 ppm or more of fluoride; sodium-free diets

NURSING CONSIDERATION
1. Note that acute fluoride overdosage can result in excessive salivation and GI disturbances. Emesis, which invariably occurs with ingestion of large amounts, serves as a protective mechanism.

PATIENT EDUCATION
1. Advise patient to use plastic container to dilute rinse or drops.
2. Instruct patient to take tablets or drops after meals but to avoid milk or dairy products with sodium fluoride tablets because GI absorption is reduced.
3. Encourage patient using rinse to apply immediately after brushing teeth and just before retiring at night. Instruct patient not to swallow while using rinse and to

(*Text continued on page 778*)

Table 75-1
Oral Nutritional Supplements

Drug	Preparations	Usual Dosage Range	Nursing Implications
Minerals and Electrolytes			
Magnesium Almora, Magonate, Magnate, Nephro-Mag, Slow-Mag	Tablets: 27 mg (as magnesium gluconate), 100 mg (as magnesium–amino acids chelate), 250 mg of magnesium carbonate Tablets (slow release): 64 mg (as magnesium chloride)	27 mg–100 mg 2–4 times a day	RDAs are 200 mg (children 4–6 yr), 300 mg to 400 mg (adults), and 450 mg (pregnant or lactating women); excessive amounts may produce diarrhea; necessary for a number of enzyme systems and for nerve conduction and muscle contraction; deficiency is rare in well-nourished persons
Manganese	Tablets: 20 mg, 50 mg	20 mg/day–50 mg/day	Need in human nutrition is not established; functions as a cofactor in many enzyme systems; localized primarily in mitochondria
Oral Electrolyte Mixture Gastrolyte Oral, Infalyte, Lytren, Pedialyte, Resol, Rehydralyte	Solution or powder (containing different electrolytes and dextrose or glucose)	Infants and young children: 1500 mL–2500 mL/m² Children (5–10 yr): 1 qt–2 qt/day Children over 10 yr and adults: 2 qt–3 qt/day (1 packet of powder is dissolved in 1 quart of water)	Used to replace water and electrolytes when food and fluid intake is sharply reduced (e.g., postoperatively, starvation) or when fluid loss is excessive (e.g., diarrhea, severe vomiting); severe, continual diarrhea requires parenteral replacement therapy; use only in recommended volumes to prevent electrolyte overload; reduce intake when other electrolytes are reinstituted; do not use in the presence of intestinal obstruction, intractable vomiting, adynamic ileus, perforated bowel, or impaired renal function; *avoid* mixing with other electrolyte-containing liquids (milk, fruit juice)
Phosphorus K-Phos Neutral, Neutra-Phos, Neutra-Phos-K, Uro-KP-Neutral	Tablets: 250 mg (with sodium and potassium) Capsules: 250 mg (with sodium and potassium) Powder for solution: 250 mg/75 mL (reconstituted solution with sodium and potassium)	1–2 tablets 4 times a day *or* Contents of 1 capsule mixed with 75 mL water 4 times a day *or* 75 mL reconstituted solution 4 times a day	Used as dietary supplement where diet is deficient, needs are increased, or GI absorption is impaired; RDAs are 800 mg (adults and children 1–10 yr) and 1200 mg (children 11–18 yr and pregnant or lactating women); phosphate can lower urinary calcium levels; a laxative effect is common early in therapy; *contraindicated* in hyperkalemia and Addison's disease
Sodium Chloride Slo-Salt	Tablets: 650 mg, 1 g, 2.25 g Tablets (slow-release): 600 mg Enteric-coated tablets: 1 g	0.5 g–1 g 3–6 times a day for prevention of dehydration and heat cramps	Used to replace excessive loss of sodium and chloride (e.g., resulting from perspiration or extreme diuresis) and to counteract excessive salt restriction; use *cautiously* in patients with congestive heart failure, renal disease, circulatory insufficiency, or electrolyte disturbances; also available with dextrose and vitamin B_1 (sodium chloride with dextrose) and in fixed combination with potassium chloride, calcium phosphate, and magnesium carbonate (Heatrol)
Sodium Bicarbonate	Tablets: 325 mg, 650 mg	325 mg to 2 g up to 4 times a day (maximum 16 g/day)	Used as a gastric, systemic, or urinary alkalinizer; *cautious use* in patients with congestive heart failure or renal impairment; 1 g provides 11.9 mEq sodium and bicarbonate; also used parenterally (*see* Table 75-2)
Zinc Sulfate Orazinc, Scrip-Zinc, Verazinc, Zinc-220, Zincate, Zinkaps (CAN) Anuzinc, PMS Egozinc **Zinc Gluconate**	Tablets: 66 mg, 200 mg, (equivalent to 15 mg and 47 mg elemental zinc, respectively) Capsules: 110 mg, 220 mg (equivalent to 25 mg and 50 mg elemental zinc, respectively) Tablets: 10 mg, 15 mg, 35 mg, 50 mg, 105 mg (equivalent to 1.4 mg, 2 mg, 5 mg, 7 mg, and 15 mg elemental zinc, respectively)	25 mg–50 mg elemental zinc a day	Important mineral for normal growth and repair of body tissues; symptoms of zinc deficiency include anorexia, loss of taste and olfactory sensation, mood changes, and growth retardation; used investigationally to treat delayed wound healing, acne, and rheumatoid arthritis, to improve the immune response in the elderly, and to delay onset of dementia in patients genetically at risk; RDAs are 10 mg (children 1–10 yr), 15 mg (adults), 20 mg–25 mg (pregnant or lactating women); excessive doses may produce severe vomiting, dehydration, and restlessness; GI upset can occur and can be minimized by taking drug with food or milk; zinc can impair absorption of tetracyclines

Continued

Table 75-1
Oral Nutritional Supplements (continued)

Drug	Preparations	Usual Dosage Range	Nursing Implications
Miscellaneous Nutritional Factors			
Bioflavonoids C Speridin, Citro-Flav, C.V.P., Flavons 500, Hesper, Pan-C-500, Peridin, Span C, Super-C	Tablets: 100 mg, 150 mg, 200 mg, 500 mg Capsules: 100 mg, 200 mg	100 mg–500 mg/day	Derived from green citrus fruits; previously used to reduce capillary fragility and referred to as vitamin P ("permeability"); no evidence that they are effective and no established need in human nutrition
Calcium Caseinate Casec	Powder: (containing 88% protein, 2% fat and 4.5% minerals)	Variable according to patient's requirements	Used as an infant formula modifier or as a diet supplement
l-Carnitine Carnitor, Vitacan	Tablets: 330 mg Capsules: 250 mg Liquid: 100 mg/mL	Adults: 1 g–3 g a day Children: 50–100 mg/kg/day	Naturally occurring amino acid derivative synthesized from methionine and lysine; acts to facilitate fatty acid metabolism and subsequent energy production; used in patients with primary carnitine deficiency, which can result in elevated triglycerides and free fatty acids and impaired ketogenesis, and, in children, reduced growth and development; GI distress is common; drug may also produce an unpleasant body odor; has been used experimentally to improve athletic performance
Choline	Tablets: 250 mg, 500 mg, 520 mg, 650 mg Powder	250 mg–1 g/day	A component of lecithin that has a lipotropic action and is essential for the formation of acetylcholine; average diet provides sufficient choline for body needs; has been used to treat fatty liver and cirrhosis, and to relieve symptoms of CNS disorders such as Huntington's disease and tardive dyskinesias; can cause GI disturbances and imparts an odor of decaying fish to the feces and occasionally the breath; used as free choline as well as bitartrate, chloride, and dihydrogen citrate salts
Corn Oil Lipomul Oral	Liquid: 10 g/15 mL	Adults: 45 mL 2–4 times a day Children: 30 mL 1–4 times a day	Used to increase caloric intake in malnourished or debilitated patients; use *cautiously* in persons with diabetes and gallbladder dysfunction; each dose contains 270 cal and 30 g fat
Glucose Polymers Moducal, Polycose, Pro-Mix, Sumacal	Liquid or powder: contains various amounts of carbohydrates, sodium, chloride, potassium, calcium and phosphorus	Add to foods or beverages and give in small, frequent feedings	Derived from cornstarch; supplies calories in patients unable to meet caloric needs with usual food intake or in patients on protein-, electrolyte-, and fat-restricted diets; *not* intended as the sole nutritional source; may be used for extended periods with diets containing all other essential nutrients
Inositol (CAN) Linodil	Tablets: 250 mg, 500 mg, 650 mg Powder	1 g–3 g/day in divided doses	An isomer of glucose possessing lipotropic activity in animals; physiologic role in humans is obscure and there is no evidence that it is clinically effective, although it has been used to treat liver disorders and disordered fat metabolism; dietary sources include mainly vegetables
Lactase Lact-Aid, Lactrase	Liquid: 1000 neutral lactase units/5-drop dose Capsules: 125 mg of standardized lactase enzyme Tablets: 3300 Lactase Units	5–10 drops per quart of milk *or* 1–2 capsules either added to a quart of milk or taken along with milk or dairy products	Powdered enzyme preparation used to facilitate digestion of milk lactose in patients with lactose intolerance
Lecithin	Capsules: 520 mg, 1.2 g Granules	1–2 capsules/day	A source of choline, inositol, phosphorus, and linoleic and linolenic acids employed as a dietary supplement (see choline, above)
l-Lysine Enisyl	Tablets: 312 mg, 325 mg, 334 mg, 500 mg	312 mg–1500 mg/day	An essential amino acid used as a dietary supplement to increase utilization of vegetable proteins; also available in combination with other amino acids, vitamins, and minerals in a variety of combination products

Continued

Table 75-1
Oral Nutritional Supplements (continued)

Drug	Preparations	Usual Dosage Range	Nursing Implications
Medium Chain Triglycerides MCT	Oil, consisting primarily of the triglycerides of C_8 and C_{10} saturated fatty acids	15 mL 3–4 times a day	A dietary supplement for persons who cannot efficiently digest and absorb conventional long-chain fatty acids; medium-chain triglycerides are more rapidly hydrolyzed than conventional food fat and are not dependent on bile salts for emulsification; may be mixed with juices, poured on salads or other foods, incorporated into sauces, or used in cooking and baking; use with *caution* in persons with hepatic cirrhosis; one dose weighs approximately 14 g and contains 115 cal
Omega-3 Polyunsaturated Fatty Acids Several manufacturers	Capsules: 500 mg, 1000 mg with vitamins, iron, and calcium	1–2 capsules 3 times a day with meals	Used as dietary supplements to *possibly* reduce cholesterol and triglyceride concentrations, prolong bleeding times, and decrease platelet aggregation; no conclusive evidence that drug decreases risk of coronary artery disease; diarrhea is common at high doses; *cautious use* in patients receiving other drugs that reduce platelet aggregation
Para-aminobenzoic Acid PABA, Potaba (CAN) Pabanol, RV Paba Stick	Tablets: 30 mg, 100 mg, 500 mg Capsules: 500 mg Powder	Adults: 12 g/day in 4–6 divided doses Children: 1 g/10 lb daily in divided doses	A substance found naturally associated with the B complex vitamins and essential for the functioning of a number of important biologic processes; considered "possibly effective" for scleroderma, dermatomyositis, morphea, pemphigus, and Peyronie's disease; dissolve tablets in liquid to minimize GI upset; drug should be taken with food; adverse reactions include anorexia, nausea, fever, and rash; use *cautiously* in patients with kidney impairment; do *not* give concurrently with sulfonamides, because PABA interferes with their antibacterial action; has no known human nutritional value; acts as a sunscreen when applied topically
Protein Hydrolysates A/G Pro, PDP Liquid Protein, Pro-Mix R.D.P., Propac	Tablets: 542 mg (45% amino acids with minerals) Capsules: 292 mg protein (with vitamins and minerals) Liquid: 15 g protein/30 mL Powder	2 tablets 3 times a day *or* 1 capsule 3 times a day *or* 30 ml liquid/day *or* 1–5 tbsp powder in liquid/day	Preparations of amino acids and peptides obtained by hydrolysis of larger proteins; used as dietary supplement to correct or prevent protein deficiency; optimum daily intake of dietary protein is 1 g/kg
Safflower Oil Microlipid	Emulsion: 50% fat	1–2 tbsp several times a day as necessary	A caloric and fatty-acid supplement used in malnourished patients and other persons with fatty-acid deficiencies; contains 4500 cal and 500 g fat per liter
l-Tryptophan Trofan, Tryptacin (CAN) Tryptan	Tablets: 300 mg, 500 mg, 667 mg, 1 g	500 mg–2 g/day in divided doses	An essential amino acid that serves as a precursor for serotonin; has been used experimentally as an antidepressant and hypnotic, although its clinical efficacy in this regard remains to be established; large doses (4 g–5 g) decrease sleep latency and increase sleep time

avoid eating or drinking for at least 30 minutes after use.
4. Instruct patient to notify drug prescriber if teeth become stained or mottled after repeated use.

PARENTERAL NUTRITIONAL SUPPLEMENTS

Parenteral nutritional supplementation is provided for a number of reasons, ranging from correction of simple acute dehydration to prolonged treatment of serious nutritional deficiencies resulting from such conditions as severe GI disorders, prolonged kidney failure, and extensive burns.

Substances provided in parenteral nutritional supplements include electrolytes, carbohydrates, fats, proteins, and vitamins. Administration of nutritional solutions via peripheral veins (i.e., peripheral parenteral nutrition) is generally adequate if caloric requirements are minimal and can be partially satisfied with oral supplements and if nutritional therapy will only be required for 1 to 2 weeks. Conversely, in severely depleted patients or in patients who will require prolonged supplemental nutrition, total parenteral nutrition (TPN) administered by a central venous catheter is usually indicated. This latter procedure, frequently termed *hyperalimentation,* is used to maintain an anabolic state when conventional oral or tube feeding is inappropriate and when peripheral IV therapy cannot meet the nutritional demands of the patient. Total parenteral nutrition is indicated following a major bowel resection, in the presence of obstructive or severe inflammatory conditions of the bowel, and in patients with prolonged paralytic ileus (such as following abdominal trauma or surgery). It is also employed to manage hypermetabolic states due to severe trauma such as extensive burns, infections, or multiple injuries; to treat malabsorption states, as, for example those resulting from hepatic or pancreatic insufficiency, and as adjunctive therapy for patients receiving chemotherapy or radiation therapy or suffering from anorexia nervosa. In general, persons requiring 1000 calories or more to maintain nutritional status are candidates for TPN.

Solutions used in TPN contain a protein source (amino acids) together with varying amounts of dextrose, vitamins, electrolytes, and trace minerals. In addition, other agents that may be added to TPN solutions include heparin, insulin, and cimetidine or another H_2 antagonist to prevent stress ulcers. Because of their high osmolarity, these solutions must be administered through a *large* vein having sufficient blood flow to provide adequate dilution so as to minimize the danger of phlebitis. For this reason, the solution is given into the superior vena cava via the subclavian vein, and the procedure is carried out by surgically implanting a catheter into the appropriate vessel. Although the technical details of the hyperalimentation procedure are not reviewed here, this form of nutritional therapy is a potentially hazardous one that requires personnel trained and experienced in the technique as well as in the care of patients undergoing the procedure.

The substances used for parenteral nutrition are considered individually; however, as previously indicated, several different kinds of nutrients are usually administered together, depending on the clinical status and nutritional requirements of the patient.

Protein (Amino Acid) Products

The protein products employed as parenteral nutrients include protein hydrolysates and mixtures of crystalline amino acids, with or without added electrolytes. Most products are used for central venous hyperalimentation, but some of the amino-acid preparations can be employed as dilute solutions for peripheral parenteral feeding. These products provide a concentrated form of utilizable amino acids for protein synthesis as well as varying amounts of electrolytes, but they require addition of sufficient dextrose to provide for full caloric energy requirements when used for long-term hyperalimentation.

Crystalline Amino-Acid Infusion

Aminosyn, FreAmine III, Novamine, ProcalAmine, Travasol, TrophAmine

Crystalline amino acids are hypertonic solutions of essential and nonessential *l*-amino acids or low-molecular-weight peptides with varying proportions of electrolytes that provide a substrate for protein synthesis and exert a protein-sparing effect. Preparations differ in degree of osmolarity, amino-acid ratios, and content of nitrogen. In addition to the general amino-acid formulations listed above, specialized formulations are available for use in patients with renal failure, hepatic failure/ encephalopathy, or acute metabolic stress. These latter products are considered after the review of the general formulations.

MECHANISM

Provide replacement of deficient amino acids and electrolytes; possess a nitrogen-sparing effect when used with a nonprotein caloric source; promote a positive nitrogen balance and increase protein synthesis

USES

Prevention of nitrogen loss or treatment of negative nitrogen balance

Adjuncts in providing adequate nutrition, as a component product of total parenteral nutrition (i.e., hyperalimentation) in full strength or peripheral parenteral nutrition in diluted form

DOSAGE

Dosage is flexible and depends on daily protein requirements, patient's clinical response, and metabolic activity; see individual package instructions; average adult dose is 2 liters/day to provide 1 g to 2 g protein/kg

> NOTE
> Solutions contain between 3% and 15% amino-acid concentration (both essential and nonessential) together with electrolytes; some solutions also contain 5% to 25% dextrose

COMMON SIDE EFFECTS

Nausea, flushing, sensation of warmth (especially with rapid infusion)

SIGNIFICANT ADVERSE REACTIONS

Vomiting, chills, headache, abdominal pain, dizziness, allergic reactions, phlebitis, venous thrombosis, skin rash, papular eruptions; metabolic disturbances include acidosis, alkalosis, hypocalcemia, hypophosphatemia, hyperglycemia, glycosuria, hypovitaminosis, and other electrolyte imbalances

CONTRAINDICATIONS

Anuria, oliguria, severe liver or kidney impairment, metabolic disorders involving impaired nitrogen utilization, decreased circulating blood volume, inborn errors of amino-acid metabolism, hepatic coma or encephalopathy, and hyperammonemia. *Cautious use* in patients with cardiac insufficiency

INTERACTIONS

Antianabolic drugs and tetracyclines may reduce the protein-sparing effects of amino acids

Addition of calcium to the infusion may precipitate the phosphate ion

NURSING CONSIDERATIONS

Nursing Alerts

- Use aseptic technique in mixing solutions and in the insertion and maintenance of central venous catheters because risk of sepsis is considerable. Use solution promptly after mixing and discard unused portion. Do not mix antibiotics with protein–carbohydrate hyperalimentation solutions.
- Infuse slowly to minimize adverse effects, particularly

> hyperglycemia and glycosuria, which can, however, be controlled with insulin if necessary.
> - In diabetics and in patients with impaired glucose tolerance, monitor results of blood sugar determinations, which should be performed frequently, and test urine for sugar often because insulin dosage may need to be adjusted.
> - When amino-acid infusions are used for prolonged hyperalimentation, ensure that sufficient dextrose (in the form of concentrated dextrose solutions) is administered to meet full caloric energy requirements.
> - Monitor results of serum electrolyte determinations. Appropriate supplemental electrolyte solutions should be provided as necessary.

1. Do *not* premix amino-acid infusions with fat emulsions. Instead, infuse simultaneously through a Y connector located near infusion site.
2. Do *not* administer simultaneously with blood through same infusion site because pseudoagglutination can occur.
3. Be alert for signs of fatty acid deficiency (flaking skin, loss of hair), and assess results of plasma lipid level determinations. Intravenous fat emulsions will correct a deficiency.
4. Do *not* administer strongly hypertonic solutions (e.g., stronger than 12.5% dextrose) by *peripheral* venous infusion. They should be given only through an indwelling central venous catheter whose tip is located in the superior vena cava.
5. Replace all IV administration sets every 24 to 48 hours.
6. Note that supplementary vitamins, minerals, electrolytes, heparin, or insulin may be administered cautiously through the indwelling catheter, but administration of any *other* medication or withdrawal or transfusion of blood by this route is *not* recommended.
7. Note that most amino-acid infusions are indicated for hyperalimentation, *except for* Aminosyn 3.5%, FreAmine III 3% w/electrolytes, ProcalAmine, and Travasol 3.5% w/electrolytes.

Amino-Acid Formulation for Renal Failure

Aminosyn-RF, Aminess, NephrAmine, RenAmin

Amino-acid formulation for renal failure is indicated to provide nutritional support for uremic patients when oral nutrition is impractical and dialysis is not feasible. The products are used in conjunction with dextrose, electrolytes, and vitamins, and are administered by central venous injection. Amino-acid formulation for renal failure supplies only essential amino acids, thus allowing urea nitrogen to be recycled to glutamate, which serves as a precursor for synthesis of nonessential amino acids. Therefore, use of these products in uremic patients promotes utilization of retained urea and amelioration of azotemic symptoms. For urea reutilization to occur, however, it is essential to provide adequate calories and to restrict intake of nonessential nitrogen.

Amino-Acid Formulation for High Metabolic Stress

Aminosyn-HBC, Branch Amin, FreAmine HBC

Amino-acid formulation for high metabolic stress is a mixture of essential and nonessential amino acids with high concentrations of the branched-chain amino acids isoleucine, leucine, and valine. Metabolic stress is often characterized by increased urinary excretion of nitrogen and by hyperglycemia, with decreased plasma levels of branched-chain amino acids. As a result, glucose utilization and fat mobilization are impaired. By supplying branched-chain amino acids, this formulation provides the substrates needed to meet the energy requirements of muscle and brain tissue.

Amino-Acid Formulation for Hepatic Failure or Hepatic Encephalopathy

HepatAmine

This formulation is very similar to that used for high metabolic stress, being a mixture of essential and nonessential amino acids with high concentrations of branched-chain amino acids. It is used for treating hepatic encephalopathy in patients intolerant of general-purpose amino acid injections. Replenishment of stores of branched-chain amino acids can reverse the abnormal plasma amino acid pattern seen in hepatic encephalopathy, with resultant improvement in mental status and EEG pattern. Nitrogen balance is also significantly improved.

Carbohydrates

Parenteral carbohydrate solutions are indicated primarily as a source of calories and fluid in patients with nutritional deficiencies who are unable to obtain the necessary nutrients orally. The available preparations include dextrose in water, alcohol in dextrose infusion, fructose in water, and invert sugar (dextrose and fructose) in water.

Dextrose in Water Injection

D-2½-W, D-5-W, D-10-W, D-20-W, D-25-W, D-30-W, D-38.5-W, D-40-W, D-50-W, D-60-W, D-70-W

Dextrose in water injection is available as solutions of varying concentrations of dextrose (D-glucose) in water for injection. Caloric content ranges from 85 cal/liter (2½%) to 2380 cal/liter (70%). The 5% solution is isotonic and along with the 2.5% and 10% solutions may be given by IV infusion into peripheral veins to provide calories when nonelectrolytic fluid is required. The 20% solution provides adequate calories in a minimal volume of water. The more concentrated solutions provide even greater caloric content with less fluid volume and may be irritating if given by peripheral infusion; they are usually administered by central venous catheters as a component of total parenteral nutrition. Dextrose is also available in several electrolyte solutions in various concentrations for IV infusion in patients having both a carbohydrate and an electrolyte deficit. Principal electrolytes used in fixed combination with dextrose are sodium, chloride, potassium, calcium, magnesium, phosphate, lactate, and acetate.

MECHANISM

Provides a source of calories and fluid volume where nutritional or fluid deficiencies (or both) exist; dextrose is oxidized to CO_2 and water and provides 3.4 cal/g of D-glucose; promotes glycogen deposition and reduces protein and nitrogen loss

USES

To provide nonelectrolytic fluid and caloric replacement (usually 5% or 10% solution)

Component of total parenteral nutrition, in conjunction with other solutions of proteins, electrolytes, fats, vitamins (usually 40%, 50%, 60%, or 70% solution)

Treatment of insulin hypoglycemia to restore blood glucose levels (50% solution)

Treatment of acute symptomatic hypoglycemia in the neonate or older infant to restore depressed blood glucose levels (25% solution)

DOSAGE

Dependent on patient's status and nutritional state

FATE

Approximately 95% is retained if infusion rate is 800 mg/kg/hr; essentially 100% retention occurs at 400 mg to 500 mg/kg/hr

SIGNIFICANT ADVERSE REACTIONS

Thrombophlebitis (with prolonged infusion), irritation, tissue necrosis, infection at injection site, hypervolemia, mental confusion, hyperglycemia, glycosuria (especially with concentrated solutions or too-rapid administration), over-hydration, congestion, and pulmonary edema

CONTRAINDICATIONS

Diabetic coma; use of concentrated solutions in patients with intracranial hemorrhage or delirium tremens. *Cautious use* in patients with renal insufficiency, cardiac decompensation, hypervolemia, carbohydrate intolerance, or urinary tract obstruction

INTERACTIONS

Dextrose infusions may alter insulin or oral hypoglycemic drug requirements and may cause vitamin B complex deficiency

Hyperglycemia and glycosuria may be intensified by diuretics that decrease glucose tolerance

NURSING CONSIDERATIONS

Nursing Alerts

- Administer concentrated (hypertonic) solutions (25% or stronger) *slowly* by central venous catheter. They are very irritating and may cause thrombosis if given into a peripheral vein.
- Observe patient for signs of hyperglycemia or hyperosmolarity (confusion, unconsciousness). If they occur, infusion should be reduced or terminated.
- Closely monitor blood and urine glucose determinations during prolonged infusions, especially with concentrated solutions. The maximum rate that dextrose can be infused without inducing glycosuria is 0.5 g/kg/hour.
- Assess patient frequently for evidence of fluid overload, which could lead to congestive heart failure and pulmonary edema.
- Discontinue hypertonic dextrose infusion gradually. If infusion is terminated abruptly, 5% dextrose should be administered to avoid rebound hypoglycemia.

1. Be prepared to add appropriate electrolytes to infusion according to patient's electrolyte status.
2. Use only clear solutions. Discard unused portions.

Alcohol in Dextrose Infusion

Alcohol in dextrose infusions are solutions of 5% dextrose in water containing 5% or 10% ethyl alcohol that provide a source of carbohydrate calories. They are not as commonly used as plain dextrose in water infusions owing to the adverse effects of alcohol in many patients.

MECHANISM

Supply a source of carbohydrate calories; may result in liver glycogen depletion and exert a protein-sparing action; alcohol can prevent premature labor, presumably by inhibiting release of oxytocin from the posterior pituitary

USES

As aid in increasing caloric intake and replenishing fluids in nutritional deficiencies

Prevention of premature labor (IV infusion of 10% solution)—investigational use only

DOSAGE

1 liter to 2 liters of a 5% solution in a 24-hour period by *slow* IV infusion

Children: 40 mL/kg/24 h

FATE

Alcohol is metabolized at a rate of 10 mL to 20 mL/hour (200 mL–400 mL of a 5% solution)

SIGNIFICANT ADVERSE REACTIONS

(Usually with too-rapid infusion) Vertigo, flushing, sedation, confusion, alcoholic odor on breath, and pain and irritation at infusion site

CONTRAINDICATIONS

Epilepsy, alcohol addiction, diabetic coma, urinary tract infections, severe kidney or liver impairment, shock. *Cautious use* in patients with diabetes or liver or renal impairment; in the presence of shock; during postpartum hemorrhage; following cranial surgery; and in pregnant or nursing women

INTERACTIONS

Alcohol may shorten the duration of effect of phenytoin, warfarin, and tolbutamide

Alcohol can potentiate the postural hypotensive effects of antihypertensive drugs, vasodilators, and diuretics

Additive CNS depressive effects can occur between alcohol and other CNS depressants, such as barbiturates, benzodiazepines, meprobamate, glutethimide, narcotics, and phenothiazines

An acute alcohol intolerance syndrome (e.g., flushing, sweating, tachycardia, nausea) has occurred with concurrent administration of disulfiram, metronidazole, moxalactam, cefamandole, cefoperazone, and sulfonylurea hypoglycemic drugs

Increased GI bleeding can occur with combined use of salicylates or other antiinflammatory drugs

NURSING CONSIDERATIONS

1. Use the largest available peripheral vein and a small-bore needle to minimize irritation. Infuse at a slow rate, and observe for signs of alcohol intoxication (slurred speech, drowsiness, flushing, dizziness).
2. Note that 10% solutions of ethyl alcohol can be used by IV infusion to delay labor, presumably by decreasing release of oxytocin from the pituitary. Commercially available alcohol and dextrose infusions are not approved by the FDA for this particular indication.
3. Avoid extravasation during IV administration. Do not inject SC.

Fructose in Water

A 10% solution of Fructose (levulose) in Water provides approximately 375 cal/liter. Unlike dextrose, it does not require insulin for ultimate conversion to utilizable glucose, and it produces lower serum and urinary glucose levels than dextrose. In addition, it is more readily converted to glycogen. Thus, it may be preferred to dextrose in diabetic patients. However, it is of no value for treating hypoglycemia. It is principally an alternative source of calories and fluid, and the dosage must be adjusted to the caloric needs of the patient. Electrolyte and vitamin supplementation should be provided as needed.

Infusion rates should not exceed 1 g/kg/hour to minimize the danger of metabolic acidosis, especially in infants and small children. Fructose should *not* be given to patients with gout, because it may increase the serum uric acid level. Use with *caution* in patients with renal insufficiency, frank cardiac decompensation, hypervolemia, or urinary tract obstruction. The suitability of long-term fructose infusions is questionable, because significant depletion of liver ATP can occur.

Invert Sugar in Water

Travert

A solution comprising equal parts of dextrose and fructose, Invert Sugar in Water, is available as a 10% concentration. The fructose reportedly enhances the utilization of dextrose and the combination represents an alternative to use of either agent alone. Refer to the respective discussions of each sugar for additional information.

Lipids

Fat emulsions designed for IV infusion are prepared from either soybean or safflower oil and contain a mixture of neutral triglycerides, which are largely polyunsaturated fatty acids. In addition, these products also contain 1.2% egg yolk phospholipids as an emulsifier and glycerin to adjust tonicity. Caloric content of the 10% IV fat emulsion is 1.1 cal/mL and that of the 20% emulsion is 2.0 cal/mL. These IV emulsions are isotonic and may be given by either peripheral or central venous routes.

Intravenous Fat Emulsion

Intralipid 10%, 20%; Liposyn 10%, 20%; Liposyn II 10%, 20%; Soyacal 10%, 20%; Travamulsion 10%, 20%

MECHANISM

Provide a source of calories and essential fatty acids in parenteral nutrition regimens

USES

Supplemental source of calories and fatty acids for patients requiring total parenteral nutrition for extended periods whose caloric requirements cannot be met by glucose
Prevention and treatment of fatty-acid deficiency states

DOSAGE

(*Note:* Fat emulsion should comprise no more than 60% of the total caloric intake of the patient.)
Total Parenteral Nutrition
Adults
10%: initially 1 mL/min for 15 to 30 minutes; gradually increase rate to 83 mL/h to 125 mL/h; infuse only 500 mL first day, then gradually increase dose
20%: initially 0.5 mL/min for 15 to 30 minutes; gradually increase rate to 62 mL/h; infuse only 250 mL first day
Do *not* exceed 3 g/kg/day
Children (see Significant Adverse Reactions)
10%: initially 0.1 mL/min for 10 to 15 minutes
20%: initially 0.5 mL/min for 10 to 15 minutes; gradually increase rate of each to 1g/kg/4 hour
Do *not* exceed 4 g/kg/day
Fatty-acid Deficiency
Supply 8% to 10% of the caloric intake by IV fat emulsion

FATE

Metabolized and utilized as a source of energy; cleared from the plasma in a manner similar to clearance of chylomicrons

SIGNIFICANT ADVERSE REACTIONS

WARNING

Infusion of IV fat emulsion in premature infants has resulted in some fatalities, presumably owing to fat accumulation in the lungs. Follow dosage guidelines strictly; infusion rate should be as slow as possible, not to exceed 1 g/kg in 4 hours. Carefully monitor the infant's ability to clear the fat from the circulation between infusions, for example, measurement of triglyceride or free fatty-acid levels. Lipemia *must* clear between daily infusions

Dyspnea, cyanosis, allergic reactions, nausea, vomiting, flushing, headache, fever, sweating, insomnia, dizziness, chest or back pain, hyperlipemia, hypercoagulability, thrombophlebitis, irritation at injection site, transient increase in liver enzymes; with prolonged administration, hepatomegaly, jaundice, leukopenia, thrombocytopenia, splenomegaly, seizures, and shock

CONTRAINDICATIONS

Disturbed fat metabolism, acute pancreatitis; in premature infants with bilirubin levels above 5 mg/dL; in patients with severe egg allergies. *Cautious use* in patients with liver damage, pulmonary disease, anemia, or coagulation disorders, or where there is danger of fat embolism

NURSING CONSIDERATIONS

Nursing Alerts

- Assess patient's liver status frequently during extended administration. Drug should be discontinued if liver dysfunction is noted.
- Monitor results of the following laboratory studies, which should be performed often: hemogram, blood coagulation, plasma, lipids, platelet count, and liver function tests. In neonates, platelet counts should be obtained daily. Infusion should be discontinued if significant abnormality occurs in any of these.

1. Use only freshly opened solutions. Store preparations at 25°C or below, but do *not* freeze.
2. Carefully avoid disturbing the emulsion when mixing with electrolyte nutrient solutions or other additive solutions, and do not use filters. Observe emulsion for any separation; do not use if it appears disturbed.
3. When administering together with carbohydrate or protein/amino-acid infusion solutions, infuse into separate peripheral site or through Y connector located near infusion site. To prevent backflow, ensure that lipid infusion line is higher than dextrose/amino-acid infusion line.
4. Expect to also administer products containing carbohydrates and amino acids because no more than 60% of patient's total caloric intake should come from IV fat emulsion.
5. Note that use of this product may cause deposition of a brown pigment in the reticuloendothelial system ("intravenous fat pigment"). The cause and significance are unknown.

(*Text continued on page 785*)

Table 75-2
Parenteral Electrolytes

Drug	Preparations	Usual Dosage Range	Nursing Implications
Ammonium Chloride	Injection: 26.75% (5 mEq/mL)	Dependent on patient's status; if edema or hyponatremia is not present, total dose is estimated as product of ECF volume (20% of body weight in kg) times serum chloride deficit in mEq/mL; initially, give one half calculated dose and check pH before giving remainder	Indicated for treatment of metabolic alkalosis or hypochloremic states severe enough to cause signs of impending tetany (severe or protracted vomiting, gastric suction); generally given with 20 mEq–40 mEq potassium/L to correct accompanying hypokalemia; *contraindicated* in severe hepatic impairment because danger of ammonia retention is present, and in patients with primary respiratory alkalosis and high CO_2; *cautious use* in renal dysfunction, cardiac edema; or pulmonary insufficiency; administer by *slow* IV infusion and observe for signs of ammonia toxicity (sweating, irregular breathing, bradycardia, vomiting, twitching, arrhythmias); do *not* give SC, intraperitoneally, or rectally; low-strength solution may be given undiluted but higher strength solution should be diluted with normal saline; may increase excretion rate of basic drugs (e.g., amphetamines, quinidine)
Calcium Chloride	Injection: 10% (1 g/13.6 mEq)	**Slow IV injection only** *Hypocalcemia:* 500 mg–1 g at 1–3-day intervals *Magnesium intoxication:* 500 mg at once; repeat as necessary *Cardiac resuscitation:* 200 mg–800 mg into the ventricular cavity *or* 500 mg–1 g IV	Indicated for treatment of hypocalcemia requiring a prompt elevation in serum calcium levels (e.g., neonatal tetany, parathyroid deficiency, alkalosis); also used to prevent hypocalcemia during exchange transfusions, as adjunctive therapy in treating serious insect bites, for managing lead colic and magnesium intoxication, and for cardiac resuscitation (calcium chloride only) when epinephrine therapy is ineffective; calcium chloride is highly irritating and severe necrosis and sloughing can occur; other calcium salts are preferred where possible; IM administration of calcium salts (except chloride—IV only) should be done only where IV administration is impractical or technically too difficult; do *not* mix calcium salts with sulfates, phosphates, carbonates, or tartrates in solution, because precipitation can occur; IV solutions should be warmed to body temperature and given slowly (0.5 mL–2 mL/min); side effects are infrequent at recommended doses; use with caution in digitalized patients and in patients with arrhythmias; calcium may antagonize the effects of verapamil
Calcium Gluceptate	Injection: 1.1 g/5 mL (1.1 g = 4.5 mEq)	*Hypocalcemia* IM: 2 mL–5 mL IV: 5 mL–20 mL *Exchange transfusions in newborn* 0.5 mL after each 100 mL of blood is exchanged	
Calcium Gluconate Kalcinate	Injection: 10% (1 g = 4.5 mEq)	*Hypocalcemia* Adults: 5 mL–20 mL as needed by IV infusion Children: 500 mg/kg/day in divided doses	
Magnesium Sulfate	Injection: 10% (0.8 mEq/mL), 12.5% (1 mEq/mL), 20% (1.97 mEq/mL), 50% (4 mEq/mL)	*Mild magnesium deficiency* 1 g (2 mL 50% solution) IM every 6 h for 4 doses *Severe magnesium deficiency* IM: 2 mEq/kg within 4 h IV: 5 g (40 mEq)/1000 mL infused over 3 h *Total parenteral nutrition* Adults: 8 mEq–24 mEq/day Infants: 2 mEq–10 mEq/day	Indicated for replacement therapy in magnesium-deficiency states, especially when accompanied by signs of tetany, and for treating hypomagnesemia resulting from hyperalimentation; may also be employed in certain acute convulsive states (e.g., toxemia, eclampsia, preeclampsia, epilepsy [1 g–4 g 10%–20% solution IV]), although other more effective and less toxic drugs are available (see Chap. 25); use with *extreme caution* in patients with renal impairment and observe closely for signs of overdosage (hypotension, respiratory depression, absence of patellar reflex); have respiratory assistance available; urine output should be maintained at a minimum of 100 mL/4 h; do *not* exceed 1.5 mL/min when infusing the 10% concentration (or equivalent volume of higher concentrations); dilute 50% solution to a concentration of 20% or less before infusing; however, the full-strength solution may be injected IM in adults; effects of CNS depressants can be potentiated by magnesium
Phosphate Potassium Phosphate, Sodium Phosphate	Injection: 3 mM phosphate/mL and either 4 mEq sodium/mL or 4.4 mEq potassium/mL	*Total parenteral nutrition* Adults: 10 mM–15 mM phosphorus (310 mg–465 mg elemental phosphorus) per liter of TPN solution Infants: 1.5 mM–2 mM/kg/day	Primarily used to prevent or correct hypophosphatemia in patients undergoing hyperalimentation; *contraindicated* in diseases with high phosphate or low calcium levels; used IV only, diluted in a larger volume of fluid and slowly infused; monitor serum phosphorus, calcium, and sodium or potassium levels depending on which phosphate salt is used; be alert for symp-

Continued

Table 75-2
Parenteral Electrolytes (continued)

Drug	Preparations	Usual Dosage Range	Nursing Implications
			toms of hypocalcemic tetany; use *cautiously* in patients with renal impairment, cardiac disease, arrhythmias, or adrenal insufficiency; symptoms of overdosage include weakness, confusion, paresthesias, hypotension, arrhythmias, flaccid paralysis, and ECG abnormalities
Potassium Chloride	Injection: 10 mEq, 20 mEq, 30 mEq, 40 mEq, 45 mEq, 60 mEq, 200 mEq in various size vials; 1,000 mEq/500 mL	Dependent on patient's status and governed by serum potassium level and ECG pattern; if serum potassium is less than 2 mEq/L, maximum infusion rate is 40 mEq/h to a total of 400 mEq/day; if serum potassium is greater than 2.5 mEq/L, maximum infusion rate is 10 mEq/h to a maximum of 200 mEq/day	Indicated for the prevention or treatment of moderate to severe potassium deficiency states and as adjunctive therapy in the management of cardiac arrhythmias, especially those due to digitalis overdosage; *contraindicated* in patients with anuria, oliguria, azotemia, adrenocortical insufficiency, acute dehydration, hyperkalemia, and severe hemolytic reactions; dilute injections with large volumes of parenteral solutions and administer *slowly* IV; direct injection of undiluted solution may be *fatal*; use *cautiously* in patients with cardiac disease, especially those taking digitalis drugs; monitor serum potassium levels, ECG, and urine flow frequently during therapy; be aware that toxic effects of potassium on the heart may be increased if serum sodium or calcium levels decrease or serum pH is reduced; most frequent adverse reactions are nausea, vomiting, diarrhea, and abdominal pain; avoid extravasation as irritation is often severe and tissue necrosis can occur
Potassium Acetate	Injection: 40 mEq, 60 mEq, 100 mEq, 200 mEq in various size vials		
Sodium Acetate	Injection: 2 mEq sodium and 2 mEq acetate/mL or 4 mEq sodium and 4 mEq acetate/ml	*Metabolic acidosis* Initially 2 mEq–5 mEq/kg by IV infusion over 4 h to 8 h; adjust dose as necessary depending on clinical response *Cardiac arrest* Adults: initially 1 mEq/kg, followed by 0.5 mEq/kg every 10 min of arrest; use 7.5% *or* 8.4% solution Children under 2 yr: initially 1 mEq–2 mEq/kg over 1 min to 2 min, followed by 1 mEq/kg every 10 min of arrest; use 4.2% solution	Indicated for acute treatment of metabolic acidosis, such as resulting from cardiac arrest, shock, or other circulatory insufficiency states, severe dehydration, or diabetic or lactic acidosis; also used to alkalinize the urine for treating certain drug intoxications and adjunctively in severe diarrhea to replace loss of bicarbonate; sodium lactate and sodium acetate are metabolized to bicarbonate, although conversion of lactate to bicarbonate is impaired in patients with hepatic disease; *contraindicated* in hypochloremia, metabolic or respiratory alkalosis, and hypocalcemia; use *cautiously* in patients with congestive heart failure, kidney impairment, edema, hypertension, or arrhythmias; do *not* exceed 8 mg/kg/day in small children, and infuse *slowly* because rapid injection or use of hypertonic solutions has resulted in decreased CSF pressure and intracranial hemorrhage; closely monitor pH and blood gases and electrolytes; avoid overdosage and subsequent production of alkalosis by giving repeated small doses; observe for signs of developing alkalosis (hyperirritability, restlessness, tetany) and discontinue drug; sodium bicarbonate is incompatible in solution with a wide variety of other drugs; administer alone to avoid undesirable interaction
Sodium Bicarbonate Neut	Injection: 4% (0.48 mEq/mL), 4.2% (0.5 mEq/mL), 5% (0.595 mEq/mL), 7.5% (0.892 mEq/mL), 8.4% (1.0 mEq/mL)		
Sodium Lactate	Injection: 0.167 mEq/mL, 5 mEq/mL		
Sodium Chloride intravenous infusion	Infusion solution: 0.2% (34 mEq/L), 0.45% (77 mEq/L), 0.9% (154 mEq/L), 3% (513 mEq/L), 5% (855 mEq/L)	(Dependent on patient's status and preparation being used) 0.9% solution: 1.5 L–3 L/24 h 0.45% solution: 2 L–4 L/24 h 3% *or* 5% solution: maximum of 100 mL over 1 h	Used IV in various concentrations as a source of fluid and electrolytes; the 0.45% solution (hypotonic) is used when fluid loss exceeds electrolyte depletion; the 0.9% solution (isotonic) is most commonly used as replacement for fluid and sodium loss and as a diluent for many other drugs and nutrients; the 3% and 5% solutions (hypertonic) are indicated for hyponatremia and hypochloremia, extreme dilution of body fluids due to excessive water intake, and treatment of severe salt depletion; use with caution in patients with congestive heart failure, severe renal impairment, and edema with sodium retention; the 3% and 5% solutions should *not* be used when plasma sodium and chloride are elevated, normal, or even slightly decreased; monitor intake–output ratio
Sodium Chloride Injection for Admixtures	Injection: 50 mEq/vial, 100 mEq/vial, 625 mEq/vial		
Sodium Chloride diluents	Injection: 0.9% in various volumes		

Continued

Table 75-2
Parenteral Electrolytes (continued)

Drug	Preparations	Usual Dosage Range	Nursing Implications
Sodium Chloride diluents (concentrated)	Injection: 14.6%, 23.4% in various volumes		and serum electrolytes; also use *cautiously* in patients with decompensated cardiovascular or nephrotic diseases and in patients receiving corticosteroids; infuse higher strength solutions very slowly to avoid pulmonary edema
Tromethamine Tham, Tham-E	Infusion solution: 18 g (150 mEq)/500 mL Powder for injection: 36 g (300 mEq)/150 mL with sodium, potassium and chloride (Tham-E)	*Acidosis associated with cardiac arrest* 2 g–6 g (62 mL–185 mL) injected into ventricular cavity *or* 3.6–10.8 g (111 mL–333 mL) injected into a large peripheral vein; additional amounts as needed *Acidosis during cardiac bypass surgery* 9.0 mL/kg (2.7 mEq/kg) to a maximum of 1000 mL in unusually severe cases *Correct acidity of ACD priming blood* 0.5–2.5 g (15 mL–77 mL) added to each 500 mL blood (usually 2 g is adequate)	A highly alkaline, sodium-free organic amine that acts as a proton acceptor, combining with hydrogen ions to prevent or correct systemic acidosis associated with, for example, cardiac arrest or cardiac bypass surgery; also added to ACD priming blood to elevate pH; may function as an osmotic diuretic and increase urine flow and excretion of fixed acids, carbon dioxide, and electrolytes; *contraindicated* in anuria or uremia; should be administered slowly IV to avoid overdosage and alkalosis; may also be given by injection into ventricular cavity during cardiac arrest and by addition to pump oxygenator ACD blood or other priming fluid; treatment should not continue longer than a 24-h period; determine blood values (pH, P_{CO_2}, P_{O_2}, glucose), electrolytes, and urinary output before treatment and frequently during drug administration to assess progress of treatment; adjust dose so that blood pH does not increase above normal (7.35–7.45); drug may depress respiration; have respiratory assistance available; avoid extravasation, because severe inflammation, vascular spasm, and tissue necrosis can result; transient hypoglycemia may occur, especially in infants; use *cautiously* in children, in patients with impaired renal function, and in pregnant women

Electrolytes

Ammonium   Phosphate
Bicarbonate   Potassium
Calcium   Sodium
Chloride   Tromethamine
Magnesium

Parenteral electrolytes are sometimes supplied individually to correct a specific known deficiency (e.g., hyponatremia, hypokalemia) but more commonly are used as combination electrolyte solutions for adjunctive treatment of nutritional disorders, dehydration, severe burns, trauma, and other emergency situations. Combined electrolyte solutions are also employed as part of the total parenteral nutrition (hyperalimentation) regimen. Serum electrolyte levels must be monitored closely during treatment, and the composition of the infusion solution as well as the rate of administration should be adjusted to provide as nearly optimal blood levels of each electrolyte as possible.

The several parenteral electrolytes are listed in Table 75-2, with available preparations, dosage, and nursing implications. Although the discussion afforded these preparations here is rather brief, anyone using these products routinely should become thoroughly familiar with their pharmacology and toxicology, because serious untoward reactions have occurred with improper selection or administration of parenteral electrolytes.

Selected Bibliography

Agranoff BW (ed): Inositol triphosphate (symposium). Fed Proc 45(11):2627, 1986

Bia MJ, DeFronzo RA: Extrarenal potassium homeostasis. Am J Physiol 240:F257, 1981

Foltz A: Evaluation of implanted infusion devices. Journal of the National Intravenous Therapy Association, January-February, 1987

Gardner C: Home I.V. therapy: Part II. Journal of the National Intravenous Therapy Association, May-June, 1986

Hutchinson MM: Administration of fat emulsions. Am J Nurs 82:275, 1982

Levander OA, Cheng L (eds): Micronutrient interactions: Vitamins, minerals and hazardous elements. Ann NY Acad Sci 355:1, 1980

Marein C et al: Home parenteral nutrition. Nutr Clin Prac August, 1986

Masoorli S: Tips for trouble-free subclavian lines. RN 38, February, 1984

Mullen JL: Consequences of malnutrition in the surgical patient. Surg Clin North Am 61:465, 1981

Munro HN (ed): Placental transport of nutrients (symposium). Fed Proc 45(10):2500, 1986

Pardridge WM (ed): Blood–brain transport of nutrients (symposium). Fed Proc 45(7):2047, 1986

Rombeau J, Caldwell M: Enteral Nutrition: Clinical Nutrition, vol I. Philadelphia, WB Saunders, 1986

Rombeau J, Caldwell M: Parenteral Nutrition: Clinical Nutrition, vol II. Philadelphia, WB Saunders, 1986

Rude RK, Singer FR: Magnesium deficiency and excess. Annu Rev Med 32:245, 1981

Wilkes G, Vannicola P, Starck P: Long-term venous access. Am J Nurs 85:793, 1985

Winters V: Implantable vascular access devices. Oncol Nurs Forum 11:25, 1984

Young DB: Relationship between plasma potassium concentration and renal potassium excretion. Am J Physiol 242:F599, 1982

SUMMARY. NUTRIENTS, MINERALS, FLUIDS AND ELECTROLYTES

Drug	Preparations	Usual Dosage Range
Oral Nutritional Supplements		
Potassium Several manufacturers	Liquid: 10 mEq/15 mL, 15 mEq/15 mL, 20 mEq/15 mL, 30 mEq/15 mL, 40 mEq/15 mL, 45 mEq/15 mL Powder: 15 mEq/dose, 20 mEq/dose, 25 mEq/dose Effervescent tablets: 20 mEq, 25 mEq, 50 mEq Oral tablets: 1 mEq, 2 mEq, 2.5 mEq, 4 mEq, 8 mEq, 10 mEq, 20 mEq, 25 mEq Controlled-release tablets: 6.7 mEq, 8 mEq, 10 mEq, 20 mEq Controlled-release capsules: 8 mEq, 10 mEq	Prevention: 16 mEq–24 mEq/day Replacement: 40 mEq–100 mEq/day
Fluoride Fluoritab, Luride, Phos-Flur, and other manufacturers	Tablets: 0.25 mg, 0.5 mg, 1 mg Capsules (controlled-release): 8 mEq Drops: 0.125 mg/mL, 0.25 mg/mL, 0.5 mg/mL Rinse: 0.01%, 0.02%, 0.09% Gel: 0.1%, 0.5%, 1.23%	Oral: 0.25 mg–1 mg/day Topical: 5 mL to 10 mL/day as a mouthwash; rinse for 1 min, then expectorate
Other oral nutritional supplements	See Table 75-1	
Parenteral Nutritional Supplements		
Proteins/Amino Acids		
Crystalline Amino-acid Infusion Aminosyn, FreAmine III, Novamine, Procalamine, Travasol, TrophAmine	Infusion solutions containing essential and nonessential amino acids with different proportions of electrolytes	Dosage must be based on daily protein requirements, clinical response, and metabolic status; see individual package instructions
Amino acid Formulation for Renal Failure Aminosyn-RF, Aminess, NephrAmine, RenAmin	Infusion solutions containing essential amino acids with different proportion of electrolytes	Dosage must be based on daily protein requirements, clinical response, and metabolic status; see individual package instructions
Amino acid Formulation for High Metabolic Stress FreAmine HBC	Infusion solution containing essential and nonessential amino acids with high concentrations of branched-chain amino acids and different proportions of electrolytes	Dosage must be based on daily protein requirements, clinical response, and metabolic status; see individual package instructions
Amino acid Formulation for Hepatic Failure or Hepatic Encephalopathy HepatAmine	Infusion solution containing essential and nonessential amino acids with high concentrations of branched-chain amino acids and different proportions of electrolytes	Dosage must be based on daily protein requirements, clinical response, and metabolic status; see individual package instructions
Carbohydrates		
Dextrose in Water Injection D-2½-W, D-5-W, D-10-W, D-20-W, D-25-W, D-30-W, D-38.5-W, D-40-W, D-50-W, D-60-W, D-70-W	Infusion solutions containing 2½%, 5%, 10%, 20%, 25%, 30%, 38.5%, 40%, 50%, 60%, 70% dextrose in water for injection	Individually calculated according to patient's clinical status and nutritional state
Alcohol in Dextrose Infusion	Infusion solutions containing either 5% or 10% ethyl alcohol in 5% dextrose in water for injection	Adults: 1 L–2 L 5% solution in a 24-h period by *slow* IV infusion Children: 40 mL/kg/24 h

Continued

SUMMARY. NUTRIENTS, MINERALS, FLUIDS AND ELECTROLYTES (continued)

Drug	Preparations	Usual Dosage Range
Fructose in Water	Infusion solution containing 10% fructose in water for injection	Must be individually calculated according to clinical status and nutritional state
Invert Sugar in Water Travert	Infusion solution containing either 5% *or* 10% invert sugar (dextrose and fructose) in water for injection	Must be individually calculated
Lipids **Intravenous Fat Emulsion** Intralipid, Liposyn, Soyacal, Travamulsion	Emulsions for infusion containing 10% *or* 20% soybean oil (Intralipid, Soyacal, Travamulsion) *or* safflower oil (Liposyn) with 1.2% egg yolk phospholipids and 2.21% to 2.5% glycerin (contain 1.1 to 2.0 calories/mL)	**Total Parenteral Nutrition** *Adults* 10%: initially 1 mL/min for 15–30 min; increase gradually to 83 mL–125 mL/h 20%: initially 0.5 mL/min for 15–30 min; increase gradually to 62 mL/h Do *not* exceed 3 g/kg/day *Children* 10%: initially 0.1 mL/min for 10–15 min 20%: initially 0.05 mL/min for 10–15 min Gradually increase to 1g/kg/4 h; *do not exceed* 4 g/kg/day **Fatty-acid deficiency** Adjust dosage to supply 8%–10% of caloric intake
Electrolytes	*See* Table 75-2	

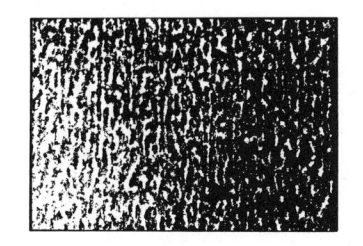

X Miscellaneous Agents

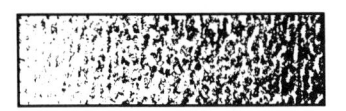

76 DIAGNOSTIC AGENTS

Effective treatment of many disease states depends upon a critical assessment of the underlying pathology. To accomplish this, a number of diagnostic agents are available that assist the clinician in evaluating the clinical status of the patient as well as the functional capacity of many body organs. In most instances, proper use of diagnostic agents requires specially trained personnel and a thorough knowledge of the agent being employed. The extensive array of available diagnostic drugs precludes an in-depth discussion of each agent in a general pharmacology text of this type. Thus, this chapter presents a brief review of the principles of diagnostic drug usage, followed by tabular listings of the categories of diagnostic agents. It is imperative, however, that health care personnel using these drugs thoroughly familiarize themselves with the pharmacology and toxicology of the particular diagnostic agent being employed.

For purposes of discussion, the various diagnostic agents can be grouped into one of the four following categories:

- *In vitro diagnostic aids:* agents usually employed at home or in the physician's office to monitor blood or urine levels of substances such as glucose, proteins, or ketones as well as pH; also included in this category are the pregnancy screening tests, as well as tests for the presence of occult blood in the urine or feces
- *Intradermal diagnostic biologicals:* agents used in skin tests for sensitivity to certain diseases, notably tuberculosis, coccidioidomycosis, histoplasmosis, and mumps
- *In vivo diagnostic aids:* agents usually employed to evaluate the functional status of body organs such as the liver, kidney, heart, pancreas, stomach, adrenal cortex, or pituitary; used in a hospital setting and require skilled personnel for administration and interpretation
- *Radiographic diagnostic agents:* opaque contrast substances, usually barium or iodinated compounds, that are impenetrable by x-rays; used to visualize internal structures such as the GI tract, kidneys, gallbladder, and bronchial tree

IN VITRO DIAGNOSTIC AIDS

A large number of preparations are used for rapid screening of the urine, feces, or blood for the presence of certain substances. These in vitro diagnostic aids commonly employ either (1) a reagent or tablet that is mixed in a test tube or on a slide with the sample to be analyzed or (2) a reagent-impregnated strip or tape that is dipped into the sample. Most are available without prescription, and complete instructions for performing the test and analyzing the results are provided with the package. A few of these aids, however, such as tests for diagnosing mononucleosis, sickle cell anemia, and the presence of beta-hemolytic streptococci, are prescription-only items and require that the user be familiar with the product to interpret the results accurately.

Another in vitro diagnostic aid is a pregnancy test that may be employed either in the home or in a care provider's office. They generally employ a reagent to be added to a urine sample. Although home test kits are certainly valuable as a preliminary screening method, confirmation of pregnancy should always be obtained professionally by use of one of the more established pregnancy-screening procedures performed in the physician's office, which measure the presence of chorionic gonadotropin in the urine.

The in vitro diagnostic aids are listed alphabetically by trade name in Table 76-1 with information regarding their dispensing status, type of preparation, and diagnostic uses.

INTRADERMAL DIAGNOSTIC BIOLOGICALS

The ability of selected biologic products to elicit a local allergic reaction following intradermal injection is used to assess sensitivity to, but not necessarily the active presence of, certain diseases. The most commonly employed skin test is the tuberculin test, although sensitivity to mumps, histoplasmosis, and coccidioidomycosis can also be determined by intradermal testing. Interpretation of the tests is based upon the appearance of a local hypersensitivity reaction at the site of intradermal injection, usually consisting of induration (tissue hardening) and, in some cases, erythema, in those patients previously exposed to the infecting organism.

Information relating to the available intradermal diagnostic drugs is presented in Table 76-2. Further information describing proper methods of administration and interpretation is provided with the individual drugs and should be consulted before performing the test.

IN VIVO DIAGNOSTIC AIDS

The diagnostic agents used to assess the functional capacity of internal body organs are termed in vivo diagnostic aids and are administered either orally or parenterally. These compounds frequently are designed to be concentrated in or excreted by the organ to be evaluated. Because they are administered systemically, a potential for untoward reactions does exist, and although these are generally mild and transient, patients should be observed carefully during, and for some time following, the testing procedure for development of more serious adverse reactions.

Several compounds that may be used for diagnostic purposes have been discussed in other chapters (e.g., edrophonium for myasthenia gravis in Chap. 10; phentolamine for pheochromocytoma in Chap. 13; radioiodide 131 for thyroid function in Chap. 40) and are not considered here. Table 76-3 lists the important in vivo diagnostic drugs, together with their preparations, uses, and pertinent remarks. It should be recognized that the consideration given to the agents in this chapter is brief and is not intended to provide comprehensive information regarding their safe and effective use. Experienced personnel and proper facilities are necessary to derive maximum benefit from use of these diagnostic agents and to deal with any untoward reaction that may occur.

RADIOGRAPHIC DIAGNOSTIC AGENTS

With the exception of barium sulfate, the substances used for radiographic diagnostic procedures are principally iodine-containing compounds. These

Table 76-1
In Vitro Diagnostic Aids

Trade Name	Preparation	Diagnostic Uses
Abbott HTLV III EIA	kit	Antibody to human T-lymphotropic virus, type III
Accussens T	liquid	Taste dysfunction
Acetest	tablets	Serum/urinary ketones
Advance-Test	reagent	Pregnancy
Albustix	strips	Urinary proteins
Answer	reagent	Pregnancy
Azostix	strips	Blood urea nitrogen
Bili-Labstix	strips	Urinary glucose, proteins, pH, blood, ketones, bilirubin
Biocult-GC	swab	Gonorrhea (cervical, pharyngeal, rectal, urethral)
CAST	kit	Human immunoglobulin E in serum
Chemstrip bG	strips	Blood glucose
Chemstrip GP	strips	Urinary glucose, protein
Chemstrip K	strips	Urinary ketones
Chemstrip LN	strips	Urinary leukocytes, nitrite
Chemstrip uG	strips	Urinary glucose
Chemstrip uGK	strips	Urinary glucose, ketones
Chemstrip 5L	strips	Urinary glucose, protein, pH, blood, ketones, leukocytes
Chemstrip 6L	strips	Urinary glucose, protein, pH, blood, ketones, bilirubin, leukocytes
Chemstrip 7L	strips	Urinary glucose, protein, pH, blood, ketones, bilirubin, urobilinogen, leukocytes
Clearblue Pregnancy	kit	Pregnancy
Clearplan	kit	Predict time of ovulation
Clinistix	strips	Urinary glucose
Clinitest	tablets	Urinary glucose
Clinitest 2-Drop	tablets	Urinary glucose
Coloscreen	kit	Fecal blood
Combistix	strips	Urinary glucose, protein, pH
CS-T ColoScreen	pad	Fecal blood
Culturette 10 min Group A Strep ID	slide	Group A streptococcal antigen
Daisy 2	reagent	Pregnancy
Dextrostix	strips	Blood glucose
Diastix	strips	Urinary glucose
Early Detector	kit	Fecal blood
Entero-Test	capsule	Upper intestinal bleeding, duodenal parasites
Entero-Test Pediatric	capsule	Screening of gastroesophageal reflux
e.p.t.	reagent	Pregnancy
EZ-Detect	pad	Fecal blood
EZ-Detect Strep-A Test	stick	Group A streptococci
Fact	reagent	Pregnancy
First Response	reagent	Pregnancy
First Response Ovulation Predictor	kit	Monoclonal immunoassay for hLH in urine
Fortel Ovulation	kit	Pregnancy
Gastroccult	reagent	Blood in gastric contents
Gastro-Test	kit	Stomach pH
Glucostix	strips	Blood glucose
Gonodecten	kit	Gonorrhea
Hema-Chek	slide	Fecal blood
Hema-Combistix	strips	Urinary glucose, protein, pH, blood
Hemastix	strips	Urinary blood
Hematest	tablets	Fecal blood
Hemoccult	slide	Fecal blood
Ictotest	reagent	Urinary bilirubin
Insta-Kit	slide	Group A streptococci
Keto-Diastix	strips	Urinary glucose, ketones
Ketostix	strips	Urinary/blood ketones
Labstix	strips	Urinary glucose, protein, pH, blood, ketones
LA-test-ASO	kit	Antistreptolysin O antibodies
LA-test-CRP	kit	C-reactive protein in serum (acute inflammation)
LA-test-RF	kit	Rheumatoid factor in blood

Continued

Table 76-1
In Vitro Diagnostic Aids (continued)

Trade Name	Preparation	Diagnostic Uses
Microstix-3	strips	Urinary nitrite, total bacteria, gram-negative bacteria
Microstix-Nitrite	strips	Urinary nitrite
MicroTrak Chlamydia	slide	*Chlamydia trachomatis* in tissue culture
MicroTrak HSV 1/HSV 2	kit	Typing of herpes simplex in tissue culture
MicroTrak *Neisseria Gonorrhoeae* Culture Test	slide	Neisseria gonorrhoeae in cervical, urethral, rectal or pharyngeal cultures
Mono-Chek	reagent	Mononucleosis
Mono-Diff Test	reagent	Mononucleosis
Monospot	reagent	Mononucleosis
Monosticon Dri-Dot	reagent	Mononucleosis
Mono-Sure	reagent	Mononucleosis
Mono-Test	reagent	Mononucleosis
MPS Papers	strips	Urinary acid mucopolysaccharides
Multistik	strips	Urinary glucose, protein, pH, blood, ketones, bilirubin, urobilinogen
Multistix SG	strips	Urinary glucose, protein, pH, blood, ketones, bilirubin, urobilinogen, specific gravity
Nimbus	liquid	Monoclonal antibody immunoassay
Nitrazine Paper	strips	Urinary pH
N-Multistix	strips	Urinary glucose, protein, pH, blood, ketones, bilirubin, urobilinogen, nitrite
N-Multistix-C	strips	As above, plus ascorbic acid
N-Multistix-SG	strips	As above, plus specific gravity
Ovu STICK Self-Test	strips	Urinary test to predict ovulation
Ovu STICK Urine hLH	strips	Monoclonal immunoassay for hLH in urine
Phenistix	strips	Phenylketonuria
Pregnolisa	reagent	Pregnancy
Pregnosis	slide	Pregnancy
Pregnospia	reagent	Pregnancy
Pregnosticon Dri-Dot	slide	Pregnancy
Rapid Test Strep	slide	Group A streptococci
Respiracult	swab	Group A beta-hemolytic streptococci
Respiralex	slide	Group A beta-hemolytic streptococci
Respirastick	strip	Group A streptococci
Rheumanosticon Dri-Dot	slide	Rheumatoid factor in blood
Rotalex	slide	Rotavirus in feces
Rubacell II	reagent	Rubella virus in serum or plasma
Sickledex Test	strips	Hemoglobin S (sickle cells)
Streptonase-B	reagent	Serum B antibodies (streptococcal infection)
Strepto-Sec	slide	Beta-hemolytic streptococci, groups A, B, C, and G
Tes-Tape	strips	Urinary glucose
UBT	strips	Blood in urine
UCG-Slide Test	slide	Pregnancy
Uricult	strips	Urinary bacteriuria/uropathogens
Uristix	strips	Urinary glucose, protein
Uroblistix	strips	Urinary urobilinogen
Visidex II	strips	Blood glucose

agents are opaque chemicals that are employed as contrast media to enhance visualization of internal structures by x-ray examination. Localization of a substance to the particular area to be visualized is accomplished either through direct instillation into an organ (e.g., uterus, colon, bronchioles, spinal column) or by incorporation of the radiopaque drug into an organic compound whose properties determine its distribution in the body (e.g., excretion by way of the bile or urine or plasma protein binding).

In addition to barium and the iodine-containing compounds, other substances used as radiolabeled agents for diagnostic purposes (with their uses in parentheses) include chromium (red cell volume), cobalt (B$_{12}$ absorption), mercury (kidney function), and technetium and phosphorus (brain tumors).

Barium Sulfate

Barium sulfate is the most commonly used substance for visualization of the GI tract. It is a highly insoluble compound; thus, only minimal amounts are absorbed systemically and toxicity is quite low. Barium sulfate can be administered orally as a thick paste for examination of the esophagus or as a more dilute suspension for visualization of the stomach and upper intestinal tract. Radiographic studies of the lower GI tract and colon may be performed following a cleansing enema and rectal instillation of barium sulfate suspension. Barium sulfate may be constipating, and complete expulsion of the suspension from the GI tract following the examination usually requires use

(*Text continued on page 799*)

Table 76-2
Intradermal Diagnostic Biologicals

Diagnostic Agent	Preparations	Uses	Nursing Implications
Coccidioidin Spherulin	Injection: 1:10, 1:100	Diagnosis of coccidioidomycosis Differentiation of coccidioidomycosis from other diseases with similar clinical findings, e.g., histoplasmosis, sarcoidosis	Diluted with sodium chloride injection; 0.1 mL of 1:10,000 is injected intradermally; if negative, repeat with 1:1000 and finally 1:100; positive reaction is appearance of area of induration measuring 5 mm or greater; erythema without induration is considered negative; reaction is readable at 24 h and maximal at 36 h and is indicative that contact with the fungus has occurred in the past although patient does not necessarily have an active infection; false positive skin reactions do *not* occur; sensitive individuals may exhibit an intense local response
Diphtheria Diphtheria Toxin for Schick Test	Injection: 1 vial of toxin and 1 vial of control	Diagnosis of serologic immunity to diphtheria	Injected intradermally on flexor surface of forearm, control solution on one arm and toxin on other arm; results are read on day 4 or 5; positive reaction is appearance of circumscribed area of redness and slight infiltration measuring 1 cm or more in diameter and indicates person has little or no antitoxin to diphtheria and is susceptible to infection; aspirate prior to injection to ensure needle is not in blood vessel
Histoplasmin Histoplasmin, Diluted; Histolyn-CYL	Injection: 1.0 mL/vial in 10 0.1-mL doses, 1.3-mL multidose vial	Diagnosis of histoplasmosis Differentiation of histoplasmosis from other mycotic or bacterial infections, e.g., coccidioidomycosis, sarcoidosis	A sterile filtrate from cultures of *Histoplasma capsulatum*; 0.1 mL is injected intradermally into flexor surface of the forearm and reaction is read in 48–72 h; induration of 5 mm or greater is considered positive and may indicate a previous mild, subacute, or chronic infection with *Histoplasma capsulatum* or immunologically related organisms; little value in diagnosing acute, fulminating infections because a negative reaction usually occurs; large doses can produce severe erythema and induration with ulceration and necrosis; systemic allergic reactions can occur; infrequently used test
Mumps Skin Test Antigen	Injection: 1 mL (10 tests)	Determination of sensitivity to mumps virus	Suspension of killed mumps virus used to determine skin sensitivity to mumps; effectiveness has not been conclusively established; may be useful in adolescence for identifying those who should be protected against the disease; however, most of the population have had contact with mumps virus and will demonstrate a delayed cutaneous hypersensitivity to the antigen; following injection of 0.1 mL intradermally on inner surface of forearm, reaction is read in 24–36 h; erythema of 1.5 cm or more indicates sensitivity to virus and probable immunity; negative reaction suggests probable susceptibility; do *not* use in persons sensitive to chicken, eggs, or feathers because preparation is cultivated in chicken embryo
Skin Test Antigens, Multiple Multitest CMI	Eight single-dose applications preloaded with seven delayed hypersensitivity skin test antigens and glycerin control	Detection of nonresponsiveness to antigens by means of delayed hypersensitivity skin testing	Applicator has 8 test heads preloaded with delayed hypersensitivity skin test antigens to tetanus toxoid, diphtheria toxoid, *Streptococcus*, old tuberculin, *Candida*, *Trichophyton*, and *Proteus*; reactivity may be reduced in patients receiving drugs that suppress immunity or in patients with acute viral infections; test results are read at 24 h and 48 h; positive reaction is induration of 2 mm or greater at antigen site provided there is *no* induration at control site; do *not* apply on infected or inflamed skin; if periodic testing is done, rotate sites of application
Tuberculin Purified Protein Derivative—Tuberculin PPD Aplisol, Tubersol	Injection: 1 U/0.1 mL, 5 U/0.1 mL, 250 U/0.1 mL	Aid in diagnosis of tuberculosis	Aqueous solution of a purified protein fraction from filtrates of cultured human strains of *Mycobacterium tuberculosis*; use only *fresh* tuberculin preparations for testing; injected intradermally (5 U) on the flexor or dorsal surface of the forearm;

Continued

Table 76-2
Intradermal Diagnostic Biologicals (continued)

Diagnostic Agent	Preparations	Uses	Nursing Implications
			reaction is read in 48–72 h; induration of 10 mm or more is a positive reaction, whereas induration of 5 mm or less is negative; erythema is not of diagnostic significance but may indicate incorrect administration; retesting is indicated if induration measures 5 mm–9 mm; positive reaction does not indicate an active infection but suggests further evaluation is necessary; positive reaction may also indicate previous BCG vaccination; preferred over old tuberculin (OT) test owing to greater purity; highly sensitive persons may experience vesiculation, ulceration, and necrosis, and persons suspected of being highly sensitive should receive an initial dose of only 1 U; the 250-U injection is used *only* for persons who do not react to 5 U, although individuals not reacting to 5 U may be considered tuberculin negative
Tuberculin PPD, Multiple Puncture Device Aplitest, Sclavo Test-PPD, Tine Test PPD	Cylindrical plastic units	*See* tuberculin PPD	A single-use device consisting of 4 stainless steel tines coated with tuberculin PPD, standardized to give reactions equivalent to 5 U of intradermal tuberculin PPD
Old Tuberculin, Multiple Puncture Devices Tuberculin Mono-Vacc Test, Tuberculin Old Tine Test	Individual units	*See* tuberculin PPD	Single-use, multiple puncture device standardized to give reactions equivalent to 5 U of standard solution of old tuberculin administered intradermally; test is read 48–96 h after administration; positive reaction is vesiculation or induration of 1 mm or greater, but further diagnostic tests are necessary to establish presence of infection; infrequently used preparation

Table 76-3
In Vivo Diagnostic Aids

Diagnostic Agent	Preparations	Uses	Nursing Implications
Aminohippurate Sodium PAH	Aqueous solution: 20%	Assessment of renal blood flow and tubular secretory mechanisms	Occasionally used to study certain aspects of kidney function; used by IV injection; not metabolized and excreted solely by the kidney; low plasma concentrations (1 mg–2 mg/dL) are used to measure renal blood flow; higher concentrations (40 mg–60 mg/dL) are employed to determine maximal tubular secretory capacity; may elicit nausea, feelings of warmth, and urge to defecate
L-arginine R-Gene 10	Solution: 10% in sterile water for injection for IV infusion	Determination of pituitary human growth hormone reserve; diagnosis of panhypopituitarism, pituitary dwarfism, pituitary trauma, and other hypopituitary conditions	Stimulates pituitary to release growth hormone; dosage is 300 mL in adults and 5 mL/kg in children; rate of false positive reactions is 32% and false negative is 27%; do *not* use in patients with strong allergic tendencies; excessive infusion rates can result in irritation, nausea, vomiting, and flushing; have antihistamine available in case of allergic reactions; do *not* use if solution is not clean or if bottle lacks a vacuum; refer to package literature for interpretation of results
Bentiromide Chymex	Solution: 500 mg/7.5 mL	Screening test for pancreatic exocrine insufficiency	A peptide containing 170 mg para-aminobenzoic acid (PABA) per 500 mg dose; following oral administration, bentiromide is hydrolyzed by pancreatic chymotrypsin, liberating PABA, which is excreted in the urine; if exocrine pancreatic function is normal, over 50% of the PABA contained in bentiromide appears in the urine within 6 h

Continued

Table 76-3
In Vivo Diagnostic Aids (continued)

Diagnostic Agent	Preparations	Uses	Nursing Implications
			and can be detected using the Smith modification of the Bratton–Marshall test for arylamines; patients should fast at least 8 h before receiving a test dose; diarrhea, headache, nausea, flatulence, and weakness can occur; instruct patient to urinate immediately before receiving bentiromide; falsely elevated readings can occur if the patient is taking other drugs metabolized to arylamines, such as acetaminophen, chloramphenicol, lidocaine, procaine, procainamide, sulfonamides, or thiazide diuretics
Benzylpenicilloyl-polylysine Pre-Pen	Ampules	Skin test for penicillin hypersensitivity in patients who have previously received penicillin and demonstrated a clinical hypersensitivity reaction	May be applied either by scratching forearm (preferred method) or by intradermal injection on upper outer arm surface; positive reaction consists of whealing, erythema, and itching; occurs usually within 10 min and is associated with an incidence of allergic reactions to systemic benzylpenicillin or penicillin G of greater than 20%; a negative skin test response predicts a less than 5% incidence of allergic complications; of doubtful value in assessing sensitivity to semisynthetic penicillins or cephalosporins; may produce an intense local inflammatory response and occasionally systemic allergic reactions
Cosyntropin Cortrosyn (CAN) Synacthen Depot	Vials with diluent: 0.25 mg with 10 mg mannitol	Diagnosis of adrenal cortical insufficiency	Synthetic subunit of human ACTH used IM or by IV infusion to differentiate primary (adrenal) from secondary (pituitary) adrenocortical insufficiency; in primary Addison's disease, 24-h urinary 17-hydroxycorticosteroid levels fail to rise following IV infusion and plasma cortisol levels do not increase significantly within 30 min following IM injection; secondary pituitary failure is characterized by a *slow increase* in urinary steroids following IV infusion; produces fewer allergic reactions than ACTH injection
Gonadorelin Factrel	Powder for injection: 100 μg/vial, 500 μg/vial	Evaluation of hypothalamic–pituitary–gonadotropic function Evaluation of residual gonadotropic function following hypophysectomy Investigational uses include induction of ovulation and treatment of precocious puberty	Synthetic luteinizing hormone–releasing hormone (LHRH) structurally identical to natural LHRH possessing a gonadotropin-releasing effect on the anterior pituitary; used SC or IV; in females, test should be performed in early follicular phase of the menstrual cycle; do *not* give concurrently with gonadal hormones, glucocorticoids or spironolactone, because pituitary secretion of gonadotropins can be affected; SC injection can result in localized pain, swelling and itching; use during pregnancy only when clearly needed; refer to package prescribing information for testing method
Histamine Phosphate	Injection: Gastric test—0.55 mg (0.2 mg base)/mL; 2.75 mg (1 mg base)/mL	Assessment of gastric acid secretory capacity	Basal acid secretion is measured, then 0.01 mg–0.04 mg histamine base/kg is injected SC and gastric contents are collected in four 15-min specimens and analyzed for volume, pH, and acidity; an antihistamine should be administered IM before histamine; many side effects noted and severe allergic reactions (e.g., asthma) can occur; largely replaced by other, safer diagnostic measures (e.g., pentagastrin)
	Pheochromocytoma: 0.275 mg (0.1 mg base)/mL	Presumptive diagnosis of pheochromocytoma	Once used for diagnosis of pheochromocytoma (positive response was at least a 60 mm/40 mm rise in blood pressure above the baseline *or* an increase of at least 20 mm/10 mm above that obtained in the cold pressor test); *very hazardous procedure*; phentolamine must be readily available to control excessive increase in blood pressure; rarely employed today with the availability of more accurate and less dangerous procedures

Continued

Table 76-3
In Vivo Diagnostic Aids (continued)

Diagnostic Agent	Preparations	Uses	Nursing Implications
Hysteroscopy Fluid Hyskon	Solution: 32% w/v dextran 70 in 10% w/v dextrose	Aid in distending the uterine cavity and visualizing its surfaces	Introduced into uterine cavity via cannula under low pressure until uterus is sufficiently distended to permit adequate visualization; volume usually required is 50 mL–100 mL; allergic reactions, including anaphylaxis, can result if drug is absorbed systemically; *do not* exceed 150 mm Hg infusion pressure
Indocyanine Green Cardio-Green	Vials: 25 mg, 50 mg Disposable units: 10 mg, 40 mg	Determination of cardiac output, hepatic function, and liver blood flow Aid in ophthalmic angiography	A water-soluble dye that is injected IV, is quickly bound to plasma proteins, and is taken up almost exclusively by hepatic parenchymal cells; dilution of dye in blood samples obtained from different sites at various times following administration is an indication of blood flow in a particular area; adverse effects are minimal; drug contains a small amount of sodium iodide and may interfere with radioactive iodine-uptake studies
Inulin	Injection: 100 mg/mL	Measurement of glomerular filtration rate	Polymer of fructose given by IV infusion; drug is rapidly filtered by the kidneys and neither secreted nor reabsorbed; following a loading dose, samples of urine are collected at regular intervals and concentration of inulin in each sample is determined colorimetrically; normal adult inulin clearance is 100 mL–160 mL/min
Mannitol	Solution: 5%, 10%, 15%, 20%, 25%	Measurement of glomerular filtration rate	An osmotic diuretic (see Chap. 37) that is also used to measure glomerular filtration rate (GFR); 100 mL of a 20% solution is diluted with 180 mg normal saline and infused at a rate of 20 mL/min; urine is collected by a catheter for a specific time period and a blood sample is drawn at the beginning and end of the collection period; mannitol concentrations (mg/mL) are determined for each sample and the GFR is calculated as mL of plasma that must be filtered to yield the amount of mannitol excreted per minute in the urine
Methacholine Provocholine	Powder for dilution: 100 mg/5-mL vial	Assessment of bronchial airway hyperactivity	Cholinergic agent that is administered by inhalation in solutions of increasing concentration; pulmonary function (forced expiratory volume—FEV) is measured after each dose; requires trained personnel and emergency equipment, and medications must be readily available; may cause headache, throat irritation, lightheadedness, and itching; do *not* inhale powder; response in patients receiving beta blockers may be exaggerated
Metyrapone Metopirone	Tablets: 250 mg	Diagnosis of hypothalamus–pituitary function	Used to test whether pituitary secretion of ACTH is adequate; ability of adrenals to respond to ACTH should be demonstrated by ACTH or cosyntropin test before giving metyrapone; following a 2-day rest period, 15 mg/kg is administered orally every 4 h for 6 doses, then urinary 17-hydroxycorticosteroids (17-OHCS) are collected for 24 h; normal pituitary function is indicated by a 2–4-fold increase in 17-OHCS over control levels obtained before drug administration; excessive excretion of 17-OHCS suggests Cushing's syndrome (adrenal hyperplasia), while subnormal excretion indicates hypopituitarism
Pentagastrin Peptavlon	Injection: 0.25 mg/mL	Evaluation of gastric and secretory capacity	Action resembles that of natural gastrin; following SC injection of 6 μg/kg, acid secretion begins within 10 min, peaks in 20–30 min, and lasts 60–90 min; elicits fewer and less intense side effects than either histamine or betazole and is the preferred drug for measuring gastric acid secretion; children's dosages have not been established; *cautious use* in patients with hepatic, biliary, or pancreatic disease

Continued

Table 76-3
In Vivo Diagnostic Aids (continued)

Diagnostic Agent	Preparations	Uses	Nursing Implications
Protirelin Relefact TRH, Thypinone	Injection: 0.5 mg/mL	Adjunct in the evaluation of thyroid function Adjunct for adjustment of thyroid hormone dosage in hypothyroid patients	Synthetic peptide similar in action to thyrotropin-releasing hormone (TRH); following IV injection (adults—500 µg; children—7 µg/kg), protirelin causes release of thyroid-stimulating hormone (TSH) from anterior pituitary; TSH blood levels are determined before injection and again 30 min after injection; thyroid function is characterized by comparing baseline TSH serum levels to those obtained following drug injection; if test is repeated, allow an interval of 7 days; discontinue thyroid drugs at least 7 days before performing test; most common side effects are nausea, urinary urgency, flushing, lightheadedness, headache, dry mouth, and abdominal discomfort; patient should be supine during testing to minimize changes in blood pressure
Secretin Secretin Ferring Powder	Powder for injection: 10 U/mL when reconstituted according to package instructions	Diagnosis of pancreatic exocrine disease or gastrinoma (Zollinger–Ellison syndrome) Aid in obtaining pancreatic cells for pathologic study	Hormone obtained from porcine duodenal mucosa that increases volume and bicarbonate content of pancreatic secretions; powder is dissolved in 10 mL sodium chloride injection and administered by slow IV injection (5 min) at a dose of 1 U–2 U/kg; samples are collected with a gastric tube and analyzed for volume, enzyme and bicarbonate content, occult blood, biliary pigment; *cautious use* in acute pancreatitis; frequently given with sincalide (see below)
Sincalide Kinevac	Injection: 5 µg/vial for reconstitution to 1 µg/mL	To stimulate pancreatic or gallbladder secretions	Synthetic subunit of cholecystokinin that produces gallbladder contraction following IV injection; also enhances pancreatic secretions when given in combination with secretin; to contract gallbladder, 0.02 µg/kg is given by rapid (30–60 sec) IV injection, which may be repeated in 15 min at 0.04 µg/kg; for secretin–sincalide test of pancreatic function, 0.02 µg/kg is infused over a 30 min period beginning 30 min after the secretion infusion; safety not established in children or pregnant women; abdominal discomfort and urge to defecate frequently occur
Teriparatide Parathar	Powder for injection: 200 U hPTH activity	Differentiation of hypoparathyroidism from pseudohypoparathyroidism	Synthetic polypeptide hormone consisting of the 1–34 fragment of human parathyroid hormone; hypercalcemia may develop; systemic allergic reactions have occurred; does *not* discriminate between hypoparathyroidism and normal
Thyrotropin Thytropar	Powder for injection: 10 IU thyrotropic activity/vial	Diffential diagnosis of thyroid failure and decreased thyroid reserve	Purified, lyophilized thyroid-stimulating hormone obtained from bovine anterior pituitary; increases iodine uptake by gland and formation and release of thyroid hormones; thyroid hyperplasia can occur; administered IM or SC (10 IU for 1–3 days), followed by radioiodine study 24 h after last dose; no response is indicative of thyroid failure; nausea, vomiting, headache, urticaria, tachycardia, and hypotension can occur, anaphylactic reactions have been reported; use *cautiously* in presence of coronary artery disease or heart disease
Tolbutamide Sodium Orinase Diagnostic	Injection: 1 g with 20 mL diluent	Diagnosis of pancreatic islet cell adenoma or diabetics	Patients with pancreatic cell insulinomas show a *sharp, intense* drop in blood glucose following IV injection of 1 g tolbutamide sodium; hypoglycemia may persist for several hours and may require treatment if symptoms are too intense; diabetic patients show a *gradual* decrease in blood glucose, whereas normal persons evidence a prompt reduction (15–20 min) associated with an elevation in serum insulin
D-xylose Xylo-Pfan	Powder	Test for intestinal malabsorption states	Nonmetabolizable sugar given orally (25 g) to assess absorptive capacity of GI tract; normal values are 5 g–8 g in urine within 5 h and 40 mg/100 mL blood within 2 h

of a laxative or an enema. The barium-containing diagnostic agents are listed in Table 76-4.

Iodinated Radiopaque Agents

A variety of iodine-containing organic compounds can be used either orally or parenterally to visualize a number of different body organs. The opacity of these agents depends upon the percentage of iodine in the molecule and the amount of drug concentrated at a particular site. Patients should be questioned concerning iodine hypersensitivity before administration of one of these compounds. Severe, *sometimes fatal,* allergic reactions have occurred with use of these agents, and patients with a history of bronchial asthma or other allergies must be closely monitored during administration and for at least 1 hour afterward. Appropriate antidotal measures, including respiratory aids, epinephrine, and corticosteroids, should be available.

Adverse reactions are uncommon, but the possibility of their occurrence must not be overlooked. Among the untoward reactions reported with use of radiographic contrast media are urticaria, wheezing, dyspnea, angioneurotic edema, laryngeal spasm, anaphylaxis, hyperthermia, headache, chest tightness, and tremor. Reactions that are probably attributable to volume, speed, and site of injection are flushing, dizziness, nausea, generalized vasodilation, and hypotension. Pain and irritation at the injection site have been noted, as well as paresthesias, numbness, hematomas, ecchymoses, and thrombophlebitis.

The iodinated radiographic contrast agents are listed in Table 76-5. Their dosage forms, iodine content, composition, and diagnostic use are given as well. Because their dosage and route of administration depend on their diagnostic intent, the information included with each drug must be consulted before administration.

An adjunctive drug that is sometimes used in lymphography to facilitate visualization of the lymphatic system is isosulfan blue (Lymphazurin 1%). Following SC injection of 0.5 mL into three interdigital spaces of each extremity per study, isosulfan is selectively concentrated in the lymphatic vessels, which it colors a bright blue. Adverse reactions are relatively infrequent (1%–2%) and are largely of an allergic nature, ranging from itching and swelling of the hands to generalized edema and respiratory distress in rare instances.

Another adjunctive agent that is used in certain radiographic studies is potassium perchlorate (Perchloracap). This agent provides perchlorate ion (ClO_4), which suppresses accumulation of pertechnetate ion ($CTcO_4$) in the choroid plexus and salivary and thyroid glands of patients receiving radioactive sodium pertechnetate (^{99m}Tc) for brain imaging or placenta localization. Perchlorate competes for plasma protein-binding sites with TcO_4, with a resultant shift of a portion of TcO_4 from the plasma to the red blood cell. The drug is given orally as capsules in a dose of 200 mg to 400 mg 30 minutes to 60 minutes before a dose of sodium pertechnetate.

Selected Bibliography

Bentiromide—A test for pancreatic insufficiency. Med Lett Drugs Ther 26:50, 1984

Berger ME, Hubner KF: Hospital hazards: Diagnostic radiation. Am J Nurs 83(8):1155, 1983

Early PJ, Sodee DB: Principles and Practice of Nuclear Medicine. St Louis, CV Mosby, 1985

Hermann CS: Performing intradermal skin tests the right way. Nursing '83 13(10):50, 1983

Rayudu CVS: Radiotracers for Medical Applications. Boca Raton, FL, CRC Press, 1983

Sincalide for cholecystography. Med Lett Drugs Ther 19:36, 1977

Synthetic LH-RH. Med Lett Drugs Ther 25:106, 1983

Table 76-4
Barium-Containing Diagnostic Agents

Trade Name	Preparations	Uses	Dosage
Baricon	Powder for suspension: 95% barium sulfate	Upper GI studies	Prepare 60% suspension
Baro-Cat	Suspension: 1.5% barium sulfate	Upper and lower GI studies	300 mL at 2 h and again at 15 min before exam
Baroflave	Powder: 100% barium sulfate	Upper and lower GI studies	50 g–500 g suspended in water
Barosperse	Powder for suspension: 95% barium sulfate in single-dose cups, disposable enemas, and air-contrast units	Esophageal, upper and lower GI, and colon studies Air-contrast studies	*Esophageal:* 45 g in 15 mL water to yield 75% suspension *Upper/lower GI, air contrast:* 225 g in 150 mL water to yield a 60% suspension *Colon:* dilute 500 mL 60% suspension with 1500 mL water to make 20% suspension; use by enema
Barosperse 110	Powder for suspension: 95% barium sulfate	Upper and lower GI and colon studies	*Upper GI/colon:* add 600 mL water to make a 60% suspension *Low-density upper GI:* add 875 mL water to make a 50% suspension

Note: Additional barium-containing diagnostic agents available in Canada include Colobar DC, Colobar-400, Epi-C, Epistat 57, Epistat-61, Esobar, Esopho-Cat, E-Z-Cat, E-Z-HD, E-Z-Jug, E-Z-Paque, Gel-Unix, Liqui-Jug, Polibar, Readi-Cat, Recto-Barium, Ultra-R, Unibar-60.

Table 76-5
Iodinated Radiographic Diagnostic Agents

Trade Name	Dosage Form	Iodine Content	Composition	Diagnostic Uses
Amipaque	Injection	48.25%	13.5%, 18.75% metrizamide	Myelography Computed tomography (CT) of intracranial subarachnoid spaces Peripheral arteriography Pediatric angiocardiography
Angio-Conray	Injection	48%	80% iothalamate	Angiocardiography Aortography
Angiovist 282	Injection	28%	60% diatrizoate meglumine	Angiography Arthrography Cholangiography Discography Excretory urography Peripheral arteriography Pyelography Splenoportography Venography
Angiovist 292	Injection	29.2%	52% diatrizoate meglumine and 8% diatrizoate sodium	See Angiovist 282
Angiovist 370	Injection	37%	66% diatrizoate meglumine and 10% diatrizoate sodium	See Angiovist 282
Bilivist	Capsules	61.4%	500 mg ipodate sodium	Cholangiography Cholecystography
Bilopaque	Capsules	57.4%	750 mg tyropanoate sodium	Cholecystography
Cholebrine	Tablets	62%	750 mg iocetamic acid	Cholecystography
Cholografin	Injection	5.1%	10.3% iodipamide meglumine	Cholecystography Cholangiography
Cholografin	Injection	26%	52% iodipamide meglumine	Cholecystography Cholangiography
Conray	Injection	28.2%	60% iothalamate meglumine	Cerebral angiography Drip infusion pyelography Peripheral arteriography Urography Venography
Conray-30	Injection	14.1%	30% iothalamate meglumine	Infusion Urography
Conray-43	Injection	20.2%	43% iothalamate meglumine	Lower extremity venography
Conray-325	Injection	32.5%	54.3% iothalamate sodium	Excretory urography
Conray-400	Injection	40%	66.8% iothalamate sodium	Angiocardiography Aortography Excretory urography IV pyelography Renal arteriography
Cysto-Conray	Instillation solution	20.2%	43% iothalamate meglumine	Cystography Cystourethrography Retrograde pyelography
Cysto-Conray II	Instillation solution	8.1%	17.2% iothalamate meglumine	Cystography Cystourethrography Retrograde pyelography
Cystografin	Instillation solution	14.1%	30% diatrizoate meglumine	Cystourethrography Retrograde pyelography
Cystografin-Dilute	Instillation solution	8.5%	18% diatrizoate meglumine	Retrograde cystourethrography
Diatrizoate-60	Injection	29.2%	52% diatrizoate meglumine and 8% diatrizoate sodium	See Angiovist 282, above Computed tomography (CT)
Diatrizoate meglumine 76%	Injection	35.8%	76% diatrizoate meglumine	Aortography Excretory urography Pediatric angiocardiography Peripheral arteriography
Ethiodol	Injection	37%	Ethiodized oil	Hysterosalpingography Lymphography
Gastrografin	Oral/rectal solution	37%	66% diatrizoate meglumine and 10% diatrizoate sodium	GI radiography

Continued

Table 76-5
Iodinated Radiographic Diagnostic Agents (continued)

Trade Name	Dosage Form	Iodine Content	Composition	Diagnostic Uses
Gastrovist	Oral/rectal solution	37%	66% diatrizoate meglumine and 10% diatrizoate sodium	GI radiography
Hexabrix	Injection	32%	39.3% ioxaglate meglumine and 19.6% ioxaglate sodium	Cerebral angiography Coronary arteriography Peripheral arteriography Visceral arteriography Digital angiography Peripheral venography Excretory urography Computed tomography (CT)
Hypaque 20%	Instillation solution	12%	20% diatrizoate sodium	Retrograde pyelography
Hypaque 25%	Injection	15%	25% diatrizoate sodium	Drip-infusion pyelography (excretory urography)
Hypaque 50%	Injection	30%	50% diatrizoate sodium	Angiography (cerebral and peripheral) Aortography Cholangiography Hysterosalpingography Intraosseous venography Splenoportography
Hypaque-M 75%	Injection	38.5%	50% diatrizoate meglumine and 25% diatrizoate sodium	Abdominal aortography Angiocardiography Arteriography (coronary, peripheral, and renal) Urography
Hypaque-M 90%	Injection	46.2%	60% diatrizoate meglumine and 30% diatrizoate sodium	Abdominal aortography Angiocardiography Arteriography (coronary and peripheral) Hysterosalpingography Urography
Hypaque-Cysto	Instillation solution	14.1%	30% diatrizoate meglumine	Retrograde cystourethrography
Hypaque Meglumine 30%	Injection	14.1%	30% diatrizoate meglumine	Infusion urography Computed tomography (CT)
Hypaque Meglumine 60%	Injection	28.2%	60% diatrizoate meglumine	Arthrography Cerebral angiography Cholangiography Discography Excretory urography Peripheral arteriography and venography Splenoportography
Hypaque Sodium	Liquid	24.9%	2.4 g diatrizoate sodium/mL	GI radiography
Hypaque Sodium	Powder for oral solution	59.8%		GI radiography
Hypaque-76	Injection	37%	66% diatrizoate meglumine and 10% diatrizoate sodium	See Angiovist 282, above
Isovue 300	Injection	30%	61% iopamidol	Angiography Arteriography IV contrast enhancement
Isovue 370	Injection	37%	75.5% iopamidol	See Isovue 300, above
Isovue-M 200	Injection	20%	40.8% iopamidol	Contrast enhancement Intrathecal neuroradiology Ventriculography
Isovue-M 300	Injection	30%	61.2% iopamidol	See Isovue-M 200, above
MD-50	Injection	30%	50% diatrizoate sodium	See Hypaque 50%, above
MD-60	Injection	29.2%	52% diatrizoate meglumine and 8% diatrizoate sodium	See Angiovist 282, above
MD-76	Injection	37%	66% diatrizoate meglumine and 10% diatrizoate sodium	See Angiovist 282, above
MD-Gastroview	Oral/rectal solution	37%	66% diatrizoate meglumine and 10% diatrizoate sodium	See Angiovist 282, above

Continued

Table 76-5
Iodinated Radiographic Diagnostic Agents (continued)

Trade Name	Dosage Form	Iodine Content	Composition	Diagnostic Uses
Omnipaque	Injection		Iohexol equivalent to 18%, 24%, 30%, or 35% iodine	Intrathecal or intravascular radiography
Oragrafin Calcium	Granules for oral suspension	61.7%	3 g ipodate calcium/8-g packet	Cholangiography Cholecystography
Oragrafin Sodium	Capsules	61.4%	500 mg ipodate sodium	Cholecystography
Renografin-60	Injection	29%	52% diatrizoate meglumine and 8% diatrizoate sodium	Arthrography Cerebral angiography Cholangiography Computed tomography (CT) Discography Excretory urography Peripheral arteriography Pyelography Splenoportography Venography
Renografin-76	Injection	37%	66% diatrizoate meglumine and 10% diatrizoate sodium	See Renografin-60, above
Reno-M-30	Instillation solution	14%	30% diatrizoate meglumine	Retrograde or ascending pyelography
Reno-M-60	Injection	28%	60% diatrizoate meglumine	Arthrography Cerebral angiography Cholangiography Discography Excretory urography Peripheral arteriography Pyelography Splenoportography Venography
Reno-M-Dip	Injection	14%	30% diatrizoate meglumine	Computed tomography (CT) Drip-infusion pyelography
Renovist	Injection	37%	34.3% diatrizoate meglumine and 35% diatrizoate sodium	Angiocardiography Aortography Excretory urography Peripheral arteriography and venography Venocavography
Renovist II	Injection	31%	28.5% diatrizoate meglumine and 29.1% diatrizoate sodium	See Renovist, above
Renovue-65	Injection	30%	65% iodamide meglumine	Excretory urography
Renovue-Dip	Injection	11.1%	24% iodamide meglumine	Excretory urography
Sinografin	Injection	38%	52.7% diatrizoate meglumine and 26.8% iodipamide meglumine	Hysterosalpingography
Telepaque	Tablets	66.7%	500 mg iopanoic acid	Cholecystography
Urovist Cysto	Instillation solution	14.1%	30% diatrizoate meglumine	Cystourethrography Retrograde pyelography
Urovist Meglumine DIU/CT	Injection	14.1%	30% diatrizoate meglumine	Drip-infusion pyelography Computed tomography (CT) Venography
Urovist Sodium 300	Injection	30%	50% diatrizoate sodium	See Hypaque 50%, above
Vascoray	Injection	40%	52% iothalamate meglumine and 26% iothalamate sodium	Angiocardiography Aortography Arteriography (coronary and renal) Excretory urography

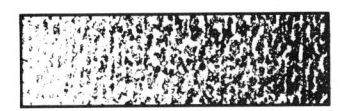

SERUMS AND VACCINES

The ability of circulating antibodies to render a person resistant to a particular disease is known as *immunity*. Immunity may be natural or acquired. Persons born with resistance to a certain disease state are said to have *natural* immunity; however, this is a relatively rare occurrence. Most types of immunity are *acquired*, that is, attained during the person's lifetime, either by production of antibodies in response to an invasion by foreign microorganisms (*active* acquired immunity) or by utilization of antibodies obtained from an animal or another human immunized against a particular disease (*passive* acquired immunity). Active immunity, therefore, is acquired through contact with the antigen itself, which stimulates the body to produce its own specific antibodies to combat it. If the antibodies develop in response to exposure to an actual disease state, whether clinical symptoms are present or not, the active immunity is said to be *naturally acquired*. Conversely, if the antibodies form in response to inoculation into the body of killed or attenuated microorganisms or their toxic by-products, the active immunity is referred to as *artificially acquired*.

The biologic preparations used to confer immunity may be categorized in the following manner:

I. Agents for active immunity
   A. Toxoids (e.g., diphtheria, tetanus)
   B. Vaccines
      1. Bacterial (e.g., BCG, cholera, hemophilus, typhoid)
      2. Viral (e.g., influenza, measles, hepatitis B, poliovirus)
II. Agents for passive immunity
   A. Antitoxins/antivenins (e.g., diphtheria, tetanus, black widow spider)
   B. Human immune serums (e.g., immune globulins)
III. Rabies prophylaxis products (e.g., antirabies serum, rabies immune globulin, rabies vaccine)

AGENTS FOR ACTIVE IMMUNITY

Agents used for active immunity contain specific antigens that induce the formation of antibodies when injected into the body. These antigenic substances are of two types, toxoids and vaccines. *Toxoids* are toxins derived from microorganisms that have been modified (i.e., detoxified), usually with formaldehyde, so that they are no longer toxic but are still antigenic, and thus are capable of stimulating antibody production. *Vaccines* are suspensions of whole microorganisms, either killed or chemically attenuated to reduce their virulence, which are capable of inducing the formation of antibodies without causing an outbreak of the disease. Active immunity with toxoids or vaccines requires several days or even weeks to develop, because sufficient antibody levels need to be attained. In some cases, more than one dose may be required. Thus, toxoids and vaccines are of limited value in treating *active* infections. Once acquired, however, active immunity can usually be made to last a lifetime, especially if reinforced by periodic "booster" doses at appropriate intervals.

Toxoids

Diphtheria	Diphtheria and tetanus toxoids and pertussis vaccine (DTP)
Diphtheria and tetanus	Tetanus

Toxoids are generally prepared by treating exotoxins with formaldehyde, which renders them nontoxic but still antigenic. Stimulation of antibody production by toxoids can be increased by precipitating the toxoid with alum or adsorbing it onto colloids such as aluminum hydroxide. The precipitated or adsorbed products are absorbed and excreted more slowly, and they persist in tissues longer than do plain toxoids, resulting in higher antibody production. The principal disadvantage of these precipitated or adsorbed toxoids is that their use is frequently associated with pain, swelling, and tenderness at the injection site, especially in older children and adults. These reactions are sometimes quite severe. The most commonly employed toxoids are diphtheria and tetanus, which are frequently given in combination with pertussis vaccine as DTP for routine immunization in preschool children. Table 77-1 lists the toxoids.

Vaccines

BCG	Mumps
Cholera	Plague
Hemophilus B	Pneumococcal
Hepatitis B	Poliovirus
Influenza virus	Rubella
Measles	Rubella and mumps
Measles and rubella	
Measles, rubella, and mumps	Staphage lysate
Meningitis	Typhoid
Mixed respiratory	Yellow fever

Vaccines are suspensions of killed or attenuated microorganisms of bacteria or viruses that are capable of stimulating antibody production but that are in themselves nonpathogenic. The live, attenuated vaccines are claimed to provide longer-lasting immunity in most cases than the killed or inactivated vaccines, although both types are quite effective in increasing antibody levels. Caution must be observed, however, in using a vaccine grown and cultivated in living tissues, for example, chick embryo, because allergic reactions can occur in patients hypersensitive to the specific animal proteins. However, influenza virus vaccine, although grown in embryonated eggs, is highly purified and is much less likely to elicit hypersensitivity reactions than other vaccines. Conversely, live viral vaccines prepared by growing viruses in human cell culture (e.g., rubella) are much less antigenic than animal-derived products.

Table 77-1
Toxoids

Preparations	Administration	Nursing Implications
Diphtheria Toxoid, Adsorbed, Pediatric	2 injections (0.5 mL) IM 6–8 wk apart, then a third dose 1 yr later *Booster:* 5–10-year intervals	Used in infants and children under 6 yr; do *not* administer subcutaneously; avoid giving during active infections or in patients receiving corticosteroids, because antibody response is diminished; *cautious use* in children with neurologic or convulsive disorders
Diphtheria and Tetanus Toxoids, Combined, Pediatric	*Infants 6 wk through 11 mo:* 3 injections (0.5 mL) IM at least 4 wk apart; a fourth injection is given after 6–12 mo *Children 1–6 yr:* 2 injections (0.5 mL) at least 4 wk apart; a third dose is given after 6–12 mo *Booster:* 0.5 mL at 4–6 yr	Used only in children 6 yr or under; indicated only where the triple antigen (DTP) is contraindicated; do *not* administer during acute infection or in patients receiving immunosuppressant drugs; note that pediatric preparation is 3–8 times as potent as adult preparation with respect to diphtheria toxoid; side effects include localized pain, swelling, and tenderness; drowsiness, fretfulness, and anorexia
Diphtheria and Tetanus Toxoids, Combined, Adult	2 injections (2 U diphtheria/0.5 mL) IM 4–6 wk apart, then a third dose 6–12 mo later *Booster* (10-yr intervals):	Reduced amount of diphtheria toxoid provides adequate immunization in adults with minimal risk of hypersensitivity reactions; tetanus toxoid content is identical in pediatric and adult preparations; *cautious use* during pregnancy and in debilitated individuals
Diphtheria and Tetanus Toxoids and Pertussis Vaccine, Adsorbed-DTP Tri-Immunol	3 injections (0.5 mL) IM at 4–8-wk intervals, beginning at 2 mo, then a fourth dose 1 yr thereafter *Booster:* at 4–6 yr of age	Most commonly used preparation for routine immunization of young children; *not* recommended in adults or children over 7 yr; use with *extreme caution* in children with history of CNS disease or convulsions because pertussis has caused neurologic side effects in a small percentage of children; *defer* administration during an acute febrile illness, shock, alterations in consciousness, extremely agitated behavior, or if patient is receiving immunosuppressive therapy; slight fever, malaise, and injection site pain frequently occur following injection
Tetanus Toxoid, Fluid or Adsorbed	Fluid: 0.5 mL at 3–8-wk intervals for 3 doses, then a fourth dose 6–12 mo later Adsorbed: 0.5 mL at 4–8-wk intervals for 2 doses, then a third dose 1 yr later *Booster:* Every 10 yr for each	Adsorbed toxoid gives higher antibody levels and longer protection than fluid toxoid and is the preferred agent; adsorbed preparation is given IM only, but fluid preparation can be administered IM or SC; do *not* use in patients with acute respiratory infection, active tetanus infection, or convulsive disorders, or in persons receiving immunosuppressive therapy; local irritation and erythema are *common*, especially in adults

Viral replication following administration of live attenuated virus vaccines may be enhanced in persons with immunodeficiency diseases or suppressed immune response, for example, persons with leukemia or other malignancies or persons receiving corticosteroids *or* cancer chemotherapeutic agents. Such patients should not be given live, attenuated virus vaccines.

In the case of certain viral vaccines, a subclinical disease state may be induced by the vaccine itself, accompanied by fever, myalgia, and other manifestations of the particular viral disease (e.g., rash, urticaria, parotitis). These symptoms are generally mild and transient and usually require nothing more than symptomatic management with medications such as antipyretics or analgesics. Vaccines do not afford immediate protection, because several days or occasionally weeks are required to produce sufficient serum antibody levels. A second and occasionally a third injection at 4- to 8-week intervals are frequently given with certain vaccines to ensure adequate antibody levels. Active or imminent infections, therefore, require administration of one of the immune serums or antitoxins.

The bacterial and viral vaccines are listed in Table 77-2, along with dosage guidelines and pertinent remarks.

In addition to the commercially available vaccines listed in Table 77-2, several other vaccines are available from the Centers for Disease Control in Atlanta for nonemergency use in persons at high risk for exposure in the laboratory. These vaccines include botulinum toxoid (pentavalent), eastern equine encephalitis (EEE) vaccine (live, attenuated), Japanese encephalitis vaccine, smallpox vaccine, tularemia vaccine (live, attenuated), and Venezuelan equine encephalitis (VEE) vaccine.

AGENTS FOR PASSIVE IMMUNITY

Substances used to confer passive immunity are termed *immune serums* and consist of preformed antibodies derived from either human or animal sources. Human immune serums contain globulins possessing antibodies against a number of bacterial and viral diseases and are derived from human serum or plasma. Conversely, immune serums obtained by actively immunizing an animal against a specific disease, then removing and purifying the serum, which contains antibodies against that disease, are generally termed *antitoxins* or *antivenins.* Although both types of immune serums are effective in protecting against certain diseases, the human immune serums are much less likely to elicit hypersensitivity reactions, inasmuch as they do not contain foreign (i.e., animal-derived) proteins.

(*Text continued on page 809*)

Table 77-2
Vaccines

Vaccine	Preparations	Administration	Nursing Implications
Bacterial			
BCG Vaccine (BCG)	Injection (intradermal): 8 million U–26 million U/mL of standardized BCG bacillus prepared from culture Injection (percutaneous): 50 mg/vial of Tice-Chicago strain	Intradermal: 0.1 mL (0.05 mL in newborns) Percutaneous: 0.2 mL–0.3 mL dropped onto skin, followed by application of a multiple-puncture disk	Live, attenuated vaccine used in tuberculin-negative patients exposed to persons with active tuberculosis; *contraindicated* in tuberculin-positive patients, burn patients, and persons receiving chronic corticosteroid therapy; low incidence of untoward reactions but can produce skin ulceration and abscesses; *sterilize unused portion* before disposal
Cholera Vaccine	Injection: suspension of killed *Vibrio cholerae* organisms	*Adults:* 0.5 mL SC or IM followed in 1–4 wk by a second 0.5-mL dose *Children:* 0.2 mL–0.3 mL SC or IM (or 0.2 mL intradermally); repeat in 1–4 wk *Booster:* 0.2 mL–0.5 mL (depending on age) given every 6 mo as long as protection is desired	Used to protect travelers to or residents of countries where cholera is endemic or epidemic or for mass immunization *prior* to a cholera outbreak; *not* indicated for treatment of acute cholera infection; vaccine does not prevent development of a carrier state; immunity is short-lived (3–6 mo); therefore repeated dosages are necessary to confer long-lasting protection; protection is not absolute, and disease can still be contacted if exposure occurs; injections *often* cause local pain, erythema, swelling, and a febrile reaction; for mass immunization during epidemics, a *single* dose of 1.0 mL can be used
Hemophilus b Polysaccharide Vaccine b-Capsa I, Hib-Immune	Powder for injection: 25 μg Hib polysaccharide/0.5 mL when reconstituted	0.5 mL (25 μg) SC; do *not* give IV or intradermally	Used for immunization of children 18 mo–6 yr against disease caused by *H. influenzae* b; younger children (under 1 yr) may not be adequately protected; acute febrile reaction, erythema, and induration of injection site can occur; do *not* give during acute febrile illness or active infection
Hemophilus b Conjugate Vaccine ProHIBiT	Powder for injection: 25 μg (with 18 μg conjugated diphtheria toxoid protein) per 0.5 mL when reconstituted		
Meningitis Vaccine Menomune-A/C/Y/W-135	Injection: suspensions of polysaccharides from *meningococcus,* groups A, C, Y, and W-135	0.5 mL SC as a single injection	Stimulates antibody production against *Neisseria meningitidis* groups A, C, Y, and W-135; used in persons 2 yr of age and older at risk in epidemic or endemic areas (e.g., travelers, medical and laboratory personnel, household or institutional contacts); do *not* give intradermally or IV; adverse reactions include chills, fever, malaise, local soreness; *contraindicated* in presence of active infections, in persons taking corticosteroids, and in pregnant women
Mixed Respiratory Vaccine (MRV)	Injection: suspensions of several strains of bacterial organisms present in common respiratory infections, including *Staphylococcus aureus, Streptococcus pneumoniae, Klebsiella pneumoniae, Branhamella catarrhalis, Hemophilus influenzae*	Initially, 0.05 mL SC; increase by 0.05 mL–0.1 mL at 4–7-day intervals until a maximum of 1 mL is given; maintenance dosage 0.5 mL every 1–2 wk	Used to prevent bacterial hypersensitization in respiratory infections that can lead to asthma, urticaria, rhinitis; effectiveness has *not* been conclusively demonstrated; repeat doses should *not* be given until all local reactions from previous dose have disappeared; frequency of administration is highly individual; children's dose is the same as adults; observe for symptoms of allergic reaction and, if severe, administer epinephrine, corticosteroids, or antihistamines; local hypersensitivity reactions are common and are not a cause for alarm
Plague Vaccine	Injection: 2 billion killed plague bacilli/mL	*Adults:* 1.0 mL IM, followed in 1–3 mo by 0.2 mL IM; third injection of 0.2 mL IM after 3–6 mo is recommended *Booster:* 0.1 mL–0.2 mL at 6-mo intervals during active exposure	Suspension of inactivated *Yersinia pestis* organisms grown in artificial media; repeated injections increase the likelihood of adverse reactions, especially local allergic effects; *common* initial side effects are malaise, headache, fever, local erythema, and mild lymphadenopathy; vaccine is recommended for those persons who must be in known plague areas (e.g., Far East, South America, China, Saudi Arabia, and parts of Western U.S.) and for persons working with the organism in laboratories or exposed to the organism in the environment

Continued

Table 77-2
Vaccines (continued)

Vaccine	Preparations	Administration	Nursing Implications
Plague Vaccine (cont'd)		*Children* Through 11 mo: one fifth adult dose 1–4 yr: two fifths adult dose 5–10 yr: three fifths adult dose	
Pneumococcal Vaccine, Polyvalent Pneumovax 23, Pnu-Imune 23	Injection: 25 µg each of 23 polysaccharide isolates derived from pneumonococci/0.5 mL	0.5 mL SC *or* IM; revaccination at not less than 5-yr intervals	Used for protection against pneumococcal pneumonia and bacteremia resulting from any of the 23 most prevalent capsular types of *pneumococci*, accounting for some 90% of all cases; indicated in persons over 2 yr of age with increased risk of morbidity or mortality (e.g., chronic debilitating disease or metabolic disorders, persons over 50, patients in chronic care facilities); also used to prevent pneumococcal otitis media in children under 2 yr who are at high risk; protection is conferred for extended periods, and too frequent revaccination results in increasingly severe local reactions; do *not* inject IV or intradermally; local soreness and induration are very common within 2 days but quickly disappear; fever and myalgia are often noted within 24 h; *not* recommended in children under 2 yr
Staphage Lysate SPL—Serologic Types I and III	Injection: 120–180 million *Staph. aureus* and 100–1000 million *Staph. bacteriophage plaque forming units*/mL	*Acute infections:* 0.05 mL–0.2 mL, followed by increases of 0.1 mL–0.2 mL at 1–2-day intervals to a maximum dose of 0.5 mL *Chronic or subacute infections:* 0.05 mL–0.1 mL followed by increases of 0.1 mL–0.2 mL at 2–4-day intervals to a maximum of 0.2 mL–0.5 mL depending on severity of disease; *Children* receive one half the adult dose	Sterile staphylococcal vaccine used to treat staphylococcal infections or polymicrobial infections with a staphylococcal component; effectiveness has *not* been conclusively demonstrated; a skin test (0.025 mL–0.05 mL intracutaneously) should be performed prior to initial use; may be administered by several routes (SC, intranasal, oral, topical, or irrigation) depending on site and severity of infection; malaise, fever, and chills can occur and local redness, itching, and swelling at injection site are common initially; following SC injection, the remaining solution in the 1-mL ampule may be given orally, topically, or intranasally to reinforce the SC dose
Typhoid Vaccine	Injection: 8 protective U/mL of a suspension of killed Ty-2 strain of *Salmonella typhosa* organisms	*Adults:* Two 0.5-mL doses SC at 4-wk intervals *Booster:* 0.5 mL SC *or* 0.1 mL intradermally every 3 yr *Children under 10 yr:* Two 0.25-mL doses, SC, at least 4 wk apart *Booster:* 0.25 mL SC *or* 0.1 mL intradermally every 3 yr	Used for immunization against typhoid fever in persons exposed to a known typhoid carrier or travelling to areas where the disease is endemic; commonly causes local erythema, tenderness, and induration as well as malaise, headache, fever, and myalgia; do *not* administer during other active infections
Viral			
Hepatitis B Vaccine Heptavax-B **Hepatitis B Vaccine, Recombinant** Recombivax HB	Injection: 20 µg hepatitis B antigen/mL Pediatric injection: 10 µg hepatitis B antigen/0.5 mL Injection: 10 µg hepatitis B antigen/mL Pediatric injection: 5 µg hepatitis B antigen/0.5 mL	*Adults:* 1.0 mL initially, IM, 1.0 mL at 1 mo, and 1.0 mL at 6 mo *Children under 10 yr:* 0.5 mL initially, 0.5 mL at 1 mo, and 0.5 mL at 6 mo *Booster:* at 5 yr to maintain immunity *Infants born to hepatitis B surface antigen–positive mothers* (see	Regular vaccine contains highly purified, formalin-inactivated hepatitis B surface antigen derived from plasma of chronic carriers of the antigen; recombinant vaccine is a genetically engineered product made by programming common yeast cells to produce large quantities of the antigen portion of the virus contained in its outer coat; therapeutically, both vaccines are equivalent—however, supply of conventional vaccine is limited; both products afford a high degree of protection (90%–95%) against hepatitis B virus, a significant health risk for health care professionals, drug

Continued

Table 77-2
Vaccines (continued)

Vaccine	Preparations	Administration	Nursing Implications
		Nursing Implications): 0.5 mL hepatitis B immune globulin at birth followed by 0.5 mL pediatric injection within 7 days, then again at 1 and 6 mo	abusers, homosexuals, patients undergoing hemodialysis or renal transplantation, cancer patients, and patients receiving multiple blood transfusions; hepatitis B infections have also been linked to hepatocellular carcinoma; effectiveness of vaccine in preventing hepatitis B when given *after* exposure to virus is not conclusively established, but vaccine has been given with hepatitis B immune globulin with no deleterious effects. Infants born to mothers who are hepatitis B surface antigen (HBsAg) positive are at high risk of becoming carriers of hepatitis B virus and of developing chronic infection sequelae; they should be treated beginning at birth according to the schedule given under Administration
Influenza Virus Vaccines Fluogen, Fluzone	Injection: suspension of inactivated influenza virus particles of the currently prevailing types	*Over 13 yr:* 0.5 mL IM in a single dose *3–12 yr:* 2 doses of 0.5 mL IM at least 4 wk apart *Under 3 yr:* 2 doses of 0.25 mL IM at least 4 wk apart	Composition of vaccine changes yearly depending on prevalent virus strains; recommended in persons at high risk for adverse reactions from lower respiratory infections, such as those with heart disease, chronic pulmonary disease, renal dysfunction, diabetes, or debilitation, *contraindicated* during first trimester of pregnancy, in persons with severe neurologic disorders, and in patients with a history of Guillain-Barré syndrome; use with caution in hypersensitive persons, because vaccine is egg-grown, although it is highly purified; *defer* immunization in patients with acute respiratory disease or other active infection; not effective against *all* influenza viruses; available as "whole-virus" or "split-virus" preparations—split virus associated with fewer adverse effects in children and is preferred in patients under 12 yr; a single dose is sufficient for persons inoculated within the previous 2 yr; vaccine may reduce elimination of drugs metabolized by cytochrome P-450 system in the liver (e.g., theophylline, warfarin)
Measles Vaccine— Rubeola Attenuvax	Injection: suspension of Enders' attenuated Edmonston strain of measles virus in single-dose vials with diluent	Administer total volume of reconstituted vaccine SC *Booster:* not necessary	Live, attenuated strain of measles virus grown in chick embryo tissue culture; most often given together with mumps and rubella vaccines as a single preparation (see below); produces a mild measles infection (e.g., fever, rash), which induces immunity in 97% of susceptible individuals; recommended in children 15 mo or older; revaccination is *not* required if child was over 12 mo when initially vaccinated; *contraindicated* in pregnancy; use *cautiously* in children with a history of febrile convulsions or cerebral injury; discard if not used within 8 h
Measles and Rubella Vaccine M-R-Vax II	Injection: single-dose vials with diluent containing a combination of live, attenuated strains of measles and rubella viruses	Administer total volume of reconstituted vaccine SC *Booster:* not necessary	Indicated for simultaneous immunization against measles and rubella (German measles) in children over 15 mo; *see* measles vaccine and rubella vaccine for additional information; most frequently given together with mumps vaccine as a single preparation (see below)
Measles, Mumps, and Rubella Vaccine M-M-R II	Injection: single-dose vials, with diluent containing live, attenuated strains of measles, mumps, and rubella viruses	Administer total volume of reconstituted vaccine SC *Booster:* not necessary	Indicated in children over 15 mo for simultaneous immunization against measles, mumps, and rubella: highly effective (95%–98% of children develop effective antibody levels to all three viruses) and generally well tolerated; widely used preparation; immunity persists for at least 8 yr to 10 yr; thus revaccination is not required; see Nursing Implications for measles, mumps, and rubella vaccines

Continued

Table 77-2
Vaccines (continued)

Vaccine	Preparations	Administration	Nursing Implications
Mumps Vaccine Mumpsvax	Injection: single-dose vials with diluent containing live, attenuated Jeryl Lynn (B) mumps virus grown in chick embryo cell cultures	Administer total volume of reconstituted vaccine SC *Booster:* not necessary	Used for immunization of children over 15 mo and adults; immunity is produced in 97% of children and 93% of adults with a single dose and persists for at least 10 yr; do *not* use in pregnant women; allergic reactions can occur (vaccine is derived from chick embryo); be prepared with epinephrine, antihistamines; fever and parotitis have occurred but are generally mild
Poliovirus Vaccine, Inactivated—IPV Poliomyelitis Vaccine	Injection: suspension of 3 types of poliovirus (types 1, 2, 3) grown in monkey kidney cell cultures	3 doses (1.0 mL each) given SC at 4–6-wk intervals, followed by a fourth dose (1.0 mL) 6–12 mo after the third dose *Booster:* every 5 yr	Indicated for polio immunization in persons with compromised immune systems; oral polio vaccine (Sabin) is vaccine of choice in other persons; dosage schedule is often integrated with that of DTP immunization and begun at 6–12 wk of age; vaccine should be clear red; do *not* use if cloudy, discolored, or precipitated; *defer* injections during periods of other active infections; hypersensitivity reactions can occur; have epinephrine injection available
Poliovirus Vaccine, Live Oral Trivalent—TOPV, Sabin Orimune	Dispettes: single-dose (0.5 mL) containing types 1, 2, and 3 poliovirus grown in monkey kidney cell cultures	3 doses (0.5 mL each) given orally at 6–12 wk of age, 8 wk later, and 8 mo after the second dose *Booster:* 5 yr of age	Vaccine of choice for primary immunization against poliovirus; advantages over Salk vaccine are ease of admnistration, longer-lasting immunity, protection against infection by wild polioviruses, and lack of need for periodic booster doses; do *not* administer if persistent vomiting or diarrhea is present; store in a freezer, thaw before use, refrigerate vial after opening, and use contents within 7 days
Rubella Vaccine Meruvax II	Injection: single-dose vials with diluent, containing Wistar RA 27/3 strain of rubella virus propagated in human diploid cell culture	Administer total volume of reconstituted vaccine SC	Live, attenuated rubella virus strains used to immunize against rubella in children from 15 mo to puberty; antibody levels persist for at least 6 yr; useful in adolescents and adults to prevent outbreaks in high risk situations; do *not* administer to pregnant women and use *cautiously* in women of childbearing age because congenital abnormalities can occur; usually given combined with measles and mumps vaccines (see MMR); side effects are uncommon but can include symptoms of the disease (rash, urticaria, sore throat, malaise, fever, headache, lymphadenopathy); arthralgia is fairly common in women (12%–20%)
Rubella and Mumps Vaccine Biavax II	Injection: single-dose vials with diluents, containing a mixture of mumps and rubella virus strains	Administer total volume of reconstituted vaccine SC	Combination vaccine yielding effective antibody levels in 97% to 100% of susceptible children; may be given as early as 1 yr of age; not as frequently used as measles, mumps, and rubella vaccine (MMR); see Nursing Implications for rubella and mumps vaccines
Yellow Fever Vaccine YF-Vax	Injection: vials with diluent for needle injection containing a live, attenuated 17D strain virus cultured in chick embryo	0.5 mL SC	Indicated for immunization of persons traveling to countries requiring vaccination against yellow fever; immunity develops within 7 days and can last for up to 10 yr; administer at least 1 mo apart from other live viruses; fever and malaise occur in about 10% of patients; keep frozen until reconstituted and then use within 1 h; do *not* use if vaccine has been exposed to temperatures above 5°C

Antitoxins/Antivenins

Black widow spider antivenin
Crotalidae antivenin
Diphtheria antitoxin
North American coral snake antivenin
Tetanus antitoxin

Antitoxins and antivenins are prepared by repeatedly inoculating an animal, usually a horse, with a toxoid (e.g., diphtheria, tetanus) or a venom (e.g., from a snake, black widow spider), then bleeding the animal and concentrating the antibody-containing fraction of the plasma. The partially purified antibodies or antitoxins can then be administered to humans to neutralize toxins produced by invading microorganisms or introduced by a bite.

It is imperative that a skin or conjunctival hypersensitivity test be performed before administering any of the horse serum antitoxins to determine if the patient might exhibit an allergic reaction to the foreign serum. Package literature describing the appropriate hypersensitivity testing procedure should always be consulted before using one of these products. Even a negative sensitivity test result, however, does not completely rule out the possibility of an allergic reaction, and epinephrine injection should always be available when an antitoxin is administered. Adverse reactions to antitoxins range from local pain and erythema at the injection site to serum sickness and anaphylaxis, the incidence of the more serious allergic reactions being approximately 5% to 10%.

Information pertaining to the commercially available antitoxins and antivenins is presented in Table 77-3. In addition, botulism equine antitoxin is available by request to the Centers for Disease Control in Atlanta.

Table 77-3
Antitoxins/Antivenins

Antitoxin/Antivenin	Preparations	Administration	Nursing Implications
Antivenins			
Black Widow Spider Species Antivenin *Antivenin Latrodectus mactans*	Injection: 6000 U/vial with diluent plus vial of normal horse serum for sensitivity testing	2.5 mL reconstituted antivenin IM *or* 2.5 mL in 10 mL–50 mL saline by IV infusion	Used to treat persons bitten by black widow spider; prompt administration yields most effective results; use of muscle relaxants appears to be most important during early reaction phase; test for sensitivity to horse serum prior to administration
Crotalidae Antivenin, Polyvalent	Injection: vial of lyophilized serum with diluent plus vial of normal horse serum for sensitivity testing	Dosage depends on severity of bite Mild: 2–4 vials IV Moderate: 5–9 vials IV Severe: 10–20 vials IV (Children and small adults may require larger doses; see Nursing Implications)	Preparation of serum globulins containing protective antibodies against a number of crotalids, including pit vipers, rattlesnakes, cottonmouths, copper heads, bushmasters (see package instructions); administer as soon as possible after bite and immobilize patient to minimize spread of venom; do *not* administer at or around the site of the bite; children have less resistance and require proportionately larger doses than adults; subsequent injections depend on clinical response; use barbiturates and narcotics with *caution*, because increased respiratory depression can result; test for sensitivity to horse serum prior to administration
North American Coral Snake Antivenin *Antivenin Micrurus fulvius*	Injection: vial with diluent	3–5 vials (30 mL–50 mL) slowly injected directly into IV infusion tubing or added to reservoir bottle of IV drip	Concentrated solution of serum globulins obtained from horses immunized against eastern coral snake venom; bitten area should be completely immobilized; first several milliliters of antivenin should be administered over a 5-min period and patient carefully observed for evidence of allergic reaction; up to 10 vials have been required in some persons with severe or multiple bites; drugs that depress respiration should be used *cautiously*, because snake venom itself produces respiratory depression and paralysis
Antitoxins			
Diphtheria Antitoxin	Injection: 10,000 or 20,000 U/vial	*Adults and children:* 20,000 U–120,000 U IM *or* IV depending on severity and duration of infection; repeat in 24 h if clinical improvement is not apparent *Prophylaxis:* 10,000 U IM if sensitivity test is negative	Concentrated solution of purified globulins obtained from the serum of horses immunized against diphtheria toxin; delay in beginning therapy increases dosage requirements and reduces beneficial effects; continue treatment until all symptoms are controlled; appropriate antimicrobial agents should be used concurrently; nonimmunized patients exposed to diphtheria should receive a low dose (see Administration) to produce a temporary passive immunity; sensitivity testing is necessary before administration
Tetanus Antitoxin	Injection: 1500 or 20,000 U/vial	*Treatment:* 50,000 U–100,000 U IV *Prophylaxis:* 1500 U–5000 U IM or SC depending on body weight	Concentrated solution of serum globulins from horses immunized against tetanus toxin; indicated *only* when tetanus immune globulin is not available; protection lasts about 2 wk with a single prophylactic dose; tetanus toxoid, adsorbed, is usually given with the antitoxin to initiate active immunization; most children are routinely immunized against tetanus and the need for the antitoxin seldom occurs

Human Immune Serums

Hepatitis B immune globulin
Immune globulin, human
Lymphocyte immune globulin
Tetanus immune globulin
Rh₀(D) immune globulin
Varicella zoster immune globulin

Immune globulins containing antibodies against certain diseases can be obtained from human serum, and these products are generally preferred over animal-derived globulins because of their lower incidence of hypersensitivity reactions. Human immune globulins may be obtained from pooled plasma of human donors, in which case the preparation contains antibodies against a number of diseases (e.g., hepatitis, rubella, varicella) or from the blood of persons recently recovered from or hyperimmunized against a *particular* disease, in which case the globulins contain high antibody titers against that particular disease. These human immune serums should be used cautiously in individuals with immunoglobulin A deficiency, thrombocytopenia, or coagulation disorders, and in pregnant women. Skin testing for hypersensitivity is meaningless with human immune serums, because intradermal injections frequently give rise to a local inflammatory response that can be misinterpreted as an allergic reaction. True hypersensitivity reactions to human immune globulins are extremely rare.

The human immune serums are listed in Table 77-4 along with dosages and other pertinent information. In addition, western equine encephalitis (WEE) immune globulin is available by request from the Centers for Disease Control in Atlanta.

Table 77-4
Human Immune Serums

Immune Serum	Preparations	Administration	Nursing Implications
Hepatitis B Immune Globulin H-BIG, Hep-B-Gamma-gee, HyperHep	Injection: 1-mL, 4-mL, 5-mL vials	0.06 mL/kg IM as soon after exposure as possible; repeat in 1 mo *Prevention of carrier state:* 0.5 mL IM no later than 24 h after birth; repeat in 3 mo *Prophylaxis of infants born to HBₛAg-positive mothers:* 0.5 mL IM at birth and again at 3 and 6 mo	Solution of immunologlobulins containing a high titer of antibodies to hepatitis B surface antigen (HBₛAg); indicated for prophylaxis following accidental oral, parenteral, or direct mucous membrane exposure to antigen-containing materials such as blood or serum; also for prophylaxis of infants born to HBₛAg-positive mothers who are at risk of being infected or becoming chronic carriers; may be given at the same time or up to 1 mo preceding hepatitis B vaccine without altering the resultant immune response; solution should be stored at 2°C–8°C but *not* frozen
Immune Globulin—Intramuscular (ISG) Gamma Globulin, Gamastan, Gammar	Injection: 2 mL, 10 mL vials	IM injection only Hepatitis A: 0.02 mL/kg Immunoglobulin deficiency: 1.3 mL/kg initially, then 0.66 mL/kg every 3–4 wk Measles: 0.25 mL/kg Rubella: 0.55 mL/kg (pregnant women *only*) Varicella: 0.6 mL–1.2 mL/kg	Solution of globulins obtained from pooled human serum, containing antibodies to a number of organisms; used to decrease the severity of certain diseases (hepatitis, measles, varicella) in persons exposed to an active infection; also indicated as replacement therapy for immunoglobulin deficiency states and as adjunctive treatment to antibiotics in severe bacterial infections or burns; may be of benefit in pregnant women exposed to rubella virus to lessen possibility of fetal damage, but routine use in early pregnancy cannot be justified; injections can be very painful
Immune Globulin, Intravenous Gamimune N, Gammagard, Sandoglobulin, Venoglobulin 1	Injection: 2.5%, 5% (in 10% maltose) Powder for injection: 1-g, 2.5-g, 3-g, 5-g, and 6-g vials with diluent	IV infusion only 100 mg/kg–300 mg/kg once a month by IV infusion (0.01 ml/kg–0.04 mL/kg/min for 30 min) *Idiopathic thrombocytopenic purpura:* 400 mg/kg for 5 consecutive days	Provides *immediate* antibody levels; half-life is about 3 wk; preferred to immune globulin, IM, in patients requiring rapid increases in IgG antibodies, in patients with a small muscle mass, and in patients with bleeding tendencies; maltose is added to stabilize the protein, reducing the incidence of adverse effects; may cause a precipitous drop in blood pressure, especially at rapid infusion rates; monitor vital signs carefully during infusion; have epinephrine available for allergic reactions

Continued

Table 77-4
Human Immune Serums (continued)

Immune Serum	Preparations	Administration	Nursing Implications
Lymphocyte Immune Globulin—Anti-thymocyte Globulin Atgam	Injection: 50 mg/mL	*IV infusion only* Adults: 10 mg/kg–30 mg/kg/day Children: 5 mg/kg–25 mg/kg/day (Given daily for 14 days, then every other day for a total of 21 doses)	A lymphocyte-selective immunosuppressant that reduces the number of circulating, thymus-dependent lymphocytes; used by *experienced personnel only* for management of allograft rejection in renal transplant patients and as an adjunct to other immunosuppressive therapy to delay onset of first rejection; *discontinue* if anaphylaxis or *severe* thrombocytopenia or leukopenia occurs; frequently encountereed adverse reactions are fever, chills, rash, pruritus, urticaria, leukopenia, and thrombocytopenia; drug must be diluted in saline before infusion; use within 12 h; do *not* dilute with dextrose solutions or highly acidic solutions because precipitation can occur; a dose should *not* be infused in less than 4 h; have resuscitative materials available (e.g., epinephrine, antihistamines, steroids, etc.)
Tetanus Immune Globulin Hyper-Tet	Injection: 250 U/vial or disposable syringe	*Treatment:* 3000 U–6000 U IM *Prophylaxis:* 250 U–500 U IM	Indicated for passive tetanus prophylaxis in persons not actively immunized or whose immunization status is uncertain; not generally necessary if person has had at least 2 doses of tetanus toxoid; produces effective levels of circulating antibodies for much longer periods than tetanus antitoxin; does not interfere with immune response to tetanus toxoid given at the same time; thorough cleansing of wounds and removal of all foreign particles is important to prevent infection; do *not* give IV
Rh$_o$(D) Immune Globulin Gamulin Rh, HypRho-D, RhoGAM (CAN) Win Rho	Injection: vial with diluent	Inject contents of 1 vial IM for every 15 mL fetal packed red cell volume within 72 h following delivery, miscarriage, abortion, or transfusion (See package instructions for mixing and injecting directions)	Used to prevent sensitization in a subsequent pregnancy to the Rh$_o$(D) factor in an Rh-negative mother who has given birth to an Rh-positive infant by an Rh-positive father; also may be employed to prevent Rh$_o$(D) sensitization in Rh-negative patients accidentally transfused with Rh-positive blood; consult product information for blood typing and drug administration procedures; do *not* give IV; also available in microdose form (MICRhoGAM, Mini-Gamulin Rh, HypRho-D Mini-Dose) to prevent maternal Rh-immunization following miscarriage or abortion up to 12 weeks' gestation
Varicella-Zoster Immune Globulin (human)—VZIG	Injection: 10% to 18% solution of the globulin fraction of human plasma containing 125 U of antibody to varicella-zoster virus in a single-dose vial	*IM only:* 125 U/10 kg body weight to a maximum of 625 U; do *not* give fractional units	Globulin fraction of adult human plasma (primarily immunoglobulin G) with high titer of varicella-zoster antibodies; used for passive immunization of *immunodeficient* children following exposure to varicella; most effective if given within 96 h after exposure; *not* indicated prophylactically; do *not* administer IV; no more than 2.5 mL should be injected at a single IM site (1.25 mL maximum if patient weighs less than 10 kg); VZIG must be requested from regional distribution centers of American Red Cross Blood Services

RABIES PROPHYLAXIS PRODUCTS

Antirabies serum, equine
Rabies immune globulin

Rabies vaccine, human diploid cell culture

Rabies is an acute viral disease of animals that can be transmitted to other animals and humans by the bite of an infected animal. Although many animals are susceptible to rabies, it occurs most commonly in dogs, cats, raccoons, skunks, coyotes, and wolves. The virus has a high affinity for the nervous system and is inevitably fatal unless appropriate immunologic therapy is instituted quickly.

Products used for rabies prophylaxis include the following:

- *Human diploid cell vaccine* (HDCV): suspension of Wistar rabies virus strain grown in human diploid cell cultures

Table 77-5
Rabies Prophylaxis Products

Immune Serum	Preparations	Administration	Nursing Implications
Antirabies Serum, Equine	Injection: 125 U/mL	40 U/kg (1000 U/55 lb) IM in a single dose. Usually given together with HDVC, although *not* at the same site nor in the same syringe	Used in conjunction with HDVC (see below) to promote passive immunity to rabies when rabies immune globulin is unavailable; delays propagation of virus, thus allowing time for rabies vaccine to induce sufficient antibodies; give as soon as possible after exposure; sensitivity testing (intradermal or conjunctival) should be done before administration; up to 50% of the dose should be infiltrated into the tissue around the wound; adverse reactions include local pain, erythema, urticaria, and frequently serum sickness
Rabies Immune Globulin, Human Hyperab, Imogam	Injection: 150 U/mL	20 U/kg (9.1 U/lb); ½ the dose IM and ½ the dose to infiltrate the wound	Used to provide rabies antibodies immediately; given in conjunction with rabies vaccine; reduced risk of serum sickness compared to equine vaccine; should be given as soon as possible following exposure, but regardless of interval, immune globulin is still recommended; do *not* give repeated doses once vaccine has been administered; muscle soreness and low grade fever can occur
Rabies Vaccine, Human Diploid Cell Cultures Intramuscular Imovax Intradermal Imovax I.D.	*IM injection:* 2.5 U rabies antigen/mL *Intradermal injection:* 0.25 U rabies antigen/unit dose	*IM* Preexposure: 3 injections, IM, of 1.0 mL each on days 0, 7, and 28 Boosters: every 2 years in high-risk individuals Postexposure: 5 injections, IM, of 1.0 mL each on days 0, 3, 7, 14, and 28 with a dose of rabies immune globulin on day 0; a sixth dose is given 90 days after the first dose *Intradermal* Preexposure *only*; 3 injections (0.1 mL) on days 0, 7, and either 21 or 28	Preferred rabies prophylaxis product; IM injection may be used either pre- or postexposure; intradermal injection is only for prophylaxis preexposure; postexposure antibody response is virtually 100% with recommended 5 doses; preexposure vaccination is indicated for persons in contact with rabid animals or patients or those handling rabies virus or contaminated articles; postexposure treatment should also include rabies immune globulin; adverse reactions to vaccine are infrequent; local swelling and erythema have occurred; corticosteroids and other immunosuppressive agents can interfere with development of active immunity to vaccine—do *not* administer together

- *Rabies immune globulin* (RIG): human immune globulin obtained from plasma of hyperimmunized donors
- *Antirabies serum, equine origin* (ARS): concentrated serum obtained from hyperimmunized horses

Postexposure treatment is best accomplished by a combination of active and passive immunization, that is, vaccine and immune globulin. For passive immunization, rabies immune globulin is the drug of choice; the equine antirabies serum should be used only when the immune globulin is unavailable. For active immunization, HDCV is used.

The rabies prophylaxis products are briefly reviewed in Table 77-5. It is important, however, that anyone using any of the products become thoroughly familiar with the indications, precautions, and general handling procedures of each particular preparation by consulting the product literature.

Selected Bibliography

Austrian R: A reassessment of pneumococcal vaccine. N Engl J Med 310:651, 1984

Bernard KW et al: Human diploid cell rabies vaccine. JAMA 247:1138, 1982

Conte JE, Barriere S: Manual of Antibiotics and Infectious Diseases. Philadelphia, Lea and Febiger, 1988

Fulginite VA: Immunization. In Kempe CH, Silver HK, O'Brien D (eds): Current Pediatric Diagnosis and Treatment, 8th ed. Los Altos, Lange Medical Publications, 1984

Gurevich J: Viral hepatitis. Am J Nurs 83(4):571, 1983

Halpern JS: Rabies vaccine: Reduced risks and fears. J Emerg Nurs 10(2):101, 1984

Immunization Practices Advisory Committee: Monovalent influenza A (HINI) vaccine, 1986–1987. MMWR 35:517, 1986

Immunization Practices Advisory Committee: Prevention and control of influenza. MMWR 35:317, 1986

Kirkman-Liff B, Dandoy S: Hepatitis B: What price exposure? Am J Nurs 84:988, 1984

Nichols AO: Taking the fear out of rabies treatment. Nursing 83 13(6):42, June, 1983

Plotkin SA, Mortimer EA: Vaccines, Philadelphia, WB Saunders, 1988

Robbins JB, Hill JC, Sadoff JC: Bacterial Vaccines. New York, Thieme-Stratton, 1987

Williams A: Hepatitis B virus vaccine. Nurse Pract 8:30, 1983

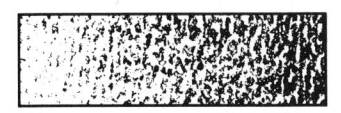

78 MISCELLANEOUS DRUG PRODUCTS

Several pharmacologic agents do not fall into one of the previously discussed categories of drugs and thus are reviewed here under a miscellaneous heading.

ALPROSTADIL

Prostin VR Pediatric

Alprostadil (prostaglandin E_1) is a solution for IV infusion that is used in neonates with congenital heart defects to temporarily maintain the patency of the ductus arteriosus until corrective surgery can be performed.

MECHANISM
Relaxes smooth muscle of the ductus arteriosus, thereby providing for adequate blood oxygenation. Other actions of PGE_1 include vasodilation, increased tone of intestinal and uterine smooth muscle, and inhibition of platelet aggregation.

USES
Palliative therapy of neonates with congenital heart defects (e.g., pulmonary stenosis, tricuspid atresia, tetralogy of Fallot, aortic coarctation) to maintain patency until corrective surgery can be performed

DOSAGE
Initially, 0.1 µg/kg/min until improvement is noted; reduce infusion rate to lowest dose that maintains the response (0.01 µg–0.05 µg/kg/min); maximum dose—0.4 µg/kg/min

FATE
Rapidly metabolized upon first pass through the lungs; metabolites are excreted primarily by the kidneys; does not appear to be retained in body tissue

COMMON SIDE EFFECTS
Fever, apnea (see Nursing Alerts), flushing, bradycardia, hypotension

SIGNIFICANT ADVERSE REACTIONS
Cardiovascular: tachycardia, edema, second-degree heart block, hyperemia, shock, congestive heart failure, ventricular fibrillation, cardiac arrest
CNS: seizures, hyperirritability, lethargy, hypothermia, cerebral bleeding, hyperextension of the neck
Hematologic: disseminated intravascular coagulation, anemia, thrombocytopenia, bleeding
GI: diarrhea, regurgitation, hyperbilirubinemia
Respiratory: wheezing, hypercapnia, respiratory depression
Other: anuria, hematuria, sepsis, peritonitis, hypokalemia, hypoglycemia, cortical proliferation of long bones

CONTRAINDICATIONS
Respiratory distress syndrome (hyaline membrane disease). *Cautious use* in neonates with bleeding tendencies, because drug inhibits platelet aggregation

NURSING CONSIDERATIONS

Nursing Alerts
- Monitor respiratory status closely during infusion, and always have respiratory assistance immediately available because apnea occurs in 10% to 20% of neonates treated with alprostadil, most often in those weighing less than 2 kg at birth.
- Assess for indications of overdosage (e.g., bradycardia, apnea, flushing, pyrexia). Infusion should be discontinued if these occur, then cautiously reinitiated when they subside.

1. Expect drug to be infused at lowest dose and for shortest time that will produce desired effect.
2. Monitor arterial pressure during drug administration. Perfusion rate should be reduced if pressure falls significantly.
3. Monitor results of blood oxygenation determinations in infants with decreased pulmonary flow and systemic blood pressure and results of blood pH determinations in infants with compromised systemic blood flow.

ANTIDOTES

Most drugs employed as specific antidotes (i.e., narcotic antagonists, acetylcysteine, protamine sulfate, vitamin K, physostigmine, leucovorin) have been considered previously in the individual chapters dealing with the pharmacologic agents that they specifically antagonize. Certain other drugs are also useful as antidotes for specific types of poisonings.

Activated Charcoal

Actidose-Aqua, Actidose with Sorbitol, Charcoaid, Liqui-Char
(CAN) SuperChar, Charcodote

Activated charcoal is a carbon residue that has a very large surface area owing to its fine networklike structure, thus providing great adsorptive capacity per unit of weight. The amount of drug or other substance that can be adsorbed by activated charcoal is approximately 100 mg to 1000 mg per gram of charcoal. The drug is used as a powder or liquid suspension for the emergency treatment of poisoning by most drugs and chemicals *except* cyanide, alkalis, and mineral acids. It is also largely ineffective against poisoning with ethanol, methanol, and iron salts.

The initial dosage would be 1 g/kg or approximately five to ten times the amount of poison ingested. The charcoal powder is given as a suspension in 6 oz to 8 oz of water, as soon as possible after the poisoning. Although the black solution does not appear palatable, it is odorless and tasteless. It may be mixed with sweet syrup to enhance palatability. Emesis should be induced if possible prior to administration of charcoal except in cases of poisoning with strong acids or alkalis, petroleum distillates, or other caustic substances. Concurrent use of syrup of ipecac or laxatives with charcoal should be avoided because charcoal can adsorb and inactivate these agents as well.

Either constipation or diarrhea may occur, and the stools will be blackened.

Heavy Metal Antagonists

Deferoxamine mesylate, Dimercaprol, Edetate calcium disodium

Several drugs have the ability to complex with various heavy metals (such as iron, lead, gold, mercury) and are employed to treat poisoning with these substances. Such poisoning can occur either from drug overdosage—for example, with use of gold salts for rheumatoid arthritis or iron for severe anemias, or from accidental ingestion of substances such as lead-containing paints, insecticides, or pesticides. Heavy metal intoxication often impairs enzymatic function; if severe, impairment can lead to cellular anoxia and possibly death.

Table 78-1 lists the heavy metal antidotes, together with their indications, dosage, and nursing implications.

BINDING/CHELATING AGENTS

Drugs capable of binding or chelating other substances, such as metals, are useful in treating certain diseases characterized by excessive body levels of these substances. One such drug, penicillamine, is an effective copper chelating agent useful in treating Wilson's disease and also in the symptomatic management of rheumatoid arthritis. It is reviewed in detail with other anti-inflammatory drugs in Chapter 19. A second chelating drug also useful in treating Wilson's disease is trientine.

Trientine

Cuprid

MECHANISM
Removes excess copper from the body by chemically complexing with the metal

USES
Treatment of patients with Wilson's disease who are intolerant of penicillamine, which is normally the drug of choice
Note: Unlike penicillamine, trientine is *not* recommended for use in cystinuria, rheumatoid arthritis, or biliary cirrhosis

DOSAGE
Adults: 750 mg to 1250 mg orally in 2 to 4 divided doses (maximum dose is 2 g/day)
Children: 500 mg to 750 mg orally in 2 to 4 divided doses (maximum dose is 1500 mg/day)

Average duration of therapy is 4 years.

SIGNIFICANT ADVERSE REACTIONS
Iron defiency, dermatitis, heartburn, epigastric distress, malaise, anorexia, cramps, muscle pain or weakness, and systemic lupus–like symptoms

CONTRAINDICATIONS
Cystinuria, rheumatoid arthritis or biliary cirrhosis. *Cautious use* in persons with iron deficiency or systemic lupus erythematosus and in pregnant or nursing women

INTERACTIONS
Concurrent administration of mineral supplements, especially iron, and trientine may retard the absorption of each

NURSING CONSIDERATION

Nursing Alerts
- Monitor results of serum copper levels, complete blood counts with differentials, and urinalyses, which should be performed prior to initiating therapy and regularly thereafter. Changes in copper level indicate drug effectiveness. Decrease in hemoglobin or hematocrit may indicate iron deficiency anemia, in which case iron supplements may be required. Appearance of urinary protein or casts may indicate early drug-induced renal changes.

PATIENT EDUCATION

1. Instruct patient to take drug at least 1 hour before or after taking any other drugs or food. If epigastric distress occurs, as it often does, instruct patient to consult drug prescriber.
2. Teach patient how to recognize and immediately report systemic lupus–like symptoms (e.g., malaise, anorexia, arthralgia, fever, decreased urinary output) because drug may need to be discontinued.
3. Encourage patient to eat iron-rich foods, including red meats, dark green vegetables, egg yolks, whole grains, legumes, raisins, prunes, brewer's yeast, and nuts. Collaborate with dietitian or refer patient for assistance as indicated.

Cellulose Sodium Phosphate

Calcibind

MECHANISM
Binds calcium by an ion-exchange mechanism, and the complex of calcium and cellulose phosphate is then excreted in the feces; also binds dietary magnesium and may increase urinary phosphorus and oxalate; no apparent alteration in serum levels of copper, zinc, or iron

USES
Treatment of absorptive hypercalciuria type 1 with recurrent calcium oxalate or calcium phosphate nephrolithiasis

DOSAGE
Initially, 5 g orally with each meal. When urinary calcium declines to less than 150 mg/day, reduce dosage to 10 g/day in three divided doses

SIGNIFICANT ADVERSE REACTIONS
Diarrhea, dyspepsia, loose bowels, bad taste in mouth

CONTRAINDICATIONS
Primary or secondary hyperparathyroidism, hypocalcemia, hypomagnesemia, osteomalacia, osteoporosis. *Cautious use* in patients with congestive heart failure or ascites (sodium content of drug is high), in pregnant women and in children

Table 78-1
Heavy Metal Antidotes

Drug	Preparations	Indications	Usual Dosage Range	Nursing Implications
Deferoxamine Mesylate *Desferal*	Powder for injection: 500 mg/vial	Acute iron intoxication; Chronic iron overload (e.g., multiple transfusions); Management of aluminum accumulation in bone in renal failure (investigational use)	*Acute intoxication* 1 g IM, followed by 0.5 g every 4 h for 2 doses, then every 4 to 12 h as needed; IV infusion: same as IM dose at rate of 15 mg/kg/h. *Chronic overload* IM: 0.5 g to 1 g/day; IV: 2 g at a rate of 15 mg/kg/h; SC: 1 g to 2 g/day over 8 to 24 h with a mini-infusion pump. *Children:* 50 mg/kg IM *or* IV every 6 h or up to 15 mg/kg/h by IV infusion	Chelates iron in the ferric state, forming a stable, water-soluble, readily excretable complex; no effect on electrolyte or trace metal excretion; *contraindicated* in severe renal disease; should be used in conjunction with other appropriate antidotal measures (emesis, lavage, correction of acidosis, control of shock, respiratory assistance); pain on injection, allergic reactions, blurred vision, diarrhea, abdominal pain, tachycardias, and fever have been reported; urine may be colored red; use an infusion pump to control drip rate and monitor BP every 5 min until stable; too-rapid infusion can cause hypotension, urticaria, erythema, and shock
Dimercaprol-BAL *Bal in Oil*	Injection: 100 mg/mL	Arsenic, gold and mercury poisoning; Acute lead poisoning (in combination with calcium EDTA)	*IM only* Arsenic/gold poisoning: 2.5 mg/kg–3 mg/kg 4 to 6 times a day for 2 days, then 2 to 4 times a day on the third day, then 1 to 2 times a day for 10 days. Mercury poisoning: 5 mg/kg initially, then 2.5 mg/kg 1 to 2 times a day for 10 days. Lead poisoning: 4 mg/kg at 4-h intervals in combination with calcium sodium EDTA at a different site	Complexes with a number of heavy metals forming stable, water-soluble chelates that are readily excreted by the kidney; sulfhydryl enzymes are thus protected from the toxic action of the metals; do *not* use in iron, cadmium, or selenium poisoning because resultant complexes are more toxic than the metals; most effective when given as soon as possible after metal ingestion; urine should be kept alkaline to minimize kidney damage as chelate is being excreted; local pain is frequent at site of injection; *contraindicated* in hepatic insufficiency; large doses may increase blood pressure and heart rate; other adverse effects include fever in children (30% frequency), nausea, vomiting, headache, burning in the mouth and throat, chest constriction, lacrimation, salivation, and paresthesias; other supportive measures are necessary (fluids, electrolytes, respiratory assistance)
Edetate Calcium Disodium *Calcium Disodium Versenate, Calcium EDTA*	Injection: 200 mg/mL	Acute and chronic lead poisoning and lead encephalopathy	IV: 1 g diluted to 250 mL to 500 mL and infused over 1 h; administer twice a day for up to 5 days, stop 2 days, then resume for another 5 days if necessary. IM (preferred in children): 50 mg to 75 mg/kg/day in 2 equally divided doses for 3 to 5 days	Calcium in the compound is displaced by a heavy metal (e.g., lead), resulting in formation of a stable metal–drug complex that is removed by the kidneys—potentially a very toxic compound; recommended dosage levels should not be exceeded; do *not* infuse rapidly in patients with lead encephalopathy; increased intracranial pressure can be fatal; IM is the preferred route of administration; procaine should be added to the solution to reduce pain on injection; closely monitor renal function; do *not* give to patients with impaired kidney function; refer to package instructions for mixing and administering directions

NURSING CONSIDERATIONS

Nursing Alerts
- Monitor intake and output, and encourage fluid intake to maintain urinary output of at least 2000 mL/day.
- Monitor results of periodic determinations of serum magnesium and parathyroid hormone, serum and urinary calcium and oxalate, and complete blood counts to detect drug effects. Urinary calcium and oxalate levels reflect responsiveness to therapy.
- Collaborate with dietitian, drug prescriber, and patient to develop acceptable dietary plan as adjunct to drug therapy. Restriction of sodium, calcium, oxalate, and ascorbic acid increases drug's effectiveness.

PATIENT EDUCATION
1. Explain that powder may be mixed with full glass of water, fruit juice, or soft drink. It is not very palatable.
2. Ensure that patient understands need to take drug with meals or at least within 30 minutes of a meal. Otherwise, it is ineffective.
3. Explain that oral magnesium supplementation, which should be administered to prevent hypomagnesemia, can be taken any time so long as it is at least 1 hour before or after cellulose sodium phosphate administration to avoid binding magnesium.
4. Verify that patient understands dietary plan. Refer patient for additional instruction as necessary.

BROMOCRIPTINE

Parlodel

An ergot derivative exhibiting dopamine agonist activity, bromocriptine markedly reduces secretion of prolactin with minimal effects on other pituitary hormones. It is used for treating amenorrhea and galactorrhea resulting from hyperprolactinemia, for suppressing postpartum lactation, and as adjunctive therapy in treating Parkinson's disease (see Chap. 26).

MECHANISM
Activates postsynaptic dopamine receptors in the tuberoinfundibular dopaminergic neuronal system, resulting in secretion of prolactin inhibitory factor (PIF) from the hypothalamus; PIF blocks liberation of prolactin from the anterior pituitary in patients with hyperprolactinemia; also stimulates dopamine receptors in the corpus striatum, thus relieving some of the symptoms of parkinsonism

USES
Short-term treatment of amenorrhea–galactorrhea associated with hyperprolactinemia, except where a demonstrable pituitary tumor is present (not indicated in patients with normal prolactin levels)
Prevention of postpartum lactation occurring after parturition, stillbirth, or abortion
Treatment of female infertility associated with hyperprolactinemia
Adjunctive treatment of parkinsonism (see Chap. 26)
Treatment of acromegaly, either alone or in conjunction with pituitary irradiation or surgery
Investigational uses include treatment of pituitary adenomas (to reduce elevated prolactin levels), neuroleptic malignant syndrome, and cocaine addiction

DOSAGE
Amenorrhea–galactorrhea: 1.25 mg to 2.5 mg daily; increase by 2.5 mg every 3 days to seven days; usual dosage range 5 mg to 7.5 mg/day
Prevention of lactation: 2.5 mg two to three times a day for 14 days to 21 days
Treatment of infertility: initially 2.5 mg once daily; increase to two to three times a day within the first week
Parkinsonism: initially 1.25 mg twice daily; increase every 2 to 4 weeks by 2.5 mg/day as necessary
Acromegaly: initially, 1.25 mg to 2.5 mg daily; increase gradually every 3 days to 7 days until optimal response; usual dosage range is 20 mg to 30 mg daily

See Chapter 26 for additional information and Nursing Consideration.

CAPSAICIN

Zostrix

Capsaicin is a plant extract that is believed to render skin insensitive to pain upon topical application. Its precise mechanism of action is not completely understood, but the drug appears to deplete substance P in peripheral sensory nerve endings. Substance P is believed to be the principal neurotransmitter in spinal cord sensory pathways that mediate pain. Capsaicin cream is indicated for temporary alleviation of pain associated with episodes of herpes zoster infections following healing of skin lesions. It is applied 3 to 4 times a day, and optimal response is usually achieved within 14 days to 28 days. Topical application can elicit a warm or burning sensation, which may be intensified by bathing. This burning sensation occurs more often when the drug is applied less than 3 or 4 times a day.

DEXPANTHENOL

Ilopan, Panol, Panthoderm

Dexpanthenol is used either by IM injection as a GI stimulant for treating adynamia, as a cream (Panthoderm) for use as an emollient to relieve skin itching and lesioning, and as oral tablets (with choline) for relieving gas distention.

MECHANISM
Not established; drug is a derivative of pantothenic acid, a precursor of coenzyme A, which serves as a cofactor in the synthesis of acetylcholine (ACh); ACh exerts a range of functions in the body, including maintenance of intestinal tone and peristalsis

USES
Prevention of paralytic ileus and intestinal atony following abdominal surgery (IM)
Treatment of adynamic ileus (IM)
Relief of itching and to assist healing of skin lesions in minor skin conditions (topical)
Relief of gas retention associated with several GI disorders, e.g., gastritis, cholecystitis, irritable colon

DOSAGE
Prevention of paralytic ileus: 250 mg to 500 mg IM; repeat in 2 hours, then every 6 hours until danger of adynamic ileus has passed

Treatment of adynamic ileus: 500 mg IM; repeat in 2 hours and again every 6 hours as needed
Skin lesions: apply topically one or two times a day
Oral: 2 to 3 tablets 3 times a day

SIGNIFICANT ADVERSE REACTIONS
(Systemic use) Itching, erythema, dermatitis, urticaria, dyspnea, intestinal colic, hypotension, vomiting, and diarrhea

CONTRAINDICATIONS
Hemophilia, ileus due to mechanical obstruction. *Cautious use* in pregnant or nursing women and in children

INTERACTIONS
Concomitant use of antibiotics, barbiturates, or narcotics may increase the likelihood of allergic reactions
Respiratory difficulty has occurred when dexpanthenol was administered following succinylcholine

NURSING CONSIDERATIONS

Nursing Alerts
- Perform complete baseline abdominal assessment before administering drug, including measurement of abdominal girth, auscultation of bowel sounds (location, frequency, pitch), and palpation for rigidity and presence and location of pain or tenderness.
- Monitor frequency of stools.

1. Seek clarification if prescribed for administration within one hour following succinylcholine use (see Interactions).
2. Withhold drug and notify prescriber if signs of hypersensitivity reaction to parenteral dexpanthenol (e.g., itching, redness, urticaria) are noted.

DIMETHYL SULFOXIDE

Rimso-50
(CAN) Kemsol

Dimethyl sulfoxide (DMSO) is a clear, colorless solvent possessing a wide range of pharmacologic actions but only a very limited clinical applicability, because the compound has not been adequately tested and its potential toxicity is rather high. It is approved for use as a bladder irrigant for the treatment of interstitial cystitis but has been used experimentally by topical application for treatment of musculoskeletal disorders and collagen diseases. Dimethyl sulfoxide can also serve as a vehicle to enhance percutaneous absorption of other drugs and has been reported to possess diuretic, local anesthetic, vasodilatory, muscle-relaxant, and bacteriostatic activity, although data to support these claims are insufficient. Principal adverse effects are a garliclike odor on the breath and skin, topical irritation, and allergic reactions due to histamine release. Ocular disturbances have been noted in experimental animals. The following discussion is limited to the use of dimethyl sulfoxide as a bladder irrigant. Its topical application should be discouraged until the efficacy and safety of the drug have been conclusively established.

MECHANISM
Not established; appears to exert anti-inflammatory, local anesthetic, diuretic, muscle-relaxing, vasodilatory, and bacteriostatic activity

USES
Symptomatic treatment of interstitial cystitis
Investigational uses include topical treatment of a variety of musculoskeletal disorders and to enhance the percutaneous absorption of other drugs

DOSAGE
Instill 50 mL into the bladder and allow to remain at least 15 minutes; repeat every 2 weeks or more as needed

COMMON SIDE EFFECTS
Garliclike taste, discomfort upon bladder instillation

SIGNIFICANT ADVERSE REACTIONS
Hypersensitivity reactions (nasal congestion, dyspnea, angioedema, pruritus, urticaria)

CONTRAINDICATIONS
No absolute contraindications. *Cautious use* in pregnant or nursing women, in children, and in patients with liver or kidney disease

PATIENT EDUCATION
1. Inform patient that garliclike odor and taste may appear within several minutes after use and persist for up to 72 hours.
2. Advise patient that periodic ophthalmic examinations and kidney and liver function tests are recommended during therapy. Changes in refractive index and lens opacities have occurred in experimental animals but not in patients receiving the drug by bladder instillation.

DISULFIRAM

Antabuse

Disulfiram is an antioxidant that blocks the oxidative metabolism of alcohol at the acetaldehyde stage. Thus, ingestion of even small amounts of alcohol in the presence of disulfiram results in a 5- to 10-fold increase in blood acetaldehyde levels, which elicits a range of unpleasant symptoms known as the disulfiram reaction or *mal rouge*. Thus, disulfiram is employed for the management of properly motivated chronic alcoholics who *desire* to be placed in a situation of enforced sobriety. The threat of illness upon consumption of alcohol is the prime deterrent with this drug. The drug is slowly absorbed and excreted, and the effects persist for up to 2 weeks after the last dose has been taken. Users must be made aware of the consequences of ingesting even small amounts of alcohol in any form whatsoever (e.g., cough syrups, mouthwashes, cold preparations, food sauces, vinegars). Also, application of alcohol-containing liniments or lotions (rubbing alcohol, colognes, toilet waters, aftershaves) should be avoided, because the alcohol may be absorbed systemically. The disulfiram–alcohol reaction consists of flushing, nausea, sweating, thirst, throbbing in the head, dyspnea, palpitations, chest pain, tachycardia, hypotension, weakness, vertigo, blurred vision, confusion, and syncope. With large amounts of alcohol, serious adverse reactions can occur, including arrhythmias, congestive heart failure, respiratory depression, convulsions, and even death. The intensity of the reaction depends on the amounts of disulfiram and alcohol ingested. Symptoms are usually fully developed at a blood alcohol level of 50 mg/dL and unconsciousness occurs at 125 mg/dL to 150 mg/dL.

MECHANISM
Blocks conversion of acetaldehyde to acetate during alcohol metabolism by inhibiting the enzyme aldehyde dehydrogenase, thereby elevating plasma levels of acetaldehyde, a toxic intermediate

USES
Adjunctive treatment of chronic alcoholism, in conjunction with supportive therapy and proper motivation

DOSAGE
Initially 500 mg/day in a single dose for 1 to 2 weeks; maintenance doses range from 125 mg to 500 mg once daily until patient is fully recovered

FATE
Rapidly and completely absorbed orally; optimal effects occur within 8 to 12 hours; highly lipid-soluble and localized initially in fatty tissue; slowly metabolized by the liver and excreted in the urine; effects persist for up to 2 weeks following withdrawal of medication

COMMON SIDE EFFECTS
Drowsiness

SIGNIFICANT ADVERSE REACTIONS
Impotence, headache, restlessness, fatigability, skin eruptions, metallic taste, optic or peripheral neuritis, polyneuritis, tremor, psychotic reactions, and arthropathy

See introductory section for disulfiram–alcohol reaction syndrome

CONTRAINDICATIONS
Severe myocardial disease, coronary occlusion, psychoses, pregnancy, and in patients who have recently received alcohol or alcohol-containing products, metronidazole, or paraldehyde. *Cautious use* in persons with epilepsy, diabetes, cerebral damage, hypothyroidism, hepatic cirrhosis, or nephritis

INTERACTIONS
Disulfiram may potentiate the effects of diazepam, chlordiazepoxide, oral anticoagulants, and phenytoin

Disulfiram plus isoniazid can result in coordination difficulties and behavioral changes

Paraldehyde is partially metabolized to acetaldehyde and can produce toxic reactions in the presence of disulfiram

Metronidazole given together with disulfiram can elicit psychotic reactions

NURSING CONSIDERATIONS

Nursing Alerts
- Ensure that patient and family are *fully* informed of rationale for therapy and consequences of ingesting or absorbing alcohol in any form (see introductory paragraph) before treatment with disulfiram is undertaken. Never administer to an intoxicated patient.
- Assist with institution of appropriate measures (e.g., oxygen, IV ascorbic acid, ephedrine, antihistamines) if severe disulfiram reactions occur.

PATIENT EDUCATION
1. Ensure that patient understands that disulfiram is not a cure for alcoholism but is merely an adjunct to other forms of therapy in managing chronic alcoholism in the person who *desires* to abstain.
2. Inform patient that tolerance does not develop with prolonged use. Instead, sensitivity to alcohol increases the longer the drug is used.
3. Instruct patient to abstain from alcohol for at least 12 hours before initiating disulfiram use.
4. Suggest that drug be taken in the morning unless sedation becomes a problem. Tablet may be crushed and mixed with a liquid if necessary.
5. Reassure patient that the side effects that may occur during the first 2 weeks of therapy (metallic taste, drowsiness, headache, weakness, skin eruptions) usually disappear with continued treatment.
6. Caution patient to exercise care in driving and performing other hazardous activities because drowsiness can occur.
7. Encourage patient to always carry identification indicating drug being taken, prescriber's name and phone number, and other pertinent information in case of an unexpected reaction. Inform patient that blood studies (CBC, SMA-12) and liver function tests are advised at regular intervals during treatment.
8. Warn patient that *mal rouge* reactions can occur up to 2 weeks after disulfiram has been discontinued if alcohol is ingested during that time.

ENZYME PREPARATIONS

Chymopapain
Chymotrypsin
Collagenase
Fibrinolysin and desoxyribonuclease
Hyaluronidase
Papain
Sutilains
Trypsin

A number of enzymes are available for either topical, intravertebral or systemic use. Most are employed topically to assist removal of excess fluids, tissue exudates, or clotted blood from ulcerated, inflamed, infected, or otherwise injured areas. Topical enzyme preparations may also be used for debriding surface ulcers, surgical or other types of wounds, and second- and third-degree burns. Systemically administered preparations may be useful in aiding the dispersion of other injected drugs or diagnostic agents, and possibly in relieving symptoms of healing surgical lesions. Finally, chymopapain is injected into herniated lumbar intervertebral disks to assist in reducing intradiskal pressure.

Since the enzyme preparations differ with regard to route of administration, indications, and precautions to be observed with their use, they are considered individually in Table 78-2.

FLAVOXATE
Urispas

MECHANISM
Exerts a direct relaxant effect on smooth muscle of the urinary tract; also possesses anticholinergic, local anesthetic, and possibly analgesic properties

Table 78-2
Enzyme Preparations

Drug	Preparations	Indications	Administration and Dosage	Nursing Implications
Topical Only				
Collagenase Biozyme-C, Santyl	Ointment: 250 U/g	Debridement of dermal ulcers and severe burns	Apply once daily	Digests collagen and promotes formation of granulation tissue and epithelization of ulcers and burns; optimal pH range for enzymatic activity is 6 to 8; cleanse lesion before application and cover wound with sterile gauze after using ointment; remove excess ointment each time dressing is changed; a suitable antibacterial ointment is used when infection is present; *avoid* soaks or washing with solutions containing metal ions or acidic substances, because they reduce enzymatic activity
Fibrinolysin and Desoxyribonuclease Elase	Ointment: 1 U fibrinolysin and 667 U DNAase per g; Powder: 25 U fibrinolysin and 15,000 U DNAase per 30-mL container	Topically: debridement of inflamed or infected lesions; Intravaginal: adjunctive treatment of vaginitis and cervicitis	Topically: apply as ointment or solution prepared from powder in the form of a spray or wet dressing; Change dressing 2 or 3 times a day, removing debris and exudates each time; Vaginally: instill 5 g of ointment or 10 mL of solution (1 vial/10 mL) deep into vagina at bedtime for 5 days	Combination of two enzymes that attack both DNA and fibrin, thus breaking down necrotic tissue and fibrinous exudates; do *not* use parenterally, because bovine fibrinolysin may be antigenic; solutions from dry powder must be used within 24 h; following instillation of solution into vagina, wait 1 to 2 min, then insert a tampon for 12 to 24 h; affected area must be cleansed and dense, dry, escharotic tissue removed before application of drug, because enzymes must be in contact with the tissue to be removed to be effective; also available as ointment with 10 mg/g chloramphenicol as Elase-Chloromycetin
Papain Panafil	Ointment: 10% with 10% urea	Debridement of surface lesions	Apply directly to lesion 1 to 2 times a day	Enzyme derived from *Carica papaya*; cover with gauze and remove accumulated necrotic tissue at each redressing; hydrogen peroxide may inactivate papain; itching or stinging can occur with topical application
Sutilains Travase	Ointment: 82,000 casein U/g	Debridement of burned areas, decubitus ulcers, incisional or traumatic wounds, and surface ulcers resulting from peripheral vascular diseases	Apply in a thin layer to moistened wound area 3 or 4 times a day	Proteolytic enzyme that digests necrotic tissue, thus facilitating formation of granulation tissue; avoid contact of ointment with eyes; a moist environment is essential for optimal enzymatic activity; action of enzyme is reduced by iodine, thimerosal, hexachlorophene, benzalkonium chloride, and nitrofurazone; side effects include mild pain, paresthesias, dermatitis, and possibly bleeding
Trypsin Granulex	Aerosol: 0.1 mg trypsin/0.82 mL with balsam of Peru and castor oil	Treatment of decubitus and varicose ulcers, wounds, and severe sunburn	Spray twice daily	Used as a spray for debriding necrotic areas

Continued

Table 78-2
Enzyme Preparations (continued)

Drug	Preparations	Indications	Administration and Dosage	Nursing Implications
Systemic Only				
Hyaluronidase Wydase (CAN) Hyalase	Injection: 150 U/mL, 1500 U/10 mL	Aid to increasing absorption and dispersion of other injected drugs and diagnostic agents Adjunct in subcutaneous urography Aid in hypodermoclysis	*Absorption of other drugs:* 150 U added to drug solution *Hypodermoclysis:* 150 U injected SC before clysis or into rubber tubing during procedure *Urography:* 75 U SC injected over each scapula	Mucolytic enzyme that hydrolyzes hyaluronic acid, thus aiding diffusion of fluids through tissues; extent of diffusion depends on amount of enzyme present and volume of solution; do *not* inject into acutely inflamed, infected, or cancerous areas; use *caution* when adding to clysis solution to prevent overhydration because enzyme can facilitate excess water absorption; monitor infusion rate carefully; preliminary skin test (0.02 mL intradermally) is often used to detect sensitive individuals; whealing and itching are positive signs of hypersensitivity
Ophthalmic Only				
Chymotrypsin Alpha Chymar, Catarase, Zolyse (CAN) Alpha Chymolean, Zonulyn	Powder for ophthalmic solution: 150 U, 300 U, 750 U	Aid in intracapsular lens extraction to facilitate enzymatic zonulysis	0.25–2.0 mL to irrigate the posterior chamber; repeat every 2 to 4 min until extraction	Proteolytic enzyme that lyses peptide bonds of amino acids in zonular fibers and ocular tissues; complete lysis occurs within 30 min; inactivated by serum, blood, alkalies, acids, antiseptics, detergents, epinephrine, chloramphenicol, and isofluorophate; may increase intraocular pressure transiently; does not lyse adhesions between lens and other ocular structures
Intravertebral Only				
Chymopapain Chymodiactin (CAN) Discase	Powder for injection: 2 U/mL after reconstitution	Treatment of documented herniated lumbar intervertebral disks whose symptoms have not responded to more conservative therapy	2 U to 4 U per disk as a single injection (maximum is 8 U in persons with multiple disk involvement)	Proteolytic enzyme that hydrolyzes the polypeptides and proteins that maintain the mucoprotein internal discal structure; compressive symptoms are thus lessened; used *only* in a hospital setting by trained personnel; paraplegia, CNS bleeding, and anaphylaxis have occurred; *avoid* intrathecal injection as drug is highly toxic by this route; risk increases with multiple injections

USES
Symptomatic relief of dysuria, urgency, nocturia, suprapubic pain, and incontinence resulting from cystitis, urethritis, prostatitis, and other genitourinary conditions

DOSAGE
100 mg to 200 mg orally three to four times/day

SIGNIFICANT ADVERSE REACTIONS
Drowsiness, dizziness, blurred vision, dry mouth, headache, nervousness, increased intraocular tension, confusion, urticaria, dermatoses, tachycardia, palpitation, hyperpyrexia, eosinophilia, and leukopenia

CONTRAINDICATIONS
Pyloric or duodenal obstruction, obstructive intestinal lesions, achalasia, and GI hemorrhage. *Cautious use* in patients with glaucoma and in pregnant women

PATIENT EDUCATION
1. Urge patient to exercise caution in driving or performing tasks requiring alertness because drowsiness, dizziness, and blurred vision may occur.
2. Teach patient interventions to alleviate dry mouth (see **Plan of Nursing Care 4**, in Chapter 14.

HEMIN
Panhematin

MECHANISM
Iron-containing metalloporphyrin that decreases the hepatic or marrow synthesis of porphyrin, probably by inhibiting an enzyme necessary for porphyrin/heme synthesis

USES
Symptomatic management of recurrent attacks of acute intermittent porphyria

DOSAGE
1 mg to 4 mg/kg/day by IV infusion over 10 to 15 minutes for 3 to 14 days. Maximum dose is 6 mg/kg/24 h

SIGNIFICANT ADVERSE REACTIONS
Phlebitis, pyrexia, leukocytosis, decreased hematocrit

CONTRAINDICATIONS
Porphyria cutanea tarda. *Cautious use* in patients with renal dysfunction, altered coagulability, thrombophlebitis; in pregnant or nursing women

INTERACTIONS
Hemin may enhance the anticoagulant effects of oral anticoagulants and heparin

The effects of hemin may be reduced by barbiturates, estrogens, and steroids, because these agents increase the activity of an enzyme that is inhibited by hemin

NURSING CONSIDERATIONS

Nursing Alert
- Monitor intake and output, particularly in patient receiving high doses. Promptly report onset of oliguria or anuria.

1. Freeze and store powder until time of use.
2. Reconstitute immediately before use (contains no preservatives). Discard unused portions.
3. Administer through large arm vein or central venous catheter to reduce risk of phlebitis.
4. To assure that no undissolved particles are injected, terminal filtration through a 0.45-μm or smaller filter is recommended.

IMMUNOSUPPRESSANTS

Drugs that suppress the immune response are extremely valuable agents in preventing rejection of transplanted tissues and in treating diseases believed to result from overactivity of the body's immune system. The clinically available immune suppressant drugs are reviewed below.

Azathioprine

Imuran

Azathioprine is an immunosuppressive agent used to prevent rejection in renal transplantations. It is a potent bone marrow depressant, and frequent blood counts are necessary during therapy. Azathioprine has been used experimentally in treating other disorders believed to be the result of altered immunologic function, such as severe rheumatoid arthritis, systemic lupus erythematosus, and idiopathic thrombocytopenic purpura.

MECHANISM
Not completely established; converted to 6-mercaptopurine, which appears to interfere with nucleic acid and protein synthesis and coenzyme function (see mercaptopurine, Chap. 72); may also alter cellular metabolism

USES
Adjunct for prevention of rejection in renal homotransplantation

Treatment of severe, active rheumatoid arthritis in patients not responsive to conventional therapy (i.e., aspirin, nonsteroidal antiinflammatory drugs, corticosteroids, gold)

Treatment of chronic ulcerative colitis (investigational use *only*)

DOSAGE
Prevention of rejection: initially 3 mg/kg to 5 mg/kg/day IV beginning at the time of transplant; switch to oral therapy as soon as feasible; usual maintenance range is 1 mg/kg to 3 mg/kg/day

Rheumatoid arthritis: initially 1 mg/kg as a single dose or two divided doses; increase stepwise in 0.5 mg/kg/day increments at 4-week to 6-week intervals if response is not satisfactory and no serious toxicity is noted; maximum dose is 2.5 mg/kg/day

FATE
Largely converted to 6-mercaptopurine following administration; most is metabolized in the liver and excreted by the kidneys; partially (30%) bound to plasma proteins

COMMON SIDE EFFECTS
Leukopenia, infections (fever, chills, sore throat, cold sores), nausea, vomiting

SIGNIFICANT ADVERSE REACTIONS
Anemia, thrombocytopenia, bleeding, jaundice, diarrhea, alopecia, oral mucosal lesions, pancreatitis, arthralgia, steatorrhea, severe secondary infections, toxic hepatitis, and biliary stasis

> **WARNING**
> Azathioprine is carcinogenic in animals and may increase the risk of neoplasia, especially in transplant recipients. The benefit:risk ratio must be carefully assessed when using azathioprine; acute myelogenous leukemia and solid tumors have occurred in rheumatoid arthritis patients receiving the drug

CONTRAINDICATIONS
Treatment of rheumatoid arthritis in pregnant women or in patients previously treated with alkylating agents. *Cautious use* in patients with liver or kidney dysfunction, during a clinically active infection, in pregnant or nursing women, and in women of childbearing potential

INTERACTIONS
Allopurinol inhibits azathioprine and mercaptopurine metabolism and can increase the toxic effects of these drugs

Azathioprine may reverse the neuromuscular blocking activity of nondepolarizing muscle relaxants (e.g., pancuronium)

NURSING CONSIDERATIONS

Nursing Alerts
- Monitor results of complete blood counts and liver and kidney function tests, which should be performed at least weekly during initial therapy and every 2 to 3 weeks during prolonged treatment. Rapid fall in leukocyte count or persistently low level mandates a dosage reduction or drug withdrawal.

- Assess patient carefully for indications of thrombocytopenia (abnormal bleeding or bruising, mucosal ulceration). Notify physician if any occur.
- Observe for indications of hepatic dysfunction (pruritus, darkened urine, light-colored stools, yellowing of skin or sclerae), and alert drug prescriber if they occur.
- Monitor intake–output ratio and renal clearance of drug to prevent cumulation toxicity.

1. Expect dosage to be reduced to one third to one fourth normal dose if azathioprine is given concurrently with allopurinol (see Interactions).

PATIENT EDUCATION

1. Teach patient interventions to reduce risk of infections; ensure that patient understands their importance. If infection develops, it should be treated immediately with appropriate drugs. In addition, the dosage of azathioprine may need to be reduced.

Cyclosporine

Sandimmune

Cyclosporine (cyclosporin A) is an immunosuppressant that may be employed to prolong and assist survival of allogeneic transplants involving the heart, kidneys, liver, and possibly also the bone marrow, pancreas, and lungs.

MECHANISM

Not completely established; appears to specifically and reversibly inhibit T lymphocytes, including the T helper cell and T suppressor cell; lymphokine production is also impaired, and release of interleukin-2 or T-cell growth factor may be reduced

USES

Prevention of organ rejection in kidney, liver, or heart transplants, in conjunction with adrenal corticosteroids
Treatment of chronic rejection in patients previously treated with other immunosuppressive drugs

DOSAGE

Oral: initially 15 mg/kg/day, 4 to 12 hours prior to transplantation; continue for 1 to 2 weeks postoperatively, then taper by 5%/week to a maintenance level of 5 mg/kg to 10 mg/kg/day
IV (see Nursing Alerts): initially 5 mg/kg to 6 mg/kg/day 4 hours to 12 hours prior to transplantation, as a slow (2–6 h) infusion of dilute solution (50 mg/20 to 100 mL of sodium chloride injection or 5% dextrose injection)

FATE

Oral absorption is erratic and incomplete; peak serum levels are attained in 3 to 4 hours; distributes to erythrocytes, granulocytes, leukocytes, and plasma, where it is approximately 90% protein-bound; extensively metabolized and excreted primarily via the bile, with only about 60% of the dose eliminated in the urine

COMMON SIDE EFFECTS

Renal dysfunction, tremor, hirsutism, hypertension, gum hyperplasia, secondary infections

SIGNIFICANT ADVERSE REACTIONS

CNS: headache, confusion, convulsions, flushing, paresthesias
GI: diarrhea, vomiting, abdominal pain, gastritis, peptic ulcer, anorexia, hepatotoxicity
Dermatologic: acne, brittle nails
Other: anxiety, depression, muscle weakness, joint pain, chest pain, visual disturbances, gynecomastia, difficulty in swallowing, upper GI bleeding, pancreatitis, mouth sores, constipation, night sweats, leukopenia, lymphoma, anemia, thrombocytopenia

CONTRAINDICATIONS

No absolute contraindications. *Cautious use* in hypertensive patients (blood pressure elevations are common); in patients with renal or liver dysfunction, seizure disorders; and in pregnant or nursing women: Although safety and efficacy have not been established in children, cyclosporine has been used in patients as young as 6 months with no apparent deleterious effects

INTERACTIONS

Cyclosporine can enhance the nephrotoxicity of aminoglycosides, loop diuretics, and other drugs that can damage the kidney
Ketoconazole and amphotericin B can elevate the plasma levels of cyclosporine
Concomitant use of cyclosporine with other immunosuppressive drugs can result in increased susceptibility to infection and possible development of lymphoma
Concurrent use of phenytoin, phenobarbital, rifampin, or sulfamethoxazole–trimethoprim may reduce plasma levels of cyclosporine

NURSING CONSIDERATIONS

Nursing Alerts

- Ensure that adequate laboratory and supportive resources are readily available and that the patient is managed only by health care personnel skilled in administering and monitoring the drug.
- With IV administration, be prepared to treat severe allergic reactions. Because the drug is highly insoluble, the IV form is prepared in a cremophor vehicle which is allergenic, and its use can result in anaphylactic reactions. Consequently, the patient should be transferred from IV to oral administration as soon as possible following surgery.
- Seek clarification if any other immunosuppressant drugs (except adrenal steroids) are prescribed because serious toxicity can result (see Interactions).
- Assess patient for occurrence of fever, sore throat, abnormal bruising, or unusual tiredness, possible early indications of a developing blood dyscrasia. Notify prescriber immediately if these occur.
- Assess renal and hepatic status regularly, and monitor results of BUN and serum creatinine, bilirubin, and liver enzyme determinations, which should be performed frequently. Although serum creatinine and BUN are commonly elevated during therapy, they usually respond to dosage reduction. If persistent elevations do not respond to a dosage alteration, it may be necessary to substitute another immunosuppressant.

1. With oral use, monitor results of cyclosporine blood level determinations, which should be obtained frequently, because oral absorption is erratic. Dosage should be adjusted as necessary to minimize toxicity due to excessive plasma levels.
2. Mix oral solution with milk or orange juice in a glass container (not styrofoam), preferably at room temperature, to mask the unpleasant taste. Stir well, and have patient drink *immediately*. Rinse mixing container with milk or juice, and have patient drink the second glass to ensure that all drug has been taken.

PATIENT EDUCATION
1. Discuss potential risks of teratogenicity should pregnancy occur during therapy.

Muromonab-CD3

Orthoclone OKT3

MECHANISM
A monoclonal antibody to the T_3 (CD3) antigen of human T cells; blocks T-cells function (which plays a major role in acute renal rejection) by reacting with and blocking the action of a molecule (CD3) in the membrane of human T cells that is essential for signal transduction; a rapid decrease in number of circulating T cells is observed within minutes after administration; reacts with most peripheral T cells in blood and body tissues

USES
Treatment of acute allograft rejection in renal transplant patients

DOSAGE
5 mg/day by IV bolus injection for 10 to 14 days, beginning once the renal rejection has been confirmed. Methylprednisolone (1 mg/kg, IV) is given before the first dose of muromonab-CD3 and hydrocortisone (100 mg, IV) is given 30 minutes after the first dose to minimize adverse reactions. Acetaminophen and antihistamines are also used to reduce early reactions.

FATE
Mean serum levels of drug will rise over the first 3 days, then level off during the remaining 7 to 10 days; antibodies to muromonab-CD3 have occurred and generally appear after approximately 21 days

COMMON SIDE EFFECTS
"First dose effects," e.g., fever, chills, wheezing, dyspnea, chest pain nausea, diarrhea, vomiting, tremor

SIGNIFICANT ADVERSE REACTIONS
Pulmonary edema, herpes infections, serum sickness, anaphylaxis

CONTRAINDICATIONS
Fluid overload. *Cautious use* in patients with fever and in pregnant women. A second course of therapy should be undertaken with caution, because drug-enduced antibody formation in the majority of patients may limit its effectiveness on repeat administration. Antibodies normally develop within several weeks of the start of therapy.

NURSING CONSIDERATIONS

Nursing Alerts
- Administer drug only in an area equipped to institute cardiac resuscitation.
- Be prepared to administer IV methylprednisolone prior to the first dose and IV hydrocortisone 30 minutes after the first dose to minimize first-dose reaction (see Dosage).
- Closely monitor patient response for 48 hours after first dose to detect symptoms of first-dose reaction (see Common Side Effects), which usually occurs within the first hour after the first dose and lasts several hours. Vital signs should be checked every 15 minutes for the first hour, every half hour for the next hour, then every 2 hours.
- Vital signs may be required every 4 hours for the duration of therapy. Temperature should be taken before treatment and several hours afterward to detect infection.
- Monitor breath sounds to detect fluid. The patient with fluid overload is particularly susceptible to acute pulmonary edema, which may be fatal.
- Implement appropriate measures for infection control. Because the drug destroys T cells, the patient is highly vulnerable to infection, particularly by viruses and opportunistic organisms.

1. When preparing injection, do not shake ampule, and draw solution into syringe through a low protein-binding filter.
2. Administer drug only by IV bolus. It should *not* be given by IV infusion or in conjunction with other drug solutions.

MESALAMINE

Rowasa

MECHANISM
Exerts an anti-inflammatory action in the colon, presumably by inhibiting production of prostaglandins and possibly leukotrienes; possesses a topical action to reduce pain and discomfort associated with chronic inflammatory bowel conditions

USES
Treatment of distal ulcerative colitis, proctitis, or other inflammatory bowel syndromes

DOSAGE
4 g once daily as a rectal suspension enema, usually at bedtime; should be retained for 8 hours; duration of treatment is 3 to 6 weeks

FATE
Poorly absorbed rectally; approximately 15% to 25% of a dose appears in the urine in 24 hours; primarily eliminated in the feces

COMMON SIDE EFFECTS
Abdominal pain, crampimg, flatulence, nausea

SIGNIFICANT ADVERSE REACTIONS

Headache, weakness, malaise, fever, diarrhea, dizziness, rectal pain, skin rash, bloating, leg pain, hemorrhoids, peripheral edema, and urinary infections

CONTRAINDICATIONS

No absolute contraindications. *Cautious use* in persons with renal dysfunction or sulfa allergies; in pregnant or nursing women; and in children

PATIENT EDUCATION

1. Teach patient proper administration and use of retention enema.
2. Inform patient that potential changes in renal function may be monitored by periodic urinalyses and BUN and serum creatinine determinations.
3. Teach patient how to recognize the acute intolerance syndrome associated with mesalamine use (e.g., cramping, bloody diarrhea, acute abdominal pain, and, sometimes, fever, headache, and rash) and to report occurrence to prescriber because the drug should be stopped promptly.
4. Warn patient hypersensitive to sulfites that the drug contains potassium metabisulfite, which may trigger the allergy.

OCTREOTIDE

Sandostatin

Octreotide is a long-acting peptide whose actions resemble those of somatostatin; therefore, it decreases secretion of many endogenous peptides, such as gastrin, vasoactive intestinal peptide (VIP), insulin, glucagon, secretin, and pancreatic polypeptide, as well as serotonin. It is used subcutaneously for the symptomatic treatment of persons with metastatic carcinoid tumors to alleviate severe diarrhea and flushing. Octreotide may also be given to reduce the profuse watery diarrhea resulting from vasoactive intestinal peptide tumors (VIPomas). Initial dosage is 50 µg SC once or twice daily; dosage may be increased thereafter depending on the response and tolerance by the patient. Octreotide has been used in a wide range of patients, from infants to the elderly. Most frequently occurring side effects are nausea, diarrhea, abdominal pain, and pain at the injection site. A wide range of other adverse reactions have been associated with octreotide, although the incidence is quite low. Like somatostatin, however, octreotide can lead to cholelithiasis, and patients must be closely monitored for gallbladder disease. Altered pancreatic and thyroid function can also occur during octreotide therapy.

PLASMA EXPANDERS

Dextran, low molecular weight (Dextran 40)
Dextran, high molecular weight (Dextran 70, 75)
Hetastarch

Dextran, a synthetic polysaccharide of varying molecular weights, and hetastarch, a chemically modified corn starch, are employed to expand reduced plasma volume, which can occur in hypovolemic shock resulting from hemorrhage, extensive burns, surgery, sepsis, or other forms of trauma. Their principal advantages over whole blood or plasma for volume replacement are their relatively low cost, wide availability, and lack of incompatibility problems, as well as the fact that they are not associated with the danger of transmitting diseases such as viral hepatitis or AIDS. However, these synthetic polysaccharides can produce allergic reactions, occasionally severe, and may also interfere with platelet function, resulting in increased bleeding tendencies. Prior IV injection of dextran-1 (Promit), a monovalent hapten, may be used to prevent severe anaphylactic reactions to dextran infusion. Plasma expanders should *not* be viewed as substitutes for whole blood or plasma proteins when such are available.

The agents used as plasma expanders are considered as a group and then are listed individually in Table 78-3

MECHANISM

Elevate the osmotic pressure of the blood, thus drawing water from extravascular spaces into the bloodstream. Plasma volume expands slightly in excess of the volume of drug solution infused. The drugs also decrease blood viscosity and reduce erythrocyte aggregation and rouleau formation, thus improving microcirculation. They reduce platelet adhesiveness and can alter the structure of fibrin clots, thus reducing the likelihood of thrombus formation. Secondary cardiovascular effects include increases in blood pressure, venous return, cardiac output, and urine flow, and decreased heart rate and peripheral resistance

USES

Adjunctive treatment of shock due to hemorrhage, burns, surgery, sepsis, or other trauma (*NOT* to be viewed as a substitute for blood or plasma)

Priming fluid in pump oxygenators during extracorporeal circulation (dextran 40 only)

Prophylaxis against venous thrombosis and pulmonary embolism in patients undergoing high-risk procedures, for example, hip surgery (dextran 40 only)

Adjunctive use in leukapheresis to increase granulocyte yield (hetastarch only)

DOSAGE

See Table 78-3

FATE

Onset of volume-expanding action varies from several minutes (dextran 40) to about 1 hour (dextran 75); hemodynamic status is improved for at least 12 hours (dextran 40) to over 24 hours (dextran 75, hetastarch) with a single infusion; molecules less than 50,000 molecular weight are eliminated by the kidneys, 40% to 75% within 24 hours; larger-molecular-weight molecules are slowly metabolized to smaller sugars and either excreted in the urine or eliminated as breakdown products (e.g., carbon dioxide and water); small amounts of drugs are excreted in the feces

SIGNIFICANT ADVERSE REACTIONS

Allergic reactions (nasal congestion, urticaria, wheezing, dyspnea, hypotension), anaphylactic reactions (rare), nausea, vomiting, headache, fever, joint pain, infection at injection site, phlebitis, hypervolemia, pulmonary edema, osmotic nephrosis, renal failure (rare), prolongation of bleeding time; *also with hetastarch*—submaxillary and parotid gland enlargement, flu-like symptoms, and edema of the lower extremities

CONTRAINDICATIONS

Severe cardiac decompensation, renal failure, and marked hemostatic defects (hyperfibrinogenemia, thrombocytopenia). *Cautious use* in patients with active hemorrhaging, liver or kidney impairment, severe dehydration, or history of allergic reactions, and in pregnant women

INTERACTIONS

Dextran may cause false elevations in blood glucose, urinary proteins, bilirubin, and total protein assays, and its use can lead to unreliable readings in blood typing and cross-matching procedures

Abnormally prolonged bleeding times can occur if plasma expanders are used together with anticoagulants or antiplatelet drugs

NURSING CONSIDERATIONS

Nursing Alerts

- Observe patient closely during infusion and discontinue drug at first sign of allergic reaction. Have resuscitative measures available (e.g., epinephrine, antihistamines, corticosteroids).
- Monitor central venous pressure during drug administration, and assess patient for signs of circulatory overload (dyspnea, wheezing, coughing, increased pulse and respiratory rate). Discontinue drug and inform physician if signs appear.
- Determine urine output and specific gravity at regular intervals. Oliguria, anuria, or altered specific gravity should be reported immediately. Marked elevations in specific gravity may indicate reduced urine flow. Recommended dosage and flow rate should not be exceeded because excessive doses can precipitate renal failure.

1. Question administration of solution containing sodium chloride to a patient with congestive heart failure or renal insufficiency or to one receiving corticosteroids.
2. Check results of hematocrit determinations, which should be obtained following administration. Advise physician if value falls below 30 mg/dL.
3. Distinguish low-molecular-weight dextran (40) from high-molecular-weight dextran (70, 75). High-molecular-weight dextran is reportedly associated with fewer adverse reactions (except allergenic) but it is slower in onset, is not cleared as rapidly, is more viscous, and exhibits much less

Table 78-3
Plasma Expanders

Drug	Preparations	Usual Dosage Range	Nursing Implications
Dextran 40—low molecular weight Gentran 40, 10% LMD, Rheomacrodex (CAN) Hyskon	Injection: 10% in either sodium chloride *or* 5% dextrose	*Shock:* 20 mL/kg/24 h by IV infusion the first day; thereafter, 10 mL/kg/day for a maximum of 5 days *Extracorporeal circulation:* 10 mL/kg–20 mL/kg added to perfusion circuit *Prophylaxis of venous thromboses:* 10 mL/kg on day of surgery, then 500 mL/day for 2 to 3 days, then 500 mL every 2 to 3 days for 2 weeks	Low-molecular-weight dextran is effective in reducing erythrocyte clumping and sludging and is reported to be able to disrupt thrombi; bleeding time can be prolonged and platelet function may be depressed by large doses; monitor coagulation time closely during therapy and observe for early signs of bleeding (epistaxis, petechiae)
Dextran 70, 75—high molecular weight Gentran 75, Macrodex	Injection: 6% in either sodium chloride *or* 5% dextrose	*Shock* Adults: 10 mL/kg to 20 mL/kg/24 h by IV infusion; usually, 500 mL is given at a rate of 20 mL to 40 mL/min for emergency treatment Children: Maximum dose 20 mL/kg	High-molecular-weight dextran is slower in onset but more prolonged acting than low-molecular-weight dextran; be alert for allergic reactions, which most often develop in first few minutes of infusion; may adversely affect capillary flow by increasing blood viscosity; can interfere with platelet aggregation and transiently prolong bleeding time
Hetastarch Hespan	Injection: 6% in sodium chloride	*Volume expansion:* 500 mL to 1000 mL/day (maximum 1500 mL/day); in acute situations, infusion rate is 20 mL/kg/h *Leukapheresis:* 250 mL to 700 mL infused at a fixed ratio (e.g., 1:8) to venous whole blood	Synthetic polymer prepared from amylopectin; similar to dextran in action and can also increase erythrocyte sedimentation rate; thus is used to improve efficiency of granulocyte collection by centrifugation; may elevate bilirubin levels; use with *caution* in patients with liver disease; during leukapheresis, hemoglobin and platelet counts may be temporarily reduced owing to volume-expanding effects of hetastarch; blood counts, hemoglobin determinations, and prothrombin times should be performed during therapy

of an effect in retarding rouleau formation and erythrocyte clumping.
4. Interpret results of the following laboratory tests cautiously because dextran may cause false elevations: blood glucose, urinary proteins, bilirubin, and total protein assays. Readings in blood typing and cross-matching procedures may also be unreliable.
5. Discard partially used containers because solution contains no bacteriostatic agent. Store at room temperature to prevent crystallization. Do not use if solution is not clear or under vacuum.

PLASMA PROTEIN FRACTIONS

Albumin, human   Plasma protein fraction

The plasma protein fractions, which are obtained by fractionating human plasma, include normal serum albumin and plasma protein fraction. These products are primarily employed to expand plasma volume, as they raise the osmotic pressure of the blood. Since they both are heat treated to destroy hepatitis B virus, they are considered somewhat safer than whole blood or plasma as volume expanders.

Normal serum albumin is available in two concentrations, a 5% solution, which is approximately osmotically and isotonically equivalent to human plasma, and a 25% solution, osmotically equivalent to five times the volume of plasma. Plasma protein fraction is a 5% solution of human plasma proteins (83%–90% albumin with small amounts of alpha and beta globulins) that is osmotically equivalent to human plasma. These albumin preparations do not appear to interfere with normal coagulation mechanisms and do not require cross-matching. The absence of cellular elements, moreover, greatly reduces the risk of sensitization with repeated administration.

The plasma protein fractions are discussed together, then listed individually in Table 78-4.

MECHANISM
Increase intravascular osmotic pressure, thereby drawing extracellular fluid into the bloodstream, expanding plasma volume; bind bilirubin in the plasma

USES
Adjunctive emergency treatment of hypovolemic shock
Temporary replacement of blood loss to prevent hemoconcentration following severe burns
Treatment of hypoproteinemia due to nephrotic syndrome, hepatic cirrhosis, toxemia of pregnancy, and tuberculosis, and in postoperative patients and premature infants
Adjunctive therapy during exchange transfusions in hyperbilirubinemia and erythroblastosis fetalis
Adjunctive treatment of acute liver failure, adult respiratory distress syndrome, acute peritonitis, pancreatitis, or mediastinitis and during cardiopulmonary bypass or renal dialysis

DOSAGE
See Table 78-4

SIGNIFICANT ADVERSE REACTIONS
Hypotension, allergic reactions (fever, chills, flushing, urticaria, rash), headache, nausea, vomiting, tachycardia, salivation, back pain, and respiratory irregularities

Table 78-4
Plasma Protein Fractions

Drug	Preparations	Usual Dosage Range	Nursing Implications
Albumin, human Albuminar, Albutein, Buminate, Plasbumin	Injection: 5%, 25%	Variable, depending upon diagnosis, severity of condition, patient's age, and concentration of solution; usually, the equivalent of 25 g to 100 g albumin per day is given by slow IV infusion (1 mL–4 mL/min depending on concentration); maximum recommended dose is 250 g/48 h	Available in two strengths, 5% and 25%, both containing 130 mEq to 160 mEq/L; the 25% solution allows administration of large amounts of albumin quickly, and 100 mL provides as much plasma protein as 500 mL plasma or 2 pints whole blood; concentrated solution usually requires supplemental fluids in dehydrated patients, thus 5% solution may be preferred for routine use because maximum osmotic effect is attained without additional fluids; preparations may cause an elevation of alkaline phosphatase levels; the 25% solution is preferred in most patients requiring sodium restriction
Plasma Protein Fraction Plasmanate, Plasma-Plex, Plasmatein, Protenate	Injection: 5%	*Hypovolemic shock* Adults: 250 mL to 500 mL by IV infusion Children: 20 mL/kg to 30 mL/kg *Hypoproteinemia:* 1000 mL to 1500 mL/day	Rate of infusion is determined by condition and patient's age and body weight; maximum infusion rate is 10 mL/min in shock and 5 mL to 8 mL/min in hypoproteinemia; do *not* give more than 250 g in 48 hours; monitor patients carefully for signs of volume overload; slow infusion if blood pressure declines; use *cautiously* in sodium-restricted patients—solution contains 130 mEq to 160 mEq/liter; if edema is present or if large amounts of protein are lost, use 25% albumin solution

Vascular overload and pulmonary edema can occur with too-rapid infusion.

CONTRAINDICATIONS
Cardiac failure, severe anemia, and normal or increased intravascular volume. In addition, plasma protein fraction is contraindicated in patients on cardiopulmonary bypass. *Cautious use* in patients with mild anemia, low cardiac reserve, hepatic or renal failure, or congestive heart failure

NURSING CONSIDERATIONS

Nursing Alerts
- Maintain a slow infusion rate (see Table 78-4) because rapid infusion may produce vascular overload and hypotension. Observe patient for signs of vascular overload (coughing, dyspnea, tachycardia, distended neck veins).
- Monitor blood pressure, pulse, and respiratory pattern during infusion.
- Be prepared to administer supplemental whole blood or plasma to satisfy large volume requirements. Albumin preparations are not a substitute for whole blood.
- Expect to administer additional fluids to patient with severe dehydration to minimize excessive depletion of tissue fluid.
- Assess patient for signs of external bleeding because blood pressure may be elevated following too-rapid administration. If bleeding is noted, be prepared to deal with new hemorrhaging or possibly shock.

1. Use *only* solutions that do not appear turbid and show no evidence of sedimentation.
2. Use promptly after opening (i.e., within 4 h), and discard unused portions because solution contains no preservatives or bacteriostatic substances.
3. Although drug solution can be added to usual IV infusion solutions, do *not* infuse together with solutions containing alcohol or protein hydrolysates because albumin may precipitate.

PIGMENTING/DEPIGMENTING AGENTS

Normal skin pigmentation is due to the presence of melanocytes in the basal layer of the epidermis. These cells have the ability to form the pigment melanin by oxidation of tyrosine. Subsequent activation of melanin occurs by exposure to radiant energy in the form of ultraviolet light.

Pigmenting Agents

PSORALENS

Methoxsalen   Trioxsalen

Two psoralen compounds, methoxsalen and trioxsalen, have the ability to increase the deposition of the pigment melanin in the skin in response to ultraviolet (UV) radiation. They may be employed either orally or topically to facilitate repigmentation in patients with vitiligo, a disorder characterized by patchy areas of nonpigmented skin. The oral dosage form of these two drugs can also be used to increase tolerance to sunlight in persons with fair complexions who suffer severe reactions upon exposure. Finally, much interest is centered on the possible beneficial effects of these drugs in treating severe psoriasis, when followed by controlled exposure to long-wave-length UV light (320 nm–400 nm). Such treatment, known as PUVA therapy, shows promise of being a very effective, albeit potentially toxic, form of therapy.

In vitiligo, repigmentation varies in time of onset, degree of completeness, and duration. Although some effect may be evident within several weeks after beginning therapy, significant repigmentation may take 6 months to 12 months. The psoralens are effective in enhancing pigmentation only when followed by exposure of affected skin areas to UV light, either artificial or natural (sunlight).

The two drugs are reviewed below, then listed individually in Table 78-5.

MECHANISM
Not established; may increase the number of functional melanocytes and activate resting or dormant cells; also initiate a local inflammatory response; can increase synthesis of melanosome and activity of tyrosinase, an enzyme involved in conversion of tyrosine to dihydroxyphenylalanine, a precursor of melanin; activity is dependent on the presence of functional melanocytes and activation of the psoralen agent by UV radiation, either artificial or sunlight

USES
Repigmentation of idiopathic vitiligo
Aid to increasing tolerance to sunlight (trioxsalen only)
Treatment of severe, recalcitrant, disabling psoriasis not responsive to other forms of therapy—given *only* in conjunction with controlled doses of long-wave UV radiation

DOSAGE
See Table 78-5

FATE
Oral absorption is 95% complete; food appears to increase serum concentrations; following oral ingestion, skin sensitivity to UV radiation is maximal in 2 hours and disappears within 8 hours; psoralens are metabolized in the liver and excreted primarily (90%) in the urine; topical application produces a rapid sensitivity

COMMON SIDE EFFECTS
Nausea, pruritus, erythema

SIGNIFICANT ADVERSE REACTIONS
WARNING
Use of psoralens together with UV radiation must be undertaken only by health care personnel experienced in photochemical treatment of psoriasis and vitiligo. Severe adverse reactions can occur (burns, ocular damage, skin aging, skin cancer) and patients must be informed of the risks inherent in such treatment

Topical: skin irritation, erythema, blistering
Oral: GI upset, nervousness, insomnia, depression, edema, dizziness, headache, hypopigmentation, vesiculation, nonspecific rash, urticaria, folliculitis, leg cramps, hypotension, severe burns from UV light, cataracts from UV exposure

Table 78-5
Psoralens

Drug	Preparations	Usual Dosage Range	Nursing Implications
Methoxsalen Oxsoralen, 8-MOP (CAN) Ultra MOP	Lotion: 1% Capsules: 10 mg	Topical: apply once weekly to small, well-defined lesions, then expose area to UV light for 1 min; subsequent exposure times should be increased with caution Oral: 2 capsules/day in a single dose, followed in 2–4 h by a 5-min exposure to UV light; gradually increase exposure time to 30–35 min	Pigmentation may begin within several weeks, but significant repigmentation may require treatment for 6–9 mo; do *not* increase dosage of oral preparation; perform liver function tests periodically during therapy and stop drug if liver impairment occurs; topical preparation is used only on small, well-defined vitiliginous lesions that can be protected from excessive exposure; use of bandages or sunscreens or both may be necessary
Trioxsalen Trisoralen	Tablets: 5 mg	*Vitiligo:* 10 mg/day, followed in 2–4 h by UV exposure ranging from 15–30 min *Sunlight tolerance:* 10 mg/day, 2 h before exposure to sun, for a maximum of 14 days	More active than methoxsalen, yet its median lethal dose is 6 times higher; do *not* increase dosage and only lengthen exposure times in gradual increments; discontinue drug if repigmentation is not evident within 3–4 mo

CONTRAINDICATIONS

Melanoma, invasive squamous cell carcinoma, aphakia, albinism, porphyria, acute lupus erythematosus, leukoderma of infectious origin; in children under 12 years of age (trioxsalen only); and concurrent use of a photosensitizing drug. *Cautious use* in patients with impaired liver function and in pregnant or nursing women

INTERACTIONS

An increased danger of severe burns exists if psoralens are used together with known photosensitizing agents, such as anthralin, coal tar derivatives, griseofulvin, nalidixic acid, phenothiazines, sulfonamides, tetracyclines, and thiazide diuretics

NURSING CONSIDERATION

Nursing Alert

- Observe patient for signs of irritation or blistering, particularly during first few days of therapy when sensitivity to light is greatest. Prescribed dosage and exposure should not be exceeded, and patient should be under *constant* supervision during therapy because overdosage or overexposure can result in severe blistering and burning.

PATIENT EDUCATION

1. Ensure that patient is aware of risks inherent in treatment (see *Warning* under Significant Adverse Reactions).
2. Instruct patient to take oral preparation with food or milk to minimize GI distress, or to divide oral dose into two portions taken one half hour apart. Topical preparations should *not* be used at home; they should be applied and monitored only by trained personnel under strictly controlled light conditions.
3. Caution patient to protect lips and eyes during UV exposure periods.
4. Instruct patient receiving topical preparation to keep treated area protected from sunlight, except for desired exposure periods, because severe burns can occur if treated area is exposed to additional UV light.
5. Inform patient that a complete blood count, an antinuclear antibody test, liver and kidney function tests, and an ophthalmologic examination are recommended prior to therapy and at 6- to 12-month intervals during prolonged therapy.

Depigmenting Agents

Two agents are available for reducing hyperpigmentation of skin, but they differ in that one of the drugs, hydroquinone, generally produces a temporary lightening of skin areas whereas the other drug, monobenzone, produces irreversible depigmentation.

Hydroquinone

Eldopaque, Esoterica Regular, Porcelana, and other manufacturers
(CAN) Eldoquin, Solaquin

Hydroquinone is capable of interfering with the formation of melanin by inhibiting the enzymatic oxidation of tyrosine. Skin color begins to lighten usually after 3 weeks to 4 weeks, but a good response may require up to 6 months. The drug may be applied twice a day as a cream (2%, 4%), lotion (2%), solution (3%), or gel (4%), often in combination with a sunscreening agent to minimize repigmentation upon exposure to sunlight. Hydroquinone should be applied only to limited areas of the face, neck, hands, or arms; the drug is *not* to be used on irritated, denuded, or damaged skin. Because the effect of the drug is temporary, treated skin areas will return to their original color when the drug is discontinued. Principal uses for hydroquinone are for reversible bleaching of hyperpigmented skin areas, such as freckles, chloasma, melasma, or senile lentigines.

Monobenzone
(CAN) Benoquin

Monobenzone is employed as a 20% cream for permanent depigmentation in patients with extensive vitiligo. It is *not* to be used on freckles, melasma, pigmented nevi, or hyperpigmentation resulting from photosensitization, inflammation, or other causes. It is a *potent* depigmenting agent. Depigmentation occurs within 1 month to 4 months after initiation of therapy. Safety for use in pregnant women, nursing mothers, and children under age 12 has not been established. The cream is applied two to three times a day. If irritation, burning, or dermatitis occurs upon application, the drug should be discontinued.

SCLEROSING AGENTS

Ethanolamine oleate **Sodium tetradecyl sulfate**
Morrhuate sodium

Sclerosing agents are injected IV and act by irritating the intimal endothelium of veins, producing a sterile inflammatory response. Ethanolamine is used to treat bleeding esophageal varices, whereas the other two agents are usually used to treat uncomplicated varicose veins of the lower extremities. The drugs are reviewed as a group, then listed individually in Table 78-6.

MECHANISM
Directly irritate the venous intimal endothelium following IV injection, resulting in development of a blood clot that occludes the vein and leads to formation of fibrous tissue and obliteration of the vein

USES
Treatment of small, uncomplicated varicose veins of the lower extremities (morrhuate sodium, sodium tetradecyl sulfate)

Supplement to venous ligation to obliterate residual varicosed veins or to reduce risk of surgery (morrhuate sodium, sodium tetradecyl sulfate)

Treatment of internal hemorrhoids (morrhuate sodium—effectiveness has not been conclusively established)

Treatment of esophageal varices that have recently bled

DOSAGE
See Table 78-6

COMMON SIDE EFFECTS
Burning and cramping at injection site

SIGNIFICANT ADVERSE REACTIONS
Urticaria, tissue sloughing and necrosis; rarely, drowsiness, headache, hypersensitivity reactions (dizziness, weakness, respiratory difficulty, GI upset, vascular collapse, anaphylaxis)

In addition, ethanolamine has caused esophageal ulcer, pyrexia, retrosternal pain, pneumonia, pleural effusion, bacteremia and acute renal failure

CONTRAINDICATIONS
Acute thrombophlebitis, uncontrolled diabetes, sepsis, blood dyscrasia, thyrotoxicosis, tuberculosis, neoplasms, asthma, acute respiratory or skin disease, varicosities due to abdominal or pelvic tumors; in bedridden patients; and persistent occlu-

---

Table 78-6
Sclerosing Agents

Drug	Preparations	Usual Dosage Range	Nursing Implications
Ethanolamine Ethamolin	Injection: 5%	1.5 mL to 5 mL injected into bleeding vein; repeat after 1 wk, 6 wk, 3 mo, and 6 mo	Mild sclerosing agent used to obliterate bleeding esophageal varices; local inflammatory reaction produces fibrosis and occlusion of the vein; *not* recommended for varicosities of the leg; rare reports of anaphylaxis and acute renal failure have been noted; severe necrosis can occur with improper injection
Morrhuate Sodium Scleromate	Injection: 50 mg/mL	50 mg to 250 mg IV (1 mL–5 mL) depending on size of vein, given as multiple injections at the same time, *or* as a single dose; repeat at 5- to 7-day intervals as needed	To determine patient sensitivity, 0.25 mL to 1 mL is given into a varicosity 24 h before administration of a large dose; vial should be warmed before injecting; use a large-bore needle to fill syringe because solution froths easily; however, a small-bore needle is used for injection; pulmonary embolism has occurred
Sodium Tetradecyl Sulfate Sotradecol (CAN) Trombovar	Injection: 10 mg/mL, 30 mg/mL	0.5 mL to 2 mL of either strength solution depending on size of varicosity	Initially 0.5 mL of 1% solution should be given to determine patient sensitivity; observe for several hours before giving a larger amount; may *permanently* discolor vein at injection site; do *not* use for injecting veins for cosmetic purposes; *caution* in patients taking oral anticoagulants

sion of deep veins. *Cautious use* in patients with local or systemic infections and in pregnant or nursing women

NURSING CONSIDERATIONS

Nursing Alert
- Have emergency measures (e.g., antihistamines, epinephrine, corticosteroids) readily available for treatment of possible allergic reactions.

1. Be prepared to assist with injection procedure. Agents should not be used unless deep vein patency has been established. A preinjection evaluation for valvular competence should be performed, and a small amount (2 mL) of drug solution should be slowly injected into the varicosity. Only clear solutions should be used. Severe ischemia may result from intra-arterial injection.

PATIENT EDUCATION
1. Warn patient that, following injection, the vein will become hard and swollen and will be tender to touch. Aching and a feeling of stiffness usually occur and may persist for 48 hours.

TIOPRONIN

Thiola

MECHANISM
Exchanges with cystine to form a mixed disulfide of tiopronin–cysteine, thus reducing the amount of sparingly soluble cystine

USES
Prevention of cystine kidney stone formation in patients with severe cystinuria who are resistant to more conservative treatment (e.g., high fluid intake, diet modification)

DOSAGE
Average adult dose: 800 mg to 1000 mg daily in 3 divided doses, given orally; adjust dosage based on urinary cystine value
Children: average dose is 15 mg/kg/day

FATE
Cystine excretion falls on the first day of therapy; effects cease as soon as drug is stopped; up to 50% of a dose appears in the urine within the first 4 hours and up to 78% within 72 hours

SIGNIFICANT ADVERSE REACTIONS
Drug fever, generalized rash, wrinkling and friability of skin, systemic lupus–like reaction, blood dyscrasias

CONTRAINDICATIONS
History of agranulocytosis, thrombocytopenia, or aplastic anemia on this medication. *Cautious use* in patients with myasthenia gravis, and in pregnant or nursing women; *not* recommended in children under 9

NURSING CONSIDERATIONS

Nursing Alerts
- Monitor results of complete blood counts with differentials, which should be performed periodically, because blood dyscrasias may occur.
- Monitor results of urinary cystine determinations. Dosage adjustments are based on these values.

PATIENT EDUCATION
1. Assist patient to develop plan to maintain high fluid intake to help deter stone formation.
2. Teach patient how to recognize symptoms of possible blood dyscrasias, which necessitate drug discontinuation, and to report them.

YOHIMBINE

Aphrodyne, Yocon, Yohimex

Yohimbine is an alkaloid that chemically resembles reserpine. The drug is primarily an alpha$_2$-adrenergic blocker and can enhance the release of presynaptic stores of norepinephrine. Yohimbine can also block peripheral serotonin receptors. In addition, it readily enters the CNS, where it elicits a complex pattern of events, including central excitation, increased blood pressure and heart rate, release of antidiuretic hormone, irritability, and tremor.

Yohimbine has no FDA-sanctioned indications but has been used with some success in overcoming male erectile impotence, as it can improve vasodilation of penile vessels, resulting in engorgement of blood in erectile tissue. The drug is used as 5.4-mg tablets in a dosage of 1 tablet three times a day if tolerated. Lower doses may be necessary. The occurrence of orthostatic hypotension does not appear to be reduced by yohimbine. The drug has also been reported to function as an aphrodisiac.

The adverse effects associated with yohimbine are largely due to the CNS actions of the drug. They include elevated blood pressure and heart rate, irritability, increased motor activity, dizziness, headache, skin flushing, sweating, nausea, and vomiting. It should not be used in persons with renal disease, in pregnant women, or in children.

Selected Bibliography

Beveridge T: Cyclosporin A: An evaluation of clinical results. Transpl Proc 15:433, 1983

Canafax DM, Ascher NC: Cyclosporine immunosuppression. Clin Pharm 2:515, 1983

Cantilena LR, Klaassen CD: The effect of chelating agents on the excretion of endogenous metals. Toxicol Appl Pharmacol 63:344, 1982

Clinical news: Enthusiastic cyclosporine consensus. Am J Nurs 85:861, 1985

Diehl JT, Lester JL, Cosgrove DM: Clinical comparison of hetastarch and albumin in postoperative cardiac patients. Ann Thorac Surg 34:674, 1982

Golden D et al: Understanding the magic of cyclosporine. RN 48(6):53, June 1985

Greenhouse AH: Heavy metals and the nervous system. Clin Neuropharmacol 5:45, 1982

Gunby P: Chymopapain: Tropical tree to surgical suite. JAMA 249:1115, 1983

Harris KR, et al.: Azathioprine and cyclosporine: Different tissue matching criteria needed. Lancet 2:802, 1985

Kahan BD (ed): First International Congress on Cyclosporine. Transplant Proc 15(Suppl 1 and 2):2207, 1983

Lafferty KJ, Borel JF, Hodgkin P: Cyclosporine-A (CsA): Models for the mechanism of action. Transplant Proc 15(Suppl 1):2230, 1983

Levy RS, Fisher M, Alter JN: Penicillamine: Review of cutaneous manifestations. J Am Acad Dermatol 8:548, 1983

Lieberman AN, Goldstein M: Bromocriptine in Parkinson disease. Pharmacol Rev 37:217, 1985

Montefusco C et al: Cyclosporine immunosuppression in organ graft recipients: Nursing implications. Crit Care Nurs 4:117, 1984

Schindler R (ed): Cyclosporin in Autoimmune Diseases. Berlin, Springer-Verlag, 1985

Sodium cellulose phosphate (Calcibind). Med Lett Drugs Ther 25:67, 1983

Thompson AW: Immunobiology of cyclosporin—A review. Aust J Exp Biol Med Sci 61:147, 1983

Wagner H: Cyclosporin A: Mechanism of action. Transpl Proc 15:523, 1983

Weil C: Cyclosporin A: Review of results in organ and bone-marrow transplantation in man. In deStevens, G (ed): Medicinal Research Reviews, vol 4, p 221. New York, John Wiley & Sons, 1984

Wenger R: Synthesis of cyclosporine and analogues: Structure activity relationships of new cyclosporine derivatives. Transplant Proc 15(Suppl 1):2230, 1983

SUMMARY. MISCELLANEOUS DRUG PRODUCTS

Drug	Preparations	Usual Dosage Range
Alprostadil Prostin VR Pediatric	Injection: 500 μg/mL	Initially 0.1 μg/kg/min until improvement is noted; reduce infusion rate to 0.01 μg/kg to 0.05 μg/kg/min; maximum dose 0.4 μg/kg/min
Antidotes		
Activated Charcoal Several manufacturers	Powder Liquid	1 g/kg as a suspension in 6 to 8 oz of water
Heavy Metal Antagonists	See Table 78-1	
Binding/Chelating Agents		
Trientine Cuprid	Capsules: 250 mg	*Adults:* 750 mg–1250 mg in 2 to 4 divided doses *Children:* 500 mg–750 mg in 2 to 4 divided doses
Cellulose Sodium Phosphate Calcibind	Powder: 2.5 g	Initially, 5 g with each meal; reduce to 10 g/day as urinary calcium declines to less than 150 mg/day
Bromocriptine Parlodel	Tablets: 2.5 mg Capsules: 5 mg	*Amenorrhea–galactorrhea:* 1.25 mg–2.5 mg daily; increase to 5 mg–7.5 mg daily as needed *Postpartum lactation:* 2.5 mg 2 to 3 times a day for 14 to 21 days *Infertility* Initially 2.5 mg once daily; increase to 2 or 3 times/day within the first week *Parkinsonism* Initially 1.25 mg twice daily; increase every 2 to 4 weeks by 2.5 mg/day *Acromegaly* Initially, 1.25 mg–2.5 mg daily; increase by 2.5 mg every 3 to 7 days; usual range is 20 mg–30 mg daily
Capsaicin Zostrix	Cream: 0.025%	Apply 3 or 4 times a day
Dexpanthenol Ilopan, Panol, Panthoderm	Injection: 250 mg/mL Tablets: 50 mg, with 25 mg choline bitartrate Cream: 2%	IM: 250 mg to 500 mg; repeat in 2 h, then every 6 h as needed Oral: 2 to 3 tablets, 3 times/day Topical: apply 1 to 2 times/day

Continued

SUMMARY. MISCELLANEOUS DRUG PRODUCTS (continued)

Drug	Preparations	Usual Dosage Range
Dimethyl Sulfoxide Rimso-50	Solution: 50%	Instill 50 mL into the bladder and retain for at least 15 min; repeat every 2 weeks or more as needed
Disulfiram Antabuse	Tablets: 250 mg, 500 mg	Initially 500 mg/day in a single dose for 2 weeks; maintenance range 125 mg–500 mg/day
Enzyme Preparations	See Table 78-2	
Flavoxate Urispas	Tablets: 100 mg	100 mg to 200 mg 3 or 4 times/day
Hemin Panhematin	Powder for injection: 313 mg/vial	1 to 4 mg/kg/day by IV infusion for 3 to 14 days
Immunosuppressants		
Azathioprine Imuran	Tablets: 50 mg Injection: 100 mg/20 mL	Initially 3 mg to 5 mg/kg/day IV; transfer to oral as soon as possible Usual maintenance dose 1 mg/kg to 3 mg/kg/day
Cyclosporine Sandimmune	Oral solution: 100 mg/mL IV solution: 50 mg/mL	Oral: initially 15 mg/kg/day, 4 h–12 h prior to transplantation; continue for 1 to 2 weeks postoperatively, then taper by 50%/week to a level of 5 mg/kg to 10 mg/kg/day IV: initially 5 mg/kg to 6 mg/kg/day 4 to 12 h prior to transplantation as a slow IV infusion
Muromonab-CD3 Orthoclone OKT3	Injection: 5 mg/5 mL	5 mg/day IV bolus for 10 to 14 days
Mesalamine Rowasa	Rectal suspension: 4 g/60 mL	4 g once daily at bedtime; retain for 8 h; continue for 3 to 6 weeks
Octreotide Sandostatin	Injection: 0.05 mg/mL, 0.1 mg/mL, 0.5 mg/mL	Initially, 50 µg SC once or twice daily; increase gradually based on patient tolerance and response
Plasma Expanders	See Table 78-3	
Plasma Protein Fractions	See Table 78-4	
Pigmenting/Depigmenting Agents		
Psoralens	See Table 78-5	
Hydroquinone Several manufacturers	Cream: 2%, 4% Lotion: 2% Solution: 3% Gel: 4%	Apply twice a day; protect treated areas from UV light
Monobenzone	Cream: 29%	Apply 2 or 3 times/day
Sclerosing Agents	See Table 78-6	
Tiopronin Thiola	Tablets: 100 mg	Adults: 800 mg–1 g daily in 3 divided doses Children: 15 mg/kg/day in divided doses
Yohimbine Aphrodyne, Yocon, Yohimex	Tablets: 5.4 mg	5.4 mg 3 times a day

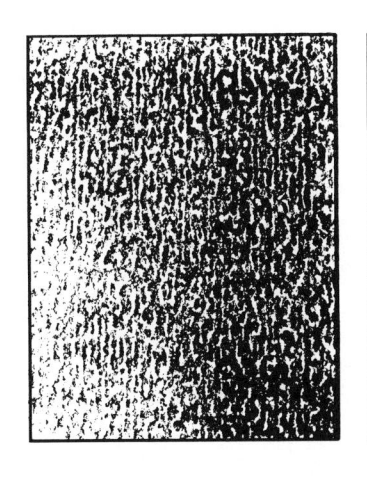

XI Drug Dependence and Addiction

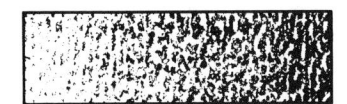

DRUGS OF ABUSE: A REVIEW

The abuse of drugs, a part of many cultures from the beginnings of recorded medical history, has in recent years reached near-epidemic proportions in certain segments of the population and shows no signs of abating. Rather, improper use of mind-altering substances, whether legally prescribed or illegally obtained, has risen significantly in the last decade, and it is likely that the incidence of drug abuse will continue to increase in the foreseeable future despite the many legal and educational efforts being made to reverse the trend.

Drug abuse is a nebulous term, broadly applied to the use of any drug in a manner that deviates from the generally accepted medicosociologic norm. The precise interpretation of this definition, however, varies from culture to culture, as do standards regarding what are considered acceptable patterns of behavior for individuals who use drugs. For example, chronic cigarette smokers are not usually viewed in the same light as chronic narcotic users in terms of drug abuse, yet both forms of behavior may be considered a misuse of a drug substance. Thus, the term *drug abuse* does not necessarily connote legally or socially unacceptable behavior, and therein frequently lies a significant deterrent to its eradication.

Drug abuse has many origins and an equal number of perpetuating factors. Precipitating circumstances include indiscriminate prescribing and inadequate monitoring of psychoactive drugs, emotional instability, peer pressure, and an environment that permits or encourages drug usage. However, a most important indicator of future substance abuse is a person's self-image. It is generally agreed by many drug counselors that those teenagers with a negative self-concept are more likely to demonstrate antisocial behavior than children who think positively about themselves. The role of the family is crucial in the development of a positive self-image; love, respect, and discipline must be provided. The compulsion to continue one's drug-taking habit may be reinforced by a number of factors, including availability, parental behavior patterns, stressful demands of everyday life, and desire for social acceptance. Drug abuse, therefore, is an extremely complex phenomenon involving environmental, sociological, and psychological aspects.

Drug testing is another complex issue. Detection of a psychoactive substance or its metabolites in urine means *only* that use has occurred at some point in the immediate past. There are, however, several problems with even this interpretation. First, a nonuser may passively inhale enough marijuana smoke of others to give a positive urine test (this is *not* likely, but it can happen). Second, because some drugs and their respective metabolites have extremely long half-lives (e.g., delta-9-THC, the major psychoactive component of marijuana, has a half-life ranging from about 25 to 60 hours), they will appear in the urine from 1 to 6 days *after* use. Third, depending on both the laboratory and the test kit being used, a 4% to 10% error rate can occur; that is, 4% to 10% of all persons tested may show up as *false* positive. Fourth, substances other than those being looked for can give a false reading of an abused substance (e.g., decongestants in over-the-counter cold medications can show up as amphetamine in some tests). Fifth, and most important, is the simple fact that the degree of impairment can be accurately correlated only to *blood* levels (or, in the case of alcohol, also to breath levels); it is scientifically invalid to measure the amount of drug in the urine and then attempt to determine the extent to which the person is impaired.

The discussion that follows focuses primarily on the pharmacology of the drugs of abuse and reviews methods for proper recognition and treatment of the drug-intoxicated state. An extensive listing of street names of abused drugs is provided at the end of this chapter to acquaint the reader with some of the terminology used by many drug abusers.

A useful, but by no means complete, classification of drugs subject to abuse is as follows:

I. CNS depressants
   A. Alcohol
   B. Barbiturates
   C. Nonbarbiturate sedatives and antianxiety agents
II. CNS stimulants
   A. Amphetamines
   B. Anorectics
   C. Cocaine
III. Narcotics
IV. Psychotomimetics (e.g., LSD, DOM, STP, psilocybin, DMT, mescaline)
V. Phencyclidine (PCP)
VI. Volatile inhalants (e.g., acetone, benzene, trichloroethylene, toluene)
VII. Marijuana
VIII. Nicotine

In discussing the drugs of abuse, frequent reference is made to the schedules in which controlled drugs are categorized. These schedules reflect the different regulations governing the prescribing and dispensing of each agent and the penalties for illegal possession. Descriptions of the schedules for controlled substances and a listing of drugs in each schedule are found in Chapter 8.

Before reviewing the pharmacology of abused drugs, it is necessary to describe briefly a few terms that appear throughout the discussion, recognizing, of course, that the following descriptions are by no means complete or universally accepted:

- *Habituation:* A pattern of repeated drug usage, although the actual physical need for the drug is minimal. There is no desire to increase the amount taken, and removal of the drug is usually not accompanied by withdrawal symptoms or by a compulsive need to obtain the drug at any cost.
- *Tolerance:* A reduced effect of a drug resulting from repeated exposure to that particular drug or to a similar drug. The latter condition is also known as *cross-tolerance.*
- *Drug dependence:* A state of reliance on a drug's effects to such an extent that absence of the drug impairs the ability to function continually in a socially acceptable manner. This term is often used interchangeably with habituation; two distinct types are recognized:
    Psychological dependence (addiction): A compulsive need to experience a pleasurable drug reaction, ranging from a mild desire for the drug on a routine basis to an overwhelming need to have the drug at any cost; similar to habituation and often used interchangeably; with many drugs, can lead to a more severe type of dependence, namely:

Physical dependence: An altered physiological state resulting from prolonged use of a drug; regular drug usage is necessary to avoid precipitation of withdrawal reactions that are often severe depending on the drug and duration of use

CNS DEPRESSANTS

Alcohol

Alcohol abuse is the major drug problem in the United States in terms of damaged health, accidents, family strife, business interruptions, and socially unacceptable behavior. The characteristics of acute alcohol intoxication depend largely on the blood level; they range from euphoria and altered judgment (50 mg/dL) to impaired motor coordination, concentration, and memory (100 mg–150 mg/dL) to profound respiratory and cardiovascular depression and coma (300 mg–400 mg/dL). More insidious and dangerous, however, are the consequences of prolonged alcohol consumption. Chronic alcohol abuse is associated with GI disturbances, liver damage, pancreatitis, neuronal damage, cardiac impairment, malnutrition, psychotic disturbances (e.g., Wernicke's encephalopathy and Korsakoff's psychosis) and cancer (liver, pancreatic, esophageal). In addition, alcohol in combination with other CNS depressants creates the most frequently observed drug-related hospital emergency and is responsible for more fatalities than any other drug or combination of drugs.

Chronic alcohol ingestion results in development of tolerance and ultimately physical dependence similar to that seen with barbiturates. Cessation of alcohol after several weeks of steady consumption may result in tremors, GI disturbances, anxiety, confusion, weakness, insomnia, and possibly delusions. Longer periods of alcohol abuse can, upon abrupt termination, lead to delirium tremens (fever, tachycardia, tremors, profuse sweating), agitation, disorientation, intense hallucinations, and convulsions.

Treatment of acute alcohol withdrawal is largely symptomatic and usually involves use of sedatives or anticonvulsants (e.g., diazepam, barbiturates) or both, along with necessary supportive therapy. Effective management of chronic alcoholism, on the other hand, often requires a combination of supportive social interaction (e.g., Alcoholics Anonymous), psychiatric counseling, and appropriate pharmacotherapy, such as antianxiety agents or disulfiram.

Barbiturates

The barbiturates, although declining in therapeutic use, remain valuable agents for induction of general anesthesia and in epilepsy. Members of the drug subculture, however, frequently employ these agents for their anxiety-reducing effects, often to quell the central excitatory action resulting from excessive stimulant abuse. The several barbiturates are classified into either schedule II, III, or IV, depending on their potency, duration of action, and tendency to produce dependence. The shorter-acting drugs (amobarbital, pentobarbital, secobarbital, and combinations thereof) are sought most by abusers because they produce a degree of euphoria following ingestion. These agents are all schedule II drugs.

Symptoms of barbiturate intoxication closely resemble those of alcohol intoxication and depend primarily on the blood level of the drug. Slurred speech, disorientation, impaired motor coordination, poor judgment, confusion, and emotional instability are frequent occurrences with excessive barbiturate usage. Serious overdosage may be associated with decreased respiration, rapid and weak pulse, cyanosis, mydriasis, and ultimately coma and respiratory paralysis. The CNS effects of barbiturates are additive to those of other CNS depressants, and combinations with alcohol or narcotics often prove fatal. Regular barbiturate use reduces the amount of time spent in rapid eye movement (REM) sleep and can lead to irritability and possibly to personality and behavioral changes.

Withdrawal reactions occur upon abrupt termination of excessive barbiturate use; these range from anxiety, weakness, confusion, anorexia, insomnia (due to rebound REM sleep), and mild tremors to delirium, disorientation, hallucinations, and convulsions. Symptoms are generally more severe with the shorter-acting derivatives. Management of the withdrawal state is symptomatic. Treatment of chronic barbiturate dependence may be accomplished by substituting phenobarbital for the barbiturate being abused at a dose that initially provides a similar effect, then gradually reducing the phenobarbital dose over a period of weeks (see also Chap. 20).

Nonbarbiturate Sedatives and Antianxiety Agents

Chronic use of a number of other hypnotic, sedative, and antianxiety drugs can result in dependence and an abstinence syndrome resembling that of the barbiturates. Glutethimide, methyprylon, and ethchlorvynol are among the hypnotic drugs employed as barbiturate alternatives, but they offer no significant advantages. Habituation commonly results from their prolonged use. Glutethimide, in particular, is an undesirable agent, inasmuch as convulsions and toxic psychoses have occurred during its continued administration, and its long duration of action makes reversal of acute overdosage extremely difficult (see also Chap. 21).

Methaqualone has been withdrawn from the market but nevertheless is still being abused by drug addicts, and medical emergencies resulting from methaqualone are still being reported. Methaqualone is used orally and produces effects resembling those of the barbiturates; in addition, paresthesias are experienced by many persons before the onset of the hypnotic effect. Although acute toxicity is usually not accompanied by severe respiratory and cardiovascular depression, other effects such as convulsions, rigidity, and coma can occur. Prolonged use invariably leads to dependence. A combination of methaqualone and the antihistamine diphenhydramine is marketed in Great Britain as Mandrax and is a more dangerous preparation than methaqualone alone, because the antihistamine can produce excitation, ataxia, and psychotic behavior in large doses. Withdrawal symptoms noted following cessation of methaqualone use include nausea, headache, cramping, insomnia, and occasionally toxic psychoses and severe convulsions.

Meprobamate is viewed as a minor tranquilizer and is used mainly for relief of anxiety, tension, and accompanying muscle spasms. It is somewhat less potent than the barbiturates and correspondingly less toxic, although tolerance occurs rather easily and physical dependence has been reported with as little as 3 g/day for several weeks. Meprobamate withdrawal is usually characterized by insomnia, anxiety, and tremors but can include hallucinations, convulsions, and coma. Fatalities have occurred with meprobamate overdosage.

The benzodiazepines are the most widely used antianxiety drugs, primarily because their margin of safety is greater than with other sedatives or hypnotics. Diazepam is the most frequently prescribed benzodiazepine and is involved in more reported emergency room cases than any other drug, with the exception of alcohol. Although not preferred as street drugs, benzodiazepines frequently are misused by patients being treated for anxiety neuroses or other psychosomatic disorders. A principal hazard with these drugs is the possibility of serious intoxication when they are combined with other depressants, most notably alcohol; deaths have resulted from this combination. Prolonged use of the benzodiazepines has resulted in both psychological and physical dependence; abrupt discontinuation of treatment (60 mg–120 mg/day) after 2 months has resulted in the appearance of cramping, sweating, agitation, disorientation, confusion, tremors, depression, auditory and visual hallucinations, and paranoia. Some patients exhibit these effects after withdrawing from even lower doses (see Chap. 23 for further discussion).

Flurazepam, temazepam, and triazolam are benzodiazepine analogs used for short-term treatment of insomnia and are claimed to have several advantages over the barbiturates (no hangover, no depression of REM sleep, greater safety margin). They are habituating drugs, nevertheless, and therefore should be accorded the same respect as any other hypnotic agent.

CNS STIMULANTS

Amphetamines

The three amphetamines (DL-amphetamine, dextroamphetamine, methamphetamine), as well as the structural analogs phenmetrazine and methylphenidate, are classified as schedule II drugs. Their approved clinical indications are limited and currently include only treatment of the attention deficit disorder syndrome in children, short-term treatment of obesity, and symptomatic control of narcolepsy. They are, however, a widely abused group of drugs; and together with the anorectics (see next discussion) are misused for their CNS-stimulating effects. Students, truck drivers, housewives, executives, athletes, and health professionals (e.g., doctors, nurses, pharmacists) have all employed amphetamines in therapeutic doses to suppress fatigue, increase alertness, enhance psychomotor performance, and generally induce a temporary state of well-being. Although potentially hazardous, and in some instances illegal, this type of amphetamine use is usually not labeled abuse. Amphetamine abuse refers to the parenteral or oral administration of large doses of the drugs to attain the intense rush or rapid high characteristic of these agents. Methamphetamine, or speed, is a favorite among drug abusers, because an IV injection elicits an almost instantaneous euphoria or orgasmic-like reaction. However, tolerance to this effect develops rapidly so that increasingly larger doses must be administered to experience the same sensation. Whereas normal therapeutic doses are in the 5-mg to 15-mg/day range, speed freaks have been known to use as much as 5000 mg/day. Obviously this behavior cannot continue for long, and after a period of several days to, occasionally, weeks, the person becomes exhausted to the point of lapsing into long periods of sleep and depression—the so-called crash.

Symptoms of mild amphetamine intoxication include insomnia, increased blood pressure and pulse rate, excitation, hyperactive reflexes, mydriasis, anorexia, and palpitations. More severe overdosage is reflected by extreme agitation, hostility, impulsiveness, hallucinations, confusion, bizarre behavior, aggressiveness, paranoid ideation, convulsions, and possibly death. The social implications of amphetamine abuse are obvious. Methamphetamine abuse, moreover, can result in cerebral vascular spasm, systemic necrotizing angiitis, cerebral hemorrhaging (cerebrovascular accident; CVA), arrhythmias, and severe abdominal pain. Effects of acute amphetamine intoxication have been treated with haloperidol, a dopamine antagonist with minimal anticholinergic effects.

Amphetamines are now believed to induce physical dependence; abrupt withdrawal results in the appearance of fatigue, muscle pain, lethargy, and depression. Withdrawal should be accomplished by allowing the patient to remain in a quiet environment and providing support of vital functions where necessary. Diazepam may be employed if sedation is needed; however, caution must be exercised to avoid adding to the subsequent depression. Acidification of the urine (e.g., with ammonium chloride) markedly increases the excretion of amphetamines and is frequently used to facilitate their removal. Conversely, the amphetamine high can be prolonged by concurrent use of urinary alkalinizers that slow renal excretion of the drug.

Although the legal production of amphetamines has been sharply curtailed, clandestine laboratories are currently providing vast amounts of these drugs, especially methamphetamine, for the street market. Amphetamine abuse remains a serious sociological and medical problem.

Phenmetrazine, an anorectic, and methylphenidate, a drug principally used in attention deficit disorder, are two structurally related compounds classified as Schedule II drugs that possess pharmacologic and toxicologic actions similar to the amphetamines. Although administered orally for their clinical indications, the tablets are frequently dissolved in water by abusers and injected IV. A major danger associated with parenteral use of these drugs is the presence of insoluble talc particles in the injection solution, which can result in circulatory impairment and talc deposits in the lungs and eye (see also Chap. 27).

Anorectics

A number of other amphetamine-related drugs termed anorectics are employed as adjuncts in the treatment of obesity and are discussed in Chapter 27. Their pharmacology in most cases is similar to that of the amphetamines, but they are less potent CNS stimulants and generally not as desirable as street drugs. They are, however, frequently misused as appetite suppressants, and chronic ingestion of these agents produces many of the symptoms of prolonged amphetamine use, namely insomnia, elevated blood pressure, tachycardia, and anxiety. Severe overdosage can result in a syndrome resembling amphetamine intoxication; these drugs should never be used continuously for longer than several weeks at a time. Most of these drugs are found in schedule III, whereas phentermine and fenfluramine are listed in schedule IV.

Cocaine

Cocaine is a natural product extracted from the leaves of the coca plant and has been employed clinically as a local anesthetic, especially for the nose and oral cavity. It is currently a popular drug of abuse; its systemic effects resemble those of amphetamine but are of much shorter duration. The powdered drug is most commonly administered by inhalation or snorting through the nasal passages, although it has been injected IV as well. Crack, a hardened form of cocaine, is heated in a glass pipe and smoked; it produces an intense euphoria within minutes. Irrespective of its mode of administration, cocaine quickly elicits a pleasurable high that may be accompanied by tachycardia, elevated blood pressure, restlessness, and mydriasis. Repeated use can lead to an overwhelming psychological dependence characterized by an extreme involvement in procuring and using the drug on a daily basis as well as to true physical dependence. Cocaine powder is commonly adulterated with various sugars as well as with local anesthetics at every level of distribution; clinical studies have shown that cocaine users are unable to distinguish between lidocaine and cocaine.

Chronic use of cocaine is associated with the following effects:

Cardiovascular
  Arrhythmias
  Acute myocardial infarction
  Rupture of the ascending aorta
  Cerebrovascular accident (CVA; stroke)
Respiratory
  Pulmonary edema
  Pneumomediastinum
  Rhinorrhea
  Rhinitis
  Ulceration and perforation of the nasal septum
Gastrointestinal
  Intestinal ischemia (may cause gangrene, requiring resection)
  Weight loss
  Nausea
Central Nervous System
  Anxiety
  Irritability
  Tactile hallucinations (imaginary skin insects, or "cocaine bugs")
  Visual disturbances (flashing lights, or "snow effect")
  Paranoia
  Insomnia
  Assertive behavior
Genitourinary
  Difficulty in maintaining erection
  Delay in orgasm for both men and women

Overdosage with cocaine can lead to arrhythmias, tremors, convulsions, respiratory failure, and death. Treatment of acute intoxication requires use of sedatives along with appropriate supportive therapy and must include careful monitoring of cardiovascular and respiratory function.

Infants born to women who used cocaine during their pregnancy show deficits in both sensory and motor functions which persist to at least 2 years of age.

Withdrawal from cocaine results in excessive fatigue, hypersomnia, depression (with possible suicidal tendencies), and extreme craving for the drug. Bromocriptine (Parlodel), a dopamine agonist, appears to be effective in reducing the latter effect.

NARCOTICS

The narcotic drugs, including the natural alkaloids of the opium plant (morphine and codeine) and the many semisynthetic and synthetic derivatives (see Chap. 18), are widely used for their potent analgesic, antitussive, and antidiarrheal actions. The alleviation of pain induced by these drugs frequently results in a temporary state of euphoria and relief from the accompanying anxiety and is a very pleasurable sensation. However, despite the fact that healthy, well-adjusted persons do not always experience the euphoric effects of opiates, it is precisely the desire to repeat this effect when it occurs that leads to opiate abuse.

Heroin, a schedule I narcotic, is a widely abused street opiate. Pure heroin is rarely obtainable, and most illicit heroin usually contains only 1% to 10% active drug, the remainder consisting of fillers such as sugars, starches, or quinine. This variable composition is a major cause of overdosage (i.e., when the percentage of opiate is significantly larger than expected). Most other narcotics are qualitatively if not quantitatively similar in their effects and are variously classified as Schedule II, III, IV, or V. Other favorite narcotics of abuse are hydromorphone (Dilaudid), a potent, short-acting opiate used either orally or parenterally, and oxycodone, available for oral administration alone or in combination with either aspirin as Percodan or acetaminophen as Percocet or Tylox.

Intravenous injection of heroin and other potent narcotics results in a sensation of exquisite pleasure (orgasmic effect, rush) and a feeling of extreme contentment. Oral use of narcotics does not produce the rush but usually leads to relaxation, euphoria, and a feeling of detachment or indifference to anxiety or pain. Other effects of narcotic drugs unrelated to their abuse potential are miosis, drowsiness, constipation, nausea, vomiting, and depression of vital functions.

Repeated use of narcotics invariably results in tolerance to the pleasurable effects of the drugs, resulting in the compulsion to continually increase the dosage. Eventually, a state of physical dependence ensues, and the abuser soon requires the drug, not to provide the euphoric effect, but to prevent development of withdrawal symptoms. Overdosage leading to respiratory paralysis is a common cause of opiate fatalities, because the dosage is pushed to extreme limits in the desire to continue to experience the rush. Other related hazards of narcotic addictions are malnutrition, infections due to unsterile injection equipment and poor hygiene, toxic reactions to contaminants injected along with the narcotic, hepatitis, vasculitis, thromboembolic complications, and AIDS (acquired immune deficiency syndrome).

Acute opiate overdosage is marked by stupor, slow and shallow respiration, pinpoint pupils (patients may present with dilated pupils due to activation of the sympathoadrenal system in cases of extreme overdosage), cold and clammy skin, hypotension, bradycardia, and possibly coma. Treatment involves a narcotic antagonist (naloxone) along with necessary supportive treatment (respiratory assistance, vasopressors). Dosage of the narcotic antagonist must be carefully controlled to avoid precipitation of acute withdrawal symptoms.

When narcotics are unavailable to a physically dependent individual, withdrawal symptoms usually begin within 8 to 12 hours, reach a maximum intensity in 36 to 72 hours, and can persist for up to 7 to 10 days. The severity of these symptoms depends on the degree of dependence, a function of the length of time the drugs have been used and the average amount administered. Initial signs of withdrawal include yawning, perspiration, lacrimation, sneezing, and restlessness. Progressively severe symptoms encompass anorexia, irritability, insomnia, anxiety, vomiting, generalized body aches, stomach cramping, diarrhea, fever, chills, tremors, jerking movements, muscle spasms, tachycardia, and elevated blood pressure. Although frightening to the patient, symptoms experienced during narcotic withdrawal are not usually life-threatening, in contrast to those associated with barbiturate withdrawal, which have resulted in fatalities.

Withdrawal symptoms can be suppressed by administration of another narcotic, frequently oral methadone, in an initial stabilizing amount, 20 mg once or twice a day, then a gradual reduction of the dose. Methadone's long duration of action (up to 24 h) also permits single daily dosing. However, it should be recognized that methadone is also a potent narcotic, and methadone abuse has now become a significant problem as well. Withdrawal from methadone is more prolonged than withdrawal from opiates, but symptoms are often less severe. Methadone and a newer chemically related compound, levo-alpha-acetylmethadol (LAAM), an even longer acting drug (48–72 h), are being used for management of narcotic addiction. This procedure involves stabilizing a patient on a regular oral dose of one of the compounds, resulting in development of cross-tolerance to the abused opiate, for example, heroin. Thus, the addict no longer experiences the rush or euphoria characteristic of heroin, and theoretically at least, can now slowly be withdrawn from methadone or LAAM.

Naltrexone (Trexan) is a long-acting antagonist that is now available for treatment of narcotic addiction; effects of heroin can be blocked for up to 3 days (depends on naltrexone dose). The patient must be narcotic-free for at least 7 days and have normal liver function prior to receiving naltrexone.

Detoxification programs work best in conjunction with psychiatric and social counseling. Because the addict's daily behavior is usually structured completely around obtaining and using narcotic drugs, withdrawal alone is rarely entirely successful in overcoming narcotic dependence.

PSYCHOTOMIMETICS

Psychotomimetic drugs, often termed hallucinogens, are a group of both naturally occurring compounds (such as psilocybin, mescaline) and synthetic compounds (e.g., LSD, DOM) capable of producing profound distortion of reality. Psychotomimetics are schedule I drugs that can cause serious psychological harm to the occasional, as well as the habitual, user. They have the capacity to distort mental function, often resulting in confusion, delirium, amnesia, and a distorted sense of direction, time, and distance. With large doses, delusions and hallucinations are common, and seriously impaired judgment and severe depression have frequently resulted from ingestion of these drugs. Although the drugs are usually employed in a desire to experience the pleasant psychic alterations such as euphoria, elation, vivid color imagery, and synesthesias (hearing colors, seeing sounds), the psychological state induced by these agents depends on many variables, the most important being the personality and expectations of the user and the environmental situation. Some persons experience the opposite type of effects, such as anxiety, dysphoria, panic, severe depression, despair, and suicidal tendencies, the so-called bad trip. These latter effects tend to occur following ingestion of large doses by inexperienced, nontolerant persons, especially those persons with preexisting psychological disturbances. Unpleasant reactions are also observed more commonly in threatening, hostile, or disturbing surroundings. Treatment of such bad trips may be accomplished by placing the patient in a nonthreatening, supportive environment and maintaining reassuring verbal contact (talking down). Mild sedatives (such as benzodiazepines) are recommended, but use of phenothiazines should be avoided.

Recurrences of the perceptual distortions are experienced by a large number of psychotomimetic drug users, especially with LSD, and can occur up to 5 years after initial usage. These flashbacks vary in duration from seconds to minutes and, although occasionally spontaneous, are most frequently triggered by periods of stress or anxiety or by use of other psychotropic drugs, such as marijuana. These flashback episodes may be potentially harmful to the person, depending on their severity and place of occurrence.

A degree of tolerance to the behavioral and psychological effects of LSD develops within a short period, but marked psychological dependence is rare, and physical dependence does not occur. There are no characteristic symptoms following abrupt discontinuation of drug usage.

Chronic episodes of psychotic behavior are not uncommon following use of psychotomimetic drugs. Most occur in persons who exhibit underlying emotional instability. The extent to which use of hallucinogens contributes to the protracted disturbed behavior of these people is difficult to assess accurately. Unfortunately, it is just such unstable persons who frequently become involved with use of psychotomimetic agents.

The most commonly used hallucinogens are the following:

- *LSD:* the most potent hallucinogen currently available; effects usually last 8 to 12 hours; tolerance develops quickly and effects usually cannot be duplicated for several days; sold as tablets, thin squares of gelatin (window panes), or impregnated paper (blotter acid); average effective oral dose is 25 μg to 50 μg.
- *Mescaline:* active ingredient of the flowering heads of the peyote cactus; oral doses of 250 mg to 500 mg produce hallucinations lasting 6 to 12 hours
- *DOM:* structural analog of mescaline, also known as STP, an acronym for serenity, tranquility, and peace; a potent, synthetic psychotomimetic producing intense, prolonged psychic alterations at a dose of 5 mg, occasionally lasting for several days following a single oral dose; frequently sold on the illicit market as mescaline
- *DMT:* a naturally occurring hallucinogen, *N, N*-dimethyltryptamine is not effective orally and must be inhaled or smoked; produces a rapid, brief alteration in perception and mood
- *Psilocybin and psilocin:* active ingredients of *Psilocybe* mushrooms, chemically related to LSD, although much less potent and shorter acting; usually administered orally

Many other substances are used for their hallucinogenic effects, many being amphetamine derivatives or centrally acting anticholinergics. One compound in particular, phencyclidine, is chemically related to the dissociative anesthetic ketamine and has become a dangerous, widely misused drug in the United States. It is discussed separately below.

Phencyclidine

Phencyclidine (PCP, angel dust), a potent psychotomimetic that is the most dangerous of all drugs of abuse, no longer is manufactured legally in the United States. Related to ketamine, PCP had been used as a veterinary anesthetic, but the PCP available on the street is a product of clandestine laboratories, is often highly contaminated, and is frequently misrepresented as LSD, THC, cocaine, or mescaline. Although occasionally administered orally or IV, it is most often used by smoking or nasal inhalation (snorting).

Effects of PCP depend on the dose and route of administration. Small amounts elicit euphoria, numbness of the extremities, and a sense of detachment. Larger amounts can result in analgesia, impaired speech, loss of coordination, agitation, muscle rigidity, tachycardia, elevated blood pressure, exaggerated gait, auditory hallucinations, acute anxiety, self-destructive behavior, and severe mood disorders, including paranoia, violent hostility, and feelings of depersonalization or doom. A psychotic state indistinguishable from paranoid schizophrenia is often a result of prolonged use of the drug but has occurred after only one dose. Delayed psychological reactions have been observed for up to several weeks following administration.

Undesirable reactions (bad trips) have become a significant problem with PCP, and the drug is capable of producing severe behavioral disturbances, frequently prolonged. Treatment of overdosage is best carried out by use of sedatives to control agitation and urinary acidifiers to facilitate excretion, and by isolation of the patient. Verbal contact should be avoided during the acute recovery stage, which frequently is accompanied by involuntary movements, facial grimacing, torticollis, and catatonic-like posturing. Although usually rapid, recovery can take several days or even weeks, and patients should be kept under close observation during this time.

VOLATILE INHALANTS

Volatile hydrocarbons such as acetone, benzene, carbon tetrachloride, trichloroethane, trichloroethylene, and toluene are present in many household products, including glue, paint, lighter fluid, nail polish remover, and varnish thinner, and are frequently abused by young persons. These volatile liquids are commonly placed on a rag or handkerchief or in a bag, and inhaled. The initial effects are CNS excitation, characterized by a sense of exhilaration, dizziness, and occasionally auditory or visual hallucinations, accompanied by tinnitus, blurred vision, slurred speech, and a staggering gait. These effects generally last 30 minutes to 60 minutes. Larger amounts of inhaled vapors can lead to drowsiness, hypotension, delirium, stupor, unconsciousness, and possibly coma. Amnesia frequently follows recovery. Fatalities have resulted, either from drug-induced respiratory failure or due to suffocation from the plastic bags placed over the face. Cardiac arrest has also been reported.

Recent reports indicate that several deaths among teenagers resulted from inhalation of correction fluid (e.g., Liquid Paper, White-Out); the halogenated hydrocarbons in these products appear to induce ventricular fibrillation.

Psychological dependence can develop, but physical dependence is rare, primarily because the duration of action is rather brief. Prolonged misuse of volatile hydrocarbons can result in significant organ damage, especially to the liver, kidneys, heart, and CNS. *Chronic* solvent inhalation can also produce cerebellar ataxia, equilibrium disorders, optic neuropathy, hearing loss, impaired memory, and a decreased ability to concentrate. These dangerous aspects of volatile inhalant abuse are overlooked by youthful users.

Treatment of acute intoxication resembles that of barbiturate overdosage and employs oxygen and respiratory assistance along with other supportive care as needed. Injections of vasopressors (such as epinephrine) should be avoided, however, because there is danger that myocardial sensitization by the volatile hydrocarbon may precipitate arrhythmias in the presence of adrenergic amines.

MARIJUANA

Marijuana is obtained from the hemp plant, *Cannabis sativa*, and constitutes a mixture of dried leaves, flowering tops, and other parts of the plant. The biologically active constituents of marijuana are termed *cannabinoids;* among the more than 60 known compounds, delta-9-tetrahydrocannabinol (THC) appears to be the major psychoactive derivative. Marijuana may be administered orally, but it is several times more potent when the powder is rolled loosely into cigarettes (joints) and smoked. Depending on the potency, peak psychopharmacologic effects occur within 10 to 20 minutes of inhalation and persist for 1 to 4 hours. The average joint contains between 2% and 4% THC (about 10 mg–20 mg), of which approximately one half is usually absorbed.

The resinous secretions from the flowering tops of the cannabis plant are also available as hashish. These secretions are usually dried and then either smoked or compressed into a variety of other dosage forms, such as cookies, cakes, or candies. Although hashish ranges in potency depending upon the source, it is generally between five and ten times more potent than marijuana itself. Hashish oil, a concentrated liquid extract of cannabis plant materials, contains a high percentage of THC (10%–50%), and several drops are equivalent to a single joint of marijuana. Hashish oil has also been administered IV, but this procedure is associated with a significant mortality.

The psychic and perceptual effects of marijuana vary widely among individuals and depend on the mental status, mood, previous experience, and expectations of the users, as well as the environment and circumstances surrounding its use. Typical psychic reactions include a sense of relaxation and well-being, perhaps even euphoria, impaired time and space orientation, altered sensory perception (especially sound and color), and spontaneous, often uncontrolled laughter. Short-term memory may be affected, psychomotor performance may be somewhat impaired and attention span can be reduced. Driving ability may be compromised—perceptual difficulties can prove hazardous to a person behind the wheel. Large doses may result in image distortion, depersonalization, disorganized thought and speech, fantasies, and, rarely, hallucinations.

Physiological changes accompanying marijuana usage can include elevated pulse rate and conjunctival congestion, which occur routinely, and erythema, enhanced appetite, disturbed equilibrium, xerostomia, oropharyngeal irritation, tinnitus, paresthesias, and vomiting, all of which may or may not be present.

Adverse reactions may appear to be minimal with occasional use in emotionally stable persons. Reported untoward reactions to marijuana comprise mild depression, anxiety, agitation, and a panic state, most frequently observed in first-time users. Acute intoxication from high doses (toxic psychoses) is manifested by hallucinations, severe agitation, and paranoia. Acute psychoses can also develop in patients with schizophrenia (known or undiagnosed), even in those currently being treated with antipsychotic medications. This condition usually resolves within 24 hours. THC can disrupt pituitary production of gonadotropic hormones and is excreted in breast milk. Further, new evidence suggests that marijuana-induced teratogenicity may occur; though these data need confirmation. Therefore, pregnant and lactating women should refrain from marijuana use.

Prolonged usage of marijuana has been implicated in pulmonary toxicity (precancerous cellular changes), suppression of cellular-mediated immune responsiveness, and personality and behavioral changes. Severe psychic disturbances, however, occur primarily in persons with preexisting emotional disorders.

Chronic use of marijuana may result in psychological dependence, but physical dependence is rare. A phenomenon of reverse tolerance has been reported in some marijuana users, whereby smaller amounts of the drug are able to elicit the desired psychic effects with repeated administration. This may be due in part to cumulation effects of the drug with frequent use.

Although acute overdosage with marijuana is rare, episodes can be managed by appropriate support of respiration, blood pressure, and other vital functions as required. A quiet environment and reassuring attitude are helpful during the acute psychotic phase, and extreme agitation is best treated with benzodiazepines such as diazepam.

Potential clinical applications are receiving much attention. Two areas of potential therapeutic benefit for the cannabinoids, especially THC, are the control of nausea and vomiting produced by chemotherapeutic agents and reduction of elevated intraocular pressure in glaucoma. Two cannabinoids (dronabinol, nabilone) are now available in the United States for the former purpose (see Chap. 52). Other properties of THC currently being investigated for possible clinical use are its analgesic, antiinflammatory, tranquilizing, bronchodilatory, and anticonvulsant actions.

NICOTINE

Nicotine is an alkaloid found in tobacco in a concentration usually between 1% and 2%. It is rapidly absorbed by the lungs and has a mild central stimulatory effect. At the same time, there is decreased skeletal muscle tone, reduced appetite, and, in novice users, occasionally nausea, vomiting, dizziness, and irritability. Tolerance usually develops to these latter effects but is of a variable nature and duration. Withdrawal from nicotine can result in nausea, diarrhea, increased appetite, headache, drowsiness, insomnia, irritability, and poor concentration. After extended abstinence, blood pressure and heart rate decrease, peripheral blood flow increases, and respiratory difficulties are reduced, but weight gain is common, because food is often used as a substitute form of oral gratification. Gradual reduction in nicotine consumption is usually less effective over the long term than abrupt cessation.

The other major risk factors associated with cigarette smoking (e.g., lung and bladder cancer, coronary artery disease, emphysema, and other chronic pulmonary disorders) cannot be exclusively linked to the nicotine content of the tobacco but probably result from constant exposure to the many carcinogenic products found in cigarette smoke.

Glossary of Street Names for Drugs of Abuse

Street Name	Drug	Street Name	Drug
Acapulco gold	Marijuana	Cube	Morphine, LSD
Acid	LSD	Cubes	LSD
Angel dust	Phencyclidine	Cyclone	Phencyclidine
Bennies	Amphetamines	Dexies	Dextroamphetamine
Big H	Heroin	Dillies	Dilaudid
Black beauties	Amphetamines	Dollies	Methadone
Black mollies	Amphetamines	Double cross	Amphetamines
Blockbusters	Barbiturates	Downers	Barbiturates
Blotter acid	LSD	Estuffa	Heroin
Blow	Cocaine	First line	Morphine
Bluebirds	Barbiturates	Flake	Cocaine
Blue devils	Barbiturates	Footballs	Amphetamines
Blues	Barbiturates	Ganga	Marijuana
Boy	Heroin	Giri	Cocaine
Brown	Heroin	Goma	Morphine
Brownies	Amphetamines	Grass	Marijuana
Brown sugar	Heroin	Green dragons	Barbiturates
Buttons	Peyote	Griffa	Marijuana
C	Cocaine	H	Heroin
Caballo	Heroin	Hash	Hashish
Cactus	Peyote	Haze	LSD
California sunshine	LSD	Hazel	Heroin
Cannabis	Marijuana	Hearts	Dextroamphetamine
Charley	Cocaine	Heaven dust	Cocaine
Christmas tree	Barbiturates	Hemp	Marijuana
Chiva	Heroin	Herb	Marijuana
Coca	Cocaine	Hero	Heroin
Coke	Cocaine	Hog	Phencyclidine, chloral hydrate
Colombian	Marijuana	Hombre	Heroin
Copilots	Amphetamines	J	Marijuana
Crack	Cocaine	Jay	Marijuana
Crank	Methamphetamines	Joint	Marijuana
Crap	Heroin	Junk	Heroin
Crossroads	Amphetamines	Lady	Cocaine
Crystal	Methamphetamine, phencyclidine	Log	Marijuana
		Ludes	Methaqualone

Continued

Glossary of Street Names for Drugs of Abuse (continued)

Street Name	Drug	Street Name	Drug
Mary Jane	Marijuana	Red devils	Barbiturates, secobarbital
Mesc	Peyote, mescaline	Reefer	Marijuana
Mescal	Peyote	Roach	Marijuana
Meth	Methamphetamine	Rock	Cocaine
Mexican mud	Heroin	Rocket fuel	Phencyclidine
Mexican reds	Barbiturates, secobarbital	Roses	Amphetamines
Microdots	LSD	Sativa	Marijuana
Minibennies	Amphetamines	Scag	Heroin
Morf	Morphine	Sleeping pills	Barbiturates
Morpho	Morphine	Smack	Heroin
Morphy	Morphine	Smoke	Marijuana
Mota	Marijuana	Snow	Cocaine
Mud	Morphine	Soapers	Methaqualone
Mujer	Cocaine	Soles	Hashish
Mutah	Marijuana	Sparklers	Amphetamines
Nebbies	Barbiturates, pentobarbital	Speed	Methamphetamine
Nimbies	Barbiturates, pentobarbital	Stick	Marijuana
Nose candy	Cocaine	Stumblers	Barbiturates
Oranges	Amphetamines	Stuff	Heroin
Panama red	Marijuana	Sunshine	LSD
Paper acid	LSD	Supergrass	Phencyclidine
Paradise	Cocaine	T's and blues	Pentazocine and tripelennamine
PCP	Phencyclidine	Tea	Marijuana
Peace pill	Phencyclidine	THC	Tetrahydrocannabinol
Pep pills	Amphetamines	Thing	Heroin
Perico	Cocaine	Thrusters	Amphetamines
Pink ladies	Barbiturates	Tic tac	Phencyclidine
Pinks	Barbiturates, secobarbital	Truck drivers	Amphetamines
Polvo	Heroin	Uppers	Amphetamines
Polvo blanco	Cocaine	Wake-ups	Amphetamines
Pot	Marijuana	Wedges	LSD
Purple haze	LSD	Weed	Marijuana
Quacks	Methaqualone	Whites	Amphetamines
Quads	Methaqualone	Window panes	LSD
Rainbows	Barbiturates, Tuinal	Yellow jackets	Barbiturates, pentobarbital
Reds and blues	Barbiturates, Tuinal	Yellows	Barbiturates, pentobarbital
Redbirds	Barbiturates, secobarbital		

Selected Bibliography

Benowitz NL, Jacob P: Daily intake of nicotine during cigarette smoking. Clin Pharmacol Ther 35:499, 1984

Chasnoff IJ, Burns WJ, Schnoll SH et al: Cocaine use in pregnancy. N Engl J Med 313:666, 1986

Cregler LL, Mark H: Medical complications of cocaine abuse. N Engl J Med 315:1495, 1986

Edwards G, Littleton J (eds): Pharmacological Treatments for Alcoholism. London, Croom Helm, 1984

Fultz JM, Senay EC, Pray BJ et al: When a narcotic addict is hospitalized. Am J Nurs 80:478, 1980

Gavin FH, Kleber HD: Cocaine abuse treatment. Open pilot trial with desipramine and lithium carbonate. Arch Gen Psychiatry 41:903, 1984

Gay GR: Clinical management of acute and chronic cocaine poisoning. Ann Emerg Med 11:562, 1982

Goldstein FJ: Cocaine: Clinical pharmacology and toxicology. Med Times 116(3):123, 1988

Goldstein FJ: Substance abuse in the health professions. Compend Contin Educat in Dentistry 8(6):438, 1987

Grabowski J (ed): Cocaine: Pharmacology, Effects, and Treatment of Abuse. National Institute of Drug Abuse Research Monograph Series, Publication 84-1326, Washington, D.C., U.S. Government Printing Office, 1984

Green PL: The impaired nurse: Chemical dependency. Focus Crit Care 11(2):42, 1984

Hollister LE: Health aspects of cannabis. Pharmacol Rev 38:1, 1986

Jacobs BL (ed): Hallucinogens: Neurochemical, Behavioral and Clinical Perspectives. New York, Raven Press, 1984

Jones RT: Cannabis and health. Annu Rev Med 34:247, 1983

Kandel DB: Marijuana users in young adulthood. Arch Gen Psychiatry 41:200, 1984

Leporati NC, Chychula LH: How can you really help the drug abusing patient? Nursing '82 12(6):46, 1982

Maykut MO: Health consequences of acute and chronic marihuana use. Prog Neuropsychopharmacol Biol Psychiatry 9:209, 1985

Mendelson JH, Mello NK (eds): The Diagnosis and Treatment of Alcoholism. New York, McGraw-Hill, 1984

Mittleman HS, Mittleman RE, Elser B: Cocaine. Am J Nurs 84:1092, 1984

Redmond DF, Krystal JH: Multiple mechanisms of withdrawal from opioid drugs. Annu Rev Neurosci 7:443, 1984

Smart RC et al (eds): Research Advances in Alcohol and Drug Problems, vol 8. New York, Plenum Press, 1984

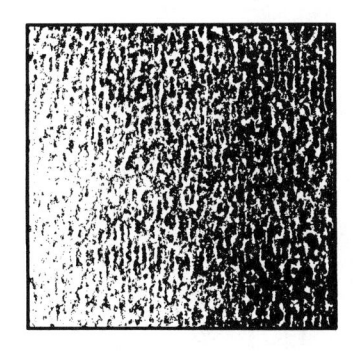

XII Appendices

COMMON ABBREVIATIONS

Common Abbreviations

aa	of each (equal parts)	FBS	fasting blood sugar	os	mouth
abd.	abdomen	Fe	iron	OS	left eye
ac	before meals	fl.	fluid	OT	occupational therapy
AD	right ear	ft	foot; feet	OU	each eye
ad	up to	FUO	fever of unknown origin	oz	ounce
ad lib	as much as needed				
Adm.	admission, admitted	g, gm	gram	pc	after meals
alb.	albumin	gal	gallon	per.	through or by
alk.	alkaline	GC	gonorrhea, gonococcus	PERLA	pupils equal and reactive to light and accommodation
AM	morning	GI	gastrointestinal		
amp.	ampule	gr	grain	PERRLA	pupils equal, round and reactive to light and accommodation
amt.	amount	gt (gtt)	drop(s)		
appt.	appointment	GU	genitourinary		
aq. (dest.)	water (distilled)	gyn	gynecology	plt.	platelet
AS	left ear			PM	afternoon; evening
AU	each (both) ear(s)	h, hr	hour	PMH	past medical history
aur.	ear	H₂O	water	PO	by mouth
		H₂O₂	hydrogen peroxide	PPD	purified protein derivative
bid	twice daily	hct	hematocrit	ppm	parts per million
bm	bowel movement	hgb	hemoglobin	prn	when necessary
BP	blood pressure	HEENT	head, eyes, ears, nose, and throat	PT	physical therapy
BR	bathroom			pulv.	a powder
BSA	body surface area	Hosp.	hospital		
BUN	blood urea nitrogen	H-S	hepato-spleno	q	every
		h.s.	hour of sleep, bedtime	q2h	every 2 hours
c̄	with	hx.	history	q4h	every 4 hours
Ca	calcium			qd	every day
Cal.	calories	IA	intra-arterial	qh	every hour
caps	capsule	i.e.	that is	qid	four times a day
CBC	complete blood count	IM	intramuscular	qod	every other day
cc	cubic centimeter	I&O, I/O	intake and output	qs	quantity sufficient
Cl	chloride	IPV	inactivated polio vaccine		
CNS	central nervous system	IV	intravenous	ⓡ	rectal
c/o	complained of			R	right
col. ct.	colony count	K	potassium	RBC	red blood cell
comp.	compound			RDA	recommended dietary allowance
conc.	concentrated	L, l	liter (quart)		
CP	cerebral palsy	Ⓛ	left	re	that is; regarding; in reference to
CPR	cardiopulmonary resuscitation	Lab.	laboratory		
		Lat.	lateral	rep.	repeat; may refill
diarr.	diarrhea	lb	pound(s)	RLQ	right, lower quadrant
dil.	dilute	LDH	lactic dehydrogenase	R/O	rule out
disch.	discharge	LE	lower extremities	ROM	range of motion
disp.	dispense	liq.	liquid; a solution	RUQ	right, upper quadrant
dist.	distilled	LLQ	left, lower quadrant	Rx	prescription
dL, dl	deciliter	LMP	last menstrual period		
DOA	date of admission	ltd.	limited	s, sec	second
DOB	date of birth	LUQ	left, upper quadrant	s̄	without
DPT, DTP	diphtheria, pertussis, tetanus immunization	mcg, μg	microgram	SC	subcutaneously
		Med.	medical	sens.	sensitive
dr.	dram	mg	milligram	SG	specific gravity
dsg./dssg.	dressing	min	minute	SGOT	serum glutamic oxaloacetic transaminase
dtd	dispense such doses	mixt	mixture		
DTR	deep tendon reflexes	mL, ml	milliliter	SGPT	serum glutamic pyruvic transaminase
Dx.	diagnosis	mo	month		
		mx.	minim	sig.	give directions; label
ECG (EKG)	electrocardiogram			sl, SL	under tongue; sublingual
ECR	emergency chemical restraint	n/c/o	no complaint of	sol.	solution
		neg.	negative	span.	spansule
ED	emergency department	Neuro.	neurology	s̄s̄	half
EEG	electroencephalogram	noct.	night	STAT	immediate
e.g.	for example	non rep., NR	do not repeat	STS	serologic test for syphilis
elix.	elixir	NPO	nothing by mouth	sub.q., SC	subcutaneous
EMG	electromyogram	Nsg.	nursing	suppos.	suppository
ENT	ear, nose, throat	NSR	normal sinus rhythm	sx.	symptoms
EOM	extraocular movements	N&V (N/V)	nausea and vomiting	syr.	syrup
ER	emergency room				
etc.	et cetera	OCP	oral contraceptive pills	t, tsp	teaspoon
eval	evaluation	OD	right eye	T, tbsp	tablespoon
ex.	example	oint.	ointment	tab.	tablet
extrem.	extremity	OPV	oral polio vaccine immunization	TB	tuberculosis
				tet-tox.	tetanus toxoid

Continued

Common Abbreviations (continued)

tid	three times daily	UA	urinalysis	VDRL	venereal disease test
TM	tympanic membrane	UE	upper extremities	V/S	vital signs
TNTC	too numerous to count	ung.	ointment	WBC	white blood cell
TPR	temperature, pulse, respirations	ut dict, UD	as directed	wk	week
tinc.	tincture	vag.	vaginal	WNL	within normal limits
tr.	trace or tincture	VD	venereal disease	w/o	without
Tx.	treatment			wt	weight

FDA PREGNANCY CATEGORIES

Category	Description
A	No demonstrated fetal risk in humans during any stage of pregnancy
B	No demonstrated fetal risk in animal studies but no adequate studies in pregnant women *or* Animal studies have shown an adverse effect but studies in pregnant women have not demonstrated a risk during any stage of pregnancy
C	Animal studies have shown an adverse effect on the fetus but there are no adequate studies in humans *or* No animal or human studies are available (use of the drug *may be acceptable* despite the risks)
D	Evidence of human fetal risk *but* the benefits from use of the drug *may be acceptable* despite the risks
X	Animal or human studies have demonstrated fetal abnormalities or adverse reaction reports give evidence of fetal risk (risk to a pregnant woman clearly outweighs the possible benefit)

DRUG COMPATIBILITY GUIDE

The following table presents a compilation of drug compatibility information obtained from several sources. It is intended to be used as a general guide to drug compatibilities rather than as a definitive information source, inasmuch as the compatibility of two or more drugs in solution depends on a number of variables, such as the solution itself, the concentration of drugs present, and the method of mixing (bottle, syringe, or Y-site).

Drugs reported to be compatible in solution are indicated by Y in the table, and drugs documented to be incompatible as reflected by the development of cloudiness, turbidity, or precipitation within the solution are indicated by an N. Where no information was found on the compatibility of two drugs, the corresponding space was left blank.

For some drug combinations, conflicting information was obtained about compatibility, especially where different parameters were used in obtaining the data. In such cases, a conservative approach was followed, and the combination was indicated as not compatible in the table, although compatibility may depend on solution strength, vehicle, time after mixing before used, or any number of other factors.

Before mixing any drugs, it is imperative that health-care personnel ascertain if a potential incompatibility problem exists by referring to an appropriate information source or by contacting the pharmacist. The accompanying table is intended solely to provide a handy guide from which one can quickly obtain a general idea of drug solution compatibility.

Bibliography

Allen LV, Levinson RS, Phisutsinthop D: Compatibility of various admixtures with secondary additives at Y-injection sites of intravenous administration sets. Am J Hosp Pharm 34:939, 1977

Allen LV, Stiles ML: Compatibility of various admixtures with secondary additives at Y-injection sites of intravenous administration sets (Part 2). Am J Hosp Pharm 38:380, 1981

Misgen R: Compatibilities and incompatibilities of some intravenous solution admixtures. Am J Hosp Pharm 22:92, 1965

Ng P: Compatibility guide for combining IV medications. Am J Nurs 79:1292, 1979

Trissel CA: Handbook of Injectable Drugs, 4th ed. Washington, DC, American Society of Hospital Pharmacists 1986.

Drug Compatibility Guide

	aminophylline	amphotericin B	ampicillin	atropine	calcium gluconate	carbenicillin	cefazolin	cimetidine	clindamycin	diazepam	dopamine	epinephrine	erythromycin	fentanyl	furosemide	gentamicin	glycopyrrolate	heparin sodium	hydrocortisone	hydroxyzine	levarterenol	lidocaine	meperidine	morphine	nitroglycerin	pentobarbital	potassium chloride	sodium bicarbonate	tetracycline	vancomycin	verapamil	vitamin B & C complex
aminophylline	*		Y		Y	N	N		N	Y	Y	N	N					Y	Y	N	N	Y	N	N	Y	Y	Y	Y	N	N	Y	N
amphotericin B		*	N		N	N		N			N					N		Y	Y		N						N	Y	N		N	
ampicillin	Y	N	*	N	N	Y	Y		N		N		N		N			Y	N			Y					Y	N	N		Y	Y
atropine			N	*			Y		N		N		Y			Y	N		Y	N		Y	Y		N	Y	N				Y	Y
calcium gluconate	Y	N	N		*	N		N		Y	N	Y						Y	Y		Y	Y					Y	N	N	Y	Y	Y
carbenicillin	N	N	Y			*	Y	Y		Y	N	N			N			Y		N	Y						Y			N	Y	N
cefazolin	N		Y	N			*	N	Y		N				N			Y	N	N		N	Y				Y	N			Y	Y
cimetidine		N		Y		Y	N	*	Y		Y	Y		Y	Y	Y	Y	Y			Y	Y			N	Y			Y	Y	Y	Y
clindamycin	N		N	Y			Y	*					Y		Y	Y						N	Y	Y						Y	Y
diazepam	Y		N		Y			*		N			N	N			N	N	N	N		N	N	N						Y	N
dopamine	Y	N	N		Y	Y				*			N		Y	Y		Y			Y		Y		Y		Y	Y	Y
epinephrine	N		N	N			Y	N		*	N		N		Y			N	N	Y			N	N				Y	Y
erythromycin	N		N	Y	N	N	Y				N	*			N	Y		Y			N	Y	Y	N	Y	Y	N
fentanyl		Y										*				Y			Y	Y		N					
furosemide						Y		N		N			Y	*	N		Y		N			Y		Y		N		Y	Y
gentamicin		N	N		N	N		Y		Y		N	*	N					Y					Y	Y
glycopyrrolate			Y					N							*		Y	Y	Y	Y		N		N			
heparin sodium	Y	Y	Y	N	Y		Y	Y	N	Y	Y	N	Y	N	*	N	N	Y	Y	N	N				Y	Y	N	N	Y	Y
hydrocortisone	Y	Y	N	Y	Y	Y		Y		Y	Y			N	*	Y	Y			N	Y	Y	Y	Y	Y
hydroxyzine	N		Y					N			Y		Y	N	*	Y	Y	Y	N				N
levarterenol	N		N	Y	N	N		N		N			N		Y	Y		*		N	Y		Y		Y	Y
lidocaine	Y	N	Y		Y	Y	N	Y		N	Y	N			Y	Y	Y		*		Y	Y	Y	Y		Y	Y
meperidine	N		Y				N		Y		Y			Y	N	Y		*	N		N		Y
morphine	N		Y				N			Y			Y	N	Y		N	*	N	Y		Y	Y
nitroglycerin	Y							Y			Y						Y		*			Y
pentobarbital	Y		N		N	N	N		N	N		N		N	N	Y	N	N	*	N	N	Y
potassium chloride	Y	N	Y	Y	Y	Y	Y	Y	Y	N	Y	N	Y		Y		Y	Y		Y				Y	Y	Y	Y	Y
sodium bicarbonate	Y	Y	N	N			Y	N		N	Y				N	Y	Y		Y	N	N		N	Y	*	N	N	Y	N
tetracycline	N	N	N		N	N	N	Y			Y	N		N				N	N		Y	Y		N	Y	*		Y
vancomycin	N		Y			Y				Y			N	Y						N	Y	N		*	Y	Y
verapamil	Y	N	Y	Y	Y	Y	Y	Y	Y	Y	Y	Y	Y		Y	Y		Y	Y		Y	Y	Y	Y	Y	Y	Y		Y	*	Y
vitamin B & C complex	N		Y	Y	Y	N	Y	Y	Y	N	Y	Y	N		Y	Y		Y	Y	N	Y	Y		Y			N	Y	Y	Y	*

GENERAL BIBLIOGRAPHY

PHARMACOLOGY AND NURSING

Abrams AC: Clinical Drug Therapy—Rationales for Nursing Practice, 2nd ed. Philadelphia, JB Lippincott, 1987

Alfaro R: Application of the Nursing Process. Philadelphia, JB Lippincott, 1986

American Drug Index (yearly): Philadelphia, JB Lippincott, 1989

Annual Review of Pharmacology and Toxicology. Palo Alto, CA, Annual Reviews (yearly).

Avery GS: Drug Treatment, 3rd ed. Baltimore, Williams & Wilkins, 1985

Bevan JA, Thompson JH (eds): Essentials of Pharmacology, 3rd ed. Philadelphia, Harper & Row, 1983

Bowman WC, Rand MJ: Textbook of Pharmacology, 2nd ed. Oxford, England, Blackwell Scientific Publications, 1980

Brunner LS, Suddarth DS: Textbook of Medical-Surgical Nursing, 5th ed. Philadelphia, JB Lippincott, 1984

Carpenito LJ: Handbook of Nursing Diagnosis, 2nd ed. Philadelphia, JB Lippincott, 1987

Clark JB, Queener SF, Karb VB: Pharmacological Basis of Nursing Practice, 2nd ed. St Louis, CV Mosby, 1986

Cooper JR, Bloom FE: The Biochemical Basis of Neuropharmacology, 5th ed. New York, Oxford University Press, 1986

Craig CR, Stitze RE (eds): Modern Pharmacology, 2nd ed. Boston, Little Brown & Co, 1986

Csaky TZ, Barnes BA: Cutting's Handbook of Pharmacology, 7th ed. New York, Appleton-Century-Crofts, 1984

Eisenhauer LA, Gerald MC: The Nurse's Guide to Drug Therapy. Englewood Cliffs, NJ, Prentice-Hall, 1984

Facts and Comparisons. Philadelphia, JB Lippincott (updated monthly)

Feldman RS, Quenzer LF: Fundamentals of Neuropsychopharmacology. Sunderland, MA, Sinauer Associates, 1984

Gahart BL: Intravenous Medications, 5th ed. St Louis, CV Mosby, 1989

Gilman AG, Goodman LS, Rall TW, Murad F (eds): The Pharmacological Basis of Therapeutics, 7th ed. New York, Macmillan, 1985

Goth A: Medical Pharmacology, 11th ed. St Louis, CV Mosby, 1984

Govoni LE, Hayes JE: Drugs and Nursing Implications, 6th ed. New York, Appleton and Lange, 1988

Haber J Leach A, Schudy S. Comprehensive Psychiatric Nursing, 3rd ed. New York, McGraw-Hill, 1987

Handbook of Nonprescription Drugs, 8th ed. Washington, DC, American Pharmaceutical Association, 1986

Hansten PD: Drug Interactions, 5th ed. Philadelphia, Lea & Febiger, 1985

Howry LB, Bindler RM, Tso Y: Pediatric Medications. Philadelphia, JB Lippincott, 1981

Jensen MD, Benson RC, Bobak IM: Maternity Care: The Nurse and the Family, 3rd ed. St Louis, CV Mosby, 1985

Katzung BC (ed): Basic and Clinical Pharmacology, 4th ed. Los Altos, CA, Appleton and Lange, 1989

Long JW: The Essential Guide to Prescription Drugs, 5th ed. New York, Harper & Row, 1989

Malseed RT, Harrigan GS: Textbook of Pharmacology and Nursing Care: Using the Nursing Process. Philadelphia, JB Lippincott, 1989

Mathewson MK (ed): Pharmacotherapeutics. Philadelphia, FA Davis, 1986

McKenry, LM, Salerno, E: Mosby's Pharmacology in Nursing, 17th ed. St Louis, CV Mosby, 1989

The Medical Letter on Drugs and Therapeutics. New Rochelle, NY, Medical Letter (biweekly)

Pagana KD, Pagana TJ: Diagnostic Testing and Nursing Implications: A Case Study Approach, 2nd ed. St Louis, CV Mosby, 1985

Pagliaro AM, Pagliaro LA: Pharmacologic Aspects of Nursing. St Louis, CV Mosby, 1986

Physicians' Desk Reference, 44th ed. Oradell, NJ, Medical Economics, 1990

Poe WD, Holloway DA: Drugs and the Aged. New York, McGraw-Hill, 1980

Rodman MJ, Karch AM, Boyd EH, Smith DW: Pharmacology and Drug Therapy in Nursing, 3rd ed. Philadelphia, JB Lippincott, 1985

Scherer JC (ed): Lippincott's Nurses' Drug Manual. Philadelphia, JB Lippincott, 1985

Schmidt RM, Margolin S: Harper's Handbook of Therapeutic Pharmacology. Philadelphia, Harper & Row, 1981

Shlafer M, Marieb EN: The Nurse, Pharmacology and Drug Therapy. Redwood City, CA, Addison-Wesley, 1989

Spencer RT, Nichols LW, Waterhouse HP et al: Clinical Pharmacology and Nursing Management. Philadelphia, JB Lippincott, 1983

United States Pharmacopeia Dispensing Information. St Louis, CV Mosby, 1987

Waechter EH, Phillips J, Holaday B: Nursing Care of Children, Philadelphia, JB Lippincott, 1985

Wardell SC, Bousard LB: Nursing Pharmacology: A Comprehensive Approach to Drug Therapy. Monterey, CA, Wadsworth, 1985

Wiener MB, Pepper GA: Clinical Pharmacology and Therapeutics in Nursing, 2nd ed. New York, McGraw-Hill, 1985

PHYSIOLOGY

Annual Review of Physiology. Palo Alto, CA, Annual Reviews (yearly)

Fox SI: Human Physiology, 2nd ed. Dubuque, IA, WC Brown, 1987

Guyton AC: Human Physiology and Mechanisms of Disease, 4th ed. Philadelphia, WB Saunders, 1987

Slaunwhite WR: Fundamentals of Endocrinology. New York, Marcel Dekker, 1988

Tortora GJ: Principles of Human Anatomy, 5th ed. New York, Harper & Row, 1989

Tortora GJ, Anagnostakos NP: Principles of Anatomy and Physiology, 5th ed. New York, Harper & Row, 1987

Wheater PR, Burkitt HG, Daniels VG: Functional Histology, 2nd ed. New York, Churchill-Livingstone, 1987

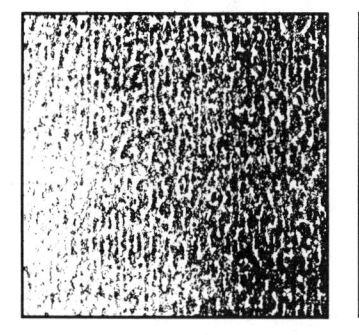

Index

INDEX

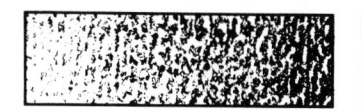

Numbers in italics indicate figures; those followed by *t* indicate tabular material.

A

Abbokinase (urokinase), 358–359, 360t
Abbott HTLV III EIA, 791, 792t
Abbreviations, 845–846
Abitrexate (methotrexate), 712, 718–719, 721–722t
Abortifacients, 470–472, 471t
Absorption, 11–13
  alterations in, drug interactions and, 28
  in children, 31
  in elderly patients, 36
  by gastrointestinal tract, 11–12, 487–488
  from parenteral sites, 12
  from skin and mucous membranes, 12–13
ABVD combination chemotherapy, 709t, 738, 740, 741t
AC-BCG combination chemotherapy, 738, 740, 741t
Accusens T, 791, 792t
Accutane (isotretinoin), 766–767
A Ce (AC) combination chemotherapy, 738, 740, 741t
ACE combination chemotherapy, 738, 740, 741t
Acebutolol (Sectral), 104–105, 105t, 106t, 108t, 109, 288t, 296–297, 303–304
Acetaminophen (Atasol; Dantril; Exdol; Robigesic; Tempra; Tylenol), 173–174
Acetazolam (acetazolamide), 250, 376–377, 378t
Acetazolamide (Acetazolam; Ak-Zol; Apo-Acetazolamide; Dazamide; Diamox), 250, 374t, 376–377, 378t
Acetest, 791, 792t
Acetohexamide (Dymelor), 431, 436–437, 438t
Acetohydroxamic acid (Lithostat), 641–642
Acetophenazine (Tindal), 205–208, 206t, 209t
Acetylcarbromal (Paxarel), 198
Acetylcholine
  intraocular (Miochol), 56
  pharmacologic effects and clinical consequences of, 56, 57t
Acetylcysteine (Airbron; Mucomyst; Mucosol; Parvolex), 541–542
Achlorhydria, 500
Achromycin (tetracycline), 609–611, 613t
Acid-base regulation, renal function in, 375
Acidulin (glutamic acid HCl), 501–502
Acilac (lactulose), 506–507, 510t
Acinetobacter, 567t, 598, 624, 625t
Aclovate (alclometasone dipropionate), 443, 445t, 445–447, 448t
ACMF combination chemotherapy, 738, 740, 741t

A-COPP combination chemotherapy, 738, 740, 741t
Acromegaly, 400
Actamer (bithionol), 672, 674, 675t, 676–680
ACTH. *See* Adrenocorticotropic hormone
Acthar (corticotropin), 407–408
ACTH Gel (repository corticotropin injection), 407–408
Acti-B$_{12}$ (hydroxocobalamin, crystalline), 349
Actidil (triprolidine), 113–114, 118t, 119
Actidose-Aqua (activated charcoal), 813–814
Actidose with Sorbitol (activated charcoal), 813–814
Actifed with Codeine, 538t
Actigall (ursodiol-ursodeoxycholic acid), 504
Actinomyces israelli, 567t
Actinomycin D (dactinomycin), 719, 722–724, 726t
Activase (alteplase, recombinant), 358–359, 360t
Activated charcoal (Actidose-Aqua; Actidose with sorbitol; Charcoaid; Charcocote; Liqui-Char; SuperChar), 813–814
Acutrim (phenylpropanolamine), 265–267, 269t
ACV combination chemotherapy, 738, 740, 741t
Acyclovir (Zovirax), 596t, 699–700
Ad-OAP (AOAP) combination chemotherapy, 738, 740, 741t
Adalat (nifedipine), 329–331, 331t, 332t
Adapin (doxepin), 227–230, 228t, 231t
AD combination chemotherapy, 738, 740, 741t
Addison's disease, 406
Additive effect, 17–18
Adenohypophysis, 395–396
  disorders of, 399–400
    hyperfunctional, 399–400
    hypofunctional, 399
  hormones of, 397–400, 407–409
Adenyl cyclase, 395
ADH. *See* Antidiuretic hormone
ADIC combination chemotherapy, 738, 740, 741t
Adipose tissue, adrenergic drug effects on, 81t
Administration routes, 3–10
  in children, 33–34
    absorption and, 31
    intramuscular, 33
    intravenous, 33
    oral, 33
    rectal, 33

topical and local, 33–34
  drug effects and, 17
  inhalation, 5–6
  ophthalmic, 4–5
  oral, 6, 33
  otic, 5
  parenteral, 6–10
    intraamniotic, 10
    intraarterial, 8
    intraarticular, 10
    intracardiac, 10
    intradermal, 10
    intramuscular, 8–10, *9*, 33
    intraperitoneal, 10
    intrapleural, 10
    intrathecal, 10
    intravenous, 6–8, *7*, 33
    subcutaneous, 8, *8*
  topical, 3–4, 33–34
    dermatologic, 3
    mucous membrane, 3–4
Administration time, drug effects and, 17
Adolescence, 31
Adrenal cortical steroids, 405, 442–453
  glucocorticoids, 443, 445–447, 448–452t
    comparative activities of, 444t
    topical, relative potencies of, 444–445t
  mineralocorticoids, 442–443
Adrenal glands, 404–406
  adrenal cortex and, 405–406
    disorders of, 406
    glucocorticoids and, 405–406
    mineralocorticoids and, 405
  adrenal medulla and, 404–405
    actions of hormones of, 404–405
    disorders of, 405
  gonadal hormones and, 406
Adrenalin (epinephrine), 79–82, 88–89, 90–91t
Adrenergic blocking drugs, 102–112
  alpha-adrenergic, 102–104
  beta-adrenergic, 104–109, 105–108t
Adrenergic drugs, 79–101
  direct-acting, 79
  dual acting, 79
  effects of, 79, 81t
  indirect acting, 79
Adrenergic nerves, 49, 51t
Adrenergic nervous system, 49
Adrenergic neuronal blockers, 102
Adrenergic receptor(s), 53, 79, 80t
Adrenergic receptor blockers, 102
Adrenocorticoids. *See* Adrenal cortical steroids
Adrenocorticotropic hormone (ACTH; corticotropin), 398, 405, 406, 407–408
  actions of, 398
  control of secretion of, 398

Adrenogenital corticoids, 442
Adrenogenital steroids, 405
Adrenogenital syndrome, 405
Adria + BCNU combination chemotherapy, 738, 740, 741t
Adriamycin-PFS (doxorubicin), 719, 722–724, 727t
Adriamycin-RDF (doxorubicin), 719, 722–724, 727t
Adrin (nylidrin), 334
Adrucil (fluorouracil), 712, 718–719, 720–721t
Adsorbents, antidiarrheal, 518
Advance-Test, 791, 792t
Adventitia, 483
Adverse drug effects, 19–25
  carcinogenicity as, 21
  classification of, 19
  disease-related, 20–21
    emotional disorders and, 21
    hepatic disease and, 20–21
    renal disease and, 21
  drug dependence as, 21
  glossary of, 22, 25
  multiple-drug reactions and, 21
  nonpharmacologic, 20
  pharmacologic, 19
    primary, 19
    secondary, 19
  teratogenicity as, 21, 21t
Advil (ibuprofen), 175, 178, 181t
Aerobacter aerogenes, 568t
AeroBid (flunisolide), 443, 445–447, 449–450t, 551–553, 552t
Aerolate (theophylline), 545–547, 549, 549t, 551
Aerolone (isoproterenol), 84–85
Aerosporin (polymyxin B sulfate), 634–635
Afferent arterioles, 371
Affinity, 16
Afrin (oxymetazoline), 88–89, 90–91t
Afrinol (pseudoephedrine), 88–89, 90–91t
Aftate (tolnaftate), 692, 696–697t, 697
Afterload, 278
Age, drug effects and, 17
Agonists, 16
Agoral Plain (mineral oil), 506–507, 509–510t
A/G Pro (protein hydrolysates), 778t
Agranulocytosis, 22
AHF (antihemophilic factor, human), 361–362
Airbron (acetylcysteine), 541–542
Ak-Chlor (chloramphenicol), 643–644
Ak-Con (naphazoline), 89, 92, 92t
Ak-Dilate (phenylephrine), 89, 92, 92t
Ak-Homatropine (homatropine hydrobromide), 76–77t
Akinesia, in Parkinson's disease, 253
Akineton (biperiden), 74–75t, 258–259, 259t
Ak-Mycin (erythromycin base), 619–620, 621t
Ak-Nefrin (phenylephrine), 89, 92, 92t
Akne-Mycin (erythromicin base, topical solution), 619–620, 621t
AK-Pentolate (cyclopentolate hydrochloride), 74–75t

Ak-Sulf (sulfacetamide), 573–575, 575–576t
Aktaine (proparacaine), 139–141, 140t, 143t
AK-Tracin (bacitracin), 632–633
Ak-Zol (acetazolamide), 250, 376–377, 378t
Alatone (spironolactone), 387–388
Alazine (hydralazine), 314–316
Albalon (naphazoline), 89, 92, 92t
Albamycin (novobiocin), 650
Albumin, human (Albuminar; Albutein; Buminate; Plasbumin), 826t, 826–827
Albuminar (albumin, human), 826t, 826–827
Albustix, 791, 792t
Albutein (albumin, human), 826t, 826–827
Albuterol (Novosalmol; Proventil; Ventolin), 94–95, 96–97t
Alcaine (proparacaine), 139–141, 140t, 143t
Alcaligenes faecalis, 567t
Alclometasone dipropionate (Aclovate), 443, 445t, 445–447, 448t
Alcohol abuse, 836
  hypoglycemia and, 403
Alcohol in dextrose infusion, 781
Alcomicin (gentamicin), 624–626, 627–628t, 630
Aldactone (spironolactone), 387–388
Aldomet (methyldopa), 311–312
Alfenta (alfentanil), 157, 158t, 159, 164t
Alfentanil (Alfenta), 157, 158t, 159, 164t
Algicon, 494–495t
Aliphatics, 205–208, 206t, 209t
Alkaban-AQ (vinblastine), 719, 722–724, 729t
Alka-Mints (calcium carbonate), 490–491, 492–493t
Alka-Seltzer, 494–495t
Alkeran (melphalan), 711–712, 717t
Alkets, 494–495t
Alkylamines, 114t
Allerdryl (diphenhydramine), 113–114, 116t, 119
Allerest (naphazoline), 89, 92, 92t
Allergic reaction. *See also* Hypersensitivity reactions
  photoallergic, 20
Allopurinol (Apo-Allopurinol; Lopurin; Noropurol; Purinol; Zurinol; Zyloprim), 188–189
Almacone, 494–495t
Almacone II, 494–495t
Alma-Mag, 494–495t
Almora (magnesium), 776t
Alopecia, 22
Alophen (phenolphthalein), 506–507, 513t
Alpha-adrenergic blocking agents, 102–104
  ergot alkaloids, 102
  prolonged-acting, noncompetitive antagonists, 102
  reversible, competitive antagonists, 102
Alpha$_1$ adrenergic receptors, 80t
Alpha$_2$ adrenergic receptors, 80t
Alpha cells, of islets of Langerhans, 402
Alpha Chymar (chymotrypsin), 818, 820t

Alpha Chymolean (chymotrypsin), 818, 820t
Alphaderm (hydrocortisone), 445t
Alphamul (castor oil), 506–507, 512t
Alpha receptor sites, 53
AlphaRedisol (hydroxocobalamin, crystalline), 349
Alphatrex (betamethasone dipropionate), 443, 444t, 445–447, 448t
Alprazolam (Xanax), 217–219, 218t, 220t
Alprostadil (Prostin VR Pediatric), 813
Alseroxylon (Rauwiloid), 313–314, 315t
Alteplase, recombinant (Activase), 358–359, 360t
ALternaGEL (aluminum hydroxide gel), 490–491, 492–493t
Alu-Cap (aluminum hydroxide gel), 490–491, 492–493t
Aludrox, 494–495t
Alumid, 494–495t
Alumid Plus, 494–495t
Aluminum carbonate gel, basic (Basaljel), 490–491, 492–493t
Aluminum hydroxide, in combination antacids, 494–497t
Aluminum hydroxide gel (ALternaGEL; Alu-Cap; Alu-Tab; Amphojel; Dialume), 490–491, 492–493t
Aluminum phosphate gel (Phosphaljel), 490–491, 492–493t
Alupent (metaproterenol), 94–95, 96–97t
Alurate (aprobarbital), 193–194, 196t, 197
Alu-Tab (aluminum hydroxide gel), 490–491, 492–493t
Alveolar ducts, 531
Alveolar sacs, 531
Alveolar ventilation, 533
Alveoli, 531
Alzapam (lorazepam), 217–219, 222t
Amantadine (Symadine; Symmetrel), 253, 255–256, 562, 569t, 700–701
Ambenonium (Mytelase), 60t, 60–61, 62–63t
Ambenyl, 538t
Ambilhar (niridazole), 672, 674, 675t, 676–680
Amcil (ampicillin), 582, 584–585, 586–587t, 595
Amcinonide (Cyclocort), 443, 444t, 445–447, 448t
Amdinocillin (Coactin), 568t, 569t, 582, 583t, 584–585, 586t, 595
Amebiasis
  extraintestinal, 681
  intestinal
    asymptomatic, 681
    symptomatic, 681
Amebicides, 681–685, 685–686t
  luminal, 681
  systemic, 681
Amen (medroxyprogesterone acetate), 456, 459, 460t, 461, 724, 730, 733t, 734–736
Amersol (ibuprofen), 175, 178, 181t
Amethopterin (methotrexate), 712, 718–719, 721–722t
Amicar (aminocaproic acid), 359, 361
Amidate (etomidate), 151

Amikacin (Amikin), 567–571t, 568–571t, 624–626, 625t, 627t, 630
Amikin (amikacin), 624–626, 627t, 630
Amiloride (Midamor), 386–387
Aminess (amino-acid formulation for renal failure), 780
Amino-acid formulation for hepatic failure or hepatic encephalopathy (HepatAmin), 780
Amino-acid formulation for high metabolic stress (Aminosyn-HBC; Branch Amin; FreAmine HBC), 780
Amino-acid formulation for renal failure (Aminosyn-RF; Aminess; NephrAmine; RenAmin), 780
Aminocaproic acid (Amicar), 359, 361
Aminoglutethimide (Cytadren), 447, 452, 724, 730, 733t, 734–736
Aminoglycoside(s), 570t, 624–626, 627–631t, 631
　administration and antimicrobial spectrum of, 625t
　resistance to, 624
Aminohippurate sodium (PAH), 791, 795t
Aminopeptidase, 488t
Aminophylline (Amoline; Corophyllin; Palaron; Phyllocontin; Somophyllin; Truphylline), 545–547, 548t, 549, 551
4-Aminoquinolines, 665, 666t
Aminosalicylic acid and salts, 655
Aminosyn (crystalline amino-acid infusion), 779–780
Aminosyn-HBC (amino-acid formulation for high metabolic stress), 780
Aminosyn-RF (amino-acid formulation for renal failure), 780
Amiodarone (Cordarone), 288t, 298–299
Amipaque, 799, 800t
Amitril (amitriptyline), 227–230, 231t
Amitriptyline (Amitril; Apo-Amitriptyline; Elavil; Emitrip; Endep; Enovil; Levate; Novotriptyn), 227–230, 228t, 231t
Ammonium chloride, 541, 783t, 785
Amobarbital (Amytal; Isobec; Novamobarb), 193–194, 195t, 197
Amodopa (methyldopa), 311–312
Amogel PG, 517t
Amoline (aminophylline), 545–547, 548t, 549, 551
Amoxapine (Asendin), 227–230, 228t, 231t
Amoxicillin (Amoxil; Apo-Amoxi; Larotid; Novamoxin; Polymox; Trimox; Utimox) 569t, 571t, 582, 583t, 584–585, 586t, 595
Amoxicillin and potassium clavulanate (Augmentin; Wymox), 567t, 569t, 570t, 571t, 582, 584–585, 586t, 595
Amoxil (amoxicillin), 582, 584–585, 586t, 595
Amphetamine(s), 262, 264–265, 266t
　abuse of, 837
Amphetamine complex (Biphetamine), 264–265, 266t
Amphetamine sulfate, 264–265, 266t
Amphojel (aluminum hydroxide gel), 490–491, 492–493t

Amphotericin B (Fungizone), 567–569t, 571t, 687–688
　topical (Fungizone), 692, 693t, 697
Ampicillin (Amcil; Ampicin; Ampliean; Apo-Ampi; Omnipen; Polycillin; Principen; Totacillin), 567–569t, 571t, 572t, 582, 583t, 584–585, 586–587t, 595
Ampicillin and sulbactam sodium (Unasyn), 582, 584–585, 587t, 595
Ampicin (ampicillin), 582, 584–585, 586–587t, 595
Ampilean (ampicillin), 582, 584–585, 586–587t, 595
Amrinone (Inocor), 285
AMV combination chemotherapy, 738, 740, 741t
Amylase
　pancreatic (amylopsin), 488t
　salivary (ptyalin), 488t
Amyl nitrite (Aspirols; Vaporole), 325–326, 327t, 329
Amylopepsin (pancreatic amylase), 488t
Amytal (amobarbital), 193–194, 195t, 197
Anabolic steroids, 474–476, 478–479t, 479
Anabolin I.M. (nandrolone phenpropionate), 474–476, 478t, 479
Anabolin L.A. (nandrolone decanoate), 474–476, 478t, 479
Anacobin (cyanocobalamin, crystalline), 348–349
Anadrol-50 (oxymetholone), 474–476, 478–479t, 479
Analeptics, 262–263
Analgesia, salicylates and, 170
Analgesics
　in combination cough mixtures, 542
　narcotic. See Narcotic analgesics
　nonnarcotic. See Nonnarcotic analgesics
　urinary, 641
Anamid (kanamycin), 624–626, 628t, 630
Anaphylactic reaction, 22
Anapolin 50 (oxymetholone), 474–476, 478–479t, 479
Anaprox (naproxen sodium), 175, 178, 183t
Anaspaz (hydroscyamine sulfate), 72–73t
Anavar (oxandrolone), 474–476, 478t, 479
Ancef (cefazolin), 598–600, 601t
Ancobon (flucytosine), 688–689
Ancotil (flucytosine), 688–689
Ancylostoma braziliense, 673t
Ancylostoma duodenale, 673t
Andro 100 (testosterone, aqueous), 474–476, 477t, 479
Andro-Cyp (testosterone cypionate), 474–476, 478t, 479, 724, 730, 731t, 734–736
Androgens, 405, 474–476, 477–478t, 479, 724, 730, 731t, 734–736
Android (methyltestosterone), 474–476, 477t, 479, 724, 730, 731t, 734–736
Android-F (fluoxymesterone), 474–476, 477t, 479, 724, 730, 731t, 734–736
Andro-L.A. (testosterone enanthate), 474–476, 478t, 479

Androlone (nandrolone phenpropionate), 474–476, 478t, 479
Androlone-D (nandrolone decanoate), 474–476, 478t, 479
Andronaq-50 (testosterone, aqueous), 474–476, 477t, 479
Andronaq-LA (testosterone cypionate), 474–476, 478t, 479
Andronate (testosterone cypionate), 474–476, 478t, 479
Andropository (testosterone enanthate), 474–476, 478t, 479
Andryl (testosterone enanthate), 474–476, 478t, 479
Andryl 200 (testosterone enanthate), 724, 730, 731t, 734–736
Anectine (succinylcholine), 132–133
Anemia, 22, 345. See also Antianemic drugs
　acute hemorrhagic, 345
　aplastic, 22, 345
　hemolytic, 22, 345
　megaloblastic (macrocytic, hyperchromic), 345
　microcytic (hypochromic), 345
Anesthesia, general, stages and characteristics of, 144, 145t
Anesthetics
　classification
　　of, 139, 140t
　general, 144–154
　　adjunctive, 144
　　inhalation, 145–149
　　intravenous, 149–153
　　postoperative, 144–145
　　preanesthetic, 144
　local, 139–141, 140–143t
　　classification of, 139, 140t
Angina. See also Antianginal agents
　classification of, 325
Angina pectoris, 275
Angio-Conray, 799, 800t
Angiostrongylus cantonensis, 673t
Angiotensin I, 373
Angiotensin II, 373
Angiotensin-converting enzyme inhibitors, 304–305, 309t
Angiovist 282, 799, 800t
Angiovist 292, 799, 800t
Angiovist 370, 799, 800t
Anhydron (cyclothiazide), 388–389, 390t, 391–392
Anisindione (Miradon), 354–356, 356t
Anisotropine, 67–70
Anisotropine methyl bromide, 74–75t
Anorectics. See Anorexiants
Anorexiants, 98–99, 262, 265–267, 268–269t
　abuse of, 837
Anorexigenics. See Anorexiants
Ansaid (flurbiprofen), 175, 178, 181t
Anspor (cephadrine), 598–600, 603t
Answer, 791, 792t
Antabuse (disulfiram), 817–818
Antacids, 490–491, 492–497t, 498
　combinations of, 494–497t
　non-receptor mediated effects of, 17
Antagonism, 18
　chemical, 18
　competitive, 18
　physiologic, 18

Antagonists, 16
Anthelmintics, 672, 673t, 674, 675t, 676–680
Antianemic drugs
  iron preparations
    oral, 345–346, 347t
    parenteral, 346–348
Antianginal agents, 325–333, 327–329t, 331t, 332t
  beta blockers, 331, 333
  calcium channel blockers, 329–331, 331t, 332t
  dipyridamole, 333
  nitrites/nitrates, 325–326, 327–329t, 329
Antianxiety drugs, 217–226
  benzodiazepines, 217–223, 218t, 220–222t
    metabolism of, 218t
  nonbarbiturates, abuse of, 836–837
  nonbarbiturate sedative-hypnotics compared with, 199t
Antiarrhythmic drugs, 287–301
  classification of, 288t
  group IA, 287–292
  group IB, 292–295
  group IC, 295–296
  group II, 296–297
  group III, 297–299
  group IV, 299–300
  pharmacokinetic and electrophysiologic properties of, 288t
Antiasthmatic drugs. See Bronchodilators
Antibiotics
  broad-spectrum, 559
  narrow-spectrum, 559
  prophylactic use of, 562
  in renal failure, 566–567
Anticholinergic/antihistaminergic agents, 253, 258–259, 259–260t
Anticholinergic drugs, 67–71, 78, 553
  antiemetic, 521t
  antimuscarinic, 67–70, 72–77t
  classification of, 69t
  in combination cough mixtures, 543
  ganglionic blockers, 67, 70–71
  neuromuscular blockers, 67
  pharmacologic actions of, 67, 68t
  quaternary amines, 67, 69t
Anticoagulant drugs, 351–358
  hemorrheologic agent, 357–358
  heparin antagonist, 354
  oral, 354–356, 356t
  oral anticoagulant antagonist, 356–357
  parenteral, 351–354
Anticonvulsants, 238–252
  acetazolamide, 250
  barbiturates, 238–240, 241t
  carbamazepine, 246–247
  clonazepam, 248–249
  diazepam, 249
  hydantoins, 240–243, 244t
  magnesium sulfate, 250–251
  oxazolidinediones, 243–245, 245t
  phenacemide, 249–250
  primidone, 240
  succinimides, 245–246, 246t
  valproic acid derivatives, 247–248
Antidepolarizing agents, 128–132

Antidepressants, 227–237
  classification of, 227
  monoamine oxidase inhibitors, 234–236, 236t
  second-generation, 230, 232–234
  tricyclic, 227–230, 228t, 231–233t
Antidiabetic agents, 429–437
  insulins and, 429–431, 430t, 435–436t
  oral, 431, 436–437, 438–439t
Antidiarrheal drugs, 514–519
  combination products, 517–518
  locally acting, 516–519
    adsorbents, 518
    antiseptics/astringents, 518
    bacterial cultures, 518–519
  systemic, 514–516
Antidiuretic hormone (ADH; vasopressin), 395, 396–397
  actions of, 396
  clinical states and, 396–397
  control of secretion of, 396
Antidotes, 813–814
  activated charcoal, 813–814
  heavy metal antagonists, 814, 815t
Antiemetics, 521t, 521–526
Antiepileptics. See Anticonvulsants
Antiflatulants, 498
Antifungal agents, 687–692, 693–697t, 697
  ophthalmic, 692
  systemic, 687–692
  topical/vaginal, 692, 693–697t, 697
Antigout drugs, 186–189
Antihemophilic factor, human (AHF; H.T. Factorate; Hemofil T; Koate-HS; Koate-HT; Kryobulin VH; Monoclate), 361–362
Antihistamines, 113–114, 114–118t, 119
  antiemetic, 521t
  classification of, 114t
  in combination cough mixtures, 543
  H_1 receptor antagonists, 113–114, 114–118t, 119
  H_2 receptor antagonists, 119, 121–122, 122t
Antihormonal agents, 724, 730, 733–734t, 734–736
Antihypertensive drugs, 302–323
  for hypertensive emergencies, 318–320
  principal sites of action of, 303t
  step 1, 303–305, 309t
  step 2, 305, 310–314, 315t
  step 3, 314–316
  step 4, 316–318
  stepped-care approach to treatment of hypertension and, 303t
Antiinfective therapy, 559–572
  adverse effects of antimicrobial drugs and, 563–566
    hypersensitivy reactions and, 563
    organ toxicity and, 563
    resistance and, 563, 566
    superinfection and, 563
  antibiotics in renal failure and, 566–567
  antimicrobial drugs of choice for common infections, 567–572t
  classification of drugs and, 559–560
  antimicrobial activity and, 559
  mechanism of action and, 559–560

spectrum of activity and, 559
combined antimicrobial therapy and, 562–563
  enhancement of antibacterial activity and, 562–563
  initial treatment of severe infections whose causative agent is unknown and, 562
  in mixed bacterial infections, 562
  postponement of emergence of resistant strains and, 562
  reduction of toxicity and, 563
dosage and duration of therapy and, 561
prophylactic use of antibiotics and, 562
selection of appropriate drug for, 560–561
  identification of pathogen and, 560
  location of infection and, 561
  necessity of therapy and, 560
  sensitivity testing and, 560–561
Antiinhibitor coagulant complex (Autoplex; Feibo VH Immuno), 362
Antilirium (physostigmine, systemic), 59
Antimalarial agents, 664–671
Antimetabolites, 712, 718–719, 720–722t
Antimicrobials
  activity of, 559
  adverse effects of, 563–566
    hypersensitivity reactions and, 563
    organ toxicity and, 563
    resistance and, 563, 566
    superinfection and, 563
  combined antimicrobial therapy with, 562–563
    enhancement of antibacterial activity and, 562–563
    initial treatment of severe infections whose causative agent is unknown and, 562
    in mixed bacterial infections, 562
    postponement of emergence of resistant strains and, 562
    reduction of toxicity and, 563
  for common infections, 567–572t
  mechanism of action of, 559–560
    alteration in cell membrane function and, 560
    inhibition of bacterial cell wall synthesis and, 559–560
    inhibition of nucleic acid metabolism and, 560
    inhibition of protein synthesis and, 560
    interference with intermediate cell metabolism and, 560
  selection of, 560–561
    identification of pathogen and, 560
    location of infection and, 561
    necessity of therapy and, 560
    sensitivity testing and, 560–561
Antiminth (pyrantel pamoate), 677–678
Antimony compounds, 672
Antimuscarinics, 67–70, 72–77t
  quaternary amine, 74–77t
Antineoplastic agents, 708–753, 709t, 710t
  alkylating agents, 711–712, 713–718t
  antimetabolites, 712, 718–719, 720–722t
  cell-cycle specific and cell-cycle nonspecific, 708, 710t

combination chemotherapy and, 738, 740, 741–753t
hormonal, antihormonal, and gonadotropin releasing-hormone analog agents, 724, 730, 731–734t, 734–736
natural products, 719, 722–724, 725–730t
Antiparkinsonian drugs, 253–261
anticholinergic/antihistaminergic agents, 253, 258–259, 259–260t
dopaminergic agents, 253–258
tertiary amine, 74–75t
Antipsychotic drugs, 205–215, 206t, 207t, 209–212t
comparison of effects of, 206t
Antipyresis, salicylates and, 170
Antirabies serum, equine, 811–812, 812t
Antiseptics/astringents, antidiarrheal, 518
Antiserotonin agents, 122, 124–126
Antithyroid drugs, 418, 420, 421t
Antitoxins, 808–809, 809t
Antitubercular agents, 655–663
Antitussives, 537–540, 538t
narcotic, 537–539
nonnarcotic, 539–540
Antivenin(s), 808–809, 809t
Antivenin *Latrodectus mactans* (black widow spider species antivenin), 808–809, 809t
Antivenin *Micrurus fulvius* (North American coral snake antivenin), 808–809, 809t
Antivert (meclizine), 113–114, 117t, 119
Antiviral agents, 699–707
Antrenyl (oxyphenonium bromide), 76–77t
Antrizine (meclizine), 113–114, 117t, 119
Antrypol (suramin), 672, 674, 675t, 676–680
Anturane (sulfinpyrazone), 188
Anuzinc (zinc sulfate), 776t
Aortic bodies, control of respiration and, 536
Aortic valve, 275
Aparkane (trihexyphenidyl hydrochloride), 74–75t, 258–259, 260t
AP combination chemotherapy, 738, 740, 741t
Aphen (trihexyphenidyl hydrochloride), 74–75t, 258–259, 260t
Aphrodyne (yohimbine), 830
A.P.L. (human chorionic gonadotropin), 469–470
Aplastic anemia, 22, 345
Aplisol (tuberculin purified protein derivative-tuberculin PPD), 791, 794–795t
Aplitest (tuberculin PPD, multiple puncture device), 791, 795t
Apneustic center, 535
Apo-Acetazolamide (acetazolamide), 250, 376–377, 378t
Apo-Allopurinol (allopurinol), 188–189
Apo-Amitriptyline (amitriptyline), 227–230, 231t
Apo-Amoxi (amoxicillin), 582, 584–585, 586t, 595

Apo-Ampi (ampicillin), 582, 584–585, 586–587t, 595
Apo-Benztropine (benztropine mesylate), 74–75t, 258–259, 259t
Apo-Bisacodyl (bisacodyl), 506–507, 511–512t
Apo-Cal (calcium carbonate), 490–491, 492–493t
Apo-Carbamazepine (carbamazepine), 246–247
Apo-Chlordiazepoxide (chlordiazepoxide), 217–219, 220–221t
Apo-Chlorpropamide (chlorpropamide), 431, 436–437, 438t
Apo-Chlorthalidone (chlorthalidone), 388–389, 390t, 391–392
Apo-Cimetidine (cimetidine), 119, 121–122, 122t
Apo-Cloxi (cloxacillin), 582, 584–585, 589t, 595
Apo-Diazepam (diazepam), 249
Apo-Erythro Base (erythromycin base), 619–620, 621t
Apo-Erythro-ES (erythromycin ethylsuccinate), 619–620, 622t
Apo-Erythro-S (erythromycin stearate), 619–620, 623t
Apo-Fluphenazine (fluphenazine), 205–208, 210t
Apo-Flurazepam (flurazepam), 198–199, 200t
Apo-Folic (folic acid), 349–350
Apo-Furosemide (furosemide), 377–378, 382–383, 384t
Apo-Guanethidine (guanethidine), 316–317
Apo-Haloperidol (haloperidol), 205–208, 212t
Apo-Hydro (hydrochlorothiazide), 388–389, 390t, 391–392
Apo-Hydroxyzine (hydroxyzine), 224–225
Apo-Imipramine (imipramine), 227–230, 231–232t
Apo-Indomethacin (indomethacin), 175, 178, 182t
Apo-ISDN (isosorbide dinitrate), 325–326, 327t, 329
Apo-Lorazepam (lorazepam), 217–219, 222t
Apo-Meprobamate (meprobamate), 225
Apo-Methyldopa (methyldopa), 311–312
Apo-Metoprolol (metoprolol), 331
Apo-Metronidazole (metronidazole), 683–685
Apomorphine, 520
Apo-Naproxen (naproxen), 175, 178, 183t
Apo-Nitrofurantoin (nitrofurantoin), 639–640
Apo-Oxazepam (oxazepam), 217–219, 222t
Apo-Oxytriphylline (oxytriphylline), 545–547, 548–549t, 549, 551
Apo-Pen-VK (penicillin V; penicillin V, potassium), 582, 584–585, 593t, 595
Apo-Perphenazine (perphenazine), 205–208, 210t
Apo-Phenylbutazone (phenylbutazone), 174–175
Apo-Piroxicam (piroxicam), 175, 178, 183t
Apo-Primidone (primidone), 240
Apo-Propranolol (propranolol), 296–297, 331

Apo-Quinidine (quinidine), 287, 289
Apo-Sulfamethoxazole (sulfamethoxazole), 573–575, 576t
Apo-Sulfisoxazole (sulfisoxazole), 573–575, 577–578t
Apo-Tetra (tetracycline), 609–611, 613t
Apo-Thioridazine (thioridazine), 205–208, 211t
Apo-Tolbutamide (tolbutamide), 431, 436–437, 439t
Apo-Trifluoperazine (trifluoperazine), 205–208, 211t
Apo-Trihex (trihexyphenidyl hydrochloride), 74–75t, 258–259, 260t
Apresoline (hydralazine), 314–316
Aprobarbital (Alurate), 193–194, 196t, 197
Aquachloral Supprettes (chloral hydrate), 199–200
AquaMEPHYTON (phytonadione; vitamin K₁), 356–357, 771t, 771–772
Aquamox (quinethazone), 388–389, 391t, 391–392
Aquasol A (vitamin A), 764–765
Aquasol E (vitamin E), 770–771
Aquatag (benzthiazide), 388–389, 390t, 391–392
Aquatensen (methyclothiazide), 388–389, 391t, 391–392
ARA-C (cytarabine), 712, 718–719, 720t
Ara-C + ADR combination chemotherapy, 738, 740, 741t
Ara-C + DNR + PRED + MP combination chemotherapy, 738, 740, 742t
Ara-C + 6-TG combination chemotherapy, 738, 740, 742t
Aralen (chloroquine), 665, 666t, 682
Aramine (metaraminol), 86–87
Arcuate arteries, 371
Arfonad (trimethaphan), 71, 320
L-Arginine (R-Gene 10), 791, 795t
Aristocort (triamcinolone), 443, 445–447, 452t
Aristocort (triamcinolone acetonide), 445t
Arlidin (nylidrin), 96–98, 334
Arm-a-Med Isoetharine (isoetharine), 94–95, 96–97t
Armour Thyroid (thyroid, dessicated), 416–418, 418t
Arrhythmias, 276. *See also* Antiarrhythmic drugs
atrial, 287
Artane (trihexyphenidyl hydrochloride), 74–75t, 258–259, 260t
Artha-G (salsalate), 170–171, 173, 177t
Arthropan (choline salicylate), 170–171, 173, 176t
Ascaris lumbricoides, 673t
Ascorbic acid (vitamin C), 758t, 761–762
Asendin (amoxapine), 227–230, 228t, 231t
Asparaginase (L-Asparaginase; Elspar), 709t, 719, 722–724, 725t
L-Asparaginase (asparaginase), 719, 722–724, 725t, 752t, 753t
Aspergillus, 567t
Aspirin, 170–171, 173, 176t
Aspirols (amyl nitrite), 325–326, 327t, 329
Asproject (sodium thiosalicylate), 170–171, 173, 177t

Astemizole (Hismanal), 113–114, 114t, 115t, 119
Asthma. *See also* Bronchodilators
  bronchial, 533
  extrinsic (atopic), 545
Asthmahaler (epinephrine), 79–82
Asthmanefrin (epinephrine), 79–82
Asthma prophylactic agent, 553–554
Astiban (stibocaptate), 672, 674, 675t, 676–680
Astramorph PF (morphine), 157, 159, 160t
Atabrine (quinacrine), 669, 678
Atarax (hydroxyzine), 224–225
Atasol (acetaminophen), 173–174
Atenolol (Tenormin), 104–105, 105t, 106t, 108t, 109, 303–304, 333
Atgam (lymphocyte immune globulin-antithymocyte globulin), 810, 811t
Atherosclerosis, 337. *See also* Hypolipemic drugs
Ativan (lorazepam), 217–219, 218t, 222t
Atracurium (Tracrium), 128–129
Atria, 275
Atrial arrhythmias, 287
Atrioventricular (AV) node, 276
Atrioventricular (AV) valves, 275
Atrocholin (dehydrocholic acid), 501
Atromid-S (clofibrate), 339–340
Atropine, 67–70, 72–73t
Atrovent (ipratropium), 76–77t, 553
A/T/S (erythromycin base, topical solution), 619–620, 621t
Attenuvax (measles vaccine-rubeola), 803–804, 807t
Augmentin (amoxicillin and potassium clavulanate), 582, 584–585, 586t, 595
Auranofin (Ridaura), 180, 184
Aureomycin (chlortetracycline), 609–611, 612t
Aurothioglucose (Solganal), 180, 184
Autonomic nervous system, 49, 50t, 51t
  sympathetic and parasympathetic divisions of, 49, 50t
Autoplex (antiinhibitor coagulant complex), 362
Autuitrin (human chorionic gonadotropin), 469–470
AV bundle, 276
AV combination chemotherapy, 738, 740, 742t
Aventyl (nortriptyline), 227–230, 228t, 232t
Avitene (microfibrillar collagen hemostat), 364
Avlosulfon (dapsone), 647–648
AV node. *See* Atrioventricular node
AV valves. *See* Atrioventricular valves
Axid (nizatidine), 119, 121–122, 122t
Ayercillin (penicillin G, procaine), 582, 584–585, 592–593t, 595
Aygestin (norethindrone acetate), 456, 459, 460t, 461
Azactam (aztreonam), 595–596
Azaline (sulfasalazine), 573–575, 577t
Azatadine (Optimine), 113–114, 114t, 115t, 119
Azathioprine (Imuran), 821–822
Azlin (azlocillin), 582, 584–585, 587–588t, 595

Azlocillin (Azlin), 567–571t, 582, 583t, 584–585, 587–588t, 595
Azmacort (triamcinolone), 443, 445–447, 452t, 551–553, 552t
Azolid (phenylbutazone), 174–175
Azostix, 791, 792t
Aztreonam (Azactam), 568t–571t, 595–596
Azulfidine (sulfasalazine), 573–575, 577t

B

Bacampicillin (Penglobe; Spectrobid), 582, 583t, 584–585, 588t, 595
Bacid, 517t
Baciguent (bacitracin), 632–633
Bacille Calmette Guérin, 741t, 744t
Bacillus anthracis, 567t
Bacitracin (AK-Tracin; Baciguent), 632–633
Baclofen (Lioresal), 134–135, 136t
BACON combination chemotherapy, 738, 740, 742t
BACOP combination chemotherapy, 709t, 738, 740, 742t
Bacteria
  alteration in cell membrane function of, 560
  inhibition of cell wall synthesis of, 559–560
  inhibition of nucleic acid metabolism of, 560
  inhibition of protein synthesis of, 560
  interference with intermediate cell metabolism and, 560
  resistance to aminoglycosides, 624
  resistance to penicillins, 582
Bacterial cultures, antidiarrheal, 518–519
Bactericidal drugs, 559
Bacteriostatic drugs, 559
Bacteroides, 567t, 598
Bacteroides fragilis, 598
Bactocil (oxacillin), 582, 584–585, 591t, 595
Bactopen (cloxacillin), 582, 584–585, 589t, 595
Bactrim (trimethoprim-sulfamethoxazole), 579–580
Balanced anesthesia, 145
Bal in Oil (dimercaprol-BAL), 814, 815t
Balminil Expectorant (guaifenesin), 540
Banflex (orphenadrine citrate), 74–75t, 134–135, 137t
Banlin (propantheline bromide), 76–77t
Banthine (methantheline bromide), 76–77t
Barbased (butabarbital), 193–194, 196t, 197
Barbiturates, 193–194, 195–196t, 197
  abuse of, 836
  anticonvulsant, 238–240, 241t
  antiemetic, 521t
  intermediate-acting, 195–196t
  long-acting, 196t
  short-acting, 195t
  ultrashort-acting, 149–151, 150t
Baricon, 793, 799, 799t
Barium sulfate, 793, 799, 799t
Baro-Cat, 793, 799, 799t
Baroflave, 793, 799, 799t
Barosperse, 793, 799, 799t

Barosperse 110, 793, 799, 799t
Basal ganglia, 54–55
Basaljel (aluminum carbonate gel, basic), 490–491, 492–493t
Bayer 205 (suramin), 672, 674, 675t, 676–680
Bay Progest (progesterone), 456, 459, 461, 461t
BCAP combination chemotherapy, 738, 740, 742t
b-Capsa (hemophilus b polysaccharide vaccine), 803–804, 805t
B-CAVe combination chemotherapy, 738, 740, 742t
BCG vaccine (BCG), 803–804, 805t
BCMF combination chemotherapy, 738, 740, 742t
BCNU (carmustine), 711–712, 713t
BCNU + 5-FU combination chemotherapy, 738, 740, 742t
B complex vitamins, 757–761, 758t
BCOP combination chemotherapy, 738, 740, 742t
BCVPP combination chemotherapy, 738, 740, 742t
B-D Glucose (glucose, oral), 437–438
B-DOPA combination chemotherapy, 738, 740, 742t
Beben (betamethasone benzoate), 443, 445–447, 448t
Beclomethasone (Beclovent; Beconase; Propaderm; Vancenase; Vanceril), 443, 445–447, 448t, 551–553, 552t
Beclovent (beclomethasone), 443, 445–447, 448t, 551–553, 552t
Beconase (beclomethasone), 443, 445–447, 448t
Beesix (vitamin B₆), 760–761
Behavior
  drug interactions and, 26
  in elderly patients, 37
Belganyl (suramin), 672, 674, 675t, 676–680
Belladonna, 67–70
Belladonna alkaloids, 67, 69t, 72–73t
  levorotatory (Bellafoline), 72–73t
Belladonna extract, 72–73t
Bellafoline (belladonna alkaloids, levorotatory), 72–73t
Bellaspaz (hyoscyamine sulfate), 72–73t
Bell/ans (sodium bicarbonate), 490–491, 494–495t
Benadryl (diphenhydramine), 113–114, 116t, 119, 258–259, 259t
Bendroflumethiazide (Naturetin), 388–389, 390t, 391–392
Benemid (probenecid), 187–188, 374t
Benisone (betamethasone benzoate), 443, 444t, 445–447, 448t
Benoquin (monobenzone), 829
Benoxinate, 139–141, 140t
Benoxinate and sodium fluorescein (Fluress), 139–141, 141t
Bensylate (benztropine mesylate), 74–75t, 258–259, 259t
Bentiromide (Chymex), 791, 795–796t
Bentyl (dicyclomine hydrochloride), 72–73t
Bentylol (dicyclomine hydrochloride), 72–73t

Index

Benuryl (probenecid), 187–188
Benylin (diphenhydramine), 539–540
Benylin DM (dextromethorphan), 539
Benzedrex (propylhexedrine), 88–89, 90–91t
Benzocaine, 139–141, 140t, 141t
Benzodiazepine antianxiety agents, 217–223, 218t, 220–222t
  metabolism of, 218t
Benzodiazepine hypnotics, 198–203
Benzomorphan, 166–167t
Benzonatate (Tessalon Perles), 539
Benzphetamine (Didrex), 265–267, 268t
Benzquinamide (Emete-Con), 521t, 522
Benzthiazide (Aquatag; Exna; Hydrex; Marazide; Proaqua), 388–389, 390t, 391–392
Benztropine mesylate (Apo Benztropine; Bensylate; Cogentin; PMS Benztropine), 67–70, 74–75t, 258–259, 259t
Benzylpenicilloylpolylysine (Pre-Pen), 791, 796t
BEP combination chemotherapy, 738, 740, 742–743t
Bestrone (estrone), 724, 730, 732t, 734–736
Beta$_1$ adrenergic receptors, 80t
Beta-2 (isoetharine), 94–95, 96–97t
Beta-adrenergic blocking agents, 104–109, 105–108t, 303–304
  approved and investigational uses for, 108t
  pharmacologic and pharmacokinetic properties of, 105t
Beta$_2$ adrenergic receptors, 80t
Beta$_2$ agonists, selective, 94–95, 96–97t
Beta blockers, 331, 333
Beta cells, of islets of Langerhans, 402
Betacort (betamethasone valerate), 443, 445–447, 448t
Betaderm (betamethasone valerate), 443, 445–447, 448t
Beta-endorphin, 156
Betagan (levobunolol), 104–105, 105t, 106t, 108t, 109
Betalin 12 (cyanocobalamin, crystalline), 348–349
Betalin S (vitamin B$_1$), 757–759, 758t
Betaloc (metoprolol), 331
Betameth (betamethasone phosphate), 443, 445–447, 448t
Betamethasone (Betnelan; Celestone), 443, 444t, 445–447, 448t
Betamethasone benzoate (Beben; Benisone; Uticort), 443, 444t, 445–447, 448t
Betamethasone dipropionate (Alphatrex; Diprolene; Diprosone; Maxivate), 443, 444t, 445–447, 448t
Betamethasone phosphate (Betameth; Betnesol; Celestone Phosphate; Cel-U-Jec; Selestoject), 443, 445–447, 448t
Betamethasone valerate (Betacort; Betaderm; Betatrex; Beta-Val; Betnovate; Celestoderm; Ectosone; Metaderm; Valisone; Valnac), 443, 444t, 445t, 445–447, 448t
Beta receptor sites, 53

Betatrex (betamethasone valerate), 443, 444t, 445t, 445–447, 448t
Beta-Val (betamethasone valerate), 443, 444t, 445t, 445–447, 448t
Betaxin (vitamin B$_1$), 757–759, 758t
Betaxolol (Betoptic), 104–105, 105t, 106t, 108t, 109
Bethanechol (Duvoid; Myotonachol; Urabeth; Urecholine), 57–58
Betnelan (betamethasone), 443, 445–447, 448t
Betnesol (betamethasone phosphate), 443, 445–447, 448t
Betnovate (betamethasone valerate), 443, 445–447, 448t
Betoptic (betaxolol), 104–105, 105t, 106t, 108t, 109
Bewon (vitamin B$_1$), 757–759, 758t
BHD combination chemotherapy, 738, 740, 743t
Biamine (vitamin B$_1$), 757–759, 758t
Biavax II (rubella and mumps vaccine), 803–804, 808t
Bicillin (penicillin G, benzathine), 582, 584–585, 592t, 595
Bicillin C-R (penicillin G, benzathine and procaine), 582, 584–585, 593t, 595
BiCNU (carmustine), 711–712, 713t
Bicuspid valve, 275
Bilarcil (metrifonate), 672, 674, 675t, 676–680
Bile acid sequestering resins, 337–339, 339t
Bile salts, 500–501
Bilharziasis, 672
Bili-Labstix, 791, 792t
Bilivist, 799, 800t
Bilopaque, 799, 800t
Bilron (ox bile extract with iron), 500–501
Biltridice (praziquantel), 677
Binding
  chemical. *See* Chemical binding
  distribution and, in children, 32
  of drugs, 13
  glomerular filtration and, 14
  plasma protein. *See* Plasma protein binding
Binding/chelating agents, 814, 816
Biocult-GC, 791, 792t
Bioflavonoids (Citro-Flav; C Speridin; C.V.P.; Flavons 500; Hesper; Pan-C-500; Peridin; Span C; Super-C), 777t
Biotransformation, 11, 13–14
  alterations in, drug interactions and, 29
  in children, 32
  in elderly patients, 36
Biozyme-C (collagenase), 818, 819t
Biperiden (Akineton), 67–70, 74–75t, 258–259, 259t
Biphetamine (amphetamine complex), 264–265, 266t
Biquin Durules (quinidine), 287, 289
Bisacodyl (Apo-Bisacodyl; Bisacolax; Bisco-Lax; Dacodyl; Deficol; Dulcolax; Fleet Bisacodyl; Laxit; Theralax), 506–507, 511–512t
Bisacodyl tannex (Clysodrast), 506–507, 512t

Bisacolax (bisacodyl), 506–507, 511–512t
Bisco-Lax (bisacodyl), 506–507, 511–512t
Bisodol, 494–495t
Bithionol (Actamer; Bitin; Lorothidol), 672, 673t, 674, 675t, 676–680
Bitin (bithionol), 672, 674, 675t, 676–680
Bitolterol (Tornalate), 94–95, 96–97t
Black-Draught (senna equivalent), 506–507, 513t
Black widow spider species antivenin (Antivenin *Latrodectus mactans*), 808–809, 809t
Bladder, urinary, 371
Blastomyces dermatidis, 567t
Blenoxane (bleomycin), 719, 722–724, 725–726t
BLEO-MTX combination chemotherapy, 738, 740, 743t
Bleomycin (Blenoxane), 709t, 710t, 719, 722–724, 725–726t, 741–746t, 748–752t
Bleph-10 (sulfacetamide), 573–575, 575–576t
Blocadren (timolol), 104–105, 105t, 108t, 109, 303–304
Blood, glucocorticoids and, 405
Blood-brain barrier, distribution and, 13
Blood dyscrasias, 22
Blood flow
  alterations in, drug interactions and, 29
  renal, control of, 373
Blood levels, glomerular filtration and, 14
Blood pressure, arterial, 279–280, *280*
Blood supply
  to lungs, 532
  renal, 371
Blood-tissue exchange of gases, 531
Blood vessels, adrenergic drug effects on, 81t
BM combination chemotherapy, 738, 740, 743t
B-MOPP combination chemotherapy, 738, 740, 743t
Body size, drug effects and, 17
Body water, distribution and, in children, 31–32
Bohr effect, 534
Bolus, for intravenous administration, 6
Bonamine (meclizine), 113–114, 117t, 119
Bone, parathyroid hormone and, 401
Bonine (meclizine), 113–114, 117t, 119
BOPP combination chemotherapy, 738, 740, 743t
Bordetella pertussis, 567t, 619
Borrelia recurrentis, 567t
Bowman's capsule, 371
Branch Amin (amino-acid formulation for high metabolic stress), 780
Branhamella catarrhalis, 567t
Breonesin (guaifenesin), 540
Brethaire (terbutaline), 94–95, 96–97t
Brethine (terbutaline), 94–95, 96–97t
Bretylate (bretylium), 297
Bretylium (Bretylate; Bretylol), 288t, 297
Bretylol (bretylium), 297
Brevibloc (esmolol), 104–105, 105t, 106t, 108t, 109
Brevicon (ethinyl estradiol/norethindrone), 463, 464t, 466–467

Index

Brevital (methohexital), 149–151, 150t
Bricanyl (terbutaline), 94–95, 96–97t
Brietal (methohexital), 149–151, 150t
Bromocriptine (Parlodel), 254, 256–257, 816
Bromo Seltzer, 494–495t
Bromphen (brompheniramine), 113–114, 115t, 119
Brompheniramine (Bromphen; Dimetane), 113–114, 114t, 115t, 119
Bronalide (flunisolide), 443, 445–447, 449–450t, 551–553, 552t
Bronchial arteries, 532
Bronchial asthma, 533
Bronchial tree, 531
Bronchial veins, 532
Bronchioles
  adrenergic drug effects on, 81t
  respiratory, 531
Bronchoconstriction, 532
Bronchodilators, 92–94, 96t, 545–555
  anticholinergics, 553
  in combination cough mixtures, 543
  inhaled corticosteroids, 551–553, 552t
  xanthine derivatives, 545–547, 546t, 548–549t, 549, 551
Bronchopulmonary segments, 531
Bronchus
  secondary (lobar), 531
  tertiary (segmental), 531
Bronitin Mist (epinephrine), 79–82
Bronkaid Mist (epinephrine), 79–82
Bronkephrine (ethylnorepinephrine), 94
Bronkodyl (theophylline), 545–547, 549, 549t, 551
Bronkometer (isoetharine), 94–95, 96–97t
Bronkosol (isoetharine), 94–95, 96–97t
Brucella, 567t
Brugia malayi, 673t
Bucladin-S (buclizine), 113–114, 115t, 119
Buclizine (Bucladin-S), 113–114, 115t, 119, 521t
Bumetanide (Bumex), 377–378, 382–383, 384t
Bumex (bumetanide), 377–378, 382–383, 384t
Buminate (albumin, human), 826t, 826–827
Bundle of His, 276
Bupivacaine (Marcaine; Sensorcaine), 139–141, 140t, 142t
Buprenex (buprenorphine), 157, 158t, 159, 165–166t
Buprenorphine (Buprenex), 157, 158t, 159, 165–166t
Bupropion (Wellbutrin), 228t, 230, 232–233
BuSpar (Buspirone), 223–224
Buspirone (BuSpar), 223–224
Busulfan (Myleran), 710t, 711–712, 713t
Butabarbital (Barbased; Butalan; Buticaps; Butisol; Day-Barb; Sarisol), 193–194, 196t, 197
Butalan (butabarbital), 193–194, 196t, 197
Butamben (Butesin), 139–141, 140t, 142t
Butazolidin (phenylbutazone), 174–175
Butesin (butamben), 139–141, 140t, 142t
Buticaps (butabarbital), 193–194, 196t, 197
Butisol (butabarbital), 193–194, 196t, 197

Butoconazole (Femstat), 687, 692, 693t, 697
Butorphanol (Stadol), 157, 158t, 159, 166t
Butyrophenone, 205–208, 206t, 212t
BVD combination chemotherapy, 738, 740, 743t

C

CAF combination chemotherapy, 738, 740, 743t
Caffedrine (caffeine), 263–264
Caffeine (Caffedrine; Dexitac; No Doz; Tirend; Vivarin), 262, 263–264
  citrated, 263–264
Caffeine and dextrose (Quick-Pep), 263–264
Caffeine and sodium benzoate, 263–264
Calan (verapamil), 299–300, 313, 329–331, 331t, 332t
Calcibind (cellulose sodium phosphate), 814, 816
Calcifediol (Calderol), 768–770, 769t
Calciferol (ergocalciferol), 768–770, 769t
Calcijex (calcitriol), 768–770, 769t
Calcilean (heparin calcium), 351–354
Calcimar (calcitonin, salmon), 424–425
Calciparine (heparin calcium), 351–354
Calcite (calcium carbonate), 490–491, 492–493t
Calcitonin (thyrocalcitonin), 400, 401, 424
  human (Cibacalcin), 424–425
  salmon (Calcimar; Miacalcin), 424–425
Calcitriol (Calcijex; Rocaltrol), 768–770, 769t
Calcium ascorbate (vitamin C), 761–762
Calcium carbonate (Alka-Mints; Apo-Cal; Calcite; Chooz; Dicarbosil; Tums), 426–427, 427t, 490–491, 492–493t
  in combination antacids, 494–497t
Calcium caseinate (Casec), 777t
Calcium channel blockers, 313, 329–331, 331t, 332t
  pharmacokinetic and pharmacologic properties of, 331t
Calcium chloride, 783t, 785
Calcium Disodium Versenate (edetate calcium disodium), 814, 815t
Calcium EDTA (edetate calcium disodium), 814, 815t
Calcium glubionate (Neo-Calglucon), 426–427, 427t
Calcium gluceptate, 783t, 785
Calcium gluconate (Kalcinate), 426–427, 427t, 783t, 785
Calcium lactate, 426–427, 427t
Calcium leucovorin (citrovorum factor), 747t, 753t
Calcium pantothenate (vitamin B$_5$), 760
Calcium salts, oral, 426–427, 427t
Calderol (calcifediol), 768–770, 769t
Caldesene (undecylenic acid and salts), 692, 697, 697t
Calicylic (salicylic acid), 170–171, 173, 177t
Calm-X (phosphorated carbohydrate solution), 525–526

Calymmato-bacterium granulomatis, 568t
Calyx, renal, 371
Camalox, 494–495t
CAM combination chemotherapy, 738, 740, 743t
CAMP combination chemotherapy, 738, 740, 743t
Cancer, 708. *See also* Antineoplastic agents
Candida, 568t
Canestan (clotrimazole), 692, 693–694t, 697
Cantil (mepenzolate), 76–77t
Capastat (capreomycin), 656–657
CAP combination chemotherapy, 738, 740, 743t
Capillaria philippinensis, 673t
Capoten (captopril), 304–305, 309t
Capreomycin (Capastat), 655, 656–657
Capsaicin (Zostrix), 816
Captopril (Capoten), 304–305, 309t
Carafate (sucralfate), 491, 498
Carbachol
  intraocular (Miostat), 56–57
  topical (Isopto carbachol), 56–57
Carbamazepine (Apo-Carbamazepine; Epitol; Mazepine; PMS Carbamazepine; Tegretol), 246–247
Carbamino compounds, 535
Carbaminohemoglobin, 535
Carbapenems, 595
Carbarsone (carbarsone), 681–682
Carbenicillin, 567t, 568t, 570t, 571t, 583t, 584
Carbenicillin disodium (Geopen; Pyopen), 582, 584–585, 588–589t, 595
Carbenicillin indanyl sodium (Geocillin), 582, 584–585, 589t, 595
Carbidopa/levodopa (Sinemet), 254–255
Carbinoxamine (Clistin), 113–114, 114t, 115t, 119
Carbocaine (mepivacaine), 139–141, 140t, 142t
Carbohydrate(s)
  absorption of, 487
  parenteral, 780–782
Carbohydrate metabolism
  glucagon and, 402
  glucocorticoids and, 405
  growth hormone and, 398
  insulin and, 402–403
Carbolith (lithium), 208, 213–214
Carbon dioxide transport, 534–535
Carbonic anhydrase, 375
Carbonic anhydrase inhibitors, 376–377, 378t
  sites of action and electrolyte disturbances and, 377t
Carboplatin (Paraplatin), 710t, 711–712, 713t, 744t, 746t, 752t
Carboprost tromethamine (Hemabate), 470–472, 471t
Carboxypeptidase (procarboxypeptidase), 488t
Carcinogenicity, 21
Cardene (nicardipine), 313, 329–331, 331t, 332t
Cardiac cycle, 277
Cardiac output, 278
Cardiac pacemaker, 276

Cardilate (erythrityl tetranitrate), 325–326, 327t, 329
Cardio-Green (indocyanine green), 791, 797t
Cardioquin (quinidine), 287, 289
Cardiotonic drugs, 281–286
　cardioactive glycosides, 281–285
　positive inotropic agents, 285
Cardiovascular system, 275–280
　acetylcholine and, pharmacologic effects and clinical consequences of, 57t
　adrenergic drug effects on, 81t
　anticholinergic drugs and, pharmacologic actions of, 68t
　arterial blood pressure and, 279–280, *280*
　cardiac cycle and, 277
　cardiac output and, 278
　conduction system and, 275–276, *277*
　coronary circulation and, 275
　electrocardiogram and, 276–277, *277*
　heart and, 275, *276*
　hemodynamics and, 278–279
　　extrinsic control of blood flow and, 279
　　intrinsic control of blood flow and, 278–279
Cardizem (diltiazem), 313, 329–331, 331t, 332t
Carfin (warfarin sodium), 354–356, 356t
Carisoprodol (Rela; Soma; Soprodol), 134–135, 136t
Carmustine (BCNU; BiCNU), 709t, 710t, 711–712, 713t, 741–743t, 746–749t, 752t
l-Carnitine (Carnitor; Vitacan), 777t
Carnitor (l-carnitine), 777t
Carotid bodies, control of respiration and, 536
Carteolol (Cartrol), 104–105, 105t, 106t, 108t, 109, 303–304
Cartrol (carteolol), 104–105, 105t, 106t, 108t, 109, 303–304
Cascara sagrada, 506–507, 512t
Casec (calcium caseinate), 777t
CAST, 791, 792t
Castor oil (Alphamul; Emulsoil; Fleet Castor Oil; Kellogg's Castor Oil; Neoloid; Purge; Unisol), 506–507, 512t
Catapres (clonidine), 310–311
Catarase (chymotrypsin), 818, 820t
Catecholamines
　endogenous, 79–84
　synthetic, 84–86
CAV combination chemotherapy, 709t, 738, 740, 743t
CAVe combination chemotherapy, 738, 740, 744t
CCNU (lomustine), 711–712, 716t
CCV-AV combination chemotherapy, 738, 740, 744t
CCV combination chemotherapy, 738, 740, 744t
CDC combination chemotherapy, 738, 740, 744t
CD combination chemotherapy, 738, 740, 744t
CDV combination chemotherapy, 738, 740, 744t

Ceclor (cefaclor), 598–600, 601t
Cedilanid-D (deslanoside), 281–283, 284t
CeeNU (lomustine), 711–712, 716t
Cefaclor (Ceclor), 569t, 598–600, 599t, 601t
Cefadroxil (Duricef; Ultracef), 598–600, 599t, 601t
Cefadyl (cephapirin), 598–600, 602–603t
Cefamandole (Mandol), 598–600, 599t, 603t
Cefazolin (Ancef; Kefzol; Zolicef), 562, 598–600, 599t, 601t
Cefixime (Suprax), 598–600, 599t, 608t
Cefizox (ceftizoxime), 598–600, 606–607t
Cefobid (cefoperazone), 598–600, 605t
Cefonicid (Monocid), 598–600, 599t, 604t
Cefoperazone (Cefobid), 570t, 598–600, 599t, 605t
Ceforanide (Precef), 598–600, 599t, 604t
Cefotan (cefotetan), 598–600, 606t
Cefotaxime (Claforan), 567t, 569–571t, 598–600, 599t, 606t
Cefotetan (Cefotan), 567t, 598–600, 599t, 606t
Cefoxitin (Mefoxin), 567t, 569t, 598–600, 599t, 604–605t
Ceftazidime (Fortaz; Magnacef; Tazicef; Tazidime), 598–600, 599t, 606t
Ceftin (cefuroxime axetil), 598–600, 605t
Ceftizoxime (Cefizox), 567t, 570t, 598–600, 599t, 606–607t
Ceftriaxone (Rocephin), 568–571t, 598–600, 599t, 607t
Cefuroxime (Kefurox; Zinacef), 567t, 569t, 570t, 598–600, 599t, 605t
Cefuroxime axetil (Ceftin), 598–600, 605t
Celestoderm (betamethasone valerate), 443, 445–447, 448t
Celestone (betamethasone), 443, 445–447, 448t
Celestone Phosphate (betamethasone phosphate), 443, 445–447, 448t
Cellular membrane permeability, insulin and, 402
Cellular respiration, 531
Cellulose, oxidized (Novocell; Oxycel; Surgicel), 364–365
Cellulose sodium phosphate (Calcibind), 814, 816
Celontin (methsuximide), 245–246, 246t
Cel-U-Jec (betamethasone phosphate), 443, 445–447, 448t
Cenolate (vitamin C), 761–762
Central nervous system, 53–55
　anticholinergic drugs and, pharmacologic actions of, 68t
Central nervous system depressants, abuse of, 836–837
Central nervous system stimulants, 98–99, 262–271
　abuse of, 837–838
　amphetamines, 264–265, 266t
　anorexiants, 265–267, 268–269t
　caffeine, 263–264
　methylphenidate, 267, 269
　pemoline, 269–270
　respiratory, 262–263
Centrax (prazepam), 217–219, 218t, 222t
CEP combination chemotherapy, 709t

Cephadrine (Anspor; Velosef), 598–600, 599t, 603t
Cephalexin (Ceporex; Keflex; Keflet; Keftab; Novolexin), 598–600, 599t, 601–602t
Cephalic phase, of gastric secretion, 484, 486
Cephalosporin(s), 568–572t, 598–600, 601–608t
　first-generation, 567t, 568t, 571t, 598–600, 601–603t
　　pharmacokinetics and bacterial spectrum of action of, 599t
　second-generation, 598–600, 603–605t
　　pharmacokinetics and bacterial spectrum of action of, 599t
　third-generation, 568t, 570t, 598–600, 605–608t
　　pharmacokinetics and bacterial spectrum of action of, 599t
Cephalothin (Ceporacin; Keflin), 598–600, 599t, 602t
Cephapirin (Cefadyl), 598–600, 599t, 602–603t
Cephulac (lactulose), 506–507, 510t
Ceporacin (cephalothin), 598–600, 602t
Ceporex (cephalexin), 598–600, 601–602t
Cerebellum, 54
Cerebral cortex, 54
Cerebral peduncles, 54
Cerespan (papaverine), 334–335
Cerubidine (daunorubicin), 719, 722–724, 726–727t
C.E.S. (estrogens, conjugated), 454–456, 457t
Cesamet (nabilone), 523–524
Cetamide (sulfacetamide), 573–575, 575–576t
CEV combination chemotherapy, 738, 740, 744t
Cevita (vitamin C), 761–762
CFB combination chemotherapy, 738, 740, 744t
CFD combination chemotherapy, 738, 740, 744t
Charcoaid (activated charcoal), 813–814
Charcoal (Charcocaps), 498
　activated (Actidose-Aqua; Actidose with Sorbitol; Charcoaid; Charcodote; Liqui-Char; SuperChar), 813–814
Charcocaps (charcoal), 498
Charcodote (activated charcoal), 813–814
Chemical binding, drug interactions and, 28
Chemoreceptors
　central, control of respiration and, 536
　peripheral, control of respiration and, 536
Chemoreceptor trigger zone (CTZ), 489
Chemotherapeutic agents, 16, 559. *See also* Antineoplastic agents
Chemotherapy. *See also* Antineoplastic agents
　combination, 738, 740, 741–753t
　neoplastic diseases showing good response to, 709t
　principles of, 708
Chemstrip bG, 791, 792t
Chemstrip GP, 791, 792t
Chemstrip K, 791, 792t
Chemstrip 5L, 791, 792t

Chemstrip 6L, 791, 792t
Chemstrip 7L, 791, 792t
Chemstrip LN, 791, 792t
Chemstrip uG, 791, 792t
Chemstrip uGK, 791, 792t
Chenex (chenodiol-chenodeoxycholic acid), 502–503
Chenodiol-chenodeoxycholic acid (Chenex), 502–503
Cheracol, 538t
Chlamydia trachomatis, 568t, 619
Chloracol (chloramphenicol), 643–644
Chloral hydrate (Aquachloral Supprettes; Noctec; Novochlorhydrate), 199–200
Chlorambucil (Leukeran), 709t, 710t, 711–712, 713–714t, 718t, 744t
Chloramphenicol (Ak-Chlor; Chloracol; Chlorofair; Chloromycetin; Chloroptic; Fenicol; Minims; Nova Phenicol; Ophthochlor; Pentamycetin), 567–572t, 643–644
Chlordiazepoxide (Apo-Chlordiazepoxide; Libritabs; Librium; Lipoxide; Medilium; Mitran; Novopoxide; Reposans-10; Solium), 217–219, 218t, 220–221t
Chloride shift, 535
Chlormezanone (Trancopal), 224
Chlorofair (chloramphenicol), 643–644
Chlorohist Long Acting (xylometazoline), 88–89, 90–91t
Chloromycetin (chloramphenicol), 643–644
Chloroprocaine (Nesacaine), 139–141, 140t, 142t
Chloroptic (chloramphenicol), 643–644
Chloroquine (Aralen), 562, 665, 666t, 681, 682
Chlorothiazide (Diachlor; Diurigen; Diuril), 374t, 388–389, 390t, 391–392
Chlorotrianisene (Tace), 454–456, 457t, 724, 730, 731t, 734–736
Chlorpazine (prochlorperazine), 205–208, 210t
Chlorphen (chlorpheniramine), 113–114, 115t, 119
Chlorphenesin (Maolate; Mycil), 134–135, 136t
Chlorpheniramine (Chlorphen; Chlor-Tripolon; Chlor-Trimeton; Novopheniram; Teldrin), 113–114, 114t, 115t, 119
Chlorpromanyl (chlorpromazine), 205–208, 209t
Chlorpromazine (Chlorpromanyl; Largactil; Novochlorpromazine; Thorazine), 205–208, 206t, 209t, 521t
Chlorpropamide (Apo-Chlorpropamide; Diabinese; Novopropamide), 431, 436–437, 438t
Chlorprothixene (Taractan; Tarasan), 205–208, 206t, 211t
Chlortetracycline (Aureomycin), 609–611, 610t, 612t
Chlorthalidone (Apo-Chlorthalidone; Hygroton; Hylidone; Novothalidone; Thalitone; Uridon), 388–389, 390t, 391–392

Chlor-Trimeton (chlorpheniramine), 113–114, 115t, 119
Chlor-Tripolon (chlorpheniramine), 113–114, 115t, 119
Chlorzoxazone (Paraflex; Parafon Forte DSC), 134–135, 136t
CHL + PRED combination chemotherapy, 738, 740, 744t
Cholac (lactulose), 506–507, 510t
Cholan-DH (dehydrocholic acid), 501
Cholebrine, 799, 800t
Cholecalciferol (Delta-D), 768–770, 769t
Choledyl (oxytriphylline), 545–547, 548–549t, 549, 551
Cholera vaccine, 803–804, 805t
Choleretics, 500–501
Cholestyramine (Questran), 337–339, 339t
Choline, 777t
Choline esters, 56–58
  for systemic application, 57–58
  for topical administration, 56–57
Cholinergic drugs, 56–65, 57t, 66t
  direct acting, 56
  indirect acting, 56
    irreversible cholinesterase inhibitors and, 56
    reversible cholinesterase inhibitors and, 56
  synthetic, pharmacologic properties of, 56, 57t
Cholinergic nerves, 49, 51t
Cholinergic nervous system, 49
Cholinergic receptors, 53
Choline salicylate (Arthropan; Teejel), 170–171, 173, 176t
Cholinesterase inhibitors
  antidote to, 64–65
  irreversible, 61–64
  reversible, 59–61
    for systemic use only, 60t, 60–61, 62t
    for topical and systemic use, 59
    for topical use only, 59–60
Cholinomimetic agents, 56
  direct-acting, 56–59
    alkaloids, 58–59
    choline esters, 56–58
  indirect-acting, 59–64
    irreversible cholinesterase inhibitors, 61–64
    reversible cholinesterase inhibitors, 59–61
Cholinomimetic alkaloids, 58–59
Cholografin, 799, 800t
Choloxin (dextrothyroxine), 340–341
Chooz (calcium carbonate), 490–491, 492–493t
CHOP-BCG combination chemotherapy, 738, 740, 744t
CHOP-Bleo combination chemotherapy, 738, 740, 744t
CHOP combination chemotherapy, 709t, 738, 740, 744t
Chophylline (oxytriphylline), 545–547, 548–549t, 549, 551
CHOR combination chemotherapy, 738, 740, 744–745t
Chorex (human chorionic gonadotropin), 469–470

Chorigon (human chorionic gonadotropin), 469–470
Choron-10 (human chorionic gonadotropin), 469–470
Chronic obstructive pulmonary diseases (COPDs), 545. *See also* Bronchodilators
Chronulac (lactulose), 506–507, 510t
Chylomicrons, 337
Chymex (bentiromide), 791, 795–796t
Chymodiactin (chymopapain), 818, 820t
Chymopapain (Chymodiactin; Discase), 818, 820t
Chymotrypsin (Alpha Chymar; Alpha Chymolean; Catarase; Chymotrypsinogen; Zolyse; Zonulyn), 488t, 818, 820t
Chymotrypsinogen (chymotrypsin), 488t
Cibacalcin (calcitonin, human), 424–425
Cibalith-S (lithium), 208, 213–214
Ciclopirox (Loprox), 687, 692, 693t, 697
Cidomycin (gentamicin), 624–626, 627–628t, 630
Cimetidine (Apo-Cimetidine; Novocimetine; Peptol; Tagamet), 119, 121–122, 122t
Cinobac (cinoxacin), 611, 614–165
Cinoxacin (Cinobac), 611, 614–165
Cin-Quin (quinidine), 287, 289
Cipro (ciprofloxacin), 568–571t, 616–617
Ciprofloxacin (Cipro), 568–571t, 616–617
Circulation, coronary, 275
Circulatory dynamics, distribution and, in children, 31
CISCA combination chemotherapy, 738, 740, 745t
CISCA$_{II}$VB$_{IV}$ combination chemotherapy, 738, 740, 745t
Cisplatin (Platinol; Platinol-AQ), 709t, 710t, 711–712, 714t, 741t, 743–747t, 749–752t
Citanest (prilocaine), 139–141, 140t, 143t
Citrated caffeine, 263–264
Citrate of Magnesia (magnesium citrate), 506–507, 510t
Citrobacter freundii, 625t
Citrocarbonate, 494–495t
Citro-Flav (bioflavonoids), 777t
Citroma (magnesium citrate), 506–507, 510t
Citro-Maq (magnesium citrate), 506–507, 510t
Citro-Nesia (magnesium citrate), 506–507, 510t
Citrovorum factor (calcium leucovorin), 747t, 752t
Citrucel (methylcellulose), 506–507, 508t
Claforan (cefotaxime), 598–600, 606t
Claripex (clofibrate), 339–340
Clark's rule, 33
Clear and Bright (tetrahydrozoline), 89, 92, 92t
Clearblue Pregnancy, 791, 792t
Clear-Eyes Comfort (naphazoline), 89, 92, 92t
Clearplan, 791, 792t
Clemastine (Tavist), 113–114, 114t, 116t, 119
Cleocin (clindamycin), 644–645, 646t

Index

Clidinium, 67–70
Clidinium bromide (Quarzan), 76–77t
Clindamycin (Cleocin; Dalacin C), 567–569t, 571t, 644–645, 646t
Clinistix, 791, 792t
Clinitest, 791, 792t
Clinitest 2-Drop, 791, 792t
Clinoril (sulindac), 175, 178, 183t
Clistin (carbinoxamine), 113–114, 115t, 119
Clobetasol (Dermovate; Temovate), 443, 445–447, 449t
Clobetasol propionate (Temovate), 444t
Clocortolone (Cloderm), 443, 445–447, 449t
Clocortolone pivalate (Cloderm), 445t
Cloderm (clocortolone pivalate), 443, 445–447, 449t, 445t
Clofazime (Lamprene), 645, 647
Clofibrate (Atromid-S; Claripex; Novofibrate), 339–340
Clomid (clomiphene), 468
Clomiphene (Clomid; Milophene; Serophene), 468
Clonazepam (Klonopin; Rivotril), 248–249
Clonidine (Catapres; Dixarit), 310–311
Clonorchis sinensis, 673t
Clopra (metoclopramide), 534–535
Clorazepate (Gen-Xene; Novoclopate; Tranxene), 217–219, 218t, 221t
Clostridium difficile, 568t
Clostridium perfringens, 568t
Clostridium tetani, 568t
Clotrimazole (Canestan; Gyne-Lotrimin; Lotrimin; Mycelex; Myclo), 568t, 692, 693–694t, 697
Cloxacillin (Apo-Cloxi; Bactopen; Cloxapen; Novocloxin; Orbenin; Tegopen), 582, 583t, 584–585, 589t, 595
Cloxapen (cloxacillin), 582, 584–585, 589t, 595
Clysodrast (bisacodyl tannex), 506–507, 512t
CMC-High dose combination chemotherapy, 738, 740, 745t
CMC-V combination chemotherapy, 738, 740, 745t
CMF combination chemotherapy, 738, 740, 745t
CMFP combination chemotherapy, 738, 740, 745t
CMFT combination chemotherapy, 738, 740, 745t
CMFVP (Cooper's regimen) combination chemotherapy, 738, 740, 745t
Coactin (amdinocillin), 582, 584–585, 586t, 595
Coagulation factors, 351, 352t
COAP combination chemotherapy, 738, 740, 745t
Cocaine, 139–141, 140t, 142t
  abuse of, 837–838
Coccidioides immitis, 568t
Coccidioidin (Spherulin), 791, 794t
Codeine (Paveral), 157, 158t, 159, 160t, 537–538, 538t
Cogentin (benztropine mesylate), 74–75t, 258–259, 259t
Colace (docusate sodium-dioctyl sodium sulfosuccinate), 506–507, 509t

Colchicine, 186–187
Colestid (colestipol), 337–339, 339t
Colestipol (Colestid), 337–339, 339t
Colistimethate (Coly-Mycin M), 567t, 632, 633
Colistin sulfate (Coly-Mycin S; polymyxin E), 632, 633–634
Collagenase (Biozyme-C; Santyl), 818, 819t
Colloid, 400
Cologel (methylcellulose), 506–507, 508t
Colonite (polyethylene glycol-electrolyte solution), 506–507, 511t
Coloscreen, 791, 792t
Coly-Mycin M (colistimethate), 633
Coly-Mycin S (colistin sulfate), 633–634
ColyMycin S Otic, 632
CoLyte (polyethylene glycol-electrolyte solution), 506–507, 511t
COMA (COMLA) combination chemotherapy, 709t, 738, 740, 745t
Combistix, 791, 792t
Compazine (prochlorperazine), 205–208, 210t
Competence, of elderly patients, 37–38
Compound W (salicylic acid), 170–171, 173, 177t
Comprehensive Drug Abuse Prevention and Control Act, 42
Conduction, neuronal, 49
Conduction system, of heart, 275–276, 277
Conjugation, biotransformation and, 14
Conn's syndrome, 406
Conray, 799, 800t
Conray-30, 799, 800t
Conray-43, 799, 800t
Conray-325, 799, 800t
Conray-400, 799, 800t
Constilac (lactulose), 506–507, 510t
Constipation. *See also* Laxatives
  acute, 506
  chronic simple, 506
Constulose (lactulose), 506–507, 510t
Contraceptives
  intrauterine progesterone system and, 467
  oral, 463, 464t, 466–467
    biphasic, 463
    hormonal balance and adverse effects of, 465t
    monophasic, 463
    triphasic, 463
Controlled drugs. *See* Narcotic drugs
Controlled Substances Act, 42, 43t
Convoluted tubule
  distal, 371
  proximal, 371
COP-BLAM combination chemotherapy, 709t, 738, 740, 746t
COP combination chemotherapy, 738, 740, 746t
COPDs. *See* Chronic obstructive pulmonary diseases
COPP (C-MOPP) combination chemotherapy, 709t, 738, 740, 746t
Cordarone (amiodarone), 298–299
Cordran (flurandrenolide), 443, 445t, 445–447, 450t
Corgard (nadolol), 104–105, 105t, 107t, 108t, 109, 303–304, 331, 333

Corgonject-5 (human chorionic gonadotropin), 469–470
Corn oil (Lipomul Oral), 777t
Coronex (isosorbide dinitrate), 325–326, 327t, 329
Corophyllin (aminophylline), 545–547, 548t, 549, 551
Corpora quadrigemina, 54
Corpus callosum, 54
Corpus striatum, 54
Corrective Mixture with Paregoric, 517t
Cortamed (hydrocortisone), 443, 445–447, 450t
Cort-Dome (hydrocortisone), 443, 445t, 445–447, 450t
Cortef (hydrocortisone), 443, 445–447, 450t
Cortex, renal, 371
Cortical stimulation, vomiting and, 489
Corticoids. *See* Adrenal cortical steroids
Corticosteroid(s), 673t
  antineoplastic, 724, 730, 733t, 734–736
  inhaled, 551–553, 552t
Corticotrophs, 396
Corticotropin. *See* Adrenocorticotropic hormone
Corticotropin injection (ACTH; Acthar), 407–408
Corticotropin zinc injection (Cortrophin-Zinc), 407–408
Cortigel (repository corticotropin injection), 407–408
Cortiment (hydrocortisone), 443, 445–447, 450t
Cortisone (Cortone), 443, 444t, 445–447, 449t
Cortone (cortisone), 443, 445–447, 449t
Cortril (hydrocortisone), 445t
Cortrophin Gel (repository corticotropin injection), 407–408
Cortrophin-Zinc (corticotropin zinc injection), 407–408
Cortropic Gel (repository corticotropin injection), 407–408
Cortrosyn (cosyntropin), 791, 796t
Corynebacterium diphtheriae, 568t, 619
Cosmegen (dactinomycin), 719, 722–724, 726t
Cosyntropin (Cortrosyn; Synacthen Depot), 791, 796t
Cotazym (pancrelipase), 502
Co-trimoxazole (trimethoprim-sulfamethoxazole), 579–580
Coughing. *See also* Antitussives; Expectorants; Mucolytics
  combination cough mixtures and, 542–543
Coumadin (warfarin sodium), 354–356, 356t
Coumarins, 354–356, 356t
Countercurrent mechanism, 375
CP combination chemotherapy, 738, 740, 746t
Creon (pancrelipase), 502
Cretinism, 400–401
Cromolyn intranasal (Nalcrom; Nasalcrom), 554
Cromolyn ophthalmic (Opticrom 4%), 554
Cromolyn sodium (Fivent; Intal), 553–554

Cross-resistance, to antimicrobials, 563
Crotalidae antivenin, polyvalent, 808–809, 809t
Cruex (undecylenic acid and salts), 692, 697, 697t
Cryptococcus neoformans, 568t
Crystalline amino-acid infusion (Aminosyn; FreAmine III; Novamine; ProcalAmine; Travasol; TrophAmine), 779–780
Crystapen (penicillin G, potassium or sodium), 582, 584–585, 591–592t, 595
Crysticillin A.S. (penicillin G, procaine), 582, 584–585, 592–593t, 595
Crystodigin (digitoxin), 281–283, 284t
C-Solve (erythromycin base, topical solution), 619–620, 621t
CS-T ColoScreen, 791, 792t
C Speridin (bioflavonoids), 777t
CT combination chemotherapy, 738, 740, 746t
CTZ. See Chemoreceptor trigger zone
Culturette 10 min Group A Strep ID, 791, 792t
Cumulative effect, drug effects and, 17
Cuprid (trientine), 814
Cuprimine (penicillamine), 185–186
Curretab (medroxyprogesterone acetate), 456, 459, 460t, 461, 724, 730, 733t, 734–736
Cushing's syndrome, 406
CVB combination chemotherapy, 738, 740, 746t
CV combination chemotherapy, 738, 740, 746t
CVI combination chemotherapy, 738, 740, 746t
C.V.P. (bioflavonoids), 777t
CVP combination chemotherapy, 738, 740, 746t
CVPP/CCNU combination chemotherapy, 738, 740, 746t
CVPP combination chemotherapy, 709t, 738, 740, 746t
CY-VA-DIC combination chemotherapy, 738, 740, 746–747t
Cyanocobalamin (vitamin B$_{12}$), 758t, 761
  crystalline (Anacobin; Betalin 12; Redisol; Rubion; Rubramin PC), 348–349
Cyclacillin (Cyclapen-W), 582, 583t, 584–585, 589t, 595
Cyclan (cyclandelate), 333–334
Cyclandelate (Cyclan; Cyclospasmol), 333–334
Cyclapen-W (cyclacillin), 582, 584–585, 589t, 595
Cyclizine (Marezine; Marzine), 113–114, 114t, 116t, 119, 521t
Cyclobenzaprine (Flexeril), 134–135, 136t
Cyclocort (amcinonide), 443, 444t, 445–447, 448t
Cyclogyl (cyclopentolate hydrochloride), 74–75t
Cyclomen (danazol), 476, 479
Cyclopentolate hydrochloride (AK-Pentolate; Cyclogyl; I-Pentolate), 67–70, 74–75t

Cyclophosphamide (Cytoxan; Neosar), 709t, 710t, 711–712, 715t, 741–753t
Cyclopropane, 146
Cycloserine (Seromycin), 569t, 570t, 655, 657
Cyclospasmol (cyclandelate), 333–334
Cyclosporin A (cyclosporine), 822–823
Cyclosporine (cyclosporin A; Sandimmune), 822–823
Cyclothiazide (Anhydron), 388–389, 390t, 391–392
Cycrin (medroxyprogesterone acetate), 456, 459, 460t, 461, 724, 730, 733t, 734–736
Cyklokapron (tranexamic acid), 361
Cylert (pemoline), 269–270
Cyproheptadine (Periactin), 114t, 124
Cyronine (liothyronine sodium-T$_3$), 416–418, 419t
Cysto-Conray, 799, 800t
Cysto-Conray II, 799, 800t
Cystografin, 799, 800t
Cystografin-Dilute, 799, 800t
Cystospaz (hyoscyamine sulfate), 72–73t
Cystospaz-M (hyoscyamine sulfate), 72–73t
Cytadren (aminoglutethimide), 447, 452, 724, 730, 733t, 734–736
Cytarabine (ARA-C; Cytosar-U; Cytosine Arabinoside), 709t, 710t, 712, 718–719, 720t, 741t, 742t, 744–747t, 749–752t
Cytomel (liothyronine sodium-T$_3$), 416–418, 419t
Cytosar-U (cytarabine), 712, 718–719, 720t
Cytosine Arabinoside (cytarabine), 712, 718–719, 720t
Cytovene (ganciclovir), 701–702
Cytoxan (cyclophosphamide), 711–712, 715t

D

Dacarbazine (DTIC-Dome), 710t, 711–712, 715t, 741–744t, 747t, 748t
Dacodyl (bisacodyl), 506–507, 511–512t
DA combination chemotherapy, 738, 740, 747t
Dactinomycin (Actinomycin D; Cosmegen), 709t, 710t, 719, 722–724, 726t, 751t, 752t
Dagenan (sulfapyridine), 573–575, 576–577t
Daisy 2, 791, 792t
Dalacin C (clindamycin), 644–645, 646t
Dalmane (flurazepam), 198–199, 200t
Danazol (Cyclomen; Danocrine), 476, 479
Danocrine (danazol), 476, 479
Danthron (Dorbane; Roydan), 506–507, 512t
Dantrium (dantrolene), 133–134
Dantrolene (Dantrium), 133–134
Dapsone (Avlosulfon), 569t, 570t, 647–648
Daranide (dichlorphenamide), 376–377, 378t
Daraprim (pyrimethamine), 667–668
Darbid (isopropamide iodide), 76–77t
Daricon (oxyphencyclimine hydrochloride), 74–75t

Darvon (propoxyphene), 157, 158t, 159, 162t
DAT combination chemotherapy, 738, 740, 747t
Datril (acetaminophen), 173–174
Daunorubicin (Cerubidine), 709t, 710t, 719, 722–724, 726–727t, 742t, 744t, 747t, 751–753t
Day-Barb (butabarbital), 193–194, 196t, 197
Dazamide (acetazolamide), 250, 376–377, 378t
DC 240 (docusate calcium-dioctyl calcium sulfosuccinate), 506–507, 509t
DC combination chemotherapy, 738, 740, 747t
DDAVP (desmopressin acetate), 411–412
DEA number, 44
Decadron (dexamethasone), 443, 445–447, 449t, 551–553, 552t
Deca-Durabolin (nandrolone decanoate), 474–476, 478t, 479
Decholin (dehydrocholic acid), 501
Declomycin (demeclocycline), 609–611, 612t
Decolone (nandrolone decanoate), 474–476, 478t, 479
Decongestants
  in combination cough mixtures, 543
  nasal, 88–89, 90t
  ophthalmic, 89, 92, 92t
Deferoxamine mesylate (Desferal), 814, 815t
Deficol (bisacodyl), 506–507, 511–512t
Degest-2 (naphazoline), 89, 92, 92t
Dehydrocholic acid (Atrocholin; Cholan-DH; Decholin; Dycholium), 500, 501
Dehydroemetine, 681
Delatest (testosterone enanthate), 474–476, 478t, 479
Delatestryl (testosterone enanthate), 474–476, 478t, 479, 724, 730, 731t, 734–736
Delaxin (methocarbamol), 134–135, 137t
Delcid, 494–495t
Delestrogen (estradiol valerate), 454–456, 458t, 724, 730, 732t, 734–736
Delsym (dextromethorphan), 539
Delta cells, of islets of Langerhans, 402
Delta-D (cholecalciferol), 768–770, 769t
Deltasone (prednisone), 724, 730, 733t, 734–736
Del-Vi-A (vitamin A), 764–765
Demecarium bromide (Humorsol), 59–60
Demeclocycline (Declomycin), 609–611, 610t, 612t
Demerol (meperidine), 157, 158t, 159, 163t
Demser (metyrosine), 320–321
Demulen 1/35 (ethinyl estradiol/ethynodiol diacetate), 463, 464t, 466–467
Demulen 1/50 (ethinyl estradiol/ethynodiol diacetate), 463, 464t, 466–467
Deoxyribonuclease, 488t
Depa (valproic acid), 247–248
Depakene (sodium valproate; valproic acid), 247–248
Depakote (divalproex sodium), 247–248
depAndro (testosterone cypionate), 474–476, 478t, 479

Depen (penicillamine), 185–186
Depestro (estradiol cypionate), 724, 730, 732t, 734–736
DepGynogen (estradiol cypionate), 724, 730, 732t, 734–736
Depigmenting agents, 828–829
Depo-Estradiol (estradiol cypionate), 454–456, 458t, 724, 730, 732t, 734–736
Depogen (estradiol cypionate), 724, 730, 732t, 734–736
Depolarizing agents, 128, 132–133
Deponit (nitroglycerin transdermal systems), 325–326, 329, 329t
Depo-Provera (medroxyprogesterone acetate), 456, 459, 460t, 461, 724, 730, 733t, 734–736
"Depot" drug form, 8
Depotest (testosterone cypionate), 474–476, 478t, 479, 724, 730, 731t, 734–736
Depo-Testosterone (testosterone cypionate), 474–476, 478t, 479, 724, 730, 731t, 734–736
Deproic (valproic acid), 247–248
Dermalar (fluocinolone), 443, 445–447, 450t
Derma-Soft (salicylic acid), 170–171, 173, 177t
Dermatitis, exfoliative, 22
Dermatologic application, 3
Dermatophytes, 568t
Dermovate (clobetasol), 443, 445–447, 449t
Deronil (dexamethasone), 443, 445–447, 449t
DES (diethylstilbestrol), 454–456, 457t, 724, 730, 731t, 734–736
Desenex (undecylenic acid and salts), 692, 697, 697t
Deserpidine (Harmonyl), 313–314, 315t
Desferal (deferoxamine mesylate), 814, 815t
DESI. See Drug Efficacy Study Implementation
Desipramine (Norpramin; Pertofrane), 227–230, 228t, 231t
Deslanoside (Cedilanid-D), 281–283, 282t, 284t
Desmopressin acetate (DDAVP; Stimate), 411–412
Desonide (Des Owen; Tridesilon), 443, 445t, 445–447, 449t
Des Owen (desonide), 443, 445t, 445–447, 449t
Desoximetasone (Topicort), 443, 444t, 445t, 445–447, 449t
Desoxyephedrine (Vicks inhaler), 88–89, 90–91t
Desoxyn (methamphetamine), 264–265, 266t
Desyrel (trazodone), 228t, 234
Detensol (propranolol), 296–297, 331
Devrom, 517t
Dexamethasone (Decadron; Deronil; Dexasone; Hexadrol), 443, 444t, 445t, 445–447, 449t, 551–553, 552t, 749t, 751t, 752t
Dexasone (dexamethasone), 443, 445–447, 449t

Dexatrim (phenylpropanolamine), 265–267, 269t
Dexchlor (dexchlorpheniramine), 113–114, 116t, 119
Dexchlorpheniramine (Dexchlor; Poladex T.D.; Polaramine; Polargen), 113–114, 114t, 116t, 119
Dexedrine (dextroamphetamine sulfate), 264–265, 266t
Dexitac (caffeine), 263–264
Dexpanthenol (Ilopan; Panol; Panthoderm), 816–817
Dextran 40-low molecular weight (Gentran 40; Hyskan; Rheomacrodex; 10% LMD), 824–826, 825t
Dextran 70, 75-high molecular weight (Gentran 75; Macrodex), 824–826, 825t
Dextroamphetamine sulfate (Dexedrine; Femdex; Oxydess II; Spancap No. 1), 264–265, 266t
Dextromethorphan (Benylin DM; Delsym; Hold; Koffex; Pertussin; Robidex; Sedatuss), 539
Dextrose in water injection (D-2½-W; D-5-W; D-10-W; D-20-W; D-25-W; D-30-W; D-38.5-W; D-40-W; D-60-W; D-70-W), 780–781
Dextrostix, 791, 792t
Dextrothyroxine (Choloxin), 340–341
Dey-Dose Isoetharine (isoetharine), 94–95, 96–97t
Dey-lute (isoetharine), 94–95, 96–97t
D.H.E. 45 (dihydroergotamine), 125
DHT (dihydrotachysterol), 768–770, 769t
Diabeta (glyburide), 431, 436–437, 439t
Diabetes, nephrogenic, 396
Diabetes insipidus, 396
Diabetes mellitus, 403–404, 404. See also Antidiabetic agents
  insulin-dependent (Type I), 403–404
  noninsulin-dependent (Type II), 404
Diabinese (chlorpropamide), 431, 436–437, 438t
Diabismul
  suspension, 517t
  tablets, 517t
Diachlor (chlorothiazide), 388–389, 390t, 391–392
Diadax (phenylpropanolamine), 265–267, 269t
Diagnostic agents, radiographic, 791, 893, 799, 799–802t
Diagnostic aids
  in vitro, 791, 792–793t
  in vivo, 791, 795–798t
Diagnostic biologicals, intradermal, 791, 794–795t
Dialose (docusate potassium-dioctyl potassium sulfosuccinate), 506–507, 509t
Dialume (aluminum hydroxide gel), 490–491, 492–493t
Diamox (acetazolamide), 250, 374t, 376–377, 378t
Diaphragm, 532
Diapid (lypressin), 412
Dia-Quel, 517t
Diar Aid, 517t

Diarrhea, 514. See also Antidiarrheal drugs
  acute, 514
  chronic, 514
Diasorb, 517t
Diastasis, 277
Diastix, 791, 792t
Diastole, 275
Diastolic pressure, 279
Diatrizoate-60, 799, 800t
Diatrizoate meglumine 76%, 799, 800t
Diazemuls (diazepam), 249
Diazepam (Apo-Diazepam; Diazemuls; E-PAM; Meval; Novodipam; Rival; Valium; Vazepam; Vivol; Zetran), 217–219, 218t, 221–222t, 249
Diazoxide
  oral (Proglycem), 440
  parenteral (Hyperstat IV), 318–319
Dibasic calcium phosphate dihydrate (dicalcium phosphate), 426–427, 427t
Dibenzoxazepine, 205–208, 206t, 212t
Dibenzyline (phenoxybenzamine), 102–103, 321
Dibucaine (Nupercainal), 139–141, 140t, 142t
Dicalcium phosphate (dibasic calcium phosphate dihydrate), 426–427, 427t
Dicarbosil (calcium carbonate), 490–491, 492–493t
Dichlorophen, 673t
Dichlorphenamide (Daranide), 376–377, 378t
Diclofenac (Voltaren), 175, 178, 181t
Dicloxacil (dicloxacillin), 582, 584–585, 589t, 595
Dicloxacillin (Dicloxacil; Dycil; Dynapen; Pathocil), 582, 583t, 584–585, 589t, 595
Dicumarol (dicumarol), 354–356, 356t
Dicyclomine hydrochloride (Bentyl; Bentylol; Lomine), 67–70, 72–73t
Didoquin (iodoquinol), 683
Didrex (benzphetamine), 265–267, 268t
Didronel (etidronate), 425–426
Diencephalon, 54
Dienestrol (DV; Estraguard; Ortho Dienestrol), 454–456, 457t
Dietary factors, drug interactions and, 26
Diethylcarbamazine (Hetrazan), 672, 673t, 674
Diethyl ether, 147
Diethylpropion (Nobesine; Propion; Tenuate; Tepanil), 265–267, 268t
Diethylstilbestrol (DES), 454–456, 457t, 463, 724, 730, 731t, 734–736
Diethylstilbestrol diphosphate (Honvol; Stilphostrol), 454–456, 457t, 724, 730, 731–732t, 734–736
Difenoxin HCl with atropine sulfate (Motofen), 514–515
Diflorasone (Florone; Flutone; Maxiflor; Psorcon), 443, 44t, 445–447, 449t
Diflunisal (Dolobid), 170–171, 173, 176t
Di-Gel, 494–495t
Di-Gel (Advanced Formula), 496–497t
Digestants, 500–502

Digestive system
  accessory organs of digestion and, 483
  anatomical and histologic features of organs of, 484t
  gastrointestinal tract and, 483, 484–486t
  major activities of, 485–486t
  major digestive enzymes and, 488t
  major hormones and regulatory peptides of, 487t
Digibind (digoxin immune Fab-ovine), 284–285
Digitalis glycosides, 281–283, 282t, 284t
Digitalization, 281
Digitoxin (Crystodigin), 281–283, 282t, 284t
Digoxin (Lanoxin; Lanoxicaps; Novo-digoxin), 281–283, 282t, 284t
Digoxin immune Fab-ovine (Digibind), 284–285
Dihydroergotamine (D.H.E. 45), 125
Dihydrotachysterol (DHT; Hytakerol), 768–770, 769t
Dihydroxyaluminum sodium carbonate (Rolaids), 490–491, 492–493t
Diiodohydroxyquin (iodoquinol), 683
Dilantin (phenytoin sodium, parenteral), 240–243, 244t, 293–294
Dilantin-125 (phenytoin), 240–243, 244t
Dilantin-30 Pediatric (phenytoin), 240–243, 244t
Dilantin Infatab (phenytoin), 240–243, 244t
Dilantin Kapseals (phenytoin sodium, extended), 240–243, 244t, 293–294
Dilaudid (hydromorphone), 157, 158t, 159, 161t
Dilor (dyphylline), 545–547, 548t, 549, 551
Dilosyn (methdilazine), 113–114, 117t, 119
Diloxanide, 681
Diltiazem (Cardizem), 313, 329–331, 331t, 332t
Dimenhydrinate (Dramamine; Gravol; Nauseatol; Travamine), 113–114, 114t, 116t, 119, 521t
Dimercaprol-BAL (Bal in Oil), 814, 815t
Dimetane (brompheniramine), 113–114, 115t, 119
Dimetane-DC, 538t
Dimethyl sulfoxide (Kemsol; Rimso-50), 817
Dinoprostone (Prostin E$_2$), 470–472, 471t
Diocto-K (docusate potassium-dioctyl potassium sulfosuccinate), 506–507, 509t
Diodrast (iodopyract), 374t
Dioval (estradiol valerate), 724, 730, 732t, 734–736
Dipeptidase, 488t
Diphenhydramine (Allerdryl; Benadryl; Benylin; Insomnal), 113–114, 116t, 119, 258–259, 259t, 539–540
Diphenidol (Vontrol), 521t, 522–523
Diphenoxylate HCl with atropine sulfate (Lomotil), 514–515
Diphenylan (phenytoin sodium, prompt), 240–243, 244t

Diphenylpyraline (Hispril), 113–114, 114t, 117t, 119
Diphtheria and tetanus toxoids
  combined, adult, 803, 804t
  combined, pediatric, 803, 804t
Diphtheria and tetanus toxoids and pertussis vaccine, adsorbed-DTP (Tri-Immunol), 803, 804t
Diphtheria antitoxin, 808–809, 809t
Diphtheria Toxin for Schick Test, 791, 794t
Diphtheria toxoid, adsorbed, pediatric, 803, 804t
Diphyllobothrium latum, 673t
Dipivefrin (Propine), 82–83
Diplococcus pneumoniae, 571t
Diprolene (betamethasone dipropionate), 443, 444t, 445–447, 448t
Diprosone (betamethasone dipropionate), 443, 444t, 445–447, 448t
Dipyridamole (Persantine), 333
Direct myotropic acting blocking agent, 133–134
Disaccharidase, 488t
Disalcid (salsalate), 170–171, 173, 177t
Discase (chymopapain), 818, 820t
Disease
  adverse drug effects related to, 20–21
  drug interactions and, 26
  in elderly patients, 37
Disipal (orphenadrine hydrochloride), 74–75t, 258–259, 259–260t
Disk diffusion method, 561
Disopyramide (Napamide; Norpace; Norpace CR; Rhythmodan), 288t, 291–292
Disorine (isoetharine), 94–95, 96–97t
Dispos-a-Med Isoetharine (isoetharine), 94–95, 96–97t
Dissociative anesthetic agents, 151–153
Distal convoluted tubule, 371
Distribution, 11, 13
  alterations in, drug interactions and, 28–29
  binding of drugs and, 13, 32
  blood-brain barrier and, 13
  in children, 31–32
    binding and, 32
    body water and, 31–32
    circulatory dynamics and, 31
    drug receptor specificity and, 32
    membrane permeability and, 32
  in elderly patients, 36
  lipid solubility and, 13
  placental barrier and, 13
Disulfiram (Antabuse), 817–818
Ditropan (oxybutynin chloride), 72–73t
Diucardin (hydroflumethiazide), 388–389, 390–391t, 391–392
Diulo (metolazone), 388–389, 391t, 391–392
Diurese (trichlormethiazide), 388–389, 391t, 391–392
Diuretics, 376–392, 377t
  carbonic anhydrase inhibitors, 376–377, 378t
  loop (high-ceiling), 377–378, 382–383, 384t
  osmotic, 383–386
    non-receptor-mediated effects of, 17
  potassium-sparing, 386–388

sites of action and electrolyte disturbances and, 377t
thiazides/sulfonamides, 388–389, 390–391t, 391–392
Diurigen (chlorothiazide), 388–389, 390t, 391–392
Diuril (chlorothiazide), 374t, 388–389, 390t, 391–392
Divalproex sodium (Depakote), 247–248
Dixarit (clonidine), 310–311
Dizmiss (meclizine), 113–114, 117t, 119
Dizymes (pancreatin), 502
DMC combination chemotherapy, 738, 740, 747t
DMT, abuse of, 839
Doan's Pills (magnesium salicylate), 170–171, 173, 176t
DOAP combination chemotherapy, 738, 740, 747t
Dobutamine (Dobutrex), 85
Dobutrex (dobutamine), 85
Docusate calcium-dioctyl calcium sulfosuccinate (DC 240; PMS-Docusate Calcium; Pro-Cal-Sof; Sulfolax; Surfak), 506–507, 509t
Docusate potassium-dioctyl potassium sulfosuccinate (Dialose; Diocto-K; Kasof), 506–507, 509t
Docusate sodium-dioctyl sodium sulfosuccinate (Colace; Doxinate; D-S-S; Laxagel; Modane Soft; Regulex), 506–507, 509t
Dolene (propoxyphene), 157, 159, 162t
Dolobid (diflunisal), 170–171, 173, 176t
Dolophine (methadone), 157, 158t, 159, 161–162t
DOM, abuse of, 839
Donnagel, 517t
Donnagel-PG, 517t
Dopamet (methyldopa), 311–312
Dopamine (Dopastat; Intropin), 79, 83–84
  adrenergic receptors for, 53
Dopaminergic agents, 253–258
Dopaminergic receptors, 80t
Dopar (levodopa), 254–255
Dopastat (dopamine), 83–84
Dopram (doxapram), 262–263
Dorbane (danthron), 506–507, 512t
Doriden (glutethimide), 201–202
Doriglute (glutethimide), 201–202
Dormarex (pyrilamine), 113–114, 118t, 119
Dosage, in children, 32–33
Dosage form, drug interactions and, 26
Down-regulation, 53
  drug interactions and, 28
Doxaphene (propoxyphene), 157, 159, 162t
Doxapram (Dopram), 262–263
Doxepin (Adapin; Sinequan; Triadapin), 227–230, 228t, 231t
Doxinate (docusate sodium-dioctyl sodium sulfosuccinate), 506–507, 509t
Doxorubicin (Adriamycin-RDF; Adriamycin-PFS), 709t, 710t, 719, 722–724, 727t, 741–752t
Doxychel (doxycycline), 609–611, 612t
Doxycycline (Doxychel; Vibramycin; Vibra Tabs), 562, 609–611, 610t, 612t

Doxylamine (Unisom), 113–114, 114t, 117t, 119
Dracunculus medinensis, 673t
Dramamine (dimenhydrinate), 113–114, 116t, 119
Drenison (flurandrenolide), 443, 445–447, 450t
Drisdol (ergocalciferol), 768–770, 769t
Dristan Long Lasting (oxymetazoline), 88–89, 90–91t
Dronabinol (Marinol), 521t, 523–524
Droperidol (Inapsine), 205, 214–215. *See also* Fentanyl/droperidol
Drug(s)
　controlled. *See* Narcotic drugs
　legend, 41
　narcotic. *See* Narcotic drugs
　official, 41
Drug abuse, 835–842
　classification of drugs and, 835
　CNS depressants and, 836–837
　　alcohol, 836
　　barbiturates, 836
　　nonbarbiturate sedatives and antianxiety agents, 836–837
　CNS stimulants and, 837–838
　　amphetamines, 837
　　anorectics, 837
　　cocaine, 837–838
　drug dependence and, 835–836
　　physical, 836
　　psychological, 835
　habituation and, 835
　marijuana and, 840–841
　narcotics and, 838–839
　nicotine and, 841
　psychotomimetics and, 839–840
　　DMT, 839
　　DOM, 839
　　LSD, 839
　　mescaline, 839
　　phencyclidine, 839–840
　　psilocin, 839
　　psilocybin, 839
　street names for drugs and, 841–842
　tolerance and, 835
　volatile inhalants and, 840
Drug compatibility guide, 848–849
Drug dependence, 21, 835–836
　physical, 836
　psychological, 835
Drug effects
　adrenergic, 79, 81t
　alterations in, drug interactions and, 27–28
　factors modifying, 17–18
　non-receptor-mediated, 17
Drug Efficacy Study Implementation (DESI), 42
Drug idiosyncrasies, drug effects and, 17
Drug interactions, 26–30
　alterations in drug effects and, 27–28
　　altered receptor sensitivity and, 27–28
　　blockade of neuronal uptake or release and, 27
　　competitive receptor antagonism and, 27
　　drugs with different pharmacologic effects and, 27
　　drugs with similar pharmacologic effects and, 27
　alterations in drug handling and, 28–30
　　absorption and, 28
　　biotransformation and, 29
　　distribution and, 28–29
　　excretion and, 29–30
　alterations in immune response and, 30
　beneficial versus adverse, 26
　classifications and mechanisms of, 27
　　in vitro, 27
　　in vivo, 27
　reasons for, 26
　residual drug effects and, 30
D-S-S (docusate sodium-dioctyl sodium sulfosuccinate), 506–507, 509t
DTIC-Dome (dacarbazine), 711–712, 715t
Dulcolax (bisacodyl), 506–507, 511–512t
Duphulac (lactulose), 506–507, 510t
Durabolin (nandrolone phenpropionate), 474–476, 478t, 479
Duracillin A.S. (penicillin G, procaine), 582, 584–585, 592–593t, 595
Dura-Estrin (estradiol cypionate), 724, 730, 732t, 734–736
Duragen (estradiol valerate), 724, 730, 732t, 734–736
Duralith (lithium), 208, 213–214
Duralutin (hydroxyprogesterone caproate), 456, 459, 460t, 461
Duramorph-PF (morphine), 157, 159, 160t
Duranest (etidocaine), 139–141, 140t, 142t
Duraquin (quinidine), 287, 289
Duratest (testosterone cypionate), 474–476, 478t, 479, 724, 730, 731t, 734–736
Durathate (testosterone enanthate), 474–476, 478t, 479
Durepam (flurazepam), 198–199, 200t
Duretic (methyclothiazide), 388–389, 391t, 391–392
Durham-Humphrey Amendment, 41
Duricef (cefadroxil), 598–600, 601t
Duvoid (bethanechol), 57–58
DV (dienestrol), 454–456, 457t
D-2½-W (dextrose in water injection), 780–781
D-5-W (dextrose in water injection), 780–781
D-10-W (dextrose in water injection), 780–781
D-20-W (dextrose in water injection), 780–781
D-25-W (dextrose in water injection), 780–781
D-30-W (dextrose in water injection), 780–781
D-38.5-W (dextrose in water injection), 780–781
D-40-W (dextrose in water injection), 780–781
D-50-W (dextrose in water injection), 780–781
D-60-W (dextrose in water injection), 780–781
D-70-W (dextrose in water injection), 780–781
Dwarfism, pituitary, 399
Dycholium (dehydrocholic acid), 501
Dycil (dicloxacillin), 582, 584–585, 589t, 595
Dyclone (dyclonine), 139–141, 140t, 142t
Dyclonine (Dyclone), 139–141, 140t, 142t
Dyflex (dyphylline), 545–547, 548t, 549, 551
Dymelor (acetohexamide), 431, 436–437, 438t
Dynapen (dicloxacillin), 582, 584–585, 589t, 595
Dynorphins, 156
Dyphilline (Dilor; Dyflex; Lufyllin; Neothylline; Protophylline), 545–547, 548t, 549, 551
Dyrenium (triamterene), 388

E

Early Detector, 791, 792t
ECG. *See* Electrocardiogram
Echothiophate (Phospholine Iodide), 61–64
Econazole (Ecostatin; Spectazole), 687, 692, 694t, 697
Ecostatin (econazole), 692, 694t, 697
Ectopic beats, 287
Ectosone (betamethasone valerate), 443, 445–447, 448t
Edecrin (ethacrynic acid), 377–378, 382–383, 384t
Edetate calcium disodium (Calcium Disodium Versenate; Calcium EDTA), 814, 815t
Edrophonium, 60t, 60–61, 62–63t
E.E.S. (erythromycin ethylsuccinate), 619–620, 622t
Efed II (ephedrine), 88–89, 90–91t
Efedron (ephedrine), 88–89, 90–91t
Effersyllium (psyllium), 506–507, 508t
Efficacy, potency versus, 16
EKG. *See* Electrocardiogram
Elase (fibrinolysin and desoxyribonuclease), 818, 819t
Elavil (amitriptyline), 227–230, 228t, 231t
Eldepryl (selegiline), 257–258
Eldopaque (hydroquinone), 828–829
Eldoquin (hydroquinone), 828–829
Electrocardiogram (ECG; EKG), 276–277, 277
Electrolyte(s)
　absorption of, 487–488
　parenteral, 783–785t, 785
Electrolyte metabolism, growth hormone and, 398
Elixophyllin (theophylline), 545–547, 549, 549t, 551
Elocon (mometasone), 443, 444t, 445–447, 451t
Elspar (asparaginase), 719, 722–724, 725t
Eltor-120 (pseudoephedrine), 88–89, 90–91t
Eltroxin (levothyroxine sodium-T$_4$), 416–418, 419t
EMCYT (Estramustine phosphate sodium), 724, 730, 732t, 734–736
Emete-Con (benzquinamide), 522
Emetics, 520–521
Emetine (emetine), 673t, 682–683

Emetrol (phosphorated carbohydrate solution), 525–526
Emex (metoclopramide), 534–535
Emitrip (amitriptyline), 227–230, 231t
Emotional disorders, adverse drug effects related to, 21
Emulsoil (castor oil), 506–507, 512t
E-Mycin (erythromycin base), 619–620, 621t
E-Mycin E (erythromycin ethylsuccinate), 619–620, 622t
Enalapril (Vasotec), 304–305, 309t
Encainide (Enkaid), 288t, 296
Endep (amitriptyline), 227–230, 231t
Endocardium, 275
Endocrine disorders, hypoglycemia and, 403
Endocrine glands, 395–406. *See also Hormone(s); specific glands and hormones*
   mechanisms of hormone action and, 395
     second messenger mechanism and, 395
   regulation of hormone secretion and, 395, *396*
   transport and metabolism of hormones and, 395
Endogenous opiates, 155–157
Endorphins, 156
Enduron (methyclothiazide), 388–389, 391t, 391–392
Enflurane (Ethrane), 146–147
Enisyl (*l*-lysine), 777t
Enkaid (encainide), 296
Enkephalins, 156
ENO, 496–497t
Enovid 5 mg (mestranol/norethynodrel), 463, 464t, 466–467
Enovid-E (mestranol/norethynodrel), 463, 464t, 466–467
Enovil (amitriptyline), 227–230, 231t
Entacyl (piperazine), 676–677
Entamoeba histolytica, 681
Enterobacter, 624, 625t, 632
Enterobacteriaceae, 568t
Enterobius vermicularis, 673t
Enterokinase, 488t
Entero-Test, 791, 792t
Entero-Test Pediatric, 791, 792t
Enulose (lactulose), 506–507, 510t
Environmental factors, drug interactions and, 26
Enzactin (triacetin), 692, 697, 697t
Enzyme(s)
   digestive, 488t
   pancreatic, 502
Enzyme acceleration, drug interactions and, 29
Enzyme induction, drug interactions and, 29
Enzyme inhibition
   drug action and, 18
   drug interactions and, 29
Enzyme preparations, 818, 819–820t
Enzyme stimulation, drug action and, 18
E-PAM (diazepam), 217–219, 221–222t, 249
Ephedrine (Efed II; Efedron; Va-Tro-Nol), 88–89, 90–91t, 93–94
Epicardium, 275
Epidural anesthetics, local, 139
Epifrin (epinephrine), 79–82

Epilepsy, 238
   classification and management of seizures in, 239t
   grand mal, 238
   petit mal, 238
   psychomotor, 238
   temporal lobe, 238
Epimorph (morphine), 157, 159, 160t
Epinal (epinephrine), 79–82
Epinephrine, 79
   inhalation (Asthmahaler; Asthmanefrin; Brontin Mist; Bronkaid Mist; Dysne-Inhal; Medihaler-Epi; Micronefrin; Primatene; Vaponefrin), 79–82
   nasal (Adrenalin), 79–82, 88–89, 90–91t
   ophthalmic (Adrenalin; Epifrin; Epinal; Eppy/N; Glaucon), 79–82, 89, 92, 92t
   parenteral (Adrenalin; Sus-Phrine), 79–82
Epithelium, of tunica mucosa, 483
Epitol (carbamazepine), 246–247
Epitrate (epinephrine), 79–82
E.P. Mycin (oxytetracycline), 609–611, 613t
Eppy/N (epinephrine), 79–82
Epsom salt (magnesium sulfate), 506–507, 511t
e.p.t., 791, 792t
Equalactin (polycarbophil calcium), 506–507, 508t
Equanil (meprobamate), 225
Ergocalciferol (Calciferol; Drisdol), 768–770, 769t. *See also* Vitamin D
Ergoloid mesylates (Gerimal; Hydergine; Hydroloid-G; Niloric), 334
Ergomar (ergotamine), 124–125
Ergonovine (Ergotrate), 413–414
Ergostat (ergotamine), 124–125
Ergotamine (Ergomar; Ergostat; Gynergen; Medihaler-Ergotamine; Wigrettes), 124–125
Ergotrate (ergonovine), 413–414
Errors, in drug administration, nurse's responsibility for, 45
Eryc (erythromycin base), 619–620, 621t
Erycette (erythromycin base, topical solution), 619–620, 621t
Eryderm (erythromycin base, topical solution), 619–620, 621t
Erymax (erythromycin base, topical solution), 619–620, 621t
Erypar (erythromycin stearate), 619–620, 623t
EryPed (erythromycin ethylsuccinate), 619–620, 622t
Ery-Tab (erythromycin base), 619–620, 621t
Erythema multiforme, 22
Erythracin (erythromycin stearate), 619–620, 623t
Erythrityl tetranitrate (Cardilate), 325–326, 327t, 329
Erythromycin(s), 567–569t, 571t, 572t, 619–620, 621–623t
Erythromycin base (Apo-Erythro Base; Ak-Mycin; E-Mycin; Eryc; Ery-Tab; Ilotycin; Novorythro Base; PCE; Robimycin), 619–620, 621t
   topical solution (Akne-Mycin; A/T/S; C-Solve; Erycette; Eryderm; Erymax; E-Solve-2; ETS-2%; Staticin; T-Stat), 619–620, 621t
Erythromycin estolate (Ilosone; Novorythro estolate), 619–620, 621–622t
Erythromycin ethylsuccinate (Apo-Erythro-ES; E.E.S; E-Mycin E; EryPed; Pediamycin; Wyamycin-E), 619–620, 622t
Erythromycin gluceptate (Ilotycin gluceptate), 619–620, 622t
Erythromycin lactobionate (Erythrocin Lactobionate-IV), 619–620, 622–623t
Erythromycin Lactobionate-IV (erythromycin lactobionate), 619–620, 622–623t
Erythromycin stearate (Apo-Erythro-S; Eramycin; Erypar; Novorythro Stearate; Wyamycin-S), 619–620, 623t
Escherichia coli, 568t, 609, 624, 625t, 632
Eserine (physostigmine, ophthalmic), 59
Esidrix (hydrochlorothiazide), 388–389, 390t, 391–392
Eskalith (lithium), 208, 213–214
Esmolol (Brevibloc), 104–105, 105t, 106t, 108t, 109
E-Solve-2 (erythromycin base, topical solution), 619–620, 621t
Esophagus
   anatomic and histologic features of, 484t
   major activities of, 485
Esoterica Regular (hydroquinone), 828–829
Espotabs (phenolphthalein), 506–507, 513t
Estinyl (ethinyl estradiol), 454–456, 459t, 724, 730, 732t, 734–736
Estrace (estradiol), 724, 730, 732t, 734–736
Estrace (estradiol, oral), 454–456, 458t
Estra-D (estradiol cypionate), 724, 730, 732t, 734–736
Estraderm (estradiol transdermal system), 454–456, 458t
Estradiol (Estrace), 724, 730, 732t, 734–736
   oral (Estrace), 454–456, 458t
Estradiol cypionate (Depo-Estradiol; Depestro; DepGynogen; Depogen; Dura-Estrin; Estra-D; Estro-Cyp; Estrofem; Estroject-LA; Estronol-LA; Hormogen-Depot), 454–456, 458t, 724, 730, 732t, 734–736
Estradiol-LA (estradiol valerate), 724, 730, 732t, 734–736
Estradiol transdermal system (Estraderm), 454–456, 458t
Estradiol valerate (Delestrogen; Dioval; Duragen; Estradiol-LA; Estraval; Femogex; Gynogen LA; Valergen), 454–456, 458t, 724, 730, 732t, 734–736
Estradurin (polyestradiol phosphate), 454–456, 459t, 724, 730, 732t, 734–736
Estraguard (dienestrol), 454–456, 457t

Estramustine phosphate sodium (EMCYT), 724, 730, 732t, 734–736
Estratab (estrogens, esterified), 454–456, 458t, 724, 730, 732t, 734–736
Estraval (estradiol valerate), 724, 730, 732t, 734–736
Estro-Cyp (estradiol cypionate), 724, 730, 732t, 734–736
Estrocon (estrogens, conjugated), 454–456, 457t
Estrofem (estradiol cypionate), 724, 730, 732t, 734–736
Estrogen(s), 405, 454–456, 457–459t, 709t, 724, 730, 731–732t, 734–736. *See also* Contraceptives, oral
  conjugated (C.E.S.; Estrocon; Premarin; Progens), 454–456, 457t, 724, 730, 732t, 734–736
  esterified (Estratab; Menest), 454–456, 458t, 724, 730, 732t, 734–736
  esters and conjugates of, 454
  natural, 454
  semisynthetic and synthetic, 454
Estroject-LA (estradiol cypionate), 724, 730, 732t, 734–736
Estrone (Bestrone; Estrone-A; Estronol; Femogen; Theelin Aqueous), 454–456, 458t, 724, 730, 732t, 734–736
Estrone-A (estrone), 724, 730, 732t, 734–736
Estronol (estrone), 724, 730, 732t, 734–736
Estronol-LA (estradiol cypionate), 724, 730, 732t, 734–736
Estropipate (Ogen), 454–456, 458t
Estrovis (quinestrol), 454–456, 459t
Etamycin (erythromycin stearate), 619–620, 623t
Ethacrynic acid (Edecrin), 377–378, 382–383, 384t
Ethambutol (Etibi; Myambutol), 569t, 655, 675–658
Ethamolin (ethanolamine), 829t, 829–830
Ethanolamine(s) (Ethamolin), 829t, 829–830
Ethaquin (ethaverine), 334–335
Ethatab (ethaverine), 334–335
Ethaverine (Ethaquin; Ethatab; Ethavex-100; Isovex), 334–335
Ethavex-100 (ethaverine), 334–335
Ethchlorvynol (Placidyl), 201
Ether (diethyl ether), 147
Ethinamate (Valmid), 201
Ethinyl estradiol (Estinyl; Feminone), 454–456, 459t, 724, 730, 732t, 734–736
Ethiodol, 799, 800t
Ethionamide (Trecator-SC), 569t, 655, 658–659
Ethon (methyclothiazide), 388–389, 391t, 391–392
Ethopropazine hydrochloride (Parsitan; Parsidol), 67–70, 74–75t, 258–259, 259t
Ethosuximide (Zarontin), 245–246, 246t
Ethotoin (Peganone), 240–243, 244t
Ethrane (enflurane), 146–147
Ethylene, 146

Ethylestrenol (Maxibolin), 474–476, 478t, 479
Ethylnorepinephrine (Bronkephrine), 94
Etibi (ethambutol), 675–658
Etidocaine (Duranest), 139–141, 140t, 142t
Etidronate (Didronel), 425–426
Etomidate (Amidate), 151
Etoposide (VePesid; VP-16-213; VP-16), 709t, 710t, 719, 722–724, 728t, 741t, 742t, 744t, 746t, 750–752t
Etretinate (Tegison), 765–766
ETS-2% (erythromycin base, topical solution), 619–620, 621t
Euglucon (glyburide), 431, 436–437, 439t
Eulexen (flutamide), 724, 730, 733–734t, 734–736
Eupnea, 533
Euthroid (liotrix), 416–418, 419t
Eutonyl (pargyline), 321
Everone (testosterone enanthate), 474–476, 478t, 479, 724, 730, 731t, 734–736
Excretion, 11, 14–15
  alterations in, drug interactions and, 29–30
  in children, 32
  in elderly patients, 36
  intestinal, 14–15
  through lungs, 15
  through mammary glands, 15
  renal, 14
    glomerular filtration and, 14
    tubular reabsorption and, 14
    tubular secretion and, 14
Exdol (acetaminophen), 173–174
Exelderm (sulconazole), 692, 696t, 697
Exfoliative dermatitis, 22
Ex-Lax (phenolphthalein), 506–507, 513t
Exna (benzthiazide), 388–389, 390t, 391–392
Exocrine glands, anticholinergic drugs and, pharmacologic actions of, 68t
Expectorants, 537, 540–541
  iodone products, 540–541
Expiratory neurons, 535
External intercostal muscles, 532
Extrapyramidal reactions, 25
Extrinsic clotting pathway, 351, 353
Eye
  adrenergic drug effects on, 81t
  anticholinergic drugs and, pharmacologic actions of, 68t
EZ-Detect, 791, 792t
EZ-Detect Strep-A Test, 791, 792t

F

FAC combination chemotherapy, 738, 740, 747t
Fact, 791, 792t
Factor IX complex, human (Konyne; Profilnine; Proplex), 362–363
Factrel (gonadorelin), 791, 796t
FAM combination chemotherapy, 738, 740, 747t
Famotidine (Pepcid), 119, 121–122, 122t
Fansidar (sulfadoxine and pyrimethamine), 668–669

FAP combination chemotherapy, 738, 740, 747t
Fasciola hepatica, 673t
Fasciolopsis buski, 673t
Fats, absorption of, 487
FCP combination chemotherapy, 738, 740, 747t
FDA. *See* U.S. Food and Drug Administration
Federal Food, Drug and Cosmetic Act, 41
  Durham-Humphrey Amendment to, 41
  Kefauver-Harris Amendment to, 41
Feen-A-Mint (phenolphthalein), 506–507, 513t
Feibo VH Immuno (antiinhibitor coagulant complex), 362
Feldene (piroxicam), 175, 178, 183t
Femazole (metronidazole), 683–685
Femdex (dextroamphetamine sulfate), 264–265, 266t
Feminone (ethinyl estradiol), 454–456, 459t, 724, 730, 732t, 734–736
Femiron (ferrous fumarate), 345–346, 347t
Femogen (estrone), 454–456, 458t
Femogex (estradiol valerate), 454–456, 458t
Femotrone (progesterone), 456, 459, 461, 461t
Femstat (butoconazole), 692, 693t, 697
Fenfluramine (Ponderal; Pondimin), 265–267, 268t
Fenicol (chloramphenicol), 643–644
Fenoprofen (Nalfon), 175, 178, 181t
Fentanyl (Sublimaze), 157, 158t, 159, 163–164t
Fentanyl/droperidol (Innovar), 152–153
Feosol (ferrous sulfate), 345–346, 347t
Feostat (ferrous fumarate), 345–346, 347t
Fergon (ferrous gluconate), 345–346, 347t
Fer-in-Sol (ferrous sulfate), 345–346, 347t
Fer-Iron (ferrous sulfate), 345–346, 347t
Fero-Gradumet (ferrous sulfate), 345–346, 347t
Fero-space (ferrous sulfate), 345–346, 347t
Ferralet (ferrous gluconate), 345–346, 347t
Ferralyn (ferrous sulfate), 345–346, 347t
Ferrous fumarate (Femiron; Feostat; Fumasorb; Fumerin; Hemocyte; Ircon; Neo-Fer-50; Novofumar; Palafer; Palmiron; Span-FF), 345–346, 347t
Ferrous gluconate (Fergon; Ferralet; Fertinic; Novoferrogluc; Simron), 345–346, 347t
Ferrous sulfate (Feosol; Fer-in-Sol; Fer-Iron; Ferralyn; Fero-Gradumet; Ferospace; Fesofor; Mol-Iron; Novoferrosulfa; Slow FE), 345–346, 347t
Fertility control
  abortifacients and, 470–472, 471t
  ovulation stimulants and, 467–470
  steroid contraceptives and, 463, 464t, 465t, 466–467
Fertinic (ferrous gluconate), 345–346, 347t
Fesofor (ferrous sulfate), 345–346, 347t
Festal II (pancrelipase), 502
Fiber-Con (polycarbophil calcium), 506–507, 508t
Fibrinolysin and desoxyribonuclease (Elase), 818, 819t

First Response Ovulation Predictor, 791, 792t
FIVB (FDVB) combination chemotherapy, 738, 740, 747t
Fivent (cromolyn sodium), 553–554
Flagyl (metronidazole), 683–685
Flavons 500 (bioflavonoids), 777t
Flavoxate (Urispas), 818, 820
Flaxedil (gallamine), 129–130
FL combination chemotherapy, 738, 740, 747t
Flecainide (Tambocor), 288t, 295–296
Fleet Babylax (glycerin), 506–507, 513t
Fleet Bisacodyl (bisacodyl), 506–507, 511–512t
Fleet Castor Oil (castor oil), 506–507, 512t
Fleet Enema (sodium phosphate and sodium biphosphate), 506–507, 511t
Fleet Mineral Oil Enema (mineral oil), 506–507, 509–510t
Flexeril (cyclobenzaprine), 134–135, 136t
Flexoject (orphenadrine citrate), 74–75t, 134–135, 137t
Flexon (orphenadrine citrate), 74–75t, 134–135, 137t
Flint SSD (silver sulfadiazine), 578–579
Florinef (fludrocortisone acetate), 442–443
Florone (diflorasone), 443, 444t, 445–447, 449t
Floropryl (isoflurophate), 64
Floxuridine (FUDR), 710t, 712, 718–719, 720t
Flucytosine (Ancobon; Ancotil), 567t, 568t, 687, 688–689
Fludrocortisone acetate (Florinef), 442–443
Fluid and electrolyte balance, alterations in, drug interactions and, 29–30
Fluid mosaic hypothesis, 11
Flunisolide (AeroBid; Bronalide; Nasalide; Rhinalar), 443, 445–447, 449–450t, 551–553, 552t
Fluocet (fluocinolone), 443, 445–447, 450t
Fluocinolone (Dermalar; Fluocet; Fluoderm; Fluolar; Fluonid; Flurosyn; Synalar; Synemol), 443, 445–447, 450t
Fluocinolone acetonide (Synalar; Synalar HP; Synemol), 444t, 445t
Fluocinonide (Lidemol; Lidex; Lidex-E; Lyderm; Topsyn), 443, 444t, 445–447, 450t
Fluoderm (fluocinolone), 443, 445–447, 450t
Fluogen (influenza virus vaccines), 803–804, 807t
Fluolar (fluocinolone), 443, 445–447, 450t
Fluonid (fluocinolone), 443, 445–447, 450t
Fluor-Op (fluorometholone), 443, 445–447, 450t
Fluoride (Fluoron; Karidium; Luride; Pediaflor; Phos-Flur), 775, 778
Fluorometholone (Flour-Op; FML Liquifilm), 443, 445–447, 450t
Fluoron (fluoride), 775, 778
Fluorouracil (Adrucil; 5-Fluorouracil; 5-FU), 709t, 710t, 712, 718–719, 720–721t, 741–745t, 747t, 749t, 751t
Fluothane (halothane), 147–148
Fluoxetine (Prozac), 228t, 233

Fluoxymesterone (Android-F; Halotestin; Ora-Testryl), 474–476, 477t, 479, 724, 730, 731t, 734–736
Fluphenazine (Apo-Fluphenazine; Modecate; Moditen; Permitil; Prolixin), 205–208, 206t, 210t
Flurandrenolide (Cordran; Drenison), 443, 445t, 445–447, 450t
Flurazepam (Apo-Flurazepam; Dalmane; Durepam; Novoflupam; PMS-Flurazepam), 198–199, 200t
Flurbiprofen (Ansaid; Ocufen), 175, 178, 181t
Fluress (benoxinate and sodium fluorescein), 139–141, 141t
Flurosyn (fluocinolone), 443, 445–447, 450t
Flutamide (Eulexin), 724, 730, 733–734t, 734–736, 747t
Flutone (diflorasone), 443, 445–447, 449t
Fluzone (influenza virus vaccines), 803–804, 807t
FML Liquifilm (fluorometholone), 443, 445–447, 450t
Folex (methotrexate), 712, 718–719, 721–722t
Folex-PFS (methotrexate), 712, 718–719, 721–722t
Folic acid (Apo-Folic; Folvite; Novofolacid), 349–350
Follicle stimulating hormone (folliculotropin; FSH), 398, 407
actions of, 398
control of secretion of, 398
Follicular cells, 400
Folliculotropin. See Follicle stimulating hormone
Follutein (human chorionic gonadotropin), 469–470
Folvite (folic acid), 349–350
FOMi combination chemotherapy, 738, 740, 747t
Forane (isoflurane), 148
Forebrain, 54
Fortaz (ceftazidime), 598–600, 606t
Fortel Ovulation, 791, 792t
Francisella tularensis, 568t, 624, 625t
FreAmine HBC (amino-acid formulation for high metabolic stress), 780
FreAmine III (crystalline amino-acid infusion), 779–780
Freezone (salicylic acid), 170–171, 173, 177t
Fried's rule, 33
Fructines-Vichy (phenolphthalein), 506–507, 513t
Fructose in water, 781–782
FSH. See Follicle stimulating hormone
5-FU (fluorouracil), 712, 718–719, 720–721t, 712, 718–719, 720–721t
FUDR (floxuridine), 712, 718–719, 720t
Fulvicin P/G (griseofulvin, ultramicrosize), 689–690
Fulvicin U/F (griseofulvin, microsize), 689–690
Fumasorb (ferrous fumarate), 345–346, 347t
Fumerin (ferrous fumarate), 345–346, 347t

Fumide (furosemide), 377–378, 382–383, 384t
Fungacetin (triacetin), 692, 697, 697t
Fungizone (amphotericin B), 687–688
Fungizone (amphotericin B, topical), 692, 693t, 697
Fungoid (triacetin), 692, 697, 697t
Furacin (nitrofurazone), 649–650
Furadantin (nitrofurantoin), 639–640
Furalan (nitrofurantoin), 639–640
Furan (nitrofurantoin), 639–640
Furanite (nitrofurantoin), 639–640
Furazolidone (Furoxone), 648–649
Furomide M.D. (furosemide), 377–378, 382–383, 384t
Furosemide (Apo-Furosemide; Fumide; Furomide M.D.; Furoside; Lasix; Luramide; Novosemide; Uritol), 377–378, 382–383, 384t
Furoside (furosemide), 377–378, 382–383, 384t
Furoxone (furazolidone), 648–649

G

Galactokinetic action, of oxytocin, 397
Gallamine (Flaxedil), 129–130
Gallstone-solubizing agents, 500, 502–504
Gamastan (immune globulin-intramuscular), 801, 810t
Gamazole (sulfamethoxazole), 573–575, 576t
Gamimune N (immune globulin, intravenous), 801, 810t
Gammagard (immune globulin, intravenous), 801, 810t
Gamma Globulin (immune globulin-intramuscular), 801, 810t
Gammar (immune globulin-intramuscular), 801, 810t
Gamulin Rh (rh$_o$[D] immune globulin), 810, 811t
Ganciclovir (Cytovene), 701–702
Ganglionic blocking agents, 70–71
Gantanol (sulfamethoxazole), 573–575, 576t
Gantrisin (sulfisoxazole), 573–575, 577–578t
Garamycin (gentamicin), 624–626, 627–628t, 630
Gardnerella, 569t
Gases, anesthetic, 145–146
Gastric acidifiers, 501–502
Gastric phase, of gastric secretion, 486
Gastrin, 486, 487t
Gastroccult, 791, 792t
Gastrografin, 799, 800t
Gastrointestinal tract, 483–489
absorption and, 11–12, 487–488
of carbohydrates, 487
of electrolytes, 487–488
of fats, 487
of proteins, 487
of vitamins, 488
of water, 487
acetylcholine and, pharmacologic effects and clinical consequences of, 57t
adrenergic drug effects on, 81t

anatomy of, 484t
anticholinergic drugs and, pharmacologic actions of, 68t
digestion and, 486, 488t
  activities of digestive tract and, 485–486t
    major hormones and regulatory peptides and, 487t
    organization of, 483
glucocorticoids and, 406
histology of, 483, 484t
motility and, 483
parathyroid hormone and, 401
secretion and, 483–484, 486
vomiting and, 488–489
Gastrolyte Oral (oral electrolyte mixture), 776t
Gastro-Test, 791, 792t
Gastrovist, 799, 801t
Gas-X (simethicone), 498
Gaviscon (liquid), 496–497t
Gaviscon (tablet), 496–497t
Gaviscon-2, 496–497t
Gaviscon Extra Strength, 496–497t
Gelatin film, absorbable (Gelfilm), 363
Gelatin powder, absorbable (Gelfoam), 364
Gelatin sponge, absorbable (Gelfoam), 363–364
Gelfilm (gelatin film, absorbable), 363
Gelfoam (gelatin powder, absorbable), 364
Gelfoam (gelatin sponge, absorbable), 363–364
Gelusil, 496–497t
Gelusil-II, 496–497t
Gelusil-M, 496–497t
Gemfibrozil (Lopid), 341–342
Gemonil (metharbital), 193–194, 196t, 197, 238–240, 241t
Genna (senna concentrate), 506–507, 513t
Genoptic (gentamicin), 624–626, 627–628t, 630
Genora 1/35 (ethinyl estradiol/norethindrone), 463, 464t, 466–467
Genora 1/50 (mestranol/norethindrone), 463, 464t, 466–467
Gentacidin (gentamicin), 624–626, 627–628t, 630
Gentafair (gentamicin), 624–626, 627–628t, 630
GentAk (gentamicin), 624–626, 627–628t, 630
Gentamicin (Alcomicin; Cidomycin; Garamycin; Genoptic; Gentacidin; Gentafair; GentAk; Jenamicin), 567–572t, 624–626, 625t, 627–628t, 630
Gentlax B (senna concentrate), 506–507, 513t
Gentle Nature (sennosides A&B-calcium salts), 506–507, 513t
Gentran 40 (dextran 40-low molecular weight), 824–826, 825t
Gentran 75 (dextran 70, 75-high molecular weight), 824–826, 825t
Gen-Xene (clorazepate), 217–219, 221t
Geocillin (carbenicillin indanyl sodium), 582, 584–585, 589t, 595
Geopen (carbenicillin disodium), 582, 584–585, 588–589t, 595

Geriatric pharmacology, 36–40, 37t
drug therapy and, 37–40
  adequacy of, 37
  competence level and, 37–38
  duration of, 37
  necessity of, 37
  variables affecting drug response and, 36–37
    absorption and, 36
    altered tissue sensitivity and, 36–37
    behavioral changes and, 37
    biotransformation and, 36
    chronic disease states and, 37
    distribution and, 36
    excretion and, 36
    hormonal changes and, 37
Gerimal (ergoloid mesylates), 334
Germanin (suramin), 672, 674, 675t, 676–680
Gesterol-50 (progesterone), 456, 459, 461, 461t
Gesterol LA (hydroxyprogesterone caproate), 724, 730, 733t, 734–736
GH. See Growth hormone
Gigantism, 399
Glands. See also specific glands
  acetylcholine and, pharmacologic effects and clinical consequences of, 57t
Glaucon (epinephrine), 79–82
Glial cells, drug distribution and, 13
Glipizide (Glucotrol), 431, 436–437, 439t
Glomerular filtration, 373–374
  drug excretion and, 14
Glucagon, 402, 438–440
  control of secretion of, 402
  major actions of, 402
Glucocorticoids, 405–406, 442, 443, 445–447, 448–452t
  comparative actions of, 444t
  control of secretion and actions of, 405–406
  topical, relative activities of, 444–445t
Glucosal (glucose, oral), 437–438
Glucose, oral (B-D Glucose; Glucosal; Glutose; Insta-Glucose; Monoject), 437–438
Glucose metabolism, disorders of, 403–404
Glucose polymers (Moducal; Polycose; ProMix; Sumacal), 777t
Glucostix, 791, 792t
Glucotrol (glipizide), 431, 436–437, 439t
Glukor (human chorionic gonadotropin), 469–470
Glutamic acid HCl (Acidulin), 501–502
Glutethimide (Doriden; Doriglute), 201–202
Glutose (glucose, oral), 437–438
Glyburide (Diabeta; Euglucon; Micronase), 431, 436–437, 439t
Glycate, 496–497t
Glycerin (Fleet Babylax; Glyrol; Osmoglyn; Sani-Supp), 383–385, 506–507, 513t
Glyceryl guaiacolate. See Guaifenesin
Glycopyrrolate (Robinul), 67–70, 76–77t
Glyrol (glycerin), 383–385
Glysennid (sennosides A&B-calcium salts), 506–507, 513t
Goiter, 400–401

Gold compounds, 178, 180, 184
Gold sodium thiomalate (Myochrysine), 180, 184
GoLYTELY (polyethylene glycol-electrolyte solution), 506–507, 511t
Gonadorelin (Factrel), 791, 796t
Gonadotrophs, 396
Gonadotropin releasing-hormone analog agent, 724, 730, 734t, 734–736
Gonic (human chorionic gonadotropin), 469–470
Gonodecten, 791, 792t
Gordofilm (salicylic acid), 170–171, 173, 177t
Granulex (trypsin), 818, 819t
Gravol (dimenhydrinate), 113–114, 116t, 119
Grifulvin V (griseofulvin, microsize), 689–690
GRIH. See Somatostatin
Grisactin (griseofulvin, microsize), 689–690
Grisactin Ultra (griseofulvin, ultramicrosize), 689–690
Griseofulvin, 568t, 687
  microsize (Fulvicin U/F; Grifulvin V; Grisactin), 689–690
  ultramicrosize (Fulvicin P/G; Grisactin Ultra; Grisovin-FP; Gris-Peg), 689–690
Grisovin-FP (griseofulvin, ultramicrosize), 689–690
Gris-Peg (griseofulvin, ultramicrosize), 689–690
Growth hormone (GH; somatotropin; STH), 397–398, 407
  actions of, 397–398
    effects on growth and, 397
    metabolic, 397–398
  secretion of, 397
    factors inhibiting, 397
    factors promoting, 397
  synthetic, 408–409
Growth hormone release-inhibiting hormone. See Somatostatin
Guaifenesin (Balminil Expectorant; Breonesin; Humibid; Resyl; Robitussin), 540
Guanabenz (Wytensin), 310–311
Guanadrel (Hylorel), 316–317
Guanethidine (Apo-Guanethidine; Ismelin), 316–317
Guanfacine (Tenex), 310–311
Guanidine, 64
Gulfasin (sulfisoxazole), 573–575, 577–578t
Gyne-Lotrimin (clotrimazole), 692, 693–694t, 697
Gynergen (ergotamine), 124–125
Gynex 0.5/35E (ethinyl estradiol/norethindrone), 463, 464t, 466–467
Gynex 1/35E (ethinyl estradiol/norethindrone), 463, 464t, 466–467
Gynogen LA (estradiol valerate), 724, 730, 732t, 734–736

H

Habituation, 835
Haemophilus vaginalis, 569t
Halazepam (Paxipam), 217–219, 218t, 222t

Halcinonide (Halog; Halog E), 443, 444t, 445t, 445–447, 450t
Halcion (triazolam), 198–199, 200t
Haldol (haloperidol), 205–208, 212t
Haldrone (paramethasone), 443, 445–447, 451t
Halog (halcinonide), 443, 444t, 445t, 445–447, 450t
Halog E (halcinonide), 443, 444t, 445–447, 450t
Haloperidol (Apo-Haloperidol; Haldol; Halperon; Novoperidol; Peridol), 205–208, 206t, 212t
Haloprogin (Halotex), 568t, 687, 692, 694t, 697
Halotestin (fluoxymesterone), 474–476, 477t, 479, 724, 730, 731t, 734–736
Halotex (haloprogin), 692, 694t, 697
Halothane (Fluothane; Somnothane), 147–148
Halperon (haloperidol), 205–208, 212t
Harmonyl (deserpidine), 313–314, 315t
Harrison Narcotic Act, 42
H-BIG (hepatitis B immune globulin), 810, 810t
HDL. *See* High-density lipoproteins
Heart, 275, *276*
 glucagon and, 402
Heavy metal antagonists, 814, 815t
Helminthiasis, 672. *See also* Antihelmintics
 classification and treatment of, 673t
Hemabate (carboprost tromethamine), 470–472, 471t
Hema-Chek, 791, 792t
Hema-Combistix, 791, 792t
Hemastix, 791, 792t
Hematest, 791, 792t
Hemin (Panhematin), 820–821
Hemoccult, 791, 792t
Hemocyte (ferrous fumarate), 345–346, 347t
Hemodynamics, 278–279
 extrinsic control of blood flow and, 279
 intrinsic control of blood flow and, 278–279
Hemofil T (antihemophilic factor, human), 361–362
Hemoglobin, oxygen transport and, 534
Hemolytic anemia, 22, 345
Hemophilus, 598
Hemophilus b conjugate vaccine (ProHIBit), 803–804, 805t
Hemophilus b polysaccharide vaccine (b-Capsa I; Hib-Immune), 803–804, 805t
Hemophilus ducreyi, 568t, 625t
Hemophilus influenzae, 569t, 625t
Hemorheologic agent, 357–358
Hemorrhagic anemia, acute, 345
Hemostatic drugs, 351, 359, 361–365
 systemic, 359, 361–363
 topical, 363–365
Hepalean (heparin calcium), 351–354
Heparin antagonist, 354
Heparin calcium (Calcilean; Calciparine; Hepalean; Minihep), 351–354
Heparin sodium (Liquaemin), 351–354
HepatAmine (amino-acid formulation for hepatic failure or hepatic encephalopathy), 780
Hepatic disease, adverse drug effects related to, 20–21
Hepatic first-pass metabolism, 14
Hepatitis B immune globulin (H-BIG; Hep-B-Gammagee; HyperHep), 810, 810t
Hepatitis B vaccine (Heptavax-B), 803–804, 806t
 recombinant, 803–804, 806–807t
Hepatotoxicity, 22
 cholestatic, 22
 hemolytic, 22
 hepatocellular, 22
Hep-B-Gammagee (hepatitis B immune globulin), 810, 810t
Heptavax-B (hepatitis B vaccine), 803–804, 806t
Herella, 567t
Hering-Breuer reflex, 536
Herpes simplex, 569t
Herplex (idoxuridine), 702
Hespan (hetastarch), 824–826, 825t
Hesper (bioflavonoids), 777t
Hetastarch (Hespan), 824–826, 825t
Hetrazan (diethylcarbamazine), 672, 674
Hexa-Betalin (vitamin B$_6$), 760–761
Hexabrix, 799, 801t
Hexadrol (dexamethasone), 443, 445–447, 449t, 445t
Hexafluorenium (Mylaxen), 133
Hexocyclium methylsulfate (Tral), 67–70, 76–77t
Hexylresorcinol, 673t
Hib-Immune (hemophilus b polysaccharide vaccine), 803–804, 805t
Hi-CP combination chemotherapy, 738, 740, 746t
High-density lipoproteins (HDL), 337
Hilus
 lungs and, 531
 renal, 371
Hindbrain, 54
Hiprex (methenamine hippurate), 637–638, 639t
Hismanal (astemizole), 113–114, 115t, 119
Hispril (diphenylpyraline), 113–114, 117t, 119
Histamine, endogenous, 113
Histamine phosphate, 791, 796t
Histantil (promethazine), 113–114, 117t, 119
Histerone (testosterone, aqueous), 474–476, 477t, 479
Histolyn-CYL (histoplasmin), 791, 794t
Histoplasma capsulatum, 569t
Histoplasmin (Histolyn-CYL; Histoplasmin, Diluted), 791, 794t
Histoplasmin, Diluted (histoplasmin), 791, 794t
Hi-Vegi-Lip (pancreatin), 502
HMG. *See* Human menopausal gonadotropin
HMS Liquifilm (medrysone), 443, 445–447, 451t
Hold (dextromethorphan), 539
Homatropine hydrobromide (Ak-Homatropine; Homatrine; Isopto Homatropine), 67–70, 76–77t
Honvol (diethylstilbestrol diphosphate), 454–456, 457t
HOP combination chemotherapy, 738, 740, 747t
Hormogen-Depot (estradiol cypionate), 724, 730, 732t, 734–736
Hormonal changes, in elderly patients, 37
Hormones. *See also specific hormones*
 adrenal, 405–406
 adenohypophyseal, 397–400, 407–410
 adrenal medulla and, 404–405
 neurohypophyseal, 396–397, 409–414
 antineoplastic, 724, 730, 731–734t, 734–736
 gonadal, 406
 mechanisms of action of, 395
 second messenger mechanism and, 395
 pancreatic, 402–404
 regulation of secretion of, 395, *396*
 sex, 405
 thyroid, 400, 416–418, 418–419t
 actions of, 400
 available preparations of, 416
 biosynthesis of, 400
 fate of, 400
 transport of, 400
 transport and metabolism of, 395
H.P. Acthar Gel (repository corticotropin injection), 407–408
H$_1$ receptor antagonists, 113–114, 114–118t, 119
H$_1$ receptor sites, 53
H$_2$ receptor antagonists, 119, 121–122, 122t
H$_2$ receptor sites, 53
H.T. Factorate (antihemophilic factor, human), 361–362
Human chorionic gonadotropin (A.P.L.; Autuitrin; Chorex; Corgonject-5; Chorigon; Choron-10; Follutein; Glukor; Gonic; Pregnyl; Profasi HP), 469–470
Human immune serums, 810, 810–811t
Human menopausal gonadotropins (HMG; Pergonal), 407, 468–469
Humatin (paromomycin), 685
Humatrope (somatrem), 408–409
Humibid (guaifenesin), 540
Humorsol (demecarium bromide), 59–60
Humulin L (insulin zinc suspension, human), 429–431, 435t
Humulin N (isophane insulin suspension, human), 429–431, 436t
Humulin R (insulin injection, human), 429–431, 435t
Humulin U (insulin zinc suspension, extended, human), 429–431, 436t
Hyalase (hyaluronidase), 818, 820t
Hyaline membrane disease, 532
Hyaluronidase (Hyalase; Wydase), 818, 820t
Hybolin (nandrolone decanoate), 474–476, 478t, 479
Hybolin Improved (nandrolone phenpropionate), 474–476, 478t, 479
Hydantoins, 240–243, 244t
Hydergine (ergoloid mesylates), 334

Hydralazine (Alazine; Apresoline), 314–316
Hydrea (hydroxyurea), 736–738, 738–739t
Hydrex (benzthiazide), 388–389, 390t, 391–392
Hydriodic Acid (hydrogen iodide), 540–541
Hydrisalic (salicylic acid), 170–171, 173, 177t
Hydrochlorothiazide (Apo-Hydro; Esidrix; Hydrodiuril; Novohydrazide), 388–389, 390t, 391–392
Hydrocholeretics, 500, 501
Hydrocodone (Robidone), 538–539
Hydrocortisone (Alphaderm; Cortamed; Cort-Dome; Cortiment; Cortef; Cortril; Hytone), 443, 444t, 445t, 445–447, 450t
Hydrocortisone valerate (Westcort), 445t
Hydrodiuril (hydrochlorothiazide), 388–389, 390t, 391–392
Hydroflumethiazide (Diucardin; Saluron), 388–389, 390–391t, 391–392
Hydrogen iodide (Hydriodic Acid), 540–541
Hydroloid-G (ergoloid mesylates), 334
Hydrolysis, biotransformation and, 14
Hydromorphone (Dilaudid), 157, 158t, 159, 161t
Hydromox (quinethazone), 388–389, 391t, 391–392
Hydroquinone (Eldopaque; Eldoquin; Esoterica Regular; Porcelana; Solaquin), 828–829
Hydroscyamine sulfate (Anaspaz; Bellaspaz; Cystospaz; Cystospaz-M; Levsin; Levsinex; Neoquess), 72–73t
Hydroxocobalamin, crystalline (Acti-B$_{12}$; AlphaRedisol), 349
Hydroxyamphetamine (Paredrine), 89, 92, 92t
Hydroxychloroquine sulfate (Plaquenil), 665, 666t
Hydroxyprogesterol caproate (Duralutin), 456, 459, 460t, 461
Hydroxyprogesterone caproate (Gesterol LA; Hylutin; Hyprogest; Hyproval PA; Hyroxon; Pro-Depo), 724, 730, 733t, 734–736
Hydroxystilbamidine, 567t, 649
Hydroxyurea (Hydrea), 710t, 736–738, 738–739t, 743t
Hydroxyzine (Apo-Hydroxyzine; Atarax; Multipax; Vistaril), 224–225, 521t
Hygroton (chlorthalidone), 388–389, 390t, 391–392
Hylidone (chlorthalidone), 388–389, 390t, 391–392
Hylorel (guanadrel), 316–317
Hylutin (hydroxyprogesterone caproate), 724, 730, 733t, 734–736
Hymenolepsis nana, 673t
Hyoscyamine, 67–70
Hypaque 20%, 799, 801t
Hypaque 25%, 799, 801t
Hypaque 50%, 799, 801t
Hypaque-76, 799, 801t
Hypaque-Cysto, 799, 801t

Hypaque-M 75%, 799, 801t
Hypaque-M 90%, 799, 801t
Hypaque Meglumine 30%, 799, 801t
Hypaque Meglumine 60%, 799, 801t
Hypaque Sodium, 799, 801t
Hyperab (rabies immune globulin, human), 811–812, 812t
Hyperaldosteronism, primary, 406
Hypercalcemia, 401, 424
Hyperchromic anemia, 345
Hyperglycemia, 402
Hyperglycemia agents, 437–440
HyperHep (hepatitis B immune globulin), 810, 810t
Hyperinsulinism, hypoglycemia and, 403
Hyperlipoproteinemia(s), 337
  classification of, 338t
Hyperparathyroidism, 401
Hypersensitivity reactions, 20
  antimicrobials and, 563
  delayed, 20
  immediate, 20
Hyperstat IV (diazoxide, parenteral), 318–319
Hypertension. *See* Antihypertensive drugs
Hypertensive emergencies, drugs for, 318–320
Hyper-Tet (tetanus immune globulin), 810, 811t
Hyperthyroidism, 400–401, 416
Hypnotic, nonbarbiturate, 151
Hypocalcemia, 401, 424
Hypochromic anemia, 345
Hypodermoclysis, 8
Hypoglycemia, 402, 403
  fasting, 403
  postprandial, 403
Hypokalemia, drug interactions and, 29–30
Hypolipemic agents, 337–344, 338t
Hypolipidemic agents. *See* Hypolipemic agents
Hypoparathyroidism, 401
Hypophysis cerebri. *See* Pituitary gland
Hypopituitarism, 399
Hypothalamohypophyseal portal system, 395
Hypothalamohypophyseal tract, 395
Hypothalamus, 54
Hypothyroidism, 400–401, 416
Hypouricemic (uricosuric) agents, anti-gout, 186
HypRho-D (rh$_o$[D] immune globulin), 810, 811t
Hyprogest (hydroxyprogesterone caproate), 724, 730, 733t, 734–736
Hyproval PA (hydroxyprogesterone caproate), 724, 730, 733t, 734–736
Hyroxon (hydroxyprogesterone caproate), 724, 730, 733t, 734–736
Hyskon (hysteroscopy fluid), 791, 797t
Hyskon (dextran 40-low molecular weight), 824–826, 825t
Hysteroscopy fluid (Hyskon), 791, 797t
Hytakerol (dihydrotachysterol), 768–770, 769t
Hytinic (polysaccharide-iron complex), 345–346, 347t
Hytone (hydrocortisone), 445t
Hytrin (terazosin), 312–313

Ibuprofen (Advil; Amersol; Motrin; Novoprofen; Nuprin), 175, 178, 181t
ICSH. *See* Luteinizing hormone
Ictotest, 791, 792t
ID combination chemotherapy, 738, 740, 748t
Idiosyncratic reaction, 20
Idoxuridine (Herplex; Stoxil), 569t, 702
Ifex (ifosfamide), 710t, 711–712, 716t, 746t, 748t
Ifosfamide (Ifex), 710t, 711–712, 716t, 746t, 748t
Ilopan (dexpanthenol), 816–817
Ilosone (erythromycin estolate), 619–620, 621–622t
Ilotycin (erythromycin base), 619–620, 621–622t
Ilotycin Gluceptate (erythromycin gluceptate), 619–620, 622t
Ilozyme (pancrelipase), 502
IMF combination chemotherapy, 738, 740, 748t
Imferon (iron dextran), 346–348
Imipenem-cilastin (Primaxin), 595
Imipramine (Apo-Imipramine; Impril; Janimine; Novopramine; Tipramine; Tofranil), 227–230, 228t, 231–232t
Immune globulin, intravenous (Gamimune N; Gammagard; Sandoglobulin; Venoglobulin 1), 801, 810t
Immune globulin-intramuscular (Gamma Globulin; Gamastan; Gammar; ISG)
Immune response, alterations in, drug interactions and, 30
Immunity, 803
  acquired, 803
    active and passive, 803
    naturally and artificially, 803
  active, agents for, 803–804
  natural, 803
  passive, agents for, 804–810
Immunologic effects, of glucocorticoids, 405
Immunosuppressants, 821–823
Imodium (loperamide), 515–516
Imodium A-D (loperamide), 515–516
Imogam (rabies immune globulin, human), 811–812, 812t
Imovax (rabies vaccine, human diploid cell cultures, intramuscular), 811–812, 812t
Imovax I.D. (rabies vaccine, human diploid cell cultures, intradermal), 811–812, 812t
Impril (imipramine), 227–230, 231–232t
Impulse conduction, disorders of, 287
Impulse formation, disorders of, 287
Imuran (azathioprine), 821–822
Inappropriate ADH syndrome, 396–397
Inapsine (droperidol), 214–215
Incompatibility, 27
  chemical, 27
  physical, 27
Indameth (indomethacin), 175, 178, 182t
Indandione, 354–356, 356t
Indapamide (Lozide; Lozol), 388–389, 391t, 391–392

Inderal (propranolol), 104–105, 105t, 107t, 108t, 109, 296–297, 303–304, 331
Inderal LA (propranolol), 331
Indocid (indomethacin), 175, 178, 182t
Indocin (indomethacin), 175, 178, 182t
Indocyanine green (Cardio-Green), 791, 797t
Indolone, 205–208, 206t, 212t
Indomethacin (Apo-Indomethacin; Indameth; Indocid; Indocin; Novomethacin), 175, 178, 182t
Infalyte (oral electrolyte mixture), 776t
Infancy, 31
Infantol Pink, 517t
Infiltration anesthetics, local, 139
"Inflation reflex," 536
Influenza A, 569t
Influenza virus vaccines (Fluogen; Fluzone), 803–804, 807t
Infundibular stalk, 395
Infusion, for intravenous administration, 6, 7, 7
INH (isoniazid), 655
Inhalation anesthetics, general, 145–149
 gases, 145–146
 volatile liquids, 146–149
Inhalation application, 5–6
Injection. *See* Parenteral administration
Inner ear disturbances, vomiting and, 489
Innovar (fentanyl/droperidol), 152–153
Inocor (amrinone), 285
Inositol (Linodil), 777t
Inotropic agents, positive, 285
Insomnal (diphenhydramine), 113–114, 116t, 119
Inspiratory neurons, 535
Insta-Glucose (glucose, oral), 437–438
Insta-Kit, 791, 792t
Insulatard NPH (isophane insulin suspension, purified), 429–431, 436t
Insulin(s), 402–403, 429–431, 435–436t
 characteristics of preparations of, 430t
 control of secretion of, 402
 "human," 429
 major actions of, 402–403
 purified, 429
 structure, biosynthesis, and secretion of, 402
Insulin injection (Regular Insulin; Regular Iletin I), 429–431, 430t, 435t
 concentrated (Regular Concentrated Iletin II), 429–431, 435t
 human (Humulin R; Novolin R; Velosulin Human), 429–431, 435t
 purified (Regular Purified Pork; Regular Iletin II; Velosulin), 429–431, 435t
Insulin zinc suspension (Lente Iletin I; Lente Insulin), 429–431, 430t, 435t
 extended (Ultralente Iletin I; Ultralente Insulin), 429–431, 430t, 436t
 human (Humulin U), 429–431, 436t
 purified (Ultralente Purified Beef), 429–431, 436t
 human (Humulin L; Novolin L), 429–431, 435t
 prompt (Semilente Iletin I; Semilente Insulin), 429–431, 430t, 435t
 purified (Lente Iletin II; Lente Purified Pork), 429–431, 435t
 purified (Semilente Purified Pork), 429–431, 435t
Intal (cromolyn sodium), 553–554
Intensity of effect, 16
Intercalated disks, 276
Intercostal muscles, external, 532
Interferon, 709t
Interferon alfa-2a, recombinant (Roferon-A), 736–738, 739t
Interferon alfa-2b, recombinant (Intron-A), 736–738, 739–740t
Interlobar arteries, 371
Interlobular arteries, 371
Interneuronal blocking agents, 134–135
Interstitial cell stimulating hormone. *See* Luteinizing hormone
Intestinal lipase, 488t
Intestinal phase, of gastric secretion, 486
Intestine. *See also* Large intestine; Small intestine
 alteration of flora of, drug interactions and, 28
 changes in motility and function of, drug interactions and, 28
 drug excretion through, 14–15
Intraamniotic administration, 10
Intraarterial administration, 8
Intraarticular administration, 10
Intrabutazone (phenylbutazone), 174–175
Intracardiac administration, 10
Intracranial pressure, vomiting and, 489
Intradermal administration, 10
Intradermal diagnostic biologicals, 791, 794–795t
Intralipid 10%, 20% (intravenous fat emulsion), 782
Intramuscular administration, 8–10, 9
 absorption and, 12
 in children, 31
 in children, 33
Intraperitoneal administration, 10
Intrapleural administration, 10
Intrapleural pressure, 532
Intrapulmonary pressure, 532
Intrathecal administration, 10
Intrauterine progesterone contraceptive system (Progestasert), 467
Intravenous administration, 6–8, 7
 absorption and, 12
 in children, 33
Intravenous anesthetics, 149–153
 dissociative agents, 151–153
 nonbarbiturate hypnotic, 151
 ultrashort-acting barbiturates, 149–151, 150t
Intravenous fat emulsion (Intralipid 10%, 20%; Liposyn 10%, 20%; Liposyn II 10%, 20%; Soyacal 10%, 20%; Travamulsion 10%, 20%), 782
Intrinsic activity, 16
Intrinsic clotting pathway, 351, *353*
Intrinsic factor, 488
Intron-A (interferon alfa-2b, recombinant), 736–738, 739–740t
Intropin (dopamine), 83–84
Inulin, 791, 797t
Inversine (mecamylamine), 70–71, 320
Invert sugar in water (Travert), 782
In vitro diagnostic aids, 791, 792–793t
In vitro drug interactions
 chemical, 27
 physical, 27
In vivo diagnostic aids, 791, 795–798t
In vivo drug interactions, 27
Involuntary nervous system, 49
Iodide, radioactive, 420–421
Iodide pump, 400
Iodide uptake, thyroid hormone biosynthesis and, 400
Iodinated glycerol (Iophen; Organidin; R-Gen Elixir), 540–541
Iodinated radiopaque agents, 799, 800–802t
Iodine/iodide compounds, 421–423, 422t
Iodine products, expectorant, 540–541
Iodochlorhydroxyquin, 687
Iodochlorhydroxyquin-clioquinol (Torofor; Vioform), 692, 694t, 697
Iodo-Niacin (potassium iodide/niacinamide), 540–541
Iodopyract (Diodrast), 374t
Iodoquinol (Diiodohydroxyquin; Diodoquin; Moebiquin; Yodoxin), 681, 683
Iodotope (radioactive sodium iodide-^{131}I), 420–421
Ion(s), renal handling of, 374
Ionamin (phentermine), 265–267, 268t
Ionization, pharmacokinetics and, 11
Iophen (iodinated glycerol), 540–541
Iosat (potassium iodide), 421–423, 422t
Ipecac syrup, 520–521
I-Pentolate (cyclopentolate hydrochloride), 74–75t
I-Picamide (tropicamide), 74–75t
Ipran (propranolol), 331
Ipratropium (Atrovent), 67–70, 76–77t, 553
Ircon (ferrous fumarate), 345–346, 347t
Iron dextran (Imferon), 346–348
Iron preparations
 oral, 345–346, 347t
 parenteral, 346–348
ISG (immune globulin-intramuscular), 801, 810t
Islets of Langerhans, 402
Ismelin (guanethidine), 316–317
Ismotic (isosorbide), 385
Isobec (amobarbital), 193–194, 195t, 197
Isocaine (mepivacaine), 139–141, 140t, 142t
Isocarboxazid (Marplan), 234–236, 236t
Isoclor Expectorant, 538t
Isoetharine (Arm-a-Med Isoetharine; Beta-2; Bronkometer; Bronkosol; Dey-Dose Isoetharine; Dey-lute; Disorine; Dispos-a Med Isoetharine), 94–95, 96–97t
Isoflurane (Forane), 148
Isoflurophate (Floropryl), 64
Isomaltase (maltase), 488t
Isoniazid (INH; Isotamine; Laniazid; Nydrazid; PMS Isoniazid; Teebaconin), 562, 569t, 655, 659–660
Isophane insulin suspension (NPH Insulin; NPH Iletin I), 429–431, 430t, 436t
 human (Humulin N; Novolin N), 429–431, 436t

purified (Insulatard NPH; NPH Iletin II; NPH Purified Pork), 429–431, 436t
Isopropamide, 67–70
Isopropamide iodide (Darbid), 76–77t
Isoproterenol
　inhalation (Aerolone; Medihaler-Iso; Norisidrine; Vapo-Iso), 84–85
　oral/parenteral (Isuprel), 84–85
Isoptin (verapamil), 299–300, 313, 329–331, 331t, 332t
Isopto carbachol (carbachol, topical), 56–57
Isopto carpine (pilocarpine), 58
Isopto Cetamide (sulfacetamide), 573–575, 575–576t
Isopto-Eserine (physostigmine, ophthalmic), 59
Isopto Frin (phenylephrine), 89, 92, 92t
Isopto Homatropine (homatropine hydrobromide), 76–77t
Isopto Hyoscine (scopolamine hydrobromide), 72–73t
Isordil (isosorbide dinitrate), 325–326, 327t, 329
Isosorbide (Ismotic), 385
Isosorbide dinitrate (Apo-ISDN; Coronex; Isordil; Novosorbide; Sorbitrate), 325–326, 327t, 329
Isotamine (isoniazid), 659–660
Isotretinoin (Accutane), 766–767
Isovex (ethaverine), 334–335
Isovue 300, 799, 801t
Isovue 370, 799, 801t
Isovue-M 200, 799, 801t
Isovue-M 300, 799, 801t
Isoxsuprine (Vasodilan; Voxsuprine), 95–96, 334
Isuprel (isoproterenol), 84–85

J

Janimine (imipramine), 227–230, 231–232t
Jaundice, 22
Jenamicin (gentamicin), 624–626, 627–628t, 630
Juxtaglomerular apparatus, 371, 373, 373
Juxtaglomerular cells, 371, 373, 373

K

K₁ (phytonadione), 356–357
Kabikinase (streptokinase), 358–359, 360t
Kainair (proparacaine), 139–141, 140t, 143t
Kalcinate (calcium gluconate), 783t, 785
Kanamycin (Anamid; Kantrex; Klebcil), 567t, 569t, 624–626, 625t, 628t, 630
Kantrex (kanamycin), 624–626, 628t, 630
Kao-tin, 518t
Kaodene Nonnarcotic, 517t
Kaodene with Paregoric, 517t
Kaopectate, 518t
Kaopectolin, 518t
Kaopectolin Gel with Belladonna, 518t
Kaopectolin PG, 518t

Kaopectolin with Paregoric, 518t
Karacil (psyllium), 506–507, 508t
Karidium (fluoride), 775, 778
Kasof (docusate potassium-dioctyl potassium sulfosuccinate), 506–507, 509t
KBP/O, 518t
K-C, 518t
Kefauver-Harris Amendment, 41
Keflet (cephalexin), 598–600, 601–602t
Keflex (cephalexin), 598–600, 601–602t
Keflin (cephalothin), 598–600, 602t
Keftab (cephalexin), 598–600, 601–602t
Kefurox (cefuroxime), 598–600, 605t
Kefzol (cefazolin), 598–600, 601t
Kellogg's Castor Oil (castor oil), 506–507, 512t
Kemadrin (procyclidine), 74–75t, 258–259, 260t
Kemsol (dimethyl sulfoxide), 817
Kenalog (triamcinolone), 443, 445t, 445–447, 452t
Keralyt (salicylic acid), 170–171, 173, 177t
Ketalar (ketamine), 151–152
Ketamine (Ketalar), 151–152
Ketoconazole (Nizoral), 567–569t, 568t, 687, 690–691, 692, 694t, 697
Keto-Diastix, 791, 792t
Ketoprofen (Orudis), 175, 178, 182t
Ketostix, 791, 792t
K-Flex (orphenadrine citrate), 74–75t, 134–135, 137t
Kidney
　adrenergic drug effects on, 81t
　control of renal blood flow and, 373
　drug excretion through, 14
　　glomerular filtration and, 14
　　tubular reabsorption and, 14
　　tubular secretion and, 14
　gross anatomy of, 371, 372
　　renal blood supply and, 371
　microscopic anatomy of, 371, 372, 373
　　juxtaglomerular apparatus and, 371, 373, 373
　parathyroid hormone and, 401
　physiology of, 373–375
　　countercurrent mechanism and, 375
　　glomerular filtration and, 373–374
　　renal function in acid-base regulation and, 375
　　renal handling of ions and water and, 374
　　renal tubular reabsorption and secretion and, 374, 374t
Kinevac (sincalide), 791, 798t
Kirby-Bauer method, 561
Klebcil (kanamycin), 624–626, 628t, 630
Klebsiella, 624, 625t, 632
Klebsiella pneumoniae, 569t, 624
Klonopin (clonazepam), 248–249
Knowledge, insufficient, drug interactions caused by, 26
Koate-HS (antihemophilic factor, human), 361–362
Koate-HT (antihemophilic factor, human), 361–362
Koffex (dextromethorphan), 539
Kolantyl, 496–497t

Konakion (phytonadione; vitamin K₁), 356–357, 771t, 771–772
Kondremul Plain (mineral oil), 506–507, 509–510t
Konsyl (psyllium), 506–507, 508t
Konyne (factor IX complex, human), 362–363
K-P, 518t
K-Pek, 518t
K-Phos Neutral (phosphorus), 776t
Kryobulin VH (antihemophilic factor, human), 361–362
Ku-Zyme HP (pancrelipase), 502

L

Labetalol (Normodyne; Trandate), 104–105, 105t, 106t, 108t, 109, 305, 310
Labstix, 791, 792t
Lact-Aid (lactase), 777t
Lactase (Lact-Aid; Lactrase), 488t, 777t
Lactinex, 518t
Lactrase (lactase), 777t
Lactrotrophs, 396
Lactulax (lactulose), 506–507, 510t
Lactulose (Acilac; Cephulac; Cholac; Chronulac; Constilac; Constulose; Duphylac; Enulose; Lactulax), 506–507, 510t
Lamina propria, 483
Lamprene (clofazime), 645, 647
Laniazid (isoniazid), 659–660
Lanoxicaps (digoxin), 281–283, 284t
Lanoxin (digoxin), 281–283, 284t
Largactil (chlorpromazine), 205–208, 209t
Large intestine
　anatomic and histologic features of, 484t
　major activities of, 486t
Largon (propiomazine), 203
Larodopa (levodopa), 254–255
Larotid (amoxicillin), 582, 584–585, 586t, 595
Lasix (furosemide), 377–378, 382–383, 384t
LA-test-ASO, 791, 792t
LA-test-CRP, 791, 792t
LA-test-RF, 791, 792t
Laxagel (docusate sodium-dioctyl sodium sulfosuccinate), 506–507, 509t
Laxatives, 506–507, 508–513t
　classification of, 506, 507t
Laxit (bisacodyl), 506–507, 511–512t
LDL. *See* Low-density lipoproteins
LE. *See* Lupus erythematosus
Lecithin, 777t
Legal aspects, 41–45
　drug legislation and, 41–44
　medication orders and, 44–45
　nurse's role in carrying out, 44–45
Legatrin (quinine sulfate), 669–670
Legend drugs, 41
Legionella pneumophila, 569t, 619
Lente Iletin I (insulin zinc suspension), 429–431, 435t
Lente Iletin I (insulin zinc suspension, purified), 429–431, 435t
Lente Insulin (insulin zinc suspension), 429–431, 435t

Lente Purified Pork (insulin zinc suspension, purified), 429–431, 435t
Leptospira, 569t
Leptotrichia buccalis, 569t
Leucovorin, 745t
Leucovorin calcium-folinic acid (Wellcovorin), 350
Leukeran (chlorambucil), 711–712, 713–714t
Leuprolide (Leupron), 724, 730, 734t, 734–736, 747t
Leupron (leuprolide), 724, 730, 734t, 734–736
Levarterenol (norepinephrine), 83
Levate (amitriptyline), 227–230, 231t
Levatol (penbutolol), 104–105, 105t, 107t, 108t, 109, 303–304
Levazine (perphenazine), 205–208, 210t
Levlen (ethinyl estradiol/levonorgestrel), 463, 464t, 466–467
Levobunolol (Betagan), 104–105, 105t, 106t, 108t, 109
Levodopa (Dopar; Larodopa; L-dopa), 253, 254–255
Levo-Dromoran (levorphanol), 157, 159, 163t
Levophed (norepinephrine), 83
Levoprome (methotrimeprazine), 215
Levorphanol (Levo-Dromoran), 157, 159, 163t
Levothroid (levothyroxine sodium-T₄), 416–418, 419t
Levothyroxine sodium-T₄ (Eltroxin; Levothroid; Levoxine; Synthroid; Synthrox; Syroxine), 416–418, 419t
Levoxine (levothyroxine sodium-T₄), 416–418, 419t
Levsin (hydroscyamine sulfate), 72–73t
Levsinex (hydroscyamine sulfate), 72–73t
LH. *See* Luteinizing hormone
Libritabs (chlordiazepoxide), 217–219, 220–221t
Librium (chlordiazepoxide), 217–219, 218t, 220–221t
Lidemol (fluocinonide), 443, 445–447, 450t
Lidex (fluocinonide), 443, 444t, 445–447, 450t
Lidex-E (fluocinonide), 443, 444t, 445–447, 450t
Lidocaine (Lidopen; Xylocaine; Xylocard), 139–141, 140t, 142t, 288t, 292–293
Lidopen (lidocaine), 292–293
Limbic system, 54
Lincocin (lincomycin), 644–645, 646t
Lincomycin (Lincocin), 644–645, 646t
Linodol (inositol), 777t
Lioresal (baclofen), 134–135, 136t
Liothyronine sodium-T₃ (Cytomel; Cyronine), 416–418, 419t
Liotrix (Euthroid; Thyrolar), 416–418, 419t
Lipase
  intestinal, 488t
  pancreatic (steapsin), 488t
Lipid(s)
  absorption of, 487
  parenteral, 782
Lipid bilayer, 11

Lipid metabolism
  glucagon and, 402
  glucocorticoids and, 405
  growth hormone and, 397
  insulin and, 403
Lipid solubility, of drugs, 13
Lipo Gantrisin (sulfisoxazole), 573–575, 577–578t
Lipogenesis, insulin and, 403
Lipolysis, insulin and, 403
Lipomul Oral (corn oil), 777t
Lipoproteins, 337
Liposyn 10%, 20% (intravenous fat emulsion), 782
Liposyn II 10%, 20% (intravenous fat emulsion), 782
Lipoxide (chlordiazepoxide), 217–219, 220–221t
Liquaemin (heparin sodium), 351–354
Liqui-Char (activated charcoal), 813–814
Liquid Pred (prednisone), 724, 730, 733t, 734–736
Lisinopril (Prinivil; Zestril), 304–305, 309t
Listeria monocytogenes, 569t
Lithane (lithium), 208, 213–214
Lithium (Carbolith; Cibalith-S; Duralith; Eskalith; Lithane; Lithizine; Lithobid; Lithonate; Lithotabs), 205, 208, 213–214
Lithizine (lithium), 208, 213–214
Lithobid (lithium), 208, 213–214
Lithonate (lithium), 208, 213–214
Lithostat (acetohydroxamic acid), 641–642
Lithotabs (lithium), 208, 213–214
Liver, adrenergic drug effects on, 81t
Liver disease, hypoglycemia and, 403
10% LMD (dextran 40-low molecular weight), 824–826, 825t
Loa loa, 673t
Loestrin 1/20 (ethinyl estradiol/norethindrone), 463, 464t, 466–467
Loestrin 1.5/30 (ethinyl estradiol/norethindrone), 463, 464t, 466–467
Lomine (dicyclomine hydrochloride), 72–73t
Lomotil (diphenoxylate HCl with atropine sulfate), 514–515
Lomustine (CCNU; CeeNU), 710t, 711–712, 716t, 742t, 744–746t, 748–751t
Loniten (minoxidil), 317–318
Loop of Henle, 371
Lo/Ovral (ethinyl estradiol/norgestrel), 463, 464t, 466–467
Loperamide (Imodium; Imodium A-D), 515–516
Lopid (gemfibrozil), 341–342
Lopressor (metoprolol), 104–105, 105t, 107t, 108t, 109, 303–304, 331
Loprox (ciclopirox), 692, 693t, 697
Lopurin (allopurinol), 188–189
Loraz (lorazepam), 217–219, 222t
Lorazepam (Alzapam; Apo-Lorazepam; Ativan; Loraz; Novolorazem), 217–219, 218t, 222t
Lorelco (probucol), 343
Lorothidol (bithionol), 672, 674, 675t, 676–680
Lotrimin (clotrimazole), 692, 693–694t, 697

Lotusate (talbutal), 193–194, 196t, 197
Lovastatin (Mevacor), 342
Low-density lipoproteins (LDL), 337
Lowsium (magaldrate), 490–491, 492–493t
Lowsium Plus, 496–497t
Loxapac (loxapine), 205–208, 212t
Loxapine (Loxapac; Loxitane), 205–208, 206t, 212t
Loxitane (loxapine), 205–208, 212t
Lozide (indapamide), 388–389, 391t, 391–392
Lozol (indapamide), 388–389, 391t, 391–392
L-PAM (melphalan), 711–712, 717t
LSD, abuse of, 839
LTH. *See* Luteotropic hormone
Ludiomil (maprotiline), 227–230, 228t, 232t
Lufyllin (dyphylline), 545–547, 548t, 549, 551
Lugol's solution (strong iodine solution), 421–423, 422t
Lungs
  anatomy and histology of, 531–532
  drug excretion through, 15
Lupus erythematosus (LE), 22, 25
Luramide (furosemide), 377–378, 382–383, 384t
Luride (fluoride), 775, 778
Luteinizing hormone (LH; luteotropin; ICSH; interstitial cell stimulating hormone), 398, 407
  actions of, 398
  control of secretion of, 398
Luteotropic hormone (LTH), 407
Luteotropin. *See* Luteinizing hormone
Lyderm (fluocinonide), 443, 445–447, 450t
Lymphocyte immune globulin-anti-thymocyte globulin (Atgam), 810, 811t
Lyphocin (vancomycin), 652–653
Lypressin (Diapid), 412
l-Lysine (Enisyl), 777t
Lysodren (mitotane), 724, 730, 734t, 734–736
Lytren (oral electrolyte mixture), 776t

M

Maalox (magnesium oxide), 490–491, 494–497t
Maalox Extra Strength, 496–497t
Maalox No. 1, 496–497t
Maalox No. 2, 496–497t
Maalox Plus, 496–497t
Maalox Plus Extra Strength, 496–497t
Maalox TC, 496–497t
MACC combination chemotherapy, 738, 740, 748t
MAC combination chemotherapy, 738, 740, 748t
MACM combination chemotherapy, 738, 740, 748t
MA combination chemotherapy, 738, 740, 748t
MACOP-B combination chemotherapy, 709t, 738, 740, 748t
Macrocytic anemia, 345

Macrodantin (nitrofurantoin macrocrystals), 639–640
Macrodex (dextran 70, 75-high molecular weight), 824–826, 825t
Macula densa, 371
Mafenide (Sulfamylon), 574t, 578
Magaldrate (Lowsium; Riopan), 490–491, 492–493t
Magan (magnesium salicylate), 170–171, 173, 176t
Magnacef (ceftazidime), 598–600, 606t
Magnate (magnesium), 776t
Magnatril, 496–497t
Magnesium (Almora; Magnate; Magonate; Nephro-Mag; Slow-Mag), 776t
Magnesium citrate (Citrate of Magnesia; Citroma; Citro-Maq; Citro-Nesia; National Laxative), 506–507, 510t
Magnesium hydroxide (Milk of Magnesia: M.O.M.), 490–491, 492–493t, 506–507, 511t
  in combination antacids, 494–497t
Magnesium oxide (Maalox; Mag-Ox 400; Par-Mag; Uro-Mag), 490–491, 494–495t
  in combination antacids, 494–497t
Magnesium salicylate (Doan's Pills; Magan; Mobidin), 170–171, 173, 176t
Magnesium sulfate (Epsom salt), 250–251, 506–507, 511t, 783t, 785
Magonate (magnesium), 776t
Mag-Ox 400 (magnesium oxide), 490–491, 494–495t
MAID combination chemotherapy, 738, 740, 748t
Malogen (testosterone, aqueous), 474–476, 477t, 479
Malogen in Oil (testosterone propionate), 474–476, 477t, 479
Malogex (testosterone enanthate), 474–476, 478t, 479
Maltase (isomaltase), 488t
Maltsupex (nondiastatic barley malt extract), 506–507, 508t
Mammary glands, drug excretion through, 15
Mandameth (methenamine mandelate), 637–638, 639t
Mandelamine (methenamine mandelate), 637–638, 639t
Mandol (cefamandole), 598–600, 603t
Manganese, 776t
Mannitol (Osmitrol), 385–386, 791, 797t
Maolate (chlorphenesin), 134–135, 136t
MAP combination chemotherapy, 738, 740, 748t
Maprotiline (Ludiomil), 227–230, 228t, 232t
Marazide (benzthiazide), 388–389, 390t, 391–392
Marbaxin-750 (methocarbamol), 134–135, 137t
Marblen, 496–497t
Marcaine (bupivacaine), 139–141, 140t, 142t
Marezine (cyclizine), 113–114, 116t, 119
Marflex (orphenadrine citrate), 74–75t, 134–135, 137t
Marijuana, 840–841

Marinol (dronabinol), 523–524
Marplan (isocarboxazid), 234–236, 236t
Marzine (cyclizine), 113–114, 116t, 119
Matulane (procarbazine), 736–738, 740t
Maxair (pirbuterol), 94–95, 96–97t
Maxeran (metoclopramide), 534–535
Maxibolin (ethylestrenol), 474–476, 478t, 479
Maxiflor (diflorasone), 443, 444t, 445–447, 449t
Maxivate (betamethasone dipropionate), 443, 444t, 445–447, 448t
Maxolon (metoclopramide), 534–535
Mazanor (mazindol), 265–267, 268t
Mazepine (carbamazepine), 246–247
Mazindol (Mazanor; Sanorex), 265–267, 268t
M-BACOD combination chemotherapy, 738, 740, 748–749t
MBD combination chemotherapy, 738, 740, 749t
MCBP combination chemotherapy, 738, 740, 749t
MCC combination chemotherapy, 738, 740, 749t
MC combination chemotherapy, 738, 740, 749t
MCP combination chemotherapy, 738, 740, 749t
MCT (medium chain triglycerides), 778t
MD-50, 799, 801t
MD-60, 799, 801t
MD-76, 799, 801t
MD-Gastroview, 799, 801t
Measles and rubella vaccine (M-R-Vax II), 803–804, 807t
Measles, mumps, and rubella vaccine (M-M-R II), 803–804, 807t
Measles vaccine-rubeola (Attenuvax), 803–804, 807t
Mebaral (mephobarbital), 193–194, 196t, 197, 238–240, 241t
Mebendazole (Vermox), 673t, 674
Mecamylamine (Inversine), 70–71, 320
Mechlorethamine (Mustargen; Nitrogen Mustard), 709t, 710t, 711–712, 716t, 742t, 743t, 749t, 750t
Meclan (meclocycline), 609–611, 613–614t
Meclizine (Antivert; Antrizine; Bonamine; Bonine; Dizmiss; Motion Cure; Ru-Vert M; Wehvert), 113–114, 114t, 117t, 119521t
Meclocycline (Meclan), 609–611, 610t, 613–614t
Meclofenamate (Meclomen), 175, 178, 182t
Meclomen (meclofenamate), 175, 178, 182t
Medication orders, 44–45
  nurse's role in carrying out, 44–45
    clarifying and evaluating written orders and, 45
    responsibility for errors in administration and, 45
    telephone orders and, 45
Medihaler-Epi (epinephrine), 79–82
Medihaler-Ergotamine (ergotamine), 124–125
Medihaler-Iso (isoproterenol), 84–85

Medilium (chlordiazepoxide), 217–219, 220–221t
Mediplast (salicylic acid), 170–171, 173, 177t
Meditran (meprobamate), 225
Medium chain triglycerides (MCT), 778t
Medrol (methylprednisolone), 443, 445t, 445–447, 451t
Medroxyprogesterone acetate (Amen; Curretab; Cycrin; Depo-Provera; Provera), 456, 459, 460t, 461, 724, 730, 733t, 734–736
Medrysone (HMS Liquifilm), 443, 445–447, 451t
Medulla, renal, 371
Medulla oblongata, 54
Medullary respiratory center, 535
Mefenamic acid (Ponstan; Ponstel), 175, 178, 182t
Mefoxin (cefoxitin), 598–600, 604–605t
Megace (megestrol acetate), 456, 459, 460t, 461, 724, 730, 733t, 734–736
Megacillin (penicillin G, potassium or sodium), 582, 584–585, 591–592t, 595
Megacillin (penicillin G, benzathine), 582, 584–585, 592t, 595
Megaloblastic anemia, 345
Megestrol acetate (Megace; Palace), 456, 459, 460t, 461, 724, 730, 733t, 734–736
Melanocyte-stimulating hormone (MSH), 398–399
  actions of, 398–399
  control of secretion of, 398
Mellaril (thioridazine), 205–208, 211t
Melphalan (Alkeran; PAM; L-PAM; Phenylalanine Mustard; L-Sarcolysin), 710t, 711–712, 717t, 748t, 749t, 753t
Membrane permeability
  distribution and, in children, 32
  drug action and, 18
Menadiol sodium diphosphate (vitamin K$_4$), 771t, 771–772
Menest (estrogens, esterified), 454–456, 458t
Meningitis vaccine (Menomune-A/C/Y/W-135), 803–804, 805t
Menomune-A/C/Y/W-135 (meningitis vaccine), 803–804, 805t
Menotropins (Pergonal), 468–469
Mepenzolate (Cantil), 67–70, 76–77t
Meperidine (Demerol; Pethadol), 157, 158t, 159, 163t
Mephentermine (Wyamine), 86
Mephenytoin (Mesantoin), 240–243, 244t
Mephobarbital (Mebaral), 193–194, 196t, 197, 238–240, 241t
Mephyton (phytonadione; vitamin k$_1$), 356–357, 771t, 771–772
Mepivacaine (Carbocaine; Isocaine; Polocaine), 139–141, 140t, 142t
Meprobamate (Apo-Meprobamate; Equanil; Meditran; Miltown; Neotran; Novomepro), 225
Mercaptopurine (6-Mercaptopurine; 6-MP; Purinethol), 710t, 712, 718–719, 742t, 749t, 750t

6-Mercaptopurine (mercaptopurine), 709t, 712, 718–719, 721t
Meruvax II (rubella vaccine), 803–804, 808t
Mesalamine (Rowasa), 823–824
Mesantoin (mephenytoin), 240–243, 244t
Mescaline, abuse of, 839
Mesencephalon, 54
Mesoridazine (Serentil), 205–208, 206t, 211t
Metaderm (betamethasone valerate), 443, 445–447, 448t
Metahydrin (trichlormethiazide), 388–389, 391t, 391–392
Metal chelating agents, non-receptor mediated effects of, 17
Metamucil (psyllium), 506–507, 508t
Metandren (methyltestosterone), 474–476, 477t, 479, 724, 730, 731t, 734–736
Metaprel (metaproterenol), 94–95, 96–97t
Metaproterenol (Alupent; Metaprel), 94–95, 96–97t
Metaraminol (Aramine), 86–87
Metaxalone (Skelaxin), 134–135, 136t
Metencephalon, 54
Methacholine (Provocholine), 791, 797t
Methacycline (Rondomycin), 609–611, 610t, 614t
Methadone (Dolophine), 157, 158t, 159, 161–163t
Methamphetamine (Desoxyn), 264–265, 266t
Methandrostenolone (methandrostenolone), 474–476, 478t, 479
Methantheline bromide (Banthine), 67–70, 76–77t
Metharbital (Gemonil), 193–194, 196t, 197, 238–240, 241t
Methazolamide (Neptazane), 376–377, 378t
Methdilazine (Dilosyn; Tacaryl), 113–114, 114t, 117t, 119
Methenamine hippurate (Hiprex; Urex), 637–638, 639t
Methenamine mandelate (Mandament; Mandelamine; Sterine), 637–638, 639t
Methergine (methylergonovine), 414
Methicillin (Staphcillin), 582, 583t, 584–585, 589–590t, 595
Methimazole (Tapazole), 418, 420, 421t
Methocarbamol (Delaxin; Marbaxin-750; Robaxin; Robomol), 134–135, 137t
Methohexital (Brietal; Brevital), 149–151, 150t
Methoscopolamine, 67–70
Methotrexate (Abitrexate; Amethopterin; Folex; Folex-PFS; Methotrexate-LPF; Mexate; Mexate-AQ; MTX; Rheumatrex DosePak), 709t, 710t, 712, 718–719, 721–722t, 741–743t, 745t, 747–751t, 753t
Methotrexate-LPF (methotrexate), 712, 718–719, 721–722t
Methotrimeprazine (Levoprome; Nozinan), 205, 215
Methoxamine (Vasoxyl), 87–88
Methoxsalen (Oxsoralen; 8-MOP; Ultra MOP), 827–828, 828t
Methoxyflurane (Penthrane), 148–149

Methscopolamine bromide (Pamine), 76–77t
Methsuximide (Celontin), 245–246, 246t
Methyclothiazide (Aquatensen; Duretic; Enduron; Ethon), 388–389, 391t, 391–392
Methylcellulose (Citrucel; Cologel), 506–507, 508t
Methyldopa (Aldomet; Amodopa; Apo-Methyldopa; Dopamet; Novomedopa; PMS Dopazide), 311–312
Methylene blue (Urolene Blue), 637, 638
Methylergobasine (methylergonovine), 414
Methylergonovine (Methergine; Methylergobasine), 414
Methylphenidate (Ritalin), 267, 269
Methylprednisolone (Medrol), 443, 444t, 445–447, 451t
Methylprednisolone acetate (Medrol), 445t
Methyl salicylate (oil of wintergreen), 170–171, 173, 177t
Methyltestosterone (Android; Metandren; Oreton; Oreton Methyl; Testred; Virilon), 474–476, 477t, 479, 724, 730, 731t, 734–736
Methyprylon (Noludar), 202
Methysergide (Sansert), 125–126
Metizole (metronidazole), 683–685
Metoclopramide (Emex; Clopra; Maxeran; Maxolon; Octamide; Reclomide; Reglan), 534–535
Metocurine (Metubine), 130
Metolazone (Diulo; Microx; Zaroxolyn), 388–389, 391t, 391–392
Metopirone (metyrapone), 791, 797t
Metoprolol (Apo-Metoprolol; Betaloc; Lopressor; Novometoprol), 104–105, 105t, 107t, 108t, 109, 303–304, 331
Metrifonate (Bilarcil), 672, 673t, 674, 675t, 676–680
Metrodin (urofollitropin), 469
Metronidazole (Apo-Metronidazole; Femazole; Flagyl; Metizole; Metro I.V.; Metro I.V. Metryl; Neo-Tric; Novonidazol; PMS Metronidazole; Protostat; Satric), 562, 568t, 681, 683–685
Metryl (metronidazole), 683–685
Metubine (metocurine), 130
Metyrapone (Metopirone), 791, 797t
Metyrosine (Demser), 320–321
Mevacor (lovastatin), 342
Meval (diazepam), 249
Mexate (methotrexate), 712, 718–719, 721–722t
Mexate-AQ (methotrexate), 712, 718–719, 721–722t
Mexiletine (Mexitil), 288t, 294–295
Mexitil (mexiletine), 294–295
Mezlin (mezlocillin), 582, 584–585, 590t, 595
Mezlocillin (Mezlin), 567–571t, 582, 583t, 584–585, 590t, 595
MF combination chemotherapy, 738, 740, 749t
Miacalcin (calcitonin, salmon), 424–425
Micatin (miconazole), 692, 695t, 697
Micelles, 487

Miconazole (Micatin; Monistat-3; Monistat 7; Monistat-Derm; Monistat I.V.), 568t, 687, 691, 692, 695t, 697
Microcytic anemia, 345
Microfibrillar collagen hemostat (Avitene), 364
Microlipid (safflower oil), 778t
Micronase (glyburide), 431, 436–437, 439t
Micronefrin (epinephrine), 79–82
Micronor (norethindrone), 456, 459, 460t, 461, 463, 464t, 466–467
Microstix-3, 791, 793t
Microstix-Nitrite, 791, 793t
Microsulfon (sulfadiazine), 573–575, 576t
MicroTrak Chlamydia, 791, 793t
MicroTrak HSV 1/HSV 2, 791, 793t
MicroTrak Neisseria Gonorrhoeae Culture Test, 791, 793t
Microx (metolazone), 388–389, 391t, 391–392
Midamor (amiloride), 386–387
Midazolam (Versed), 219, 222–223
Midbrain, 54
Milkinol (mineral oil), 506–507, 509–510t
Milk of Magnesia (magnesium hydroxide), 490–491, 492–493t, 506–507, 511t
Milontin (phensuximide), 245–246, 246t
Milophene (clomiphene), 468
Miltown (meprobamate), 225
Mima, 567t
Mineralocorticoids, 405
Mineral oil (Agoral Plain; Fleet Mineral Oil Enema; Kondremul Plain; Milkinol; Neo-Cultol; Zymenol), 506–507, 509–510t
Minihep (heparin calcium), 351–354
Minipress (prazosin), 312–313
Minocin (minocycline), 562, 567t, 570t, 609–611, 610t, 614t
Minocycline (Minocin), 562, 567t, 570t, 609–611, 610t, 614t
Minoxidil (Loniten), 317–318
Mintezol (thiabendazole), 678
Minute respiratory volume, 533
Miocarpine (pilocarpine), 58
Miochol (acetylcholine, intraocular), 56
Miostat (carbachol, intraocular), 56–57
Miradon (anisindione), 354–356, 356t
Mithracin (plicamycin), 426, 719, 722–724, 729t
Mitomycin (Mutamycin), 719, 722–724, 728t, 741t, 743t, 747–751t, 753t
Mitotane (Lysodren), 724, 730, 734t, 734–736
Mitoxantrone (Novantrone), 709t, 710t, 719, 722–724, 728t, 749t
Mitran (chlordiazepoxide), 217–219, 220–221t
Mitrolan (polycarbophil calcium), 506–507, 508t, 518t
Mixed respiratory vaccine (MRV), 803–804, 805t
M-M-R II (measles, mumps, and rubella vaccine), 803–804, 807t
Moban (molindone), 205–208, 212t
MOB combination chemotherapy, 738, 740, 749t

Mobenol (tolbutamide), 431, 436–437, 439t
Mobidin (magnesium salicylate), 170–171, 173, 176t
Moctanin (monoctanoin), 503–504
Modane (phenolphthalein), 506–507, 513t
Modane Soft (docusate sodium-dioctyl sodium sulfosuccinate), 506–507, 509t
Modecate (fluphenazine), 205–208, 210t
Moderil (rescinnamine), 313–314, 315t
Modicon (ethinyl estradiol/norethindrone), 463, 464t, 466–467
Moditen (fluphenazine), 205–208, 210t
Moducal (glucose polymers), 777t
Moebiquin (iodoquinol), 683
Molecular size, glomerular filtration and, 14
Molindone (Moban), 205–208, 206t, 212t
Mol-Iron (ferrous sulfate), 345–346, 347t
M.O.M. (magnesium hydroxide), 490–491, 492–493t, 506–507, 511t
Mometasone (Elocon), 443, 444t, 445–447, 451t
Monistat-3 (miconazole), 692, 695t, 697
Monistat 7 (miconazole), 692, 695t, 697
Monistat-Derm (miconazole), 692, 695t, 697
Monistat I.V. (miconazole), 691
Monoamine oxidase inhibitors, 234–236, 236t
Monobactam(s), 595–596
Monobenzone (Benoquin), 829
Mono-Chek, 791, 793t
Monocid (cefonicid), 598–600, 604t
Monoclate (antihemophilic factor, human), 361–362
Monoctanoin (Moctanin), 503–504
Mono-Diff Test, 791, 793t
Mono-Gesic (salsalate), 170–171, 173, 177t
Monoject (glucose, oral), 437–438
Monospot, 791, 793t
Monosticon Dri-Dot, 791, 793t
Mono-Sure, 791, 793t
Mono-Test, 791, 793t
8-MOP (methosalen), 827–828, 828t
MOPP-LO BLEO combination chemotherapy, 738, 740, 749t
MOPP combination chemotherapy, 709t, 738, 740, 749t
Moranyl (suramin), 672, 674, 675t, 676–680
Morphine (Astramorph PF; Duramorph-PF; Epimorph; Morphitec; M.O.S.; MS Contin; MSIR; Roxanol; Roxanol SR; RMS; Statex), 157, 158t, 159, 160t
Morphitec (morphine), 157, 159, 160t
Morrhuate sodium (Scleromate), 829t, 829–830
M.O.S. (morphine), 157, 159, 160t
Motion Cure (meclizine), 113–114, 117t, 119
Motofen (difenoxin HCl with atropine sulfate), 514–515
Motrin (ibuprofen), 175, 178, 181t
Moxalactam (Moxam), 598–600, 607–608t
Moxam (moxalactam), 598–600, 607–608t
6-MP (mercaptopurine), 712, 718–719, 721t

MP combination chemotherapy, 738, 740, 749t
MPL + PRED (MP) combination chemotherapy, 738, 740, 749t
M-2 Protocol combination chemotherapy, 738, 740, 748t
MPS papers, 791, 793t
MRV (mixed respiratory vaccine), 803–804, 805t
M-R-Vax II (measles and rubella vaccine), 803–804, 807t
MS Contin (morphine), 157, 158t, 159, 160t
MSIR (morphine), 157, 159, 160t
M sites, 53
MTX (methotrexate), 712, 718–719, 721–722t
MTX + MP combination chemotherapy, 738, 740, 749t
MTX + MP + CTX combination chemotherapy, 738, 740, 750t
Mucin, 483
Mucolytics, 541–542
Mucomyst (acetylcysteine), 541–542
Mucor, 569t
Mucosal edema, 532
Mucosol (acetylcysteine), 541–542
Mucous membrane(s), absorption from, 12–13
Mucous membrane application, 3–4
Multipax (hydroxyzine), 224–225
Multiple-drug reactions, 21
Multistik, 791, 793t
Multistix SG, 791, 793t
Multitest CMI (skin test antigens, multiple), 791, 794t
Mumps skin test antigen, 791, 794t
Mumps vaccine (Mumpsvax), 803–804, 808t
Mumpsvax (mumps vaccine), 803–804, 808t
Murine 2 (tetrahydrozoline), 89, 92, 92t
Muromonab-CD3 (Orthoclone OKT3), 823
Muro's Opcon (naphazoline), 89, 92, 92t
Muscularis externa, 483
Muscularis mucosa, 483
Mustargen (mechlorethamine), 711–712, 716t
Mutamycin (mitomycin), 719, 722–724, 728t
M-VAC combination chemotherapy, 738, 740, 750t
MV combination chemotherapy, 738, 740, 750t
MVPP combination chemotherapy, 738, 740, 750t
MVVPP combination chemotherapy, 738, 740, 750t
Myambutol (ethambutol), 675–658
Myasthenia-like reaction, 25
Mycelex (clotrimazole), 692, 693–694t, 697
Mycifradin (neomycin), 624–626, 628–629t, 630
Myciguent (neomycin), 624–626, 628–629t, 630
Mycil (chlorphenesin), 134–135, 136t
Myclo (clotrimazole), 692, 693–694t, 697
Mycobacterium, 569t

Mycobacterium leprae, 569t
Mycobacterium tuberculosis, 569t, 625t, 655
Mycoplasma hominis, 569t
Mycoplasma pneumoniae, 569t, 609, 619
Mycostatin (nystatin), 692, 695–696t, 697
Mydfrin (phenylephrine), 89, 92, 92t
Mydriacyl (tropicamide), 74–75t
Myelencephalon, 54
Myidil (triprolidine), 113–114, 118t, 119
Myidone (primidone), 240
Mykinac (nystatin), 692, 695–696t, 697
Mylanta, 496–497t
Mylanta II, 496–497t
Mylaxen (hexafluorenium), 133
Myleran (Busulfan), 711–712, 713t
Mylicon (simethicone), 498
Myocardial infarction, 275
Myocardium, 275
Myochrysine (gold sodium thiomalate), 180, 184
Myoepithelial cells, 397
Myolin (orphenadrine citrate), 74–75t, 134–135, 137t
Myotonachol (bethanechol), 57–58
Myproic acid (sodium valproate), 247–248
Mysoline (primidone), 240
Mytelase (ambenonium), 60t, 60–61, 62–63t
Myxedema, 400–401

N

Nabilone (Cesamet), 521t, 523–524
Nadolol (Corgard), 104–105, 105t, 107t, 108t, 109, 303–304, 331, 333
Nadostine (nystatin, oral), 692
Nafazair (naphazoline), 89, 92, 92t
Nafcil (nafcillin), 582, 584–585, 590–591t, 595
Nafcillin (Nafcil; Nalipen; Unipen), 582, 583t, 584–585, 590–591t, 595
Nafrine (oxymetazoline), 88–89, 90–91t
Naftifine (Naftin), 687, 692, 695t, 697
Naftin (naftifine), 692, 695t, 697
Naganol (suramin), 672, 674, 675t, 676–680
Nalbuphine (Nubain), 157, 158t, 159, 165t
Nalcrom (cromolyn intranasal), 554
Naldecon-CX, 538t
Nalfon (fenoprofen), 175, 178, 181t
Nalidixic acid (Neg Gram), 615–616
Nalipen (nafcillin), 582, 584–585, 590–591t, 595
Naloxone (Narcan), 167–168
Naltrexone (Trexan), 168
Nandrobolic (nandrolone phenpropionate), 474–476, 478t, 479
Nandrobolic L.A. (nandrolone decanoate), 474–476, 478t, 479
Nandrolone decanoate (Anabolin L.A.; Androlone-D; Deca-Durabolin; Decolone; Hybolin; Nandrobolic L.A.; Neo-Durabolic), 474–476, 478t, 479
Nandrolone phenpropionate (Anabolin I.M.; Androlone; Durabolin; Hybolin Improved; Nandrobolic), 474–476, 478t, 479

Index

Napamide (disopyramide), 291–292
Naphazoline (Ak-Con; Albalon; Allerest; Clear-Eyes Comfort; Degest-2; Muro's Opcon; Nafazair; Naphcon; privine; VasoClear; Vasocon), 88–89, 90–91t, 92, 92t
Naphcon (naphazoline), 89, 92, 92t
Naphuride (suramin), 672, 674, 675t, 676–680
Naprosyn (naproxen), 175, 178, 183t
Naproxen (Apo-Naproxen; Naxen; Naprosyn; Novonaprox), 175, 178, 183t
Naproxen sodium (Anaprox), 175, 178, 183t
Naqua (trichlormethiazide), 388–389, 391t, 391–392
Narcan (naloxone), 167–168
Narcotic drugs
  abuse of, 838–839
  analgesics, 155, 158t, 160–167t
    agonist-antagonists, 157, 158t, 159–160, 165–167t
    agonists, 157, 158t, 160–165t
    classification of, 155
    endogenous opiates and, 155–157
    long-term use of, 157
    pharmacologic actions of, 155, 156t
  antagonists, 167–168
  antitussive, 537–539
  Controlled Substances Act and, 42, 43t
  Harrison Narcotic Act and, 42
  nurse's role in administration of, 44
    in healthcare institutions, 44
    in home-care settings, 44
  prescribing and dispensing, 42–44
    emergency dispensing of Schedule II drugs and, 43–44
    nonprescription dispensing of Schedule V drugs and, 44
    partial distribution and, 43
Nardil (phenelzine), 234–236, 236t
Nasal administration, in children, 33–34
Nasalcrom (cromolyn intranasal), 554
Nasal decongestants, 88–89, 90t
Nasalide (flunisolide), 443, 445–447, 449–450t
Nasal mucosa, mucosal application and, 4
Natacyn (natamycin), 692
Natamycin (Natacyn), 687, 692
National Formulary (NF), 41
National Laxative (magnesium citrate), 506–507, 510t
Naturetin (bendroflumethiazide), 388–389, 390t, 391–392
Naus-A-Way (phosphorated carbohydrate solution), 525–526
Nauseatol (dimenhydrinate), 113–114, 116t, 119
Nausetrol (phosphorated carbohydrate solution), 525–526
Navane (thiothixene), 205–208, 212t
Naxen (naproxen), 175, 178, 183t
Nebcin (tobramycin), 624–626, 630, 630t
NebuPent (pentamidine), 650–651
Necator americanus, 673t
N.E.E. (ethinyl estradiol/norethindrone), 463, 464t, 466–467
Negatan (negatol), 364
Negatol (Negatan), 364

Neg Gram (nalidixic acid), 615–616
Neisseria, 598
Neisseria gonorrhoeae, 569t, 625t
Neisseria meningitidis, 570t, 609
Nelova 0.5/35E (ethinyl estradiol/norethindrone), 463, 464t, 466–467
Nelova 1/35E (ethinyl estradiol/norethindrone), 463, 464t, 466–467
Nelova 10/11 (ethinyl estradiol/norethindrone), 463, 464t, 466–467
Nemasol (para-aminosalicylate sodium), 655–656
Nembutal (pentobarbital), 193–194, 195t, 197
Neo-Calglucon (calcium glubionate), 426–427, 427t
Neo-Cultol (mineral oil), 506–507, 509–510t
Neocyten (orphenadrine citrate), 134–135, 137t
Neo-Durabolic (nandrolone decanoate), 474–476, 478t, 479
Neo-Fer-50 (ferrous fumarate), 345–346, 347t
Neoloid (castor oil), 506–507, 512t
Neomycin (Mycifradin; Myciguent), 624–626, 625t, 628–629t, 630
Neonatal period, 31
Neoquess (hydroscyamine sulfate), 72–73t
Neosar (cyclophosphamide), 711–712, 715t
Neo-Spray Long Acting (xylometazoline), 88–89, 90–91t
Neostigmine, 60t, 60–61, 62–63t
Neo-Synephrine (phenylephrine), 89, 92, 92t
Neo-Synephrine (phenylephrine parenteral), 88
Neo-Synephrine 12 Hour (oxymetazoline), 88–89, 90–91t
Neo-Synephrine II (xylometazoline), 88–89, 90–91t
Neo-Synephrinol (pseudoephedrine), 88–89, 90–91t
Neo-Tetrine (tetracycline), 609–611, 613t
Neothylline (dyphylline), 545–547, 548t, 549, 551
Neotran (meprobamate), 225
Neo-Tric (metronidazole), 683–685
Neotrizine (sulfonamides, multiple), 573–575, 578t
NephrAmine (amino-acid formulation for renal failure), 780
Nephro-Mag (magnesium), 776t
Nephronex (nitrofurantoin), 639–640
Nephrotoxicity, 25
Neptazane (methazolamide), 376–377, 378t
Nervous system, 49–55
  central. *See* Central nervous system
  neurohormonal function and, 49–50, 52
    sequence of neurotransmission and, 50, 52
  peripheral, 49, 50t
    autonomic branch of, 49, 50t, 51t
    mechanism of drug action on, 52–53
    somatic branch of, 49
Nesacaine (chloroprocaine), 139–141, 140t, 142t
Nestrex (vitamin B_6), 760–761
Net filtration pressure (NFP), 373

Netilmicin (Netromycin), 567–571t, 624–626, 625t, 629t, 630
Netromycin (netilmicin), 624–626, 629t, 630
Neurohormones, 49–50, 52
  biosynthesis of, 50
  drug action and, 18
  inactivation of, 52
  interaction with postsynaptic membrane, 52
  release of, 50, 52
  repolarization of synaptic membrane and, 52
  sequence of neurotransmission and, 50, 52
  storage of, 50
Neurohypophysis, 395
  hormones of, 396–397, 409–414
Neuromuscular blocking agents, 128–133
  antidepolarizing, 128–132
  depolarizing, 132–133
  plasma cholinesterase inhibitor, 133
Neuron(s), 49
  expiratory, 535
  inspiratory, 535
Neuronal release, blockade of, drug interactions and, 27
Neuronal uptake, blockade of, drug interactions and, 27
Neurotoxicity, 25
Neurotransmitters. *See* Neurohormones
Neut (sodium bicarbonate), 784t, 785
Neutra-Phos (phosphorus), 776t
Neutra-Phos-K (phosphorus), 776t
NF. *See National Formulary*
NFP. *See* Net filtration pressure
Niac (vitamin B_3), 759–760
Niacels (vitamin B_3), 759–760
Niacin (nicotinic acid), 758t, 760
Niazide (trichlormethiazide), 388–389, 391t, 391–392
Nicardipine (Cardene), 313, 329–331, 331t, 332t
Niclocide (niclosamide), 674, 676
Niclosamide (Niclocide), 673t, 674, 676
Nico-400 (vitamin B_3), 759–760
Nicobid (vitamin B_3), 759–760
Nicolar (vitamin B_3), 759–760
Nicotine, 841
Nicotinex (vitamin B_3), 759–760
Nicotinic acid (niacin; vitamin B_3), 758t, 759–760
Nicotinic acid-niacin, 342–343
Nifedipine (Adalat; Procardia), 329–331, 331t, 332t
Niferex (polysaccharide-iron complex), 345–346, 347t
Niloric (ergoloid mesylates), 334
Nilstat (nystatin), 692, 695–696t, 697
Nimbus, 791, 793t
Nimodipine (Nimotop), 329–331, 331t, 332t
Nimotop (nimodipine), 329–331, 331t, 332t
Nipride (nitroprusside), 319–320
Niridazole (Ambilhar), 672, 673t, 674, 675t, 676–680
Nitrazine Paper, 791, 793t
Nitrites/nitrates, 325–326, 327–329t, 329

Nitro-Bid (nitroglycerin, topical ointment), 435–436, 328t, 329
Nitro-Bid (nitroglycerin, sustained release), 435–436, 328t, 329
Nitro-Bid IV (nitroglycerin, injection), 325–326, 328–329t, 329
Nitro-Dur (nitroglycerin transdermal systems), 325–326, 329, 329t
Nitrocine (nitroglycerin transdermal systems), 325–326, 329, 329t
Nitrodisc (nitroglycerin transdermal systems), 325–326, 329, 329t
Nitrofan (nitrofurantoin), 639–640
Nitrofurantoin (Apo-Nitrofurantoin; Furadantin; Furalan; Furan; Furanite; Nephronex; Nitrofan; Novofuran), 571t, 637, 639–640
Nitrofurantoin macrocrystals (Macrodantin), 639–640
Nitrofurazone (Furacin), 649–650
Nitrogard (nitroglycerin, transmucosal), 435–436, 328t, 329
Nitrogen Mustard (mechlorethamine), 711–712, 716t
Nitroglycerin
  injection (Nitrostat IV; Nitro-Bid IV; Tridil), 325–326, 328–329t, 329
  sublingual (Nitrostat), 325–326, 327t, 329
  sustained release (Nitro-Bid; Nitrospan; Nitrostat SR), 435–436, 328t, 329
  topical ointment (Nitro-Bid; Nitrol; Nitrong; Nitrostat), 435–436, 328t, 329
  translingual (Nitrolingual), 325–326, 327–328t, 329
  transmucosal (Nitrogard), 435–436, 328t, 329
Nitroglycerin transdermal systems (Deponit; Nitrocine; Nitrodisc; Nitro-Dur; Transderm-Nitro), 325–326, 329, 329t
Nitrol (nitroglycerin, topical ointment), 435–436, 328t, 329
Nitrolingual (nitroglycerin, translingual), 325–326, 327–328t, 329
Nitrong (nitroglycerin, topical ointment), 435–436, 328t, 329
Nitropress (nitroprusside), 319–320
Nitroprusside (Nipride; Nitropress), 319–320
Nitrospan (nitroglycerin, sustained release), 435–436, 328t, 329
Nitrostat (nitroglycerin, sublingual), 325–326, 327t, 329
Nitrostat (nitroglycerin, topical ointment), 435–436, 328t, 329
Nitrostat IV (nitroglycerin, injection), 325–326, 328–329t, 329
Nitrostat SR (nitroglycerin, sustained release), 435–436, 328t, 329
Nitrous oxide, 146
Nizatidine (Axid), 119, 121–122, 122t
Nizoral (ketoconazole), 690–691, 692, 694t, 697
N-Multistix, 791, 793t
N-Multistix-C, 791, 793t
N-Multistix-SG, 791, 793t
Nobesine (diethylpropion), 265–267, 268t

Nocardia, 570t
Noctec (chloral hydrate), 199–200
Nodose ganglion, vomiting and, 489
No Doz (caffeine), 263–264
Nolestrin 1/50 (ethinyl estradiol/norethindrone), 463, 464t, 466–467
Noludar (methyprylon), 202
Nolvadex (tamoxifen), 724, 730, 734t, 734–736
Nondiastatic barley malt extract (Maltsupex), 506–507, 508t
Nonnarcotic analgesics, 170–175
  para-aminophenol derivatives, 173–174
  pyrazolones, 174–175
  salicylates, 170–171, 172, 173, 176–177t
Nonsteroidal antiinflammatory drugs (NSAIDs), 175, 178, 181–183t
Norcept-E 1/35 (ethinyl estradiol/norethindrone), 463, 464t, 466–467
Norcuron (vecuronium), 131–132
Nordette (ethinyl estradiol/levonorgestrel), 463, 464t, 466–467
Norepinephrine (Levarterenol; Levophed), 79, 83
Norethin 1/35E (ethinyl estradiol/norethindrone), 463, 464t, 466–467
Norethin 1/50M (mestranol/norethindrone), 463, 464t, 466–467
Norethindrone (Micronor; Norlutin; Nor-Q.D.), 456, 459, 460t, 461
Norethindrone acetate (Aygestin; Norlutate), 456, 459, 460t, 461
Norflex (orphenadrine citrate), 74–75t, 134–135, 137t
Norflex (orphenadrine HCl), 258–259, 259–260t
Norfloxacin (Noroxin), 568–571t, 616
Norgestrel (Ovrette), 456, 459, 460t, 461
Norinyl 1 + 35 (ethinyl estradiol/norethindrone), 463, 464t, 466–467
Norinyl 1 + 50 (mestranol/norethindrone), 463, 464t, 466–467
Norinyl 1 + 80 (mestranol/norethindrone), 463, 464t, 466–467
Norinyl 2 mg (mestranol/norethindrone), 463, 464t, 466–467
Norisodrine (isoproterenol), 84–85
Norlestrin 2.5/50 (ethinyl estradiol/norethindrone), 463, 464t, 466–467
Norlutate (norethindrone acetate), 456, 459, 460t, 461
Norlutin (norethindrone), 456, 459, 460t, 461
Normodyne (labetalol), 104–105, 105t, 106t, 108t, 109, 305, 310
Noropurol (allopurinol), 188–189
Noroxin (norfloxacin), 616
Norpace (disopyramide), 291–292
Norpace CR (disopyramide), 291–292
Norpanth (propantheline bromide), 76–77t
Norpramin (desipramine), 227–230, 228t, 231t
Nor-Q.D. (norethindrone), 456, 459, 460t, 461, 463, 464t, 466–467
North American coral snake antivenin (Antivenin *Micrurus fulvius*), 808–809, 809t
Nortriptyline (Aventyl; Pamelor), 227–230, 228t, 232t

Nosocomial infections, 563
Novafed (pseudoephedrine), 88–89, 90–91t
Novahistine Expectorant, 538t
Novamine (crystalline amino-acid infusion), 779–780
Novamobarb (amobarbital), 193–194, 195t, 197
Novamoxin (amoxicillin), 582, 584–585, 586t, 595
Novantrone (mitoxantrone), 719, 722–724, 728t
Nova Phenicol (chloramphenicol), 643–644
Nova-Rectal (pentobarbital), 193–194, 195t, 197
Novobiocin (Albamycin), 650
Novobutamide (tolbutamide), 431, 436–437, 439t
Novobutazone (phenylbutazone), 174–175
Novocain (procaine), 139–141, 140t, 143t
Novocell (oxidized cellulose), 364–365
Novochlorhydrate (chloral hydrate), 199–200
Novochlorpromazine (chlorpromazine), 205–208, 209t
Novocimetine (cimetidine), 119, 121–122, 122t
Novoclopate (clorazepate), 217–219, 221t
Novocloxin (cloxacillin), 582, 584–585, 589t, 595
Novodigoxin (digoxin), 281–283, 284t
Novodipam (diazepam), 217–219, 221–222t, 249
Novoferrogluc (ferrous gluconate), 345–346, 347t
Novoferrosulfa (ferrous sulfate), 345–346, 347t
Novofibrate (clofibrate), 339–340
Novoflupam (flurazepam), 198–199, 200t
Novofolacid (folic acid), 349–350
Novofumar (ferrous fumarate), 345–346, 347t
Novofuran (nitrofurantoin), 639–640
Novohexidyl (trihexyphenidyl), 74–75t, 258–259, 260t
Novohydrazide (hydrochlorothiazide), 388–389, 390t, 391–392
Novolexin (cephalexin), 598–600, 601–602t
Novolin L (insulin zinc suspension, human), 429–431, 435t
Novolin N (isophane insulin suspension, human), 429–431, 436t
Novolin R (insulin injection, human), 429–431, 435t
Novolorazem (lorazepam), 217–219, 222t
Novomedopa (methyldopa), 311–312
Novomepro (meprobamate), 225
Novomethacin (indomethacin), 175, 178, 182t
Novometoprol (metoprolol), 331
Novomucilax (psyllium), 506–507, 508t
Novonaprox (naproxen), 175, 178, 183t
Novoniacin (vitamin B_3), 759–760
Novonidazol (metronidazole), 683–685
Novopen-VK (penicillin V; penicillin V, potassium), 582, 584–585, 593t, 595
NovopenG (penicillin G, potassium or sodium), 582, 584–585, 591–592t, 595

Novopentobarb (pentobarbital), 193–194, 195t, 197
Novoperidol (haloperidol), 205–208, 212t
Novopheniram (chlorpheniramine), 113–114, 115t, 119
Novopirocam (piroxicam), 175, 178, 183t
Novopoxide (chlordiazepoxide), 217–219, 220–221t
Novopramine (imipramine), 227–230, 231–232t
Novopranol (propranolol), 296–297, 331
Novoprofen (ibuprofen), 175, 178, 181t
Novopropamide (chlorpropamide), 431, 436–437, 438t
Novopropanthil (propantheline bromide), 76–77t
Novopropoxyn (propoxyphene), 157, 159, 162t
Novoquinidin (quinidine), 287, 289
Novoquinine (quinine sulfate), 669–670
Novoreserpine (reserpine), 313–314, 315t
Novoridazine (thioridazine), 205–208, 211t
Novorythro Base (erythromycin base), 619–620, 621t
Novorythro Estolate (erythromycin estolate), 619–620, 621–622t
Novorythro Stearate (erythromycin stearate), 619–620, 623t
Novosalmol (albuterol), 94–95, 96–97t
Novosemide (furosemide), 377–378, 382–383, 384t
Novosorbide (isosorbide dinitrate), 325–326, 327t, 329
Novosoxazole (sulfisoxazole), 573–575, 577–578t
Novospiroton (spironolactone), 387–388
Novotetra (tetracycline), 609–611, 613t
Novothalidone (chlorthalidone), 388–389, 390t, 391–392
Novotriphyl (oxytriphylline), 545–547, 548–549t, 549, 551
Novotriptyn (amitriptyline), 227–230, 231t
Novoxapam (oxazepam), 217–219, 222t
Nozinan (methotrimeprazine), 215
NPH Iletin I (isophane insulin suspension), 429–431, 436t
NPH Iletin II (isophane insulin suspension, purified), 429–431, 436t
NPH Insulin (isophane insulin suspension), 429–431, 436t
NPH Purified Pork (isophane insulin suspension, purified), 429–431, 436t
NSAIDs. See Nonsteroidal antiinflammatory drugs
N sites, 53
Nubain (nalbuphine), 157, 158t, 159, 165t
Nuclease (nucleotidase), 488t
Nucleotidase (nuclease), 488t
Nucofed, 538t
Nu-Iron (polysaccharide-iron complex), 345–346, 347t
Numorphan (oxymorphone), 157, 158t, 159, 161t
Nupercainal (dibucaine), 139–141, 140t, 142t
Nuprin (ibuprofen), 175, 178, 181t
Nurse(s)
 role in administration of controlled drugs, 44
 in healthcare institutions, 44
 in home-care settings, 44
 role in carrying out medication orders, 44–45
 clarifying and evaluating written orders and, 45
 responsibility for errors in administration and, 45
 telephone orders and, 45
Nursing care plan
 for patient compliance with prescribed drug regimen, 38–39
 for patients treated with antibacterial drugs, 564–566
 for patients treated with antidiabetic agents, 432–435
 for patients treated with antihistamine drugs, 120–121
 for patients treated with benzodiazepine antianxiety drugs, 219-220
 for patients treated with beta-adrenergic blockers, 109–111
 for patients treated with diuretic drugs, 379–382
 for patients treated with H$_2$-receptor antagonists, 123
 for patients treated with methylxanthine bronchodilators, 550–551
 for patients treated with nondiuretic antihypertensive drugs, 306–309
 for patients treated with nonsteroidal antiinflammatory drugs, 179–180
 for patients whose knowledge of drug regimen is deficient, 23–25
Nutritional supplements
 oral, 774–775, 776–778t, 778
 parenteral, 778–782, 783–785t
Nyaderm (nystatin), 692, 695–696t, 697
Nydrazid (isoniazid), 659–660
Nylidrin (Adrin; Arlidin; PMS Nylidrin), 96–98, 334
Nystatin (Mycostatin; Mykinac; Nilstat; Nyaderm; Nystex; O-V Statin), 568t, 687, 692, 695–696t, 697
 oral (Mycostatin; Nadostine; Nilstat), 692
Nystex (nystatin), 692, 695–696t, 697
Nytilax (sennosides A&B-calcium salts), 506–507, 513t

O

OAP combination chemotherapy, 738, 740, 750t
Occlusal (salicylic acid), 170–171, 173, 177t
OCL (polyethylene glycol-electrolyte solution), 506–507, 511t
Octamide (metoclopramide), 534–535
Octreotide (Sandostatin), 824
Ocufen (flurbiprofen), 175, 178, 181t
Ocular toxicity, 25
Ocusert Pilo (pilocarpine ocular therapeutic system), 58–59
Off-Ezy (salicylic acid), 170–171, 173, 177t
O'Flex (orphenadrine citrate), 74–75t, 134–135, 137t
Ogen (estropipate), 454–456, 458t
Oil of wintergreen (methyl salicylate), 170–171, 173, 177t
Omega-3 polyunsaturated fatty acids, 778t
Omnipaque, 799, 802t
Omnipen (ampicillin), 582, 584–585, 586–587t, 595
Onchocerca volvulus, 673t
Oncovin (vincristine), 719, 722–724, 730t
Ophthacet (sulfacetamide), 573–575, 575–576t
Ophthaine (proparacaine), 139–141, 140t, 143t
Ophthalmic administration, 4–5
 in children, 33–34
Ophthalmic decongestants, 89, 92, 92t
Ophthetic (proparacaine), 139–141, 140t, 143t
Ophthochlor (chloramphenicol), 643–644
Opiate(s). See Narcotic drugs
Opiate receptors, 155, 156t
Opisthorchis viverrini, 673t
Opium (Paregoric; Pantopan), 157, 159, 161t
Opium tincture, camphorated (Paregoric), 516
Opt-Ease (tetrahydrozoline), 89, 92, 92t
Opticrom 4% (cromolyn ophthalmic), 554
Optimine (azatidine), 113–114, 115t, 119
Ora-Testryl (fluoxymesterone), 474–476, 477t, 479, 724, 730, 731t, 734–736
Oragrafin Calcium, 799, 802t
Oragrafin Sodium, 799, 802t
Oral administration, 6
 absorption and, in children, 31
 in children, 33
Oral calcium salts, 426–427, 427t
Oral electrolyte mixture (Gastrolyte Oral; Infalyte; Lytren; Pedialyte; Resol; Rehydralyte), 776t
Oral mucosa, mucosal application and, 4
Oral nutritional supplements, 774–775, 776–778t, 778
Oramide (tolbutamide), 431, 436–437, 439t
Orap (pimozide), 214
Orasone (prednisone), 724, 730, 733t, 734–736
Orazinc (zinc sulfate), 776t
Orbenin (cloxacillin), 582, 584–585, 589t, 595
Oreton (methyltestosterone), 474–476, 477t, 479
Oreton Methyl (methyltestosterone), 724, 730, 731t, 734–736
Organ function, changes in, with age, 36, 37t
Organidin (iodinated glycerol), 540–541
Organ toxicity, of antimicrobials, 563
Orimune (poliovirus vaccine, live oral trivalent-TOPV, Sabin), 803–804, 808t
Orinase (tolbutamide), 431, 436–437, 439t
Orinase Diagnostic (tolbutamide sodium), 791, 798t
Orphanate (orphenadrine citrate), 134–135, 137t
Orphenadrine citrate (Banflex; Flexon; Flexoject; K-Flex; Marflex; Myolin; Neo-

cyten; Norflex; O'Flex; Orphanate), 67–70, 74–75t, 134–135, 137t
Orphenadrine hydrochloride (Disipal; Norflex), 74–75t, 258–259, 259–260t
Orthoclone OKT3 (muromonab-CD3), 823
Ortho Dienestrol (dienestrol), 454–456, 457t
Ortho-Novum 1/35 (ethinyl estradiol/norethindrone), 463, 464t, 466–467
Ortho-Novum 1/50 (mestranol/norethindrone), 463, 464t, 466–467
Ortho-Novum 7/7/7 (ethinyl estradiol/norethindrone), 463, 464t, 466–467
Ortho-Novum 10/11 (ethinyl estradiol/norethindrone), 463, 464t, 466–467
Orudis (ketoprofen), 175, 178, 182t
Osmitrol (mannitol), 385–386
Osmoglyn (glycerin), 383–385
Osmotics, 383–386
  sites of action and electrolyte disturbances and, 377t
OTC. *See* Over-the-counter drugs
Otic administration, 5
  in children, 33–34
Ototoxicity, 25
Otrivin (xylometazoline), 88–89, 90–91t
Ovcon-35 (ethinyl estradiol/norethindrone), 463, 464t, 466–467
Ovcon-50 (ethinyl estradiol/norethindrone), 463, 464t, 466–467
Over-the-counter (OTC) drugs, patient education for, 6
Ovol (simethicone), 498
Ovral (ethinyl estradiol/norethindrone), 463, 464t, 466–467, 463, 464t, 466–467
Ovrette (norgestrel), 456, 459, 460t, 461, 463, 464t, 466–467
O-V Statin (nystatin), 692, 695–696t, 697
Ovulation stimulants, 467–470
Ovulen (mestranol/ethynodiol diacetate), 463, 464t, 466–467
Ovu STICK Self-Test, 791, 793t
Ovu STICK Urine hLH, 791, 793t
Oxacillin (Bactocil; Prostaphlin), 582, 583t, 584–585, 591t, 595
Oxamniquine (Vansil), 673t, 676
Oxandrolone (Anavar), 474–476, 478t, 479
Oxazepam (Apo-Oxazepam; Novoxapam; Ox-Pam; Serax; Zapex; Zaxopam), 217–219, 218t, 222t
Oxazolidinediones, 243–245, 245t
Ox bile extract, 500–501
Ox bile extract with iron (Bilron), 500–501
Oxiconazole (Oxistat), 687, 692, 696t, 697
Oxidation, biotransformation and, 14
Oxidized cellulose (Novocell; Oxycel; Surgicel), 364–365
Oxistat (oxiconazole), 692, 696t, 697
Ox-Pam (oxazepam), 217–219, 222t
Oxsoralen (methoxsalen), 827–828, 828t
Oxybutazone (oxyphenbutazone), 174–175
Oxybutynin chloride (Ditropan), 67–70, 72–73t
Oxycel (oxidized cellulose), 364–365
Oxyclean (salicylic acid), 170–171, 173, 177t
Oxycodone (Roxicodone; Supeudol), 157, 158t, 159, 161t

Oxydess II (dextroamphetamine sulfate), 264–265, 266t
Oxygen transport, 534
Oxymetazoline (Afrin; Dristan Long Lasting; Nafrine; Neosynephrine 12 Hour; Sinex Long Lasting), 88–89, 90–91t
Oxymetholone (Anadrol-50; Anapolin 50), 474–476, 478–479t, 479
Oxymorphone (Numorphan), 157, 158t, 159, 161t
Oxyphencyclimine hydrochloride (Daricon), 74–75t
Oxyphenbutazone (Oxybutazone; Tandearil), 174–175
Oxyphencyclimine, 67–70
Oxyphenonium bromide (Antrenyl), 67–70, 76–77t
Oxytetracycline (E.P. Mycin; Terramycin; Uri-Tet), 609–611, 610t, 613t
Oxytocics, nonhypophyseal, 413–414
Oxytocin, 395, 397
  control of secretion and actions of, 397
  galactokinetic action and, 397
  oxytocic action and, 397
  nasal (Syntocinon), 412–413
  parenteral (Pitocin; Syntocinon), 412–413
Oxytriphylline (Apo-Oxytriphylline; Choledyl; Chophylline; Novotriphyl), 545–547, 548–549t, 549, 551

P

P-50 (penicillin G, potassium or sodium), 582, 584–585, 591–592t, 595
PABA (para-aminobenzoic acid), 778t
Pabanol (para-aminobenzoic acid), 778t
PAC-5 combination chemotherapy, 738, 740, 750t
Pacemaker, cardiac, 276
PA combination chemotherapy, 738, 740, 750t
Paget's disease, 424
PAH (para-aminohippuric acid), 374t, 791, 795t
Pain, sensation and perception of, narcotic analgesics and, 156
Palace (megestrol acetate), 456, 459, 460t, 461
Palafer (ferrous fumarate), 345–346, 347t
Palaron (aminophylline), 545–547, 548t, 549, 551
Palmiron (ferrous fumarate), 345–346, 347t
PAM (pralidoxime chloride), 65
PAM (melphalan), 711–712, 717t
Pamelor (nortriptyline), 227–230, 228t, 232t
Pamine (methscopolamine bromide), 76–77t
Panafil (papain), 818, 819t
Pan-C-500 (bioflavonoids), 777t
Pancreas, 402–404
  adrenergic drug effects on, 81t
  disorders of glucose metabolism and, 403–404
  hormones of, 402–403

Pancrease (pancrelipase), 502
Pancreatic amylase (amylopepsin), 488t
Pancreatic enzymes, 502
Pancreatic lipase (steapsin), 488t
Pancreatin (Dizymes; Hi-Vegi-Lip), 502
Pancrelipase (Cotazym; Creon; Festal II; Ilozyme; Ku-Zyme HP; Pancrease; Viokase), 502
Pancuronium (Pavulon), 130–131
Panhematin (hemin), 820–821
Panmycin (tetracycline), 609–611, 613t
Panol (dexpanthenol), 816–817
Panthoderm (dexpanthenol), 816–817
Pantopan (opium), 157, 159, 161t
Pantothenic acid (vitamin B$_5$), 758t, 760
Panwarfin (warfarin sodium), 354–356, 356t
Papain (Panafil), 818, 819t
Papaverine (Cerespan; Pavabid; Paverolan), 334–335
Papilla, renal, 371
Para-aminobenzoic acid (PABA; Pabanol; Potaba; RV Paba Stick), 778t
Para-aminohippuric acid (PAH), 374t
Para-aminophenol derivatives, 173–174
Para-aminosalicylate sodium (Nemasol; PAS; P.A.S. Sodium; Teebacin), 655–656
l-Paracaine (proparacaine), 139–141, 140t, 143t
Paradione (paramethadione), 243–245, 245t
Paraflex (chlorzoxazone), 134–135, 136t
Parafollicular cells, 400
Parafon Forte DSC (chlorzoxazone), 134–135, 136t
Paragonimus westermani, 673t
Paral (paraldehyde), 202–203
Paraldehyde (Paral), 202–203
Paralysis agitans, 253. *See also* Antiparkinsonian drugs
Paramethadione (Paradione), 243–245, 245t
Paramethasone (Haldrone), 443, 444t, 445–447, 451t
Paraplatin (carboplatin), 711–712, 713t
Parasympathetic division, of autonomic nervous system, 49, 50t, 51t
Parathar (teriparatide), 791, 798t
Parathyroid drugs, 424–428
Parathyroid glands, 401
  disorders of, 401
Parathyroid hormone (PTH), 401, 424
Paraventricular nuclei, 395
Paredrine (hydroxyamphetamine), 89, 92, 92t
Paregoric (opium tincture, camphorated), 157, 159, 161t, 516
Parenteral administration, 6–10
  absorption and, 12
  intraamniotic, 10
  intraarterial, 8
  intraarticular, 10
  intracardiac, 10
  intradermal, 10
  intramuscular, 8–10, *9*
  intraperitoneal, 10
  intrapleural, 10
  intrathecal, 10
  intravenous, 6–8, *7*
  subcutaneous, 8, *8*

Parenteral nutritional supplements, 778–782, 783–785t
Parepectolin, 518t
Pargyline (Eutonyl), 321
Parkinson's disease, 253. *See also* Antiparkinsonian drugs
Parlodel (bromocriptine), 256–257, 816
Par-Mag (magnesium oxide), 490–491, 494–495t
Parnate (tranylcypromine), 234–236, 236t
Paromomycin (Humatin), 673t, 681, 685
Parsidol (ethopropazine), 74–75t, 258–259, 259t
Parsitan (ethopropazine), 74–75t, 258–259, 259t
Pars nervosa, 395
Partial pressure, 534
Particle size, inhalation application and, 5
Parvolex (acetylcysteine), 541–542
PAS (para-aminosalicylate sodium), 655–656
P.A.S. Sodium (para-aminosalicylate sodium), 655–656
Pastuerella multocida, 570t
Pasteurella pestis, 572t
Pathilon (tridihexethyl chloride), 76–77t
Pathocil (dicloxacillin), 582, 584–585, 589t, 595
Pathologic conditions, drug effects and, 17
Pavabid (papaverine), 334–335
Paveral (codeine), 157, 159, 160t, 537–538
Paverolan (papaverine), 334–335
Pavulon (pancuronium), 130–131
Paxarel (acetylcarbromal), 198
Paxipam (halazepam), 217–219, 218t, 222t
PBZ (tripelennamine), 113–114, 118t, 119
PCE (erythromycin base), 619–620, 621t
PCV combination chemotherapy, 738, 740, 750t
PDP Liquid Protein (protein hydrosylates), 778t
PEB combination chemotherapy, 738, 740, 750t
PectoKay, 518t
Pediaflor (fluoride), 775, 778
Pedialyte (oral electrolyte mixture), 776t
Pediamycin (erythromycin ethylsuccinate), 619–620, 622t
Pediatric pharmacology, 31–34
 administration route and, 33–34
  intramuscular, 33
  intravenous, 33
  oral, 33
  rectal, 33
  topical and local, 33–34
 drug dosage and, 32–33
 factors affecting therapeutic response and, 31–32
  absorption and, 31
  biotransformation and, 32
  distribution and, 31–32
  excretion and, 32
Pedicels, 371
Peganone (ethotoin), 240–243, 244t
Pelamine (tripelennamine), 113–114, 118t, 119
Pemoline (Cylert), 269–270
Penbutolol (Levatol), 104–105, 105t, 107t, 108t, 109, 303–304

Penglobe (bacampicillin), 582, 584–585, 588t, 595
Penicillamine (Cuprimine; Depen), 185–186
Penicillin(s), 374t, 582, 584–586, 586–594t
 antipseudomonal, 570t
 bacterial resistance to, 582
 broad-spectrum, 584
 extended-spectrum, 584
 general characteristics of, 583t
 natural, 582
 penicillinase-resistant, 571t, 584
 semisynthetic derivatives, 582, 584
Penicillin G, 562, 567–572t, 582, 583t
 benzathine (Bicillin; Megacillin; Permapen), 582, 584–585, 592t, 595
 benzathine and procaine (Bicillin C-R), 582, 584–585, 593t, 595
 procaine (Ayercillin; Crystocillin A.S.; Duracillin A.S.; Pfizerpen-AS; Wycillin), 582, 584–585, 592–593t, 595
 potassium or sodium (Crystapen; Megacillin; Novopen G; P-50; Pentids; Pfizerpen G), 582, 584–585, 591–592t, 595
Penicillin V (Apo-Pen-VK; Novopen-VK; Pen-Vee K; V-Cillin K), 571t, 582, 583t, 584–585, 593t, 595
 potassium (Apo-Pen-VK; Novopen-VK; Pen-Vee K; V-Cillin K), 582, 584–585, 593t, 595
Pentaerythritol tetranitrate (P.E.T.N.; Peritrate), 325–326, 329, 329t
Pentagastrin (Peptavlon), 791, 797t
Pentam 300 (pentamidine), 650–651
Pentamidine (NebuPent; Pentam 300), 570t, 650–651
Pentamycetin (chloramphenicol), 643–644
Pentazocine (Talwin), 157, 159, 166–167t
Penthrane (methoxyflurane), 148–149
Pentids (penicillin G, potassium or sodium), 582, 584–585, 591–592t, 595
Pentobarbital (Nembutal; Nova-Rectal; Novopentobarb; Pentogen), 193–194, 195t, 197
Pentogen (pentobarbital), 193–194, 195t, 197
Pentothal (thiopental), 149–151, 150t
Pentoxifylline (Trental), 357–358
Pen-Vee K (penicillin V; penicillin V, potassium), 582, 584–585, 593t, 595
Pepcid (famotidine), 119, 121–122, 122t
Pepsin (pepsinogen), 488t, 500
Pepsinogen (pepsin), 488t
Peptavlon (pentagastrin), 791, 797t
Pepto-Bismol, 518t
Peptol (cimetidine), 119, 121–122, 122t
Pergolide (Permax), 258
Pergonal (human menopausal gonadotropins), 468–469
Periactin (cyproheptadine), 124
Peridin (bioflavonoids), 777t
Peridol (haloperidol), 205–208, 212t
Peripheral nervous system, 49, 50t
 mechanism of drug action on, 52–53
 receptor concept and, 52t, 53
 types of drug action and, 52–53

Peritrate (pentaerythritol tetranitrate), 325–326, 329, 329t
Peritubular capillaries, 371
Permapen (penicillin G, benzathine), 582, 584–585, 592t, 595
Permax (pergolide), 258
Permitil (fluphenazine), 205–208, 210t
Perphenazine (Apo-Perphenazine; Phenazine; PMS Levazine; Trilafon), 205–208, 206t, 210t, 521t
Persantine (dipyridamole), 333
Pertofrane (desipramine), 227–230, 228t, 231t
Pertussin (dextromethorphan), 539
Pethadol (meperidine), 157, 158t, 159, 163t
P.E.T.N. (pentaerythritol tetranitrate), 325–326, 329, 329t
Pfizerpen-AS (penicillin G, procaine), 582, 584–585, 592–593t, 595
Pfizerpen G (penicillin G, potassium or sodium), 582, 584–585, 591–592t, 595
pH
 gastric, alterations in, drug interactions and, 28
 urinary, alterations in, drug interactions and, 29
Pharmacodynamic agents, 16
Pharmacodynamics, 16–18
 factors modifying drug effects and, 17–18
 mechanism of drug action and, 18
 non-receptor-mediated drug effects and, 17
 potency versus efficacy and, 16
 therapeutic index and, 16–17
Pharmacogenetics, 20
Pharmacokinetics, 11–15
 absorption and, 11–13
 biotransformation and, 11, 13–14
 distribution and, 11, 13
 excretion and, 11, 14–15
Pharynx, major activities of, 485
Phazyme (simethicone), 498
Phenacemide (Phenurone), 249–250
Phenanthrenes, 160–161t, 165–166t
Phenazine (perphenazine), 205–208, 210t
Phenazo (phenazopyridine), 641
Phenazopyridine (Phenazo; Pyridium; Pyronium), 637, 641
Phenbuff (phenylbutazone), 174–175
Phencyclidine, 839–840
Phendimetrazine, 265–267, 268t
Phenelzine (Nardil), 234–236, 236t
Phenergan (promethazine), 113–114, 117t, 119
Phenergan VC with Codeine, 538t
Phenergan with Codeine, 538t
Phenindamine, 114t
Phenistix, 791, 793t
Phenmetrazine (Preludin), 265–267, 268t
Phenobarbital, 193–194, 196t, 197, 238–240, 241t
Phenolphthalein (Alophen; Espotabs; Ex-Lax; Feen-A-Mint; Fructines-Vichy; Modane), 506–507, 513t
Phenol red (phenolsulfonphthalein), 374t
Phenolsulfonphthalein (Phenol red; PSP), 374t

Phenothiazines, 114t, 205–208, 206t, 209–211t
  antiemetic, 521t
Phenoxybenzamine (Dibenzyline), 102–103, 321
Phensuximide (Milontin), 245–246, 246t
Phentermine (Ionamin), 265–267, 268t
Phentolamine (Regitine; Rogatine), 103, 321
Phenurone (phenacemide), 249–250
Phenylalanine Mustard (melphalan), 711–712, 717t
Phenylbutazone (Apo-Phenylbutazone; Azolid; Butazolidin; Intrabutazone; Novobutazone; Phenbuff), 174–175
Phenylephrine (Ak-Dilate; Ak-Nefrin; Isopto Frin; Mydfrin; Neo-Synephrine), 88–89, 90–91t, 92, 92t
  parenteral (Neo-Synephrine), 88
Phenylpiperidines, 163–165t
Phenylpropanolamine (Acutrim; Dexatrim; Diadax; Prolamine; Propagest; Rhindecon; Sucrets Cold Decongestant Lozenge), 88–89, 90–91t, 265–267, 269t
Phenytoin (Dilantin; Dilantin Infatab; Dilantin-30 Pediatric; Dilantin-125; Diphenylan), 240–243, 244t, 288t, 293–294
Phenytoin sodium
  extended (Dilantin Kapseals), 240–243, 244t
  parenteral (Dilantin), 240–243, 244t
  prompt (Diphenylan), 240–243, 244t
Pheochromocytoma, 405
Phos-Flur (fluoride), 775, 778
Phosphaljel (aluminum phosphate gel), 490–491, 492–493t
Phosphate (potassium phosphate; sodium phosphate), 783–784t, 785
Phospholine Iodide (echothiophate), 61–64
Phosphorated carbohydrate solution (Calm-X; Emetrol; Naus-A-Way; Nausetrol), 525–526
Phosphorus (K-Phos Neutral; Neutra-Phos; Neutra-Phos-K; Uro-KP-Neutral), 776t
Phospho-Soda (sodium phosphate and sodium biphosphate), 506–507, 511t
Photoallergic reaction, 20
Photosensitivity, 20, 25
Phototoxic reaction, 20
Phyllocontin (aminophylline), 545–547, 548t, 549, 551
Physical dependence, 836
Physiological state, drug interactions and, 26
Physiologic dead space, 533
Physostigmine
  ophthalmic (Eserine; Isopto-Eserine), 59
  systemic (Antilirium), 59
Phytonadione (AquaMEPHYTON; K₁; Konakion; Mephyton; vitamin K₁), 356–357, 771t, 771–772
Pigmenting agents, 827–828, 828t
Pilocar (pilocarpine), 58
Pilocarpine (Isopto Carpine; Miocarpine; Pilocar), 58

Pilocarpine ocular therapeutic system (Ocusert Pilo), 58–59
PIMA (potassium iodide), 421–423, 422t, 540–541
Pimozide (Orap), 205, 214
Pindolol (Visken), 104–105, 105t, 107t, 108t, 109, 303–304
Piperacillin (Pipracil), 567–571t, 582, 583t, 584–585, 593–594t, 595
Piperazine(s) (Entacyl; Vermizine), 114t, 205–208, 206t, 209–211t, 673t, 676–677
Piperidines, 114t, 205–208, 206t, 211t
Pipobroman (Vercyte), 710t, 711–712, 717t
Pipracil (piperacillin), 582, 584–585, 593–594t, 595
Pirbuterol (Maxair), 94–95, 96–97t
Piroxicam (Apo-Piroxicam; Feldene; Novopirocam), 175, 178, 183t
Pitocin (oxytocin, parenteral), 412–413
Pitressin Synthetic (vasopressin), 410–411
Pitressin Tannate in Oil (vasopressin tannate), 410–411
Pitrex (tolnaftate), 692, 696–697t, 697
Pituitary dwarfism, 399
Pituitary gland, 395–400
  adenohypophysis of, 395–396
    hormones of, 397–400
  anatomy of, 395–396, 396
  neurohypophysis of, 395
    hormones of, 396–397
Pituitary insufficiency, 399
Pituitrin-S (posterior pituitary injection), 410
Placental barrier, distribution and, 13
Placidyl (ethchlorvynol), 201
Plague vaccine, 803–804, 805–806t
Plaquenil (hydroxychloroquine sulfate), 665, 666t
Plasbumin (albumin, human), 826t, 826–827
Plasma cholinesterase inhibitor, 133
Plasma expanders, 824–826, 825t
Plasmanate (plasma protein fraction), 826t, 826–827
Plasma-Plex (plasma protein fraction), 826t, 826–827
Plasma protein binding
  competition for, drug interactions and, 28–29
  glomerular filtration and, 14
Plasma protein fraction(s) (Plasmanate; Plasma-Plex; Plasmatein; Protenate), 826t, 826–827
Plasmatein (plasma protein fraction), 826t, 826–827
Plasmodium falciparum, 664
Plasmodium malariae, 664
Plasmodium ovale, 664
Plasmodium vivax, 664
Platelet(s), adrenergic drug effects on, 81t
Platelet aggregation, salicylates and, 170
Platinol (cisplatin), 711–712, 714t
Platinol-AQ (cisplatin), 711–712, 714t
Pleura
  parietal, 531
  visceral, 531
Pleural cavity, 531
Plexus of Auerbach, 483

Plexus of Meissner, 483
Plicamycin (Mithracin), 426, 719, 722–724, 729t
PMS Benztropine (benztropine mesylate), 74–75t, 258–259, 259t
PMS Carbamazepine (carbamazepine), 246–247
PMS Docusate Calcium (docusate calcium-dioctyl calcium sulfosuccinate), 506–507, 509t
PMS Dopazide (methyldopa), 311–312
PMS Egozinc (zinc sulfate), 776t
PMS Flurazepam (flurazepam), 198–199, 200t
PMS Isoniazid (isoniazid), 659–660
PMS Metronidazole (metronidazole), 683–685
PMS Nylidrin (nylidrin), 96–98, 334
PMS Procyclidine (procyclidine), 74–75t, 258–259, 260t
PMS Propranolol (propranolol), 296–297, 331
PMS Pyrazinamide (pyrazinamide), 660–661
PMS Sulfasalazine (sulfasalazine), 573–575, 577t
PMS Theophylline (theophylline), 545–547, 549, 549t, 551
PMS Thioridazine (thioridazine), 205–208, 211t
Pneumococcal vaccine, polyvalent (Pneumovax 23; Pnu-Imune 23), 803–804, 806t
Pneumocystis carinii, 570t
Pneumotaxic center, 535
Pneumovax 23 (pneumococcal vaccine, polyvalent), 803–804, 806t
Pnu-Imune 23 (pneumococcal vaccine, polyvalent), 803–804, 806t
POCC combination chemotherapy, 738, 740, 750t
Podocytes, 371
Poladex (dexchlorpheniramine), 113–114, 116t, 119
Polaramine (dexchlorpheniramine), 113–114, 116t, 119
Polargen T.D. (dexchlorpheniramine), 113–114, 116t, 119
Poliomyelitis Vaccine (poliovirus vaccine, inactivated-IPV), 803–804, 808t
Poliovirus vaccine
  inactivated-IPV (Poliomyelitis Vaccine), 803–804, 808t
  live oral trivalent-TOPV, Sabin (Orimune), 803–804, 808t
Polocaine (mepivacaine), 139–141, 140t, 142t
Polycarbophil calcium (Fiber-Con; Mitrolan; Equalactin), 506–507, 508t
Polycillin (ampicillin), 582, 584–585, 586–587t, 595
Polycose (glucose polymers), 777t
Polydipsia, in diabetes mellitus, 403
Polyestradiol phosphate (Estradurin), 454–456, 459t, 724, 730, 732t, 734–736
Polyethylene glycol-electrolyte solution (Colonite; CoLyte; GoLYTELY; OCL), 506–507, 511t

Polymox (amoxicillin), 582, 584–585, 586t, 595
Polymyxin(s), 632
Polymyxin B, 567t, 632
Polymyxin B sulfate (Aerosporin), 634–635
Polymyxin E (colistin sulfate), 632
Polypeptides, 632–636
Polyphagia, in diabetes mellitus, 403
Polysaccharide-iron complex (Hytinic; Niferex; Nu-Iron), 345–346, 347t
Polysynaptic blocking agents, 134–135
Polythiazide (Renese), 388–389, 391t, 391–392
Polyunsaturated fatty acids, omega-3, 778t
Polyuria, in diabetes mellitus, 403
POMP (low dose) combination chemotherapy, 738, 740, 750t
Ponderal (fenfluramine), 265–267, 268t
Pondimin (fenfluramine), 265–267, 268t
Pons, 54
Ponstan (mefenamic acid), 175, 178, 182t
Ponstel (mefenamic acid), 175, 178, 182t
Pontine respiratory centers, 535
Pontocaine (tetracaine), 139–141, 140t, 143t
Porcelana (hydroquinone), 828–829
Positive inotropic agents, 285
Posterior pituitary injection (Pituitrin-S), 410
Posture (tricalcium phosphate), 426–427, 427t
Potaba (para-aminobenzoic acid), 778t
Potassium, 774–775
Potassium acetate, 784t, 785
Potassium chloride, 784t, 785
Potassium iodide (Iosat; PIMA; Thyro-Block), 421–423, 422t, 540–541, 571t
 saturated solution (SSKI), 421–423, 422t
Potassium iodide/niacinamide (Iodo-Niacin), 540–541
Potassium phosphate, 783–784t, 785
Potency, efficacy versus, 16
Potentiation, 18
PP cells, of islets of Langerhans, 402
Pralidoxime chloride (PAM; Protopam), 65
Pramegel (pramoxine), 139–141, 140t, 143t
Pramoxine (Pramegel; Prax; Proctofoam; Tronothane), 139–141, 140t, 143t
Prax (pramoxine), 139–141, 140t, 143t
Prazepam (Centrax), 217–219, 218t, 222t
Praziquantel (Biltricide), 673t, 677
Prazosin (Minipress), 312–313
Preanesthetic medication, 144
Precef (ceforanide), 598–600, 604t
Prednisolone, 443, 445–447, 451t, 444t, 751t
Prednisone (Deltasone; Liquid Pred; Prednisone Intensol; Orasone), 443, 445–447, 451t, 444t, 709t, 724, 730, 733t, 734–736, 741–750t, 752t, 753t
Prednisone Intensol (prednisone), 724, 730, 733t, 734–736
Pregnancy, FDA categories of, 847
Pregnolisa, 791, 793t
Pregnosis, 791, 793t
Pregnospia, 791, 793t

Pregnosticon Dri-Dot, 791, 793t
Pregnyl (human chorionic gonadotropin), 469–470
Preload, 278
Preludin (phenmetrazine), 265–267, 268t
Premarin (estrogens, conjugated), 454–456, 457t
Pre-Pen (benzylpenicilloylpolylysine), 791, 796t
Preschool age, 31
Presynaptic membrane, depolarization of, 50
Prilocaine (Citanest), 139–141, 140t, 143t
Primaquine (primaquine phosphate), 667
Primaquine phosphate (Primaquine), 667
Primatene (epinephrine), 79–82
Primaxin (imipenem-cilastin), 595
Primidone (Apo-Primidone; Myidone; Mysoline; Sertan), 240
Principen (ampicillin), 582, 584–585, 586–587t, 595
Prinivil (lisinopril), 304–305, 309t
PR interval, 276
Prinzmetal's angina, 325
Priscoline (tolazoline), 103–104, 374t
Privine (naphazoline), 88–89, 90–91t
PRL. *See* Prolactin
Proaqua (benzthiazide), 388–389, 390t, 391–392
Probalon (probenecid), 187–188
Pro-Banthine (propantheline bromide), 76–77t
Probenecid (Benemid; Benuryl; Probalon), 187–188, 374t
Probucol (Lorelco), 343
Procainamide (Procan SR; Promine; Pronestyl; Pronestyl-SR; Procamide SR; Rhythmin), 288t, 289–291
Procaine (Novocain), 139–141, 140t, 143t
ProcalAmine (crystalline amino-acid infusion), 779–780
Pro-Cal-Sof (docusate calcium-dioctyl calcium sulfosuccinate), 506–507, 509t
Procamide SR (procainamide), 289–291
Procan SR (procainamide), 289–291
Procarbazine (Matulane), 709t, 710t, 736–738, 740t, 741–743t, 746t, 749t, 750t
Procarboxypeptidase (carboxypeptidase), 488t
Procardia (nifedipine), 329–331, 331t, 332t
Prochlorperazine (Chlorpazine; Compazine; Stemetil), 205–208, 206t, 210t, 521t
Proctofoam (pramoxine), 139–141, 140t, 143t
Procyclid (procyclidine), 74–75t, 258–259, 260t
Procyclidine (Kemadrin; PMS Procyclidine; Procyclid), 67–70, 74–75t, 258–259, 260t
Pro-Depo (hydroxyprogesterone caproate), 724, 730, 733t, 734–736
Pro-drugs, 13–14
Profasi HP (human chorionic gonadotropin), 469–470
Profene 65 (propoxyphene), 157, 159, 162t
Profilnine (factor IX complex, human), 362–363

Progens (estrogens, conjugated), 454–456, 457t
Progestaject (progesterone), 456, 459, 461, 461t
Progestasert (intrauterine progesterone contraceptive system), 467
Progesterone (Bay Progest; Femotrone; Gesterol-50; Progestaject), 456, 459, 461, 461t
Progestin(s), 405, 456, 459, 460–461t, 461, 709t, 724, 730, 733t, 734–736. *See also* Contraceptives, oral
Proglycem (diazoxide, oral), 440
ProHIBit (hemophilus b conjugate vaccine), 803–804, 805t
Proinsulin, 402
Proklar (sulfamethizole), 573–575, 576t
Prolactin (PRL), 398, 407
 actions of, 398
 control of secretion of, 398
Prolamine (phenylpropanolamine), 265–267, 269t
Prolixin (fluphenazine), 205–208, 210t
Proloid (thyroglobulin), 416–418, 418t
Proloprim (trimethoprim), 640–641
ProMACE-MOPP combination chemotherapy, 709t, 738, 740, 750–751t
Promazine (Sparine; Prozine), 205–208, 206t, 209t
Promethazine (Histantil; Phenergan), 113–114, 114t, 117t, 119, 521
Promine (procainamide), 289–291
Pro-Mix (glucose polymers), 777t
Pro-Mix R.D.P. (protein hydrosylates), 778t
Pronestyl (procainamide), 289–291
Pronestyl-SR (procainamide), 289–291
Propac (protein hydrosylates), 778t
Propaderm (beclomethasone), 443, 445–447, 448t
Propagest (phenylpropanolamine), 88–89, 90–91t
Propanthel (propantheline bromide), 76–77t
Propantheline bromide (Banlin; Norpanth; Novopropanthil; Pro-Banthine; Propanthel), 67–70, 76–77t
Proparacaine (Aktaine; Alcaine; l-Paracaine; Kainair; Ophthaine; Ophthetic), 139–141, 140t, 143t
Propine (dipivefrin), 82–83
Propiomazine (Largon), 203
Propion (diethylpropion), 265–267, 268t
Proplex (factor IX complex, human), 362–363
Propoxyphene (Darvon; Dolene; Doxaphene; Novopropoxyn; Profene 65; 642), 157, 158t, 159, 162t
Propranolol (Apo-Propranolol; Detensol; Inderal; Inderal LA; Ipran; Novopranol; PMS Propranolol), 104–105, 105t, 107t, 108t, 109, 288t, 296–297, 303–304, 331
Proprionibacterium acnes, 609
Propylhexedrine (Benzedrex), 88–89, 90–91t
Propylthiouracil (Propyl-Thyracil), 418, 420, 421t
Propyl-Thyracil (propylthiouracil), 418, 420, 421t

Prostaglandin abortifacients, 470–472, 471t
Prostaphlin (oxacillin), 582, 584–585, 591t, 595
Prostin E₂ (dinoprostone), 470–472, 471t
Prostin VR Pediatric (alprostadil), 813
Protamine (protamine zinc insulin suspension), 429–431, 436t
Protamine sulfate, 354
Protamine zinc insulin suspension (Protamine; Zinc and Iletin I), 429–431, 430t, 436t
  purified (Protamine; Zinc and Iletin II), 429–431, 436t
Protein(s), absorption of, 487
Protein (amino acid) supplements, 779–780
Protein hydrosylates (A/G Pro; PDP Liquid Protein; Pro-Mix R.D.P.; Propac), 778t
Protein metabolism
  glucagon and, 402
  glucocorticoids and, 405
  growth hormone and, 397
  insulin and, 403
Protenate (plasma protein fraction), 826t, 826–827
Proteus, 570t, 624, 625t
Proteus mirabilis, 570t
Protirelin (Relefact TRH; Thypinone), 791, 798t
Protopam (pralidoxime chloride), 65
Protophylline (dyphylline), 545–547, 548t, 549, 551
Protostat (metronidazole), 683–685
Protriptyline (Triptil; Vivactil), 227–230, 228t, 232t
Protropin (somatrem), 408–409
Proventil (albuterol), 94–95, 96–97t
Provera (medroxyprogesterone acetate), 456, 459, 460t, 461, 724, 730, 733t, 734–736
Providencia, 624, 625t
Providencia stuartii, 570t
Provocholine (methacholine), 791, 797t
Proximal convoluted tubule, 371
Prozac (fluoxetine), 228t, 233
Prozine (promazine), 205–208, 209t
Pseudoephedrine (Afrinol; Eltor-120; Neosynephrinol; Novaphed; Pseudofrin; Robidrine; Sudafed), 88–89, 90–91t
Pseudofrin (pseudoephedrine), 88–89, 90–91t
Pseudomonas, 598, 624, 632
Pseudomonas aeruginosa, 570t, 624, 625t
Pseudomonas mallei, 570t, 624
Pseudomonas pseudomallei, 570t
Psilocin, 839
Psilocybin, 839
Psoralens, 827–828, 828t
Psorcon (diflorasone diacetate), 443, 444t, 445–447, 449t
PSP (phenolsulfonphthalein), 374t
Psychological dependence, 835
Psychological factors
  drug effects and, 17
  vomiting and, 489
Psychotomimetics, abuse of, 839–840
Psyllium (Effersyllium; Karacil; Konsyl; Metamucil; Novomucilax; Serutan), 506–507, 508t

PTH. *See* Parathyroid hormone
Ptyalin (salivary amylase), 488t
Pulmonary exchange of gases, 531
Pulmonary veins, 532
Pulmonary ventilation, 531, 532–533
  respiratory compliance and, 532–533
    resistance to airflow and, 532–533, *533*
    surface tension and, 532
    volumes of air exchanged and, 533
Pulmonic valve, 275
Pulmophylline (theophylline), 545–547, 549, 549t, 551
Pulse pressure, 279
Pure Food and Drug Act, 41
  Sherley Amendment to, 41
Purge (castor oil), 506–507, 512t
Purinethol (mercaptopurine), 712, 718–719, 721t
Purkinje fibers, 276
Purpura, 25
PVB combination chemotherapy, 738, 740, 751t
P wave, 276
Pyopen (carbenicillin disodium), 582, 584–585, 588–589t, 595
Pyramids, renal, 371
Pyrantel pamoate (Antiminth; Reese's Pinworm), 673t, 677–678
Pyrazinamide (PMS Pyrazinamide; Tebrazid), 569t, 660–661, 655
Pyrazolones, 174–175
Pyribenzamine (tripelennamine), 113–114, 118t, 119
Pyridium (phenazopyridine), 641
Pyridostigmine, 60t, 60–61, 62–63t
Pyridoxine (vitamin B₆), 758t, 760–761
Pyrilamine (Dormarex), 113–114, 114t, 118t, 119
Pyrimethamine (Daraprim), 667–668, 751t
Pyronium (phenazopyridine), 641
Pyroxine (vitamin B₆), 760–761

Q

QRS complex, 276
QT interval, 276–277
Quarzan (clidinium bromide), 76–77t
Quelicin (succinylcholine), 132–133
Questran (cholestyramine), 337–339, 339t
Quiagel, 518t
Quiagel PG, 518t
Quick-Pep (caffeine and dextrose), 263–264
Quinacrine (Atabrine), 669, 678
Quinaglute Dura-Tabs (quinidine), 287, 289
Quinamm (quinine sulfate), 669–670
Quinate (quinidine), 287, 289
Quinatime (quinidine), 287, 289
Quine (quinine sulfate), 669–670
Quinestrol (Estrovis), 454–456, 459t
Quinethazone (Aquamox; Hydromox), 388–389, 391t, 391–392
Quinidex Extentabs (quinidine), 287, 289
Quinidine (Apo-Quinidine; Biquin Durules; Cardioquin; Cin-Quin; Duraquin; Novoquinidin; Quinaglute Dura-Tabs; Quinate; Quinatime;

Quinidex Extentabs; Quinora; Quin-Release), 287, 288t, 289
Quinine sulfate (Legatrin; Novoquinine; Quinamm; Quine; Quiphile; Strema), 669–670
Quinolone(s), 611, 614–617
Quinora (quinidine), 287, 289
Quin-Release (quinidine), 287, 289
Quinsana (undecylenic acid and salts), 692, 697, 697t
Quiphile (quinine sulfate), 669–670

R

Rabies immune globulin, human (Hyperab; Imogam), 811–812, 812t
Rabies prophylaxis products, 811–812, 812t
Rabies vaccine, human diploid cell cultures
  intradermal (Imovax I.D.), 811–812, 812t
  intramuscular (Imovax), 811–812, 812t
Radioactive sodium iodide-^{131}I (Iodotope), 420–421
Radiographic diagnostic agents, 791, 893, 799, 799–802t
Radiopaque agents, iodinated, 799, 800–802t
Ranitidine (Zantac), 119, 121–122, 122t
Rapid Test Strep, 791, 793t
Rate theory, of intensity of effect, 16
Raudixin (rauwolfia whole root), 313–314, 315t
Rauwiloid (alseroxylon), 313–314, 315t
Rauwolfia alkaloids, 313–314, 315t
Rauwolfia whole root (Raudixin), 313–314, 315t
Razepam (temazepam), 198–199, 200t
RDAs. *See* Recommended dietary allowances
Rebound congestion, mucosal application and, nasal, 4
Receptor(s), 16
  adrenergic, 53, 78, 79, 80t
  cholinergic, 53
  opiate, 155, 156t
  of peripheral nervous system, mechanism of drug action and, 52t, 53
  up-regulation and down-regulation and, 53
Receptor antagonism, competitive, drug interactions and, 27
Receptor occupation theory, 16
Receptor sensitivity, drug interactions and, 27–28
Receptor specificity, distribution and, in children, 32
Reclomide (metoclopramide), 534–535
Recommended dietary allowances (RDAs), 757
Rectal administration, in children, 33
Rectal mucosa, mucosal application and, 4
Redisol (cyanocobalamin, crystalline), 348–349
Red nucleus, 54
Reduction, biotransformation and, 14
Reese's Pinworm (pyrantel pamoate), 677–678
Reflex regulation, of respiration, 536
Regitine (phentolamine), 103, 321
Reglan (metoclopramide), 534–535

Regular Concentrated Iletin II (insulin injection, concentrated), 429–431, 435t
Regular Iletin I (insulin injection), 429–431, 435t
Regular Iletin II (insulin injection, purified), 429–431, 435t
Regular Insulin (insulin injection), 429–431, 435t
Regular Purified Pork (insulin injection, purified), 429–431, 435t
Regulex (docusate sodium-dioctyl sodium sulfsuccinate), 506–507, 509t
Rehydralyte (oral electrolyte mixture), 776t
Rela (carisoprodol), 134–135, 136t
Relefact TRH (protirelin), 791, 798t
Remegel, 496–497t
Renal arteries, 371
Renal (malpighian) corpuscle, 371
Renal disease, adverse drug effects related to, 21
Renal failure, antibiotics in, 566–567
Renal pelvis, 371
Renal threshold, 374
Renal tubular reabsorption, 374
Renal tubular secretion, 374, 374t
RenAmin (amino-acid formulation for renal failure), 780
Renese (polythiazide), 388–389, 391t, 391–392
Renin-angiotensin-aldosterone system, 279–280, *280*
Renografin-60, 799, 802t
Renografin-76, 799, 802t
Reno-M-30, 799, 802t
Reno-M-60, 799, 802t
Reno-M-Dip, 799, 802t
Renoquid (sulfacytine), 573–575, 576t
Renovist, 799, 802t
Renovist II, 799, 802t
Renovue-65, 799, 802t
Renovue-Dip, 799, 802t
Repeated dosage, drug effects and, 17
Reposans-10 (chlordiazepoxide), 217–219, 220–221t
Repository corticotropin injection (ACTH Gel; Cortigel; Cortrophin Gel; Cortropic Gel; H.P. Acthar Gel), 407–408
Rescinnamine (Moderil), 313–314, 315t
Reserfia (reserpine), 313–314, 315t
Reserpine (Novoreserpine; Reserfia; Serpasil), 313–314, 315t
Residual drug effects, drug interactions and, 30
Resistance
  to antimicrobials, 562, 563, 566
    acquired, 563
    natural, 563
  drug effects and, 17
  to penicillins, 582
Resol (oral electrolyte mixture), 776t
Respiracult, 791, 793t
Respiralex, 791, 793t
Respirastick, 791, 793t
Respiration
  cellular, 531
  phases of, 531
  regulation of, 535–536

chemical, 536
neural, 535
reflex, 536
Respiratory bronchioles, 531
Respiratory compliance, 532–533
  resistance to airflow and, 532–533, *533*
  surface tension and, 532
Respiratory defense mechanisms, 532
Respiratory distress syndrome, 532
Respiratory division, 531
Respiratory rate, 533
Respiratory stimulants. *See* Analeptics
Respiratory system, 531–536
  anatomy and histology of, 531–532
    blood supply and, 532
    conducting division and, 531
    nerve supply and, 532
    respiratory division and, 531–532
  exchange and transport of respiratory gases and, 534–535, *535*
    carbon dioxide transport and, 534–535
    oxygen transport and, 534
  phases of respiration and, 531
  pulmonary ventilation and, 532–533
    respiratory compliance and, 532–533
    volumes of air exchanged and, 533
  regulation of respiration and, 535–536
    chemical, 536
    neural, 535
    reflex, 536
  respiratory defense mechanisms and, 532
Respiratory tree, anatomy and histology of, 531
Restoril (temazepam), 198–199, 200t
Resyl (guaifenesin), 540
Reticular formation, 54
Retin-A (tretinoin), 767–768
Retinoic acid (tretinoin), 767–768
Retrovir (zidovudine), 705–706
Rexolate (sodium thiosalicylate), 170–171, 173, 177t
R-Gene 10 (L-arginine), 791, 795t
R-Gen Elixir (iodinated glycerol), 540–541
Rheaban, 518t
Rheomacrodex (dextran 40-low molecular weight), 824–826, 825t
Rheumanosticon Dri-Dot, 791, 793t
Rheumatrex DosePak (methotrexate), 712, 718–719, 721–722t
Rhinalar (flunisolide), 443, 445–447, 449–450t, 551–553, 552t
Rhindecon (phenylpropanolamine), 88–89, 90–91t
RhoGAM (rh₀[D] immune globulin), 810, 811t
Rh₀(D) immune globulin, (Gamulin Rh; HypRho-D; RhoGAM; Win Rho), 810, 811t
Rhythmin (procainamide), 289–291
Rhythmodan (disopyramide), 291–292
Ribavarin (Virazole), 702–703
Riboflavin (vitamin B₂), 758t, 759
Ribonuclease, 488t
Rickettsia, 570t
Ridaura (auranofin), 180, 184
Rifadin (rifampin), 661–662
Rifampin (Rifadin; Rimactane; Rofact), 562, 569t, 570t, 571t, 655, 661–662
Rigidity, in Parkinson's disease, 253

Rimactane (rifampin), 661–662
Rimso-50 (dimethyl sulfoxide), 817
Riopan (magaldrate), 490–491, 492–493t
Riopan Extra Strength, 496–497t
Riopan Plus, 496–497t
Riopan Plus 2, 496–497t
Ritalin (methylphenidate), 267, 269
Ritodrine (Yutopar), 98
Rival (diazepam), 249
Rivotril (clonazepam), 248–249
RMS (morphine), 157, 159, 160t
Robaxin (methocarbamol), 134–135, 137t
Robidex (dextromethorphan), 539
Robidone (hydrocodone), 538–539
Robidrine (pseudoephedrine), 88–89, 90–91t
Robigesic (acetaminophen), 173–174
Robimycin (erythromycin base), 619–620, 621t
Robinul (glycopyrrolate), 76–77t
Robitussin (guaifenesin), 540
Robitussin A-C, 538t
Robomol (methocarbamol), 134–135, 137t
Rocaltrol (calcitriol), 768–770, 769t
Rocephin (ceftriaxone), 598–600, 607t
Rofact (rifampin), 661–662
Roferon-A (interferon alfa-2a, recombinant), 736–738, 739t
Rogatine (phentolamine), 321
Rolaids (dihydroxyaluminum sodium carbonate), 490–491, 492–493t
Ronase (tolazamide), 431, 436–437, 438t
Rondomycin (methacycline), 609–611, 614t
Rotalex, 791, 793t
Rowasa (mesalamine), 823–824
Roxanol (morphine), 157, 158t, 159, 160t
Roxanol SR (morphine), 157, 159, 160t
Roxicodone (oxycodone), 157, 159, 161t
Roydan (danthron), 506–507, 512t
Rubacell II, 791, 793t
Rubella and mumps vaccine (Biavax II), 803–804, 808t
Rubella vaccine (Meruvax II), 803–804, 808t
Rubion (cyanocobalamin, crystalline), 348–349
Rubramin PC (cyanocobalamin, crystalline), 348–349
Rulox No. 1, 496–497t
Rulox No. 2, 496–497t
Ru-Vert M (meclizine), 113–114, 117t, 119
RV Paba Stick (para-aminobenzoic acid), 778t

S

S-60 (sodium salicylate), 170–171, 173, 177t
Safflower Oil (Microlipid), 778t
St. Joseph Antidiarrheal, 518t
Salacid (salicylic acid), 170–171, 173, 177t
Salazopyrin (sulfasalazine), 573–575, 577t
Salflex (salsalate), 170–171, 173, 177t
Salicylamide, 170–171, 173
Salicylates, 170–171, *172*, 173, 176–177t, 374t

Salicylic acid (Calicylic; Compound W; Derma-Soft; Freezone; Gordofilm; Hydrisalic; Keralyt; Mediplast; Occlusal; Off-Ezy; Oxyclean; Salacid; Saligel; Salonil; Sebcur; Soluver; Wart-off), 170–171, 173, 177t
Saligel (salicylic acid), 170–171, 173, 177t
Salivary amylase (ptyalin), 488t
Salmonella, 571t, 598, 625t, 632
Salmonella typhi, 571t
Salonil (salicylic acid), 170–171, 173, 177t
Salsalate (Artha-G; Disalcid; Mono-Gesic; Salsitab; Salflex)
Salsitab (salsalate), 170–171, 173, 177t
Saluron (hydroflumethiazide), 388–389, 390–391t, 391–392
Sandimmune (cyclosporine), 822–823
Sandoglobulin (immune globulin, intravenous), 801, 810t
Sandostatin (octreotide), 824
Sani-Supp (glycerin), 506–507, 513t
SA node. *See* Sinoatrial node
Sanorex (mazindol), 265–267, 268t
Sansert (methysergide), 125–126
Santyl (collagenase), 818, 819t
L-Sarcolysin (melphalan), 711–712, 717t
Sarisol (butabarbital), 193–194, 196t, 197
S.A.S.-500 (sulfasalazine), 573–575, 577t
Satric (metronidazole), 683–685
Saturated solution potassium iodide (SSKI), 421–423, 422t
SCAB combination chemotherapy, 738, 740, 751t
Schedules, for controlled substances, 42, 43t
 prescribing and dispensing and, 42–44
Schistosoma haematobium, 673t
Schistosoma japonicum, 673t
Schistosoma mansoni, 673t
Schistosoma mekongi, 673t
Schistosomiasis, 672
Sclavo Test-PPD (tuberculin PPD, multiple puncture device), 791, 795t
Scleromate (morrhuate sodium), 829t, 829–830
Sclerosing agents, 829t, 829–830
Scopolamine, 67–70, 521t
Scopolamine hydrobromide (Isopto Hyoscine), 72–73t
Scopolamine transdermal therapeutic system (Transderm-Scop), 72–73t
Scrip-Zinc (zinc sulfate), 776t
Sebcur (salicylic acid), 170–171, 173, 177t
Sebizon Lotion (sulfacetamide), 573–575, 575–576t
Secobarbital (Seconal), 193–194, 195t, 197
Seconal (secobarbital), 193–194, 195t, 197
Secretin (Secretin Ferring Powder), 791, 798t
Secretin Ferring Powder (secretin), 791, 798t
Secretion
 of digestive system, 483–484, 486
 gastric, control of, 484, 486, 487t
Sectral (acebutolol), 104–105, 105t, 106t, 108t, 109, 296–297, 303–304
Sedative(s)
 antiemetic, 521t
 nonbarbiturate, abuse of, 836–837

Sedative-hypnotics
 barbiturate. *See* Barbiturates
 nonbarbiturate, 193, 198–204
 antianxiety drugs compared with, 199t
 benzodiazepine hypnotics, 198–203
Sedatuss (dextromethorphan), 539
Seizures. *See* Anticonvulsants; Epilepsy
Seldane (terfenadine), 113–114, 118t, 119
Selegiline (Eldepryl), 254, 257–258
Selestoject (betamethasone phosphate), 443, 445–447, 448t
Semilente Iletin I (insulin zinc suspension, prompt), 429–431, 435t
Semilente Insulin (insulin zinc suspension, prompt), 429–431, 435t
Semilente Purified Pork (insulin zinc suspension, prompt, purified), 429–431, 435t
Semilunar valves, 275
Semisynthetic antiinfectives, 559
Senexon (senna concentrate), 506–507, 513t
Senna concentrate (Genna; Gentlax B; Senexon; Senokot; Senna-Gel; Senolax; X-Prep), 506–507, 513t
Senna equivalent (Black-Draught), 506–507, 513t
Senna-Gen (senna concentrate), 506–507, 513t
Sennosides A&B-calcium salts (Gentle Nature; Glysennid; Nytilax), 506–507, 513t
Senokot (senna concentrate), 506–507, 513t
Senolax (senna concentrate), 506–507, 513t
Sensitivity testing, antimicrobials and, 560–561
Sensorcaine (bupivacaine), 139–141, 140t, 142t
Septra (trimethoprim-sulfamethoxazole), 579–580
Sequestration, drug interactions and, 28
Serax (oxazepam), 217–219, 218t, 222t
Serentil (mesoridazine), 205–208, 211t
Seromycin (cycloserine), 657
Serophene (clomiphene), 468
Serpasil (reserpine), 313–314, 315t
Serratia, 571t, 598, 624, 625t
Sertan (primidone), 240
Serutan (psyllium), 506–507, 508t
Sex, drug effects and, 17
Sex hormones, 405
Sherley Amendment, 41
Shigella, 571t, 625t, 632
Sickledex Test, 791, 793t
Side effects. *See* Adverse drug effects
Silain (simethicone), 498
Silain-Gel, 496–497t
Silvadene (silver sulfadiazine), 578–579
Silver sulfadiazine (Flint SSD; Silvadene), 574t, 578–579
Simethicone (Gas-X; Mylicon; Ovol; Phazyme; Silain), 498
 in combination antacids, 494–497t
Simron (ferrous gluconate), 345–346, 347t
Sincalide (Kinevac), 791, 798t
Sincomen (spironolactone), 387–388
Sinemet (carbidopa/levodopa), 254–255

Sinequan (doxepin), 227–230, 228t, 231t
Sinex Long Lasting (oxymetazoline), 88–89, 90–91t
Sinoatrial (SA) node, 276
Sinografin, 799, 802t
642 (propoxyphene), 157, 159, 162t
Skelaxin (metaxalone), 134–135, 136t
Skeletal muscle relaxants, 128–138
 centrally acting, 134–135, 136–137t
 peripherally acting, 128–134
 direct myotropic acting blocking agent, 133–134
 neuromuscular blocking agents, 128–133
Skin
 absorption from, 12–13
 adrenergic drug effects on, 81t
Skin test antigens
 multiple (Multitest CMI), 791, 794t
 mumps, 791, 794t
Slo-Phyllin (theophylline), 545–547, 549, 549t, 551
Slo-Salt (sodium chloride), 776t
Slow FE (ferrous sulfate), 345–346, 347t
Slow-Mag (magnesium), 776t
Small intestine
 anatomic and histologic features of, 484t
 major activities of, 486t
SMF (FMS) combination chemotherapy, 738, 740, 751t
Smooth muscle
 acetylcholine and, pharmacologic effects and clinical consequences of, 57t
 anticholinergic drugs and, pharmacologic actions of, 68t
Smooth muscle relaxants, 67, 95–98
Soda Mint (sodium bicarbonate), 490–491, 494–495t
Sodium, renal reabsorption of, 374
Sodium acetate, 784t, 785
Sodium ascorbate (Cenolate; Cevita; vitamin C), 761–762
Sodium bicarbonate (Bell/ans; Neut; Soda Mint), 490–491, 494–495t, 776t, 784t, 785
Sodium chloride (Slo-Salt), 776t
Sodium chloride, 20% solution, 472
Sodium chloride diluents, 784–785t, 785
Sodium chloride injection for admixtures, 784t, 785
Sodium chloride intravenous infusion, 784t, 785
Sodium iodide, 421–423, 422t
 radioactive (Iodotope), 420–421
Sodium lactate, 784t, 785
Sodium phosphate, 783–784t, 785
Sodium phosphate and sodium biphosphate (Fleet Enema; Phospho-Soda), 506–507, 511t
Sodium salicylate (Uracel; S-60), 170–171, 173, 177t
Sodium Sulamyd (sulfacetamide), 573–575, 575–576t
Sodium tetradecyl sulfate (Sotradecol; Trombovar), 829t, 829–830
Sodium thiosalicylate (Asproject; Rexolate; Tusal), 170–171, 173, 177t
Sodium valproate (Depakene; Myproic acid), 247–248

Sofarin (warfarin sodium), 354–356, 356t
Solaquin (hydroquinone), 828–829
Solganal (aurothioglucose), 180, 184
Solium (chlordiazepoxide), 217–219, 220–221t
Soluver (salicylic acid), 170–171, 173, 177t
Soma (carisoprodol), 134–135, 136t
Somatic nervous system, 49
Somatomedins, 397
Somatostatin (GRIH; growth hormone release-inhibiting hormone; SRIH), 403
  actions of, 403
Somatotropin. See Growth hormone
Somatrem (Humatrope; Protropin), 408–409
Somatrophs, 396
Somnothane (halothane), 147–148
Somophyllin (aminophylline), 545–547, 548t, 549, 551
Somophyllin (theophylline), 545–547, 549, 549t, 551
Soothe Eye (tetrahydrozoline), 89, 92, 92t
Soprodol (carisoprodol), 134–135, 136t
Sorbitrate (isosorbide dinitrate), 325–326, 327t, 329
Sotradecol (sodium tetradecyl sulfate), 829t, 829–830
Soyacal 10%, 20% (intravenous fat emulsion), 782
Span C (bioflavonoids), 777t
Spancap No. 1 (dextroamphetamine sulfate), 264–265, 266t
Span-FF (ferrous fumarate), 345–346, 347t
Span-Niacin (vitamin B_3), 759–760
Sparine (promazine), 205–208, 209t
Spectazole (econazole), 692, 694t, 697
Spectinomycin (Trobicin), 569t, 651–652
Spectrobid (bacampicillin), 582, 584–585, 588t, 595
Spherulin (coccidioidin), 791, 794t
Spinal anesthetics, local, 139
Spirillum minus, 571t
Spironolactone (Alatone; Aldactone; Novo-spiroton; Sincomen), 387–388
SPL-Serologic Types I and III (staphage lysate), 803–804, 806t
Sporothrix schenckii, 571t
S-P-T (thyroid, dessicated), 416–418, 418t
SRIH. See Somatostatin
SSKI (saturated solution potassium iodide), 421–423, 422t
Stadol (butorphanol), 158t
Stanozolol (Winstrol), 474–476, 479, 479t
Staphage lysate (SPL-Serologic Types I and III), 803–804, 806t
Staphcillin (methicillin), 582, 584–585, 589–590t, 595
Staphylococcus, 625t
Staphylococcus aureus, 571t
Starling's Law of the Heart, 278
Statex (morphine), 157, 159, 160t
Staticin (erythromycin base, topical solution), 619–620, 621t
Status epilepticus, 238
Steady state plasma level, drug effects and, 17
Steapsin (pancreatic lipase), 488t
Stelazine (trifluoperazine), 205–208, 211t

Stemetil (prochlorperazine), 205–208, 210t
Sterine (methenamine mandelate), 637–638, 639t
Steroids, anabolic, 474–476, 478–479t, 479
Stevens-Johnson syndrome, 22
STH. See Growth hormone
Stibocaptate (Astiban), 672, 673t, 674, 675t, 676–680
Stie VAA (tretinoin), 767–768
Stilphostrol (diethylstilbestrol diphosphate), 454–456, 457t, 724, 730, 731–732t, 734–736
Stimate (desmopressin acetate), 411–412
Stimulants. See Central nervous system stimulants
Stomach
  achlorhydria and, 500
  alterations in pH of, drug interactions and, 28
  anatomic and histologic features of, 484t
  major activities of, 485
Storage depots, displacement from, drug interactions and, 29
Stoxil (idoxuridine), 702
Street names, for drugs of abuse, 841–842
Strema (quinine sulfate), 669–670
Streptase (streptokinase), 358–359, 360t
Streptobacillus moniliformis, 571t
Streptococcus, 571t, 572t, 625t
Streptococcus bovis, 571t
Streptococcus faecalis, 571t
Streptococcus pneumoniae, 571t, 609
Streptococcus pyogenes, 571t, 572t
Streptokinase (Kabikinase; Streptase), 358–359, 360t
Streptomycin (Streptomycin), 567–572t, 624–626, 625t, 629–630t, 630, 655, 661
Streptonase-B, 791, 793t
Strepto-Sec, 791, 793t
Streptozocin (Zanosar), 710t, 711–712, 717t, 751t
Stretching, for intramuscular administration, 9
Stroke volume, 278
Strong iodine solution (Lugol's solution), 421–423, 422t
Strongyloides stercoralis, 673t
Subcutaneous administration, 8, 8
Sublimaze (fentanyl), 157, 158t, 159, 163–164t
Substantia nigra, 54
Succinimides, 245–246, 246t
Succinylcholine (Anectine; Quelicin; Sucostrin; Sux-Cert), 132–133
Sucostrin (succinylcholine), 132–133
Sucralfate (Carafate; Sulcrate), 491, 498
Sucrase, 488t
Sucrets Cold Decongestant Lozenge (phenylpropanolamine), 88–89, 90–91t
Sudafed (pseudoephedrine), 88–89, 90–91t
Sufenta (sufentanil), 157, 158t, 159, 164–165t
Sufentanil (Sufenta), 157, 158t, 159, 164–165t
Sulconazole (Exelderm), 687, 692, 696t, 697
Sulcrate (sucralfate), 491, 498

Sulf-10 (sulfacetamide), 573–575, 575–576t
Sulfabenzamide, 574t
Sulfacetamide (Ak-Sulf; Bleph-10; Cetamide; Isopto Cetamide; Minims; Ophthacet; Sebizon Lotion; Sodium Sulamyd; Sulfair-15; Sulfex; Sulf-10; Sulten-10), 573–575, 574–576t
Sulfacytine (Renoquid), 573–575, 574t, 576t
Sulfadiazine (Microsulfon), 573–575, 574t, 576t
Sulfadoxine and pyrimethamine (Fansidar), 668–669
Sulfair-15 (sulfacetamide), 573–575, 575–576t
Sulfamerazine, 574t
Sulfamethazine, 574t
Sulfamethizole (Proklar; Thiosulfil Forte), 573–575, 574t, 576t
Sulfamethoxazole (Apo-Sulfamethoxazole; Gamazole; Gantanol; Urobak), 573–575, 574t, 576t. See also Trimethoprim-sulfamethaxazole
Sulfamylon (mafenide), 578
Sulfapyridine (Dagenan), 573–575, 574t, 576–577t
Sulfasalazine (Azaline; Azulfidine; PMS Sulfasalazine; Salazopyrin; S.A.S.-500), 573–575, 574t, 577t
Sulfation factor, 397
Sulfex (sulfacetamide), 573–575, 575–576t
Sulfinpyrazone (Anturane), 188
Sulfisoxazole (Apo-Sulfasoxazole; Gantrisin; Gulfasin; Lipo Gantrisin; Novosoxazole), 573–575, 574t, 577–578t
Sulfolax (docusate calcium-dioctyl calcium sulfosuccinate), 506–507, 509t
Sulfonamide(s), 568t, 569t, 570t, 573–575, 575–578t, 578–581. See also Thiazides/sulfonamides
  multiple (Neotrizine; Sul-Trio MM; Terfonyl; Triple Sulfa), 573–575, 578t
Sulindac (Clinoril), 175, 178, 183t
Sulten-10 (sulfacetamide), 573–575, 575–576t
Sul-Trio MM (sulfonamides, multiple), 573–575, 578t
Sumacal (glucose polymers), 777t
Sumycin (tetracycline), 609–611, 613t
Super-C (bioflavonoids), 777t
SuperChar (activated charcoal), 813–814
Superinfection, antimicrobials and, 563
Supeudol (oxycodone), 157, 159, 161t
Supraoptic nuclei, 395
Suprax (cefixime), 598–600, 608t
Suprazine (trifluoperazine), 205–208, 211t
Suramin (Antrypol; Bayer 205; Belganyl; Germanin; Moranyl; Naganol; Naphuride), 672, 673t, 674, 675t, 676–680
Surface anesthetics, 139
Surface area method, dosage and, 33
Surface tension, respiratory compliance and, 532
Surfactant, 532
Surfak (docusate calcium-dioctyl calcium sulfosuccinate), 506–507, 509t
Surgicel (oxidized cellulose), 364–365

Index

Surital (thiamylal), 149–151, 150t
Surmontil (trimipramine), 227–230, 228t, 232t
Sus-Phrine(epinephrine), 79–82
Sutilains (Travase), 818, 819t
Sux-Cert (succinylcholine), 132–133
Symadine (amantadine), 255–256
Symmetrel (amantadine), 255–256, 700–701
Sympathetic division, of autonomic nervous system, 49, 50t, 51t
Sympathomimetic drugs. *See* Adrenergic drugs
Synacthen Depot (cosyntropin), 791, 796t
Synalar (fluocinolone acetonide), 443, 445–447, 445t, 450t
Synalar HP (fluocinolone acetonide), 444t
Synaptic junction, 49
Syncytium, 276
Synemol (fluocinolone acetonide), 443, 445–447, 445t, 450t
Synergism, drug effects and, 17–18
Synkayvite (vitamin K$_4$), 771t, 771–772
Synophylate (theophylline sodium glycinate), 545–547, 549, 549t, 551
Synthetic growth hormone, 408–409
Synthroid (levothyroxine sodium-T$_4$), 416–418, 419t
Synthrox (levothyroxine sodium-T$_4$), 416–418, 419t
Syntocinon (oxytocin, nasal), 412–413
Syntocinon (oxytocin, parenteral), 412–413
Syroxine (levothyroxine sodium-T$_4$), 416–418, 419t
Systole, 275
Systolic pressure, 279

T

T-2 protocol combination chemotherapy, 738, 740, 751t
Tacaryl (methdilazine), 113–114, 117t, 119
Tace (chlorotrianisene), 454–456, 457t, 724, 730, 731t, 734–736
Taenia saginata, 672, 673t
Taenia solium, 672, 673t
Tagamet (cimetidine), 119, 121–122, 122t
Talbutal (Lotusate), 193–194, 196t, 197
Talwin (pentazocine), 157, 158t, 159, 166–167t
Tambocor (flecainide), 295–296
Tamoxifen (Nolvadex), 709t, 724, 730, 734t, 734–736, 745t
Tandearil (oxyphenbutazone), 174–175
Tao (troleandomycin), 620, 623
Tapazole (methimazole), 418, 420, 421t
Taractan (chlorprothixene), 205–208, 211t
Tarasan (chlorprothixene), 205–208, 211t
Tavist (clemastine), 113–114, 116t, 119
Tazicef (ceftazidime), 598–600, 606t
Tazidime (ceftazidime), 598–600, 606t
TC, 496–497t
Tebrazid (pyrazinamide), 660–661
Teebacin (para-aminosalicylate sodium), 655–656
Teebaconin (isoniazid), 659–660
Teejel (choline salicylate), 170–171, 173, 176t
Tegison (etretinate), 765–766

Tegopen (cloxacillin), 582, 584–585, 589t, 595
Tegretol (carbamazepine), 246–247
Teldrin (chlorpheniramine), 113–114, 115t, 119
Telencephalon, 54
Telepaque, 799, 802t
Temaril (trimeprazine), 126
Temaz (temazepam), 198–199, 200t
Temazepam (Razepam; Restoril; Temaz), 198–199, 200t
Temovate (clobetasol propionate), 443, 444t, 445–447, 449t
Tempo, 496–497t
Tempra (acetaminophen), 173–174
Tenex (guanfacine), 310–311
Tenormin (atenolol), 104–105, 105t, 106t, 108t, 109, 303–304, 333
Tenuate (diethylpropion), 265–267, 268t
Tepanil (diethylpropion), 265–267, 268t
Teratogenicity, 21, 21t
Terazol 7 (terconazole), 692, 696t, 697
Terazosin (Hytrin), 312–313
Terbutaline (Brethaire; Brethine; Bricanyl), 94–95, 96–97t
Terconazole (Terazol 7), 687, 692, 696t, 697
Terfenadine (Seldane), 113–114, 114t, 118t, 119
Terfonyl (sulfonamides, multiple), 573–575, 578t
Teriparatide (Parathar), 791, 798t
Terpin hydrate, 541
Terpin Hydrate with Codeine, 538t
Terramycin (oxytetracycline), 609–611, 613t
Tertiary amine(s), 67
  antiparkinsonian agents, 69t
  antispasmodics, 69t, 72–75t
  mydriatics, 69t, 74–75t
Tes-Tape, 791, 793t
Teslac (testolactone), 724, 730, 731t, 734–736
Tessalon Perles (benzonatate), 539
Testa-C (testosterone cypionate), 474–476, 478t, 479
Testadiate-Depo (testosterone cypionate), 474–476, 478t, 479
Testamone 100 (testosterone, aqueous), 474–476, 477t, 479
Testaqua (testosterone, aqueous), 474–476, 477t, 479
Testex (testosterone propionate), 474–476, 477t, 479, 724, 730, 731t, 734–736
Testoject (testosterone, aqueous), 474–476, 477t, 479
Testoject (testosterone cypionate), 724, 730, 731t, 734–736
Testoject-LA (testosterone cypionate), 474–476, 478t, 479
Testolactone (Teslac), 724, 730, 731t, 734–736
Testone L.A. (testosterone enanthate), 474–476, 478t, 479
Testosterone, aqueous (Andronaq-50; Andro 100; Histerone; Malogen; Testamone 100; Testaqua; Testoject), 474–476, 477t, 479

Testosterone cypionate (Andro-Cyp; Andronate; Andronaq-LA; dep-Andro; Depotest; Depo-Testosterone; Duratest; Testa-C; Testadiate-Depo; Testoject; Testoject-LA; Testred), 474–476, 478t, 479, 724, 730, 731t, 734–736
Testosterone enanthate (Andro-L.A.; Andropository; Andryl; Andryl 200; Delatest; Delatestryl; Durathate; Everone; Malogex; Testone L.A.; Testrin-P.A.), 474–476, 478t, 479, 724, 730, 731t, 734–736
Testosterone propionate (Malogen in Oil; Testex), 474–476, 477t, 479, 724, 730, 731t, 734–736
Testred (methyltestosterone), 474–476, 477t, 479, 724, 730, 731t, 734–736
Testred (testosterone cypionate), 474–476, 478t, 479
Testrin-P.A. (testosterone enanthate), 474–476, 478t, 479, 724, 730, 731t, 734–736
Tetanus antitoxin, 808–809, 809t
Tetanus immune globulin (Hyper-Tet), 810, 811t
Tetanus toxoid, fluid or adsorbed, 803, 804t
Tetracaine (Pontocaine), 139–141, 140t, 143t
Tetrachloroethylene, 673t
Tetracon (tetrahydrozoline), 89, 92, 92t
Tetracycline(s) (Achromycin; Apo-Tetra; Neo-Tetrine; Novotetra; Panmycin; Sumycin), 567–572t, 609–611, 612–614t
  characteristics of, 610t
Tetrahydrozoline (Clear and Bright; Murine 2; Opt-Ease; Soothe Eye; Tetracon; Tetrasine; Tyzine; Visine), 88–89, 90–91t, 92, 92t
Tetrasine (tetrahydrozoline), 89, 92, 92t
TG (thioguanine), 712, 718–719, 722t
Thalamus, 54
Thalitone (chlorthalidone), 388–389, 390t, 391–392
Tham (tromethamine), 785, 785t
Tham-E (tromethamine), 785, 785t
Theelin Aqueous (estrone), 454–456, 458t, 724, 730, 732t, 734–736
Theo-Dur (theophylline), 545–547, 549, 549t, 551
Theophylline (Aerolate; Bronkodyl; Elixophyllin; Pulmophylline; PMS Theophylline; Slo-Phyllin; Somaphyllin; Theo-Dur), 545–547, 549, 549t, 551
  in xanthine derivatives, 546, 546t
Theophylline sodium glycinate (Synophylate), 545–547, 549, 549t, 551
Theralax (bisacodyl), 506–507, 511–512t
Therapeutic index (TI), 16–17
Thiabendazole (Mintezol), 673t, 678
Thiamine (vitamin B$_1$), 757–759, 758t
Thiamylal (Surital), 149–151, 150t
Thiazides/sulfonamides, 388–389, 390–391t, 391–392
  sites of action and electrolyte disturbances and, 377t

Thiethylperazine, 521t
Thioguanine (TG; 6-Thioguanine), 710t, 712, 718–719, 722t, 742t, 746t, 747t, 751t, 752t
6-Thioguanine (thioguanine), 712, 718–719, 722t
Thiola (tiopronin), 830
Thiopental (Pentothal), 149–151, 150t
Thioridazine (Apo-Thioradizine; Mellaril; Novoridazine; PMS Thioridazine), 205–208, 206t, 211t
Thiosulfil Forte (sulfamethizole), 573–575, 576t
Thiotepa (triethylene-thiophosphoramide), 711–712, 717t
Thiothixene (Navane), 205–208, 206t, 212t
Thioxanthenes, 205–208, 206t, 211–212t
Thorazine (chlorpromazine), 205–208, 209t
Thrombin, topical (Thrombinar; Thrombostat), 365
Thrombinar (thrombin, topical), 365
Thrombocytopenia, 22
Thrombolytic drugs, 351, 358–359, 360t
Thrombostat (thrombin, topical), 365
Thypinone (protirelin), 791, 798t
Thyrar (thyroid, dessicated), 416–418, 418t
Thyro-Block (potassium iodide), 421–423, 422t
Thyrocalcitonin. See Calcitonin
Thyroglobulin (Proloid), 400, 416–418, 418t
Thyroid, dessicated (Armour Thyroid; S-P-T; Thyrar), 416–418, 418t
Thyroidectomy, 422
Thyroid gland, 400–401
  anatomy of, 400
  disorders of, 400–401
  function of, 416. See also Antithyroid drugs; Thyroid hormones
    laboratory parameters for assessment of, 416
    radioactive iodide and, 420–421
Thyroid hormones, 416–418, 418–419t. See also specific hormones
  actions of, 400
  available preparations of, 416
    biosynthesis of, 400
    fate of, 400
    transport of, 400
Thyroid stimulating hormone (thyrotropin; Thytropar; TSH), 398, 407, 409, 791, 798t
  actions of, 398
  control of secretion of, 398, 399
Thyrolar (liotrix), 416–418, 419t
Thyrotoxicosis, 400–401
Thyrotrophs, 396
Thyrotropin. See Thyroid stimulating hormone
Thyroxine, 416
Thyroxine-binding globulin, 400
Thyroxine-binding prealbumin, 400
Thytropar (thyrotropin), 409, 791, 798t
TI. See Therapeutic index
Ticar (ticarcillin), 582, 584–585, 594t, 595
Ticarcillin (Ticar), 567t, 568t, 570t, 571t, 582, 583t, 584–585, 594t, 595
Ticarcillin and potassium clavulanate (Timentin), 582, 584–585, 594t, 595

Tidal volume, 533
Tigan (trimethobenzamide), 526
Timentin (ticarcillin and potassium clavulanate), 582, 584–585, 594t, 595
Timolol (Blocadren), 303–304
  ophthalmic (Timoptic), 104–105, 105t, 108t, 109
  oral (Blocadren), 104–105, 105t, 108t, 109
Timoptic (timolol), 104–105, 105t, 108t, 109
Tinactin (tolnaftate), 692, 696–697t, 697
Tindal (acetophenazine), 205–208, 209t
Tine Test PPD (tuberculin PPD, multiple puncture device), 791, 795t
Ting (undecylenic acid and salts), 692, 697, 697t
Tiopronin (Thiola), 830
Tipramine (imipramine), 227–230, 231–232t
Tirend (caffeine), 263–264
Tissue sensitivity, in elderly patients, 36–37
Titralac, 496–497t
Tobramycin (Nebcin; Tobrex), 567–570t, 568t, 569t, 571t, 624–626, 625t, 630, 630t
Tobrex (tobramycin), 624–626, 630, 630t
Tocainide (Tonocard), 288t, 293
TODD combination chemotherapy, 738, 740, 751t
Toddler period, 31
Tofranil (imipramine), 227–230, 228t, 231–232t
Tolamide (tolazamide), 431, 436–437, 438t
Tolazamide (Ronase; Tolamide; Tolinase), 431, 436–437, 438t
Tolazoline (Priscoline), 103–104, 374t
Tolbutamide (Apo-Tolbutamide; Mobenol; Novobutamide; Oramide; Orinase), 431, 436–437, 439t
Tolbutamide sodium (Orinase Diagnostic), 791, 798t
Tolectin (tolmetin), 175, 178, 183t
Tolerance, 835
  drug effects and, 17
Tolinase (tolazamide), 431, 436–437, 438t
Tolmetin (Tolectin), 175, 178, 183t
Tolnaftate (Aftate; Pitrex; Tinactin), 568t, 687, 692, 696–697t, 697
Tonocard (tocainide), 293
Topical administration, 3–4
  in children, 33–34
    absorption and, 31
  dermatologic, 3
  mucous membrane, 3–4
Topicort (desoximetasone), 443, 444t, 445t, 445–447, 449t
Topsyn (fluocinonide), 443, 445–447, 450t
Tornalate (bitolterol), 94–95, 96–97t
Torofor (iodochlorhydroxyquin-clioquinol), 692, 694t, 697
Totacillin (ampicillin), 582, 584–585, 586–587t, 595
Toxoids, 803, 804t
Tracrium (atracurium), 128–129
Tral (hexocyclium methylsulfate), 76–77t
TRAMPCO(L) combination chemotherapy, 738, 740, 751–752t
Trancopal (chlormezanone), 224

Trandate (labetalol), 104–105, 105t, 106t, 108t, 109, 305, 310
Tranexamic acid (Cyklokapron), 361
Transderm-Nitro (nitroglycerin transdermal systems), 325–326, 329, 329t
Transderm-Scop (scopolamine transdermal therapeutic system), 72–73t
Transport maximum, 374
Tranxene (clorazepate), 217–219, 218t, 221t
Tranylcypromine (Parnate), 234–236, 236t
TRAP combination chemotherapy, 738, 740, 752t
Travamine (dimenhydrinate), 113–114, 116t, 119
Travamulsion 10%, 20% (intravenous fat emulsion), 782
Travase (sutilains), 818, 819t
Travasol (crystalline amino-acid infusion), 779–780
Travert (invert sugar in water), 782
Trazodone (Desyrel), 228t, 234
Trecator-SC (ethionamide), 569t, 655, 658–659
Tremor, in Parkinson's disease, 253
Trental (pentoxifylline), 357–358
Treponema pallidum, 572t
Treponema pertenue, 572t
Tretinoin (Retin-A; retinoic acid; Stie VAA; Vitamin A Acid), 767–768
Trexan (naltrexone), 168
Triacetin (Enzactin; Fungacetin; Fungoid), 687, 692, 697, 697t
Triadapin (doxepin), 227–230, 231t
Triaderm (triamcinolone), 443, 445–447, 452t
Trialadine, 234
Triamcinolone (Aristocort; Azmacort; Kenalog; Triaderm; Triamcort), 443, 444t, 445–447, 452t, 551–553, 552t
Triamcinolone acetonide (Aristocort; Kenalog), 445t
Triamcort (triamcinolone), 443, 445–447, 452t
Triamterene (Dyrenium), 388
Triazolam (Halcion), 198–199, 200t
Tri-B3 (vitamin B$_3$), 759–760
Tricalcium phosphate (Posture), 426–427, 427t
Trichinella spiralis, 673t
Trichlormethiazide (Diurese; Metahydrin; Naqua; Niazide; Trochlorex), 388–389, 391t, 391–392
Trichlorex (trichlormethiazide), 388–389, 391t, 391–392
Trichuris trichiura, 673t
Tricuspid valve, 275
Tricyclic antidepressants, 227–230, 228t, 231–233t
Tridesilon (desonide), 443, 445t, 445–447, 449t
Tridihexethyl chloride (Panthilon), 76–77t
Tridil (nitroglycerin, injection), 325–326, 328–329t, 329
Tridione (trimethadione), 243–245, 245t
Trientine (Cuprid), 814
Triethylene-thiophosphoramide (Thiotepa), 710t, 711–712, 717t

Trifluoperazine (Apo-Trifluoperazine; Stelazine; Suprazine), 205–208, 206t, 211t
Triflupromazine (Vesprin), 205–208, 206t, 209t
Trifluridine (Viroptic), 569t, 703–704
Triglycerides, medium chain (MCT), 778t
Trihexane (trihexyphenidyl hydrochloride), 74–75t, 258–259, 260t
Trihexidyl (trihexyphenidyl hydrochloride), 74–75t, 258–259, 260t
Trihexy (trihexyphenidyl hydrochloride), 74–75t, 258–259, 260t
Trihexyphenidyl hydrochloride (Aparkane; Aphen; Apo-Trihex; Artane; Novohexidyl; Trihexane; Trihexidyl; Trihexy), 67–70, 74–75t, 258–259, 260t
Tri-Immunol (diphtheria and tetanus toxoids and pertussis vaccine, adsorbed-DTP), 803, 804t
Triiodothyronine, 416
Trilafon (perphenazine), 205–208, 210t
Tri-Levlen (ethinyl estradiol/levonorgestrel), 463, 464t, 466–467
Trimeprazine (Temaril), 114t, 126
Trimethadione (Tridione), 243–245, 245t
Trimethaphan (Arfonad), 71, 320
Trimethobenzamide (Tigan), 521t, 526
Trimethoprim (Proloprim; Trimpex), 640–641
Trimethoprim-sulfamethoxazole (Bactrim; Septra), 562, 567–572t, 579–580, 637
Trimipramine (Surmontil), 227–230, 228t, 232t
Trimox (amoxicillin), 582, 584–585, 586t, 595
Trimpex (trimethoprim), 640–641
Tri-Norinyl (ethinyl estradiol/norethindrone), 463, 464t, 466–467
Trioxsalen (Trisoralen), 827–828, 828t
Tripelennamine (Pyribenzamine; Pelamine; PBZ), 113–114, 114t, 118t, 119
Triphasil (ethinyl estradiol/levonorgestrel), 463, 464t, 466–467
Triple Sulfa (sulfonamides, multiple), 573–575, 578t
Triprolidine (Actidil; Myidil), 113–114, 114t, 118t, 119
Triptil (protriptyline), 227–230, 232t
Trisoralen (trioxsalen), 827–828, 828t
Trisulfpyramidines, 570t
Trobicin (spectinomycin), 651–652
Trofan (l-tryptophan), 778t
Troleandomycin (Tao), 619, 620, 623
Trombovar (sodium tetradecyl sulfate), 829t, 829–830
Tromethamine (Tham; Tham-E), 785, 785t
Tronothane (pramoxine), 139–141, 140t, 143t
TrophAmine (crystalline amino-acid infusion), 779–780
Trophozoites, 664
Tropicacyl (tropicamide), 74–75t
Tropicamide (I-Picamide; Mydriacyl; Tropicacyl), 67–70, 74–75t
Truphylline (aminophylline), 545–547, 548t, 549, 551

Trypsin (Granulex), 818, 819t
Trypsin (trypsinogen), 488t
Trypsinogen (trypsin), 488t
Tryptacin (l-tryptophan), 778t
Tryptan (l-tryptophan), 778t
l-Tryptophan (Trophan; Tryptacin; Tryptan), 778t
TSH. See Thyroid stimulating hormone
T-Stat (erythromycin base, topical solution), 619–620, 621t
Tubarine (tubocurarine), 131
Tuberculin PPD, multiple puncture device (Aplitest; Sclavo Test-PPD; Tine Test PPD), 791, 795t
Tuberculin purified protein derivative-tuberculin PPD (Aplisol; Tubersol), 791, 794–795t
Tubersol (tuberculin purified protein derivative-tuberculin PPD), 791, 794–795t
Tubocurarine (Tubarine; Tubocurarine), 131
Tubular mechanisms, competition for, drug interactions and, 29
Tubular resorption, drug excretion and, 14
Tubular secretion, drug excretion and, 14
Tumors, extrapancreatic, hypoglycemia and, 403
Tums (calcium carbonate), 490–491, 492–493t
Tunica mucosa, 483
Tunica muscularis, 483
Tunica serosa, 483
Tunica submucosa, 483
Tusal (sodium thiosalicylate), 170–171, 173, 177t
Tussar-2, 538t
Tussi-Organidin, 538t
T wave, 276, 277
Tylenol (acetaminophen), 173–174
Typhoid vaccine, 803–804, 806t
Tyzine (tetrahydrozoline), 88–89, 90–91t

U

UBT, 791, 793t
UCG-Slide Test, 791, 793t
Ultracef (cefadroxil), 598–600, 601t
Ultralente Iletin I (insulin zinc suspension, extended), 429–431, 436t
Ultralente Insulin (insulin zinc suspension, extended), 429–431, 436t
Ultralente Purified Beef (insulin zinc suspension, extended, purified), 429–431, 436t
Ultra MOP (methoxsalen), 827–828, 828t
Unasyn (ampicillin and sulbactam sodium), 582, 584–585, 587t, 595
Undecylenic acid and salts (Caldesene; Cruex; Desenex; Quinsana; Ting), 687, 692, 697, 697t
Unipen (nafcillin), 582, 584–585, 590–591t, 595
Unisol (castor oil), 506–507, 512t
Unisom (doxylamine), 113–114, 117t, 119
U.S. Food and Drug Administration (FDA), 41
United States Pharmacopeia (USP), 41
Unstable angina, 325

Up-regulation, 53
drug interactions and, 28
Urabeth (bethanechol), 57–58
Uracel (sodium salicylate), 170–171, 173, 177t
Uracil mustard, 711–712, 718t
Urea (Ureaphil), 386
Ureaphil (urea), 386
Urease inhibitor, 641–642
Urecholine (bethanechol), 57–58
Urex (methenamine hippurate), 637–638, 639t
Uri-Tet (oxytetracycline), 609–611, 613t
Uricult, 791, 793t
Uridon (chlorthalidone), 388–389, 390t, 391–392
Urinary analgesic, 641
Urinary antiinfectives, 637–642
Urinary bladder, 371
Urinary tract
acetylcholine and, pharmacologic effects and clinical consequences of, 57t
anticholinergic drugs and, pharmacologic actions of, 68t
Urine, alterations in pH of, drug interactions and, 29
Urispas (flavoxate), 818, 820
Uristix, 791, 793t
Uritol (furosemide), 377–378, 382–383, 384t
Urobak (sulfamethoxazole), 573–575, 576t
Uroblistix, 791, 793t
Urofollitropin (Metrodin), 469
Urokinase (Abbokinase), 358–359, 360t
Uro-KP-Neutral (phosphorus), 776t
Urolene Blue (methylene blue), 638
Uro-mag (magnesium oxide), 490–491, 494–495t
Urovist Cysto, 799, 802t
Urovist Meglumine DIU/CT, 799, 802t
Urovist Sodium, 799, 802t
Ursodiol-ursodeoxycholic acid (Actigall), 504
USP. See *United States Pharmacopeia*
Uterus, adrenergic drug effects on, 81t
Uticort (betamethasone benzoate), 443, 444t, 445–447, 448t
Utimox (amoxicillin), 582, 584–585, 586t, 595

V

Vaccines, 803–804, 805–808t
bacterial, 803–804, 805–806t
viral, 803–804, 806–808t
VAC combination chemotherapy, 709t, 738, 740, 752t
VAC Pulse combination chemotherapy, 738, 740, 752t
VAC Standard combination chemotherapy, 738, 740, 752t
VAD combination chemotherapy, 738, 740, 752t
Vagal reflex, 536
Vaginal mucosa, mucosal application and, 4
Valergen (estradiol valerate), 724, 730, 732t, 734–736

Valisone (betamethasone valerate), 443, 445–447, 448t, 444t
Valium (diazepam), 217–219, 218t, 221–222t, 249
Valmid (ethinamate), 201
Valnac (betamethasone valerate), 443, 445–447, 448t
Valproic acid (Depa; Depakene; Deproic), 247–248
Valproic acid derivatives, 247–248
Vancenase (beclomethasone), 443, 445–447, 448t
Vanceril (beclomethasone), 443, 445–447, 448t, 551–553, 552t
Vancocin (vancomycin), 652–653
Vancoled (vancomycin), 652–653
Vancomycin (Lyphocin; Vancocin; Vancoled), 568t, 571t, 572t, 652–653
Vansil (oxamniquine), 676
VAP combination chemotherapy, 738, 740, 752t
Vapo-Iso (isoproterenol), 84–85
Vaponefrin (epinephrine), 79–82
Vaporole (amyl nitrite), 325–326, 327t, 329
Vasa recta, 371
Vascoray, 799, 802t
VasoClear (naphazoline), 89, 92, 92t
Vasocon (naphazoline), 89, 92, 92t
Vasodilan (isoxsuprine), 95–96, 334
Vasodilators, 325
  peripheral, 333–335
Vasopressin (Pitressin Synthetic), 409–411
Vasopressin tannate (Pitressin Tannate in Oil), 410–411
Vasopressor amines, 86–88
Vasospastic angina, 325
Vasotec (enalapril), 304–305, 309t
Vasoxyl (methoxamine), 87–88
Va-Tro-Nol (ephedrine), 88–89, 90–91t
Vazepam (diazepam), 249
VBAP combination chemotherapy, 738, 740, 752t
VBD combination chemotherapy, 738, 740, 752t
VBP combination chemotherapy, 738, 740, 752t
VCAP combination chemotherapy, 738, 740, 752t
VC combination chemotherapy, 738, 740, 752t
V-Cillin K (penicillin V; penicillin V, potassium), 582, 584–585, 593t, 595
VCR-MTX-CF (VMC) combination chemotherapy, 738, 740, 753t
Vecuronium (Norcuron), 131–132
Velban (vinblastine), 719, 722–724, 729t
Velosef (cephadrine), 598–600, 603t
Velosulin (insulin injection, purified), 429–431, 435t
Velosulin Human (insulin injection, human), 429–431, 435t
Velsar (vinblastine), 719, 722–724, 729t
Venoglobulin 1 (immune globulin, intravenous), 801, 810t
Ventolin (albuterol), 94–95, 96–97t
Ventricles, 275
Ventricular rhythm, 287
Venules, lungs and, 532
VePesid (etoposide), 719, 722–724, 728t

Verapamil (Calan; Isoptin), 288t, 299–300, 313, 329–331, 331t, 332t
Verazinc (zinc sulfate), 776t
Vercyte (pipobroman), 711–712, 717t
Vermizine (piperazine), 676–677
Vermox (mebendazole), 674
Versed (midazolam), 219, 222–223
Very low density lipoproteins (VLDL), 337
Vesprin (triflupromazine), 205–208, 209t
Vibramycin (doxycycline), 609–611, 612t
Vibra Tabs (doxycycline), 609–611, 612t
Vibrio cholerae, 572t
Vicks inhaler (desoxyephedrine), 88–89, 90–91t
Vidarabine (Vira-A), 569t, 704–705
Villi, intestinal, absorption and, 11
Vinblastine (Alkaban-AQ; Velban; Velsar), 710t, 719, 722–724, 729t, 741t, 742t, 744–746t, 750–753t
Vincasar PFS (vincristine), 719, 722–724, 730t
Vincristine (Oncovin; Vincasar PFS), 709t, 710t, 719, 722–724, 730t, 741–753t
Vioform (iodochlorhydroxyquin-clioquinol), 692, 694t, 697
Viokase (pancrelipase), 502
Vira-A (vidarabine), 704–705
Virazole (ribavarin), 702–703
Virilon (methyltestosterone), 474–476, 477t, 479, 724, 730, 731t, 734–736
Viroptic (trifluridine), 703–704
Visceral pleura, 531
Visceral stimulation, vomiting and, 489
Visidex II, 791, 793t
Visine (tetrahydrozoline), 89, 92, 92t
Visken (pindolol), 104–105, 105t, 107t, 108t, 109, 303–304
Vistaril (hydroxyzine), 224–225
Vitacan (l-carnitine), 777t
Vitamin(s), 757
  absorption of, 488
  fat-soluble, 764–773, 765t
    vitamin A, 764–765, 765t
    vitamin A analogs, 765–768
    vitamin D preparations, 765t, 768–770, 769t
    vitamin E, 765t, 770–771
    vitamin K, 765t, 771t, 771–772
  water-soluble, 757–763, 758t
    B complex, 757–761, 758t
    vitamin C, 758t, 761–762
Vitamin A (Aquasol A; Del-Vi-A), 764–765, 765t
Vitamin A Acid (tretinoin), 767–768
Vitamin A analogs, 765–768
Vitamin B₁ (Betalin S; Betaxin; Bewon; Biamine; thiamine), 757–759, 758t
Vitamin B₂ (riboflavin), 758t, 759–760
Vitamin B₃ (Niac; Niacels; Niacin; Nico-400; Nicobid; Nicolar; Nicotinex; nicotinic acid; Novoniacin; Span-Niacin; Tri-B3), 758t, 759–760
Vitamin B₅ (calcium pantothenate; pantothenic acid), 758t, 760
Vitamin B₆ (Beesix; Hexa-Betalin; Nestrex; pyridoxine; Pyroxine), 758t, 760–761

Vitamin B₁₂ (cyanocobalamin), 348–349, 758t, 761
Vitamin C (ascorbic acid; calcium ascorbate; sodium ascorbate), 758t, 761–762
Vitamin D, 424, 765t, 768–770, 769t
Vitamin E (Aquasol E), 765t, 770–771
Vitamin K, 765t, 771t, 771–772
Vitamin K₁ (AquaMEPHYTON; Konakion; Mephyton; phytonadione), 771t, 771–772
Vitamin K₄ (menadiol sodium diphosphate; Synkayvite), 771t, 771–772
Vivactil (protriptyline), 227–230, 228t, 232t
Vivarin (caffeine), 263–264
Vivol (diazepam), 249
VLDL. *See* Very low density lipoproteins
VM combination chemotherapy, 738, 740, 753t
VMCP combination chemotherapy, 738, 740, 753t
Volatile inhalants, 840
Volatile liquids, anesthetic, 146–149
Voltaren (diclofenac), 175, 178, 181t
Voluntary nervous system, 49
Vomiting, 488–489. *See also* Antiemetics; Emetics
  chemoreceptor trigger zone and, 489
  cortical stimulation and, 489
  inner ear disturbances and, 489
  nodose ganglion and, 489
  visceral stimulation and, 489
Vontrol (diphenidol), 522–523
Voxsuprine (isoxsuprine), 334
VP-16 (etoposide), 719, 722–724, 728t
VP-16-213 (etoposide), 719, 722–724, 728t
VP combination chemotherapy, 738, 740, 753t
VP-L-Asparaginase (VPAsp) combination chemotherapy, 738, 740, 753t
VP plus Daunorubicin combination chemotherapy, 738, 740, 753t

W

Warfarin sodium (Carfin; Coumadin; Panwarfin; Sofarin; Warfilone), 354–356, 356t
Warfilone (warfarin sodium), 354–356, 356t
Wart-off (salicylic acid), 170–171, 173, 177t
Water
  absorption of, 487
  renal handling of, 374
Wehvert (meclizine), 113–114, 117t, 119
Weight, drug effects and, 17
Wellbutrin (bupropion), 228t, 230, 232–233
Wellcovorin (leucovorin calcium-folinic acid), 350
Westcort (hydrocortisone valerate), 445t
Wigrettes (ergotamine), 124–125
Wiley-Heyburn Act, 41
Win-Gel, 496–497t
Win Rho (rh₀[D] immune globulin), 810, 811t
Winstrol (stanozolol), 474–476, 479, 479t

Wuchereria bancrofti, 673t
Wyamine (mephentermine), 86
Wyamycin-E (erythromycin ethylsuccinate), 619–620, 622t
Wyamycin-S (erythromycin stearate), 619–620, 623t
Wycillin (penicillin G, procaine), 582, 584–585, 592–593t, 595
Wydase (hyaluronidase), 818, 820t
Wymox (amoxicillin), 582, 584–585, 586t, 595
Wytensin (guanabenz), 310–311

X

Xanax (alprazolam), 217–219, 218t, 220t
Xanthine derivatives, 545–547, 548–549t, 549, 551
   theophylline content of, 546, 546t
Xylocaine (lidocaine), 139–141, 140t, 142t, 292–293
Xylocard (lidocaine), 139–141, 140t, 142t, 292–293
Xylometazoline (Chlorohist Long Acting; Neo Spray Long Acting; Neo-Synephrine II; Otrivin), 88–89, 90–91t
Xylo-Pfan (D-xylose), 791, 798t
X-Prep (senna concentrate), 506–507, 513t
D-Xylose (Xylo-Pfan), 791, 798t

Y

Yellow fever vaccine (YF-Vax), 803–804, 808t
Yersinia pestis, 572t, 624, 625t
YF-Vax (yellow fever vaccine), 803–804, 808t
Yocon (yohimbine), 830
Yodoxin (iodoquinol), 683
Yohimbine (Aphrodyne; Yocon; Yohimex), 830
Yohimex (yohimbine), 830
Young's rule, 32
Yutopar (ritodrine), 98

Z

Zanosar (streptozocin), 711–712, 717t
Zantac (ranitidine), 119, 121–122, 122t
Zapex (oxazepam), 217–219, 222t
Zarontin (ethosuximide), 245–246, 246t
Zaroxolyn (metolazone), 388–389, 391t, 391–392
Zaxopam (oxazepam), 217–219, 222t
Zestril (lisinopril), 304–305, 309t
Zetran (diazepam), 217–219, 221–222t
Zidovudine (Retrovir), 705–706
Zinacef (cefuroxime), 598–600, 605t
Zinc-220 (zinc sulfate), 776t
Zinc and Iletin I (protamine zinc insulin suspension), 429–431, 436t
Zinc and Iletin II (protamine zinc insulin suspension, purified), 429–431, 436t
Zincaps (zinc sulfate), 776t
Zincate (zinc sulfate), 776t
Zinc gluconate, 776t
Zinc sulfate (Anuzinc; Orazinc; PMS Egozinc; Scrip-Zinc; Verazinc; Zinc-220; Zincate; Zinkaps), 776t
"Z" method, for intramuscular administration, 9
Zolicef (cefazolin), 598–600, 601t
Zolyse (chymotrypsin), 818, 820t
Zonulyn (chymotrypsin), 818, 820t
Zostrix (capsaicin), 816
Zovirax (acyclovir), 699–700
Z-track method, 9
Zurinol (allopurinol), 188–189
Zyloprim (allopurinol), 188–189
Zymenol (mineral oil), 506–507, 509–510t